THE ART AND SCIENCE OF
OPERATIVE DENTISTRY

THE ART AND SCIENCE OF
OPERATIVE DENTISTRY

SENIOR EDITOR   **CLIFFORD M. STURDEVANT, D.D.S.**

Professor Emeritus
Department of Operative Dentistry
University of North Carolina School of Dentistry
Chapel Hill, North Carolina

CO-EDITORS   **THEODORE M. ROBERSON, B.S., D.D.S.**

Professor
Department of Operative Dentistry
University of North Carolina School of Dentistry
Chapel Hill, North Carolina

HARALD O. HEYMANN, D.D.S., M.Ed.

Associate Professor
Department of Operative Dentistry
University of North Carolina School of Dentistry
Chapel Hill, North Carolina

JOHN R. STURDEVANT, D.D.S.

Associate Professor
Department of Operative Dentistry
University of North Carolina School of Dentistry
Chapel Hill, North Carolina

THIRD EDITION   *WITH 2497 ILLUSTRATIONS*

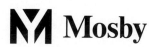 **Mosby**

St. Louis Baltimore Berlin Boston Carlsbad Chicago London Madrid
Naples New York Philadelphia Sydney Tokyo Toronto

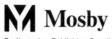
Mosby
Dedicated to Publishing Excellence

Editor: Linda L. Duncan
Developmental Editor: Jo Salway
Project Manager: Gayle May Morris
Production Editors: Deborah L. Vogel, Lisa Nomura
Manufacturing Supervisor: John E. Babrick
Design Manager: Susan Lane
Cover Designers: C.M. Sturdevant and E. Rohne Rudder

THIRD EDITION

Printed in the United States of America
Composition by Clarinda Company
Printing/Binding by Von Hoffman Press, Inc.

Mosby–Year Book, Inc.
11830 Westline Industrial Drive
St. Louis, Missouri 63146

Library of Congress Cataloging-in-Publication Data

The art and science of operative dentistry / senior editor, Clifford
    M. Sturdevant ; co-editors, Theodore M. Roberson, Harald O. Heymann,
    John R. Sturdevant. --3rd ed.
        p.   cm.
    Includes bibliographical references and index.
    ISBN 0-8016-6366-0
    1. Dentistry, Operative.   I. Sturdevant, Clifford M.
RK501.A78   1994
617.6'05—dc20   94-7883
                                                  CIP

98 99 / 9 8 7 6 5

Contributors

STEPHEN C. BAYNE, M.S., Ph. D.
Professor
Section Head of Biomaterials
Department of Operative Dentistry
School of Dentistry
University of North Carolina
Chapel Hill, North Carolina

JAMES J. CRAWFORD, M.A., Ph.D.
Professor, Coordinator for Infection Control
Director, Oral Microbiology Diagnostic Laboratory
School of Dentistry
University of North Carolina
Chapel Hill, North Carolina

VAN B. HAYWOOD, D.M.D.
Associate Professor
Department of Operative Dentistry
School of Dentistry
University of North Carolina
Chapel Hill, North Carolina

HARALD O. HEYMANN, D.D.S., M.Ed.
Associate Professor and Chair
Department of Operative Dentistry
School of Dentistry
University of North Carolina
Chapel Hill, North Carolina

THOMAS F. LUNDEEN, D.M.D., M.S.
Associate Professor
Department of Operative Dentistry
School of Dentistry
University of North Carolina
Chapel Hill, North Carolina

KENNETH N. MAY, Jr., D.D.S.
Associate Professor
Department of Operative Dentistry
Director of Admissions and Student Affairs
School of Dentistry
The University of North Carolina
Chapel Hill, North Carolina

THEODORE M. ROBERSON, D.D.S.
Professor
Department of Operative Dentistry
School of Dentistry
University of North Carolina
Chapel Hill, North Carolina

DANIEL A. SHUGARS, D.D.S., Ph.D., M.P.H.
Professor
Department of Operative Dentistry
University of North Carolina
Chapel Hill, North Carolina

DIANE C. SHUGARS, D.D.S., M.P.H., Ph.D.
Adjunct Assistant Professor
Department of Dental Ecology
School of Dentistry
University of North Carolina
Chapel Hill, North Carolina

TROY B. SLUDER, Jr., D.D.S., M.S.
Professor
Department of Operative Dentistry
School of Dentistry
University of North Carolina
Chapel Hill, North Carolina

GREGORY E. SMITH, D.D.S., M.S.D.
Professor and Chair
Department of Operative Dentistry
College of Dentistry
University of Florida
Gainesville, Florida

CLIFFORD M. STURDEVANT, D.D.S.
Professor Emeritus
Department of Operative Dentistry
School of Dentistry
University of North Carolina
Chapel Hill, North Carolina

JOHN R. STURDEVANT, D.D.S.
Associate Professor
Department of Operative Dentistry
School of Dentistry
University of North Carolina
Chapel Hill, North Carolina

DUANE F. TAYLOR, B.S.E., M.S.E., Ph.D.
Professor
Department of Operative Dentistry
School of Dentistry
University of North Carolina
Chapel Hill, North Carolina

ALDRIDGE D. WILDER, Jr., D.D.S.
Associate Professor
Department of Operative Dentistry
University of North Carolina
Chapel Hill, North Carolina

We dedicate this book to the betterment of operative dentistry.
The central motivating factor of the authors/editors is to provide a book
that is worthy for use by our teaching colleagues.
May students present, past, and future benefit from these pages.

We further dedicate this book to our spouses and families for their continual love,
understanding, and support through the trying times of this revision.

Foreword

Dentistry is undergoing enormous changes at the present time, and the field of operative dentistry is in the very forefront of that transformation. No dental educator can fail to notice that varying restorative dental technologies, some only 15 years old, are becoming obsolete, and that today's students and practitioners alike must incorporate new paradigms in their approach to providing the care that our patients require and demand. This third edition of *The Art and Science of Operative Dentistry* is an exemplary attempt to codify the principles of operative dentistry pertinent to the education in and practice of operative dentistry in the twenty-first century.

The contents of this book advance an approach to teaching operative dentistry that has evolved and progressed in a highly dynamic fashion. Indeed, at the University of North Carolina the subject matter in operative dentistry is constantly tested and must repeatedly survive what may be called the challenge of pedagogical Darwinism. That is, the concepts that constitute operative dentistry practice and teaching are continually evaluated against the unrelenting stream of information flowing from the basic and clinical sciences that shape everything we do in the health care field. What is outdated is discarded; what remains applicable is updated; and what is new and necessary is incorporated. Only the best information and technologies survive to guide our teaching and practice of operative dentistry. We could call this process *the survival of excellence.*

Dental caries is not a lesion, it is a disease. This book is written with the explicit assumption that the disease of dental caries must be exquisitely understood if efforts at its prevention and treatment are to improve in the future. Paradoxically, the advent of modern microbiology and molecular biology has led to such an explosion in the field of cariology that it is virtually impossible to provide more than a cursory overview within the covers of the present volume. The molecular mechanisms of dental decay lead to definable stages of caries initiation, some of which can be treated with nonsurgical techniques, others with varying sealant technologies, and still others with a wide variety of restorative approaches. The molecular basis of pulpal reponse, not only to the caries process, but also to restorative procedures and materials, must be understood. Marginal leakage, pulpal inflammation, and recurrent caries—major problems in operative dentistry—are also initiated at the molecular level.

During the last 20 years dental caries prevalance and severity have declined in most of the highly industrialized world. However, taking a more global perspective, it is known that dental caries prevalance is increasing in many industrializing countries, and in many highly populated mid-tier countries caries is still a largely untreated condition. It cannot be overlooked that in such countries the challenges facing dental educators, students, and practitioners are enormous. *The Art and Science of Operative Dentistry* is expressly written for the dental schools and offices that represent the loci for excellence in operative dentistry in those countries. The modern fundamental principles of operative dentistry have universal application in the treatment of dental caries.

Among the most illustrative examples of the changes facing the dental profession are the emerging field of esthetic dentistry and the beginning application of computer assisted design and computer assisted machining (CAD/CAM) in dentistry. For operative dentistry, both of these endeavors represent the pinnacle of high technology and convincingly demonstrate operative dentistry's skill in dealing with the larger issue of technology transfer into its discipline. I am particularly pleased that the third edition of *The Art and Science of Operative Dentistry* incorporates these new developments into its pages. The authors of this text have substantial experience in these new technologies, and they give an excellent account of what will surely become an essential component of operative dentistry in the twenty-first century. Learn and enjoy as much as I did from this outstanding text.

John W. Stamm, D.D.S.
Dean
School of Dentistry
University of North Carolina

Preface

Revision of the second edition of *The Art and Science of Operative Dentistry* was a major undertaking because dentistry has undergone major changes since 1984. Those changes relating to operative dentistry include: (1) the emphasis on and necessity for improved infection control; (2) the increased importance of early diagnosis of communicable diseases, especially dental caries; (3) the improvements in esthetic restorative materials and conservative esthetic restorative techniques, resulting in increased demand for esthetic dental care; and (4) the significant advancements in the ability to bond various restorative materials to tooth structure.

Chapter 1, "Introduction to Operative Dentistry," continues to emphasize the biological basis of operative dentistry; the prevention of dental disease; the conservation of tooth structure; the impact of an ever-increasing aging population; the increasing need and demand for conservative dental restorations, as well as replacement dentistry; and the public's increasing knowledge of and desire for esthetic treatments of the teeth.

Chapter 2, "Clinical Significance of Dental Anatomy, Histology, Physiology, and Occlusion," includes expanded sections on the pulp-dentin complex and occlusion. The biological aspects of dentin are presented in relationship to the health of the pulp and the dentinal adhesive systems. Extensive new artwork in the presentation of occlusal relationships and chewing movements should aid the assessment of occlusion and the provision of acceptable occlusion in restorations.

Chapter 3, "Cariology, the Lesion, Etiology, Prevention, and Control," explains cariology on an ecological basis. It emphasizes (1) the potential for remineralization of incipient enamel lesions under favorable conditions, (2) the histological observations that support the clinical division of the dentinal lesion into an inner affected portion and an outer infected portion, (3) the modalities of prevention, (4) the caries control restoration, and (5) the importance, during examination, of discriminating between the high-risk patient and low-risk patient. The micro-histology of enamel and the micro-features of growing plaque are illustrated by new artwork. Carious lesions are uniquely presented by new

prints accompanied by matching line drawings. Commensurate with the importance of oral hygiene in preventive dentistry the section on this subject is expanded and includes illustrations.

Chapter 4, "Infection Control," is an extensive addition to the text. This chapter integrates applicable topics regarding infectious diseases, epidemiology, and infection control procedures recommended by the AADS (American Association of Dental Schools). These topics also are integrated with OSHA (Occupational Safety and Health Administration) infection control regulations, as well as with requirements from the ADA (American Dental Association) and the CDC (Centers for Disease Control and Prevention). Practical instructions are presented on infection control procedures.

Chapter 5, "Patient Assessment, Examination and Diagnosis, and Treatment Planning," provides a ready reference for the practitioner and/or student. A new section discusses contagious diseases of particular concern in dentistry and further summarizes the discussion in a two-page reference format. Also, a new color plate shows intraoral and extraoral manifestations associated with some communicable diseases. There is new updated information for caries detection on occlusal surfaces, interpretation of diagnostic tests, prescription of dental radiographs, risk assessment, the patient in pain, and the management and prevention of caries.

Chapter 6, "Dental Materials," is a new chapter presenting essential information regarding dental materials used in operative dentistry. The chapter's four sections are (I) Introduction—for presentation of materials science definitions and the biomechanics for restorative dentistry; (II) Direct Restorative Dental Materials—for discussion of dental amalgam, liners and bases, dental adhesion (including contemporary bonding), pit-and-fissure sealants, dental composites, glass ionomer cements, and direct filling gold; (III) Indirect Restorative Dental Materials—for discussion of impression materials, cast restorations, dental cements, and machined restorations, and (IV) Safety and Efficacy Issues—a presentation of the national and global standards programs and the safety programs of OSHA and EPA (Environmental Protection Agency) for the protection of both the patient and office personnel from chemical and environmental hazards.

Chapter 7, "Fundamentals in Cavity Preparation," has undergone a major revision and includes many new illustrations. A significant feature is the presentation of the information as the stages and steps of cavity preparation. For efficiency in cavity preparation, as well as to best manage cavity preparation in the teaching clinic, the procedure is divided into two stages, with each stage having several steps. Steps 1 to 4 comprise the "Initial cavity preparation stage," namely: (1) establishing outline form and initial pulpal depth, (2) primary resistance forms, (3) primary retention form, and (4) convenience form, aud steps 5 to 9 comprise the "Final cavity preparation stage," namely: (5) removing remaining infected dentin and/or defective old restorative material, (6) pulp protection, (7) secondary resistance and retention forms, (8) finishing external margins, and (9) final procedures. For each step detailed definitions and descriptions of factors and features are presented. The "Nomenclature" section is reorganized and expanded. Traditional use of liners, bases, and varnishes is discussed; however, dentin bonding agents are recognized as beneficial for dentinal sealing. The chapter closes by recognizing that increased bond strengths of adhesive systems are likely to result in significant future emphasis on *bonded restorations,* and the use of these likely will alter significantly the entire cavity preparation procedure.

Chapter 10, "Pain Control," discusses the principles and technique in the use of local anesthesia by needle injection for most operative dentistry procedures. Such anesthesia, when profound, favors excellence in operative dentistry due to a resulting near cessation of salivation. Emphasis is given to the psychology in administering local anesthesia, the prevention of needle-stick injury, avoidance of intravascular deposition, elimination of any patient sensations during the injection, and *slow* deposition.

Chapter 11, "Isolation of the Operating Field," em-phasizes the merits of isolation by proper use of the rubber dam. A new section presents the principles of isolation using retraction cord, along with profound anesthesia of the operating site.

Chapters on amalgam restorations **(Chapters, 12, 13, 14, and 15)** have new discussions and illustrations relating to proper pulpal floor depths, additional secondary retention form features, and proper wedging techniques for matrixing systems. Additional emphasis is also placed on slot retention form for complex amalgam restorations. Bonding systems reduce microleakage and may reinforce tooth structure.

Chapters on tooth-colored restorations **(Chapters 16, 17, and 18)** present new concepts in both cavity preparations and restoration that result from improvements in both enamel/dentin bonding systems and restorative materials. The use of glass ionomers is also detailed in this section. Chapter 16 expands the concept of modified cavity preparations for Classes III, IV, and V restorations, and Chapter 17 advocates the use of composite in many Class I and Class II restorations. A new section, "Indirect Tooth-Colored Inlays and Onlays," describes laboratory-processed composite inlays, some types of ceramic inlays, and a new system, the CEREC® system,* which fabricates chairside indirect computer-generated ceramic restorations. Chapter 18 has been updated to include information on basic artistic concepts, as well as new information on a variety of esthetic treatments including vital bleaching, microabrasion, macroabrasion, etched porcelain veneers, and all-porcelain pontics.

Successful bonding significantly reduces microleakage and often provides substantial tooth reinforcement with tooth-colored restorations. These qualities, along with the improved physical properties of tooth-colored materials, should translate into greater conservation of tooth structure and general acceptance of tooth-colored restorations when isolation of the operating site is possible.

*CEREC® system, Pelton and Crane, Siemens Product Division, Charlotte, NC.

Chapter 19, "Cast Metal Restorations for Class II Cavity Preparations," has been updated in materials and procedures used for bases, interocclusal records, temporization, and the final impression.

Chapter 20 presents general concepts and techniques for gold foil preparations and restorations.

In addition to *teaching* operative dentistry, the contributors *practice* the principles and techniques presented in this book on a weekly, scheduled basis in a group private practice conducted in the dental school. In this practice there is peer review of the *quality of service* and periodic projection and review of individual *productivity*. Thus the authors regularly demonstrate that the advocated procedures are worthy of application to the private practice of dentistry.

The authors also engage in clinical (or laboratory) *research* on a weekly, scheduled basis in school facilities. The restorative concepts presented in this book are suported by sound clinical and laboratory studies, not only from the University of North Carolina School of Dentistry and its Dental Research Center, but also from many other sources.

The authors and editors thank Warren McCollum, Director of the Learning Resources Center of the University of North Carolina School of Dentistry, and his staff for outstanding cooperation and diligence in the production of illustrations. We also thank Pam Fogleman, Marie Roberts, and Brenda Haithcock for their capable assistance. Indeed we were fortunate benefactors of the diligence and ability of Ms. Fogleman, who processed almost all of the text material resulting in a manuscript having consistent format and terminology.

The reader will notice bold italicized words in the text material. These are words that (1) are very important, (2) are not found in a heading, and (3) are in the index. Conversely, when the user desires to know what is in this text regarding a certain word (or subject) and finds it in the index (with indicated page[s]), the word (or subject) usually will be found on the page either in bold italics or in a heading.

Although Drs. Barton, Sockwell, and Strickland (editors/authors in the second edition) were not active in this edition, we express our appreciation for their past contributions in both the first and second editions, and we gratefully acknowledge the use of portions of those contributions in this edition.

Clifford M. Sturdevant, Chair, 1959-1979
Theodore M. Roberson, Chair, 1979-88
Harald O. Heymann, Chair, 1988 to present

Department of Operative Dentistry
School of Dentistry
University of North Carolina-Chapel Hill

Contents

5   Patient assessment, examination and diagnosis, and treatment planning, 168

Daniel A. Shugars
Diane C. Shugars

6   Dental materials, 206

Stephen C. Bayne
Duane F. Taylor

7   Fundamentals in cavity preparation, 289

Theodore M. Roberson
Clifford M. Sturdevant
Roger E. Barton
Joe T. Wall

8   Instruments and equipment for tooth preparation, 325

Duane F. Taylor
Stephen C. Bayne
Clifford M. Sturdevant

9   Preliminary considerations for operative dentistry, 361

Kenneth N. May, Jr.
Aldridge D. Wilder, Jr.
Roger E. Barton

10   Pain control, 366

Clifford M. Sturdevant

11   Isolation of the operating field, 378

Aldridge D. Wilder, Jr.
Kenneth N. May, Jr.
William D. Strickland

12   Amalgam restorations for Class I cavity preparations, 406

Aldridge D. Wilder, Jr.
Kenneth N. May, Jr.
William D. Strickland

13   Amalgam restorations for Class II cavity preparations, 434

Aldridge D. Wilder, Jr.
Kenneth N. May, Jr.
William D. Strickland

14   Amalgam restorations for Classes III, V, and VI cavity preparations, 476

Kenneth N. May, Jr.
Aldridge D. Wilder, Jr.
William D. Strickland

18   Additional conservative esthetic procedures, 627

Harald O. Heymann
Clarence L. Sockwell
Van B. Haywood

19   Cast metal restorations for Class II cavity preparations, 688

John R. Sturdevant
Clifford M. Sturdevant

CHAPTER 1

Introduction to operative dentistry

Theodore M. Roberson

DEFINITION AND HISTORY
Definition

Operative dentistry is the art and science of the diagnosis, treatment, and prognosis of defects of teeth which do not require full coverage restorations for correction; such treatment should result in the restoration of proper tooth form, function, and esthetics while maintaining the physiological integrity of the teeth in harmonious relationship with the adjacent hard and soft tissues; all of which enhance the general health and welfare of the patient.

History

Although *operative dentistry was once considered to be the entirety of the clinical practice of dentistry,* today many of the past subject areas in operative dentistry have become specialty areas. As information increased and the need for other complex treatment was recognized, areas such as endodontics, prosthodontics, and orthodontics became dental specialties. Operative dentistry has been recognized as the foundation of dentistry and the base from which most other aspects of dentistry evolved.

In the United States dentistry originated in the seventeenth century when several "barber-dentists" were sent from England. The practice of these early dentists consisted mainly of tooth extractions. Many practiced dentistry while pursuing other livelihoods and some traveled from one area to another to provide their dental services. These early dentists learned their "trade" by serving apprenticeships under more experienced practitioners. Consequently, much of the practice of dentistry during the founding years of this country was not based on scientific knowledge. Disputes often arose regarding treatment techniques and materials. One such dispute concerning use of early amalgam material played some part in the establishment of the Baltimore College of Dental Surgery in 1840,[20] which marked the official birth of formal dental education as a discipline. In 1867, 27 years later, Harvard University established the first university-affiliated dental program.[15]

It was in this same period in France that Louis Pasteur discovered the role of microorganisms in disease,[19] a finding that would have a significant impact on the developing dental and medical professions. Also during this time, contributions in the United States by G.V. Black[4] became the foundation of the dental profession. *Black,* who had both honorary dental and medical degrees, *related the clinical practice of dentistry to a scientific basis.* This scientific foundation for operative dentistry was further expanded by Black's son, Arthur Black. Studies commissioned by the Carnegie Foundation, the Flexner report[11] in 1910, and the Gies report[13] in 1926 further identified the need for establishing dental and medical educational systems on a firm scientific foundation. The primary needs reported by these studies were relating clinical practice to the basic sciences, prescribing admissions and curriculum criteria, and promoting university-based programs.

Thus the early days of itinerant, often uneducated dentists ended. Dentists began to be educated in the basic sciences and clinical dentistry, resulting in practitioners who possessed and demonstrated intellectual and scientific curiosity. The heritage of operative dentistry is filled with such practitioners. In addition to the Blacks, others such as Charles E. Woodbury, E.K. Wedelstaedt, Waldon I. Ferrier, and George Hollenback made significant contributions in the early development of operative dentistry.

The contributions of many practitioners, educators, and researchers throughout the world have resulted in operative dentistry being recognized today as a scientifically based discipline that plays an important role in enhancing dental health. Although segments of early operative dentistry have now branched into dental specialties, operative dentistry today continues to be a most active component of most dental practices.[14,27] Moreover, epidemiological studies project that demand for operative dentistry will not decrease in the foreseeable future.[27] It is cardinal that treatment of a defective tooth will never be obsolete.

FACTORS AFFECTING OPERATIVE TREATMENT
Indications

The indications for operative procedures are numerous. However, they can be categorized into three primary treatment needs: (1) caries; (2) malformed, discolored, or fractured teeth; and (3) restoration replacement or repair. The specific procedures associated with these treatment indicators are covered in subsequent chapters.

Considerations

There are also a number of considerations that usually must be undertaken before any operative treatment: (1) an understanding of and appreciation for infection control to safeguard health service personnel and the patients (see Chapter 4); (2) a thorough examination of not only the affected tooth but also the oral and systemic health of the patient; (3) a diagnosis of the dental problem that recognizes the interaction of the affected area with other bodily tissues; (4) a treatment plan that has the potential to return the affected area to a state of health and function, thereby enhancing the overall health and well-being of the patient; (5) an understanding of the material to be used to restore the affected area to a state of health and function with a realization of both the material's limitations and demands; (6) an understanding of the oral environment into which the restoration will be placed; (7) the biological knowledge necessary to make the previously mentioned determinations; (8) an understanding of the biological basis and function of the various tooth components and supporting tissues; (9) an appreciation for and knowledge of correct dental anatomy; and (10) the effect of the operative procedure on the treatments of other disciplines. Subsequent chapters will amplify these factors in relation to specific operative procedures.

In summary, the placement of a restoration in a tooth requires the dentist to practice applied human biology and microbiology, use principles of mechanical engineering, possess highly developed technical skills, and demonstrate artistic abilities.

Conservative approach

Although cavity preparations for operative procedures originally adhered to the concept of "extension for prevention," increased knowledge of prevention methods, advanced techniques, and improved restorative materials have now provided a more conservative approach to the restoration of teeth. This newer concept is a result of the reduction in the incidence of caries because of increased preventive emphasis, use of multiple fluoride applications, and proper sealant application. The benefits of the supragingival placement of restoration margins, whenever possible, have also been recognized.

Ongoing research efforts in operative dentistry have provided other benefits. For example, high-copper amalgam restorations demonstrate significant improvements in early strength, corrosion resistance, marginal integrity, and longevity. In addition, the bonding of materials to tooth structure has made possible dramatic improvements in composite, ceramic, and glass ionomer restorations and the development of expanded restorative applications of these materials. More conservative approaches are now available for many typical restorative procedures (Classes I, II, III, IV, and V); diastema closure procedures; the esthetic and/or functional correction of malformed, discolored, or fractured teeth; and the actual replacement of teeth. When compared with past treatment modalities, these newer approaches result in significantly less removal of tooth structure.

Although these are only several examples, they demonstrate the current emphasis on conservation. *The primary result of conservative treatment is the retention of more intact tooth structure and less trauma to the pulp tissue and contiguous soft tissue.* Not only will the remaining tooth structure be stronger but also the restoration should be more easily retained, offer greater esthetic potential, and cause less alteration in intraarch and interarch relationships.

Efforts for the conservative restoration of teeth are ongoing. Research activity is progressing toward the development of materials and techniques to completely bond restorative materials to tooth structure, the result being to significantly reduce the necessity for extensive cavity preparations. Such activity will be vigorously pursued in the future, and continued advances in operative dentistry will occur. These efforts will ultimately have the impact of benefiting the oral health of the public.

Dynamics of operative dentistry

In the future, advances in treatment techniques, philosophies, and materials almost certainly will be developed, just as in the past several decades technological and scientific advances have occurred that have dramatically affected the need for, demand for, and delivery of restorative services. Such past and future developments illustrate the dynamics of operative dentistry, a constantly changing and advancing discipline.

The development of the *high-speed handpiece* played a dramatic role in the more conservative and efficient removal of tooth structure for restorative procedures. The use of the high-speed instrumentation along with the acknowledged benefits of water coolants also led to the concept of *four-handed dentistry*. Major changes in operatory equipment design followed, which resulted in a more comfortable, efficient, and productive setting for the delivery of dental care.

The mechanical bonding of restorations to tooth structure by etching enamel and using dentin bonding agents has led to the development of many new composite restorative materials, as well as *conservative restorative bonding techniques*. Studies on filler composition and polymerization methodology for these *composite materials* have led to both increased esthetic qualities and resistance to wear. Similarly, the benefits of *sealants* have been widely accepted for the prevention of pit and fissure caries.

The increased knowledge of the carious process and the beneficial effects of multiple fluoride application have resulted in a significant decrease in caries incidence. Likewise, the increasing professional *emphasis on prevention* is as important as the recent technological and scientific advancements. The recognition that *most dental disease is preventable* has resulted in better patient self-care and more conservative efforts by dentists in treatment.

Increased research on biomaterials has led to the introduction of *vastly improved dental materials*. Developments in impression materials and gold foil, as well as advancements in knowledge about bases and varnishes, are other factors that have resulted in better care and treatment for patients. Advances in metallurgy have resulted in a variety of improved alloys that are either already available or are being developed. Corrosion-resistant amalgam alloys have been developed that will enhance the oral health of the population by providing longer-lasting restorations.

All of the factors previously mentioned have played an important role in the development of operative dentistry. They have resulted in a reduction of the incidence of caries and a more conservative and effective approach toward treatment, with the ultimate result of improved oral health for all populations.

FACTORS AFFECTING THE FUTURE DEMAND FOR OPERATIVE DENTISTRY

Because of the dynamic status of operative dentistry, many developments and advancements will occur in the future. These advances in technology, science, and materials will have a significant impact on the future practice of and demand for operative dentistry. Additionally, there are other factors which will affect the future.

To project the future demand for operative dentistry treatment, both current and projected dental health in the United States must be identified. This first necessitates a projection of demographic changes, economic factors, and dental health and the impact of these projections on the future demand for dental services.

Demographics

The population of the United States will increase from 241 million in 1986 to 268 million by the year 2000.[8] This represents a 12% increase which will result from increased numbers of immigrants, higher birth rates of immigrants and minorities, and the Baby Boom Echo, a short-lived birth rate increase brought about by the 75 million Baby Boomers (those born between 1946 and 1964) going through the U.S. society. Between 1991 and 2030 the population is projected to increase by 61 million people (to a total of 310 million)[31] and the composition of the American population then will be different: one third of the population will consist of minorities, and the numbers of elderly will be significantly higher. These population changes will affect the entire professional life of most of today's dental school graduates.

The percentage of *elderly in the population will increase* substantially in the next 40 years. This increase will occur primarily as a result of the aging of the Baby Boomers (the first of whom will turn 50 years old on January 1, 1996) as well as the increased life expectancy for U.S. residents. As a result of these factors, the 65-year-old and older age group will be 20% of the population by the year 2030; while that age group was only 4% of the population in 1900 and 7% in 1940.[33] The 65-year-old and older age group (senior adults) makes up the fastest growing segment of society, growing twice as fast as the general population. Two thirds of all people in the United States who have lived to the age of 65 are alive today.

Because of the increased life expectancy, the Baby Boomers will grow older than the previous elderly segments. Many of the Baby Boomers were not exposed to fluoridated water during their formative years and consequently have had extensive restorative dental care. But this large segment of the population along with other-age cohorts, except the current elderly, have developed an appreciation for dental health and practice reasonable dental self-care. Since most of these individuals also will retain more of their teeth as they age, *they will create a continuing demand for dental services* because they not only will want to keep their teeth, but also they will experience a standard of living which will permit a degree of discretionary income for health care expenditures.

Because of the aging of the U.S. population, emphasis will shift from the needs of the young to the concerns and demands of the middle-aged and elderly. Although the absolute numbers of children will not decrease substantially in the next 40 years, their percentage in the population and relative importance in health care policies will decrease. On the other hand, the elderly will increase in both absolute size and importance.[8] Already the elderly are receiving a much higher percentage of health care benefits than is their percentage of society. Such benefits will increase as the political and economic clout of the elderly increases.

Economic factors

No one can accurately project the economic status for the future. While the U.S. economy will be part of a more global, world-wide economy, the economic projections for the United States appear bright. The national deficit may not be eliminated but will become a lesser and lesser percentage of the Gross National Product. The annual improvement of both the Gross National Product and productivity growth is projected to be at least equal to earlier periods in U.S. history that are considered to have been good economic times. If inflation and unemployment continue at reasonable levels, there will be more discretionary income available in the future; and discretionary income is generally that which is utilized for dental health expenditures.

Thus it appears that the economic forecast for the United States is good. With more discretionary income and more health care benefits for the adult segment of society, *the demand for future dental services should increase.*

Health of the population, general and dental

In considering the current and projected dental health of the U.S. population, a brief assessment of the general health of the population is necessary.

General health. The general health of the U.S. population is good. The ability to prevent or cure infectious disease has led to an increase in life expectancy. The ability to control, partially or fully, some of the chronic diseases is resulting in a larger proportion of elderly persons in the population. Life expectancy rates in 1991 were 80 years for males and 84 years for females,[5] as compared to 1776 when the Declaration of Indepen-

dence was signed and life expectancy was only 35 years.[32]

In 1990, Americans spent \$662.2 billion on health care.[34] Yet, access to and financial resources for health care are problems for some segments of society. More than 30 million Americans do not have health insurance[17] and the elderly (over 65) have four fifths of nursing home costs and one third of all health expenditures and fees to physicians.[37]

Dental health. Americans are in good dental health. They know the benefits of good dental health and practice good oral homecare. Except for many of the current elderly, most Americans do not believe that the eventual loss of teeth is inevitable. Consequently, they are willing to invest their resources for dental health care. In 1990, \$34 billion was spent on dental care in the United States[34] which represented a 7½% increase over 1989 dental expenditures. This percentage increase was less than the increase in total health care spending (10½%) but greater than the growth rate of the economy (5.1%).[34] Over 100 million Americans have dental insurance, which in 1989 covered approximately 43% (\$14 billion) of all dental care costs.[30]

Yet, a significant increase in dental insurance coverage for those not currently enrolled is not expected. Even though the dental care expenditure for 1990 was 5.1% of the total health care expenditure,[34] that was a decrease compared to the 1987 level of 6.5%.[17] Furthermore, it is projected that in the year 2000, dental care spending will be \$63 billion yet will represent only 4.3% of total health care spending.[34] Thus, *the financing of dental care will require more attention in the future.*

In considering the future demand for operative dentistry, an assessment of the current and projected status of caries, missing teeth, and periodontal health will be presented briefly, followed by a projection of the increased numbers of teeth that will be at risk to dental disease in the future.

Caries. The incidence of caries has decreased. This reduction in caries is a result of increased usage of sealants and antibiotics as well as improved homecare efforts, but primarily is a result of increased exposure to fluoride. Fluoridation of community water systems began in Grand Rapids, Michigan, in 1945. By 1980, 106 million Americans in 8000 communities had the benefits of adjusted fluoridated water[38] and, additionally, 9.8 million Americans in 3000 communities had naturally fluoridated water.[18] The expanded use of dietary fluoride supplements, school-based fluoride mouth-rinse programs, professional topical fluoride applications, and fluoride toothpastes have also contributed to this reduction.[3] For example, over one fourth of the school districts in the United States offer schoolchildren the opportunity to participate in a fluoride mouth-rinse program.[29]

Children are experiencing less caries. A 1986 survey[23] revealed that 50% of all children (age 5 to 17) were caries-free. This compared with 37% caries-free in 1980 and 28% in 1972.[36] Yet the caries-free children were the very young and the incidence of caries increased with age. By age 17, 84% of the population has had caries, averaging 11 decayed or filled surfaces.[24] Lastly, this same survey revealed that in 1986, children had an average of 3.07 decayed, missing, or filled surfaces (DMFS) compared to a 1979-80 survey in which children had a 4.77 DMFS.[5] Thus, while the incidence of caries in children has decreased, caries remains a problem for this age group.

The most recent survey on caries activity in *adults* was presented by the National Institutes of Health (NIH) in 1987.[25] This data, which separated adults into younger (or employed) adults (age 18 to 64) and senior adults (65 and older), revealed that adults had many decayed or filled surfaces. The *younger adults* averaged 23 decayed or filled surfaces (DFS) and *21% had root caries*. The 40- to 50-year age group had the highest decayed and filled ratio of the younger adult cohort, and 16.2% of the filled surfaces in this age group had recurrent caries that required replacement restorations.[25] This same age group had a DFS score of 31 while 18- and 19-year-olds had a DFS score of only 12. Less than 5% of the 18 to 64 age group had no caries.[25]

Per 100 teeth, the *senior adults* had a higher incidence of caries than either the younger adults or children.[6] The senior adults averaged 20 DFS (a lower average because 42% of the elderly had no teeth) and *2 out of 3 seniors had root caries*. Although most of the coronal caries had been filled, only half of the root caries lesions were restored. From the 1987 NIH survey, the DMFS scores for senior adults did not decline and was slightly higher than for younger adults.

Missing teeth. From this same 1987 NIH survey, it was also noted that even though **partial edentulism** *will continue in the adult population,* total edentulism (no teeth) is decreasing dramatically in the elderly population. In 1987 42% of the senior adults were edentulous as compared to 50% in 1972 and 60% in 1958. Only 4% of the younger adults were edentulous in 1987. As these younger adults age, it is projected that, as senior adults, their edentulism rate will be very low. However, 45% of the 35- to 45-year-old group did have tooth loss patterns that were consistent with the need for complete dentures, partial dentures, or fixed bridges.[22] This age group will be dental patients for the next 30 to 50 years. Thus, fewer current elderly are edentulous than previous elderly and the trend in retaining more teeth is expected to continue in the future. Also, partial edentu-

lism will continue and therefore be a source of demand for dental care in the future.

Periodontal status. The 1987 NIH survey also assessed periodontal status, and showed that half of the adults had some gingival bleeding, more than three fourths had calculus, and periodontal attachment loss was evident in 77% of the younger adults (age 18 to 64) and 95% of the senior adults. The attachment loss was much more severe in the senior adults. The attachment loss and associated gingival recession is a major factor in the development of root caries.

Teeth at risk to dental disease. Reinhardt and others[27] have used some of these 1987 NIH survey results in combination with other studies and Bureau of Census population projections to determine and predict how many teeth are at risk to dental disease. Their findings demonstrate that in 1980 there were 2.8 billion teeth at risk to dental disease and that number will increase to 4.0 billion by 1990, 4.4 billion by 2000, and 5.0 billion by 2030.[27] Thus between 1990 and 2030 there will be an increase of 1 billion teeth at risk to dental disease. This increase will occur because of a decreased rate of tooth loss combined with the aging of the Baby Boomers. Between 1990 and 2030, there will be a 73% increase in the 45-and-older age group and a 104% increase in the senior adults, thereby resulting in 90% more teeth in the 45-and-older age group and 153% more teeth in the senior adult group.[27]

*The **future demand for operative dentistry** care will increase.* As previously noted, the population will increase with the greatest increase occurring in the elderly component of society. Because these increased numbers of adults will retain more teeth, there will be more teeth at risk to dental disease and many of these teeth will require operative care. In exploring these expectations further, several other factors must be addressed.

Dental manpower

In 1990 there was a total of 18,000 enrolled dental students, which was an 18% decrease in enrollment since the late 1970s.[1] Likewise, the first-year dental school enrollment for 1993 was projected to be only 3450, approximately one-half of the highest first-year enrollment level of 1978.[28] Even though dental school enrollment has decreased, there was a 400% increase in the number of female dentists in the 1980s. It is projected there will be 24,000 female dentists, representing 15% of all dentists by the year 2000.[1]

Because of the dramatic proliferation of dental schools and dental school enrollments in the 1960s and 1970s, the number of dentists increased from 75,000 in 1950 to 121,200 in 1980, and the number of dentists is projected to be 156,300 by the year 2000.[28] These numbers will result in the dentist-to-population ratio (DDS/

100,000 people) increasing from 53.5 in 1980 to 59.0 in 2000.[8] However, when the projected increased number of teeth at risk to dental disease is considered, the dentist-to-teeth ratio (DDS/1,000,000 teeth) is decreased from 43.3 in 1980 to 35.5 in 2000.[8] Because of the decrease in dental school enrollment, it is projected that the number of dentists will decrease to 135,000 by 2020 and the dentist-to-population ratio will only be 43.5. Thus, there will be fewer dentists per teeth at risk in the future, which will increase the demand for operative dentistry on those dentists.

Projected hours of need for operative dentistry

Douglas and others[9] projected that the hours of needed operative dentistry treatment in the year 2000 will be 36 million hours more than the hours needed in the early 1970s. This projection included a perceived reduction in the number of hours of operative dentistry needed for children; but the dramatic increase in need for adults more than offsets that reduction. Another study[27] showed a 20% increase in the number of needed operative hours from 125 million in 1972 to 150 million in 1990. Furthermore, it projected 192 million hours of operative treatment will be needed by 2030. This would be 65 million hours more than in 1972, representing a 54% increase.

The increased *number of hours needed for operative care in the future* will be for the following operative procedures: (1) restorations for restoring teeth with new carious lesions; (2) restorations to restore teeth with root caries; (3) restorations to replace existing, faulty restorations; and (4) restorations to enhance the esthetic appearance of patients.

New caries. New caries will continue to occur. Even though 50% of children (age 5 to 17) are caries-free, the remaining 50% have caries. Seventeen-year-olds have 11 decayed or filled surfaces and are estimated to have 32 million carious permanent tooth surfaces needing restoration.[5] Yet, overall, the need for operative services for children is expected to decrease.[8] *Adults, especially older adults, have high caries rates.* The 45- to 49-year-old age group had 31 decayed or filled surfaces[5] and the senior adults had a higher incidence of caries than the younger adult groups. Less than 5% of the 18- to 64-year-old age group had no caries.[5]

Root caries. Root caries will increase due to the increased number of elderly who will retain more teeth and experience more gingival recession. Additionally, many of the elderly may have systemic problems which may directly or indirectly alter normal salivary functioning, thus increasing the potential for root caries formation. The 1987 NIDR survey reported root caries in 63% of the senior adults. With more teeth retained by the future elderly, a greater incidence of root caries can be expected.

Replacement restorations. Replacement restorations will also stimulate much future demand. There is a large need for replacement dentistry. It has been estimated that at any given time approximately one third of existing restorations need replacement.[10,16] The knowledge that the "baby boom" generation is middle-aged, which has the highest number of decayed and filled tooth surfaces of any age group, documents the continuing need for restorative care in the future. Currently more than 50% of the income from restorative procedures is from the replacement of restorations in patients older than 40.[21]

Esthetic restorations. The public has come to appreciate the possibilities of esthetic enhancements from dental treatment due to the publicity about bonding. Such publicity has occurred in the form of magazine articles, television shows, and special news programs. It is now estimated that 10% of a dentist's gross income is derived from esthetic treatment on non-carious teeth.[26] With more teeth being retained in the future, more people are likely to seek appearance enhancements, especially when most such treatments are relatively simple, non-invasive, and non-stressful.

Public's perception of dentistry

The public's perception about dentistry is another factor which will influence whether or not the increased numbers of teeth and increased need for operative services will be converted to increased demand. Fortunately, the public considers dentists and dentistry very positively. The public ranks a dentist as one of the most respected members of the community and dentistry has the highest satisfaction rating by the public when assessing the services they receive. Lastly, the public not only thinks highly of the profession, but also appreciates the benefits of good dental health. All of this suggests a continuing demand for operative services.

Patient visits

Because of the significant increase in the number of adults in the future, it is important to consider their past use of dental services as well as their potential economic status. In 1970, 25.8% of the senior adults visited a dentist annually. That percentage had increased to 38.6% by 1983.[12] While prior to 1983 this group averaged only 1.5 visits to the dentist per year,[2] they increased their dental visits by 29% between 1983 and 1986.[21] Currently they make more visits to a dentist than any other age group.[35] The economic status of the adults will affect their future dental demand. With dental expenditures considered as discretionary, the availability of discretionary income will influence the amount of dental care sought. One study showed that over one half of the elderly with annual incomes below $10,000 had not seen a dentist for 5 years; while only

18% of those with incomes over $35,000 had not seen a dentist during the same time period.[21] Overall, the elderly (over 55) currently have 77% of the financial assets in the United States, 68% of all money market funds, and 80% of all money in savings and loans institutions. Additionally, 75% own their on home with 84% of the mortgages already paid off.[32] *Therefore the new elderly and the future elderly will not only possess positive perceptions about dentistry and dental health but also will have the economic means to secure the dental care they need.*

These factors affecting the demand for operative dentistry point to an *increase in operative treatment in the future.* The increased number of elderly, the increased number of teeth, the increased affluence of the population, the positive image of dentistry, and the projected increased hours of operative need all support this increased demand.

THE FUTURE OF OPERATIVE DENTISTRY

"Research is the primary catalyst to professional growth and has greatly added to the understanding of the etiology, diagnosis, and treatment of dental diseases."[3] Exciting research is occurring that will have an additional impact on the future of operative dentistry. "New knowledge in molecular and cellular biology, genetics, pharmacology, radiation biology, radiation physics and technology, including tomography, dental materials based on polymer chemistry and ion exchange, microbiology, immunology, and behavioral science are all relevant to the understanding and clinical management of dental problems."[19] "In terms of future scientific achievement, it is not difficult to predict startling new advances due to the application of recombinant DNA technology, the application of space age technology, and the general advancement of scientific methodology. Advances in these areas can have direct impact on dental practice through the development of new treatments and preventive modes, new biomaterials applicable to dental practice, and more sophisticated techniques to measure the health status of individuals."[7]

Research in operative dentistry is now occurring in a number of fields. The use of lasers in dentistry may lead to a new mechanism for welding dental alloys or altering tooth structure in cavity preparation. Already, lasers are used in etching enamel and making enamel more resistant to demineralization. Extended uses of acid etch techniques and further developments in composite restorative materials may lead to even more conservative restorative techniques. The beneficial use of composites in posterior teeth has become more evident. Much research and clinical testing also is being done on castable ceramic materials. The introduction of computer-generated restorations has stimulated much interest, and fur-

ther refinement of such technology is anticipated. *Improvements in composites, castable ceramics, and computer-generated restorations could result in a significant decrease in the use of metal alloy systems in operative dentistry.* Also, the increasing *concern about potential toxicity* of some components of current alloy systems, such as mercury and nickel, may result in decreased use of these systems in the future. Likewise, significant *environmental concerns* are surfacing regarding the disposal of certain materials used in dentistry, especially mercury.

Efforts are also being made to develop an anticaries vaccine. Even if developed, the widespread use of such an agent may not occur in the foreseeable future in the United States because of the already documented caries reduction from multiple fluoride use, limitations imposed by regulatory agencies, and concern about possible side effects.[3] Whereas use of such an agent in developing countries may provide greater immediate benefits, its use in the United States may be confined to high-risk patients.

In the future the method to adhesively bond composite materials to dentin will improve. Such a development will have dramatic effects on the practice of operative dentistry, resulting in minimal tooth preparation. *Effective dentinal bonding* could significantly increase tooth conservation while potentially reducing patient anxiety. Techniques used for such bonding procedures may also increase productivity.

Finally, the *developing concepts in cariology* may have major implications in dealing with dental caries. The increased knowledge about factors involved in the carious process should place an emphasis on treating the carious lesion by other than restorative techniques. It seems possible to foresee a time when diagnosis and treatment techniques are so refined as to preclude the necessity of cavity preparation to control some carious activity. The remineralization of a tooth surface affected by a beginning carious lesion may not only decrease the need for restorative care but also result in a tooth surface that will be more resistant to subsequent carious attacks. The development of appropriate fluoride applications and techniques to produce this remineralization appears to be a reality in the near future.

All of these potential developments and changes will occur in a future environment of increased need for operative treatment because of more people, especially adults, who will retain more of their teeth. *The emphasis of the profession will shift to care for the senior adult segment of the population.* This population will require significant dental care due not only to replacement needs for existing restorations but also to development of new caries, especially root caries. Increased understanding of treatment methods for the elderly will be required as well as improved knowledge of information pertaining to their overall medical health. Dental research efforts will continue in seeking treatment methods which will be more efficient and less stressful for these patients. Bonded restorations, both amalgam and composite, may provide benefits in treating this segment of the population as compared to current treatment modalities requiring more complex and time-consuming techniques such as pin amalgam or cast restorations.

SUMMARY

Many thoughts have been presented in this chapter, some of which will be expanded in other chapters of this book. *The objective has been to indicate the factors that influence operative dentistry both today and in the future.* Certainly changes in our society, changes in the future oral health of the U.S. population, and developments within the discipline of operative dentistry will affect the future practice of operative dentistry.

Many exciting advances have already been made, and others are expected in the future. Important progress is being made toward the time when caries and periodontal disease will no longer be major public health problems. "As part of their professional responsibilities, dentists have an obligation to monitor the dental welfare of the public and adjust their patterns of treatment accordingly. Professional ethics dictate that dentists must embrace new and accepted dental treatment, materials and devices, and, at the same time, discard outmoded treatment and techniques in pursuit of optimal oral health for the public"[3]

Dental education should strive to produce practitioners who can think critically using the scientific method so they can be in a position to evaluate future claims related to advancing the profession.

Dentistry must also continue to broaden its knowledge of the biological basis on which it is founded. Practitioners must continually familiarize themselves with the advances being made. Increased research activity and continued practitioner adaptability will result in improved oral health of populations throughout the world.

REFERENCES

1. American Association of Dental Schools: 1988 *Dean's briefing book,* 1987-88 academic year, Washington, DC.
2. American Dental Association, Bureau of Economic Research and Statistics: *Utilization of dental services by the elderly population,* Chicago, 1980.
3. American Dental Association: Interim report of the American Dental Association's special committee on the future of dentistry: issue papers on dental research, manpower, education, practice and public and professional concerns, *J Am Dent Assoc,* Sept 1982.
4. Black CE, Black BM: *From pioneer to scientist,* St Paul, Minn, 1940, Brace Publishing.
5. Bowen WH: Dental caries: is it an extinct disease?, *J Am Dent Assoc* 122:49-52, Sept 1991.
6. Chauncey et al: The effects of age and dentition status on caries incidence in adults, *J Dent Res* 69:212, 1990 (abstract).
7. DePaola DP: Application of basic and medical sciences in the dental curriculum, *J Dent Educ* 45:685, 1981.
8. Douglass CW, Furino A: Balancing dental service requirements and supplies: epidemiologic and demographic evidence, *J Am Dent Assoc* 121:587-592, Nov 1990.
9. Douglass CW, Gammon MD: The epidemiology of dental caries and its impact on the operative dentistry curriculum, *J Dent Educ* 48:547-555, 1984.
10. Elderton RJ: The cause of failure of restorations: a literature review, *J Dent* 4:257, 1976.
11. Flexner A: *Medical education in the United States and Canada, a report to the Carnegie Foundation for the Advancement of Teaching,* New York, 1910, Carnegie Foundation.
12. Giangrego E: Dentistry and the older adult, *J Am Dent Assoc* 114:299-307, March 1987.
13. Gies WJ: *Dental education in the United States and Canada, a report to the Carnegie Foundation for the Advancement of Teaching,* New York, 1926, Carnegie Foundation.
14. Heymann HO, Roberson TM: Operative dentistry in North Carolina: a survey, *N C Dent Gazette* 3(6):10, 1981.
15. Horner HH: *Dental education today,* Chicago, 1947, University of Chicago Press.
16. Lavelle CI: A cross-sectional longitudinal survey into the durability of amalgam restorations, *J Dent* 4:139, 1976.
17. Levit KR, Freeland MS: National medical care spending, *Health Aff* 7:124-136, 1988.
18. Loe H: The fluoridation status of US public water supplies, *Public Health Rep* 101:157-162, March/April 1986.
19. Loe H: The impact of research and technological advances on dental education, *J Dent Educ* 45:670, 1981.
20. McCluggage RW: *A history of the American Dental Association,* Chicago, 1959, American Dental Association.
21. Meskin LH et al: Economic impact of dental service utilization by older adults, *J Am Dent Assoc* 120:665-668, June 1990.
22. Meskin LH et al: Patterns of tooth loss and accumulated prosthetic treatment potential in U.S. employed adults and seniors, *Gerondontics* 4:126-135, 1986.
23. National Institute of Dental Research. National survey of oral health in school children 1986-87. Tables from the NIDR released data on the survey (unpublished).
24. National Institute of Dental Research, U.S. Department of Health and Human Services, *NIDR Research News* 173:2, May 1982.
25. National Institutes of Health. Oral Health of United States adults. The national survey of oral health in U.S. employed adults and seniors: 1985-1986. National findings. Washington, DC: U.S. Government Printing Office, 1987; *NIH publication no. 87-2868.*
26. Reinhardt JW, Capilouto ML: Composite resin esthetic dentistry survey in New England, *J Am Dent Assoc* 120:541-544, May 1990.
27. Reinhardt JW, Douglass CW: The need for operative dentistry services: projecting the effects of changing disease patterns, *Operative Dentistry* 14:114-120, 1989.

28. Schwab P: Medical and dental manpower projections of the Health Resources and Services Administration. Office of Data Analysis and Management, the Division of Medicine and Division of Associated and Dental Health Professions (to the American Association of Dental Schools Council of Deans), November 1988.

29. Silversin JB, Coombs JA, Drolette ME: Achievements of the seventies: self-applied fluorides, *J Public Health Dent* 40:256, 1980.

30. Sorian R, Firshein J: Dentistry wrestles with change, *Perspectives,* supplement to *Medicine and Health,* Sept 1991.

31. Spencer G: *1984 population estimates and projections: projections of the population of the United States by age, sex, and race: 1983 to 2080,* U.S. Department of Commerce, May 1984.

32. Truono EJ: The aging population and its impact on the future of dentistry—a symposium, *J Am Coll Dent* 58(2):14-16, Summer 1991.

33. U.S. Bureau of Census. Decennial census and current population, *Report Series II;* 1987:25.

34. U.S. Department of Health and Human Services, Health Care Financing Administration, *Health Care Financing Review,* Fall 1991.

35. U.S. Department of Health and Human Services: Use of dental services and dental health, United States, 1986, Washington, DC, U.S. Government Printing Office, 1988. *DHHS publication no. 88-1593.*

36. U.S. Department of Health and Human Services: The prevalence of dental caries in United States children, NIDR, Washington, DC, Dec 1981, *NIH Pub. No. 82-2245.*

37. Waldo DR, Levit KR, Lazenby H: National health expenditures, 1985, *Health Care Financing Rev* 8:1-43, 1986.

38. Waldron HB: Dentists and dentistry changed in the 1980s, *J Am Coll Dent* 56(4):4-13, Winter 1989.

CHAPTER 2

Clinical significance of dental anatomy, histology, physiology, and occlusion

Thomas F. Lundeen

John R. Sturdevant

Troy B. Sluder, Jr.

INTRODUCTION

Dental anatomy, histology, physiology, and occlusion are interrelated disciplines that are prerequisites for success in restorative procedures. In addition to the instruments and materials used to prepare and restore the teeth, the relationships of internal and external tooth anatomy to function and restorative procedures must be understood. A knowledge of the various structures of the teeth (enamel, dentin, cementum, and pulp) and their relationships to each other and of the supporting structures is necessary for excellence in the performance of operative dental procedures. (See Fig. 2-3 for illustration of these structures.)

A basic understanding of proper anatomical form is essential in the restoration of either a single tooth or a group of teeth, because function depends on form. *The individual form of a tooth and the contour relationships with adjacent and opposing teeth are major determinants of function in mastication, esthetics, speech, and protection.* The protective function of tooth form applies both to the contiguous investing tissues (osseous and mucosal) and to the pulp. Proper tooth form usually is a factor contributing to a healthy state of the investing tissues, with a critical balance of protection (e.g., of interproximal tissues) and stimulative massage from the passage of food during mastication (see Figs. 2-37, 2-38, and 2-39). Certainly the soft pulp is protected by the hard, overlying tooth structures of dentin, enamel, and cementum. Also, knowing the usual form of the pulp cavity, chamber, and canal(s), is an essential factor for determining the materials and procedures best suited for restoring the protective function of the tooth's hard tissues lost due to disease or trauma. This knowledge is helpful in maintaining health of the pulp.

The tooth is an organ of mastication and must be treated as such in restoring it to proper form and function and preventing further insult to it and its investing tissues. A high degree of manipulative skill is required in the fabrication of a restoration to replace lost tooth structure and to prevent further damage to the tooth and supporting structures. *Supporting tissues of the teeth are an important consideration in operative procedures* since the attachment apparatus must be treated with care and respect to prevent periodontal disease.

TEETH AND INVESTING TISSUES
Dentitions

Normally, in the human dentition two sets of teeth erupt during the life cycle from childhood to adult. The first set is the ***primary dentition*** which consists usually of 10 maxillary and 10 mandibular teeth. The second set usually is referred to as the ***permanent dentition,*** normally consisting of 16 maxillary and 16 mandibular teeth.

Classes of human teeth—form and function

Human teeth are divided into classes on the basis of form and function. Both the primary and permanent dentitions include incisors, canines, and molars. The fourth class, the premolars, is found only in the permanent dentition (Fig. 2-1). The form predicts the function of teeth, and therefore class traits are the characteristics that place teeth into functional categories. Since the diet of humans consists of both animal and vegetable foods, the human dentition is called ***omnivorous.***

Incisors. The incisors are located near the entrance of the oral cavity and function as cutting or shearing instruments for food (Fig. 2-1). From a proximal view the crowns of these teeth have a triangular shape with a narrow incisal surface, including the incisal edge, and a broad cervical base (see Fig. 2-47, *D*.) The incisors contribute significantly to function, esthetics, and phonetics.

Canines. The canines possess the longest roots of all teeth and are located at the corners of the dental arch. They function in the seizing, piercing, and tearing of food, as well as in cutting. From a proximal view the crown also has a triangular shape with a thick incisal ridge. The stocky anatomical form of the crown and length of the root are reasons why these teeth are strong, stable abutment teeth for a fixed or removable prosthesis. The canines serve as important guides in occlusion because of their anchorage and strategical position in the dental arches (see Figs. 2-1 and 2-60).

Premolars. The premolars serve a dual role in function in that they act like the canines in the tearing of

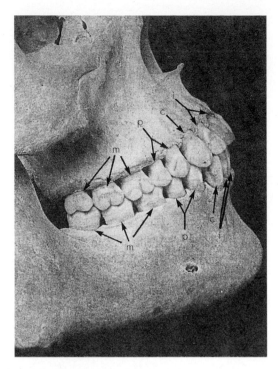

Fig. 2-1. Maxillary and mandibular teeth in centric occlusion. The classes of teeth are incisors *(i)*, canines *(c)*, premolars *(p)*, and molars *(m)*. Note that cusps of mandibular teeth are one-half cusp anterior of corresponding cusps of teeth in maxillary arch. (From Shankle RJ: Clinical dental anatomy, physiology, and histology. In Sturdevant CM et al, editors: *The art and science of operative dentistry,* ed 1, New York, 1968, McGraw-Hill.)

food and are similar to molars in the grinding of food. Whereas the first premolars are angular with their facial cusps resembling the canines, the lingual cusps of the maxillary premolars and molars have a more rounded anatomical form (see Figs. 2-1 and 2-40). The occlusal surfaces present a series of curves that are in the form of concavities and convexities. This form of rounded ideal anatomical shape should be maintained through life for correct occlusal contacts and function.

Molars. The molars are large, multicusped, strongly anchored teeth located nearest the temporomandibular joint, which serves as the fulcrum during function (see Fig. 2-54). These teeth have a major role in the crushing, grinding, and chewing of food to the smallest dimensions suitable for deglutition. The occlusal surfaces of both the premolars and molars act as a myriad of shears that function in the final mastication of food. The premolars and molars are also important in maintaining the vertical dimension of the face (see Figs. 2-1 and 2-2).

Structures of the teeth

The teeth are composed of enamel, pulp-dentin complex, and cementum (Fig. 2-3). Each of these structures will be discussed individually.

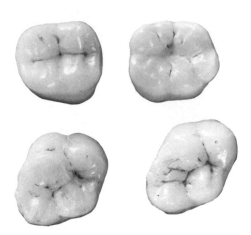

Fig. 2-2. Occlusal surfaces of maxillary and mandibular first and second molars after several years of use showing rounded curved surfaces and minimal wear.

Enamel. Enamel is formed by cells called *ameloblasts,* which originate from the embryonic germ layer known as *ectoderm.* Ameloblasts have short extensions toward the dentinoenamel junction and these are termed *Tomes processes.* Enamel covers the *anatomical crown of the tooth* and varies in *thickness* in different areas of a tooth (see Fig. 2-14). The enamel is thicker at the incisal and occlusal areas of a tooth and becomes progressively thinner until it terminates at the cementoenamel junction. The thickness also varies from one class of tooth to another, averaging 2 mm at the incisal ridges of incisors, and varying from 2.3 to 2.5 mm at the cusps of premolars and 2.5 to 3 mm at the cusps of molars. Enamel usually decreases in thickness toward the junction of the developmental cuspal lobes of the posterior teeth (premolars and molars) sometimes nearing zero where the junction is fissured (non-coalesced) (see Figs. 2-12 and 2-14.)

Because enamel is mostly gray and is semitranslucent, the color of the tooth depends upon the color of

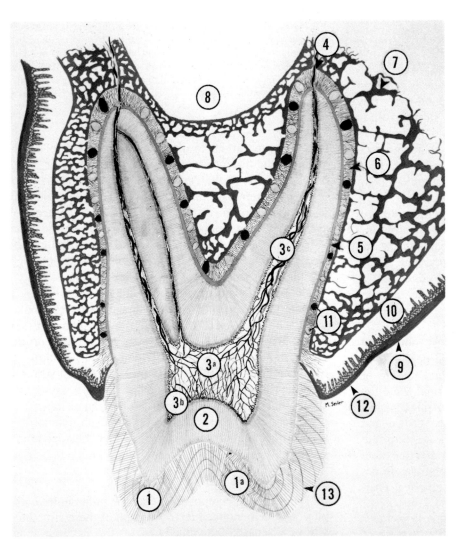

Fig. 2-3. Schematic drawing illustrating cross section of maxillary molar and its supporting structures. *1,* enamel; *1a,* gnarled enamel; *2,* dentin; *3a,* pulp chamber; *3b,* pulp horn; *3c,* pulp canal; *4,* apical foramen; *5,* cementum; *6,* periodontal fibers in periodontal ligament; *7,* alveolar bone; *8,* maxillary sinus; *9,* mucosa; *10,* submucosa; *11,* blood vessels; *12,* gingiva; *13,* lines of Retzius. (From Brauer JC, Richardson RE: *The dental assistant,* ed 3, New York, 1964, McGraw-Hill. Reproduced with permission.)

the underlying dentin, the thickness of the enamel, and the amount of stain in the enamel. The amount of *translucency* of enamel is related to variations in the degree of calcification and homogeneity. Abnormal conditions of enamel usually result in aberrant color. Enamel becomes temporarily whiter within minutes when the tooth is isolated from the moist oral environment by rubber dam or absorbents. Thus the shade must be determined before isolation and preparation of the tooth for a tooth-colored restoration. This change in color is explained by the temporary loss of loosely bound (or exchangeable) water (less than 1% by weight). (For details refer to the discussion of optical properties in Chapter 6, section titled, Physical Properties.)

Chemically, enamel is a highly mineralized crystalline structure containing from 95% to 98% inorganic matter by weight. *Hydroxyapatite,* in the form of a crystalline lattice, is the largest mineral constituent and is present 90% to 92% by volume. Other minerals and trace elements are contained in smaller amounts. The remaining *constituents of tooth enamel* are an organic content of about 1% to 2% and a water content of about 4% by weight, and these total approximately 6% by volume.

Structurally, enamel is composed of millions of enamel *rods* or *prisms,* which are the largest structural components, as well as rod sheaths and a cementing interrod substance in some areas. (Interrod substance, or sheath, may be the increased spacing between crystallites oriented differently where the "tail" portion of one rod meets the "head" portion of another. This spacing apparently is partially organic material. Ed. C. Sturdevant. See Fig. 3-6.) The rods vary in number from approximately 5 million for a mandibular incisor to about

12 million for a maxillary molar. The rods are densely packed and intertwined in a wavy course, and each extends from the dentinoenamel junction to the external surface of the tooth. In general the rods are aligned perpendicularly to both the dentinoenamel junction and the tooth surface in the primary and permanent dentitions, except in the cervical region of permanent teeth where they are oriented outward in a slightly apical direction. In the primary dentition the enamel rods in the cervical and central parts of the crown are nearly perpendicular to the long axis of the tooth, and are similar in their direction to the permanent teeth in the occlusal two thirds of the crown. Enamel rods measure in diameter near the dentinal borders about 4 μm and about 8 μm near the surface; this difference accommodates the larger outer surface of the enamel crown compared to the dentinal surface at the dentinoenamel junction.

The hardest substance of the human body is enamel. Hardness may vary over the external tooth surface according to the location of the area; also, it decreases inward, with hardness lowest at the dentinoenamel junction. The density of enamel also decreases from the surface to the dentinoenamel junction. Enamel is a very brittle structure having a high elastic modulus and low tensile strength, which indicates it is a rigid structure. However, dentin is a highly compressive tissue that acts as a cushion for the enamel. Enamel requires a base of dentin to withstand masticatory forces. Enamel rods that fail to possess a dentin base because of caries or improper cavity design are easily fractured away from neighboring rods. For maximal strength in cavity preparation all enamel rods should be supported by dentin (Fig. 2-4).

Human enamel is composed of rods that in transverse

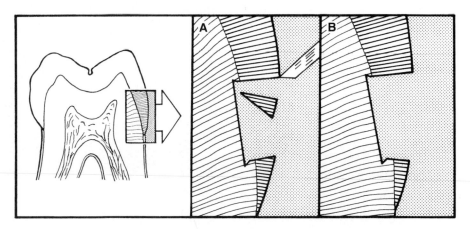

Fig. 2-4. A, Enamel rods unsupported by dentin base are fractured away readily by pressure from hand instrument. **B,** Cervical preparation showing enamel rods supported by dentin base. (From Shankle RJ: Clinical dental anatomy, physiology, and histology. In Sturdevant CM et al, editors: *The art and science of operative dentistry,* ed 1, New York, 1968, McGraw-Hill.)

section are shaped with a rounded *head* or body section and a *tail* section, which forms a repetitive series of interlocking prisms. The rounded head portion of each prism (5 μm wide) lies between the narrow tail portions (5 μm long) of two adjacent prisms (Fig. 2-5; see also Fig. 3-6). Generally, the rounded head portion of the prism is oriented in the incisal or occlusal direction, and the tail section is oriented cervically.

The structural components of the enamel prism are millions of small elongated apatite crystallites that are variable in size and shape. The crystallites are tightly packed in a distinct pattern of orientation that gives strength and structural identity to the enamel prisms. The long axis of the apatite crystallites within the central region of the head (body) is aligned almost parallel to the rod long axis, and they incline with increasing angles up to 65 degrees to the prism axis in the tail region. The susceptibility of these crystallites to acid, either with an etching procedure or caries, appears to be correlated with their orientation. Whereas the dissolution process occurs more in the head regions of the rod, the tail regions and the periphery of the head regions are relatively resistant to acid attack. The crystallites are irregular in shape with an average length of about 1600 Å and an average width of about 200 to 400 Å. Each apatite crystallite is composed of thousands of unit cells that have a highly ordered arrangement of atoms. A crystallite may be 300 unit cells long, 40 cells wide, and 20 cells thick in a hexagonal configuration (Fig. 2-6).

An organic *matrix* or prism *sheath* also surrounds in-

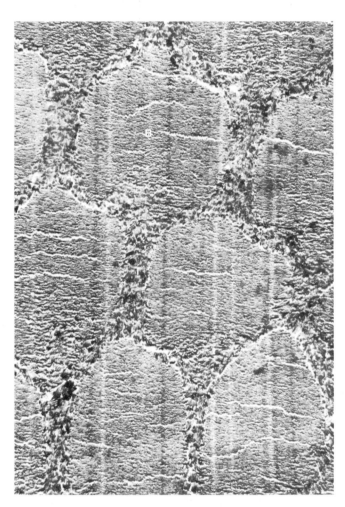

Fig. 2-5. Electron micrograph of cross section of rods in mature human enamel. Crystal orientation is different in "bodies" *(B)* than in "tails" *(T)*. (Approximately × 5000.) (Reprinted with permission from *Arch Oral Biol,* vol 10, AH Meckel, WJ Griebstein, RJ Neal, Structure of mature human dental enamels observed by electron microscopy, Copyright 1965, Pergaman Press, Ltd.)

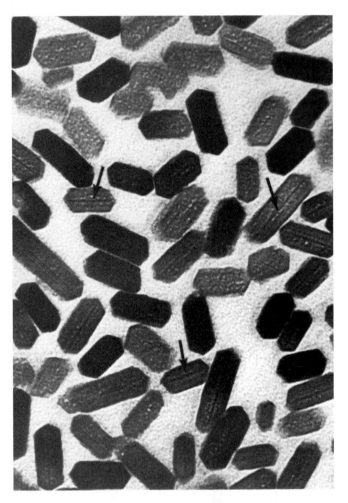

Fig. 2-6. Electron micrograph of mature, hexagonally shaped enamel crystallites *(arrows).* (Approximately × 350,000.) (From Nylen MU, Eanes ED, Omnell KÅ. Reproduced from *The Journal of Cell Biology,* 1963, vol 18, p 109, by copyright permission of The Rockefeller University Press.)

dividual crystals, and it appears to be an organically rich interspace rather than a structural entity.

Enamel rods follow a wavy, spiraling course, producing an alternating arrangement for each group or layer of rods as they change direction in progressing from the dentin toward the enamel surface where they end a few microns short of the tooth surface. Enamel rods rarely run a straight radial course because it appears there is an alternating clockwise and counterclockwise deviation of the rods from the radial course at all levels of the crown. They initially follow a curving path through one third of the enamel next to the dentinoenamel junction. Then the rods usually follow a more direct path to the enamel surface in the remaining two thirds of the enamel. There are groups of enamel rods that may entwine with adjacent groups of rods, and they follow a curving irregular path toward the tooth surface. These comprise what is termed *gnarled enamel,* and it occurs near the cervical regions and the incisal and occlusal areas (Fig. 2-7). Gnarled enamel is not subject to cleavage as is the more regular enamel. This type of enamel formation does not yield readily to the pressure of bladed, hand cutting instruments in cavity preparation.

The changes in direction of enamel prisms that minimize cleavage in the axial direction produce an optical appearance called *Hunter-Schreger bands* (Fig. 2-8). These bands appear to be composed of alternate light and dark zones of varying widths that have slightly different permeability and organic content. These bands are found in different areas of each class of teeth. Since the enamel rod orientation varies in each tooth, Hunter-Schreger bands have a variation in the number present in each tooth. In the anterior teeth they are located near the incisal surfaces. They increase in numbers and areas of the teeth from the canines to the premolars. In the molars these bands occur from near the cervical region to the cusp tips. The orientation of the enamel rod heads and tails and the gnarling of enamel rods provide strength by resisting impact forces and distributing and dissipating these forces.

Enamel tufts are hypomineralized structures of enamel rods and interrod substance that project between adjacent groups of enamel rods from the dentinoenamel junction (Fig. 2-9). These projections arise in the dentin, extend into enamel in the direction of the long axis of the crown, and may play a role in the spread of dental caries. *Enamel lamellae* are thin, leaflike faults be-

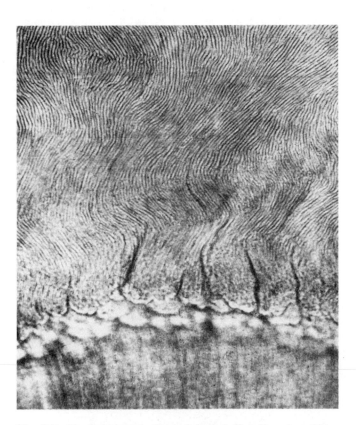

Fig. 2-7. Gnarled enamel. (From Schour I: *H.J. Noyes' oral histology and embryology,* Philadelphia, 1960, Lea & Febiger.)

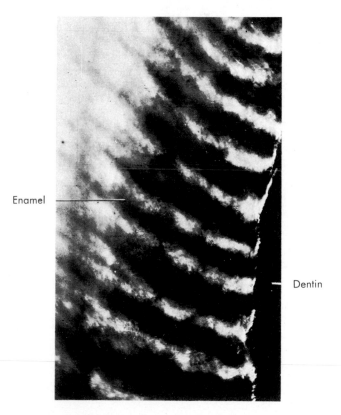

Enamel

Dentin

Fig. 2-8. Longitudinal ground section through enamel photographed by reflected light of Hunter-Schreger bands. (From Yaeger JA: Enamel. In Bhaskar SN, editor: *Orban's oral histology and embryology,* ed 9, St Louis, 1980, Mosby.)

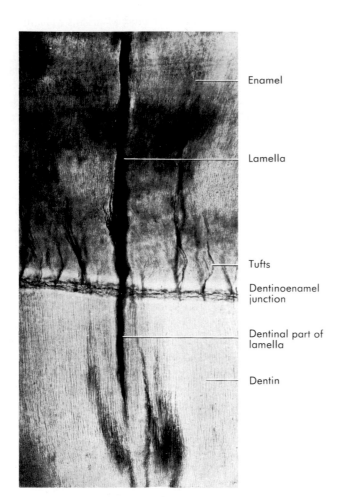

Fig. 2-9. Transverse ground section through lamella that goes from enamel surface into dentin. Note enamel tufts. (From Yaeger JA: Enamel. In Bhaskar SN, editor: *Orban's oral histology and embryology,* ed 9, St Louis, 1980, Mosby.)

Fig. 2-10. Ground section. Odontoblastic processes extend into enamel as enamel spindles. (From Yaeger JA: Enamel. In Bhaskar SN, editor: *Orban's oral histology and embryology,* ed 9, St Louis, 1980, Mosby.)

tween enamel rod groups that extend from the enamel surface toward the dentinoenamel junction, sometimes extending into the dentin (Fig. 2-9). They contain mostly organic material, which is a weak area predisposing the tooth to entry of bacteria and dental caries. Odontoblastic processes sometimes cross the dentinoenamel junction into the enamel, and they are termed *enamel spindles* when their ends are thickened (Fig. 2-10). They may serve as pain receptors, thereby explaining the enamel sensitivity experienced by some patients during cavity preparation.

Enamel rods are formed linearly by successive apposition of enamel in discrete increments. The resulting variations in structure and mineralization are called the *incremental striae of Retzius* and can be considered as growth rings (see Figs. 2-3 and 3-6, *A* and *B*). In transverse sections of a tooth the striae of Retzius appear as concentric circles. In longitudinal sections the lines transverse the cuspal and incisal areas in a symmetrical arc pattern descending obliquely to the cervical region and terminating at the dentinoenamel junction (see Fig. 2-3). When these circles are incomplete at the enamel surface, a series of alternating grooves, which are called the *imbrication lines of Pickerill,* are formed. The elevations between the grooves are called *perikymata* (see Figs. 3-6, *B*, and 3-7). They are continuous around a tooth and usually lie parallel to the cementoenamel junction and to each other.

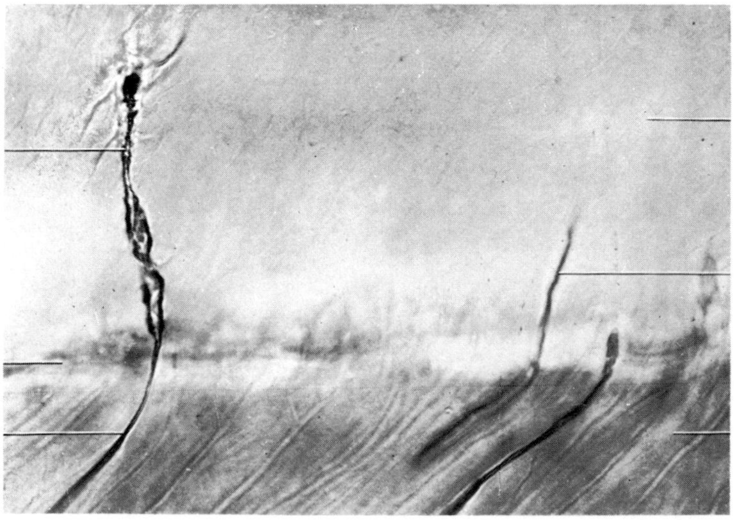

There is a *structureless outer layer of enamel* about 30 μm thick found most commonly toward the cervical area and less often on cusp tips. There are no prism outlines visible, and all the apatite crystals are parallel to one another and perpendicular to the striae of Retzius. It appears that this layer is more heavily mineralized. Microscopically, the enamel surface initially has circular depressions indicating where the enamel rods end (see Fig. 3-6, *B*). These concavities vary in depth and shape, and they may contribute to the adherence of plaque material with a resultant caries attack, especially in young people. However, the dimpled surface anatomy of the enamel gradually wears smoother with age.

The interface of the enamel and dentin is called the **dentinoenamel junction** (DEJ) (Fig. 2-11). It is scalloped or wavy in outline with the crest of the waves penetrating toward the enamel. The rounded projections of enamel fit into the shallow depressions of dentin. This interdigitation seems to contribute to a firm attachment between the dentin and enamel. The dentinoenamel junction is also a hypermineralized zone that is about 30 μm thick.

Recall that deep invaginations occur in pit and fissure areas of the occlusal surfaces of premolars and molars that decrease enamel thickness in these areas. These *fissures* act as food and bacterial traps that may predispose the tooth to dental caries (Fig. 2-12). Occlusal *grooves,* which are sound, serve an important function as an escapeway for the movement of food to the facial and lingual surfaces during mastication. A functional cusp that opposes a groove occludes on the enamel inclines on each side of the groove and not in the depth of the groove. Therefore this arrangement leaves a *V-shaped escapeway* between the cusp and its opposing groove for the movement of food during chewing.

Grooves/fissures are formed at the junction of the developmental lobes of the enamel. *Sound coalescence of the lobes results in grooves; faulty coalescence results in fissures.*

Enamel is incapable of repairing itself once it is destroyed, because the ameloblast cell degenerates following the formation of the enamel rod. The final act of the ameloblast cell is secretion of a membrane covering the end of the enamel rod. This layer is referred to as the **Nasmyth membrane,** or the **primary enamel cuticle.** This membrane covers the newly erupted tooth and is worn away by mastication and cleaning. The membrane is replaced by an organic deposit called a **pellicle,** which appears to be a precipitate of salivary proteins. Microorganisms invade the pellicle to form bacterial plaque, which is a precursor to dental disease.

Although enamel is a very hard and dense structure, it is **permeable** to certain ions and molecules, permitting partial and complete penetration. The route of passage appears to occur through structural units that are hypomineralized and rich in organic content such as rod sheaths, enamel cracks, and other defects. It appears that water plays an important role as a transporting medium through small intercrystalline spaces. Enamel permeability decreases with age because of changes in the enamel matrix, although basic permeability is main-

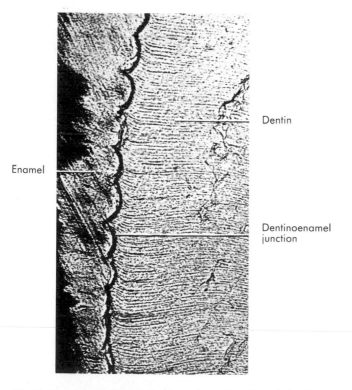

Fig. 2-11. Longitudinal ground section of scalloped dentinoenamel junction. (From Yeager JA: Enamel. In Bhaskar SN, editor: *Orban's oral histology and embryology,* ed 9, St Louis, 1980, Mosby.)

Enamel

Dentin

Dentinoenamel junction

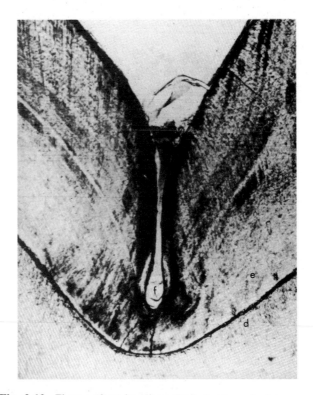

Fig. 2-12. Fissure *(f)* at junction of lobes acts as food trap predisposing tooth to dental caries. *e,* enamel; *d,* dentin. (From Gilling B, Buonocure M: *J Dent Res* 40:119, Jan-Feb 1961.)

tained. This decrease is referred to as ***enamel maturation.***

Enamel is *soluble* when exposed to an acid medium, although the dissolution is not uniform. Solubility of enamel increases from the enamel surface to the dentinoenamel junction. When fluorides are present during enamel formation or are topically applied to the enamel surface, the solubility of surface enamel is decreased. Fluoride concentration decreases toward the dentinoenamel junction. Fluoride additions can affect the chemical and physical properties of the apatite mineral and influence the hardness, chemical reactivity, and stability of enamel while preserving the apatite structures. Trace amounts of fluoride stabilize enamel by lowering acid solubility, by decreasing the rate of demineralization, and by enhancing the rate of remineralization. In addition, there is evidence that topical fluorides alter the oral bacterial flora, thereby increasing resistance to dental caries.

An established operative technique involves acid etching the enamel surface for the micro-mechanical "bonding" of composite restorative materials or pit and fissure sealants directly to the etched surface. The etchant usually is a 35% to 50% solution of phosphoric acid. This etching produces an irregular and pitted surface with numerous microscopic undercuts by an uneven dissolution of enamel rod heads and tails. Composite or pit and fissure sealant is bonded to the enamel surface by resin tags formed in the acid etched enamel rod structures (see Figs. 6-41 and 16-9). Therefore it is apparent that the structure of enamel can be an asset when it is subjected to purposeful and controlled acid dissolution of the enamel rods to provide this microretention for composite or sealant.

Pulp-dentin complex. Dentin and pulp tissues are specialized connective tissues of mesodermal origin and are formed from the dental papilla of the tooth bud. These two tissues are considered by many investigators as a single tissue, thus forming the pulp-dentin complex, with mineralized dentin comprising the mature end product of cell differentiation and maturation. Dentin is formed by cells called ***odontoblasts.*** Odontoblasts are considered part of both dentin and pulp tissues since their cell bodies are in the pulp cavity but their long, slender cytoplasmic cell processes ***(Tomes fibers)*** extend well into the tubules in the mineralized dentin (Fig. 2-13). It is because of these odontoblastic cell processes that dentin is considered a living tissue, with the capa-

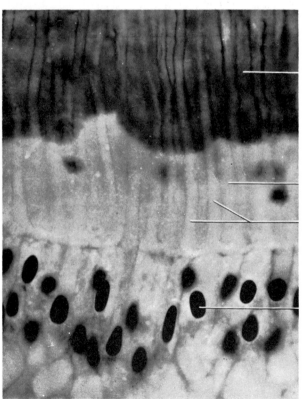

Calcified dentin

Uncalcified dentin (predentin)

Odontoblastic processes

Bodies of odontoblasts

Fig. 2-13. Odontoblastic processes (Tomes fibers), lying in dentinal tubules, extend from odontoblasts into dentin. (From Avery JK: Dentin. In Bhaskar SN, editor: *Orban's oral histology and embryology,* ed 9, St Louis, 1980, Mosby.)

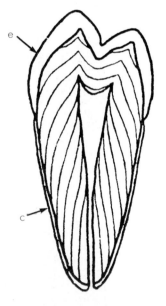

Fig. 2-14. Pattern of formation of primary dentin. (From Scott JH, Symons NBB: *Introduction to dental anatomy,* ed 7, Edinburgh, 1974, Churchill Livingstone.) (This figure also shows the enamel *(e)* covering the anatomical crown of the tooth and cementum *(c)* covering the anatomical root.)

bility to react to physiological and pathological stimuli. Such stimuli can result in changes throughout the life of the tooth, such as secondary dentin, reparative dentin, sclerotic dentin, and dead tracts. The dentin and pulp are discussed separately in the following sections.

Dentin. Dentin forms the largest portion of tooth structure, extending almost the full length of the tooth. Externally dentin is covered by enamel on the anatomical crown and by cementum on the anatomical root. Internally dentin forms the walls of the pulp cavity (*pulp chamber* and *pulp canal[s]*) (Fig. 2-14).

The odontoblasts begin dentin formation immediately before enamel formation by the ameloblasts. **Dentinogenesis** begins with the odontoblasts laying down a collagen matrix, moving from the dentinoenamel junction inward towards the pulp. Mineralization of the collagen matrix gradually follows its secretion. The most recently formed layer of dentin is always on the pulpal surface. This unmineralized zone of dentin is immediately next to the cell bodies of the odontoblasts and is called **predentin.** Dentin formation begins at areas subadjacent to the cusp tip or incisal ridge and gradually spreads to the apex of the root (Fig. 2-14). Unlike enamel, dentin formation continues after tooth eruption and throughout the life of the pulp. The dentin forming the initial shape of the tooth is called **primary dentin,** and is usually completed 3 years after tooth eruption (for permanent teeth).

The **dentinal tubules** are small canals that extend across the entire width of dentin, from the dentinoenamel or dentinocemental junction to the pulp (Fig. 2-15; see also Fig. 2-21). Each tubule contains the cytoplasmic cell process (Tomes fiber) of an odontoblast. Each dentinal tubule is lined with a layer of **peritubular dentin,** which is much more mineralized than the surrounding **intertubular dentin** (Fig. 2-16).

The surface area of dentin is much larger at the dentinoenamel or dentinocemental junction than it is on the pulp cavity side. Since the odontoblasts form dentin progressing inward toward the pulp, the tubules are forced closer together. The number of tubules increases from 15,000 to 20,000/mm^2 at the dentinoenamel junction to 45,000 to 65,000/mm^2 at the pulp.[5] The lumen of the tubules varies from the dentinoenamel junction to the pulp surface as well. In coronal dentin, the average diameter of tubules at the dentinoenamel junction is 0.5 to 0.9 μm, but increases to 2 to 3 μm at the pulp (Fig. 2-17).

The course of the dentinal tubules is in a slight S-curve in the tooth crown, but the tubules are straighter in the incisal ridges, cusps, and root areas (Fig. 2-18). The ends of the tubules are perpendicular to the dentinoenamel and dentinocemental junctions. Along the tubule walls are small lateral openings called **canaliculi.** As the odontoblastic process proceeds from the cell in the pulp to the dentinoenamel junction, lateral secondary branches extend into the canaliculi and appear to communicate with lateral extensions of adja-

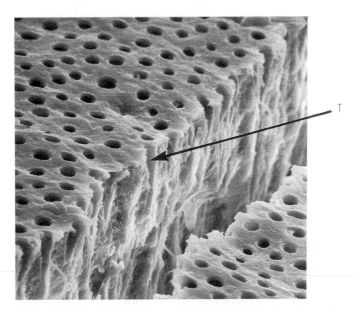

Fig. 2-15. Ground dentinal surface, acid-etched for 5 seconds with 37% phosphoric acid. The artificial crack shows part of the dentinal tubules, *T*. The tubule apertures are opened and widened by acid application. (From Brännström M: *Dentin and pulp in restorative dentistry,* London, 1982, Wolfe Medical Publications.)

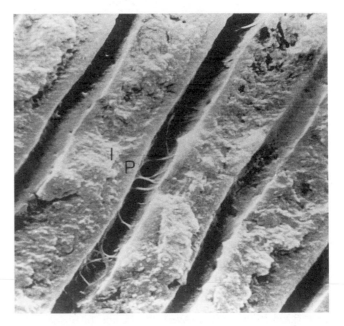

Fig. 2-16. Dentinal tubules in cross section, 1.2 mm from pulp. Peritubular dentin, *P*, is more mineralized than intertubular dentin, *I*. (From Brännström M: *Dentin and pulp in restorative dentistry,* London, 1982, Wolfe Medical Publications.)

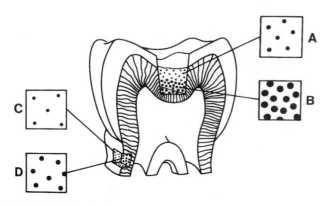

Fig. 2-17. Tubules in superficial dentin close to the dentinoenamel junction, *A,* are smaller and more sparsely distributed compared to deep dentin, *B.* The tubules in superficial root dentin, *C,* and deep root dentin, *D,* are smaller and less numerous than those in comparable depths of coronal dentin. (From Trowbridge HO: *Dentistry '82,* 2:22, 1982; modified by Pashley DH.)

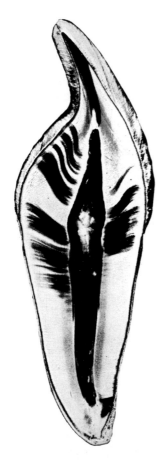

Fig. 2-18. Ground section of human incisor. Course of dentinal tubules is in a slight S-curve in crown but rather straight at incisal tip and in root. (From Avery JK: Dentin. In Bhaskar SN, editor: *Orban's oral histology and embryology,* ed 9, St Louis, 1980, Mosby.)

cent odontoblastic processes. Near the dentinoenamel junction the tubules (with processes seen in young teeth) divide into several terminal branches, thus forming an intercommunicating and anastomosing network (Fig. 2-19).

After the primary dentin is formed, dentin deposition continues at a reduced rate even without obvious external stimuli, though the rate and amount of this physiological *secondary dentin* varies considerably between individuals. In secondary dentin the tubules take a slightly different directional pattern in contrast to primary dentin (Fig. 2-20). Secondary dentin forms on all internal aspects of the pulp cavity, but in the pulp chamber in multi-rooted teeth it tends to be thicker on the roof and floor than on the side walls.[20]

Reparative dentin (tertiary dentin) is formed by replacement odontoblasts (termed ***secondary odontoblasts***) in response to moderate-level irritants, such as attrition, abrasion, erosion, trauma, moderate-rate dentinal caries, and some operative procedures. It usually appears as a localized dentin deposit on the wall of the pulp cavity immediately sub-adjacent to the area on the tooth that has received the injury (a dentin deposit underneath the affected tubules) (Fig. 2-21). For example, reparative dentin usually is formed when cavities are prepared within 1.5 mm from the pulp.[21] The cut fibers (odontoblastic processes) die along with the corresponding odontoblasts, leaving dead tracts that are described in the next paragraph. New odontoblasts are differentiated from mesenchymal cells of the pulp (in about 15 days), and these replacement odontoblasts lay down the reparative dentin. It is confined to the localized irritated area of the pulp cavity wall, becomes apparent microscopically about 1 month from inception of stimulus, is structurally and chemically different from primary and secondary dentin, and being highly atubular is impervious to most irritants. Reparative or

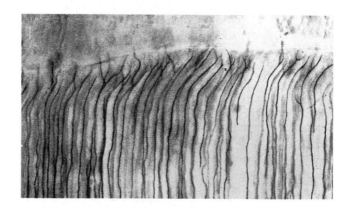

Fig. 2-19. Ground section showing dentinal tubules and their lateral branching close to dentinoenamel junction. (From Scott JH, Symons NBB: *Introduction to dental anatomy,* ed 7, Edinburgh, 1974, Churchill Livingstone.)

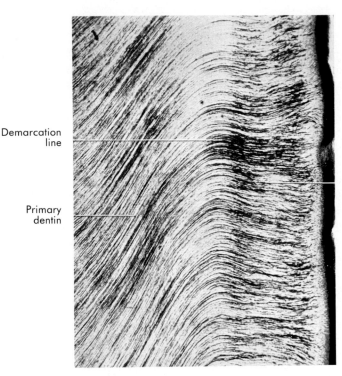

Demarcation line

Primary dentin

Secondary dentin

Fig. 2-20. Ground section of dentin with pulpal surface at right. Dentinal tubules curve sharply as they move from primary to secondary dentin. Dentinal tubules are more irregular in shape in secondary dentin. (From Avery JK: Dentin. In Bhaskar SN, editor: *Orban's oral histology and embryology,* ed 9, St Louis, 1980, Mosby.)

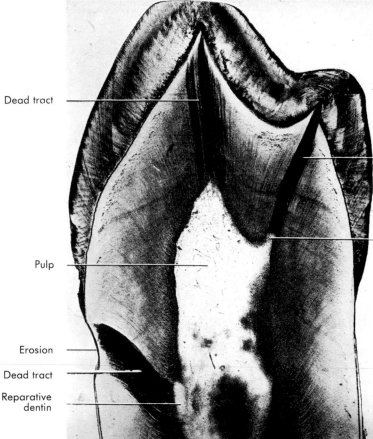

Dead tract

Dead tract

Reparative dentin

Pulp

Erosion

Dead tract

Reparative dentin

Fig. 2-21. Cross section illustrating dead tracts and reparative dentin caused by degeneration of odontoblasts in pulpal horns and exposure of dentinal tubules to erosion on root surface, respectively. (From Avery JK: Dentin. In Bhaskar SN, editor: *Orban's oral histology and embryology,* ed 9, St Louis, 1980, Mosby.)

tertiary dentin is a defense reaction to an area of moderate-intensity injury.

Stating again, when moderate-level stimuli are applied to dentin, such as moderate-rate caries or attrition, the affected odontoblastic processes may die as well as the associated odontoblasts. These areas of dentin are called *dead tracts* and extend from the external dentin surface to the pulp. The tubules are empty, and thus appear black when ground sections of dentin are viewed microscopically with transmitted light. Dead tracts are sealed off at the pulpal surface by reparative dentin formed by replacement odontoblasts. While dead tracts are commonly associated with areas of caries or attrition, they have occurred in unerupted incisors and in teeth that show little if any obvious external defects. Dead tracts may be considered in some circumstances a form of age change that is associated with the death of odontoblasts. Usually this occurs in areas of the pulp where the odontoblasts have been crowded into narrow pulp horns (Fig. 2-21). In dried ground sections of normal teeth the odontoblastic processes contract and may allow the tubules to fill with air, giving the appearance of a dead tract. However, a true dead tract can be distinguished by a deposit of reparative dentin on the pulpal surface.[20]

Sclerotic dentin results from aging or mild irritation (such as slowly advancing caries) and causes a change in the composition of the primary dentin. The peritubular dentin becomes wider, gradually filling the tubules with calcified material, progressing from the dentinoenamel junction pulpally (Fig. 2-22). These areas are harder, denser, less sensitive, and more protective of the pulp against subsequent irritations. Sclerosis resulting from aging is *physiological dentin sclerosis,* and that resulting from a mild irritation is *reactive dentin sclerosis.* Reactive dentin sclerosis often can be seen radiographically in the form of a more radiopaque (lighter) area in the S-shape of the tubules. *Eburnated dentin* is a term referring to the outward (exposed) portion of reactive sclerotic dentin where slow caries has destroyed formerly overlying tooth structure, leaving a hard, darkened, cleanable surface (see Fig. 5-19, *A* and *B).*

The *composition of human dentin* is approximately 75% inorganic material, 20% organic material, and 5% water and other materials. Dentin is less mineralized than enamel but more mineralized than cementum or bone. The mineral content of dentin increases with age. This mineral phase is composed primarily of hydroxyapatite crystallites, which are arranged in a less systematic manner than enamel crystallites. Dentinal crystallites are smaller than enamel crystallites, having a length of 200 to 1000 Å and a width of about 30 Å, similar to the sizes seen in bone and cementum.[20] The organic phase of dentin consists primarily of collagen.

Dentin is significantly softer than enamel but harder than bone or cementum. The *hardness of dentin* averages about one fifth that of enamel. The hardness of dentin near the dentinoenamel junction is about three times greater than the value near the pulp. Dentin becomes harder with increasing age, due primarily to increases in mineral content. While dentin is a hard, mineralized tissue, it is somewhat flexible, with a *modulus of elasticity* of 1.67×10^6 PSI. This flexibility of dentin helps it to support the more brittle, nonresilient enamel. Often small "craze lines" are seen in enamel that indicate minute fractures of that structure. These craze lines usually are not clinically significant unless they are associated with cracks in the underlying dentin. In general, dentin is not as prone to cleavage as is the enamel rod structure. The *tensile strength of dentin* is approximately 40 MPa (6000 PSI), which is less than cortical bone and approximately one-half that of enamel. The *compressive strength of dentin* is much higher at 266 MPa (40,000 PSI).[8]

During cavity preparation, dentin is usually distin-

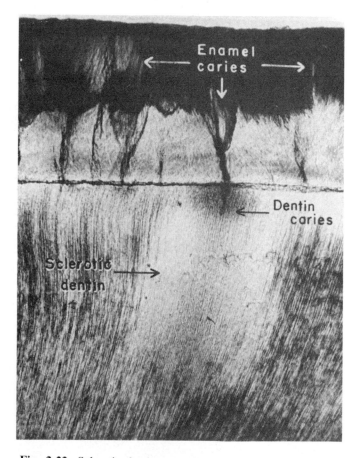

Fig. 2-22. Sclerotic dentin occurring under enamel caries with early penetration of dentin caries along enamel lamella. (From Schour I: *Noyes oral histology and embryology,* Philadelphia, 1960, Lea & Febiger.)

guished from enamel by its (1) *color,* (2) *reflectance,* (3) *hardness,* and (4) *sound.* Dentin is normally yellow-white and slightly darker than enamel. In older patients dentin is darker, and can become brown or black in cases where it has been exposed to oral fluids, old restorative materials, or slowly advancing caries. Dentin surfaces are more opaque and dull, being less reflective to light than similar enamel surfaces which appear shiny. Dentin is softer than enamel and will provide greater yield to the pressure of a sharp explorer tine, which tends to catch and hold in dentin. When moving an explorer tine over the tooth, enamel surfaces will provide a sharper, higher-pitched sound than dentin surfaces.

Sensitivity is encountered whenever odontoblasts and their processes are stimulated during operative procedures even though the pain receptor mechanism appears to be within the dentinal tubules near the pulp. A variety of physical, thermal, chemical, bacterial, and traumatic stimuli are transmitted through the dentinal tubules, although the precise mechanism of the transmissive elements of sensation has not been established conclusively. The most accepted theory of pain transmission is the *hydrodynamic theory.* This theory accounts for pain transmission by the small, rapid movements of fluid that occur within the dentinal tubules.[2] Because many tubules contain mechanoreceptor nerve endings near the pulp, small fluid movements in the tu-

bules arising from cutting, drying, pressure changes, osmotic shifts, or changes in temperature account for the majority of pain transmission (Fig. 2-23).

Dentinal tubules are normally filled with odontoblastic processes and *dentinal fluid,* a transudate of plasma. When enamel or cementum is removed during cavity preparation, the external seal of dentin is lost, and the tubules become fluid-filled channels from the cut surface directly to the pulp. Fortunately pulpal fluid has a slight positive pressure that forces fluid outward toward any breach in the external seal. *Permeability* studies of dentin indicate that tubules are functionally much smaller than would be indicated by their measured microscopic dimensions, as a result of numerous constrictions along their paths (see Fig. 2-16).[15] Dentin permeability is not uniform throughout the tooth. Coronal dentin is much more permeable than root dentin. There are also differences within coronal dentin (Fig. 2-24).[22] Dentin permeability is primarily dependent on the remaining dentin thickness (length of the tubules), and the diameter of the tubules. Since the tubules are shorter, become more numerous, and increase in diameter closer to the pulp, deep dentin is a less effective barrier than is superficial dentin near the dentinoenamel or dentinocemental junctions (Fig. 2-25).

Dentin must be treated with great care during restorative procedures to minimize damage to the odontoblasts and the pulp. Air-water spray should be used whenever cutting with high-speed handpieces to avoid heat build up. The dentin should not be dehydrated by compressed air blasts, ideally always having the dentin with its normal fluid content (Fig. 2-26). Protection is also provided by the judicious use of cavity liners, bases, dentin bonding agents, and nontoxic restorative

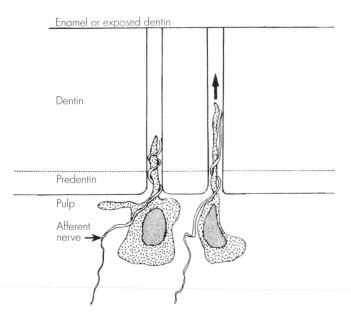

Fig. 2-23. Stimuli which induce fluid movements in dentinal tubules distort odontoblasts and afferent nerves *(arrow),* leading to sensation of pain. Many operative procedures such as cutting or air-drying induce such fluid movement. (From Brännström M: *Dentin and pulp in restorative dentistry,* London, 1982, Wolfe Medical Publications.)

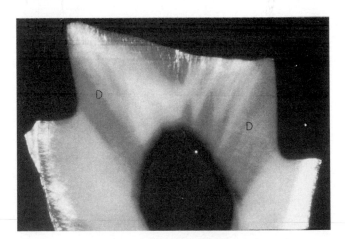

Fig. 2-24. Ground section of mesioocclusodistal (MOD) cavity preparation on third molar. Dark blue dye was placed in pulp chamber under pressure after cavity preparation. Dark areas of dye penetration, *D,* show that dentinal tubules of axial walls are much more permeable than those of pulpal floor of cavity preparation.

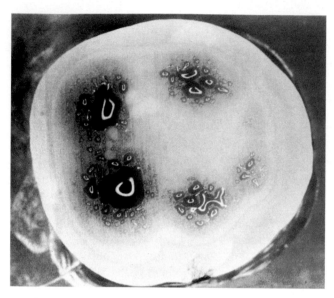

Fig. 2-25. Horizontal section in occlusal third of molar crown. Dark blue dye was placed in pulp chamber under pressure. Deep dentin areas (over pulp horns) are much more permeable than superficial dentin. (Reprinted from *Arch Oral Biol* 32:7, Pashley DH, et al. Regional variability in the permeability of human dentin, 519-523, 1987, with permission from Pergaman Press Ltd, Headington Hill Hall, Oxford 0X3 0BW, UK.)

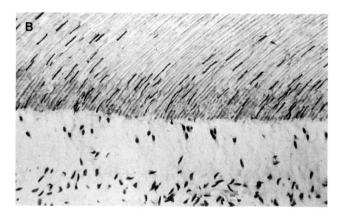

Air blast

Removal of fluid = rapid outward flow due to capillary force

Aspiration of cells and nerves = stretching and/or disruption of nerves

materials. Restorations must adequately seal the cavity to avoid microleakage and bacterial penetration (Fig. 2-27).

When a deep carious lesion occurs and there are no clinical or radiographic indications of irreversible pulp damage (see *reversible pulpitis* in later section, Pain from Pulpal Inflammation), the tooth may be treated by a procedure termed ***indirect pulp capping.*** This procedure involves the removal of infected dentin except for the deepest, last small amount, which if removed might expose the pulp. Subsequent placement of restorative materials must *adequately seal the cavity* and provide thermal, mechanical, and chemical protection. If the pulp is healthy, secondary odontoblasts will differentiate and form a layer of reparative dentin for further protection. The decision on whether to re-enter the cavity at a later time (at least 6 months) is based on how much infected dentin was left behind during the indirect pulp capping procedure. This decision must consider the possibility for further injury to the pulp from additional operative procedures. (See further details regarding indirect pulp capping in Caries Control Technique, in Chapter 3.)

If a small pulpal exposure occurs during cavity preparation and is not due to caries (mechanical pulp exposure), ***direct pulp capping*** with a dressing of calcium hydroxide may help stimulate the pulp to form secondary odontoblasts, which can produce a ***dentin bridge*** across the exposure site. Direct pulp capping is most successful in young patients who have healthy pulps, in

Fig. 2-26. A, Excessive drying of cavity preparations can cause odontoblasts to be aspirated into dentinal tubules. **B,** Nuclei are seen as dark rods in dentinal tubules. (From Brännström M: *Dentin and pulp in restorative dentistry,* London, 1982, Wolfe Medical Publications.)

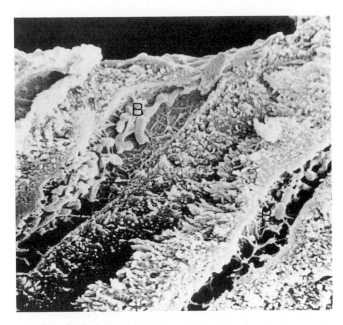

Fig. 2-27. Cross section of dentin showing an acid etched cavity left unsealed intraorally for one week. Micro-organisms *(B)* can be seen in longitudinally fractured, widened dentinal tubules. Peritubular zone has been removed. (From Olgart L, Brännström M, Johnson G: Invasion of bacteria into dentinal tubules, *Acta Odontol Scand* 32:61-70, 1974.)

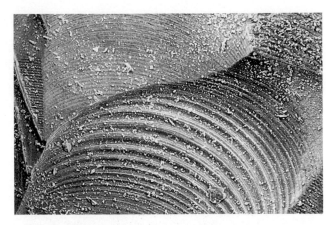

Fig. 2-28. Smear layer on cut dentin cavity surface. Swirls on surface are from end of a carbide bur. (From Marshall GW, Marshall SJ, Bayne SC: Restorative dental materials: Scanning electron microscopy and x-ray microanalysis, *Scanning Microsc* 2(4):2007-2028, 1988.)

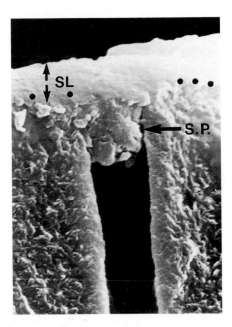

Fig. 2-29. Smear layer, *SL*, in cross section. Smear plugs, *SP*, are formed from cutting debris forced into tubules. Smear layer and smear plugs greatly reduce permeability of cut dentin surface. (From Pashley DH: Dentin: a dynamic substrate, *Scanning Microsc* 3(1):161-176, 1989.)

small exposure sites (<0.5 mm), if bleeding at the site of the exposure is easily controlled, if the exposure has not been contaminated by saliva, and if there has been little or no mechanical damage to the pulp tissue.

Whenever dentin has been cut or abraded, a thin altered surface is created called the **smear layer.** The smear layer is only a few micrometers in thickness and is composed of denatured collagen, hydroxyapatite, and other cutting debris (Fig. 2-28). The smear layer acts like a natural bandage over the cut surface since it occludes many of the dentinal tubules with debris called **smear plugs** (Fig. 2-29). While the smear layer is a good protective barrier, it is relatively weak and subject to dissolution by acids.

Reliable **dentin bonding** of composite resin restorations has been an elusive goal for dental manufacturers. While some manufacturers claim their products create chemical bonds to dentin, most experts agree that the majority of the bond strengths are formed by mechanical interlocking. Most dentin bonding systems have acidic "conditioners" that remove the smear layer and partially demineralize the intertubular dentin. In most systems these acidic components are weaker than the 37% phosphoric acid commonly used to etch enamel surfaces. When viewed under high magnification, dentin without a smear layer provides many opportunities for micromechanical retention (Fig. 2-30). Ideally, such etchants would remove the smear layer but leave the

smear plugs, since they greatly reduce dentin permeability and sensitivity. Etchants should not excessively damage exposed collagen fibers, since much of the bond strength develops from resin encapsulating these fibers.[23] After the acid conditioners, hydrophilic resin "bonding agents" are applied that can adapt to the inherently moist dentin surfaces and co-polymerize with the composite resin restoration.[16,17] While some of the bond forms from resin "tags" extending into the den-

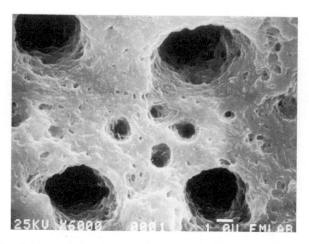

Fig. 2-30. Smear layer removed from deep human dentin with 0.5M EDTA (ethylene diamine tetracetic acid). (Courtesy DH Pashley.)

tinal tubules, most of the bond strength develops from resin penetrating and adapting to the demineralized intertubular dentin and exposed collagen fibers. The resultant resin interdiffusion zone is often termed the "hybrid layer" (Figs. 2-31 and 2-32).

While dentin bond strengths have improved, they are quite variable due to the variability of the dentin substrate. Bond strengths for superficial dentin close to the dentinoenamel or dentinocemental junctions are greater than those for deep dentin. In deep dentin the greater number of tubules and the larger diameter of tubules reduce the amount of intertubular dentin available for bonding.[18]

An important aspect of current dentin bonding agents

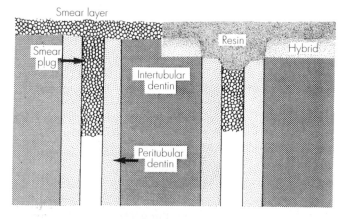

Fig. 2-31. Most dentin bonding systems remove or solubilize smear layer, allowing resins to penetrate and form "hybrid layer" with dentin structures. Ideally, smear plugs would not be removed. (From Pashley DH: The effects of acid etching on the pulpodentin complex, *Oper Dent* 17(6):229-242, 1992.)

is their ability to seal cut dentinal surfaces and thus reduce permeability and microleakage. Many dentists use dentin bonding products to seal and desensitize dentin surfaces in all cavity preparations, as well as in unrestored Class V cervical abrasion/erosion defects (Fig. 2-33).

Pulp. The ***dental pulp*** occupies the pulp cavity in the tooth. Each pulp organ is circumscribed by the dentin and is lined peripherally by a cellular layer of odontoblasts adjacent to the dentin. Anatomically the pulp organ is divided into (1) the *coronal pulp* located in the *pulp chamber* in the crown portion of the tooth, including the pulp *horns* that are directed toward the incisal ridges and cusp tips; and (2) the *radicular pulp* located

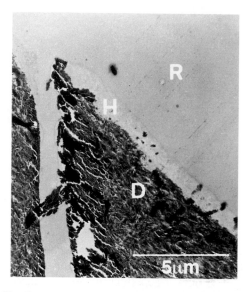

Fig. 2-32. Cross-sectional transmission electron micrograph of resin restoration bonded to dentin. Dentin bonding agent has extensive penetration into dentin structures. Hybrid layer *(H)* in middle, with resin *(R)* above, and dentin *(D)* below. (From Nakabayashi N, Takarada K: Effect of HEMA on bonding to dentin, *Dent Mater* 8(2):125-130, 1992.)

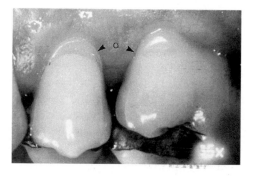

Fig. 2-33. As an alternative to restoration, sensitivity from exposed and abraded root surfaces, *(a),* can be reduced by the application of dentin bonding agents.

in the *pulp canal(s)* in the root portion of the tooth. The radicular pulp is continuous with the periapical tissues by connecting through the *apical foramen* or foramina of the root. *Accessory canals* may extend from the pulp canal(s) laterally through the root dentin to the periodontal tissues. The shape of each pulp conforms generally to the shape of each of the respective teeth (see Fig. 2-3).

The dental pulp is composed of myelinated and unmyelinated nerves, arteries, veins, lymph channels, connective tissue cells, intercellular substance, odontoblasts, fibroblasts, macrophages, and collagen and fine fibers. The central area of the pulp contains the large blood vessels and nerve trunks. The pulp is circumscribed peripherally by a specialized odontogenic area made up of (1) the odontoblasts, (2) the cell-free zone, and (3) the cell-rich zone.

The pulp is a unique, specialized organ of the human body serving four functions: (1) formative or developmental, (2) nutritive, (3) sensory or protective, and (4) defensive or reparative. The *formative function* is the production of primary and secondary dentin by the odontoblasts. The *nutritive function* supplies nutriments and moisture to the dentin through the blood vascular supply to the odontoblasts and their processes. The *sensory function* provides sensory nerve fibers within the pulp to mediate the sensation of pain. Dentin receptors are unique because various stimuli elicit only pain as a response. The pulp usually does not differentiate between heat, touch, pressure, or chemicals. *Motor* fibers initiate reflexes to the muscles of the blood vessel walls for the control of circulation in the pulp.

The *defensive function* of the pulp is related primarily to its response to irritation by mechanical, thermal, chemical, or bacterial stimuli. Such irritants can cause the degeneration and death of the involved odontoblastic processes and corresponding odontoblasts and the formation by the pulp of replacement odontoblasts (from undifferentiated mesenchymal cells) that lay down irregular or reparative dentin. The deposition of reparative dentin by the replacement odontoblasts lining the pulp cavity acts as a protective barrier against caries and various other irritating factors. This is a continuous but relatively slow process, taking 100 days to form a reparative dentin layer 0.12 mm thick. In cases of severe irritation the pulp responds by an *inflammatory reaction* similar to any other soft tissue injury. However, the inflammation may become irreversible and can result in the death of the pulp because the confined, rigid structure of the dentin limits the inflammatory response and the ability of the pulp to recover.

If, however, the irritant is very mild, such as cutting the odontoblastic processes more than 1.5 mm peripheral of the pulp at high speed with air-water coolant during cavity preparation, and although the processes and corresponding odontoblasts then die, *no replacement odontoblasts are formed and thus no reparative dentin.*[21] Therefore, there is no barrier (except for the smear layer) between the dead tracts remaining and the pulp. This may explain why many teeth have pulpal problems following cavity preparation and restoration. Newer dentin bonding agents are promising for sealing the cut dentinal surfaces.

A knowledge of the contour and size of the pulp cavity is essential during cavity preparation. In general, the pulp cavity is a miniature contour of the external surface of the tooth. The size varies among the various teeth in the same mouth and among individuals. With advancing age, the pulp cavity usually decreases in size. Radiographs are an invaluable aid in determining the size of the pulp cavity and an existing pathological condition (Fig. 2-34). Also with advanced age, the pulp generally becomes more fibrous because of episodes of irritation and may contain pulp stones or denticles. The latter are nodular, calcified masses usually appearing in the pulp chamber but also may be in the pulp canal (see Fig. 5-13, *A*). These may be attached to the pulp cavity wall or free in the mass of pulp tissue. Timely root canal therapy is advised before a stone is formed since it can be a significant problem for the root canal therapist.

Pain from pulpal inflammation. Clinical interpretation of pain from pulpal inflammation is somewhat empirical, but is nonetheless important to the successful practice of operative dentistry. One of the primary services rendered by the dentist is diagnosis and relief of pain of pulpal origin.

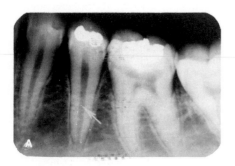
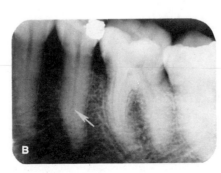

Fig. 2-34. Pulp cavity size. **A,** Premolar radiograph of young person. **B,** Premolar radiograph of older person. Note difference in size of pulp cavity. (From Shankle RJ: Clinical dental anatomy, physiology, and histology. In Sturdevant CM et al, editors: *The art and science of operative dentistry,* ed 1, New York, 1968, McGraw-Hill.)

When an irritant, such as sugar, cold, or acid from caries, first contacts dentin, the patient may be alerted by a twinge of pain. This pain is usually only momentary, ceasing if the irritant is removed. If such an irritant continues or is applied repeatedly, *hyperemia* (increased blood flow and volume) and inflammation of the pulp can result; and the pain elicited from the irritation will linger a few seconds. The reaction is because the pulp is contained by unyielding dentinal walls, and thus drainage of the increased blood is limited by the constricted apical foramen. As long as an irritant, such as touching an "ice stick" to the tooth, *causes pain that lingers no more than 10 to 15 seconds after removal of the irritant, resolution of the hyperemia by immediate restorative treatment is a possibility*. Thus such hyperemia is termed *reversible pulpitis.*

When pulpal pain, either spontaneous or elicited by an irritant, lingers more than 15 seconds, infection of the pulp often has occurred and resolution by operative dentistry treatment is usually doubtful; root canal therapy is advised for this pulpal condition termed *irreversible pulpitis,* if the tooth is to be maintained in the dentition. When this condition is untreated, suppuration and then *pulpal necrosis* follows, typified by spontaneous, continuous throbbing pain or pain elicited by heat that can be relieved by cold, and then, later, with no response to any stimulus. Pulpal necrosis is treated by root canal therapy or tooth extraction.

A primary objective during operative procedures must be the preservation of the health of the pulp. The successful management of the disease process by proper treatment of the pulp organ is discussed further in Chapters 3, 6, and 7, as well as in the chapters on restorations.

Cementum. Cementum is the hard dental tissue covering the *anatomical roots of teeth* and is formed by cells known as *cementoblasts,* which develop from undifferentiated mesenchymal cells in the connective tissue of the dental follicle. Cementum is slightly softer than dentin and consists of about 45% to 50% inorganic material (hydroxyapatite) by weight and 50% to 55% organic matter and water by weight. The organic portion is primarily composed of collagen and protein polysaccharides. *Sharpey's fibers* are the portions of the collagenous *principal fibers of the periodontal ligament* embedded in both the cementum and alveolar bone to attach the tooth to the alveolus (Fig. 2-35). Cementum is avascular. (The periodontal ligament is presented in a later section, Attachment Apparatus.)

The cementum is light yellow and slightly lighter in color than dentin. It has the highest fluoride content of all the mineralized tissue. Cementum is also permeable to a variety of materials. Cementum is formed continuously through life, because a new layer of cementum is deposited to keep the attachment intact as the superficial layer of cementum ages. *Two kinds of cementum are*

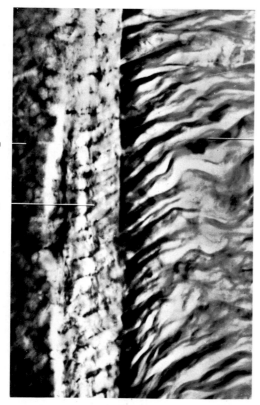

Dentin

Cementum

Fibers of periodontal ligament

Fig. 2-35. Principal fibers of periodontal ligament continue to course into surface layer of cementum as Sharpey's fibers. (From Armitage GC: Cementum. In Bhaskar SN, editor: *Orban's oral histology and embryology,* ed 9, St Louis, 1980, Mosby.)

formed: acellular and *cellular*. The **acellular layer of cementum** is a living tissue that does not incorporate cells in its structure and usually predominates on the coronal half of the root; **cellular cementum** occurs more frequently on the apical half. Cementum on the root end surrounds the apical foramen and may extend slightly onto the inner wall of the pulp canal. Cementum thickness can increase on the root end to compensate for attritional wear of the occlusal/incisal surface and passive eruption of the tooth.

The cementodentinal junction is a relatively smooth area in the permanent tooth, and the attachment of cementum to the dentin is firm but not understood completely. The cementum joins the enamel to form the cementoenamel junction, which is referred to as the *cervical line*. In about 10% of teeth, enamel and cementum do not meet, and this can result in a sensitive area. Abrasion, erosion, caries, scaling, and the procedures of finishing and polishing may result in denuding the dentin of its cementum covering, which can cause the dentin to be sensitive to several types of stimuli such as heat, cold, and sweet and sour substances. Cementum is capable of repairing itself to a limited degree and is not resorbed under normal conditions. Some resorption of the apical portion of the root often occurs during physiological tooth movement (Fig. 2-36).

Physiology of tooth form

Function. The teeth serve four main *functions*: (1) *mastication*, (2) *esthetics*, (3) *speech*, and (4) *protection of the supporting tissues*. Normal tooth form and proper alignment ensure efficiency in the incising and reduction of food with the various tooth classes—incisors, canines, premolars, and molars—performing specific functions in the masticatory process. In esthetics the form and alignment of the anterior teeth are important to a person's physical appearance. The form and alignment of the anterior and posterior teeth assist in the ar-

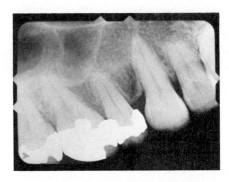

Fig. 2-36. Radiograph showing root resorption on lateral incisor following orthodontic tooth movement.

ticulation of certain sounds that can have a significant effect on speech. Finally, the form and alignment of the teeth assist in sustaining the teeth in the dental arches by assisting in the development and protection of the gingival tissues and alveolar bone that support them.

Contours. The facial and lingual surfaces possess some degree of convexity that affords protection along with stimulation to the supporting tissues during mastication. This convexity is located generally at the cervical third of the crown on *facial surfaces* of all teeth and the *lingual surfaces* of the incisors and canines. The lingual surfaces of the posterior teeth usually have their height of contour in the middle third of the crown. *Normal tooth contours* act in deflecting food only to the extent that the passing food stimulates by gentle massage the investing tissues rather than irritates them. If these curvatures are too great, the tissues usually receive inadequate stimulation by the passage of food. Too little contour may result in trauma to the attachment apparatus. These tooth contours must be considered in the performance of operative dental procedures. Improper location and degree of *facial or lingual convexities* can result in serious complications, as illustrated in Fig. 2-37,

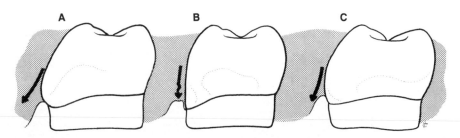

Fig. 2-37. Contours. Arrows show pathways of food passing over facial surface of mandibular molar during mastication. **A,** Overcontour deflects food from gingiva and results in understimulation of supporting tissues. **B,** Undercontour of tooth may result in irritation of soft tissues. **C,** Correct contour permits adequate stimulation for supporting tissues, resulting in healthy condition. (From Brauer JC, Richardson RE: *The dental assistant,* ed 3, New York, 1964, McGraw-Hill. Reproduced with permission.)

where the proper facial contour is disregarded in the placement of a cervical restoration on a mandibular molar. *Overcontouring is the worst offender, usually resulting in flabby, red-colored, chronically inflamed gingiva and increased plaque retention.*

Proper form of the *proximal surfaces of the teeth* is just as important to the maintenance of the periodontal tissues as proper form of the facial and lingual surfaces. The proximal height of contour serves to provide (1) *contacts* with the proximal surfaces of the adjacent teeth, which prevents food impaction; and (2) adequate

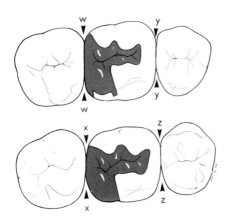

Fig. 2-38. Portion of skull showing triangular spaces beneath proximal contact areas. These spaces are occupied by soft tissue and bone for support of teeth. (From Shankle RJ: Clinical dental anatomy, physiology, and histology. In Sturdevant CM et al, editors: *The art and science of operative dentistry,* ed 1, New York, 1968, McGraw-Hill.)

embrasure space gingivally of the contacts for the gingival tissue, the supporting bone, blood vessels, and nerves that serve the supporting structures (Fig. 2-38).

Proximal contact area. The *proximal contact area* is the term used to denote the area of proximal height of contour of the mesial or distal surface of a tooth that touches (contacts) its adjacent tooth in the same arch. When teeth erupt to make proximal contact with previously erupted teeth, there is initially a contact point. The contact point becomes an area due to wear of one proximal surface against another during physiological tooth movement (Figs. 2-39 and 2-40).

The physiological significance of properly formed and properly located proximal contacts cannot be overemphasized because they promote normal healthy interdental papillae filling the interproximal spaces. Improper contacts can result in food impaction between the teeth, producing periodontal disease, carious lesions, and possible movement of the teeth. In addition, the retention of food is objectionable by its physical presence and by the halitosis that results from food decomposition. The proximal contacts along with interdigitation of the teeth through occlusal contacts stabilizes and maintains the integrity of the dental arches.

The proximal contact area is located in the incisal third of the approximating surfaces of the maxillary and mandibular central incisors (Fig. 2-41). It is positioned

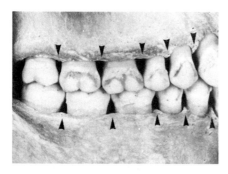

Fig. 2-39. Embrasure form. *w,* Improper embrasure form caused by overcontouring of restoration resulting in unhealthy gingiva from lack of stimulation; *x,* good embrasure form; *y,* frictional wear of contact area has resulted in decrease of embrasure dimension; *z,* when embrasure form is good, supporting tissues receive adequate stimulation from foods during mastication. (From Brauer JC, Richardson RE: *The dental assistant,* ed 3, New York, 1964, McGraw-Hill. Reproduced with permission.)

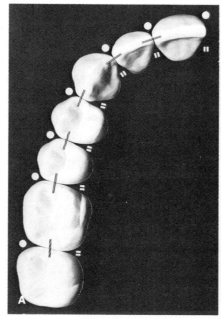
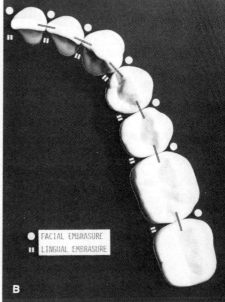

Fig. 2-40. Proximal contact area. Double black lines show positions of contacts faciolingually. **A,** Maxillary teeth. **B,** Mandibular teeth. Facial and lingual embrasures are indicated. (From Shankle RJ: Clinical dental anatomy, physiology, and histology. In Sturdevant CM et al, editors: *The art and science of operative dentistry,* ed 1, New York, 1968, McGraw-Hill.)

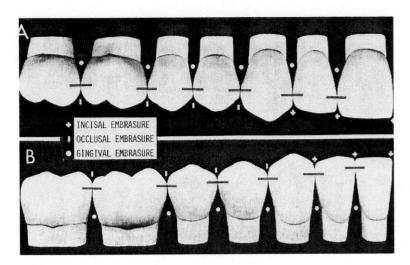

INCISAL EMBRASURE
OCCLUSAL EMBRASURE
GINGIVAL EMBRASURE

Fig. 2-41. Proximal contact area. Double black lines show positions of contacts incisogingivally and occlusogingivally. Incisal, occlusal, and gingival embrasures are indicated. **A,** Maxillary teeth. **B,** Mandibular teeth. (From Shankle RJ: Clinical dental anatomy, physiology, and histology. In Sturdevant CM et al, editors: *The art and science of operative dentistry,* ed 1, New York, 1968, McGraw-Hill.)

slightly facial to the center of the proximal surface faciolingually (see Fig. 2-40). Proceeding posteriorly from the incisor region through all the remaining teeth, the contact area is located near the junction of the incisal (or occlusal) and middle thirds or in the middle third. Because of these contacts being positioned progressively lower cervically (Fig. 2-41), larger incisal or occlusal embrasures result. Restorative procedures require maintenance of correct proximal contact relationships between teeth, which results in correct embrasures.

Embrasures. Embrasures are V-shaped spaces that originate at the proximal contact areas between adjacent teeth and are named for the direction toward which they radiate. These ***embrasures*** are (1) facial, (2) lingual, (3) incisal or occlusal, and (4) gingival (see Figs. 2-40 and 2-41).

Initially the interdental papilla fills the gingival embrasure. In a mouth where tooth form and function are ideal and optimal oral health is maintained, the interdental papilla may continue in this position throughout life. When the gingival embrasure is filled by the papilla, the trapping of food in this region is prevented. In a faciolingual longitudinal section the papilla may be triangular between anterior teeth, whereas in the posterior teeth the papilla may be shaped like a mountain range, with facial and lingual peaks and the *col* ("valley") lying beneath the contact area (Fig. 2-42). This col, or central faciolingual concave area beneath the contact, is more vulnerable to periodontal disease from incorrect contact and embrasure form because it is covered by nonkeratinized epithelium.

The correct relationship of embrasures, cusps to sulci, marginal ridges, and grooves of adjacent and opposing teeth provides for the escape of food from the occlusal surfaces during mastication (Fig. 2-43). When an embrasure is decreased in size or absent, additional stress is created in the teeth and the supporting struc-

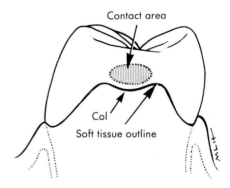

Contact area

Col
Soft tissue outline

Fig. 2-42. Relationship of ideal interdental papilla to molar contact area. (From Shankle RJ: Clinical dental anatomy, physiology, and histology. In Sturdevant CM et al, editors: *The art and science of operative dentistry,* ed 1, New York, 1968, McGraw-Hill.)

tures during mastication. Embrasures that are too large provide little protection to the supporting structures as food is forced into the interproximal space by an opposing cusp. A prime example is the failure to restore the distal cusp of a mandibular first molar when placing a restoration (Fig. 2-44). The lingual embrasures are usually larger than the facial embrasures to allow more of the food to be displaced lingually, since the tongue can return the food to the occlusal surface easier than if the food is displaced facially into the buccal vestibule (see Fig. 2-40).

The marginal ridges of adjacent posterior teeth should be at the same height to have proper contact and embrasure forms. When this relation is absent, there is an increase in the problems associated with weak contacts and faulty embrasure form.

The preservation of the curvatures of the opposing cusps and surfaces in function maintains masticatory efficiency throughout life (see Fig. 2-2). The correct ana-

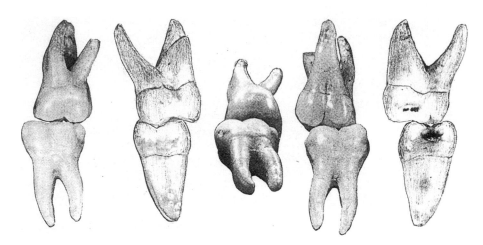

Fig. 2-43. Maxillary and mandibular first molars in centric occlusal relationship. Note grooves for escape of food.

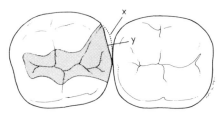

Fig. 2-44. Embrasure form. *x,* Portion of tooth that offers protection to underlying supporting tissue during mastication; *y,* restoration fails to establish adequate contour for good embrasure form. (From Brauer JC, Richardson RE: *The dental assistant,* ed 3, New York, 1964, McGraw-Hill. Reproduced with permission.)

tomical form renders the teeth more self-cleansing because of the smoothly rounded contours that are more exposed to the cleansing action of foods and fluids and the frictional movement of the tongue, lips, and cheeks. Failure to understand and adhere to correct anatomical form in the performance of restorative procedures can contribute to the breakdown of the stomatognathic system (Fig. 2-45). The importance of providing correct anatomical features in restorative dentistry cannot be overemphasized.

Maxilla and mandible

The human maxilla is formed by two bones, the *maxilla proper* and the *premaxilla.* The two maxillae form the bulk of the upper jaw and the major portion of the hard palate and help to form the floor of the orbit and the sides and base of the nasal cavity. They contain

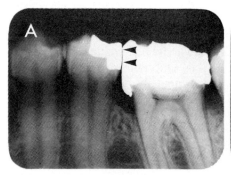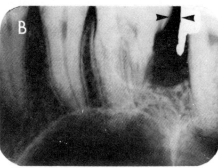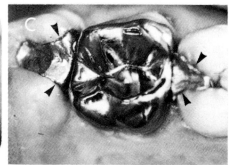

Fig. 2-45. Poor anatomical restorative form. **A,** Radiograph of flat contact and amalgam gingival excess. **B,** Radiograph of restoration with amalgam gingival excess and absence of contact resulting in trauma to supporting tissue. **C,** Poor occlusal margins. (From Shankle RJ: Clinical dental anatomy, physiology, and histology. In Sturdevant CM et al, editors: *The art and science of operative dentistry,* ed 1, New York, 1968, McGraw-Hill.)

the 10 maxillary primary teeth initially and later the 16 maxillary permanent teeth in the *alveolar process (bone)* (see Figs. 2-1 and 2-3, *label 7*).

The mandible is a bilateral bone structure that forms the lower jaw (Fig. 2-52, *F*). It is a horseshoe-shaped bone attached to the skull on either side by a nonbony union called the *temporomandibular joint* (Fig. 2-52, *B*). It is the heaviest and strongest bone of the head. The mandible is composed of a *body,* composed of two horizontal portions joined at the midline *symphysis mandibulae,* and the *rami,* the vertical parts. The *coronoid process* and *condyle* make up the superior border of each ramus. The mandible initially contains the 10 mandibular primary teeth and later the 16 mandibular permanent teeth in the *alveolar process.*

The maxillary and mandibular bones consist of about 65% inorganic and 35% organic material. The inorganic portion is hydroxyapatite, and the organic part is primarily collagen.

Oral mucosa

The oral mucosa is the mucous membrane which covers all oral structures except the clinical crowns of the teeth. It is composed of *two layers,* (1) the *stratified squamous epithelium* and (2) a supporting connective tissue, the *lamina propria.* (See lamina propria of the gingiva in Fig. 2-46, *arrow 8.)* The epithelium may be *keratinized, parakeratinized,* or *nonkeratinized* depending upon its location. The lamina propria varies in thickness and supports the epithelium. It may be attached to the periosteum of the alveolar bone, or it may be interposed over the submucosa, which may vary in different regions of the mouth such as the floor of the mouth and the soft palate. The *submucosa* consists of connective tissues varying in density and thickness and attaches the mucous membrane to the underlying bony structures. The submucosa contains glands, blood vessels, nerves, and adipose tissue.

The oral mucosa may be divided into *three major functional types:* (1) masticatory mucosa, (2) lining or reflective mucosa, and (3) specialized mucosa.

The masticatory mucosa is composed of the free and attached gingivae (see arrows labelled 6 and 9 in Fig. 2-46) *and the mucosa of the hard palate.* The epithelium of these tissues is keratinized, and the lamina propria is a dense, thick, firm connective tissue containing collagenous fibers. The hard palate has a distinct submucosa except for a few narrow specific zones. The dense lamina propria of the attached gingiva is connected to the cementum and the periosteum of the bony alveolar process (see Fig. 2-46, *arrow 8*).

The lining or reflective mucosa covers the inside of the lips, cheek, vestibule, lateral surfaces of the alveolar process (except the mucosa of the hard palate), *floor*

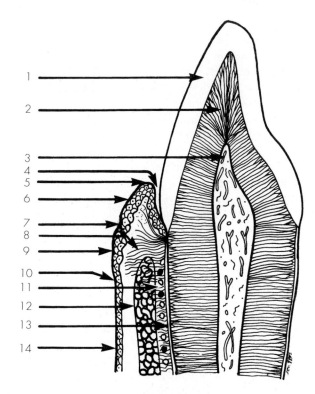

Fig. 2-46. Longitudinal section of maxillary incisor illustrating supporting structures: *1,* enamel; *2,* dentin; *3,* pulp; *4,* gingival sulcus; *5,* free gingival margin; *6,* free gingiva; *7,* free gingival groove; *8,* lamina propria of gingiva; *9,* attached gingiva; *10,* mucogingival junction; *11,* periodontal ligament; *12,* alveolar bone; *13,* cementum; *14,* alveolar mucosa.

of the mouth, soft palate, and inferior surface of the tongue. Lining mucosa is a thin, *movable* tissue with a relatively thick, nonkeratinized epithelium and a thin lamina propria. The submucosa is composed mostly of thin, loose connective tissue with muscle and collagenous and elastic fibers with different areas varying from one another in their structure. The junction of lining mucosa with masticatory mucosa is the *mucogingival junction,* which is located at the apical border of the attached gingiva facially and lingually in the mandibular arch and facially in the maxillary arch (see Fig. 2-46, *arrow 10*).

The specialized mucosa covers the dorsum of the tongue and the taste buds. The epithelium is nonkeratinized except the covering of the dermal filiform papillae.

Periodontium

The periodontium consists of the oral hard and soft tissues that invest and support the teeth. It can be divided into (1) the *gingival unit* consisting of free and attached *gingivae* and the *alveolar mucosa* and (2) the *attachment apparatus* consisting of the *cementum, periodontal ligament,* and *alveolar process* (Fig. 2-46). The periodontium, a connective tissue structure with its stratified squamous epithelium, attaches the teeth to the maxilla and the mandible and provides a continually adapting structure for the support of the teeth during function. The periodontium has two mineralized connective tissues, *cementum* and *alveolar bone,* and two fibrous connective tissues, the *periodontal ligament* and the *lamina propria* of the gingiva. The periodontium is attached to the jaws by alveolar bone and to the dentin of the tooth root by cementum.

Gingival unit

Gingivae. As stated previously the *free* and *attached gingivae* are masticatory mucosa. The *free gingiva* is the gingiva from the marginal crest to the level of the base of the gingival sulcus (see Fig. 2-46, *arrows 4 and 6*). The *gingival sulcus* is the space between the tooth and the free gingiva. The outer wall of the sulcus (inner wall of the free gingiva) is lined with a thin, nonkeratinized epithelium. The outer aspect of the free gingiva in each gingival embrasure is called the *gingival* or *interdental papilla.* The *free gingival groove* is a shallow groove that runs parallel to the marginal crest of the free gingiva and usually indicates the level of the base of the gingival sulcus (see Fig. 2-46, *arrow 7*).

The *attached gingiva,* a dense connective tissue with its keratinized stratified squamous epithelium, extends from the level of the depth of the gingival sulcus (free gingival groove) to the *mucogingival junction.* A dense network of collagenous fibers connects the attached gingiva firmly to the cementum and the periosteum of the alveolar process (bone).

Alveolar mucosa. The alveolar mucosa is a thin soft tissue that is loosely attached to the underlying alveolar bone (see Fig. 2-46, *arrows 12 and 14*). It is covered by a thin, nonkeratinized epithelial layer. The underlying submucosa contains loosely arranged collagen fibers, elastic tissue, fat, and muscle tissue. The alveolar mucosa is delineated from the attached gingiva by the mucogingival junction and continues apically to the *vestibular fornix* and then the inside of the cheek.

Attachment apparatus. The tooth root is attached to the alveolus (bony socket) by the *periodontal ligament* (Fig. 2-46, *arrow 11*). The ligament is a complex, soft, connective tissue containing numerous cells, blood vessels, nerves, and extracellular substance consisting of fibers and ground substance. The majority of the fibers are collagen, and the ground substance is composed of a variety of proteins and polysaccharides. The periodontal ligament serves the following functions: (1) *attachment* and *support,* (2) *sensory,* (3) *nutritive,* and (4) *homeostatic.* Bundles of the collagen fibers, known as the **principal fibers of the ligament,** serve to attach the cementum to the alveolar bone and act as a cushion to suspend and support the tooth. The portions of the principal fibers embedded in the cementum and alveolar bone are called ***Sharpey's fibers.*** The sensory function is provided by the nerve supply through an efficient proprioceptive mechanism. The blood vessels supply the attachment apparatus with nutritive substances. Specialized cells of the ligament function to resorb and replace the cementum, periodontal ligament, and alveolar bone.

Cementum is a hard tissue with a calcified intercellular substance covering the anatomical roots of teeth and has been discussed previously in this chapter.

The ***alveolar process,*** a part of the maxilla and mandible, forms, supports, and lines the sockets into which the roots of the teeth fit. Anatomically, no distinct boundary exists between the body of the maxilla or the mandible and the alveolar process. The tissue elements of the alveolar process are the same as for bone found elsewhere. The alveolar process is thin, compact bone with many small openings through which blood vessels, lymphatics, and nerves pass. As previously stated, both cementum and the alveolar bone contain Sharpey's fibers, the ends of the principal fibers of the periodontal ligament. The inner wall of the bony socket consists of the thin lamella of bone that surrounds the root of the tooth (and gives attachment to Sharpey's fibers). It is termed the *alveolar bone proper.* The second part of the bone is called *supporting alveolar bone,* which surrounds the alveolar bone proper and supports the socket. Supporting bone is made up of two parts: (1) the cortical plate that consists of compact bone and forms the inner (lingual) and outer (facial) plates of the alveolar process and (2) the spongy base that fills the area between the plates and the alveolar bone proper. Bone is composed of about 65% inorganic and 35% organic material. The inorganic material is hydroxyapatite, and the organic material is primarily type I collagen (88% to 89%), which is surrounded by a ground substance of glycoproteins and proteoglycans.

Clinically the level of the gingival attachment and the gingival sulcus is an important factor in restorative dentistry. The soft tissue health must be maintained by the teeth having correct form and position if apical recession of the gingivae and possible abrasion and erosion of the roots are to be prevented. *The margin of a cavity preparation should not be positioned subgingivally (at levels between the marginal crest of the free gingiva and the base of the sulcus) unless dictated by caries, previous restoration, or esthetics.*

OCCLUSION
Introduction to dental occlusion

Occlusion literally means closing; *in dentistry the word **occlusion** means the contact of teeth in opposing dental arches when the jaws are closed (**static occlusal relationships**) and during various jaw movements (**dy-**

namic occlusal relationships). The size of the jaws and arrangement of the teeth within the jaws are subject to a wide range of variation in humans. The locations of contacts between opposing teeth *(occlusal contacts)* vary as a result of differences in the size and shape of the teeth and the jaws as well as the relative position of the jaws. A wide variety of occlusal schemes can be found in healthy individuals. Consequently, definition of an ideal occlusal scheme is fraught with difficulties.[3] Despite repeated attempts to describe an ideal occlusal scheme, descriptions of ideal occlusion become so restrictive that few individuals can be found to fit the criteria. Failing to find a single adequate definition of an ideal occlusal scheme, Carlsson et al. concluded that "in the final analysis, optimal function and the absence of disease is the principal characteristic of a good occlusion."[3] The dental relationships described in this section conform to the concepts of normal or usual occlusal schemes and include common variations of tooth and jaw relationships. Fortunately, the masticatory system is highly adaptable and can function successfully over a wide range of differences in jaw size and tooth alignment. *Despite this great adaptability, many patients are highly sensitive to abrupt changes in tooth contacts often brought about by restorative dental procedures.* Some patients will complain and seek correction of even very minor vertical discrepancies in occlusal contacts. *Thus the operative dentist must understand the precise details of occlusion.*

Occlusal contact patterns vary with position of the mandible. *Static occlusion* is further defined by use of reference positions that include fully closed, terminal hinge closure, retruded, and right and left lateral extremes. The number and location of occlusal contacts between opposing teeth have important effects on the amount and direction of force applied during mastication and other mandibular clenching *(bruxing)* activities. In extreme cases, the forces can cause damage to the teeth or their supporting tissues. Forceful tooth contact occurs routinely very near the limits or borders of mandibular movement, thus providing the relevance of these reference positions.[6]

As stated previously, tooth contact during mandibular movement is termed the *dynamic occlusal relationship*. Gliding or sliding contacts occur during mastication and other mandibular movements. Gliding contacts may be advantageous or disadvantageous depending on the teeth involved and the position of the contacts. *The design of the restored tooth surface can have important effects on the number and location of occlusal contacts and must take into consideration both static and dynamic relationships.* The following sections will discuss the common arrangements of the teeth and masticatory system as well as the more common variations. Mastication and the contacting relationships of anterior and

posterior teeth are described with reference to the potential restorative needs of the teeth.

General description of dental occlusion

Tooth alignment and dental arches. In Fig. 2-47, *A*, *cusps* are drawn as blunt, rounded, or pointed projections of the crowns of the teeth. The posterior teeth have one, two, or three cusps near the facial and lingual surfaces of each tooth. Cusps are separated by distinct **developmental grooves** and sometimes have additional supplemental grooves on the cusp inclines. The facial cusps are separated from the lingual cusps by a deep groove termed the *central groove*. If a tooth has multiple facial cusps or multiple lingual cusps, then the cusps are separated by facial or lingual developmental grooves respectively. Depressions between the cusps are termed **fossae** (singular form—*fossa*). Recall that grooves having non-coalesced enamel are termed **fissures** and non-coalesced enamel in a fossa is termed a **pit.** Cusps in both jaws are aligned in a roughly parabolic curve. Usually the maxillary arch is larger than the mandibular arch, resulting in the maxillary cusps overlapping the mandibular cusps when the arches are in maximal occlusal contact (Fig. 2-47, *B*). In Fig. 2-47, *A*, two curved lines are drawn over the teeth to aid in the visualization of the arch form. These curved lines identify the alignment of similarly functioning cusps or fossae. On the left side of the arches, an imaginary arc connecting the row of facial cusps in the mandibular arch is drawn and labeled the **facial occlusal line.** Above that, an imaginary line connecting the maxillary central fossae is labeled the **central fossa line.** The mandibular facial occlusal line and the maxillary central fossa line coincide exactly when the mandibular arch is fully closed into the maxillary arch. On the right side of the dental arches the maxillary lingual occlusal line and mandibular central fossa line are drawn and labeled. These lines also coincide when the mandible is fully closed.

In Fig. 2-47, *B*, the dental arches are fully interdigitated. Note again that the maxillary dental arch is larger than the mandibular, so the maxillary teeth overlap the mandibular teeth. The overlap of the maxillary cusps can be observed directly when the jaws are closed. *Intercuspal position—IP* (or *centric occlusion—CO*) is the position of the mandible when the teeth are brought into full interdigitation with the maximal number of teeth contacting. Synonyms for IP include: acquired occlusion, habitual occlusion, and convenience occlusion.

In Fig. 2-47, *C*, a proximal view, the mandibular facial occlusal line and the maxillary central fossa line can be seen to coincide exactly. In a similar manner, the maxillary lingual occlusal line and the mandibular central fossa line, identified in Fig. 2-47, *A*, also are coincident. Cusps that contact the opposing teeth along the central fossa line are termed **supporting cusps (cen-**

A Dental arch cusp and fossa alignment

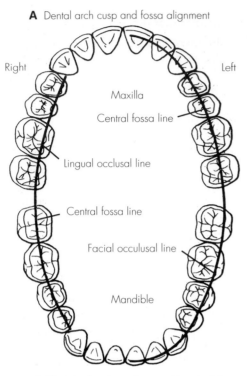

1. The maxillary lingual occusal line and the mandibular central fossa line are coincident.
2. The mandibular facial occlusal line and the maxillary central fossa line are coincident.

B Intercuspal position (IP): the teeth in opposing arches are in maximal contact

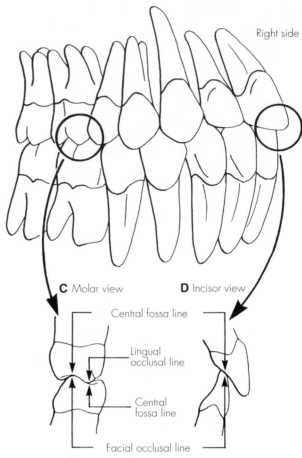

C Molar view   **D** Incisor view

E Facial view of anterior-posterior variations

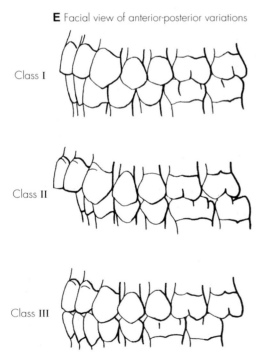

F Molar Class I, II, and III relationships

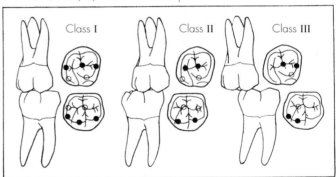

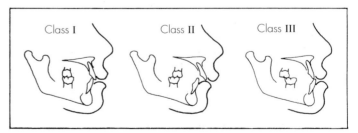

G Skeletal Class I, II, and III relationships

Fig. 2-47. Dental arch relationships.

tric, holding, or stamp cusps), and the cusps that overlap the opposing teeth are termed ***non-supporting cusps (non-centric or gliding cusps).*** For example, the mandibular facial occlusal line identifies the mandibular supporting cusps while the maxillary facial cusps are non-supporting cusps. These terms are usually applied only to posterior teeth to distinguish the difference in function between the two rows of cusps. In some circumstances the functional role of the cusps can be reversed as illustrated in Fig. 2-48, *C-2. The posterior teeth are well suited to crushing food because of the mutual cusp-fossa contacts* (see Fig. 2-49, *D*).

In Fig. 2-47, *D,* the anterior teeth are seen to have a different relationship in intercuspal position (IP) but also show the characteristic maxillary overlap. *The incisor teeth are best suited to shearing food because of their overlap and the sliding contact* on the lingual surface of the maxillary teeth. In IP the mandibular incisors and canines contact the respective lingual surfaces of their maxillary opponents. *The amount of horizontal (overjet) and vertical (overbite) overlap* (Fig. 2-48, *A-2) can significantly influence mandibular movement and thus influence the cusp design of restorations of posterior teeth* as discussed subsequently. Variations in growth (development) of the jaws and position of the anterior teeth result in openbite when vertical or horizontal discrepancies prevent the teeth from contacting (see Fig. 2-48, *inset A-3).*

Anterior-posterior interarch relationships. In Fig. 2-47, *E,* the cusp interdigitation pattern of the first molar teeth is used to classify anterior-posterior arch relationships using a system developed by Edward Angle.[1] During eruption of the teeth, the tooth cusps and fossae guide the teeth into maximal contact. Three interdigitated relationships of the first molars are commonly observed. See Fig. 2-47, *F* for an illustration of the occlusal contacts that result from the different molar positions. *The location of the mesiofacial cusp of the maxillary first molar in relation to the mandibular first molar is used as a marker in this classification.* The most common molar relationship finds the maxillary mesiofacial cusp located in the mesiofacial developmental groove of the mandibular first molar. This relationship is termed ***Angle Class I,*** abbreviated as Cl I. Slight posterior positioning of the mandibular first molar results in the mesiofacial cusp of the maxillary molar settling into the facial embrasure between the mandibular first molar and the mandibular second premolar. This is termed ***Class II (Cl II)*** and occurs in approximately 20% of the population in the United States. Anterior positioning of the mandibular first molar relative to the maxillary first molar is termed ***Class III (Cl III)*** and is least common. In Cl III relationships, the mesiofacial cusp of the maxillary first molar settles into the distofacial groove of the mandibular first molar. This occurs in 3% of the popu-

lation of the United States. Significant differences in these percentages occur in other countries and in different racial and ethnic groups.

Although the Angle classification is based on the relationship of the cusps, Fig. 2-47, *G* illustrates that *it is the location of the tooth roots in the alveolar bone that determines the relative positions of the crowns and cusps.* When the mandible is proportionally similar in size to the maxilla, the Class I molar relationship is formed. When the mandible is proportionally smaller than the maxilla, a Class II relationship is formed; and when the mandible is relatively greater than the maxilla, a Class III relationship is formed.

Interarch tooth relationships. Fig. 2-48 illustrates the occlusal contact relationships of individual teeth in more detail. In Fig. 2-48, *A-2, incisor overlap* is illustrated. The overlap is characterized in two dimensions, ***horizontal overlap (overjet)*** and ***vertical overlap (overbite).*** Differences in the size of the mandible and maxilla can result in clinically significant variations in incisor relationships including (1) openbite due to mandibular deficiency, (2) excessive eruption of the posterior teeth, or (3) mandibular growth excess (Fig. 2-48, *A-3).* These variations have significant clinical effects on the contacting relationships of the posterior teeth during various jaw movements, because the anterior teeth do not provide gliding contact. See Fig. 2-58, *E* to *G,* for more details on the effects of the ***lack of anterior guidance.***

Fig. 2-48, *B-1,* illustrates the normal Cl I occlusion in which each mandibular premolar is located one-half a tooth width anterior to its maxillary antagonist. This relationship results in the mandibular facial cusp contacting the maxillary premolar mesial marginal ridge, and the maxillary premolar lingual cusp contacting the mandibular distal marginal ridge. Because only one antagonist is contacted, this is termed a ***tooth-to-tooth relationship.*** The most stable relationship results from the contact of the supporting cusp tips against two marginal ridges, termed a ***tooth-to-two tooth contact.*** Variations in the mesial-distal root position of the teeth will produce different relationships (see Fig. 2-48, *B-2).* When the mandible is slightly distal to the maxilla, termed a Cl II tendency, each supporting cusp tip will occlude in a stable relationship with the opposing mesial or distal fossa. This relationship is termed *cusp-fossa contact.*

Fig. 2-48, *C,* illustrates Class I molar relationships in more detail. Fig. 2-48, *C-1,* shows how cutting away the facial half of the maxillary molar reveals the mandibular facial cusp tips contacting the maxillary marginal ridges and the central fossa triangular ridges. A facial-lingual longitudinal section reveals how the supporting cusps contact the opposing fossae and also the effect of the developmental grooves on reducing the height of the non-supporting cusps opposite to the sup-

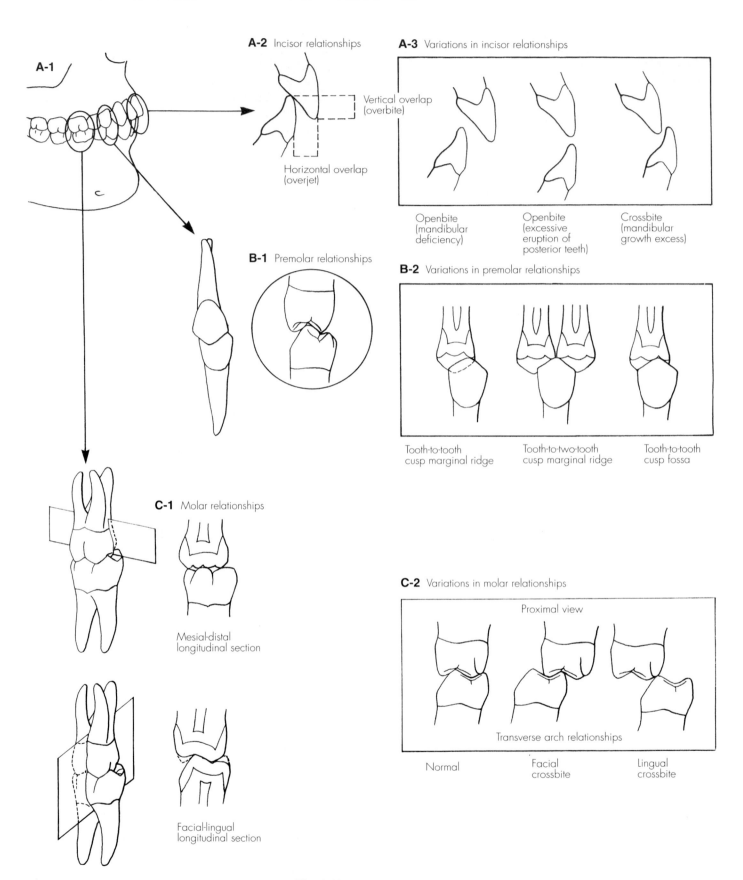

A-1

A-2 Incisor relationships

Vertical overlap (overbite)

Horizontal overlap (overjet)

A-3 Variations in incisor relationships

Openbite (mandibular deficiency)

Openbite (excessive eruption of posterior teeth)

Crossbite (mandibular growth excess)

B-1 Premolar relationships

B-2 Variations in premolar relationships

Tooth-to-tooth cusp marginal ridge

Tooth-to-two-tooth cusp marginal ridge

Tooth-to-tooth cusp fossa

C-1 Molar relationships

Mesial-distal longitudinal section

Facial-lingual longitudinal section

C-2 Variations in molar relationships

Proximal view

Transverse arch relationships

Normal

Facial crossbite

Lingual crossbite

Fig. 2-48. Tooth relationships.

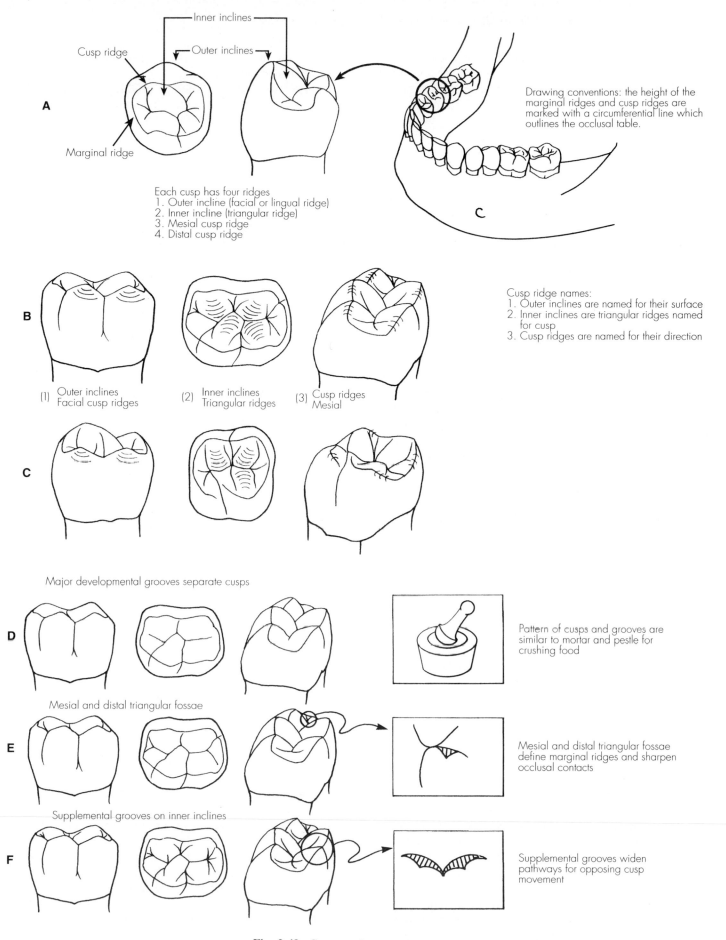

Inner inclines

Cusp ridge

Outer inclines

Marginal ridge

A

Drawing conventions: the height of the marginal ridges and cusp ridges are marked with a circumferential line which outlines the occlusal table.

C

Each cusp has four ridges
1. Outer incline (facial or lingual ridge)
2. Inner incline (triangular ridge)
3. Mesial cusp ridge
4. Distal cusp ridge

B

(1) Outer inclines
Facial cusp ridges

(2) Inner inclines
Triangular ridges

(3) Cusp ridges
Mesial

Cusp ridge names:
1. Outer inclines are named for their surface
2. Inner inclines are triangular ridges named for cusp
3. Cusp ridges are named for their direction

C

Major developmental grooves separate cusps

D

Pattern of cusps and grooves are similar to mortar and pestle for crushing food

Mesial and distal triangular fossae

E

Mesial and distal triangular fossae define marginal ridges and sharpen occlusal contacts

Supplemental grooves on inner inclines

F

Supplemental grooves widen pathways for opposing cusp movement

Fig. 2-49. Common features of all posterior teeth.

porting cusp tips. During lateral movements the supporting cusp can move through the facial and lingual developmental groove spaces. Facial-lingual position variations are possible in molar relationships due to differences in growth of the width of the maxilla or the mandible. Fig. 2-48, *C-2*, illustrates normal molar contact position, facial crossbite, and lingual crossbite relationships. Facial crossbite in the posterior teeth is characterized by contact of the maxillary facial cusps in the opposing mandibular central fossae and the mandibular lingual cusps in the opposing maxillary central fossae. Facial crossbite (also termed *buccal crossbite*) results in reversal of the role of the cusps of the involved teeth. In this reversal example, the mandibular lingual cusps and maxillary facial cusps become supporting cusps and the maxillary lingual cusps and mandibular facial cusps become non-supporting cusps. Lingual crossbite results in a very poor molar relationship that provides little functional contact.

Posterior cusp characteristics. Four *cusp ridges* can be identified as common features of all cusps. The outer incline of a cusp faces either the facial (or the lingual) surface of the tooth and is named for its respective surface. In the example using a mandibular second premolar (see Fig. 2-49, *A*) the *facial cusp ridge* of the facial cusp is indicated by the line that points to the outer incline of the cusp. The inner inclines of posterior cusps face the central fossa or the central groove of the tooth. The inner incline cusp ridges are widest at the base and become narrower as they approach the cusp tip. For this reason, they are termed *triangular ridges*. The triangular ridge of the facial cusp of the mandibular premolar is indicated by the arrow to the inner incline. Triangular ridges are usually set off from the other cusp ridges by one or more supplemental groves. In Figs. 2-49, *B (1)* and *C (1)*, the outer inclines of the facial cusps of the mandibular and maxillary first molars are highlighted. In Fig. 2-49, *B (2)* and *C (2)*, the triangular ridges of the facial and lingual cusps are highlighted.

The *mesial* and *distal cusp ridges* extend from the cusp tip mesially and distally and are named for their direction. The mesial and distal cusp ridges extend downward from the cusp tips forming the characteristic facial and lingual profiles of the cusps as viewed from the facial or lingual aspect. At the base of the cusp, the mesial or distal cusp ridge either abuts to another cusp ridge, forming a developmental groove/fissure, or the cusp ridge turns toward the center line of the tooth and fuses with the marginal ridge. *Marginal ridges* are elevated rounded ridges located on the mesial and distal edges of the tooth's occlusal surface (Fig. 2-49, *A*). The *occlusal table* of posterior teeth is the area contained within the mesial and distal cusp ridges and marginal ridges of the tooth. The occlusal table limits are indicated in the tooth drawings by a circumferential line

connecting the highest point of curvature of these cusp ridges and marginal ridges.

Some cusps are modified to produce the characteristic form of individual posterior teeth. Mandibular first molars have extra-long triangular ridges on the distofacial cusps causing a deviation of the central groove/fissure (Fig. 2-49, *B [2]*). The mesiolingual cusp of a maxillary molar is much larger than the mesiofacial cusp. The distal cusp ridge of the maxillary first molar mesiolingual cusp curves facially to fuse with the triangular ridge of the distofacial cusp (Fig. 2-49, *C [2]*). This junction forms the oblique ridge, which is characteristic of the maxillary molars. The transverse groove crosses the oblique ridge where the distal cusp ridge of the mesiolingual cusp meets the triangular ridge of the distofacial cusp. Textbooks on dental anatomy should be consulted for more detailed discussions of individual cusp variations.

Supporting cusps. Note in Fig. 2-50 that the lingual occlusal line of the maxillary teeth and the facial occlusal line of the mandibular teeth mark the locations of the supporting cusps (also termed: stamp cusps, centric holding cusps, holding cusps). These cusps contact the opposing teeth in their corresponding faciolingual center on a marginal ridge or a fossa. Supporting cusp-central fossa contact has been compared to a mortar and pestle because the supporting cusp cuts, crushes, and grinds fibrous food against the ridges forming the concavity of the fossa (Fig. 2-49, *D*). Natural tooth form has multiple ridges and grooves that seem to be ideally suited to aid in the reduction of the food bolus during chewing. *During chewing, the highest forces and longest duration of contact occur at intercuspal position (IP). Supporting cusps also serve to prevent drifting and passive eruption of the teeth, hence the term holding cusp.*

Supporting cusps (Fig. 2-50) can be identified by *five common characteristic features*[9]:

1. They contact the opposing tooth in IP.
2. They support the vertical dimension of the face.
3. They are nearer the faciolingual center of the tooth than non-supporting cusps.
4. Their outer incline has the potential for contact.
5. They have broader, more rounded cusp ridges than non-supporting cusps.

Because the maxillary arch is larger than the mandibular arch, the supporting cusps are located on the maxillary lingual occlusal line (Fig. 2-50, *D*), while the mandibular supporting cusps are located on the mandibular facial occlusal line (Fig. 2-50, *A* and *B*). The supporting cusps of both arches are *more robust and better suited to crushing food* than the non-supporting cusps. The *lingual tilt of the posterior* teeth increases the relative height of the supporting cusps with respect to the non-supporting cusps (Fig. 2-50, *C*). The central fossa

Synonyms for supporting
cusps include:
1. Centric cusps
2. Holding cusps
3. Stamp cusps

A Mandibular arch

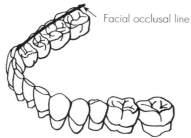

Facial occlusal line

The mandibular arch is smaller than the
maxillary arch so the supporting cusps are
located on the facial occlusal line. The
mandibular lingual cusps that overlap the
maxillary teeth are non-supporting cusps.

B Mandibular right quadrant

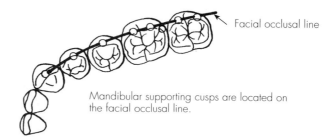

Facial occlusal line

Mandibular supporting cusps are located on
the facial occlusal line.

C Proximal view of molar
teeth in occlusion

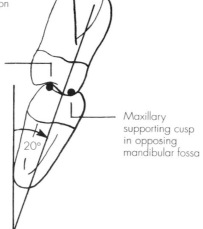

Mandibular
supporting cusp
in opposing
maxillary fossa

20°

Maxillary
supporting cusp
in opposing
mandibular fossa

D Maxillary right quadrant

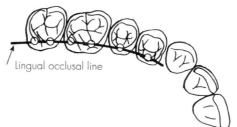

Lingual occlusal line

Supporting cusps are located on the lingual
occlusal line in maxillary arch

E Lingual view of left dental arches in
occlusion

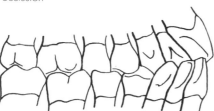

F Facial view of left dental arches in
occlusion

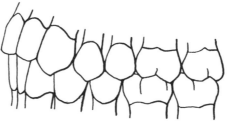

Supporting cusp features:
1. Contact opposing tooth in IP
2. Support vertical dimension
3. Nearer faciolingual center of tooth
   than non-supporting cusps
4. Outer incline has potential for
   contact
5. More rounded than non-supporting
   cusps

G Mandibular non-supporting cusps
removed

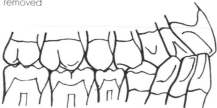

Maxillary supporting cusps occluding in
opposing fossae and on marginal ridges

H Maxillary non-supporting cusps removed

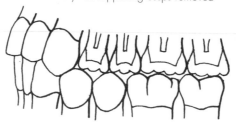

Mandibular supporting cusps occluding in
opposing fossae and on marginal ridges

Fig. 2-50. Supporting cusps.

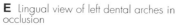
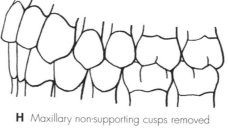

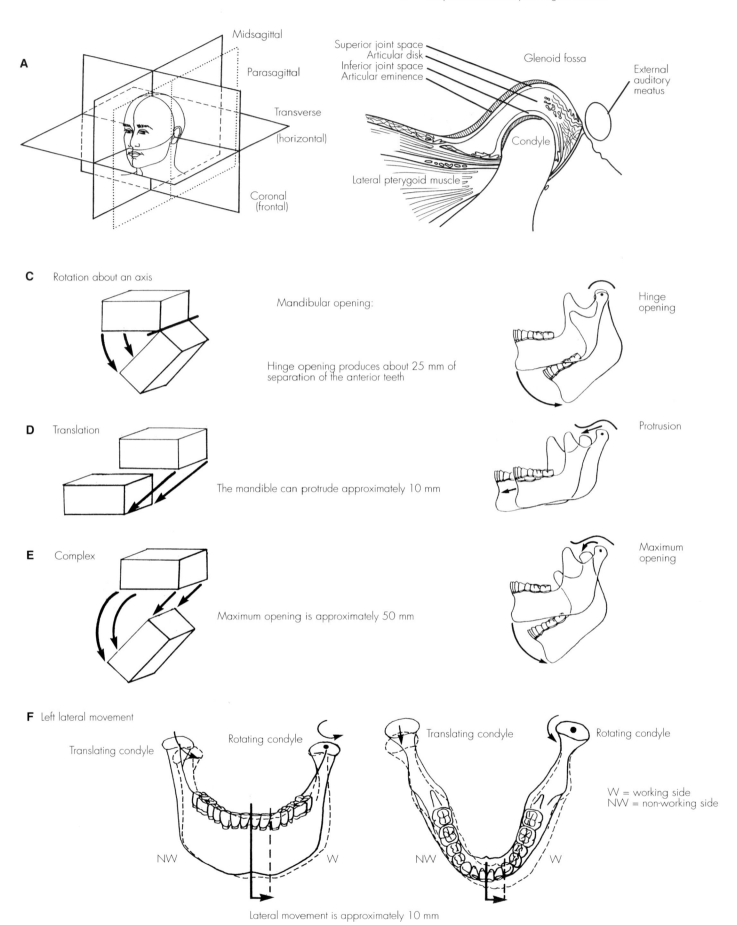

A Midsagittal, Parasagittal, Transverse (horizontal), Coronal (frontal)

B Temporomandibular joint sagittal section

Superior joint space
Articular disk
Inferior joint space
Articular eminence
Glenoid fossa
External auditory meatus
Condyle
Lateral pterygoid muscle

C Rotation about an axis

Mandibular opening:

Hinge opening produces about 25 mm of separation of the anterior teeth

Hinge opening

D Translation

The mandible can protrude approximately 10 mm

Protrusion

E Complex

Maximum opening is approximately 50 mm

Maximum opening

F Left lateral movement

Translating condyle
Rotating condyle
Translating condyle
Rotating condyle

W = working side
NW = non-working side

NW   W   NW   W

Lateral movement is approximately 10 mm

Fig. 2-52. Types and directions of motion of the mandible.

mandible is free to move in three planes providing six degrees of freedom of movement. This freedom of motion is greatest at the teeth and occurs to a lesser degree in the condyles. To describe mandibular motion, its direction and length must be specified in three mutually perpendicular planes. By convention these planes are: sagittal, coronal (frontal), and transverse (horizontal) (Fig. 2-52, A). The *mid-sagittal plane* is a vertical (longitudinal) plane that passes through the center of the head in an anterior-posterior direction. A vertical plane off the center line, such as a section through the TMJ, is termed a *para-sagittal plane*. The *coronal plane* is a vertical plane perpendicular to the sagittal plane. The *transverse plane* is a horizontal plane that passes from anterior to posterior and is perpendicular to both the sagittal and frontal planes. Mandibular motion will be described in each of these planes.

Types of motion. *Rotation* is a simple motion of an object around an axis (Fig. 2-52, C). The mandible is capable of rotation about an axis through centers located in the condyles. The attachments of the disks to the poles of the condyles permit the condyles to rotate under the disks. *Rotation with the condyles stabilized under the disks superiorly positioned in the fossae in healthy TMJs is termed* **terminal hinge (TH) movement.** TH is used in dentistry as a reference movement for construction of restorations and dentures. Contact of the teeth during a TH closure provides a reference point, termed **retruded contact point (RCP)** or occasionally **centric relation (CR).** Maximum rotational opening is limited to approximately 25 mm measured between the incisal edges of the anterior teeth.

Translation is the bodily movement of an object from one place to another (Fig. 2-52, D). The mandible is capable of translation by movement anteriorly of the disk-condyle complex from the closed position over the articular eminence and back. Simultaneous, direct anterior movement of both condyles, or mandibular thrusting, is termed **protrusion.** The pathway followed by the anterior teeth during protrusion may not be smooth or straight because of contact between the anterior teeth and sometimes the posterior teeth. (See superior border of Posselt's diagram in Fig. 2-53, A.) Protrusion is limited to approximately 10 mm by the ligamentous attachments of the masticatory muscles and the TMJs.

Fig. 2-52, E, illustrates **complex motion** combining rotation and translation in a single movement. Most mandibular movement during speech, chewing, and swallowing consists of rotation and translation. The combination of rotation and translation allows the mandible to open 50 mm or more.

Fig. 2-52, F, illustrates **lateral movement** of the mandible. Left lateral movement of the mandible is illustrated. It is the result of forward translation of the right condyle and rotation of the left condyle. Right lateral movement of the mandible is the result of forward translation of the left condyle and rotation of the right condyle.

The capacity of motion of the mandible

In 1952 Ulf Posselt described the capacity of motion of the mandible.[19] Using a system of clutches and flags, he was able to record the motion of the mandible. The resultant diagram has been termed **Posselt's diagram** in some texts (Fig. 2-53, A). By necessity the original recordings of mandibular movement were done outside of the mouth, and this magnified the vertical dimension but not the horizontal dimension. Modern systems using digital computer techniques can record mandibular motion in real time and dimension, and then compute and draw the motion as it occurred at any point in the mandible and teeth.[7] This makes it possible to accurately reconstruct mandibular motion simultaneously at several points. Three of these points are particularly significant clinically — the incisor point, molar point, and condyle point (see Fig. 2-54, A, i, m, c.).[6] **Incisor point** is located on the midline of the mandible at the junction of the facial surface of the mandibular central incisors and the incisal edge. **Molar point** is the tip of the mesiofacial cusp of the mandibular first molar on a specified side. **Condyle point** is the center of rotation of the mandibular condyle on the specified side.

The limits of mandibular motion: the borders. In Fig. 2-53, A, the limits for movement of the incisor point are illustrated in the sagittal plane. The mandible is not drawn to scale with the drawing of the sagittal borders. The starting point for the diagram is intercuspal position (IP), the position where the teeth best interdigitate and there is maximal contact of the teeth. The posterior border of the diagram from IP to *a* in Fig. 2-53, A, is formed by rotation of the mandible around the condyle points. This border from IP to *a* is termed **terminal hinge (TH)** movement. *Hinge axis is the term used to describe an imaginary line connecting the centers of rotation in the condyles (condyle points) and is useful for reference to articulators.* Hinge axis closure is a reference movement used in prosthetic dentistry, and is only valid when the disks are properly positioned in the fossae. The inferior limit to this hinge opening occurs at approximately 25 mm, and is indicated by *a* in Fig. 2-53, A. The superior limit of the posterior border occurs at the first tooth contact and is identified by **RCP (retruded contact point).** *In most healthy adults, a sliding tooth contact movement positions the mandible slightly anteriorly from RCP into IP* (Fig. 2-54, B).

Centric relation (CR) is a term used to describe the position of the condyles that occurs when terminal hinge closure permits the teeth to close directly into intercuspal position (IP). CR is often incorrectly used to identify retruded contact point (RCP). CR is a term sur-

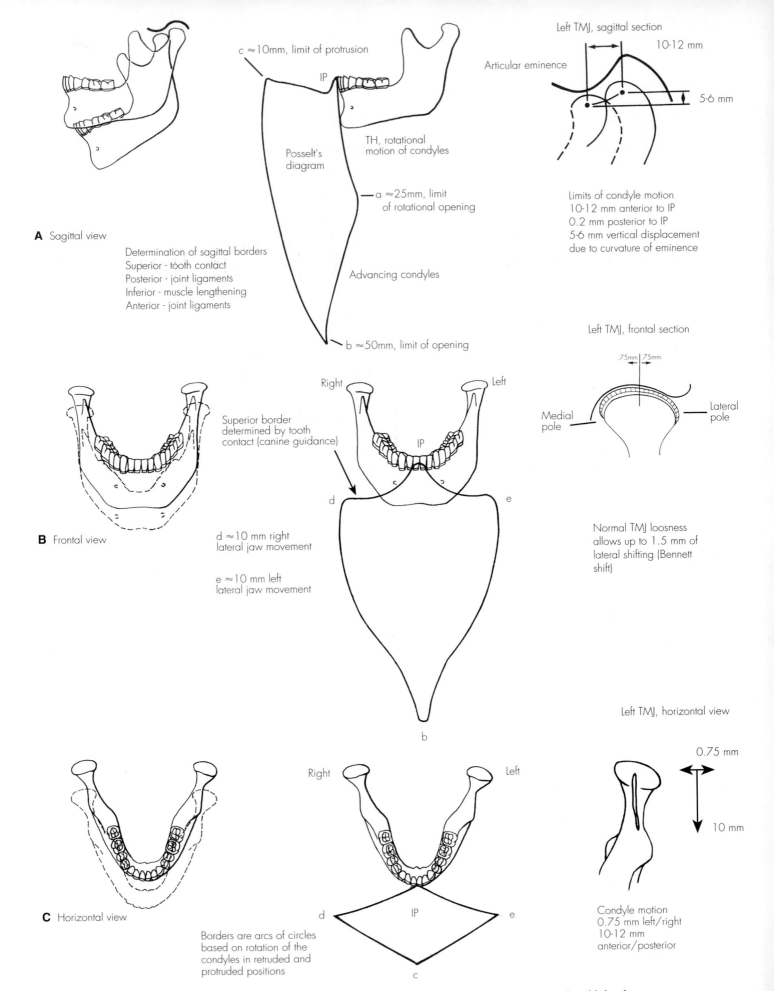

A Sagittal view

c ≈10mm, limit of protrusion

IP

Posselt's diagram

TH, rotational motion of condyles

a ≈25mm, limit of rotational opening

Advancing condyles

b ≈50mm, limit of opening

Determination of sagittal borders
Superior - tooth contact
Posterior - joint ligaments
Inferior - muscle lengthening
Anterior - joint ligaments

Left TMJ, sagittal section

10-12 mm

Articular eminence

5-6 mm

Limits of condyle motion
10-12 mm anterior to IP
0.2 mm posterior to IP
5-6 mm vertical displacement
due to curvature of eminence

B Frontal view

Right   Left

Superior border determined by tooth contact (canine guidance)

IP

d

e

d ≈10 mm right lateral jaw movement

e ≈10 mm left lateral jaw movement

b

Left TMJ, frontal section

.75mm .75mm

Medial pole   Lateral pole

Normal TMJ loosness allows up to 1.5 mm of lateral shifting (Bennett shift)

C Horizontal view

Right   Left

d

IP

e

c

Borders are arcs of circles based on rotation of the condyles in retruded and protruded positions

Left TMJ, horizontal view

0.75 mm

10 mm

Condyle motion
0.75 mm left/right
10-12 mm anterior/posterior

Fig. 2-53. Capacity of motion of the mandible. (Mandible drawings are not to scale with border diagrams.)

rounded by controversies.[4] Many unresolved issues remain concerning this concept. Some examples of the controversies include the following questions. Is CR a strained or unstrained position? Should the mandible be guided into this position by the dentist? If so, how should the mandible be grasped, shoved, supported, et cetera into position? Or should only the patient's muscles be used to guide the mandible into position? Should mechanical devices such as jigs, tongue blades, or plastic shims be used to guide the mandible into position? How is CR defined in disease states such as degenerative joint disease, arthritic remodeling, or disk displacements? *In order to avoid entanglements with these controversies, the simple descriptive terms IP and RCP will be used to describe mandibular positions associated with tooth contact.*

At point *a* in Fig. 2-53, *A*, further rotation of the condyles is impossible due to the limits of stretch of the joint capsule, ligamentous attachments to the condyles, and the mandible-opening muscles. The limit of pure rotational opening is very close to 25 mm in adults. Further opening can be achieved only by **translation of the condyles anteriorly,** producing the line *a-b*. Maximum opening, point *b*, in adults is approximately 50 mm. These measures are important diagnostically. For example, mandibular opening limited to 25 mm suggests blockage of condylar translation that is usually the result of disk disorders. Limitation of opening in the 35 to 45 mm range is suggestive of muscular limitation. *Changes in mandibular opening are useful measures of the course of disorders involving the TMJs and the muscles of mastication.* The line *IP-a-b* represents the maximum retruded opening path. This is the **posterior border,** or the posterior limit of mandibular opening. The line *b-c* represents the **maximum protruded closure.** This is achieved by a forward thrust of the mandible that keeps the condyles in their maximum anterior positions while arcing the mandible closed.

Retrusion, or posterior movement of the mandible, results in the irregular line *c-IP*. The irregularities of the superior border are due to tooth contacts and thus *the* **superior border** *is a tooth-determined border.* **Protrusion** is a reference mandibular movement starting from *IP* and proceeding anteriorly to point *c*. Protrusive mandibular movements are used by dentists to evaluate occlusal relationships of the teeth and restorations. The complete diagram, *IP-a-b-c-IP*, represents the maximum possible motion of the incisor point in all directions in the sagittal plane. *The area of most interest to dentists is the superior border produced by tooth contact.* Mandibular movement in the sagittal plane is illustrated in more detail in Fig. 2-54.

The motion of the condyle point during chewing is strikingly different from the motion of the incisor point. *Motion of the condyle point is a curved line that follows*

the **articular eminence***.* The maximum protrusion of the condyle point is 10 to 12 mm anteriorly while following the downward curve of the articular eminence. *It is notable that the condyle point does not drop away from the eminence during mandibular movements.* Thus, chewing movements in the sagittal plane are characterized by a nearly vertical up and down motion of the incisor point while the condyle points move anteriorly and then return posteriorly over a curved surface (see Fig. 2-54, *B*).

In the frontal view shown in Fig. 2-53, *B*, the incisor point and the chin are capable of moving about 10 mm to the left or right. This lateral movement (sometimes termed an *excursion)* is indicated by the lines *IP-d* to the right and *IP-e* to the left. Points *d* and *e* indicate the limit of lateral motion of the incisor point. **Lateral movement** is often described with respect to only one side of the mandible for the purpose of defining the relative motion of the mandibular to the maxillary teeth. For example, in a left lateral movement, the left mandibular teeth move away from the midline while the right mandibular teeth move toward the midline. Mandibular pathways directed away from the midline are termed **working** (synonyms include: laterotrusion and function), and mandibular pathways directed toward the midline are termed **non-working** (synonyms include: mediotrusion, non-function, and balancing). The terms working and non-working are based on observations of chewing movements where the mandible is seen to shift during closure toward the side of the mouth containing the food bolus. Thus the working side is used to crush food while the non-working side is without a food bolus.

The *left* lateral mandibular motion indicated by the line *IP-e* (Fig. 2-53, *B*) is the result of rotation of the left condyle (working side condyle) and translation of the right condyle (non-working side condyle) to its anterior limit (also see Fig. 2-52, *F*). The translation of the non-working condyle in a *right* lateral motion of the mandible can be seen in the horizontal view in Fig. 2-55, *A* and *B*. The line *e-b* in Fig. 2-53, *B*, is completed by mandibular opening that is the result of rotation of both condyles and translation of the working condyle to its maximum anterior position. Line *b-d-IP* represents similar motions on the right side.

The vertical displacement in the incisor point line from *IP* to *e* or *d*, shown in Fig. 2-53, *B*, is the result of the teeth, usually the canines, gliding over each other. The vertical displacement of the mandible due to gliding contact of the canine teeth is termed **canine guidance** and has significance for restorative procedures. *The gliding tooth contact supplied by canine guidance provides some of the vertical separation of the posterior teeth during lateral jaw movements and prevents potentially damaging collisions of their cusps.* When the ca-

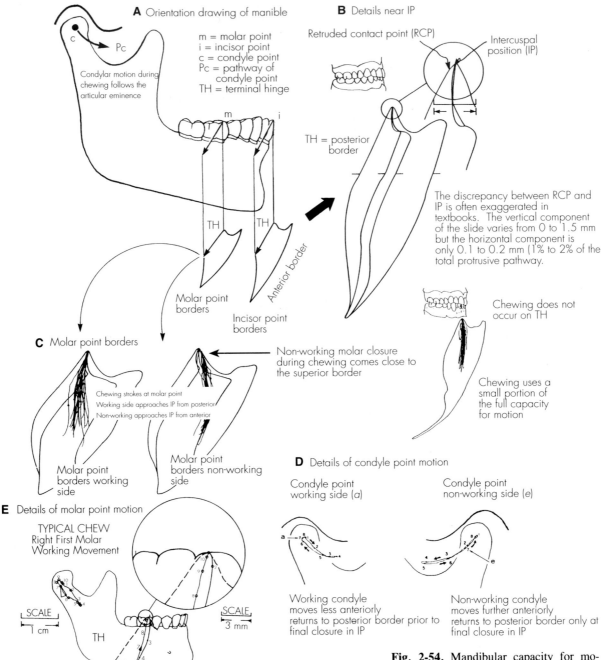

A Orientation drawing of manible

m = molar point
i = incisor point
c = condyle point
Pc = pathway of
      condyle point
TH = terminal hinge

Condylar motion during chewing follows the articular eminence

B Details near IP

Retruded contact point (RCP)

Intercuspal position (IP)

TH = posterior border

The discrepancy between RCP and IP is often exaggerated in textbooks. The vertical component of the slide varies from 0 to 1.5 mm but the horizontal component is only 0.1 to 0.2 mm (1% to 2% of the total protrusive pathway.

Chewing does not occur on TH

Chewing uses a small portion of the full capacity for motion

Molar point borders

Incisor point borders

Non-working molar closure during chewing comes close to the superior border

C Molar point borders

Chewing strokes at molar point
Working side approaches IP from posterior
Non-working approaches IP from anterior

Molar point borders working side

Molar point borders non-working side

D Details of condyle point motion

Condyle point working side (a)

Condyle point non-working side (e)

Working condyle moves less anteriorly returns to posterior border prior to final closure in IP

Non-working condyle moves further anteriorly returns to posterior border only at final closure in IP

E Details of molar point motion

TYPICAL CHEW
Right First Molar
Working Movement

SCALE
1 cm

SCALE
3 mm

TH

Fig. 2-54. Mandibular capacity for motion: sagittal view. (**B** to **D,** from Gibbs CH, Lundeen HC: Jaw movements and forces during chewing and swallowing and their clinical significance. In Lundeen HC, Gibbs CH, editors: *Advances in occlusion,* Bristol, 1982, John Wright PSG.)

Lateral movement is produced by
anterior translation of one condyle,
producing rotation about the center in the
opposite condyle.

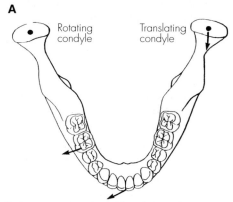

A

Rotating
condyle

Translating
condyle

Test movements such as this right lateral movement
are made in the direction opposite to the
corresponding chewing closure illustrated in *B*.

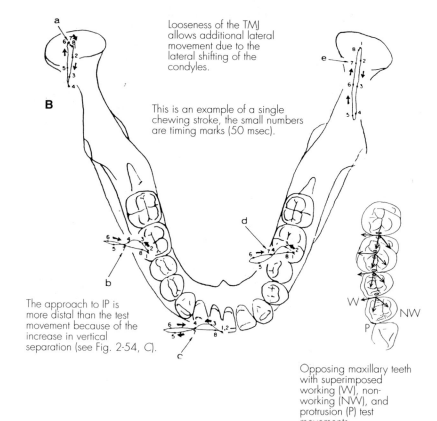

Looseness of the TMJ
allows additional lateral
movement due to the
lateral shifting of the
condyles.

B

This is an example of a single
chewing stroke, the small numbers
are timing marks (50 msec).

The approach to IP is
more distal than the test
movement because of the
increase in vertical
separation (see Fig. 2-54, *C*).

W

NW

P

Opposing maxillary teeth
with superimposed
working (W), non-
working (NW), and
protrusion (P) test
movements.

Non-working condyle movement
1. Condylar translation with rotation about the center
   of the opposite condyle
2. Solid line indicates the change in the condylar path
   due to progressive shifting of the center of rotation in
   the opposite condyle
3. Solid line indicates the condylar path resulting from
   immediate shifting of the center of rotation of the
   opposite condyle
4. Observed motion of the condyle during chewing:
   note shifting as closing is initiated and the return to
   normal position at the end of closure

Effect of shifting at first molar
1. Little change on working side
2. Wide lateral motion on non-working side

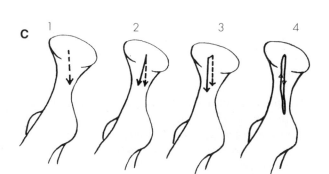

C   1   2   3   4

Left lateral movement with shifting

D

The non-working pathway
of the maxillary
mesiolingual cusp makes a
wider path over the
mandibular molar,
compare with Fig. 2-59, *E*
and *F*.

Fig. 2-55. Mandibular capacity for motion: horizontal view. (**B** used with permission from Gibbs
CH, Lundeen HC: Jaw movements and forces during chewing and swallowing and their clinical
significance. In Lundeen HC, Gibbs CH, editors: *Advances in occlusion,* Bristol, 1982, John
Wright PSG.)

nine guidance is shallow, the occlusal surface of the posterior teeth must be altered to prevent potentially damaging contacts in lateral movements. The articulator aids in the evaluation of the posterior tooth relationships during construction of posterior restorations.

There is some laxity in the TMJs and consequently the condyles can move slightly to the working side during the closing stroke. This lateral shift of the condyle points, illustrated in the frontal view of a right TMJ in Fig. 2-53, *B*, is termed **Bennett shift** or **lateral shift.** This shift is variable from patient to patient, and is a measure of the looseness of the TMJs (Fig. 2-55, *B* to *D*). The magnitude of the shift in normal TMJs varies from 0 to 1.5 mm and normally has little effect on the posterior teeth. Excessive lateral shift is associated with morphologic changes of the TMJs. Excessive lateral condylar shifting coupled with shallow canine guidance poses a significant problem for restorative procedures. In this circumstance lateral mandibular movements are very flat, and consequently little separation of the posterior teeth occurs (see Figs. 2-57 to 2-60).

In Fig. 2-53, *C*, the horizontal view illustrates the capability of the mandible to translate anteriorly. Extreme left lateral motion is indicated by *IP-e* produced by rotation of the left condyle (working side condyle) and translation of the right condyle (non-working condyle) to its anterior limit. From point *e*, protrusion of the left condyle will move the incisor point to *c*, the maximum protruded position. If there is looseness in the TMJs, the lateral shift of the mandible will be seen in this view as well. Lateral shifting can be seen in normal chewing movements in Figs. 2-55 and 2-56.

Sagittal view. In Fig. 2-54 the drawing of the mandible is used to orient the sagittal border diagrams. Projected below the mandible are diagrams of the incisor point *(i)* and molar point *(m)* borders (see Fig. 2-54, *A*). The molar point borders are similar to the incisor point diagram but are shorter in the vertical dimension because the molar point is closer to the TMJ. Closure of the jaw on the posterior border is termed **terminal hinge (TH) closure.** Terminal hinge closure is a simple arc of a circle with a radius equal to the length from incisor point to the center of hinge axis (condyle point *c*). The area near IP is shown enlarged to illustrate the details of the terminal hinge closure (see Fig. 2-54, *B*). RCP and IP are located in very close proximity. In the magnified view, *the teeth can be seen to guide the mandible from RCP to IP.* The gliding (sliding) contact typically occurs on the first premolars and is 1 to 2 mm long. *The horizontal component of this slide is only a few tenths of a millimeter in healthy joints.* However, this has been exaggerated in many textbooks, and many dentists do not recognize that the horizontal component of the slide is much smaller than the observed diagonal slide. Traditionally, the discrepancy between IP and RCP has been

the source of debate in dentistry, resulting in extensive literature on the topic.[4] This IP-RCP controversy is the result of misinterpretation of the inherent resiliency or looseness of normal, healthy TMJs. Failure to recognize that some patients have damaged TMJs can further add to the confusion concerning the significance of the IP-RCP controversy. *Damage to the TMJs as a consequence of arthritic processes or internal derangements increases the looseness of the joints and changes the relationship of IP to RCP.*

Chewing movements at the incisor point involve almost vertical opening and then a loop slightly to the posterior on closing, using only a small percentage of the total area of the sagittal border diagram. During chewing, the only border contact occurs at IP. The closing strokes never approach TH (terminal hinge), indicating that at least one condyle (the non-working side) remains advanced during the closing stroke. The condyle point moves along the pathway *Pc* during all movements other than TH. In contrast to the nearly vertical closing strokes at incisor point, the sagittal *closing* strokes at the molar point involve an anterior component on the working side and a posterior component on the non-working side. This difference in molar point movement is due to the deviation of the jaw to the working side during closure. This is illustrated by the difference in motion of the working and non-working side condyles. *The non-working side closing strokes closely approach the superior border, indicating the potential for undesirable contact on the non-working side* (Fig. 2-54, *C*).

Horizontal view. Fig. 2-55, *A*, shows a horizontal view (or occlusal view when referring to the teeth) of the mandible with superimposed incisor, molar, and condyle point test movements. Chewing movements are characterized by wide lateral movement of the mandible to the working side during closure (Fig. 2-55, *B*). When viewed from above, the pathways of the molar and incisor points are typically in a figure-eight pattern with an S-shaped lateral opening motion and a straight medial closing stroke. There are important differences in the directions of closure for the molar point on the working and non-working sides. During closure on the working side (labeled *b* in Fig. 2-55, *B*), the mandibular teeth approach medially the maxillary teeth from a slightly posterior position and move slightly anteriorly into IP. On the contralateral side (non-working side labeled *d* in Fig. 2-55, *B*), the mandibular molar teeth during closure approach in a medial-to-lateral direction the maxillary teeth from a slightly anterior position and move slightly posteriorly into IP. The closing strokes are the same pathways that are generated by guided (test) lateral mandibular movements used to check the occlusion, except the directions traveled are opposite (see Fig. 2-55, *B, inset*). On the inset drawing of the

The superior border of the incisor point tracing is determined by the canine teeth, but the molar point superior border is influenced by the pathway of the condyle point. Canine guidance and articular eminence slope are mechanically coupled to produce the superior border of the molar point tracing but they do not contribute equally. The canine is primarily responsible for the superior border of molar point on the working pathway (away from the midline). The non-working side articular eminence has the dominant influence on the non-working pathway (toward the midline) on the molar point superior border.

If the molar cusps are higher than the border then they will collide during chewing. This is more likely to occur on the non-working side.

In this right lateral movement, the canine controls the final closing path on the working side as indicated by the coincidence of the closure tracing and the superior border.

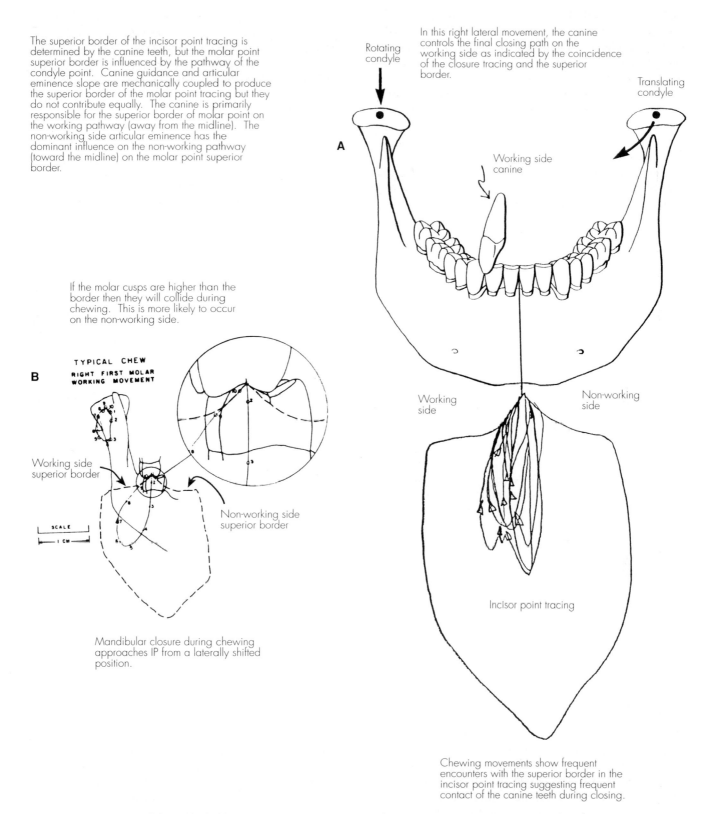

Mandibular closure during chewing approaches IP from a laterally shifted position.

Chewing movements show frequent encounters with the superior border in the incisor point tracing suggesting frequent contact of the canine teeth during closing.

Fig. 2-56. Mandibular capacity for motion: frontal view. (**B** used with permission from Gibbs CH, Lundeen HC: Jaw movements and forces during chewing and swallowing and their clinical significance. In Lundeen HC, Gibbs CH, editors: *Advances in occlusion,* Bristol, 1982, John Wright PSG.)

maxillary left teeth in Fig. 2-55, the working, non-working, and protrusive pathways are marked *W, NW,* and *P* respectively. *These are the guided test movements employed by dentists to assess the occlusal function of the teeth.*

The horizontal, enlarged view of the mandible showing *condyle point movement* (working side labeled *a* and non-working side labeled *e*) *during chewing is important because it illustrates the lateral shift of the condyles during the closing stroke* (Fig. 2-55, *B*). Opening, in the typical chew illustrated, involves movement of both condyle points on the mid-sagittal path, producing the vertical drop in the incisor point seen in the sagittal view. Lateral opening may be seen in normal children and adults with worn and flattened teeth. As closing is initiated, the mandible shifts laterally moving both condyle points to the working side. The non-working condyle movement closely approaches its medial border during the closing stroke (Fig. 2-55, *C*). During final closure, when the teeth are bought into IP, the condyle points return to their starting positions. *Contact and gliding on the inclines of the teeth are responsible for bringing the mandible into its final, fully closed position (IP).*

Allowance for lateral displacement of the condyles during lateral jaw movements is built into semiadjustable articulators. In older models, this usually takes the form of a Bennett angle or progressive lateral shift adjustment. The progressive lateral shift allows the condyles to shift gradually during lateral mandibular movement. As a result of mandibular movement studies, more *recent articulator models have replaced the progressive lateral shift with immediate shift.* (For more details on setting the medial wall of the condylar housing, see Fig. 2-59 and a later section, Articulators and Mandibular Movements.) Shifting of the mandible, as depicted by the shift in the condyle points, results in a similar shift at the teeth that cannot be simulated by progressive shift (see Fig. 2-55, *C*).

Frontal view. Note in Fig. 2-56, *A,* that lateral movement of the mandible on the superior border is controlled by three elements: the rotating condyle, the translating condyle, and the working side canine. During chewing closures the mandibular teeth approach the maxillary teeth from a lateral position. Frequent contact with the border occurs in the incisor and molar point tracings, indicating that lateral tooth gliding is common during chewing. This gliding contact occurs on the teeth having the highest projecting cusps that form the superior border; usually these are the canine teeth.

The incisor point tracing is projected below the drawing of the mandible in Fig. 2-56, *A.* The chewing strokes show the gliding contact on the border. The incisor point superior border is shaped by the lingual surfaces of the guiding teeth, which most frequently are the maxillary canine teeth. In Fig. 2-56, *B,* the lateral

side of the molar point superior border is shaped by the working-side tooth guidance, which is usually the maxillary canine. The medial side of the molar point superior border is predominately formed by the non-working condyle moving over the articular eminence. The shape of the superior border at the molar point is the critical factor for determining the location and height of the molar cusps during restorative procedures. It is easy to visualize the effect of changes in cusp height when viewing the closeup of the molar teeth in the magnified inset.

Articulators and mandibular movements

Figs. 2-57 to 2-60 illustrate the scientific basis for the use of articulators to aid in diagnostic evaluation of the occlusion and the fabrication of dental restorations. In these figures, the characteristics of chewing movements and dentist-guided test movements are compared with the characteristics of movements produced by simple articulators. This can be done by comparing cusp movement near IP produced by the articulator with the cusp movement observed in chewing studies or guided movements. Additionally the changes in cusp movement near IP due to variation in the adjustment of articulators are discussed with respect to their effects on dental restorations.

Fig. 2-57 illustrates the relationship between condylar movement and articulator settings. Together, the horizontal condylar guidance setting and the medial wall setting of an articulator supply sufficient information to simulate the condyle point movement near IP. The **horizontal condylar guidance setting** *approximates the slope of the articular eminence,* and the **medial wall setting** *approximates the lateral shift. Collectively these two settings are termed the* **posterior guidance.**

Posterior guidance alone is not sufficient to simulate mandibular movements near IP because tooth guidance is also involved in forming the superior border. Full-arch casts mounted in the articulator supply the information concerning **anterior guidance** from the canine and the incisor teeth. The mechanical coupling of the anterior guidance and the posterior guidance settings provides sufficient information to simulate movement of the posterior teeth on the superior border. *The articulator can then be used to diagnose the need to alter the anterior guidance and to design restorations that avoid cusp collisions in mandibular movements.*

In Fig. 2-58 **horizontal condylar guidance** is the term used to describe *the shape of the pathway of condyle point movement in the anterior-posterior direction.* The condyles move in contact with the curved surface of the articular eminence. Recent designs of semi-adjustable articulators have adopted curved surfaces to simulate the curvature of the articular eminence. Rotation of the condylar housing downward increases the slope of the guiding surface of the articulator. The

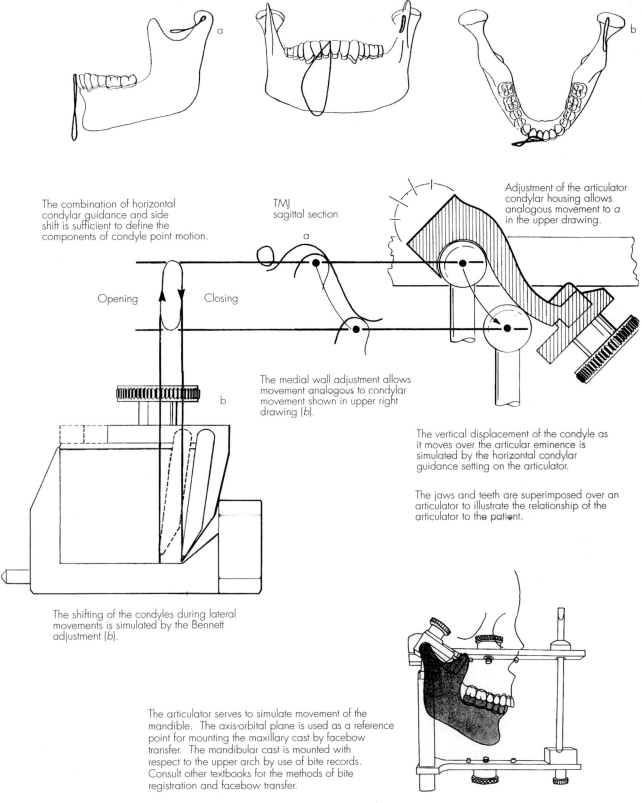

The combination of horizontal condylar guidance and side shift is sufficient to define the components of condyle point motion.

Opening   Closing

b

The shifting of the condyles during lateral movements is simulated by the Bennett adjustment (b).

TMJ sagittal section

a

The medial wall adjustment allows movement analogous to condylar movement shown in upper right drawing (b).

Adjustment of the articulator condylar housing allows analogous movement to a in the upper drawing.

The vertical displacement of the condyle as it moves over the articular eminence is simulated by the horizontal condylar guidance setting on the articulator.

The jaws and teeth are superimposed over an articulator to illustrate the relationship of the articulator to the patient.

The articulator serves to simulate movement of the mandible. The axis-orbital plane is used as a reference point for mounting the maxillary cast by facebow transfer. The mandibular cast is mounted with respect to the upper arch by use of bite records. Consult other textbooks for the methods of bite registration and facebow transfer.

Fig. 2-57. The relationship between condylar motion and articulator settings.

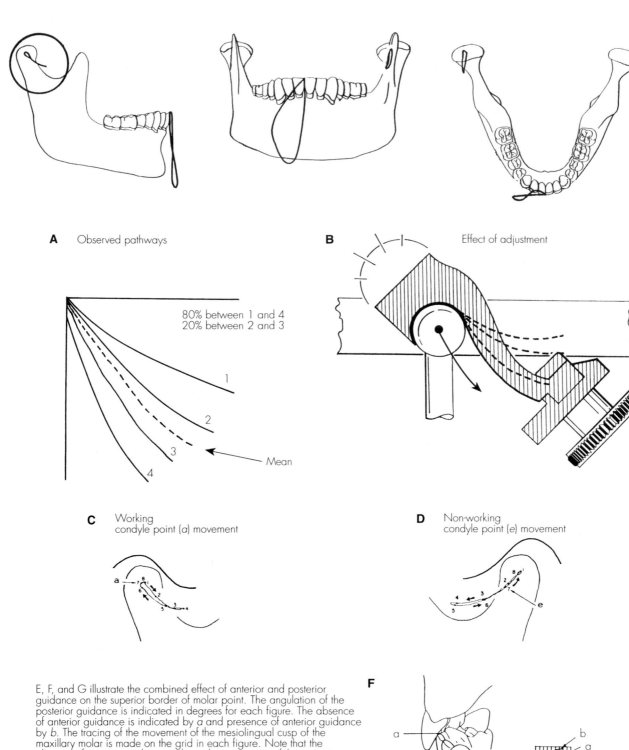

A Observed pathways

B Effect of adjustment

80% between 1 and 4
20% between 2 and 3

1

2

3

Mean

4

C Working
condyle point (a) movement

D Non-working
condyle point (e) movement

E, F, and G illustrate the combined effect of anterior and posterior guidance on the superior border of molar point. The angulation of the posterior guidance is indicated in degrees for each figure. The absence of anterior guidance is indicated by a and presence of anterior guidance by b. The tracing of the movement of the mesiolingual cusp of the maxillary molar is made on the grid in each figure. Note that the absence of anterior guidance reduces the separation of the posterior teeth, but has the greatest effect when the posterior guidance is shallow.

F

30°

E

20°

G

50°

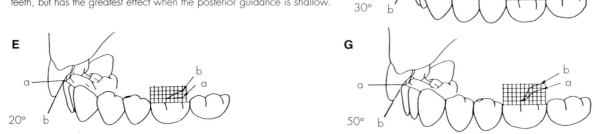

Fig. 2-58. Horizontal condylar guidance. (**A,** modified from Lundeen HC, Wirth CG: Condylar movement patterns engraved in plastic blocks, *J Prosthet Dent* 30:866-875, 1973; **E** to **G,** modified from Lundeen HC, Shryock EF, Gibbs CH: *J Prosthet Dent* 40:442-452, 1978.)

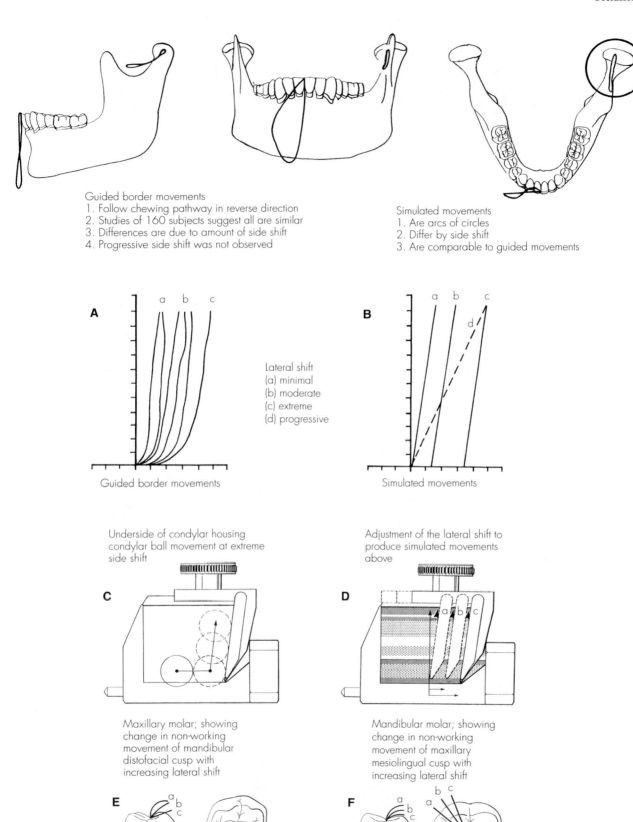

Guided border movements
1. Follow chewing pathway in reverse direction
2. Studies of 160 subjects suggest all are similar
3. Differences are due to amount of side shift
4. Progressive side shift was not observed

Simulated movements
1. Are arcs of circles
2. Differ by side shift
3. Are comparable to guided movements

A

a   b   c

Guided border movements

B

a   b   c

d

Simulated movements

Lateral shift
(a) minimal
(b) moderate
(c) extreme
(d) progressive

Underside of condylar housing
condylar ball movement at extreme
side shift

C

Adjustment of the lateral shift to
produce simulated movements
above

D

a b c

Maxillary molar; showing
change in non-working
movement of mandibular
distofacial cusp with
increasing lateral shift

E

a b c

a b c

Mandibular molar; showing
change in non-working
movement of maxillary
mesiolingual cusp with
increasing lateral shift

F

a b c

b c a

Fig. 2-59. Lateral condylar guidance: the medial wall. (**A** and **B,** based on data from Lundeen HC, Wirth CG: *J Prosthet Dent* 30:866-875, 1973.)

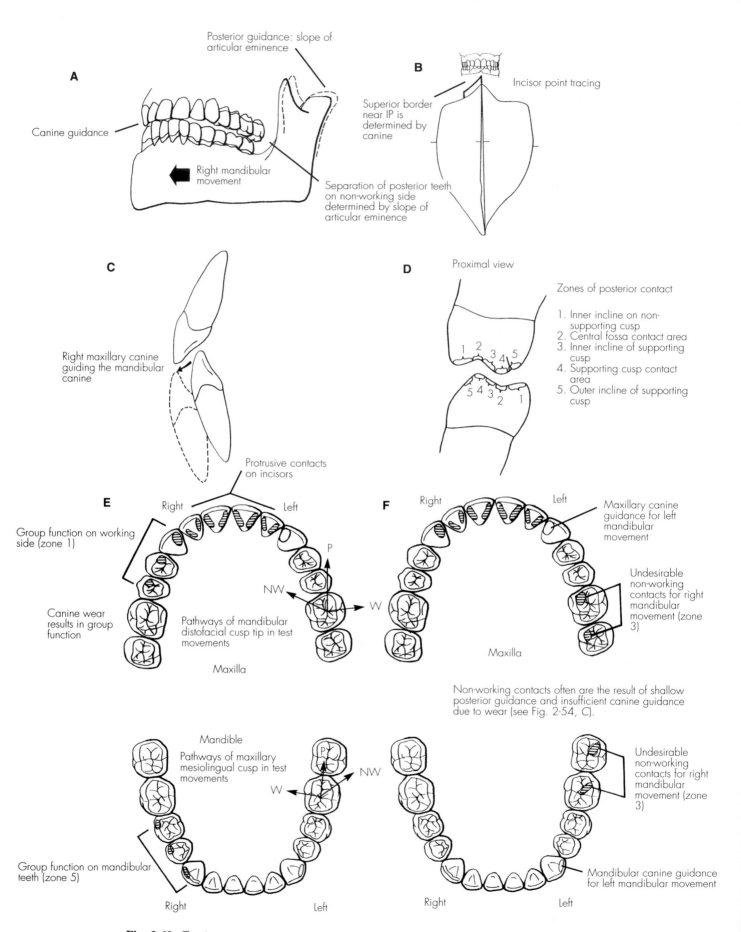

A

Posterior guidance: slope of articular eminence

Canine guidance

Right mandibular movement

Separation of posterior teeth on non-working side determined by slope of articular eminence

B

Incisor point tracing

Superior border near IP is determined by canine

C

Right maxillary canine guiding the mandibular canine

D

Proximal view

Zones of posterior contact

1. Inner incline on non-supporting cusp
2. Central fossa contact area
3. Inner incline of supporting cusp
4. Supporting cusp contact area
5. Outer incline of supporting cusp

Protrusive contacts on incisors

E

Right   Left

Group function on working side (zone 1)

Canine wear results in group function

Pathways of mandibular distofacial cusp tip in test movements

P

NW   W

Maxilla

F

Right   Left

Maxillary canine guidance for left mandibular movement

Undesirable non-working contacts for right mandibular movement (zone 3)

Non-working contacts often are the result of shallow posterior guidance and insufficient canine guidance due to wear (see Fig. 2-54, C).

Maxilla

Mandible

Pathways of maxillary mesiolingual cusp in test movements

P

NW

W

Group function on mandibular teeth (zone 5)

Right   Left

Undesirable non-working contacts for right mandibular movement (zone 3)

Mandibular canine guidance for left mandibular movement

Right   Left

Fig. 2-60. Tooth contacts during mandibular movement. (**B,** from Gibbs CH, Lundeen HC: Jaw movements and forces during chewing and swallowing and their clinical significance. In Lundeen HC, Gibbs CH, editors: *Advances in occlusion,* Bristol, 1982, John Wright PSG.)

range of adjustment of horizontal condylar inclination is well within the range of measured movements in human subjects (see Fig. 2-58, *A* and *B*).[12] Although there may be differences in the relative anterior movement of the two condyles (Fig. 2-58, *C* and *D*), only the first few millimeters of movement have significant effects on the posterior teeth.

Horizontal condylar guidance and anterior guidance (supplied by the mounted casts) are mechanically coupled to produce separation of the posterior teeth. The *combined guidance determines the amount of (or lack of) vertical separation of the posterior teeth as the mandible leaves or enters IP during **protrusion** and lateral movements.*

Lateral mandibular movements also produce separation of the posterior teeth. Horizontal guidance of the non-working condyle coupled with working-side canine guidance determines the amount of *vertical separation of the posterior teeth on both sides as the mandible leaves or enters IP during **lateral movements*** (see Fig. 2-56 for details). This information can be used to design restorations with the proper cusp location and height to avoid collisions during chewing and other mandibular movements.

The slope of the articular eminence varies considerably among individuals. The effect of different slopes can be evaluated by altering the horizontal condylar guidance on articulators. Increasing the horizontal condylar guidance increases the steepness of the mandibular molar movement (molar point) in protrusion. The movement of the maxillary mesiolingual cusp relative to the mandibular molar is plotted in Fig. 2-58, *E* to *G*, for 20-, 30-, and 50-degree slopes.[11] The effect of removing the anterior guidance *(a)* is also drawn on the same grid. Note that the loss of anterior guidance has the greatest effect when the horizontal condylar guidance is shallow (20 degrees) and has the least effect when the horizontal condylar guidance is steep (50 degrees). *Anterior guidance has an additive effect on the molar pathway at all degrees of horizontal guidance. This is an important observation because anterior guidance often can be changed by the dentist.* The anterior guidance can be increased by restorative or orthodontic means to facilitate separation of the posterior teeth in patients who have shallow horizontal guidance.

Fig. 2-59 *(**lateral condylar guidance:** the medial wall)* illustrates how setting the articulator simulates the looseness of the TMJs. TMJ laxity can be measured and transferred to the articulator by use of dentist-guided bite registration records, pantographic tracings, or a clutch and flag system. Bite registrations consistently produce lower values for the lateral shift because tooth contact tends to center the condyles.[14] A clutch and flag system can produce results comparable to a pantographic tracing used to set fully-adjustable articulators.[13] A series of tracings of guided movements from different patients is presented in Fig. 2-59, *A*.[12] All of the tracings are parallel after the first few millimeters of movement. The only difference from one patient to the next is due to the amount of lateral shift. Fig. 2-59, *B*, illustrates simulations of arcs at different degrees of lateral shift; note the similarity of lines *a, b,* and *c* to the lines similarly marked in Fig. 2-59, *A*. Note also that none of the tracings of lateral condylar movement exhibited the "progressive" lateral shift indicated by the dashed line *d* in Fig. 2-59, *B*. Fig. 2-59, *C*, illustrates the underside of a condylar housing of an articulator. Shifting the medial wall simulates the TMJ laxity and allows movements similar to those illustrated in Fig. 2-59, *A*. Fig. 2-59, *D*, illustrates how movements *a, b,* and *c* were made for Fig. 2-59, *B*, by shifting the medial wall of the condylar box.

Increasing laxity of the TMJ, indicated by increasing lateral shift, results in significant changes in movement of the molar point near IP (see Fig. 2-59, *E*). The working-side movement is least affected because it is already a directly lateral movement. The non-working molar point movement is changed in both the lateral and horizontal components. The lateral pathway is extended progressively more laterally in patients with excessive lateral looseness of the TMJs. The horizontal effect is a "flattening" of the pathway by reduction of the vertical separation. These effects are illustrated by tracings of molar point movement on an articulator as the amount of lateral shift is increased from 0 to 3.5 mm. The effect of increasing looseness is to increase the likelihood of collisions of the mesiolingual cusp of the maxillary molars with the mandibular distofacial cusps of the molars on the non-working side (see Figs. 2-59, *E* and *F*). *This type of undesirable contact between the opposing supporting cusps is termed **non-working interferences.***

Tooth contacts during mandibular movements

Operative dentists must design restorations that are capable of withstanding the forces of mastication and clenching. The choice of restorative material and the design of the restoration are frequently highly influenced by the need to withstand the forceful contact with the opposing teeth. *Thus evaluation of the location, direction, and area of tooth contacts during various mandibular movements is an essential part of the preoperative evaluation of teeth to be restored.* The anterior teeth support gliding contacts while the posterior teeth support the heavy forces applied during chewing and clenching. Fig. 2-60 shows a variety of tooth contact relationships. In Fig. 2-60, *A*, a right mandibular movement is illustrated, showing the separation of the posterior teeth on the left or non-working side. The separation of the posterior teeth results from the combined effects of the canine guidance and the slope of the articular eminence on the non-working side. The effect of the canine guidance is illustrated in the incisor point tracing in Fig. 2-60, *B*. The superior border on either side of IP is determined by the shape of the lingual surfaces of the maxillary canine teeth. Guiding contact between the right canines is illustrated in Fig. 2-60, *C*.

A variety of areas on the posterior teeth may contact the opposing tooth during mandibular movements. In Fig. 2-60, *D*, the **opposing surfaces of the molar teeth** are **divided into five areas:**

1. Inner incline of non-supporting (non-centric) cusp. This area sometimes participates in working-side movements by contacting the outer aspect of the supporting (centric) cusp (area 5).
2. Fossa or marginal ridge contact area. This is the main holding contact (or centric stop) area for the opposing supporting cusp.
3. Inner incline of the supporting (centric holding) cusp. This is the area where there is the potential for undesirable contact to occur during non-working movements.
4. Contact area of the supporting (centric holding) cusp. This is the main cusp contact area.
5. Outer aspect of the supporting (centric holding) cusp. This area sometimes participates in working-side movements by contacting the inner incline of the non-supporting (non-centric) cusp (area 1).

Anterior tooth contacts. During anterior movement of the mandible—protrusion—the lower anterior teeth glide along the lingual surfaces of the maxillary anterior teeth (Fig. 2-60, *E* and *F*). Multiple contacts between the opposing dental arches on the anterior teeth are desirable in protrusion and lateral mandibular movements. In protrusion multiple contacts serve to prevent excessive force on any individual pair of gliding teeth. Posterior tooth contact during protrusion is not desirable because it may overload the involved teeth. The combination of the anterior guidance (slope and vertical overlap of the anterior teeth) and the slope of the articular eminence (horizontal condylar guidance on the articulator) determines the amount of vertical separation of the posterior teeth as the mandible moves anteriorly. Some texts refer to this separation as **disocclusion** or **disclusion** of the posterior teeth. Articulator-mounted casts can be used to assess the superior border near IP, which is the critical zone for tooth contact. This information is extremely useful during the fabrication of ceramic and cast metallic restorations because the position and height of the restored cusps can be evaluated and adjusted in the laboratory, which minimizes the time and effort required to adjust the completed restorations at chairside.

Posterior tooth contacts. In idealized occlusal schemes designed for restorative dentistry, *the posterior teeth should contact only in IP*. Any movement of the mandible should result in separation of the posterior teeth by the combined effects of anterior guidance and the slope of the articular eminence (horizontal condylar

guidance on the articulator). Forceful contact or collisions of individual posterior tooth cusps during chewing and clenching may lead to patient discomfort or damage to the teeth. *Patients with shallow anterior guidance or openbite are more difficult to restore without introduction of undesirable tooth contacts. Articulator-mounted casts may be used to assess and solve restorative problems that are difficult to achieve by direct intraoral techniques.*

The side of the jaw where the bolus of food is placed is termed the **working side**. Working side is also used in reference to the jaws or teeth when the patient is not chewing (e.g., in guided test movements directed laterally). The term can also identify a specific side of the mandible (i.e, the side toward which the mandible is moving). During chewing the working-side closures start from a lateral position and are directed medially to IP. Test movements are used by dentists to assess the occlusal contacts on the working side. For convenience, these movements are started in IP and move laterally. Thus, *the working-side test movement follows the same pathway as the working-side chewing closure but occurs in the opposite direction. The preferred occlusal relationship, for restorative purposes, is to limit the working-side contact to the canine teeth. Tooth contact posterior to the canine on the working side may occur naturally in worn dentitions.* As the canine teeth are shortened by wear, the separation of the posterior teeth diminishes. Lateral mandibular movements in worn dentitions bring into contact successively more posterior teeth as the height of the canines decreases. Multiple tooth contacts during lateral jaw movement is termed **group function.** Right-sided group function is illustrated in Fig. 2-60, *E*. Compare this with left canine guidance contact in Fig. 2-60, *F*. Because the amount of torque and wear imposed on teeth increases closer to the muscle attachments on the mandible, molar contact in group function is undesirable. Group function occurs naturally in a worn dentition; however, group function can be a therapeutic goal where the bony support of the canine teeth is compromised by periodontal disease or in Cl II occlusions where canine guidance is impossible.

The **non-working side** is opposite to the working side, and normally does not contain a food bolus during chewing. During chewing closures, the mandibular teeth on the non-working side close from a medial and anterior position and approach IP by moving laterally and posteriorly. *Test movements on the non-working side are made from IP in a medial and anterior direction. Thus the test movements and the chewing strokes are made in opposite directions along the same pathway.* Voluntary lateral movements may not fully approach the borders and thus *it is recommended that the dentist guide the patient in these test movements.* Contact of the molar cusps on the non-working side may overload the teeth or the TMJs. Undesirable non-working contacts are illustrated in Fig. 2-60, F. *Avoidance of contacts on the non-working side is an important goal for restorative procedures on the molar teeth.*

Neurological correlates and control of mastication

This summary of neurological control is based on an excellent review by Lund.[10] The control of mastication is dependent on sensory feedback. *Sensory feedback serves to control the coordination of the lips, tongue, and mandibular movement* during manipulation of the food bolus through all stages of mastication and preparation for swallowing. *Physiologists divide an individual chewing cycle into three components: opening, fast closing, and slow closing.* The *slow closing segment* of chewing is associated with the increased forces required for crushing food. The central nervous system receives several types of feedback from muscle spindles, periodontal receptors, and touch receptors in the skin and mucosa. This feedback controls the mandibular closing muscles during the slow closing phase of mastication. Often sensory feedback results in inhibition of movement, for example due to pain. During mastication some sensory feedback from the teeth is excitatory causing an increase in the closing force as the food bolus is crushed. However, there must be an upper limit where inhibition occurs, which prevents the build-up of excessive forces on the teeth during the occlusal stage.

A group of neurons in the brainstem produces bursts of discharges at regular intervals when excited by oral sensory stimuli. These bursts drive motor neurons to produce contractions of the masticatory muscles at regular intervals, resulting in rhythmic mandibular movement. *The cluster of neurons in the brainstem that drives the rhythmic chewing is termed the central pattern generator (CPG).* Oral sensory feedback can modify the basic CPG pattern and is essential for coordination of the lips, tongue, and mandible. Sensory input from the periodontal and mucosal receptors keeps the rhythmical chewing going. During opening, the mandibular opening muscles are contracted and the closing muscles are inhibited. During closing, the mandibular closing muscles are activated but the opening muscles are not inhibited. *The coactivation of the opening and closing muscles makes the mandible more rigid and probably serves to brace the condyles while the food is crushed.* This coactivation of the opening and closing muscles probably contributes to the rigidity noticed by clinicians attempting to manipulate the mandible.

Chewing cycles illustrated in Figs. 2-54 to 2-56 are due to CPG rhythms. Gliding tooth contact occurs frequently during chewing on the working side. These contacts probably cause an increase in the closing force. Working-side contacts are forceful and represent about 11% of the maximum possible bite force. The borders of mandibular function are relevant to construction of dental restorations because forceful contacts occur regu-

larly during chewing. When the mandibular closure results in molar contact on the non-working side, opposite the food bolus, the teeth or TMJs may be overloaded.

REFERENCES

1. Angle EH: Classification of malocclusion, *Dent Cosmos* 41:248-264, 350-357, 1899.
2. Brännström M: *Dentin and pulp in restorative dentistry,* London, 1982, Wolfe Medical Publications.
3. Carlsson GE, Haraldson T, Mohl ND: The dentition. In Mohl ND et al, editors: *A textbook of occlusion,* Chicago, 1988, Quintessence Publishing.
4. Celenza FV, Nasedkin JN: *Occlusion the state of the art,* Chicago, 1978, Quintessence Publishing.
5. Garberoglio R, Brännström M: Scanning electron microscopic investigation of human dentinal tubules, *Arch Oral Biol* 21:355-362, 1976.
6. Gibbs CH, Lundeen HC: Jaw movements and forces during chewing and swallowing and their clinical significance. In Lundeen HC, Gibbs CH, editors: *Advances in occlusion,* Bristol, 1982, John Wright PSG.
7. Gibbs CH et al: Functional movements of the mandible, *J Prosthet Dent* 26:601-610, 1971.
8. Jordan RE, Abrams L, Kraus BS: *Kraus' dental anatomy and occlusion,* ed 2, St Louis, 1992, Mosby.
9. Kraus BS, Jordan RE, Abrams L: *Dental anatomy and occlusion,* ed 1, p 234, Baltimore, 1969, Williams & Wilkins.
10. Lund JP: Mastication and its control by the brain stem, *Crit Rev Oral Biol Med* 2:33-64, 1991.
11. Lundeen HC, Shryock EF, Gibbs CH: An evaluation of mandibular border movements: their character and significance, *J Prosthet Dent* 40:442-452, 1978.
12. Lundeen HC, Wirth CG: Condylar movement patterns engraved in plastic blocks, *J Prosthet Dent* 30:866-875, 1973.
13. Lundeen TF, Mendosa MA: Comparison of Bennett shift measured at the hinge axis and an arbitrary hinge axis position, *J Prosthet Dent* 51:407-410, 1984.
14. Lundeen TF, Mendosa MA: Comparison of two methods for measurement of immediate Bennett shift, *J Prosthet Dent* 51:243-245, 1984.
15. Michelich V, Pashley DH, Whitford GM: Dentin permeability: comparison of function versus anatomic tubular radii, *J Dent Res* 57:1019-1024, 1978.
16. Nakabayashi N, Takarada K: Effect of HEMA on bonding to dentin, *Dent Mater* 8(2):125-130, 1992.
17. Pashley DH: The effects of acid etching on the pulpodentin complex, *Oper Dent* 17(6):229-242, 1992.
18. Pashley DH: Clinical correlations of dentin structure and function, *J Prosthet Dent* 66(6):777-781, 1991.
19. Posselt U: Studies in the mobility of the mandible, *Acta Odont Scand* 10 (Suppl 10), 1952.
20. Scott JH, Symons NBB: *Introduction to dental anatomy,* ed 7, Edinburgh, 1974, Churchill Livingstone.
21. Stanley HR: *Human pulp response to operative dental procedures,* Gainesville, Fla, 1976, Sorter Printing.
22. Sturdevant JR, Pashley DH: Regional dentin permeability of Class I and II cavity preparations, *J Dent Res* (abstract No. 173) 68:203, 1989.
23. Van Meerbeek M et al: Comparative SEM and TEM examination of the ultrastructure of the resin-dentin interdiffusion zone, *J Dent Res* 72(2):495-501, 1993.

CHAPTER 3

Cariology: the lesion, etiology, prevention, and control

Thomas F. Lundeen

Theodore M. Roberson

INTRODUCTION AND DEFINITIONS

Dental caries (tooth decay) (Figs. 3-1 to 3-5) and periodontal disease are probably the most common chronic diseases in the world. Although caries has affected humans since prehistorical times, the prevalence of this disease has greatly increased in modern times on a worldwide basis, and the increase is strongly associated with dietary change. There is now evidence that this trend peaked and began to decline in the late 1970s and early 1980s, and the decline was most marked in certain segments of the population of the United States, western Europe, New Zealand, and Australia[26] (see Table 3-1). The exact cause of the decline is unknown but is attributed to the addition of trace amounts of fluoride ion to public drinking water. Trace amounts of fluoride

Table 3-1. The decline in caries

Country	Age	Time period	Change in %
Denmark	Military recruits	1972-1982	39
UK	12	1970-1980	23
Ireland	13-14	1961-1980	42
The Netherlands	12	1967-1980	31
New Zealand	12-13	1950-1982	35
Norway	16	1970-1979	55
Scotland	11-12	1970-1980	28
Sweden	15	1973-1978	51
USA	16	1972-1980	36

Modified from Carlos JP: In Guggenheim B, editor: *Cariology today,* Basel, 1984, Karger.

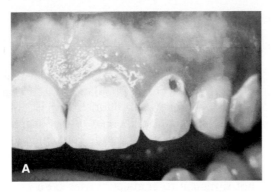 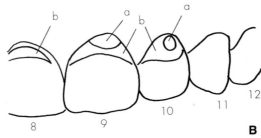

Fig. 3-1. A, A young adult with multiple active carious lesions involving teeth No. 8 to No. 12. B, Cavitated areas *(a)* are surrounded by areas of extensive demineralization that are chalky and opaque *(b)*. Some areas of incipient caries have superficial stain.

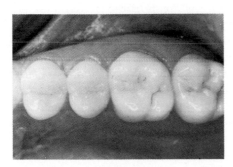 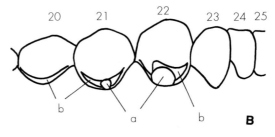

Fig. 3-2. Extensive active caries in a young adult (same patient as in Fig. 3-1). A, Mirror view of teeth No. 20 to No. 25. B, Cavitated lesions *(a)* are surrounded by extensive areas of chalky, opaque demineralized areas *(b)*. The presence of smooth surface lesions like these is associated with rampant caries. Occlusal and interproximal smooth surface caries usually occur in advance of facial smooth surface lesions. The presence of these types of lesions should alert the dentist to the possibility of extensive caries activity elsewhere in the mouth. The interproximal gingiva is swollen red and will bleed easily upon probing. These gingival changes are the consequence of long-standing irritation from the plaque adherent to the teeth.

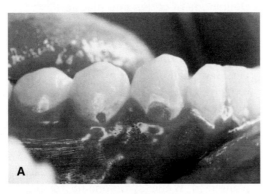 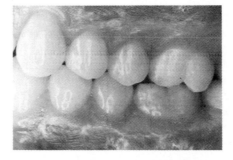 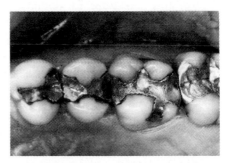

Fig. 3-3. Occlusal, mirror view of teeth No. 2 to No. 5. These healthy teeth have few suitable habitats for plaque populations. Note that many of the grooves on the occlusal surfaces are coalesced. There are some areas of stain, particularly in the distal oblique fissure (noncoalesced groove) of the first molar. This superficial stain is typically found in caries-free fissures and should not be confused with other color changes in enamel associated with caries. Compare this with Figs. 3-23 to 3-26.

Fig. 3-4. Facial view of teeth in Fig. 3-3. Note healthy gingiva and translucent enamel, especially along the crest of the gingiva. Compare this photo to Fig. 3-2 showing inflamed gingival tissues. Compare the enamel characteristics to Fig. 3-28.

Fig. 3-5. Occlusal view of restored teeth with corroded, ditched margins. These teeth provide numerous retentive habitats for plaque communities. Note poor interproximal contours associated with broad, rough contact areas. The corrosion and breakdown at the tooth-restoration interface (margin) produces small V-shaped defects (ditches) that become new habitats for cariogenic bacteria.

were discovered to have a marked limiting effect on the progression of caries lesions originating on the adjacent contacting, or proximal, surfaces of teeth. This discovery lead to widespread addition of fluoride to public water supplies in the 1950s and 1960s and the addition of fluoride to a variety of oral hygiene products, especially toothpaste. By 1984, 94% of the toothpaste products contained added fluoride.[64]

The decline in caries in these developed countries, such as the United States, has been most prominent in the upper and middle classes, while the lower socioeconomic and rural classes have retained a high prevalence of tooth decay. For example, the National Preventive Dentistry Program found that 60% of the caries occurred in 20% of the children, who were frequently in lower socioeconomic groups or minorities.[7] This effect has been characterized as a "polarization" of caries, where a limited segment of the population experiences most of the disease. A similar polarization is occurring on a worldwide basis where the prevalence of caries is declining in developed countries, is increasing in less developed countries, and is epidemic in countries with emerging economies. Thus caries is increasingly being localized in segments of populations that can least afford the necessary dental treatment.

The cost of caries to society is enormous. The bill for dental care in the United States alone was $27 billion in 1985.[101] This represents probably less than half the actual need considering that only 40% to 50% of the public regularly seek dental care. This published cost represents only the direct expense of the dental care services. The total indirect costs, such as loss of time from work and the training of dentists, are also substantial. Tooth loss resulting in diminished chewing ability, which can lead to nutritional disorders, is a significant problem in the lower socioeconomic groups, where replacement may not be available for economic reasons. In addition, caries results in other significant, although intangible, costs in the form of pain, suffering, and cosmetic defects. In 1986, Walter Loesche described caries and periodontal disease as ". . . *perhaps the most expensive infections that most individuals have to contend with during a lifetime.*"[53] That statement remains correct in the 1990s, with perhaps the exception of HIV infection.

Considering the magnitude and almost universal impact of caries, it is remarkable that a public-supported program for the eradication of the disease never developed as did programs against polio and smallpox. Caries eradication is dependent on the availability of four factors: (1) a potent eradicator weapon (vaccine), (2) strong and efficient public health service support, (3) popular support for the program, and (4) an efficient surveillance system to monitor caries activity on a population level.[61] Caries eradication is not yet achievable

because these four basic requirements have not been met. In particular, the vaccine is not available. The single most effective population-based caries control method, public water fluoridation, is not sufficient to prevent pit and fissure caries of the posterior teeth. Water fluoridation and fluoride-containing dentifrices are not sufficient to prevent caries in individuals with poor dietary and oral hygiene practices. While knowledge is not sufficient to eradicate caries on a population level, individuals under professional supervision having good dietary and oral hygiene practices can indeed live a lifetime caries free.[36]

Definitions of caries and plaque

Dental caries is an infectious microbiological disease of the teeth that results in localized dissolution and destruction of the calcified tissues. It is essential to understand that cavitations in teeth (destruction of the tooth surface, creating a cavity) are signs of bacterial infection. In clinical practice, it is possible to lose sight of this fact and focus entirely on the restorative treatment of the lesions, thereby failing to treat the underlying cause of the disease. (See Chapter 5 for a thorough discussion of clinical diagnosis of caries and treatment planning.) While symptomatic treatment is important, *failure to identify and treat the underlying cause (i.e., the infection of the tooth from odontopathic [causing disease to the teeth] bacteria) will allow the disease to continue.* The preventive section of this chapter emphasizes the components of an antibacterial treatment program that controls the infection by regulation of the oral ecological conditions.

Caries activity, as evidenced by demineralization and loss of tooth structure, is highly variable; and therefore the course of individual lesions is not always predictable. Carious lesions only occur under a mass of bacteria capable of producing a sufficiently acidic environment to demineralize tooth structure. *A gelatinous mass of bacteria adhering to the tooth surface is termed dental plaque.* The plaque bacteria metabolize refined carbohydrates for energy and produce organic acids as a by-product. The acids produced may then cause a carious lesion by dissolution of the tooth's crystalline structure. Caries *lesions progress as a series of exacerbations and remissions as the pH at the tooth surface varies with the changes in plaque metabolism.* The availability of simple carbohydrates, such as sucrose, greatly stimulates plaque metabolism. Exacerbations of caries activity are characterized by periods of high bacterial metabolic activity and low pH in the plaque near the tooth surface. During intervening episodes when few carbohydrates are available, there is little bacterial metabolic activity, and the pH rises near the surface of the tooth. *Remineralization of the damaged tooth structure occurs as the local pH rises above 5.5.* Saliva contains high concentrations of calcium and phosphate ions in solution which serve as a supply of raw material for the remineralization process. Acid attack on tooth surfaces continually occurs throughout an individual's life. Virtually all of the interproximal (adjacent contacting) surfaces of teeth are attacked by acid produced by plaque and are partially demineralized. Fortunately, relatively few tooth surfaces partially demineralized by plaque acids progress to cavitation. Understanding the balance between demineralization and remineralization is the key to enlightened caries management.

The evidence for the role of bacteria in the genesis of caries is overwhelming. Animal and human models have been used in an extensive series of studies leading to the following conclusions[71]:

1. Teeth free from infection with bacteria, either in germ-free animals or unerupted teeth in humans, do not develop caries.
2. Antibiotics are effective in reducing caries in animals and humans.
3. Oral bacteria can demineralize enamel in vitro and produce lesions similar to naturally occurring caries.
4. Specific bacteria can be isolated and identified from plaque over various carious lesions.

While the role of bacterial activity in the genesis of carious lesions is well defined, establishing a cause-and-effect relationship between an individual organism in the oral flora and caries has not been completely successful. Oral bacteria do not occur as solitary colonies, but as members of a complex community of many species contained as a mass of tightly packed cells held together by the sticky matrix of polymerized glucose. There are some 200 to 300 species of bacteria, yeast, and even protozoa that appear to be indigenous to the human oral cavity.[70,87] It is the metabolic activity of the complex community of bacteria which form plaque that determines the presence or absence of disease of the adjacent hard and soft tissues. Assessing the contribution of an individual species to the pathology associated with a complex plaque community has proven to be very difficult in in vivo systems. It has become clear, however, in recent years that a relatively small group of bacteria are primarily responsible for production of the two major oral diseases, namely, caries and periodontal disease. One group of bacteria which consists of eight *Streptococcus mutans* serotypes has been associated with caries. The serotypes have been labeled *a* through *h*. Several serotypes have been elevated to species status and given names: *S. rattus* (serotype b), *S. cricetus* (serotype a), *S. ferus* (serotype c), and *S. sobrinus* (serotypes d, g, and h). All *S. mutans* serotypes have been demonstrated to have significant potential to cause caries; but because of their significant genetic and biochemical differences, they should not be simply referred

to as the single species *S. mutans*. This text will use the term **mutans streptococci** as a collective term for all the serotypes. *Mutans streptococci and lactobacilli can produce great amounts of acids (acidogenic), are tolerant of acidic environments (aciduric), are vigorously stimulated by sucrose, and appear to be the primary organisms associated with caries in man. Organisms which cause caries are termed* **cariogenic.** *The degree to which a tooth is likely to become carious is described as its* **cariogenicity potential.** Mutans streptococci are present as a pandemic infection in humans; that is, mutans streptococci are found in everyone regardless of race, ethnic background, or geographical origin. Normally mutans streptococci exist in the mouth as an insignificantly small component of the oral flora. In patients with multiple active carious lesions, mutans streptococci have become a dominant member of the plaque flora. Recent evidence suggests that mutans streptococci are most strongly associated with the onset of caries while lactobacilli are associated with active progression of cavitated lesions.[53]

Epidemiology of caries

Dental caries has been studied extensively during the last 50 years in North America and Europe. These epidemiological studies have been very useful in determination of the extent of the need for, and effectiveness of, dental treatment. Originally, epidemiology focused on the study of epidemics, but in modern times epidemiology has expanded to cover any aspect of health needs of a population. A *population* consists of all individuals located in a prescribed area. The number of individuals in a population having a disease at a specific point in time is known as the *prevalence* of the disease. The number of individuals developing new cases of disease in a population over a specific period of time, usually 1 year, is the *incidence* of the disease. The length or duration of the disease has an important effect on the measures of prevalence and incidence. For short duration diseases, such as the flu, the incidence and the prevalence are nearly identical. For diseases that persist over long periods (years or decades), the prevalence will be much higher than the incidence.

The most common epidemiological measure of caries is the **DMF.** This is a measure of the number of teeth that are *diseased, missing,* or *filled* (DMF). DMF may be reported as the number of teeth *(DMFT)* or surfaces affected *(DMFS).* This measure is cumulative because it totals the number of restorations and extractions in addition to the number of teeth having active caries. It is presumed that the restored or extracted teeth were treated because of caries at some point in time prior to the epidemiological survey. Once the tooth is restored or removed, it becomes a permanent measure for the life of the patient. The *M* and *F* components are therefore historical markers of the presence of past disease and should not be confused with the *D,* active disease, component. Thus *DMF* rates are not the equivalent to a true measure of caries prevalence, and in fact, overestimate the prevalence of active caries. Having noted the problems with *DMF* measures of caries, it is important to recognize the importance of *DMF* to making decisions concerning changes in caries in populations. Table 3-1 lists the reported changes in *DMF* rates in 9 countries in the last decade. The important observation is that children in the 1980s have less total caries experience than their predecessors in the 1960s and 1970s. The trend, however, indicates the DMF rate will increase over an individual's life.

The effects of the changes in caries pattern in the developed countries will be dramatic on the nature of operative dentistry practiced in the near future. The populations in many of these countries are aging. Thus in the United States, for example, the percentage of the population over the age of 65 will double from the year 1980 to the year 2000 and will comprise one fifth of the population by the year 2030. Thus there will be more elderly people and they will have more teeth than any preceding generation. This large elderly population will be at increased risk for caries, especially on exposed root surfaces. Little is known about the caries risk in adults, particularly with regard to root caries, except that the risk increases with age. *It is expected that root caries will increase over the next several decades. Furthermore, both maintenance of teeth with existing restorations (replacement needs) and new dental disease will increase the demand for operative dentistry* despite the decline of caries in children.[15]

The status of caries in third-world countries represents the greatest challenge to dental science. In developing economies there is minimal income for basic health care needs, including dental care. Staggering DMF increases, such as three- to five-fold increases in children, are reported in widely diverse regions, including Uganda, Chile, Mexico, Lebanon, and Thailand.[84] It is widely believed that the cause of this increase is due to a substantial rise in dietary sucrose that was previously unavailable to these populations. Paradoxically, in these countries it is the higher social classes, with greater exposure to dietary sucrose, that are frequently the most affected. Unfortunately, there are many barriers to treating these populations. In addition to minimal income, social and cultural norms often do not allow ready acceptance of new oral care and hygiene procedures. The costs of fluoride toothpaste and simple materials for a school-based fluoride rinse program often are prohibitive. There usually are few trained dentists and hygienists in these countries to deliver such simple care as sealants and fluoride treatments. Public water supply fluoridation would be the best and the least expensive treatment method, but it can only be applied if adequate public water distribution exists and if culturally acceptable, neither of which typically exists.

Hypothesis concerning etiology of caries

Two basic yet opposing hypotheses concerning the pathogenicity of plaque have been proposed.[56,58] The older and more accepted hypothesis recognizes the universal presence of potential pathogens in plaque and therefore assumes that all accumulations of plaque are pathogenic. The alternative hypothesis is based on the observation that accumulation of plaque is not always associated with disease. Under the latter hypothesis, accumulation of plaque could be regarded as normal in the absence of disease. *Plaque is assumed to be pathogenic only when signs of disease are present.* The difference between these two hypotheses has been clearly identified and discussed by Walter Loesche, who, although studying periodontal disease, applied these concepts equally well to caries. The first hypothesis, which assumes all plaque is pathogenic, is termed the **nonspecific plaque hypothesis.** The alternative, or **specific plaque hypothesis,** recognizes plaque as pathogenic only when signs of associated disease are present.[57]

The problem with the *nonspecific plaque hypothesis* is that it requires a therapeutic goal which completely eliminates plaque in *all* patients. This goal is unrealistic and not achievable even in the most dedicated patients. Treatment under the nonspecific plaque hypothesis requires an open-ended regimen of continuous therapy directed at total plaque elimination. Dentists trying to achieve such ambitious goals have inevitably become frustrated by repeated failure of their patients to achieve total plaque control and have abandoned such "preventive practices."

The *specific plaque hypothesis* provides a new scientific basis for the treatment of caries that has radically altered caries treatment (Tables 3-2 and 3-3). *Plaques can be identified as pathologic when they are associated with clinical disease.* Because only a limited number of microorganisms are capable of caries production, specific plaque hypothesis treatment is aimed at elimination

Table 3-2. The new caries treatment based on the medical model

Etiology	*Mutans streptococci* infection
Symptoms	Demineralization lesions in teeth
Treatment, symptomatic	Restoration of cavitated lesions
Treatment, therapeutic	Eliminate *Mutans streptococci* infection
Post-treatment assessment, symptomatic	Examine teeth for new lesions
Post-treatment assessment, therapeutic	Bacteriologic testing for *Mutans streptococci*

Table 3-3. Comparison of traditional versus new caries treatment

	Traditional	New
Diagnosis	Not required, plaque is universal	Diagnosis is essential, only some plaques are pathologic
Target population	The entire population must be treated	Treatment is necessary only for infected or high-risk individuals
Treatment goal	Removal of all plaque	Elimination of infection
Purpose of recall	Determine need for restoration	Determine if infection has been eliminated
Responsibility for outcome	Treatment failure primarily is the patient's fault	Treatment failure primarily is the dentist's fault

Modified from: Anderson MH, Bales DJ, Omnell, K-A: *J Am Dent Assoc* 124:37-44, 1993.

of the specific pathogenic organisms, but not total plaque elimination. To quote from Loesche[53]:

> The goal of therapy is to suppress the cariogenic plaques and to replace them with pathogen-free plaques. This therapeutic goal may be realized if antimicrobial modalities, such as mechanical debridement and chemical agents, can be applied with sufficient intensity so as to achieve for short periods of time on the tooth surface some semblance of "sterility." If such "sterility" can be obtained, then the newly forming plaque will be derived from organisms in the bathing saliva and will contain high proportions of *Streptococcus sanguis* and *Streptococcus mitis*, and low proportions of *S. mutans* . . .

The subsequent plaque, dominated by non-cariogenic bacteria will have little or no cariogenic potential.

Ecological basis of caries

The basic premise of this chapter is that development and growth of plaque on teeth is a normal phenomenon. The plaque community structure undergoes a succession of changes during periods of unrestricted growth. These changes in the community structure consequently change the overall metabolism and other characteristics of the plaque. Community structural changes are predictable and are governed by general principles of *ecology*,[2] *which is the science of interactions between organisms and their environment*. Unrestricted plaque growth produces local environmental conditions that may selectively promote the accumulation of pathogenic bacterial species.

High frequency sucrose exposure may be the single most important factor in producing a cariogenic plaque. Frequent sucrose ingestion begins a series of changes in the local tooth environment that promotes the growth of highly acidogenic bacteria and eventually leads to caries. In contrast, when sucrose is severely restricted or absent, plaque growth typically does not lead to caries. *Dietary sucrose plays a leading role in the development of pathogenic plaques and may be the single most important factor in disruption of the normal healthy ecology of dental plaque communities*.

Multiple factors determine the characteristics of plaque. The factors that control the presence of individual species in plaque are termed *ecological determi-*

nants. These can be divided into several broad interrelated categories: host resistance, extent and nature of shelter for bacteria, host diet, oral hygiene, status of the dentition, and composition of the oral flora. These various factors can be viewed as links in a chain of reactions eventually leading to caries.

The decline in caries in developed countries is widely believed to be due primarily to the increased use of fluorides in public water supplies and oral hygiene products. Improvements in oral hygiene, diet, and other factors have been considered to be of much less importance to the general decline in caries worldwide. However, analysis of the observed caries reduction based on detailed data from studies of children in Zurich[65] found that an average of 40% of the reduction was not explained by fluoride use (in all of its forms). Changes in dietary habits and better oral hygiene were assumed to have been responsible for the additional caries reduction. Yet total sucrose consumption for the Zurich community had remained steady at 39 to 46 kg/person/year for the past 30 years, including the period of caries decline, and there were no suggestions that the Zurich children consumed less sugar during this study period. This study is representative in indicating that the mechanism of caries reduction is not entirely understood and apparently not fully explained by either the use of fluoride or a reduction in sucrose consumption. Thus the other factors once considered to be of little importance, in fact, may have a considerable impact on caries. Whatever the cause, the children of the '90s in developed countries tend to have less pathogenic plaque than their parents. This is a consequence of a change in the oral ecology of these children.

ETIOLOGICAL AGENT OF CARIES: PATHOGENIC BACTERIAL PLAQUE
Introductory description of plaque

As previously stated, the soft, translucent, and tenaciously adherent material accumulating on the surface of teeth is commonly called *plaque*. It is more accurately described as *bacterial plaque* because it is composed almost completely of bacteria and their by-products (Figs. 3-6 to 3-10). Plaque is neither adherent food debris, as is widely and erroneously thought, nor does it

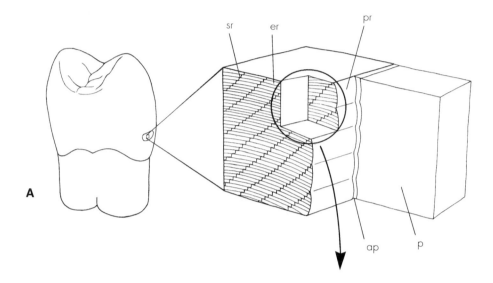

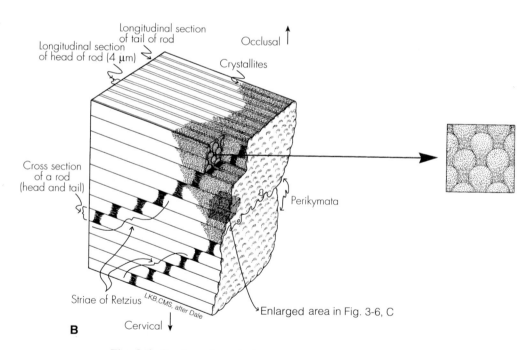

Fig. 3-6. For legend see facing page.

C

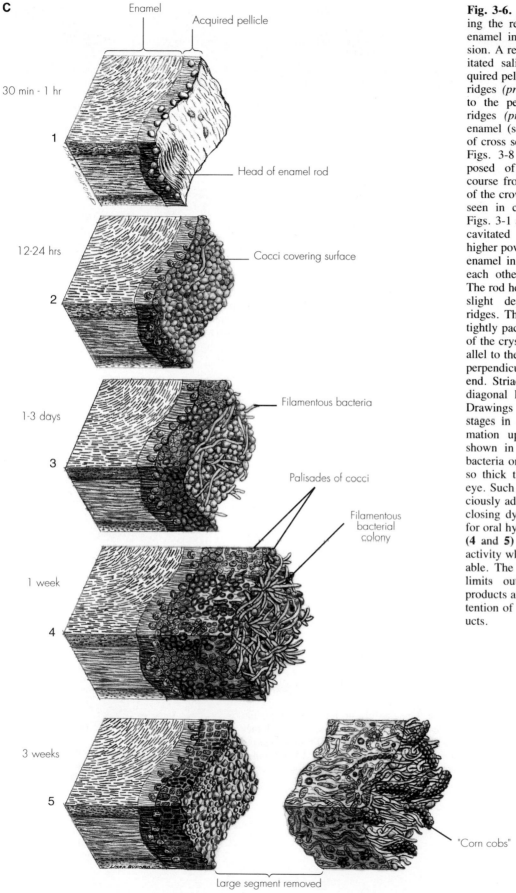

Enamel

Acquired pellicle

30 min - 1 hr

1

Head of enamel rod

12-24 hrs

2

Cocci covering surface

1-3 days

3

Filamentous bacteria

1 week

4

Palisades of cocci

Filamentous bacterial colony

3 weeks

5

"Corn cobs"

Large segment removed

Fig. 3-6. A, Composite diagram illustrating the relationship of plaque *(p)* to the enamel in a smooth surface incipient lesion. A relatively cell-free layer of precipitated salivary protein material, the acquired pellicle *(ap),* covers the perikymata ridges *(pr)*. The plaque bacteria attaches to the pellicle. Overlapping perikymata ridges *(pr)* can be seen on surface of enamel (see Fig. 3-7). Photomicrographs of cross sections of plaque can be seen in Figs. 3-8 to 3-10. The enamel is composed of rod-like structures *(er)* that course from the inner DEJ to the surface of the crown. Striae of Retzius *(sr)* can be seen in cross sections of enamel. (See Figs. 3-1 and 3-2 for typical incipient and cavitated smooth surface lesions.) **B,** A higher power view of the cutout portion of enamel in **A.** Enamel rods interlock with each other in a head-to-tail orientation. The rod heads are visible on the surface as slight depressions on the perikymata ridges. The enamel rods are composed of tightly packed crystallites. The orientation of the crystallites changes from being parallel to the rod in the head region to being perpendicular to the rod axis in the tail end. Striae of Retzius form a descending diagonal line, descending cervically. **C,** Drawings **1** to **5** illustrate the various stages in colonization during plaque formation upon the shaded enamel block shown in **B.** The accumulated mass of bacteria on the tooth surface may become so thick that it is visible to the unaided eye. Such plaques are gelatinous and tenaciously adherent; they readily take up disclosing dyes, aiding in their visualization for oral hygiene instruction. Thick plaques **(4 and 5)** are capable of great metabolic activity when sufficient nutrients are available. The gelatinous nature of the plaque limits outward diffusion of metabolic products and thus serves to prolong the retention of organic acid metabolic by-products.

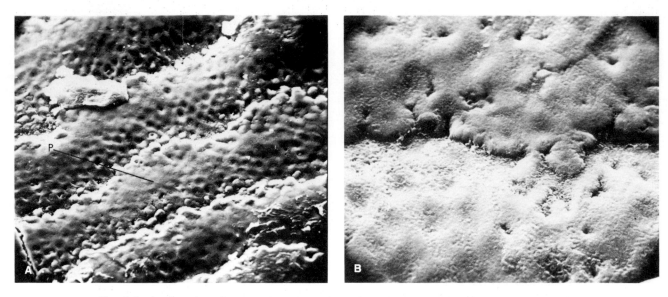

Fig. 3-7. A, Scanning electron microscope view of overlapping perikymata *(p)* in sound enamel from unerupted molar (× 600). **B,** Higher power view of overlapped site rotated 180 degrees (× 2300). Surface of incipient enamel lesions has "punched out" appearance. (From Hoffman S: Histopathology of caries lesions. In Menaker L, editor: *The biologic basis of dental caries,* New York, 1980, Harper & Row, Publishers.)

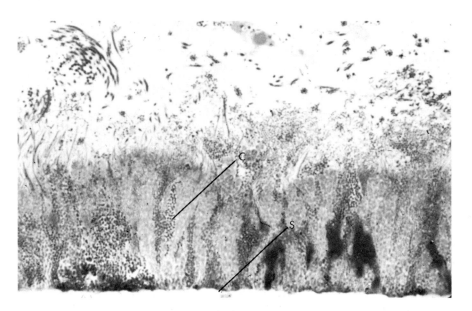

Fig. 3-8. A photomicrograph of bacterial plaque. One-day plaque formation in patient who is a heavy plaque former. This plaque consists primarily of columnar microcolonies of cocci **(C)** growing perpendicular to crown surface **(S)** (× 1350). (From Listgarten MA, Mayo HE, Tremblay R: *J Periodontol* 46(1):19, 1975. Copyright 1975 Munksgaard International Publishers Ltd, Copenhagen, Denmark.)

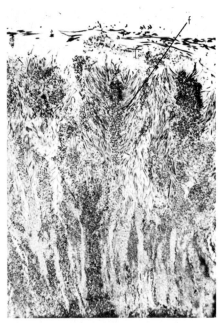

Fig. 3-9. Plaque formation at 1 week. Filamentous bacteria *(f)* appear to be invading cocci microcolonies. Plaque near gingival sulcus has fewer coccal forms and more filamentous bacteria (× 860). (From Listgarten MA, Mayo HE, Tremblay R: *J Periodontol* 46(1):10, 1975. Copyright 1975 Munksgaard International Publishers Ltd, Copenhagen, Denmark.)

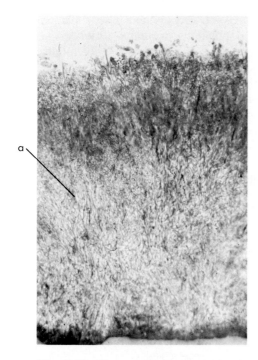

Fig. 3-10. Three-week-old plaque is almost entirely composed of filamentous bacteria. Heavy plaque formers have spiral bacteria *(a)* associated with subgingival plaque (× 660). (From Listgarten MA, Mayo HE, Tremblay R: *J Periodontol* 46(1):10, 1975. Copyright 1975 Munksgaard International Publishers Ltd, Copenhagen, Denmark.)

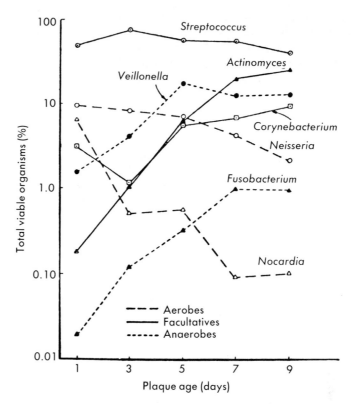

Fig. 3-11. Succession in plaque communities results from shift to predominantly anaerobic conditions within mass of plaque. Note that over a period of 9 days relative proportions of aerobic and anaerobic species change dramatically. (From HL Ritz: *Arch Oral Biol,* vol 12, copyright 1967, Pergamon Press.)

result from the haphazard collection of opportunistic microorganisms. Actually *the accumulation of plaque on teeth is a highly organized and ordered sequence of events.* Many of the organisms found in the mouth are not found elsewhere in nature. *Survival of microorganisms in the oral environment depends on their ability to adhere to a surface.* Free-floating organisms are rapidly cleared from the mouth by salivary flow and frequent swallowing. Only a few specialized organisms, primarily streptococci, are able to adhere to oral surfaces such as the mucosa and tooth structure. These adherent bacteria have special receptors for adhesion to the tooth surface and also produce a sticky *matrix* that allows them to cohere to each other. This adherence and coherence allows the bacteria to successfully colonize the tooth surface. Once they are attached, these pioneering organisms proliferate and spread laterally to form a mat-like covering over the tooth surface (see Fig. 3-6, *C*). Further growth of bacteria produces a vertical growth away from (external to) the tooth surface. The resulting mixed streptococcal mat allows the adherence of other organisms, such as filamentous and spiral bacteria, that

otherwise are unable to adhere directly to the tooth surface (see Figs. 3-6, *C* and 3-8 to 3-10). Thus the formation of a mature plaque community involves a succession of changes (Fig. 3-11), and each change depends on the preceding stage preparing the local environment for the next stage (Table 3-4).

Plaque communities and habitats

There are significant differences in the plaque communities found in various habitats (ecological environments) within the oral cavity (Fig. 3-12). The oral mucosa is populated by organisms with receptors specialized for attachment to the surface of epithelium. The dorsum of the tongue has a plaque community dominated by *Streptococcus salivarius.* The teeth normally have a plaque community dominated by *S. sanguis* and *S. mitis.* The population size of *mutans streptococci* on teeth is highly variable. Normally it is a very small percentage of the total plaque population but can be as large as one-half the facultative streptococcal flora in other plaques.

Many distinct habitats may be identified on individual teeth, with each habitat containing a unique plaque community (Table 3-5). While the pits and fissures on the crown may harbor a relatively simple population of streptococci, the root surface in the gingival sulcus may harbor a very complex community dominated by filamentous and spiral bacteria. Facial and lingual smooth surfaces and proximal surfaces also may harbor vastly different plaque communities.[30] For example the mesial surface of a molar may be carious and have a plaque dominated by large populations of *mutans streptococci* and *lactobacilli,* while the distal surface may totally lack these organisms and be caries-free. Therefore, generalization about plaque communities is difficult. Nevertheless, the general activity of plaque growth and maturation is predictable and sufficiently well-known to be of therapeutic importance in the prevention of caries.

Table 3-4. Analysis of two-species population interactions: Effect on population growth and survival of two populations, A and B*†

Type of interaction	When not interacting		When interacting		General result of interaction
	A	B	A	B	
Neutralism (A and B independent)	0	0	0	0	Neither population affects the other
Competition (A and B competitors)	0	0	−	−	Population most affected eliminated from niche
Mutualism (A and B partners or symbionts)	−	−	+	+	Interaction obligatory for both
Protocooperation (A and B cooperators)	0	0	+	+	Interaction favorable to both but not obligatory
Commensalism (A commensal; B host)	−	0	+	0	Obligatory for A; B not affected
Amensalism (A amensal; B inhibitor or antibiotic)	0	0	−	0	A inhibited; B not affected
Parasitism (A parasite; B host)	−	0	+	−	Obligatory for A; B inhibited
Predation (A predator; B prey)	−	0	+	−	Obligatory for A; B inhibited

From *Fundamentals of ecology,* Third Edition by Eugene P. Odum, copyright © 1971 by W.B. Saunders Company, Reprinted by permission of CBS College Publishing.
*Interactions among plaque organisms are very complex and can change over time. Careful use of ecological terminology can facilitate the description of various population interactions.
†*Key:* +, Population growth increased; −, population growth decreased; 0, population growth not affected.

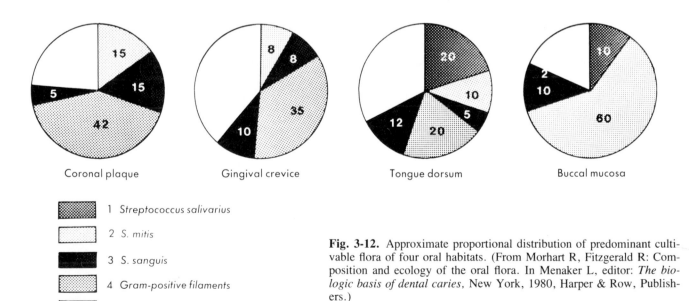

Coronal plaque   Gingival crevice   Tongue dorsum   Buccal mucosa

1 *Streptococcus salivarius*

2 *S. mitis*

3 *S. sanguis*

4 *Gram-positive filaments*

5 *Veillonella* sp.

6 Other species

Fig. 3-12. Approximate proportional distribution of predominant cultivable flora of four oral habitats. (From Morhart R, Fitzgerald R: Composition and ecology of the oral flora. In Menaker L, editor: *The biologic basis of dental caries,* New York, 1980, Harper & Row, Publishers.)

Table 3-5. Oral habitats*

Habitat	Predominant species	Environmental conditions within plaque
Mucosa	S. mitis	Aerobic
	S. sanguis	pH—approximately 7
	S. salivarius	Oxidation-reduction potential—positive
Tongue	S. salivarius	Aerobic
	S. mutans	pH—approximately 7
	S. sanguis	Oxidation-reduction potential—positive
Teeth (noncarious)	S. sanguis	Aerobic
		pH—5.5
		Oxidation-reduction—negative
Gingival crevice	Fusobacterium species	Anaerobic
	Spirochaeta species	pH—variable
	Actinomyces species	Oxidation-reduction—very negative
	Veillonella species	
Enamel caries	S. mutans	Anaerobic
Dentin caries	S. mutans	pH—< 5.5
	Lactobacillus species	Oxidation-reduction—negative
Root caries	Actinomyces species	

*The microenvironmental conditions in the habitats associated with host health are generally aerobic, near neutrality in pH, and positive in oxidation-reduction potential. Significant microenvironmental changes are associated with caries and periodontal disease. The changes are the result of the plaque community metabolism.

Development of bacterial plaque: an ecological phenomenon

The complex and dynamic relationships among bacterial plaque, the host, and dental disease are best understood by viewing dental disease as a result of the functioning of an ecological system that operates on widely known and accepted ecological principles. An **ecosystem** is a circumscribed area occupied by a biological community. The oral cavity is a well-defined ecosystem because it has recognized geographical limits and the general composition of the biological community is known. Within the oral ecosystem are distinct habitats (see Table 3-5) such as the dorsum of the tongue, oral mucosa, gingival sulcus, and various tooth locations including pits, fissures, and certain smooth surface areas. These habitats have unique environmental conditions and harbor markedly different communities of microorganisms (see Figs. 3-3 to 3-5). Within each habitat, special combinations of food and shelter are available to support particular species of oral bacteria. *This special combination of food and shelter is termed an **ecological niche**.*

A particular niche is generally occupied by a single, best adapted species. Thus for each habitat, a dental fissure for example, a limited number of niches are available to the oral flora. The niches will be occupied by the organisms present in the greatest numbers in the saliva. If the niches on the teeth are already occupied by an organism, new opportunistic organisms will be excluded and prevented from becoming a part of the plaque. This process can prevent pathologic organisms (*mutans streptococci)* from being established on already covered plaque surfaces. Thus plaques dominated by

normal oral flora, such as *S. sanguis,* may be considered to be desirable because of their ability to control or prohibit the introduction of more pathogenic organisms.

As a plaque community develops on a tooth surface, eventually all the available niches will become occupied. When *niche saturation* occurs, only very competitive microorganisms can displace the indigenous bacteria from the community. Niche saturation provides inherent stability to plaque communities. Although large numbers of foreign organisms pass through the oral cavity, it is rare for any to become established as permanent residents.[82] Niche saturation may be the mechanism that prevents these multitudes of exogenous organisms from becoming established in the mouth. This homeostatic mechanism has been termed **colonization resistance.** Colonization resistance can be quantified by measuring the threshold dose (number of organisms) required to establish a new resident population.[98] *Mutans streptococci* have a very high threshold dose because they must compete with *S. sanguis* for niches. *S. sanguis* is more efficient in adhering to tooth surfaces than *mutans streptococci* and, thus, is more rapidly established in the local community.[100] Thus the threshold dose (the total number of bacteria inoculated into the mouth) is a critical factor for establishment of an organism in plaque communities. This concept forms the basis for bacteriologic testing of saliva to determine caries risk (Table 3-6).

In normal healthy circumstances, the oral flora capable of colonizing the teeth are not capable of causing disease. In order for *mutans streptococci* to spread to other tooth surfaces, they must be present in sufficient numbers in the saliva to overcome the colonization re-

Table 3-6. Significance of odontopathic bacteria in the saliva*

Stimulated saliva sample colony forming units per ml of saliva	Interpretation of results
Mutans streptococci > 10^6 *Lactobacilli* > 10^5	**High risk**—high counts suggest there already exists cariogenic plaques and good potential to infect other sites by overcoming colonization resistance
Mutans streptococci < 10^5 *Lactobacilli* < 10^3	**Low risk**—lower counts suggest insufficient numbers to overcome colonization resistance and therefore reduced risk of infection

Saliva collected while chewing wax (see Table 3-9 for method) is plated on selective media by standard methods. The number of colonies growing on the plates is an estimate of the number of odontopathic bacteria free-floating in the saliva. *Mutans streptococci* are strongly adherent to the teeth and accumulate in sheltered sites. *Lactobacilli* are not able to adhere, but are residents in cavitation. Thus only a limited number of these pathogens can be liberated by chewing. It is possible to have a low count and still have cariogenic plaque, but high counts are good indicators of extensive caries potential.

sistance afforded by the normal oral flora. Therefore it should be noted that an active carious lesion can serve as a reservoir of *mutans streptococci* and *lactobacilli,* providing the large threshold dose necessary to establish infections on other tooth surfaces. Millions of *mutans streptococci* and *lactobacilli* are continually lost from the surface of active carious lesions. Consequently, it is essential to eliminate carious lesions because they may become the source for pathogenic infection of non-cariogenic plaques. *Restoration of carious lesions has significant beneficial clinical effects in addition to the benefit of restoration of the damaged tooth structure and maintenance of pulpal vitality because the restorative process also effectively removes a nidus of infection.*

Some strains of *mutans streptococci* are easier to establish in a host than other strains. This difference may be due in part to their ability to produce proteins called **bacteriocins,** which are lethal to closely related bacteria. Bacteriocin production is an ecological adaptation that allows an organism to be more effective in competition with similar bacteria for the same niche.[28] Thus, bacteriocin production is an important ecological determinant. Persistent colonization of the teeth by bacteriocin-producing *mutans streptococci* has been demonstrated.[33,34] Bacteriocin production by itself is probably insufficient to allow *mutans streptococci* to become a dominant plaque species. However, a combination of bacteriocin-producing *mutans streptococci* with poor diet and oral hygiene can lead to a very extensive and persistent infection.[33,34]

Addition of another isolated and purified bacteriocin (known to inhibit *mutans streptococci)* to the diet of rats had little effect when the availability of sucrose was good, but when sucrose was limited, the bacteriocin killed *mutans streptococci* and related streptococci.[76] This suggests a possible therapeutic role for bacteriocins. Many oral bacteria produce bacteriocins that are effective against *mutans streptococci* and it is possible that some bacterial strains could give the host some immunity to caries when they are present. As already mentioned, bacteriocins effective against *mutans streptococci* have been identified and purified.[60] Therefore, an effective therapeutic treatment for caries could be the replacement of normal inhabitants of the oral cavity with strains having enhanced bacteriocin activity against the more pathogenic organisms (such as *mutans streptococci).*[39]

Some habitats on the teeth encourage caries by virtue of their physical shape. The pits and fissures of teeth are the most susceptible areas to caries and the most favorable habitat for *mutans streptococci*. These deep recesses not only shelter bacteria residing in them but also limit access of salivary factors that attenuate and repair demineralization. Obturation of these anatomical faults by occlusal sealants or amalgam restorations prevents caries and greatly reduces the numbers of *mutans streptococci* in the mouth. This is an excellent example of ecological control of an undesirable plaque organism without wholesale disruption of the remainder of the oral flora. *Sealing the pits and fissures eliminates a habitat of **mutans streptococci** and is an example of disease prevention based on sound ecological principles.*

Plaque growth. As previously stated, the growth of plaque is not the result of a random accumulation of opportunistic organisms passing through the oral cavity. Rather, what occurs is an orderly sequence of replacement communities occupying the tooth surface, each community modifying the local environment of that site. The available niches, the limiting factors, and the environment conditions change as a result of the biological activity of each plaque community. This process of mutual change of the community and its environment is called *ecological succession* (see Fig. 3-11). Individual stages in a succession sequence are known as *seres* and the final stage of succession is a stable biological community termed the *climax community.*[2] Two different types of succession occur and both can be identified in the oral cavity. In general ecology, *primary succession* occurs as the process of development of a biological community where none previously existed. Applied to the oral cavity, primary succession is the process of normal change in the oral flora occurring over the lifetime of an individual host. *Secondary succession* is the process of restoration of the climax community after a disruption in the community structure. Secondary succession as it applies to the teeth is the process of plaque regrowth after the tooth surface is cleaned. If the environmental conditions remain the same, secondary succession will result in an identical climax community. Thus a similar plaque will reform on the teeth after prophylaxis if there is no other change in the oral environmental conditions.

Primary succession occurs over the lifetime of the host. For example, a newborn's mouth is rapidly occupied by skin bacteria and *Streptococcus salivarius*. Newborns lack teeth and therefore cannot harbor organisms adapted to tooth habitats. Transient organisms, such as *Escherichia coli*, may be noted, but they fail to establish a permanent residence in the oral cavity. Major changes in the species composition of the oral cavity occur with the eruption of teeth because the teeth supply new habitats. In the adult, the general composition of a well-established oral flora remains relatively stable if there are no major changes in the health of the host. Loss of all teeth in elderly patients results in the loss of organisms specialized for tooth attachment and, consequently, the oral flora reverts to a composition similar to that of a newborn.

Plaque growth first consists of surface attachment and then lateral spreading as the attached organisms multiply (Fig. 3-13). When the entire surface is covered, growth of the colonies increases the thickness of the plaque. As the original colonizing organisms proliferate, their progeny produce vertical columns of cells called *palisades* (see Figs. 3-6, *C* and 3-8 to 3-10). The palisades can be invaded by filamentous bacteria that otherwise could not exist on the tooth surface. Proliferation of the new, invading bacteria produce tangled masses of filaments extending upward, away from the surface of the tooth. Plaques may grow to become many thousands of cells thick, resulting in interesting plaque structures such as "corn cobs," which consist of filaments with cocci attached (see Fig. 3-6, *C, e*). These probably indicate preferential attachment of two types of organisms that each derive some benefit from the attachment.

Early stages of plaque succession. Professional tooth cleaning is a practice that is intended to control plaque and prevent disease. After professional removal of all organic material and bacteria from a tooth surface, a new coating of organic material begins to accumulate immediately. Within 2 hours a cell-free, struc-

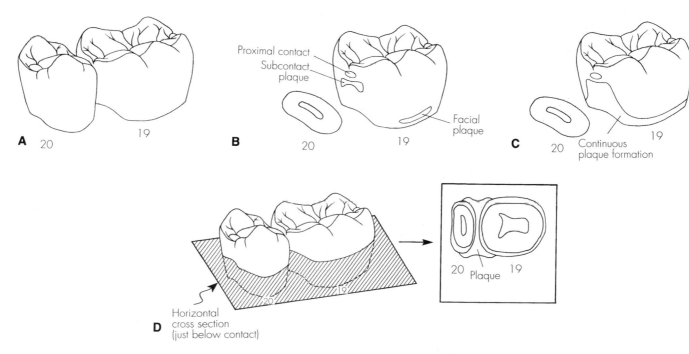

Fig. 3-13. Plaque formation on posterior teeth and associated carious lesions. **A,** Teeth No. 19 and No. 20 in contacting relationship. **B,** The crown of tooth No. 20 has been removed at the cervix. The proximal contact and subcontact plaque can be seen on the mesial surface of No. 19. A facial plaque is also illustrated. **C,** During periods of unrestricted growth, the mesial and facial plaques become part of a continuous ring of plaque around the teeth. Continuous rings of carious lesions can be seen in Fig. 3-28. **D,** A horizontal cross section through teeth No. 19 and No. 20 with heavy plaque. The inset shows the interproximal space below the contact area filled with gelatinous plaque. This mass of interproximal plaque concentrates the effects of plaque metabolism on the adjacent tooth smooth surfaces. All interproximal surfaces are subject to plaque accumulation and acid demineralization. In patients exposed to fluoridated water, most interproximal lesions become arrested at a stage prior to cavitation.

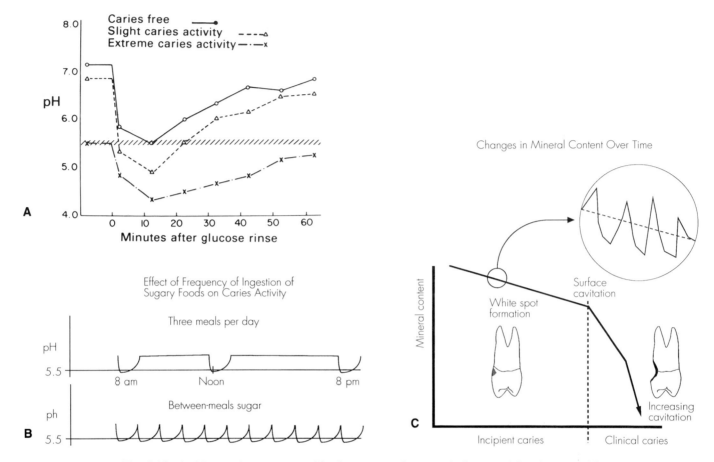

Fig. 3-15. A, Mature plaque communities have tremendous metabolic potential and are capable of very rapid anaerobic metabolism of any available carbohydrates. Classic studies by Stephan[90] demonstrate this metabolic potential by severe pH drops at plaque-enamel interface following glucose rinse. It is generally agreed that pH of 5.5 is *threshold for enamel demineralization*. Note than exposure to glucose rinse for extreme caries activity plaque results in sustained period of demineralization (pH 5.5). Recording from slight caries activity plaque demonstrates much shorter period of demineralization. **B,** The frequency of sucrose exposure for cariogenic plaque greatly influences the progress of tooth demineralization. The top line illustrates Ph depression, patterned after the Stephan's curves in **A.** Three meals per day results in three exposures of plaque acids, each lasting approximately 1 hour. The plaque pH depression is relatively independent of the quantity of sucrose ingested. Between-meal snacks or the use of sweetened breath mints results in many more acid attacks, as illustrated at the bottom. The effect of frequent ingestion of small quantities of sucrose results in a nearly continuous acid attack on the tooth surface. The clinical consequences of this behavior can be seen in Fig. 3-38. **C,** In active caries there is a progressive loss of mineral content subjacent to the cariogenic plaque. The inset illustrates that the loss is not a continuous process. Instead, there are alternating periods of mineral loss (demineralization) with intervening periods of remineralization. The critical event for the tooth is cavitation of the surface, marked by the vertical dashed line. This event marks an acceleration in caries destruction of the tooth and irreversible loss of tooth structure. For these reasons restorative intervention is required. (**A** modified from Stephan RM: *J Dent Res* 23(4):257, 1944.)

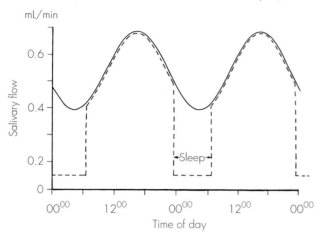

Fig. 3-16. Diurnal salivary flow variation. This illustrates the importance of sleep in the promotion of caries. The extreme decline in salivary flow during sleep promotes the prolongation of acid attack during sleep. For this reason, brushing and flossing prior to going to bed is highly recommended. (From Dawes C: Unpublished data [used with permission]).

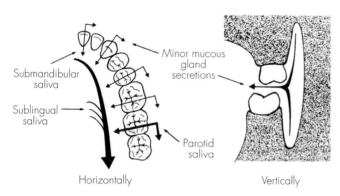

Fig. 3-17. Salivary flow direction over the teeth. Saliva flows as a thin film (0.1 mm) over the teeth and oral mucosa in the mouth. This figure illustrates the net directions of salivary flow around the teeth. The velocity is estimated to vary between 1 and 8 mm/min in normal adults. The velocity of salivary flow has important site-specific effects on the clearance of substrate and acids. Areas where the velocity of salivary flow is low will be subject to increased caries risk. It was observed that the flow rates on the lingual surfaces of the lower anterior teeth and the lingual surfaces of the maxillary posterior teeth were much higher than the flow on the facial surfaces of the mandibular anterior teeth and the maxillary anterior teeth. This finding correlates well with the observation that the facial surfaces of the maxillary and mandibular anterior teeth have a higher prevalence of caries than the lingual surfaces. (From Lecomte P, Dawes C: *J Dent Res* 66:1614-1618, 1987.)

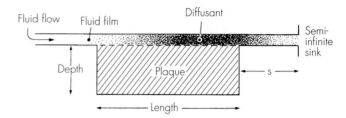

Fig. 3-18. Diagrammatic representation of model used by Dawes[13a] to calculate the effects of different salivary flow rates. (From Dawes C: *J Dent Res* 68:1483-1488, 1989.)

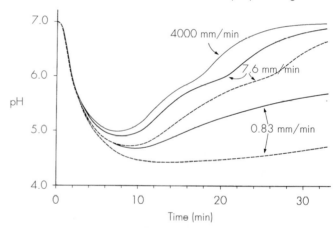

Fig. 3-19. Predicted effects of three different film velocities on Stephan curves for plaque 0.5 mm thick and 6 mm wide (see model in Fig. 3-18). The salivary film flow is assumed to be unidirectional. The dashed lines give the predicted pH values at the enamel surface under the plaque that first comes into contact with the saliva, and the solid lines represent the values for the exit side of the plaque. The lower flow rate has the effect of greatly extending the duration of the pH depression in the plaque. (From Dawes C: *J Dent Res* 68:1483-1488, 1989.)

rough topography provides additional shelter not available on the mucosal surface. *S. salivarius* and *Micrococcus mucilaginous* are two species commonly found on the tongue but rarely found on teeth.[45]

The prevailing environmental conditions on both the mucosa and the tongue are largely determined by the saliva. Both of these habitats are aerobic, have neutral pH, and are positive in oxidation-reduction potential, and yet they harbor different communities of organisms.

Tooth habitats for pathogenic plaque. The tooth surface is unique because it is not protected by the surface shedding mechanisms (continual replacement of epithelial cells) used throughout the remainder of the alimentary canal. The tooth surface is stable and covered with the pellicle of precipitated salivary glycoproteins, enzymes, and immunoglobulins. It is the ideal surface for the attachment of many oral streptococci. If left undisturbed, plaque will rapidly build up to sufficient depth to produce an anaerobic environment adjacent to the

tooth surface. Tooth habitats that are favorable for harboring pathogenic plaque include: (1) pits and fissures; (2) the smooth enamel surfaces both immediately gingival to the proximal contacts and in the gingival one-third of the facial and lingual surfaces of the clinical crown; (3) root surfaces, particularly near the cervical line; and (4) subgingival areas (Fig. 3-20, *A* to *C*). These sites correspond to the locations where caries is most frequently encountered.

Pits and fissures. Pit and fissure caries has the highest prevalence of all dental caries (Figs. 3-20 to 3-26). The *pits and fissures provide excellent mechanical shelter for organisms* and harbor a community dominated by *S. sanguis* and other streptococci.[40] The relative proportion of *mutans streptococci* most probably determines the cariogenic potential of the pit and fissure community. Complex communities dominated by filamentous bacteria, such as those in the gingival crevice, apparently fail to develop in the pit and fissure habi-

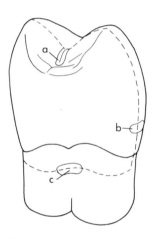

Fig. 3-20. A, There are many distinct sites where caries may originate: pits and fissures *(a);* smooth surface of crown *(b);* root surface *(c).* Proximal surface lesion of crown is not illustrated here because it is a special case of smooth surface lesion. Histopathology and progress of both facial (or lingual) and proximal lesions are identical. Dotted line indicates cut used to reveal cross sections illustrated in Figs. 3-20, *B* and *C.*

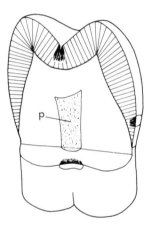

Fig. 3-20. B, In cross section the three types of lesions demonstrate different rates of progression and different morphology. Lesions illustrated here are intended to be representative of each type. No particular association between three lesions is implied. Pit and fissure lesions have small site of origin visible on occlusal surface but have wide base. Overall shape of pit and fissure lesion is inverted V. In contrast, smooth surface lesion is V-shaped with wide area of origin and apex of V directed toward pulp *(p).* Root caries begins directly on dentin. Root surface lesions can progress rapidly, since dentin is less resistant to caries attack.

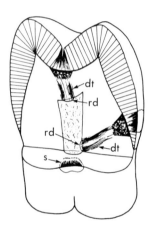

Fig. 3-20. C, Advanced carious lesions produce considerable histological change in enamel, dentin, and pulp. Bacterial invasion of lesion results in extensive demineralization and proteolysis of the dentin. Clinically this necrotic dentin appears soft, wet, and mushy. Deeper pulpally, dentin is demineralized but not invaded by bacteria and is structurally intact. This tissue appears to be dry and leathery in texture. Two varieties of pulp-dentin response are illustrated. Under pit and fissure lesion and smooth surface lesion, odontoblasts have died, leaving empty tubules called dead tracts *(dt).* New odontoblasts have been differentiated from pulp mesenchymal cells. These new odontoblasts have then produced reparative dentin *(rd),* which seals off dead tracts. Another type of pulp-dentin reaction is sclerosis *(s)*—occlusion of the tubules by peritubular dentin. This is illustrated under root caries lesion.

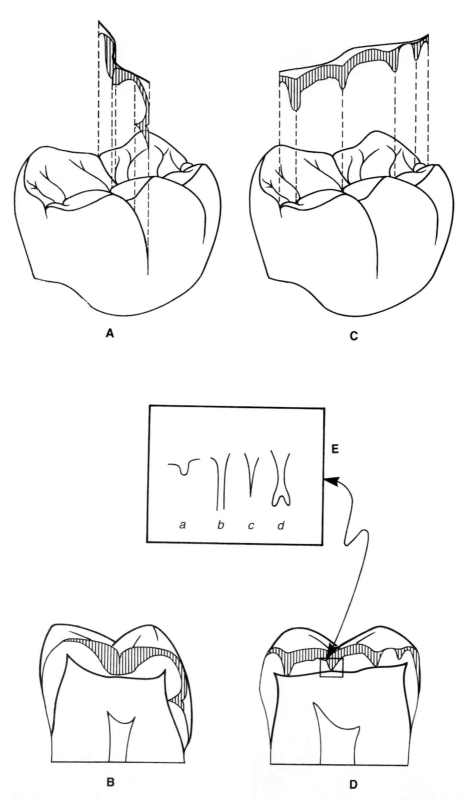

Fig. 3-21. Developmental pits, grooves, and fissures on the crowns of the teeth can have complex and varied anatomy. **A** and **B,** The facial developmental groove of the lower first molar often terminates in a pit. The depth of the groove and the pit is highly variable. **C** and **D,** The central groove extends from the mesial pit to the distal pit. Sometimes grooves extend over the marginal ridges. **E,** The termination of pits and fissures may vary from a shallow groove *(a)* to complete penetration of the enamel *(b)*. The end of the fissure may end blindly *(c)* or open into an irregular chamber *(d)*.

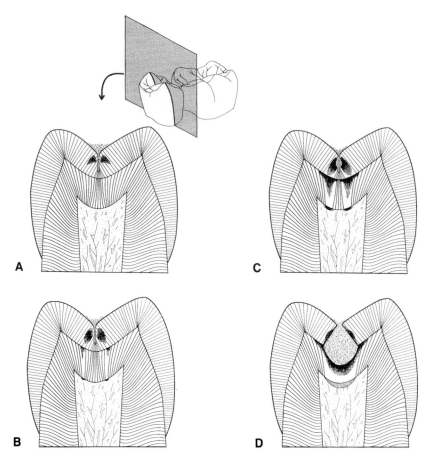

Fig. 3-22. Progression of caries in pits and fissures. **A,** The initial lesions develop on the lateral walls of the fissure. Demineralization follows the direction of the enamel rods, spreading laterally as it approaches the DEJ. **B,** Soon after the initial enamel lesion occurs, a reaction can be seen in the dentin and pulp. Forceful probing of the lesion at this stage can result in damage to the weakened porous enamel and accelerate the progression of the lesion. Clinical detection at this stage should be based on observation of discoloration and opacification of the enamel adjacent to the fissure. These changes can be observed by careful cleaning and drying of the fissure. **C,** Initial cavitation of the opposing walls of the fissure cannot be seen on the occlusal surface. Opacification can be seen that is similar to the previous stage. Remineralization of the enamel because of trace amounts of fluoride in the saliva may make progression of pit and fissure lesions more difficult to detect. **D,** Extensive cavitation of the dentin and undermining of the covering enamel will darken the occlusal surface (see Fig. 3-23).

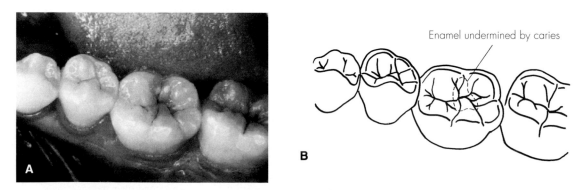

Fig. 3-23. A, Mandibular first molar has undermined discolored enamel due to extensive pit and fissure caries. Lesion began as illustrated in Fig. 3-22 and has progressed to stage illustrated in Fig. 3-22, *D*. **B,** Discolored enamel is outlined by broken line in the central fossa region.

tat.[19] The appearance of *mutans streptococci* in pits and fissures is usually followed by caries, 6 to 24 months later. *Sealing the pits and fissures just after tooth eruption may be the single most important event in providing their resistance to caries* (see later section, Pit and Fissure Sealants).

Smooth enamel surfaces. The **proximal enamel surfaces** *immediately gingival of the contact area are the second most susceptible areas to caries* (see Figs. 3-20, 3-25, 3-27, and 3-29). These areas also are protected physically and are relatively free from the effects of mastication of food, tongue movement, and salivary flow. The amount and types of organisms making up the proximal surface plaque community are variable. Important ecological determinants for the plaque community on the proximal surfaces are the topography of the tooth surface, the size and shape of the gingival papillae, and the oral hygiene of the patient. A rough surface (caused by caries, a poor quality restoration [new or old], or a structural defect) restricts adequate plaque removal. This results in retention of a more advanced successional plaque stage, favoring the occurrence of caries or periodontal disease at the site.

In very young patients the gingival papilla completely fills the interproximal space under a proximal contact and is termed a *col* (see Chapter 2 for illustration and definition of col). Thus the proximal surfaces of very young patients are in crevicular spaces which are less favorable habitats for *mutans streptococci*. Consequently, proximal caries is less likely to develop where this favorable soft tissue architecture exists. Conversely, apical migration of the papillae creates more habitats in more exposed environments for tooth surface colonizing bacteria. Increasing the exposed surface area has a stimulating effect on the growth of *mutans streptococci*.[83] Therefore poor soft tissue form tends to stimulate plaque growth in the sheltered proximal areas, rendering them more susceptible to both caries and periodontal disease. More vigorous and conscientious oral hygiene practices will be required to keep these open proximal regions free of disease.

Often the gingival aspect of the **facial and lingual smooth enamel surface** that is supragingival but gingival of the occlusogingival height of contour is neither rubbed daily by the bolus of food nor cleaned daily by the toothbrush. Therefore these surface areas are habi-

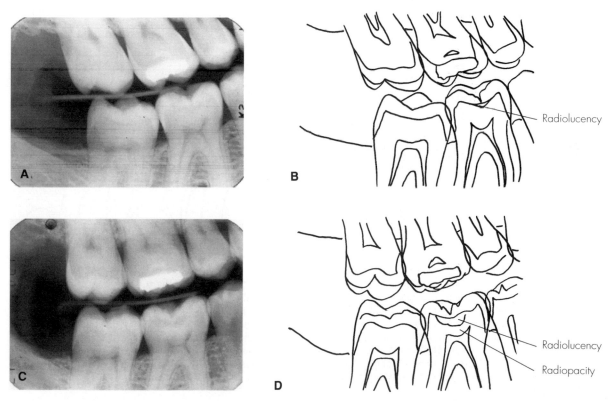

Fig. 3-24. Progression of pit and fissure caries. **A,** The mandibular right first molar (No. 30) was sealed in 1985. Note radiolucent areas under the occlusal enamel in **A** and **B.** The seal failed and caries progressed slowly, the only symptom was occasional biting-force pain. **C** and **D,** Note the extensive radiolucency under the enamel and an area of increased radiopacity below the lesion, suggesting sclerosis.

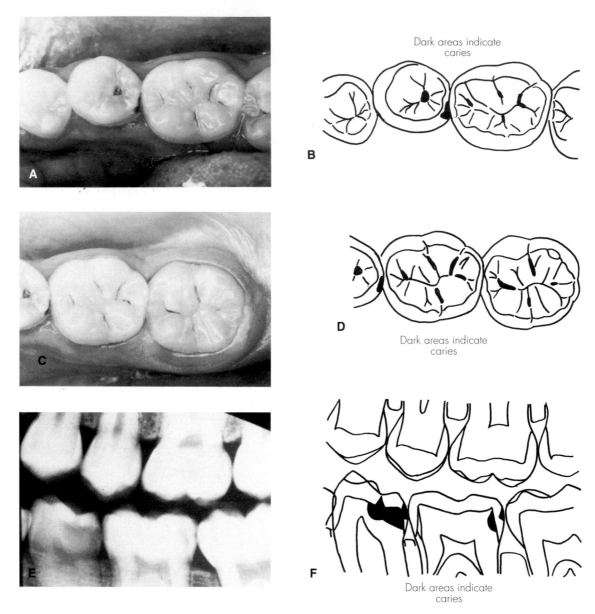

Fig. 3-25. A young patient with extensive caries. **A** and **B,** The occlusal pits of the first molar and second premolar are carious. There is an interproximal carious lesion on the second premolar. The second premolar is rotated almost 90 degrees bringing the lingual surface into contact with the mesial surface of the first molar. Normally the lingual surfaces of the mandibular teeth are rarely attacked by caries, but here, the tooth rotation makes the lingual surface a proximal contact and, consequently, produces an interproximal habitat which increases the susceptibility of the surface to caries. **C** and **D,** The first and second molars have extensive caries in the pits and fissures. On the bitewing radiograph (**E** and **F**), not only can the extensive nature of the caries in the second premolar be seen, but also seen is a lesion on the distal aspect of the first molar, which is not visible clinically.

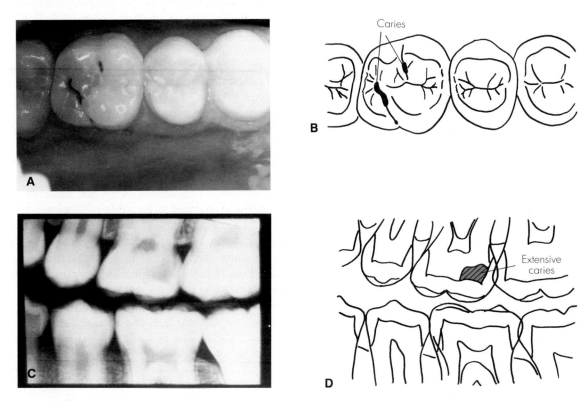

Fig. 3-26. Example of occlusal caries that is actually much more extensive than is apparent clinically. **A** and **B,** Clinical example. **C** and **D,** A bitewing radiograph further reveals an extensive area of demineralization undermining the distofacial cusp.

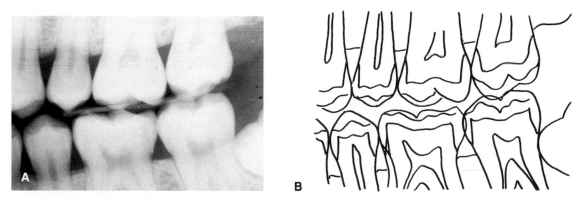

Fig. 3-27. Bitewing radiograph of normal teeth, free from caries. Note the uniform density of the enamel on the interproximal surfaces. There is a third molar impacted on the distal aspect of the lower second molar. The interproximal bone levels are uniform and located slightly below the cementoenamel junctions, suggesting a healthy periodontium.

tats for the caries-producing mature plaque. The presence of caries in these areas usually is indicative of a caries-active mouth (see Figs. 3-1, 3-2, 3-28, and 3-44).

Root surfaces. The proximal root surface, particularly near the cervical line, is often unaffected by the action of hygiene procedures such as flossing because it may have concave anatomic surface contours (fluting) and occasional roughness at the termination of the enamel. These conditions, when coupled with exposure to the oral environment (as a result of gingival recession), favor the formation of mature, caries-producing plaque and proximal *root surface caries.* Likewise the facial or lingual root surfaces (particularly near the cervical line) when exposed to the oral environment (due to gingival recession) are often both neglected in hygiene procedures and usually not rubbed by the bolus of food. Consequently, these root surfaces also frequently harbor caries-producing plaque. Root surface caries is more common in older patients because of niche availability and other factors sometimes associated with senescence, such as decreased salivary flow and poor oral hygiene due to lowered digital dexterity and decreased motivation. Caries originating on the root is alarming because: (1) it has a comparatively rapid progression,

(2) it is often asymptomatic, (3) it is closer to the pulp, and (4) it is more difficult to restore.

Subgingival areas. The gingival sulcus (or crevice) habitat is unique. The initial occupants of the sulcus are merely an extension of the plaque community on the immediately adjacent surface of the tooth.[97] Metabolites released from plaque easily penetrate the thin epithelial lining of the sulcus, inducing a strong inflammatory reaction. The capillaries dilate and become very permeable, resulting in the leakage of blood plasma into the tissue. Some metabolites have chemotactic properties that induce infiltration of white blood cells into the region. The gingival inflammatory reaction results in the sulcular tissue release of plasma-like fluid-containing immunoglobulins, polymorphonuclear leukocytes, albumins, and hemins. These immunological materials may change some characteristics of the adjacent plaque by removing the most susceptible organisms. New niches then become available because of the loss of some species and the availability of new nutrients. The plaque community changes progressively from masses of cocci in the supragingival plaque to a community dominated by filamentous bacteria and spirochetes in the subgingival habitat.[51] As previously stated, *Bacteroides melaninogenicus* can exploit this habitat, since proteins and

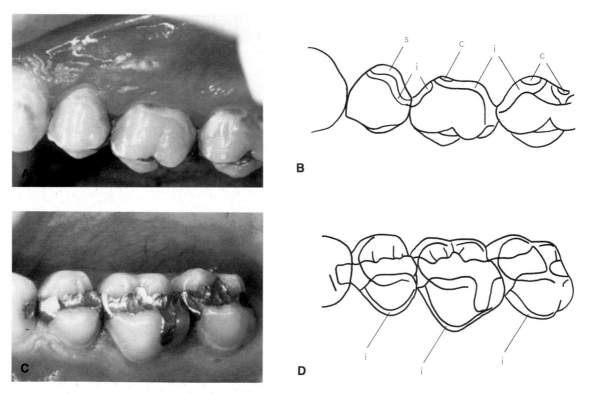

Fig. 3-28. Facial and lingual smooth surface caries. This patient has very high caries activity with rapidly advancing caries lesions. Plaque, containing *mutans streptococci,* extends entirely around the cervical areas of the posterior teeth. Several levels of caries involvement can be seen including: cavitation *(c),* incipient white spot lesions *(i),* and stained, roughened, partially remineralized incipient lesions *(s).*

iron-containing compounds (hemins) are available. The establishment of a sizable population of *B. melaninogenicus* results in a very pathogenic plaque, since this organism produces a number of enzymes capable of destroying the gingival epithelium.

Oral hygiene. Another ecological determinant is oral hygiene. Careful cleaning of the teeth mechanically disrupts the bacterial plaque and leaves a clean enamel surface. The recolonization of the tooth surface occurring after tooth cleaning is properly termed *secondary succession*. This process is much more rapid than primary succession, since all the normal residents of the climax community of plaque are already present in the oral cavity. The cleaning process does not actually destroy most of the oral bacteria but merely removes them from the surfaces of the teeth. Large numbers of these bacteria are subsequently removed from the oral cavity during rinsing and swallowing after flossing and brushing, but sufficient numbers remain to recolonize the teeth. Some fastidious organisms and obligate anaerobes may in fact be killed by exposure to oxygen during tooth cleaning. However, no single species is likely to be entirely eliminated. Although all the species that make up mature plaque will continue to be present, most of these are unable to initiate colonization on the clean tooth surface. To return to the climax community of plaque, the tooth surface must be sequentially colonized, and the local environment must be returned to the climactic condition.

Until the environment of the climax community of plaque is restored, many of its residents are unable to grow. The pioneering organisms can have an important effect on the nature of the climax community. In experimental studies, the initial colonization of artificial fissures has been shown to depend on the relative abundance of organisms in the saliva.[92] *Mutans streptococci* and *S. sanguis* are competitive pioneering organisms. Only when *mutans streptococci* are present in great numbers in the saliva can the organism establish itself as a significant member of the resulting mature plaque. It is of obvious benefit to the host to favor the establishment of large populations of *S. sanguis* on the teeth because *mutans streptococci* are considerably more cariogenic than *S. sanguis*. Simple oral hygiene procedures—flossing and brushing—help to achieve this desired result by frequently disrupting the plaque succession (see oral hygiene procedures in later section, Diagnosis and Prevention). In the absence of a high-sucrose diet, this frequent disruption will favor the preferential growth of *S. sanguis* rather than *mutans streptococci*.

Available nutrients. The nutrients necessary for plaque growth are considered ecological determinants. The nutritional requirements of plaque organisms can vary from simple to complex. All living organisms maintain themselves by two basic antagonistic processes: *catabolic and anabolic reactions*. Catabolic reactions break down complex molecules, such as carbohydrates and proteins, and release useful energy. Anabolic reactions require energy to build complex cellular molecules from simple precursors. The pioneering or initiating organisms that first colonize a tooth surface must, by necessity, have simple nutritional requirements. They must be able to catabolize almost any available energy-containing molecule. Furthermore, since they rely on the host for diet and salivary flow, they must be able to produce anabolically all necessary cellular components from relatively simple precursors. For example, *mutans streptococci* and *S. sanguis* can produce all their amino acid needs from the metabolism of normally available salivary proteins. Organisms with complex nutritional requirements cannot occupy a tooth surface until such specific nutrients become available.

The nature and quality of the nutrient supply vary significantly from habitat to habitat. Supragingival areas on teeth characteristically have high oxygen concentrations, good carbohydrate availability, and are continually bathed in saliva. These areas are characteristically inhabited by facultative streptococci using carbohydrates as their primary energy source. Sucrose in the diet of the host strongly favors the establishment of *mutans streptococci* as a predominant member of the supragingival plaque.[99] The subgingival habitat on the same tooth has low oxygen saturation, low carbohydrate availability, and few salivary components. Both hemorrhage and released sulcular tissue fluid in the subgingival habitat provide a rich variety of proteins and other complex molecules as nutrients. Thus there is a strong selection pressure in the subgingival habitat for anaerobic bacteria that use proteins as their primary energy source. As stated previously, *B. melaninogenicus* is an obligate anaerobe that requires hemins and albumins for its growth and primarily depends on proteins as a source of energy. This particular organism can establish residency in a subgingival plaque only after the plaque has caused both an anaerobic interior environment and gingival bleeding. *B. melaninogenicus* produces strong proteolytic enzymes, including hyaluronidase and collagenase, and is thought to be one of the primary causative agents of periodontal disease. Its presence in plaque is largely controlled by the availability of its special nutritional requirements. Therefore by keeping the plaque at an earlier aerobic successional stage and eliminating periodontal pockets, it is possible to prevent *B. melaninogenicus* from becoming a threat to the periodontium.

Fig. 3-14 illustrates *energy flow* through a hypothetical plaque ecosystem. Four sources of energy are listed. The host's diet frequently supplies the majority of the energy requirements of the plaque community in the form of fermentable carbohydrates. As previously noted, the plaque community can also be entirely supported by the host's saliva. Sulcular fluid and desquamated epithelial cells may play small, but important roles in supporting plaque residents such as *B. melaninogenicus.*[83]

The *energy input* to plaque supports a large number of organisms. The energy trapped in their cell bodies can be considered stored. Because of the inherent unreliability of the host's diet, it is expected that these plaque organisms have mechanisms to store carbohydrates intracellularly or extracellularly. The intracellular storage mechanism is the storage of glycogen-like granules that can be demonstrated by iodine staining. The extracellular storage mechanism is in the form of a variety of polysaccharides. These extracellular polysaccharides also serve other functions for the organism such as adhesion, diffusion limitation, and protection. Other energy-containing materials are trapped within the plaque matrix and make a small addition to the total stored energy.

There are four *energy outputs* from the plaque. First is the energy lost during metabolic processes of contained organisms. The second and largest energy output is in the production of metabolites. These are generally small molecules such as lactic, formic, and acetic acids that provide some residual energy content which the largely anaerobic plaque community is unable to metabolize. The deepest cells in the plaque may be literally starved to death and thus small amounts of large molecules such as enzymes, cell wall components, and toxins are released from the plaque. These act as strong immunogens and can produce potent reactions from the host. The other two losses of energy include viable cells and extracellular polysaccharides that are mechanically dislodged from the plaque.

From a clinical viewpoint the energy output side of the plaque community is of prime importance. *If the plaque community is producing large amounts of organic acids, caries will develop subjacent to the plaque.* If the output is largely toxins, proteolytic enzymes, and other antigenic materials, periodontal disease will result. This output can be controlled by regulating the input side, the habitat, or the successional stage of the plaque community.

Sulcular fluid. In the early stages of gingival inflammation a serous exudate is produced from the sulcular epithelium. This may occur after only 2 to 4 days of gingival tissue exposure to undisturbed plaque. This sulcular fluid contains serum proteins such as immunoglobulins, complement, fibrin, and white blood cells. Immunoglobulins of the IgG class can activate the complement system to produce a number of very destructive enzymes capable of lysing gram-negative bacteria and inducing phagocytosis of gram-positive bacteria. This

system is therefore capable of very effective control of many microorganisms and, consequently, represents a very strong immunological challenge to bacterial invasion of the sulcular epithelium. Actual invasion of the epithelium is only seen in acute ulcerative necrotizing gingivitis. Many organisms reside in the gingival crevice. Over long periods of residence they can produce destruction of periodontal tissues but do not normally produce caries. The effects of the immunological controls exerted by the sulcular fluid are likely to be limited to the immediate area of the gingival crevice. Outside the crevice the immunoglobulins and other immunological defenses are diluted and washed away rapidly by the saliva.

Saliva. Saliva is the primary means by which the host (patient) exerts control over its parasites (oral flora). The normal oral flora is beneficial to the host. It must be recognized that the oral flora and the host have co-evolved to provide a mutually satisfactory relationship. The fact that many normal residents of the oral flora are not found to occur naturally in any other place is strong evidence of this evolution. A parasite that rapidly destroys its host is not likely to have long-term success! However, the host can derive benefits from the parasite if that parasite occupies a niche that would otherwise be available to a more damaging parasite. The apparent result of long-term co-evolution is a system in which the host cultivates a limited and specialized oral flora that, in turn, protects the host from many potential pathogens that pass through the oral cavity. The dependent relationship of the resident oral flora is demonstrated by its ability to subsist entirely on nutrients available in saliva, whereas nonresident organisms are strongly inhibited by the many antimicrobial components of saliva. Many medications are capable of reducing salivary flow and thus increasing caries risk (Table 3-8). This importance of saliva in the maintenance of the normal oral flora is dramatically illustrated by ob-

Table 3-8. Medications that can reduce salivary flow

Medication class	Example
Antispasmodic	Belladonna alkaloids
Antidepressant	Amitriptyline
Antipsychotic	Chlorpromazine
Skeletal muscle relaxant	Cyclobenzaprine
Parkinsonian	Benztropine
Arrhythmia medications	Disopyramide
Antihistamine	Chlorpheniramine
Appetite depressant	Chlorphentermine
Anticonvulsant	Carbamazepine
Anxiolytic	Alprazolam
Antihypertensive	Atenolol
Diuretic	Hydrochlorothiazide
Miscellaneous	Isotretinoin

serving changes in the oral flora following therapeutic radiation to the head and neck. Post radiation, the salivary glands become fibrotic and produce little or no saliva giving the patient an extremely dry mouth, a condition termed *xerostomia*[12,16] (xero—dry, stoma—mouth). Such patients may experience near total destruction of the teeth in just a few months following radiation treatment.

Salivary protective mechanisms[62] that maintain the normal oral flora and maintain tooth surface integrity include: (1) bacterial clearance, (2) direct antibacterial activity, (3) buffers, and (4) remineralization.

Bacterial clearance. Secretions from the various salivary glands pool in the mouth to form whole or mixed saliva (see Fig. 3-17). The amount of saliva secreted varies greatly over time (see Fig. 3-16). Once secreted, saliva remains in the mouth for a short period prior to being swallowed. While in the mouth, saliva lubricates the oral tissues and bathes both the teeth and the plaque. The secretion rate of saliva may have a bearing on caries susceptibility and calculus formation (see Fig. 3-19). Adults produce 1 to 1.5 liters of saliva a day, very little of which occurs during sleep. The *flushing effect* of this salivary flow is, by itself, adequate to remove virtually all microorganisms not adherent to an oral surface (see Figs. 3-17 and 3-18). The flushing is most effective during mastication or oral stimulation, both of which produce large volumes of saliva. Large volumes of saliva also can dilute and buffer plaque acids.

Direct antibacterial activity. Potential pathogens are continually introduced to the oral cavity from food, hands, eating utensils, or virtually anything placed in the mouth. Upon entry into the oral cavity, these organisms must first resist being washed away by the saliva. If they encounter oral surfaces, they usually find them either coated with toxic enzymes or already occupied by other organisms. Even if the new organism can survive the initial defenses and establish some adhesion to a tooth surface, it must then compete with the other oral flora organisms for nutrients. Because the normal resident oral flora is well-adapted to the oral conditions and is extremely competitive, a new organism cannot successfully compete unless it is introduced in very large numbers.

Salivary glands produce an impressive array of *antimicrobial products* (see Table 3-1). For example, lysozyme, lactoperoxidase, lactoferrin and agglutinins possess antibacterial activity. These salivary proteins are not part of the immune system but are part of an overall protection scheme for mucous membranes that occurs in addition to immunological control. These protective proteins are present continuously at relatively uniform levels, have a broad spectrum of activity, and do not possess the "memory" of immunological mechanisms. The normal resident oral flora apparently has developed resistance to most of these antibacterial mechanisms.

While the antibacterial proteins in saliva play an important role in protection of the soft tissues in the oral cavity from infection by pathogens, they have little effect on caries since similar levels of antibacterial proteins can be found in both caries-active and caries-free individuals.[4,63] This suggests that *caries susceptibility in healthy individuals is not related to saliva composition.* However, *individuals with decreased salivary production* (due to illness, medication, or irradiation) *may have significantly higher caries susceptibility* (see Table 3-8).

Buffers. The volume and *buffering capacity* of saliva available to tooth surfaces has a major role in caries protection. The buffering capacity of saliva is primarily determined by the concentration of bicarbonate ion.[13] Buffering capacity can be estimated by titration methods and may be a useful method for assessment of saliva in caries-active patients. The benefit of the buffering is to reduce the potential for acid formations.

In addition to buffers, saliva contains molecules that contribute to plaque pH rise.[43] These include urea and sialin (which is a tetrapeptide that contains lysine and arginine). Hydrolysis of either of these basic compounds results in production of ammonia, causing the pH to rise.[38]

Because saliva is very important in controlling both the oral flora and the mineral content of the teeth, salivary testing should be done on patients with high caries activity (Table 3-9). A portion of the salivary sample also may be used for bacteriologic testing.

Table 3-9. Evaluation of saliva

Secretion rate	Technique
Patient directions: Chew 5 minutes	Supply patient with paraffin wax to chew—time with stopwatch
Empty saliva into funnel	Collect in graduated cylinder
Results	**Observed secretion rate**
Normal	1-2 ml/min
Low	0.1-.9 ml/min
Xerostomia	<0.1 ml/min

Buffering capacity	Technique
Titration	Add 3 ml of 0.005 N HCl to 1 ml saliva—measure resulting pH
Results	**Observed pH**
Normal	5-7
Borderline	4-5
Low	<4

Adapted from: Krassa B: *Caries risk,* Chicago, 1985, Quintessence Publishing.

Remineralization. Saliva and plaque fluid are super-saturated with calcium and phosphate ions.[32] Without a means to control precipitation of these ions, the teeth would become literally encrusted with mineral deposits. Fortunately, saliva contains statherin, a proline-rich peptide that is capable of stabilizing calcium and phosphate ions and thus prevents excessive deposition of these ions on the teeth.[31] Yet, this supersaturated state of the saliva provides constant opportunity for *remineralizing enamel* and thus can help protect the teeth in times of cariogenic challenges.

When the local pH is high (above 5.5) and calcium and phosphate ions are present, the demineralization of the carious process is reversed by remineralization of the damaged tooth structure. This reversal can occur at any stage of the caries lesion. If it occurs before cavitation, the external surface of the tooth may show evidence of the carious episode by the presence of discoloration (usually brownish) resulting from incorporation of exogenous pigmented material. If remineralization occurs after cavitation, the remaining exposed surface becomes harder and often becomes dark brown or black in color. Either surface is termed *arrested caries* and is often more resistant to future cariogenic challenge. If caries becomes arrested on a dentinal surface, it is referred to as *eburnated dentin* (see Figs. 5-14, *C [brown spot]* and 5-19).

Pathophysiology of caries. The primary damaging action of caries is demineralization and dissolution of tooth structure. This results from (1) a highly localized drop in the pH at the plaque-tooth interface and (2) tooth demineralization. The local pH drop occurs as the result of plaque metabolism (see Fig. 3-15); but only plaque communities with high concentrations of *mutans streptococci* and *Lactobacillus* can produce a sufficiently low pH to cause demineralization of teeth. A single exposure of sucrose solution to a cariogenic plaque results in rapid metabolism of the nutrients to organic acids. The organic acids (primarily lactic acid) dissociate to lower the local pH (see Fig. 3-15). Single events of lowered pH are not sufficient to produce significant changes in the mineral content of the surfaces of the teeth. However, many episodes of long-duration demineralization (lowered pH), occurring over long periods of time, will produce the characteristic lesions of caries. *Frequent sucrose exposure is the single most important factor in maintenance of pH depression at the tooth surface.*

The output (production) of acid from caries-active plaques is twice that of caries-inactive plaques per milligram wet weight of plaque.[68] The production of acid from a caries-active plaque can overcome the buffering capacity of salivary bicarbonate available at the tooth plaque interface, causing the local pH to fall. Once the pH falls below 5.5, tooth mineral is dissolved. In car-ies-active individuals, the pH at the tooth surface remains below the critical pH (5.5) for 20 to 50 minutes following a single exposure to sucrose. Thus it should be noted that sweet snacks between meals can result in almost continuous acid attack on the tooth surface.

Below the critical pH (5.5), the tooth mineral acts like a buffer and loses calcium and phosphate ions into the plaque. This tooth buffering capacity maintains the local pH at approximately 5.0, which is responsible for the characteristic histological form of carious lesions described in the subsequent section. At lower pH values, such as 3.0 or 4.0, the surface of enamel is etched and roughened. At 5.0 pH, the surface remains intact while the subsurface mineral is lost. *This initial carious lesion limited to the enamel is* **incipient caries** *and is characterized by a virtually intact surface, but a porous subsurface.* The intact surface and subsurface porosity are responsible for the clinical characteristics of incipient lesions: smooth intact surfaces that become chalky white opacities when dried. When the porous body of an incipient lesion is hydrated, the lesion is not detectable clinically because the porous area remains translucent. But desiccation (drying) of the tooth with a stream of compressed air removes the subsurface water, leaving air-filled voids which render the area opaque and white. Incipient lesions may be reversed by remineralization, restoring the enamel to a sound state. When fluoride ion is part of the remineralization process, the enamel will not only be restored to soundness but also increase its resistance to further caries attacks.

The intact surface over incipient lesions is critical to the process of potential remineralization because it protects the etched hydroxyapatite crystals in the enamel from being coated by salivary proteins. The etched crystal lattice remains open and can readily precipitate more hydroxyapatite when the local environmental conditions change and calcium and phosphate ions are provided to the area from saliva. Cavitation of the surface occurs when the subsurface demineralization is so extensive that the tooth structure surface collapses. *Cavitation of enamel is not reversible and is usually associated with an acceleration in the process of carious destruction of the tooth.* It occurs when a series of demineralization (pH drop) and remineralization (salivary ions) episodes are dominated by the demineralization process.

CLINICAL CHARACTERISTICS OF THE LESION

Recall that a plaque community of sufficient mass (thickness) to become anaerobic at the tooth surface has the potential to be cariogenic. A large population of *mutans streptococci* virtually assures this occurrence. A sucrose-rich diet gives a selective advantage to *mutans streptococci* and allows the organism to accumulate in large numbers in the plaque community. The sucrose-rich environment also allows *mutans streptococci* to produce large quantities of *extracellular polysaccharides* (dextrans and insoluble mutans). These form a gelatinous material that produces a **diffusion-limiting barrier** in the plaque. The combination of limited diffusion and tremendous metabolic activity makes the local environment anaerobic and very acidic and, thus, an ideal environment for dissolution of the subjacent tooth surface.

Once the tooth surface becomes cavitated, a more retentive surface area is available to the plaque community. This allows filamentous bacteria that have poor adhesion abilities, such as *Lactobacillus,* to become established in the lesion. In the absence of change in the host's diet and oral hygiene practices, the cavitation of the tooth surface produces a synergistic acceleration of the growth of the cariogenic plaque community and expansion of the cavitation. This results in a rapid and progressive destruction of tooth structure. Once enamel caries penetrates to the dentinoenamel junction (DEJ), rapid lateral expansion of the carious lesion takes place, since dentin is much less resistant to caries attack. This internal sheltered, highly acidic, and anaerobic environment provides an ideal niche for *Lactobacillus* species. This organism was previously thought to be the primary etiological agent of caries, but it has no ability to adhere to the tooth surface and therefore is unlikely to be a factor in the initiation of caries. *Mutans streptococci are probably the most important organisms in the initiation of enamel caries, and A. viscosus is the most likely organism to initiate root caries.*[82] After caries initiation, *Lactobacillus* organisms then become important residents of the carious lesion, once their niche is available. Because of their acidogenic potential and aciduric lifestyle, *Lactobacillus species are probably very important in the progression of dentinal caries.*

Clinical sites for caries initiation

The characteristics of a carious lesion vary with the nature of the surface on which the lesion develops. There are three distinctly different clinical sites for caries initiation, as follows (see Fig. 3-20, *A to C):*

1. The first and most susceptible site is in the recesses of **developmental pits and fissures** of enamel.
2. The second site is on certain areas of the **smooth enamel surfaces** where contour or tooth position protects (shelters) plaque against the rubbing action of some foods and often from being loosened by the toothbrush. These include the areas of the *contacting proximal surfaces* which are gingival of the contact and thereby highly susceptible to caries because of shelter afforded to plaque. (Only proper daily application of dental floss [or

dental tape] to such surfaces can disrupt the plaque's successional change.) Plaque on *noncontacting proximal surfaces* may also be sheltered due to tooth surface contour or position (e.g., the distal surface of the most posterior tooth). Other susceptible smooth enamel surfaces are those *areas gingival to the height of contour of the facial and lingual surfaces* where, again, the plaque is sheltered from the rubbing of food and often, as well, from the toothbrush due to improper brushing technique (see later section, Oral Hygiene, for discussion of flossing and brushing).
3. The third site where caries may attack is the **root surface.**

Each of these areas has distinct surface topography and environmental conditions. Consequently, each area has a distinct plaque population. The diagnosis, treatment, and prevention of these different lesion types should take into account the different etiological factors operating at each site.

Pits and fissures. The pits and fissures of newly erupted teeth are rapidly colonized by bacteria. These early colonizers form a "bacterial plug" that remains in the site for a long time, perhaps even the life of the tooth. The type and nature of the organisms prevalent in the oral cavity determine the type of organisms colonizing the pits and fissures and therefore are instrumental in determining the outcome of the colonization. There are large variations in the microflora found in pits and fissures, suggesting that each site can be considered a separate ecological system. Large numbers of gram-positive cocci, especially *S. sanguis,* are found in the pits and fissures of newly erupted teeth, while large numbers of *mutans streptococci* are usually found in carious pits and fissures.

The shape of the pits and fissures contributes to their high susceptibility to caries. The long narrow orifice prevents examination visually and tactilely (see Fig. 3-21). There is considerable morphological variation in these structures. Some pits and fissures end blindly, others open near the dentin, and others penetrate entirely through the enamel.

Pit and fissure caries expands as it penetrates into the enamel. Thus the entry site may appear much smaller than the actual lesion, making clinical diagnosis difficult. Carious lesions of pits and fissures develop from attack on their walls (see Fig. 3-22, *A to C).* The progress of dissolution of the walls of a pit or fissure lesion is similar in principle to that of the smooth surface lesion, as there is a wide area of surface attack extending inward, paralleling the enamel rods. The occlusal enamel rods bend down and terminate on the dentin immediately below the developmental enamel fault. Thus a lesion originating in a pit or fissure affects a greater area of the DEJ than does a comparable smooth

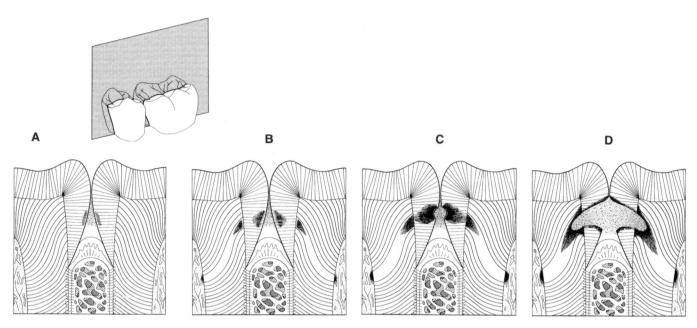

Fig. 3-29. Longitudinal sections (see *inset* in **A**) showing initiation and progression of caries on interproximal surfaces. **A,** Initial demineralization (indicated by the shading in the enamel) on the proximal surfaces is not detectable clinically or radiographically. All proximal surfaces are demineralized to some degree, but most are remineralized and become immune to further attack. The presence of small amounts of fluoride in the saliva virtually ensures that remineralization and immunity to further attack will occur. **B,** When proximal caries first becomes detectable radiographically, the enamel surface is likely to still be intact. An intact surface is essential for successful remineralization and arrest of the lesion. Demineralization of the dentin (indicated by the shading in the dentin) occurs prior to cavitation of the surface of the enamel. Treatment designed to promote remineralization can be effective up to this stage. **C,** Cavitation of the enamel surface is a critical event in the caries process in proximal surfaces. Cavitation is an irreversible process and requires restorative treatment/correction of the damaged tooth surface. Cavitation can only be diagnosed by clinical observation. The use of a sharp explorer to detect cavitation is problematic because excessive force in application of the explorer tip during inspection of the proximal surfaces can damage weakened enamel and accelerate the caries process by creating cavitation. Separation of the teeth can be used to provide more direct visual inspection of suspect surfaces. Fiber optic illumination and dye absorption are also promising new evaluation procedures, but neither is specific for cavitation. **D,** Advanced cavitated lesions require prompt restorative intervention to prevent pulpal disease, limit tooth structure loss, and remove the nidus of infection of odontopathic organisms.

surface lesion. *In cross section, the gross appearance of a pit and fissure lesion is of an inverted V with a narrow entrance and a progressively wider area of involvement closer to the DEJ* (see Fig. 3-22, *D*).

Smooth enamel surfaces. The smooth enamel surfaces of the teeth present a less favorable site for plaque attachment. Plaque usually develops only on those smooth surfaces that are near the gingiva or are under proximal contacts. The proximal surfaces are particularly susceptible to caries because of the extra shelter provided to resident plaque due to the proximal contact area immediately occlusal to the plaque. Lesions starting on smooth enamel surfaces have a broad area of origin and a conical, or pointed, extension toward the DEJ. The path of ingress of the lesion is roughly parallel to the long axes of the enamel rods in the region. *A cross section of the enamel portion of a smooth surface*

lesion shows a V shape with a wide area of origin and the apex of the V directed toward the DEJ. After caries penetrates the dentinoenamel junction, softening of the dentin spreads rapidly laterally and pulpally (see Fig. 3-29).

Root surface. The root surface is rougher than enamel and readily allows plaque formation in the absence of good oral hygiene. The cementum covering the root surface is extremely thin and provides little resistance to caries attack. *Root caries lesions have less well-defined margins, tend to be U-shaped in cross section, and progress more rapidly due to the lack of protection from an enamel covering.* In recent years there has been a notable increase in the prevalence of root caries, probably due to the increasing number of older persons who experience gingival recession and usually have cariogenic plaque on the exposed root surfaces.

Progression of carious lesions

The progression and morphology of the carious lesion is variable depending on the site of origin and the conditions in the mouth (see Figs. 3-20, 3-22, and 3-29). The time for progression from incipient caries to clinical caries (cavitation) on smooth surfaces is estimated to be 18 months, plus or minus 6 months.[77] Peak rates for the incidence of new lesions occurs 3 years after the eruption of the tooth. Occlusal pit and fissure lesions develop in less time than smooth surface caries. Both poor oral hygiene and frequent exposures to sucrose-containing food can produce incipient (white spot) lesions (first clinical evidence of demineralization) in as little as 3 weeks. Radiation-induced xerostomia (dry mouth) can lead to clinical caries development in as little as 3 months from the onset of the radiation. Thus caries development in healthy individuals is usually slow in comparison to the rate possible in compromised persons.

HISTOPATHOLOGY OF CARIES
Enamel caries

Histology of enamel. Enamel is composed of very tightly packed hydroxyapatite *crystallites,* organized into long columnar *rods (prisms).* The rods are somewhat key-shaped in cross section as described in Chapter 2. Individual enamel rods are formed by the activity of *ameloblasts.* Each rod starts at the DEJ and extends as a wavy, continuous column to the surface of the crown. The mineralization process is apparently somewhat discontinuous and is characterized by alternating phases of high and low activity. Periods of low activity create "rest" lines within the rods. These rest lines, in combination with similar lines in neighboring rods, form a structure visible in mounted cross sections of enamel and are named the **striae of Retzius.** The striae are regions characterized by relatively higher organic content (see Fig. 3-6, *B).* Both the striae and the inherent spaces in prism boundaries provide sufficient porosity to allow movement of water and small ions, such as hydrogen ions. Thus enamel is capable of acting as a molecular sieve by allowing free movement of small molecules and blocking the passage of larger molecules and ions. *The sieve-like behavior of enamel also explains why even incipient caries of enamel can produce a pulpal response prior to penetration of bacteria.* The movement of ions through carious enamel can result in acid dissolution of the underlying dentin before actual cavitation of the enamel surface. This acid attack at the external ends of the dentinal tubules initiates a pulpal response by unknown mechanisms. Since the striae form horizontal lines of greater permeability in the enamel, they probably contribute to the lateral spread of smooth surface lesions. The decreased mineral content of the striae in incipient lesions is illustrated in Figs. 3-30 and 3-31. Indeed the striae appear to be accentuated in early lesions. In the occlusal enamel, the striae of Retzius and the enamel rod directions are mutually perpendicular. On the axial surfaces of the crown, the striae course diagonally and terminate on the surface as slight depressions. The surface manifestations of the

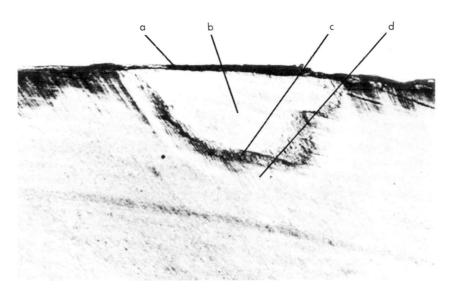

Fig. 3-30. Cross section of small carious lesion in enamel examined in quinoline by transmitted light. Surface *(a)* appears to be intact. Body of lesion *(b)* shows enhancement of striae of Retzius. Dark zone *(c)* surrounds body of lesion while translucent zone *(d)* is evident over entire advancing front of lesion ($\times$ 100). (From Silverston LM. In Silverston LM et al, editors: *Dental caries,* London and Basingstoke, 1981, Macmillan, Ltd.)

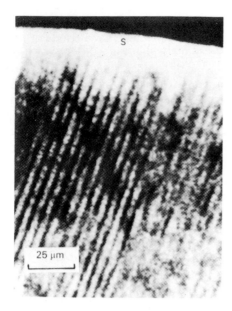

Fig. 3-31. Microradiograph of cross section of small carious lesion in enamel. Well-mineralized surface *(s)* is evident. Alternating radiolucent and radiopaque lines indicate demineralization between enamel rods (× 150). (From Silverston LM. In Silverston LM et al, editors: Dental caries, London and Basingstoke, 1981, Macmillan, Ltd.)

striae are the ***imbrication lines of Pickerel*** that lie between the ***perikymata ridges*** (see Fig. 3-7). Caries preferentially attacks the cores of the rods and the more permeable striae of Retzius, which promotes lateral spreading and undermining of the adjacent enamel.

Clinical characteristics of enamel caries; the incipient smooth surface lesion. Caries-prone patients usually have extensive deposits of plaque on the teeth which must be removed prior to clinical examination. On clean, dry teeth, the earliest evidence of caries on the smooth enamel surface of a crown is a *white spot* (see Figs. 3-1, 3-2, 3-28, and 5-5, *D).* These lesions are usually observed on the facial and lingual surfaces of the teeth. White spots are chalky white, opaque areas that are revealed only when the tooth surface is desiccated (dried), and are termed ***incipient caries.*** These areas of enamel lose their translucency because of the extensive subsurface porosity caused by demineralization. *Care must be exercised to distinguish white spots of in-cipient caries from developmental white spot hypocalcifications of enamel (see Fig. 5-10). Incipient caries will partially or totally disappear visually when the enamel is hydrated (wet), while hypocalcified enamel is unaffected by drying and wetting* (Table 3-10). Hypocalcified enamel does not represent a clinical problem except when its appearance is objectionable esthetically. The surface texture of an incipient lesion is unaltered and is undetectable by tactile examination with an explorer. A more advanced lesion develops a rough surface that is softer than the unaffected, normal enamel. Softened chalky enamel that can be chipped away with an explorer is a sign of active caries. Similar incipient lesions occur on the proximal smooth surfaces but usually are undetectable by visual or tactile (explorer) examination. Incipient lesions sometimes can be seen on radiographs as a faint radiolucency, limited to the superficial enamel. When a proximal lesion is clearly visible radiographically, the lesion has advanced significantly and histological alteration of the underlying dentin has already occurred (see Fig. 3-40).

It has been shown experimentally and clinically that *incipient caries of enamel can remineralize.*[5,86] Tables 3-10 and 3-11 list the characteristics of enamel at various stages of demineralization. Noncavitated enamel lesions retain most of the original crystalline framework of the enamel rods and the etched crystallites serve as nucleating agents for remineralization. Calcium and phosphate ions from saliva can then penetrate the enamel surface and precipitate on the highly reactive crystalline surfaces in the enamel lesion. The supersaturation of the saliva with calcium and phosphate ion serves as the driving force for the remineralization process. Both artificial and natural carious lesions of human enamel have been shown to regress to earlier histological stages after exposure to conditions that promote remineralization. Furthermore, the presence of trace amounts of fluoride ions during this remineralization process greatly enhances the precipitation of calcium and phosphate, resulting in the remineralized enamel becoming more resistant to subsequent caries attack due to the incorporation of more acid-resistant fluorapatite (see Fig. 3-43). ***Arrested (remineralized) lesions*** can be observed clinically as intact, but discolored, usually brown or black spots (see Fig. 5-14, *C).* The change in

Table 3-10. Clinical characteristics of normal and altered enamel

	Hydrated	Desiccated	Surface texture	Surface hardness
Normal enamel	Translucent	Translucent	Smooth	Hard
Hypo-calcified enamel	Opaque	Opaque	Smooth	Hard
Incipient caries	Translucent	Opaque	Smooth	Softened
Active caries	Opaque	Opaque	Cavitated	Very soft
Arrested caries	Opaque, dark	Opaque, dark	Roughened	Hard

Table 3-11. Clinical significance of enamel lesions

	Plaque	Enamel structure	Anti-microbial treatment	Restorative treatment
Normal enamel	Normal	Normal	Not indicated	Not indicated
Hypo-calcified enamel	Normal	Abnormal, but not weakened	Not indicated	Only for esthetics
Incipient caries	Pathogenic	Porous, weakened	Yes	Not indicated
Active caries	Pathogenic	Cavitated, very weak	Yes	Yes
Arrested caries	Normal	Remineralized, strong	Not indicated	Only for esthetics

color is presumably due to trapped organic debris and metallic ions within the enamel. *These discolored, remineralized, arrested caries areas are intact and are more resistant to subsequent caries attack than the adjacent unaffected enamel. They should not be restored unless they are esthetically objectionable.*

Zones of incipient lesion. Considerable research has been applied to producing carious lesions in simplified systems.[85,86] The first attempts to produce artificial lesions used strong organic acids. These failed because the strong acids aggressively attacked the surface of enamel producing a damaged surface similar to that produced by the acid etch technique now used for tooth-colored restorations. However, when acidified gels were used over a very long exposure time (10 to 12 weeks), artificial carious lesions could be produced that were histologically identical to natural, incipient lesions. The success of this technique illustrates the importance of the diffusion-limiting nature of plaque described earlier (see Clinical Characteristics of the Lesion). The ability to artificially produce natural enamel lesions has resulted in an identification of a detailed description of the *early stages of caries in enamel*. Figs. 3-30 and 3-32 il-

lustrate the *four regularly observed zones in a sectioned incipient lesion: (1) the translucent zone, (2) the dark zone, (3) the body of the lesion, and (4) the surface zone.*

Zone 1, the translucent zone. The deepest zone is the translucent zone (see Fig. 3-32, *C*) and represents the advancing front of the enamel lesion. The name refers to its structureless appearance when perfused with quinoline solution and examined with polarized light. In this zone the pores or voids form along the enamel prism (rod) boundaries presumably because of the ease of hydrogen ion penetration during the carious process. When these boundary area voids are filled with quinoline solution, which has the same refractive index as enamel, the features of the area disappear. The pore volume of the translucent zone of enamel caries is 1%, 10 times greater than normal enamel.

Zone 2, the dark zone. The next deepest zone is known as the dark zone because it does not transmit polarized light. This light blockage is caused by the presence of many tiny pores too small to absorb quinoline. These smaller air- or vapor-filled pores make the region opaque. The total pore volume is 2% to 4%. There is

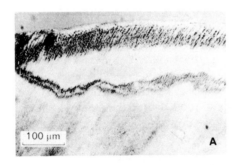
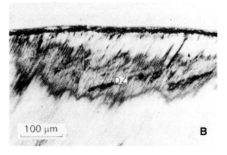
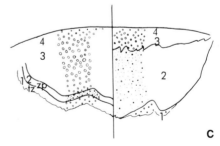

Fig. 3-32. A, Cross section of small carious lesion in enamel examined in quinoline with polarized light. Advancing front of lesion appears as dark band below body of lesion (× 100). **B,** Same section after exposure to artificial calcifying solution examined in quinoline and polarized light. Dark zone *(DZ)* covers much greater area after remineralization has occurred (× 100). **C,** Schematic diagram of Figs. 3-32, *A* and *B*. Left side indicates small extent of zones 1 and 2 before remineralization. Small circles indicate relative sizes of pores in each zone. Right side indicates increase in zone 2, the dark zone, following remineralization. This micropore system must have been created where previously the pores were much larger. (From Silverston LM. In Silverston LM et al, editors: *Dental caries,* London and Basingstoke, 1981, Macmillan, Ltd.)

some speculation that the dark zone is not really a stage in the sequence of the breakdown of enamel; rather the dark zone may be formed by deposition of ions into an area previously only containing large pores. *It must be remembered that caries is an episodic disease with alternating phases of demineralization and remineralization.* Experimental remineralization has demonstrated increases in the size of the dark zone at the expense of the body of the lesion (see Fig. 3-32, *C).* There is also a loss of crystalline structure in the dark zone, suggestive of the process of demineralization and remineralization. The size of the dark zone is probably an indication of the amount of remineralization that has recently occurred.

Zone 3, the body of the lesion. The body of the lesion is the largest portion of the incipient lesion while in a demineralizing phase. It has the largest pore volume, varying from 5% at the periphery to 25% at the center. The striae of Retzius are well marked in the body of the lesion, indicating preferential mineral dissolution along these areas of relatively higher porosity. The first penetration of caries enters the enamel surface via the striae of Retzius. The interprismatic areas and these cross-striations provide access to the rod (prism) cores, which are then preferentially attacked. Bacteria may be present in this zone if the pore size is large enough to permit their entry. Studies using transmission electron microscopy (TEM) and scanning electron microscopy (SEM) demonstrate the presence of bacteria invading between the enamel rods (prisms) in the body zone.[10,20]

Zone 4, the surface zone. The surface zone is relatively unaffected by the caries attack. It has a lower pore volume than the body of the lesion (less than 5%) and a radiopacity comparable to unaffected adjacent enamel (see Fig. 3-31). The surface of normal enamel is hypermineralized by contact with saliva and has a greater concentration of fluoride ion than the immediately subjacent enamel. It has been hypothesized that hypermineralization and increased fluoride content of the superficial enamel are responsible for the relative immunity of the enamel surface. However, removal of the hypermineralized surface by polishing fails to prevent the reformation of a typical, well-mineralized surface over the carious lesion. Thus the intact surface over incipient caries is a phenomenon of the caries demineralization process rather than any special characteristics of the superficial enamel. Nevertheless, the importance of the intact surface can not be over-emphasized, because it serves as a barrier to bacterial invasion. As the enamel lesion progresses, conical-shaped defects in the surface zone can be seen by SEM. These are probably the first sites where bacteria can gain entry into a carious lesion. Arresting the caries process at this stage results in a hard surface that may at times be rough, though cleanable (see Fig. 5-19, *C).*

Dentinal caries

Histology of dentin. Dentin is the hard portion of the tooth that is covered by enamel on the crown and cementum on the root. Dentin is the calcified product of the odontoblasts which line the inner surface of the dentin within the periphery of the external pulp tissue. Each odontoblast has an extension (termed **Tomes' fiber** in older texts) into a dentinal tubule. The tubules transverse the entire thickness of dentin from the pulp to the dentinoenamel junction (Fig. 3-33, *A).* Filling the space between the tubules is the **intertubular dentin,** a rigid bone-like material composed of hydroxyapatite crystals embedded in a network of collagen fibers. The walls of the tubules are lined with a smooth layer of mineral termed **peritubular dentin.** A thin membrane is always observed lining the tubule in normal dentin. There remains controversy concerning the nature of this lining membrane: it may be a true plasma membrane of the odontoblast or simply a limiting membrane similar to that found on the surface of bone.[102] The material within the membrane is odontoblastic cytoplasm if the membrane is part of the odontoblast, or a plasma-like exudate if the membrane is not a part of the odontoblast. In either case, the tubule allows fluid movement and ion transport necessary for remineralization of intertubular dentin, apposition of peritubular dentin, and/or perception of pain.

The dentin and the pulp are morphologically and embryologically a single unit. Teeth are formed early during development of the mandible and maxilla. A sheet of epithelial tissue grows inward and condenses with the underlying mesenchymal tissue in the developing jaws. This condensed ball of cells, called the dental papilla, differentiates to form dentin- and enamel-forming tissues. The surrounding epithelial cells form the enamel organ by differentiating into ameloblasts. On the inside of the bell-shaped tooth bud, the mesenchymal cells immediately adjacent to the developing ameloblasts transform into odontoblasts. The two tissues, dentin and enamel, grow away from their original junction zone to form the structure of the tooth. The *DEJ (dentinoenamel junction)* is the remnant of the bell stage of the tooth bud. The odontoblasts lay down dentin and move toward the center of the tooth, while the ameloblasts lay down enamel and move outward, away from the tooth bud center. In the process of dentinogenesis (formation of dentin), the odontoblasts' cell bodies are pushed further and further inward. As they move inward, they leave a tubule behind. Thus each odontoblast is a pulp cell that is associated with a tubule extending to the external periphery of the dentin. Because of the intimate relationship between the odontoblasts and the dentin, *the pulp and the dentin should be regarded as a single functional unit.* More detail of the histology of dentin is presented in Chapter 2.

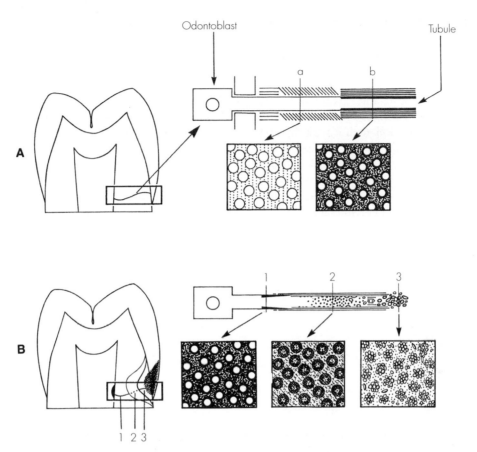

Fig. 3-33. Normal and carious dentin. Normal dentin (**A**) has characteristic tubules that follow a wavy path from the external surface of the dentin, below the enamel or cementum, to the inner surface of the dentin in the pulp tissue of the pulp chamber or pulp canal. Dentin is formed from the external surface and grows inward (see text). As the dentin grows, the odontoblasts become increasingly compressed in the shrinking pulp chamber and the number of associated tubules becomes more concentrated per unit area. The more recently formed dentin near the pulp *(a)* has both large tubules with little or no peritubular dentin and calcified intertubular dentin filled with collagen fibers. The older dentin, closer to the external surface *(b),* is characterized by smaller, more widely separated tubules and a greater mineral content in the intertubular dentin. The older dentin tubules are lined by a uniform layer of mineral termed peritubular dentin. These changes occur gradually from the inner surface to the external surface of the dentin. Horizontal lines indicate predentin; diagonal lines indicate increasing density of minerals; darker horizontal lines indicate densely mineralized dentin and increased thickness of peritubular dentin. The transition in mineral content is gradual as indicated in Fig. 3-32. Carious dentin (**B**) undergoes a number of changes. The most superficial **infected** zone of **carious dentin** *(3)* is characterized by bacteria filling the tubules, and granular material in the intertubular space. The granular material contains very little mineral and lacks characteristic cross-banding of collagen. Pulpal of (below) the infected dentin is a zone where the dentin appears transparent in mounted whole specimens. This zone *(2)* is **affected** (not infected) **carious dentin** and is characterized by loss of mineral in the intertubular and peritubular dentin. Many crystals can be detected in the lumen of the tubules in this zone. The crystals in the tubule lumen render the refractive index of the lumen similar to that of the intertubular dentin, making the zone transparent. Normal dentin *(1)* is found pulpal of (below) the transparent dentin.

Clinical and histological characteristics of dentinal caries; acid levels; reparative responses. Progression of caries in dentin is different from progression in the overlying enamel because of the structural differences of dentin (Figs. 3-33 to 3-36). There is much less mineral in dentin and it possesses microscopic tubules that provide a freeway for the ingress of acids and egress of mineral. The dentinoenamel junction has the least resistance to caries attack and allows rapid lateral spreading once caries has penetrated the enamel (see Figs. 3-22 and 3-29). Because of these characteristics, *dentinal caries* is V-shaped in cross section with a wide base at the DEJ, and the apex directed pulpally. *Caries advances more rapidly in dentin than in enamel because dentin provides much less resistance to acid attack.* Caries produces a variety of responses in dentin, including pain, demineralization, and remineralization.

Often, pain is not reported even when caries invades dentin, except when deep lesions bring the bacterial infection close to the pulp. Episodes of short duration pain may be felt occasionally during earlier stages of dentin caries. These pains are due to stimulation of pulp tissue by movement of fluid through dentinal tubules that have been opened to the oral environment by cavitation. Once bacterial invasion of the dentin is close to the pulp, toxins and possibly even a few bacteria enter the pulp, resulting in inflammation of the pulpal tissues. Initial pulpal inflammation is thought to be evident clinically by production of sharp pains, with each pain lingering only a few seconds (10 or less) in response to a thermal stimulus. A short, painful response to cold suggests *reversible pulpitis* or pulpal *hyperemia.* Reversible pulpitis, as the name implies, is a limited inflammation of the pulp from which the tooth can recover if the caries producing the irritation is eliminated by timely operative treatment. When the pulp becomes more severely inflamed, a thermal stimulus will produce pain that continues after termination of the stimulus,

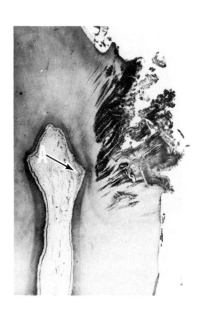

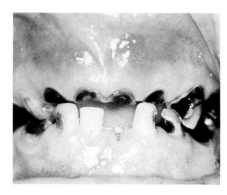

Fig. 3-34. Cross section of demineralized specimen of advanced caries in dentin. Reparative dentin *(A)* can be seen adjacent to most advanced portion of lesion. (From Boyle P: Kornfeld's histopathology of the teeth and their surrounding structures, Philadelphia, 1955, Lea & Febiger.

Fig. 3-35. Rampant caries in 10-year-old boy.

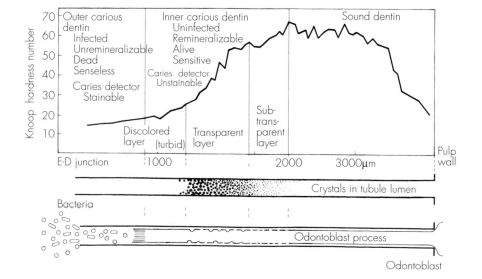

Fig. 3-36. Schematic illustration of the relationship of dentin hardness, crystal deposition, and condition of the odontoblastic process. According to Fusayama and coworkers, the odontoblastic process extends into the turbid layer but disappears prior to the advancing front of the bacterial invasion. Crystals are deposited in the lumen in the transparent layer and the subtransparent layer. The area of crystal deposition corresponds to the area of damage to the odontoblast process membrane. For orientation of layers on tooth, see Fig. 3-37. (Courtesy Dr. T. Fusayama. Copyright Ishiyaku EuroAmerica, Inc. Tokyo, 1993.)

typically longer than 10 seconds. This clinical pattern suggests *irreversible pulpitis,* when the pulp is unlikely to recover after removing the caries. Pulp extirpation and root canal filling usually are necessary in addition to the restorative treatment in order to save the tooth. Throbbing, continuous pain suggests partial or total pulp necrosis that is treated only by root canal therapy or extraction. While these clinical characteristics are useful as guidelines for pulp treatment, it is emphasized that pulp symptoms can vary widely and are not always predictive of the histologic status of the tooth pulp. (See Chapter 5 for more details regarding pulpal diagnosis.)

The pulp-dentin complex reacts to caries attacks by attempting to initiate remineralization and blocking off the open tubules. These reactions result from odontoblastic activity as well as the physical process of demineralization and remineralization. Three *levels of dentinal reaction to caries* can be recognized: (1) reaction to a long-term, low-level acid demineralization associated with a slowly advancing lesion; (2) reaction to a moderate-intensity attack; and (3) reaction to severe, rapidly advancing caries characterized by very high acid levels. The dentin can react defensively (by repair) to low- and moderate-intensity caries attack as long as the pulp remains vital and has an adequate blood circulation.

In slowly advancing caries, a vital pulp can repair demineralized dentin by remineralization of the intertubular dentin and by apposition of peritubular dentin. Early stages of caries or mild caries attacks produce long-term, low-level acid demineralization of dentin. Direct exposure of the pulp tissue to microorganisms is not a prerequisite for an inflammatory response. Toxins and other metabolic by-products, especially hydrogen ion, can penetrate via the dentinal tubules to the pulp. Even when the lesion is limited to the enamel,[6,10] the pulp can be shown to respond with inflammatory cells. Dentin responds to the stimulus of its first caries demineralization episode by deposition of crystalline material in both the lumen of the tubules and the intertubular dentin of affected dentin in front of the advancing infected dentin portion of the lesion (see Fig. 3-33, *B*). Hypermineralized areas may be seen on radiographs as zones of increased radiopacity (often S-shaped following the course of the tubules) ahead of the advancing, infected portion of the lesion. This repair only occurs if the tooth pulp is vital.[95] Dentin that has more mineral content than normal dentin is termed *sclerotic dentin.* Sclerotic dentin formation occurs ahead of the demineralization front of a slowly advancing lesion and may be seen under an old restoration. Sclerotic dentin is usually shiny and darkly colored, but feels hard to the explorer tip. By comparison, normal freshly cut dentin lacks a shiny, reflective surface and allows some penetration from a sharp explorer tip. The apparent function of sclerotic dentin is to wall off a lesion by blocking (sealing) the tubules. The permeability of sclerotic dentin is greatly reduced in comparison to normal dentin because of the decrease in the tubule lumen diameter.[78]

There is also crystalline precipitate in the lumen of the dentinal tubules in the advancing front of a demineralization zone (affected dentin). Once these affected tubules become completely occluded by the mineral precipitate, they appear clear when a section of the tooth is evaluated. This portion of dentin has been termed the *transparent zone of dentin* (see next section, Zones of Dentinal Caries) and, again, is the result of both mineral loss in the intertubular dentin and precipitation of this mineral in the tubule lumen. Consequently, translucent dentin is softer than normal dentin (Fig. 3-37).[73]

The second level of dentinal response is to moderate-intensity (or intermediate) irritants. More intense caries activity results in bacterial invasion of the dentin. The infected dentin contains a wide variety of pathogenic materials or irritants, including high acid levels, hydrolytic enzymes, bacteria, and bacterial cellular debris. These materials can cause the degeneration and death of the odontoblasts and their tubular extensions below the lesion, as well as a mild inflammation of the pulp. Groups of these dead, empty tubules are termed *dead tracts.* The pulp may be irritated sufficiently from high acid levels or bacterial enzyme production to cause the formation (from undifferentiated mesenchymal cells) of replacement odontoblasts (secondary odontoblasts). These cells produce *reparative dentin (reactionary dentin)* on the affected portion of the pulp chamber wall (see Fig. 3-33, *B* and 3-37). This dentin is different from the normal dentinal apposition that occurs throughout the life of the tooth by primary (original) odontoblasts. The structure of reparative dentin can vary from well-organized tubular dentin (less often) to very

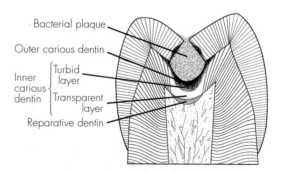

Fig. 3-37. Cross section of occlusal caries. The occlusal enamel appears intact, with a small opening in the occlusal fissure. The enamel is darkened where it is undermined by demineralization. The surface of the enamel is unaffected. The cavity is filled with a bacterial plug containing high numbers of *mutans streptococci* and *lactobacilli.* The dentin is infected below the plug. The deeper dentin is not infected but is extensively demineralized. Reparative dentin is being formed below the lesion.

irregular atubular dentin (more often), depending on the severity of the stimulus. Reparative dentin is a very effective barrier to diffusion of material through the tubules and is an important step in the repair of dentin. Severe stimuli can also result in the formation within the pulp chamber of unattached dentin, termed *pulp stones,* in addition to reparative dentin.

The success of dentinal reparative responses, either by remineralization of intertubular dentin and apposition of peritubular dentin or by reparative dentin, depends on the severity of the caries attack and the ability of the pulp to respond. The pulpal blood supply may be the most important limiting factor to the pulpal responses.

The third level of dentinal response is to severe irritation. Acute, rapidly advancing caries with very high levels of acid production overpowers dentinal defenses and results in infection, abscess, and death of the pulp. In comparison to other oral tissues, the pulp is poorly tolerant of inflammation. Small, localized infections in the pulp produce an inflammatory response involving capillary dilation, local edema, and stagnation of blood flow. Since the pulp is contained in a sealed chamber and its blood is supplied through very narrow root canals, any stagnation of blood flow can result in local anoxia and necrosis. The local necrosis leads to more inflammation, edema, and stagnation of blood flow in the immediately adjacent pulp tissue, which then becomes necrotic in a cascading process that rapidly spreads to involve the entire pulp.[88]

Maintenance of pulp vitality is dependent on the adequacy of pulpal blood supply. Recently erupted teeth with large pulp chambers and short, wide canals, with large apical foramina have a much more favorable prognosis for surviving pulpal inflammation than fully formed teeth with small pulp chambers and small apical foramina.

Zones of dentinal caries. Caries advance in dentin proceeds through three changes[22]: (1) weak organic acids demineralize the dentin; (2) the organic material of the dentin, particularly collagen, is degenerated and dissolved; and (3) the loss of structural integrity is followed by invasion of bacteria. Five different zones have been described in carious dentin (see Table 3-10).[21] The zones are most clearly distinguished in slowly advancing lesions. In rapidly progressing caries the difference between the zones becomes less distinct.

Zone 1, normal dentin. Normal dentin has tubules with odontoblastic processes that are smooth, and no crystals are in the lumens. The intertubular dentin has normal cross-banded collagen and normal dense apatite crystals. There are no bacteria in the tubules. Stimulation of the dentin (e.g., by osmotic gradient [from applied sucrose or salt], a drill, a dragging instrument, or desiccation from heat or air), produces a sharp pain.

Zone 2, sub-transparent dentin. The sub-transparent layer is a zone of demineralization (by acid from caries) of the intertubular dentin and initial formation of very fine crystals in the tubule lumen at the advancing front. Damage to the odontoblastic process is evident, however, no bacteria are found in the zone. Stimulation of the dentin produces pain, and the dentin is capable of remineralization.

Zone 3, transparent dentin. The transparent layer is a zone of carious dentin that is softer than normal dentin and shows further loss of mineral from the intertubular dentin and many large crystals in the lumen of the dentinal tubules. Stimulation of this region produces pain. There are no bacteria present. While organic acids attack both the mineral and organic content of the dentin, the collagen cross-linking remains intact in this zone.[75] The intact collagen can serve as a template for remineralization of the intertubular dentin, and thus this region remains capable of self-repair provided the pulp remains vital.[42,69]

Zone 4, turbid dentin. Turbid dentin is the zone of bacterial invasion and is marked by widening and distortion of the dentinal tubules which are filled with bacteria. There is very little mineral present and the collagen in this zone is irreversibly denatured. The dentin in this zone will not self-repair. This zone cannot be remineralized and must be removed prior to restoration.

Zone 5, infected dentin. The outermost zone, infected dentin, consists of decomposed dentin that is teeming with bacteria. There is no recognizable structure to the dentin and there seems to be an absence of collagen and mineral. Great numbers of bacteria are dispersed in this granular material. Removal of infected dentin is essential to sound, successful restorative procedures as well as prevention of spreading the infection.

Advanced carious lesions. Increasing demineralization of the body of the enamel lesion results in the weakening and eventual collapse of the surface covering. The resulting cavitation provides an even more protective and retentive habitat for the cariogenic plaque, thusly accelerating the progression of the lesion. The DEJ provides less resistance to the carious process than either the enamel or the dentin. The resultant lateral spread of the lesion at the DEJ produces the characteristic second cone of caries activity in the dentin. Figs. 3-33 to 3-35, and 3-51 illustrate advanced lesions with infected dentin.

Necrotic dentin is recognized clinically as a wet, mushy, easily removable mass. This material is structureless or granular in histologic appearance and contains masses of bacteria. Occasionally remnants of dentinal tubules may be seen in histological preparations. Removal of the necrotic material uncovers deeper infected dentin (zone 4) which appears dry and leathery. The leathery dentin is easily removed by hand instruments and flakes off in layers parallel to the DEJ. Microscopic examination of this material reveals distorted dentinal tubules engorged with bacteria. Clefts coursing perpendicular to the tubules are also seen in leathery dentin. Apparently these clefts represent the rest lines formed during the original deposition of the dentin and are more susceptible to caries attack. Further excavation will uncover harder and harder dentin. *If the lesion is progressing slowly, there may be a zone of hard, hypermineralized sclerotic dentin which is the result of remineralization of what formerly was transparent dentin* (zone 3). When sclerotic dentin is encountered, it is the ideal final excavation depth because it is a natural barrier that blocks the penetration of toxins and acids.

Removal of the bacterial infection is an essential part of all operative procedures. Because bacteria never penetrate as far as the advancing front of the lesion,[25] it is not necessary to remove all the dentin that has been affected by the caries process. In operative procedures, it is convenient to term dentin as either infected, and thus requires removal, or affected, and does not require removal.[24] *Affected dentin* is softened, demineralized dentin that is not yet invaded by bacteria (zones 2 and 3). *Infected dentin* (zones 4 and 5) is both softened and contaminated with bacteria. It includes the superficial, granular necrotic tissue and the softened, dry, leathery dentin. Significant new research supports this empirically derived clinical concept of two layers of carious dentin.[21] The outer layer (infected dentin) can be selectively stained in vivo by 1% acid red 52 (acid rhodamine B or food red 106) in propylene glycol.[23] This solution stains the irreversibly denatured collagen in the outer carious layer but not the reversibly denatured collagen in the inner carious layer.[48] Using this staining technique clinically may provide a more conservative preparation of a tooth, since the boundary between two layers differentiated by this technique cannot easily be detected tactilely.[25]

In slowly advancing lesions it is expedient to remove softened dentin until the readily identifiable zone of sclerotic dentin is reached. In rapidly advancing lesions (see Figs. 3-38 and 3-51), there is little clinical evidence (as determined by texture or color change) to indicate the extent of the infected dentin. For very deep lesions, this lack of clinical evidence may result in an excavation that risks pulp exposure. In a tooth with a deep carious lesion but no history of spontaneous pain,

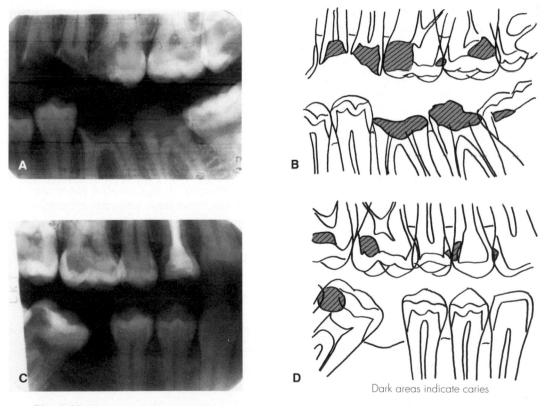

Dark areas indicate caries

Fig. 3-38. Rampant caries in a 21-year-old man. While both occlusal and interproximal lesions exist in the patient, it is the progress of the occlusal lesions that produced the most tooth destruction. The potential for developing occlusal lesions could have been reduced by earlier application of sealants. This extensive amount of caries was the result of the patient's excessive fear of bad breath. In an attempt to keep his breath fresh-smelling, he kept sugar-containing breath mints in his mouth most of the day.

normal responses to thermal stimuli, and a vital pulp (demonstrated by electric testing), a deliberate, incomplete caries excavation may be indicated. A calcium hydroxide liner is placed on the thin layer of questionable dentin remaining over the pulp. This procedure is termed *indirect pulp capping*. A *direct pulp cap* is when calcium hydroxide is placed directly on exposed pulpal tissue (a pulpal exposure) and the surrounding deeply excavated dentinal area. The techniques of indirect and direct pulp capping stimulate the formation of reparative dentin and are discussed in a later section, Caries Control Restoration.

The restorative procedures involving pulpal therapy are rapidly changing. Recent research indicates that an excellent bond and seal against microleakage can be achieved by acid etching or conditioning the dentinal (as well as enamel) walls of the cavity preparation. This conditioning typically is followed by application of a suitable bonding adhesive resin. Conventional liners and bases are not required except when protection of the pulp thermally or mechanically (against pressure) is indicated.[24]

CARIES DIAGNOSIS AND PREVENTIVE TREATMENT

The process of caries diagnosis involves both risk assessment and the application of diagnostic criteria in order to determine the disease state of a tooth. Caries treatment includes preventive measures, temporary caries control restorations (see Caries Control Restoration), and "permanent" restorations. For individuals at low risk for caries, preventive measures may be limited to oral hygiene; for those at high risk, extensive preventive measures are required, often including control restorations.

Preventive treatment methods are designed to limit tooth demineralization caused by cariogenic bacteria, thereby preventing cavitated lesions. They include: (1) limiting pathogen growth and metabolism and (2) increasing the resistance of the tooth surface to demineralization. Caries control methods are operative procedures used both to stop the advance of individual lesions and to prevent the spread of pathogenic bacteria to other tooth surfaces; and in this sense they are preventive procedures. These operative procedures remove irreversibly damaged tooth structure and the associated pathogenic bacterial infection. Caries control methods are most effective if all active, cavitated lesions can be treated in a very short time, even in a single appointment. Control procedures also include medication of the tooth and restoration of the damaged tooth surface to appropriate anatomic contours and function. New restorative treatment methods have rendered the distinction between preventive and control methods less distinct. Fluoride treatment is capable of rendering tooth surfaces acid-resistant and in some circumstances may also arrest active caries. Sealants were designed as a preventive measure, yet studies have shown that deliberately sealing active carious lesions effectively arrests the caries progress by cutting off the nutrient supply to the pathogenic plaque trapped under the sealant.[27]

Caries diagnosis

Caries diagnosis and treatment has traditionally been limited to the detection and restoration of cavitated lesions. This "drill and fill" approach is simply symptomatic treatment and fails to deal with the underlying etiological factors. Undoubtedly, unaffected teeth are superior to restored teeth. *Therefore, early detection of incipient caries and limitation of caries activity prior to significant tooth destruction are primary goals of an effective diagnosis and treatment program.* Cavitation of the tooth surface is a late event in the carious process. Cavitation is preceded by a lengthy period of subsurface demineralization that presents the dentist an opportunity to detect the disease and start preventive measures prior

Table 3-12. Comparison of the structure and characteristics of three layers of dentin of carious teeth and their diagnosis

| Traditional pathology layers by Furrer | Dentin reactions | | | | Dentin structure | | | |
| | Caries detector staining | Vital reaction | | Bacterial invasion | Apatite crystals | | Collagen | |
		Sensitivity	Remineralization		Periodic on collagen	Normal formation	Cross-banding	Cross-linking
Bacteria rich Few bacteria Pioneer bacteria	+	−	−	+	−	−	−	−
Turbid Transparent Vital Reaction	−	+	+	−	+	+	+	+/−
Normal	−	+	+	−	+	+	+	+

(Modified from: Fusayama A: *J. Biol. Buccale* 19(261), 1991.)

to the advent of significant tooth damage. A variety of diagnostic methods are available to detect caries activity at early stages. These include: (1) identification of subsurface demineralization (inspection, radiographic, and dye uptake methods), (2) bacterial testing, and (3) assessment of environmental conditions such as pH, salivary flow, and salivary buffering. Since no single test has been developed that is 100% predictive of later development of cavitated lesions,[1,14,82] a concept of *caries risk* has been promoted. Once identified, patients at high risk for caries can be treated with preventive methods that reduce their likelihood of developing cavitated lesions in the future.[47]

If failure to detect caries in its earliest stage (incipient lesion) occurs, caries is diagnosed by the presence of cavitation of the tooth surface. The tooth surface is examined visually and tactilely. Visual evidence of caries includes cavitation, surface roughness, opacification, and discoloration. Tactile evidence of caries includes roughness and softness of the tooth surface. Roughness and softening are determined by probing the suspected areas with a sharp explorer. Both penetration and resistance to removal of an explorer tip (a "catch") have been interpreted as evidence of demineralization and weakening of tooth structure (a carious lesion). However, many years of using an explorer for caries diagnosis is being replaced by visual and other diagnosis methods. Even though radiolucent areas in the proximal surfaces and below the occlusal enamel are interpreted as evidence of caries (demineralization), they do not indicate whether the surface has been cavitated.

A single test for caries diagnosis usually cannot be used alone because such tests may not be sufficient for accurate caries diagnosis. Particularly the use of the explorer is an unreliable procedure, because mechanical binding (a "catch") can be caused by factors other than the presence of caries. The use of only radiographs for caries diagnosis is also unreliable because of technical difficulties which might include exposure, angulation, tooth position, the presence of restorations, and interpretation bias. Demineralization in enamel that is visible radiographically may not be indicative of active caries and is not necessarily an indication for restoration because radiolucency is visible on proximal enamel surfaces prior to surface cavitation. Furthermore, there are differences in caries susceptibility of persons based on age, geographical origin, ethnic background, and fluoride exposure. For example, in communities with fluoridated water supplies, susceptibility to proximal caries is greatly reduced. *Therefore, multiple criteria must be used and the diagnostic criteria should be adjusted according to the patient's overall risks (age, gender, fluoride exposure history, general health, and ability to maintain good oral hygiene)* (Tables 3-12 to 3-16).

Pits and fissures. Caries cavitation is difficult to detect in pits and fissures because it is difficult to distinguish from the normal anatomical form of these features (Table 3-17). Cavitation at the base of a pit or fissure sometimes can be detected tactilely as softness or by binding of the explorer tip. However, mechanical binding of an explorer in the pits or fissures may be due to non-carious causes such as (1) the shape of the fissure, (2) the sharpness of the explorer, or (3) the force of application. *Thus, explorer tip binding is not, by itself, a sufficient indication to make a caries diagnosis. Discoloration of pits and grooves,* limited to the depth of the fissure or pit, is almost a universal finding in normal healthy teeth of adults and, thus, *as an isolated finding is not a sufficient indication for a diagnosis of caries.* Because of these confounding factors, additional criteria have been developed by the U.S. Public Health Service for pit and fissure caries diagnosis. These factors are (1) softening at the base of the pit or fissure; (2) opacity surrounding the pit or fissure, indicating undermining or demineralization of the enamel; and (3) softened enamel that may be flaked away by the explorer. Actual penetration of the enamel by an explorer tip at the base of a pit or fissure suggests extensive demineralization and weakening of the enamel. Porous enamel (resulting from demineralization) appears chalky, or opaque, when dried with compressed air. Once caries penetrates to the dentin, demineralization rapidly spreads laterally through the less-resistant DEJ. Lateral-spreading caries undermines more enamel and may be seen clinically as a brown-gray discoloration that radiates away from the pit or fissure. Discolored enamel due to undermining caries is easily distinguished from superficial staining because it is more diffuse and does not affect the surface of the enamel. On bitewing radiographs, evidence of dentinal caries may be seen as a radiolucent area spreading laterally under the occlusal enamel from a pit or fissure.

Dentinal tubule			Clinical Diagnosis
Odontoblast process	Crystals in lumen	Discoloration	Three layers
absent	−	+	Infected dentin
damaged	+	+/−	Affected dentin
normal	−	−	Normal dentin

Table 3-13. Medical history factors that are associated with increased caries risk

History factor	Risk-increasing observation
Age	Childhood, adolescence, senescence
Gender	Women are at slightly greater risk
Fluoride exposure	No flouride in public water supply
Smoking	Risk increases with amount smoked
Alcohol	Risk increases with amount consumed
General health	Chronic illness, debilitation decrease ability to give self-care
Medication	Medications that reduce salivary flow

Table 3-14. Clinical examination findings that are associated with increased caries risk

Clinical examination	Risk-increasing findings
General appearance	Appears sick, obese, or malnourished
Mental or physical disability	Patients who are unable or unwilling to comply with dietary and oral hygiene instruction
Mucosal membranes	Dry red, glossy mucosa suggests decreased salivary flow
Active carious lesions	Cavitation and softening of enamel and dentin, circumferential chalky opacity at gingival margins,
Plaque	High plaque scores
Gingiva	Puffy, swollen, inflamed, bleeds easily
Existing restorations	Large numbers indicate past high caries rate; poor quality indicates increased habitat for cariogenic organisms

Table 3-15. Caries activity tests*

Test	Principle and result
Buffering capacity	Titrates a saliva sample to estimate buffering capacity
Dewar	Similar to Fosdick
Fosdick	Measures capacity of saliva sample to dissolve powdered enamel
Lactobacillus count	Estimates the number of bacteria in saliva by counting colonies on a selective media plate.
Reductase	Measures activity of reductase enzyme from a saliva sample
Rickles	Measures the rapidity of acid formation from a saliva sample in culture medium
Snyder	Measures the rapidity of acid formation from a saliva sample in culture medium
Mutans streptococci screening	Estimates the number of colony-forming bacteria in saliva by use of selective culture media (several variations of this test are available)

Adapted from Newburn E: *Cariology*, Chicago, 1989, Quintessence Publishing.

*A wide variety of caries activity tests have been proposed. Most tests lack sufficient predictive value to be clinically useful for individual patients. The microbiologic tests are the most useful for monitoring caries treatment progress. Monitoring salivary *Mutans streptococci* levels is an essential test for evaluation of the effectiveness of antimicrobial treatment of caries.

Table 3-16. Pit and fissure caries treatment decision making*

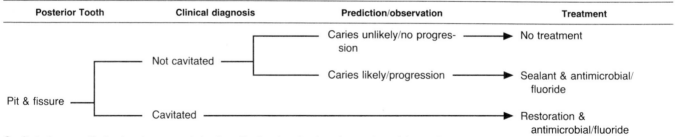

Cavitated means that extensive enamel demineralization has lead to destruction of the walls of the pit or fissure and bacterial invasion has occurred. Demineralization of the underlying dentin is usually extensive by the time the cavitation has occurred.

Not cavitated: (caries-free) pits and fissures:
• No radiolucency below occlusal enamel
• Deep grooves may be present
• Superficial staining may be present in grooves
• Mechanical binding of explorer may occur

Cavitated (diseased) pits and fissures:
• Chalkiness of enamel on walls and base of pit or fissure
• Softening at the base of a pit or fissure
• Brown-gray discoloration under enamel adjacent to pit or fissure
• Radiolucency below occlusal enamel

*If a cavitated lesion exists in a pit or fissure it must be restored. If the pit or fissure is not cavitated, but at risk then it should be sealed. The pits and fissures of molar teeth in children should be sealed routinely as soon as possible after eruption. Pits and fissures in adults should be sealed if the adult is found to have multiple active lesions or is found to be at high risk.

Table 3-17. Proximal caries treatment decision making*

Posterior tooth	Clinical diagnosis	Prediction/observation	Treatment
Proximal surface	Not cavitated	Caries unlikely/no progression	No treatment
		Caries likely/progression	Antimicrobial/fluoride
	Cavitated		Restoration & antimicrobial/fluoride

Not cavitated:
- Surface intact—use of explorer to judge surface must be done with caution because excessive force can cause penetration of intact surface over demineralized enamel
- Opacitiy of proximal enamel may be present
- Radiolucency may be present
- Marginal ridge is not discolored
- Opaque area may be seen in enamel by translumination

Cavitated:
- Surface broken, detectable visually or tactilely—temporary mechanical separation of the teeth may aid diagnosis
- Marginal ridge may be discolored
- Opaque area in dentin on translumination
- Radiolucency is present

*Proximal surfaces are difficult to judge clinically. The critical event in the caries process is surface cavitation. A cavitated surface must be restored while a demineralized noncavitated surface can be treated only by antimicrobial and fluoride agents. Bitewing radiographs can reveal a decrease in density, but radiolucencies alone are not diagnostic of cavitation. Restoration of all radiolucent surfaces results in excessive, unnecessary restorative treatment.

Box 3-1. Clinical risk assignment for caries

A patient is at high risk for the development of new cavitated lesions if either of the following is present:
1. High *Mutans streptococci* counts are found
   Bacteriologic testing *(Mutans streptococci)* should be done when:
   The patient has one or more medical health history risk factors
   After antimicrobial therapy
   The patient presents with new incipient lesions
   Undergoing orthodontic care
   The patient's treatment plan calls for extensive restorative dental work
2. Any two of the following factors are present:
   Two or more active carious lesions
   Large number of restorations
   Poor dietary habits
   Low salivary flow

Smooth surfaces. Bitewing radiographs are the most effective method for evaluation of the proximal smooth surfaces for evidence of demineralization because these areas are not readily assessed visually or tactilely (see Table 3-17). An early lesion is detectable radiographically as a localized decrease in the density of the enamel immediately below the proximal contact, resulting in a radiolucent area on the radiograph. *Proximal radiolucencies detectable on bitewing radiographs should be examined clinically because not all proximal radiolucencies are associated with cavitation of the surface and therefore are not conclusive evidence of the need for restorative treatment.* A common diagnostic error concerning proximal caries diagnosis may result from an extensive superficial enamel incipient lesion that wraps around the proximal surface and extends onto the facial and lingual surfaces. Such a lesion produces a well-defined radiolucent area that appears (by overlapped images) to penetrate through the enamel, when, in fact, the lesion is only minimally extended into the enamel (see Figs. 3-28 and 3-39).

A proximal incipient enamel lesion that is detectable as a faintly visible radiolucency on a bitewing radiograph is unlikely to have a cavitated surface (Fig. 3-40). Newer high-speed radiographic film and lower kV exposures provide a wide range of densities on radiographs that seem to require greater skill in interpretation than the older, higher-contrast films. Studies comparing the diagnostic information available from the two film types show them to be equal.[3] One study demonstrated a small (2%) reduction in ability to detect caries on the higher-speed film.[94] Most incipient proximal lesions in healthy patients end up as arrested lesions (see Clinical Characteristics of Enamel Caries; the Incipient Smooth Surface Lesion). Therefore, restoration of incipient proximal lesions should be delayed to allow time to observe whether or not it progresses. *Arrested lesions are routinely found on proximal surfaces and are visible clinically as slightly discolored, hard spots in older persons after extraction of an adjacent tooth has occurred* (see Fig. 5-14, *C).* However, since ar-

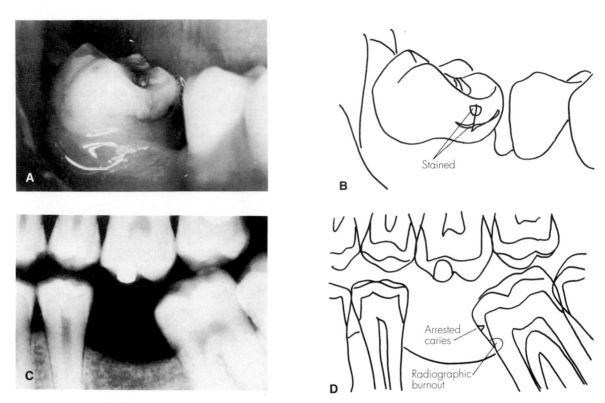

Fig. 3-39. Example of arrested caries on the mesial surface of a mandibular second molar. The area below the proximal contact (**A** and **B**, mirror view of No. 18) can be seen to be partly opaque and stained. Clinically the surface is hard and intact, yet the area is more radiolucent than the enamel above or below the stain. Caries diagnosis based only on the radiograph (**C** and **D**) would lead to a false positive diagnosis (i.e., caries present when it is not). The radiolucency is due to the broad area of subsurface demineralization that extends from the facial to the lingual line angles. The x-ray beam path was directed parallel to the long axis of demineralization and consequently produced a sharply demarked zone of radiolucency in the enamel. This example illustrates the shortcomings of radiographic diagnosis. Were there not visual access to the mesial surface of the second molar, it would be very easy to incorrectly diagnose active caries and consequently restore the tooth.

rested lesions may have a decreased radiographic density that is not distinguishable from new, active caries, radiographs cannot be used solely for complete caries diagnosis without additional clinical examination and history.

The overall accuracy (sensitivity [see Chapter 5 for a discussion of sensitivity and specificity]) of bitewing radiographs to detect caries is estimated to be 40% to 65%.[18,67] Combination of different radiographic procedures does not seem to improve the overall sensitivity. Panoramic radiographic sensitivity for caries is 18%, but is 41% when combined with bitewing radiographs. This is low when compared with a full mouth series, which has an overall sensitivity of 70%.[41] The accuracy of the diagnosis of healthy surfaces (specificity) is much better, varying from 98% to 99% from panoramic, bitewing, or full series radiographs. Thus, when radiolucencies are absent, there is a high likelihood that caries is absent; but when radiolucencies are present, there is

only a small increase in the likelihood of caries being present. A diagnosis of caries based only on radiographs is likely to be correct between 4 of 10 times (less than chance) and 7 of 10 times. When the surfaces are clear of radiolucencies, it is highly likely (98 of 100 times) that these surfaces are caries-free. In clinical practice, therefore, the finding of a radiolucency should be followed by careful clinical assessment of the patient.

It is equally important to detect smooth surface lesions on facial or lingual surfaces as soon as possible, because lesions on these surfaces are almost always seen in individuals with high caries activity. As stated earlier, incipient caries consists of opaque, chalky white areas (white spots) that appear when the tooth surface is dried. The diagnosis is confirmed when the affected area is rehydrated (wetted) and the chalky area partially or totally disappears. These incipient lesions have intact surfaces and care should be given to avoid damaging

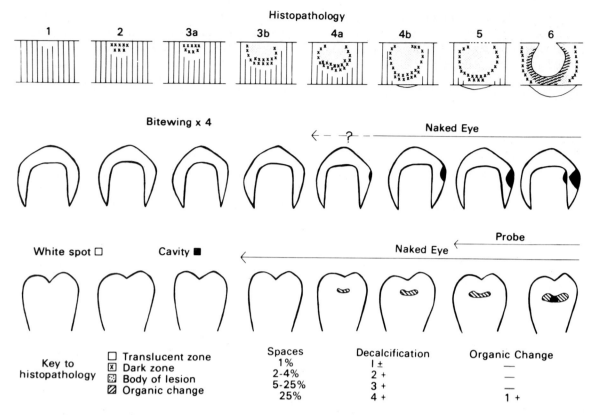

Fig. 3-40. Schematic representation of developmental stages of enamel carious lesion correlated with radiographic and clinical examination. Note that cavitation occurs very late in development of lesion and before cavitation remineralization is possible. (From Darling AI: *Brit Dent J* 107:287, 1959.)

the surface with an explorer. The progress of incipient lesions can be reversed by remineralization when appropriate preventive procedures are instituted. However, once cavitation of the surface has occurred, either by natural causes or by overzealous application of an explorer tip, treatment by cavity preparation and restoration is usually advocated. Sometimes, in selected circumstances, slight surfacing/smoothing of the area by rotary stone or disc followed by fluoride application may be sufficient to arrest the lesion.

Children and adolescents living in communities lacking fluoridated water will have much higher caries rates on smooth surfaces than their peers who have the benefit of fluoridated water. While traditional diagnostic methods for caries should continue to be used for patients living in these nonfluoridated regions, more aggressive treatment with topical fluorides, sealants, and earlier operative intervention is likely to be needed in this higher-risk group.

Root surfaces. Root surfaces exposed to the oral environment, usually due to gingival recession, are at risk for caries and should be examined visually and tactilely. Discoloration of such areas is common and usually is associated with remineralization. Generally, the darker

the discoloration, the greater the remineralization. On the other hand, active, progressing root caries shows little discoloration and is primarily detected by the presence of softness and cavitation.

Caries activity tests. A number of caries activity tests have been developed to help detect the presence of oral conditions associated with increased risk of caries (see Table 3-15). For individual patients, currently no single caries activity test can be relied upon to predict caries with a high degree of confidence. Since many of these tests rely on samples of salivary bacteria, the reliability of such tests is limited because bacteria that are free-floating in the saliva may not be necessarily representative of the bacteria in plaque. Other tests measure the plaque index (amount of plaque present) but also are not sufficient for complete assessment of caries risk.[47] A good caries risk assessment program has been published in a book by Krasse.[47] This program not only consists of microbiological testing for the presence of *S. mutans* and *Lactobacillus* but also is supplemented with analyses of diet and saliva. This combined approach has more promise for accuracy than any single caries activity test. Individual caries activity tests, despite their limitations, can be a useful adjunct to the clinical practitioner by guiding the clinician in making decisions concerning the need for control measures, the timing of recall appointments, the types of indicated restorative procedures and materials, and the determination of a prognosis.[71] The test results also can be used to motivate patients and to determine patient compliance with treatment regimens.

Caries preventive treatment

Caries (cavitated lesions) preventive treatment is a complex process involving multiple interrelated factors (Tables 3-18 and 3-19). Prevention should start with a consideration of the overall resistance of the patient to infection by cariogenic bacteria. The general health of the patient, the exposure history to fluoride, and function of the immune system have a significant impact on the patient's caries risk, but are factors over which the patient has little control. On the other hand, the patient usually is capable of controlling other factors such as diet, oral hygiene, and dental care. This section presents a variety of *factors that may have an impact on the prevention of caries.*

Host resistance. Every patient has a very effective surveillance and destruction system for "foreign" bacteria. The effectiveness of a patient's immunological system is highly dependent on overall health status. Patients undergoing radiation or chemotherapy treatment have significantly decreased immunocompetence and are at risk for increased caries.

General health. The general health of the patient has a significant impact on overall caries risk. Declining health signals the need for increased preventive measures including more frequent recalls. Medically ill patients should be examined for changes in the following: plaque index, salivary flow, oral mucosa, gingiva, and teeth. Early signs of increased risk include increased plaque, puffy bleeding gingivae, dry mouth with red glossy mucosa, and demineralization of the teeth. Decreased saliva flow is very common during acute and chronic systemic illnesses and is responsible for the dramatic increase in plaque. Ambulatory patients with chronic illnesses often take multiple medications, which individually or in combination may significantly reduce salivary flow (see Table 3-8). The saliva should be

Table 3-18. Methods of caries treatment by the medical model (mutans streptococci [MS])

Method and indications	Rationale	Techniques or material
A. Limit substrate		
Indications:	Reduce number, duration, and intensity of acid attacks	Eliminate sucrose from between-meal snacks
Frequent sucrose exposure		Substantially reduce or eliminate sucrose from meals
Poor quality diet	Reduce selection pressure for mutans streptococci (MS)	
B. Modify microflora		
Indications:	Intensive antimicrobial treatment to eliminate MS from mouth	Bactericidal mouthrinse—chlorhexidine
High *MS* counts		Topical fluoride treatments
High *Lactobacillus* counts	Select against reinfection by MS	Antibiotic treatment—vancomycin, tetracycline
C. Plaque disruption		
Indications:	Prevents plaque succession,	Brushing
High plaque scores	Decreases plaque mass	Flossing
Puffy red gingiva	Promotes buffering	Other oral hygiene aids as necessary
High bleeding point score		
D. Modify tooth surface		
Indications:	Increase resistance to demineralization	Systemic fluorides
Incipient lesions	Decrease plaque retention	Topical fluorides
Surface roughening		Smooth surface
E. Stimulate saliva flow		
Indications:	Increases clearance of substrate and acids	Eat non-cariogenic foods that require lots of chewing
Dry mouth, little saliva	Promotes buffering	
Red mucosa		Sugarless chewing gum
Medication that reduces salivary flow		Medications to stimulate salivary flow
F. Restore tooth surfaces		
Indications:	Eliminate nidus of MS and *Lactobacillus* infection	Restore all cavitated lesions
Cavitated lesions		Seal pits and fissures at caries risk
Pits and fissures at caries risk	Deny habitat for MS for reinfection	Correct all defects—marginal crevices, proximal overhangs, etc.
Defective restorations		

Table 3-19. Treatment strategies

Examination findings	Nonrestorative treatment	Restorative treatment	Follow-up
Normal No lesions	None	None	1 year Clinical examination
Hypocalcified enamel (developmental white spot)	None for nonhereditary lesions Hereditary lesions (dentinogenesis imperfecta) may require special management	Treatment is elective Esthetics—restore defects	1 year Clinical examination

Incipient enamel lesions only
  Bitewing radiographs indicated
  (demineralized white spot)
	Techniques *A* to *E* in Table 3-18 as indicated	Seal defective pits and fissures as indicated	3 months
			Evaluate:
			  Oral flora, *MS* counts
			  Progression of white spots
			  Presence of cavitations

Cavitated lesions (Active caries), other incipient lesions may be present
Bitewing radiographs indicated
	Techniques *A* to *E* in Table 3-18 as indicated	Technique *F* (restorations, sealants) in Table 3-18 as indicated	3 months
			Evaluate:
			  Oral flora, *MS* counts
			  Progression of white spots
			  Presence of new cavitations
			  Pulpal response

Arrested caries
  No active (new cavitations) or
  incipient lesions
	None	Treatment is elective
		Esthetics—restore defects
			1 year
			Clinical examination

tested for both flow and buffering capacities when changes are detected from an oral examination.

Fluoride treatment. Fluoride in trace amounts increases the resistance of tooth structure to demineralization and is therefore a particularly important consideration for caries prevention (Fig. 3-41). Fluoride appears to be an essential nutrient for humans that is required only in very small quantities. Laboratory animals fed on a completely fluoride-free diet develop anemias and reduced reproduction after four generations. When available to humans, *fluoride produces spectacular decreases in the caries rate. The availability of fluoride for humans to reduce caries risk is primarily achieved by fluoridated community water systems but also may occur from fluoride in the diet, toothpastes, mouth rinses, and topical applications. **The optimal fluoride levels for public water supplies** is about 1 part per million (PPM).*[35] At 0.1 PPM and below, the preventive effect is lost and the caries rate is higher for such populations lacking sufficient fluoride exposure. Excessive fluoride exposure (10 PPM or more) results in *fluorosis,* a brownish discoloration of enamel, termed *mottled enamel* (Fig. 3-42).

Fluorides exert their anticaries effect by three different mechanisms.[46] First, the presence of fluoride ion greatly enhances the precipitation into tooth structure of *fluorapatite* from calcium and phosphate ions present in saliva. This insoluble precipitate replaces the soluble salts containing manganese and carbonate which were lost due to bacterial-mediated demineralization. This exchange process results in the enamel becoming more

Postoperative changes in dental enamel:
the fate of Class V lesions

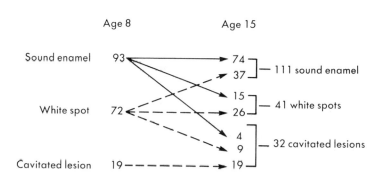

Fig. 3-41. White spot lesions of enamel (stage 3 in Fig. 3-40) may remineralize, remain unchanged, or progress to cavitated lesions. In this study, done in community with fluoridated public water supply, only 9 of 72 incipient lesions became cavitated. Over one half of incipient lesions (37 of 72) actually regressed to become indistinguishable from normal enamel. (From Baker-Dirts O: *J Dent Res* 45:503, 1966.)

acid resistant (Fig. 3-43). Second, incipient, noncavitated, carious lesions are remineralized by the same process. Third, fluoride has antimicrobial activity.[59] In low concentrations fluoride ion inhibits the enzymatic production of *glucosyltransferase.* Glucosyltransferase prevents glucose from forming extracellular polysaccharides, and this reduces bacterial adhesion and slows ecological succession. Intracellular polysaccharide formation is also inhibited, preventing storage of carbohy-

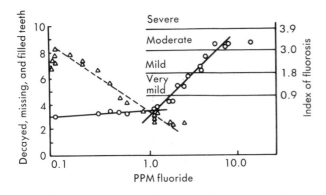

Fig. 3-42. Optimal public water fluoridation levels appear to be approximately 1 ppm when DMF rates are plotted against incidence of fluorosis of teeth. (From Hodge HC: J Am Dent Assoc 40:436, 1950. Copyright by the American Dental Association.)

Fig. 3-43. Diagrammatic representation of enamel adaptation reaction. Enamel interacts with its fluid environment in periods of undersaturation and supersaturation, presented here as periodic cycles. Undersaturation periods dissolve most soluble mineral at the site of cariogenic attack, whereas periods of supersaturation deposit most insoluble minerals if their ionic components are present in immediate fluid environment. As a result, under favorable conditions of remineralization, each cycle could lead toward higher enamel resistance to a subsequent challenge. (From Koulouirides T. In Menaker L, editor: *The biologic basis of dental caries,* New York, 1980, Harper & Row, Publishers.)

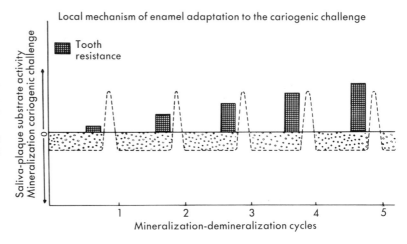

drates by limiting microbial metabolism between the host's meals. Thus, the duration of caries attack is limited to periods during and immediately after eating. In high concentrations (12,000 PPM) used in topical fluoride treatments, fluoride ion is directly toxic to some oral microorganisms, including *mutans streptococci*. Suppression of growth of *mutans streptococci* following a single topical fluoride treatment may last several weeks.[93] It is possible to greatly lengthen this suppression by a change in dietary habits (especially eliminating sucrose) and by the patient's conscientious application of a good oral hygiene program.

There are a variety of methods for fluoride treatment (Table 3-20). All are effective to some degree. The clinician's goal is to choose the most effective combination for each patient. This choice must be based on the patient's age, caries experience, general health, and oral hygiene. *Children with developing permanent teeth benefit most from systemic fluoride treatments via the public water supply.* In regions without adequate fluoride in the water supply, ***dietary supplementation of fluoride*** is indicated for children and sometimes for adults. The amount of fluoride supplement must be individually determined. This is of particular importance in rural areas with individual wells, since the fluoride content of the

well water can vary greatly over short distances. *Accepted Dental Therapeutics* should be consulted for the prescription of dietary supplements of fluoride.

Topical application of fluoride should be done semi-annually for children as well as for adults who are at high risk for caries development. The teeth must be cleaned free of plaque before the application of topical fluorides. Flossing and then tooth brushing are recommended for this purpose. Pumicing the teeth (professional prophylactics) can remove a considerable amount of the fluoride-rich surface layer of enamel and therefore can be counter-productive.[89] Acidulated phosphate fluoride (APF) is the most effective and least objectionable topical agent. APF is available in thixotropic gels and has a long shelf life. Stannous fluoride (8% F), another option, has a very bitter, metallic taste, may burn the mucosa, and has a short shelf life. While the tin ion in stannous fluoride may be responsible for staining the teeth, it may be beneficial for arresting root caries. Topical fluoride agents should be applied according to the manufacturer's recommendations.

Self-administered ***fluoride rinses*** have an additive effect (about 20% reduction) when used in conjunction with topical or systemic fluoride treatment. Fluoride rinses are indicated in high-risk patients and those pa-

Table 3-20. Fluoride treatment modalities*

Route	Method of delivery	Concentration (ppm)	Caries reduction (%)
Systemic	Public water supply	1	50-60
Topical	*Self-application*		
	Low-dose/high-frequency rinses (0.05% sodium fluoride daily)	225	30-40
	High-potency/low-frequency rinses (0.2% sodium fluoride weekly)	900	30-40 after 2 yr
	Fluoridated dentrifices (daily)	1000	20
	Professional application		
	Acidulated phosphate fluoride gel (1.23%) annually or semi-annually	12,300	40-50
	Sodium fluoride solution (2%)	20,000	40-50
	Stannous fluoride solution (8%)	80,000	40-50

*Caries reduction estimates for topically administered fluorides indicate their effectiveness when used individually. When they are combined with systemic fluoride treatment, they can provide some additional caries protection.

tients exhibiting a recent increase in caries activity. There are two varieties of fluoride rinses that have similar effectiveness: high dose/low frequency and low dose/high frequency. The high-dose (0.2% F)/low-frequency rinses are probably best used in supervised weekly rinsing programs based in public schools.[79] The low-dose (0.05% F)/high-frequency rinses are best used by individual patients at home. The high-risk or caries-active patient should be advised to use the rinse daily. The optimal application time is in the evening after flossing and brushing. The rinse should be forced between the teeth many times and then expectorated, not swallowed. Eating and drinking should be avoided after the rinse.

Immunization. Bacteria passing through the mouth into the stomach and intestines come into contact with specialized lymphoid tissue located in Peyer's patches along the intestinal walls. Certain T and B cells in Peyer's patches become sensitized to the new bacteria. The sensitized T and B cells migrate through the lymphatic system to the bloodstream and eventually settle in glandular tissues, including the salivary glands in the oral cavity. There, these sensitized cells produce IgA class immunoglobulins that are secreted in the saliva. These IgA antibodies are capable of agglutination (clumping) of oral bacteria. This prevents their adherence to the teeth and other oral structures, and they are more easily cleared from the mouth by swallowing. For patients with high concentrations of *mutans streptococci*, agglutinating IgA may have an important anti-caries effect. This immunological occurrence promotes the possibility of further *vaccination against caries.* Studies in rats and primates already have demonstrated the feasibility of such immunization attempts.[49,96] However, it is known that the procedure is more effective against smooth surface lesions than pit and fissure lesions.

Even with the development of an anti-caries vaccine, there are remaining concerns that may affect its widespread use. First, potential side effects of a vaccine must be identified. The safety of such a vaccine has not yet been demonstrated, and, in fact, there are concerns of a possible cross-reaction with human heart tissue. Second, its cost must be compared with that of public water fluoridation, which is inexpensive and already very effective at reducing caries. Vaccination may be no more effective than fluoride therapy, which has a proven safety record. However, it may be practical to use a caries vaccine when public water fluoridation is impractical or in developing third world countries. Third, limitations imposed by governmental regulatory agencies may affect the widespread use of an anti-caries vaccine.

Diet. *Dietary sucrose* has two important detrimental effects on plaque. First, frequent ingestion of foods containing sucrose provides a stronger potential for colonization by *mutans streptococci*, enhancing the caries potential of the plaque. Second, mature plaque exposed frequently to sucrose rapidly metabolizes it into organic acids, resulting in a profound and prolonged drop in plaque pH. *Caries activity is most strongly stimulated by the frequency, rather than the quantity, of sucrose ingested.* The message that excessive and frequent sucrose intake can cause caries has been widely disseminated and has become part of popular culture. Despite this knowledge, dietary modification for the purpose of caries control has failed as a public health measure. However, for an individual patient, dietary modification can be effective if the patient is motivated and supervised. Evidence of new caries activity in adolescent and adult patients indicates the need for dietary counseling. *The goals of dietary counseling should be to identify the sources of sucrose in the diet and reduce the frequency of its ingestion.* Minor dietary changes such as substitution of sugar-free foods for snacks are more likely to be accepted than more dramatic changes. *Rampant (or acute) caries* (a rapidly invading infectious process usually involving several teeth) is a sign of gross dietary inadequacy, a complete absence of oral hygiene practice, or systemic illness. The presence of rampant caries is an indication of the need for comprehensive patient evaluation. Textbooks on nutrition and medicine should be consulted. Acute caries treatment is discussed in this chapter's last section, Caries Control Restorative Treatment.

Oral hygiene. Plaque-free tooth surfaces do not decay! Daily removal of plaque by dental flossing, tooth brushing, and rinsing is the single best measure for preventing both caries and periodontal disease (Figs. 3-44 and 3-45). Loe[52] and others have established supragingival plaque as the etiological agent of gingivitis. Longstanding gingivitis can lead to damage of the epithelial attachment and progression to a more serious periodontal disease. *Effective plaque control by oral hygiene measures results in both resolution of the gingival inflammation and remineralization of the enamel surface.* Pits and fissures are not accessible to toothbrush bristles because of the small diameter of their orifices, thus these areas are highly susceptible to caries. Obturation of pits and fissures by sealants is a highly effective method for caries prevention (see next section, Pit and Fissure Sealants).

Mechanical plaque removal by brushing and flossing has the advantage of not eliminating the normal oral flora. Topical antibiotics, on the other hand, could control plaque, but long-term use predisposes the host to infection by antibiotic-resistant pathogens such as *Candida albicans*. Frequent mechanical plaque removal does not engender the risk of infection of opportunistic organisms. It does change the species composition of plaque in both the selection for pioneering organisms as well as the denial of habitat to potential pathogens. Thus the oral flora on the teeth of patients with good plaque control will have a high percentage of *S. sanguis* or *S. mitis* and will be much less cariogenic than older, mature plaque communities, which have a significant higher percentage of *mutans streptococci*.

Krasse has demonstrated that a combination of oral hygiene and diet counseling is effective in children.[47] In this classic study, children in two schools were monitored for *Lactobacillus* levels. The children in one school were given both feedback about the results of the studies and proper preventive oral hygiene and dietary instruction. After 18 months, the children in the school receiving preventive counseling had an average of 3.3

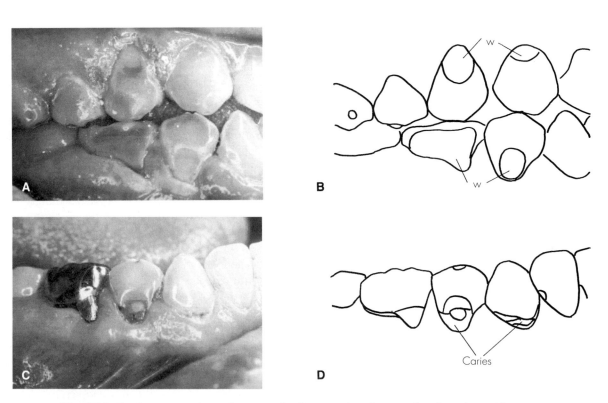

Fig. 3-44. Erosion wear and poor homecare leading to caries. A young female patient with severe wear on the facial surfaces of the posterior teeth. This patient was subsequently found to have a hiatal hernia with frequent regurgitation of stomach acids. Too vigorous brushing and acid demineralization of the teeth accelerated the loss of tooth structure (**A** and **B**). Areas of severe wear *(w)* exhibit dentin hypersensitivity. The dentin pain was the symptom that caused the patient to seek dental care. Advising the patient to reduce the vigorous tooth brushing unfortunately resulted in cessation of all brushing. Caries activity rapidly occurred (**C** and **D**).

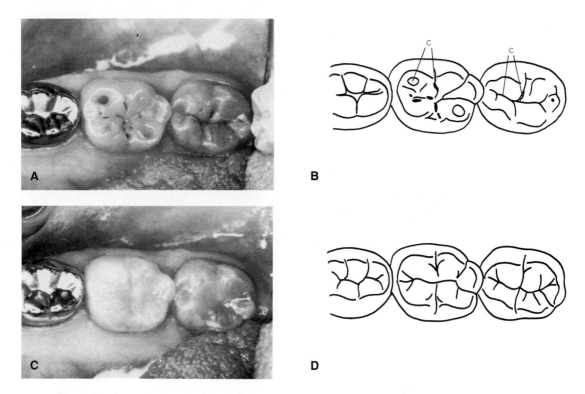

Fig. 3-45. A and **B,** Photograph of the occlusal surfaces of the teeth illustrated in Fig. 3-44, **C.** Following cessation of oral hygiene procedures, caries *(c)* rapidly developed in the exposed dentin and fissures on the occlusal surfaces. **C** and **D,** This was conservatively treated by excavation of the softened dentin and restoration of the excavations and fissures with a highly-filled visible light-cured composite.

new restorations; while the control school children who received no counseling averaged 8.2 new restorations. This is an excellent demonstration that good oral hygiene and dietary improvements can be effective when using microbiological testing as a motivational tool.

Rigid oral hygiene programs should be prescribed only to high-risk persons with evidence of active disease. Overzealous, universal application of oral hygiene training programs are frustrating to both dentists and their patients. High-risk patients should receive intensive oral hygiene training, dietary instruction, and preventive dental treatment as necessary to control the progress of the disease. Plaque removal in high-risk patients should be done frequently. Flossing, brushing, and thorough rinsing after every meal is indicated for this group. Patients without active disease do not need intensive intervention in their self-care program. However, they should still be counseled to optimize their results. Adults with a low caries experience probably only require flossing, brushing, and rinsing once a day, and the best time for this is in the evening before going to bed. During sleep, salivary flow is greatly reduced, limiting the anti-caries benefits of saliva and, therefore, allowing unrestricted plaque metabolism and growth (see Fig. 3-16).

Plaque control requires a little dexterity and a lot of motivation. Some knowledge of tooth contours, embrasure form, proximal contacts, and tooth alignment is helpful to optimal plaque control. Instruction should include both the selection and use of mechanical aids, based on the patient's needs. The primary impediment to patient acceptance of flossing, as a part of routine oral hygiene procedures, is the difficulty of passing the floss through tight proximal contacts. Damage to the interproximal papilla and/or tearing or shredding of the floss are the usual reasons cited by patients for failure to use this technique.

To prepare for *flossing the teeth,* lightly wind one end of a 60 cm length (approximately 2 feet) of ribbon or Teflon floss twice around the ring finger of the dominant hand, anchoring this end by the second loop overlapping the first. The remaining length of floss is around the ring finger of the other hand and serves as a spool of clean floss. The section of floss remaining between the hands should be approximately 15 cm (6 inches). The middle 2 to 3 cm (1/2 inch) is held taut between the tips of the thumbs and first fingers (Fig. 3-46, *A).*

A braced technique is necessary for passing the floss through contacts atraumatically. The first finger of the nondominant hand is used to brace the floss in the facial

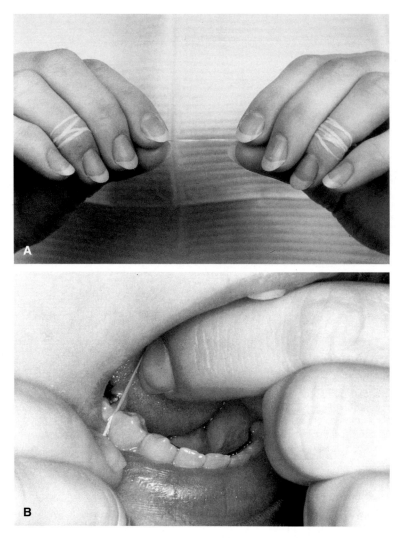

Fig. 3-46. Flossing. **A,** Fingers positioning the floss. **B,** The **braced** flossing technique prevents damage to the interproximal gingiva. The index finger braces the floss in the embrasure while the other hand presses the floss diagonally through the contact.

embrasure adjacent the contact to be cleaned (Fig. 3-46, *B*). With the floss pressed against the embrasure area, the free end of the floss is passed diagonally through the contact. A sliding motion helps to introduce the floss into the contact area without sudden uncontrolled movement of the floss which might injure the gingiva. Once through the contact, the floss is wrapped over a proximal surface and moved up and down to remove the adherent plaque. The adjacent proximal surfaces must be cleaned individually. Fig. 3-46, *C,* illustrates cleaning the distal surface of the approximating pair of teeth. Damage to the papilla when changing surfaces is avoided by gently lifting the floss to the underside of the contact and moving it to the adjacent proximal surface. The floss is wrapped around the opposite (mesial in this example) surface by pressing distally and moving the floss up and down (Fig. 3-46, *D*). *The purpose of routine flossing is not to remove debris from the inter-proximal space (although it is ideally suited for removal of fibrous food caught in contacts), but rather, it is for the removal of plaque from proximal tooth surfaces.* The floss can be removed from the interproximal space by either simultaneously pulling both ends *facially* (Fig. 3-46, *E)* or releasing one end and gently pulling the length out through the interproximal space.

With experience, satisfactory flossing can be completed in 3 or 4 minutes. Whether to use waxed or unwaxed floss is controversial, although not highly significant. The benefits from good flossing technique are much more important than the choice of floss. Every effort should be made to encourage good flossing. Gingival bleeding may occur even with good flossing technique when the gingiva is inflamed. Patients should be advised that gingival bleeding is a sign of gingival inflammation, not the result of damage caused by the flossing or toothbrushing. As good oral hygiene contin-

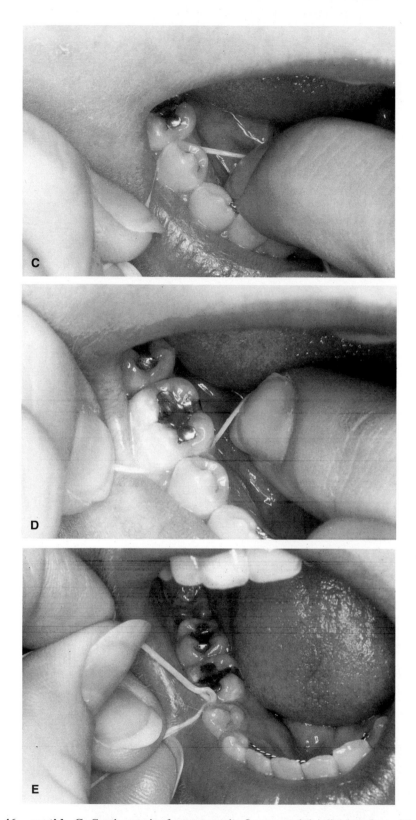

Fig. 3-46—cont'd. C, Gentle anterior force wraps the floss around the distal surface of the more anterior tooth of the contacting pair of teeth. The floss is moved superiorly and inferiorly over the tooth surface from the inferior side of the contact to the depth of the gingival sulcus. **D,** The floss is lifted over the papilla and gently positioned posteriorly to wrap over the mesial surface of the more posterior tooth of the contacting pair. The tooth surface is cleaned of plaque by the same superior/inferior motion. **E,** Removing the floss **facially** through contact.   *Continued.*

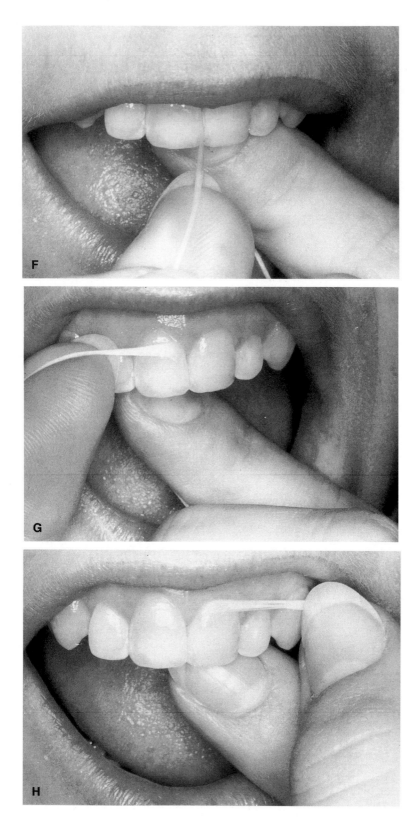

Fig. 3-46—cont'd.   F to **H,** Passing floss through contact of maxillary central incisors **(F)** and flossing the mesial surfaces and mesial transitional angles **(G, H).**

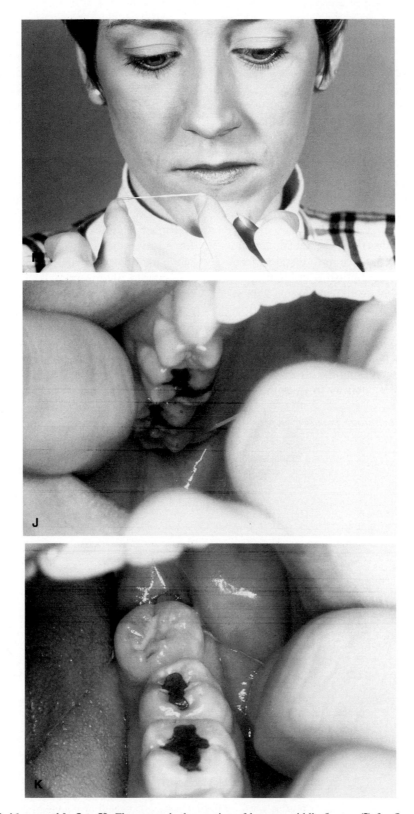

Fig. 3-46—cont'd. I to **K,** Floss stretched over tips of longer, middle fingers **(I)** for flossing the most posterior distal surfaces **(J, K).**

ues, this inflammation will resolve. Within days the gingiva will change from slightly red and glossy to light pink and stippled. The healthy gingiva will become "tough" and will no longer bleed when brushed or flossed.

Each contact can be cleaned with a fresh section of the floss (Fig. 3-46, *F* to *H)* by unwinding the floss from the spool finger and taking-up the increased length by winding onto the take-up finger. For flossing the distal surface of the most posterior tooth of each quadrant, it may be necessary to use the tips of the longer, middle fingers (Fig. 3-46, *I* to *K)*. It is important to floss these surfaces because they are not easily reached by the toothbrush.

Flossing is followed by *brushing* the facial, lingual, and occlusal surfaces, as well as the most distal surfaces (Fig. 3-47, *A* to *D)*. A soft toothbrush with blunt-tipped nylon bristles is applied to the teeth and gingiva with vibrating technique (see Fig. 3-47, *A* and *B)*. A rapid anterior-posterior sawing motion severely abrades tooth surfaces and is not effective for interproximal plaque removal. A small amount of fluoride-containing dentifrice on the brush is useful for increasing the effectiveness of stain and plaque removal as well as to treat the teeth with fluoride.

The sulcular-brushing technique is superior to previously advocated methods. The bristles are held at a 45-degree angle to the tooth surface and vibrated into the gingival sulcus and embrasure. The end of the brush can be applied to the lingual of the anterior teeth (Fig. 3-47, *E)* as well as the non-contacting distal surfaces (Fig. 3-47, *F)*. For these surfaces the toothbrush handle must be raised at a 45-degree angle (or more) to the occlusal plane. During sulcular brushing, the tips of the bristles should be forced to enter the gingival sulcus and the embrasures as far as possible. After brushing the teeth, gently brush the top (dorsal) surface of the *tongue*. This reduces the debris and plaque that otherwise accumulate on this rough surface.

Rinsing follows flossing and brushing. Rinse water is forced over the teeth by tongue and cheek movements while the lips are closed. Rinsing should force the water through the interproximal spaces. Rinsing is repeated until the expectorated rinse water is clear.

Professional tooth cleaning also has an important effect on caries reduction.[44] One study divided grade school students into three treatment groups: control, monthly professional cleaning, and twice-a-month professional cleaning. In students with low *mutans streptococci* levels, the once-a-month cleaning group had half as many new carious surfaces (0.8 surfaces/student) as did the control group (1.8 surfaces/student). In the high *mutans streptococci* group, the control group had the most new caries (2.5 surfaces/student) while the once-a-month cleaning group had similar levels (0.96 surfaces/student) to the low *mutans streptococci* group, and the

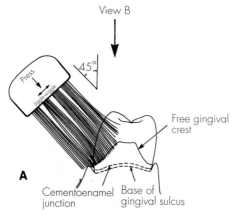

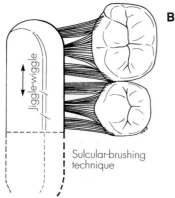

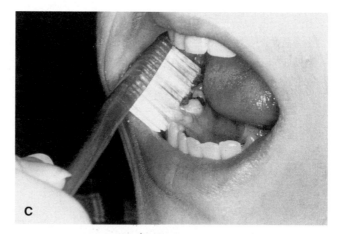

Fig. 3-47. Brushing. **A** and **B, Sulcular-brushing technique** for toothbrush applied to facial tooth surfaces with bristles directed 45 degrees gingivally (same gingival tilt of bristles when on lingual surfaces). Length of double-headed arrows indicates the short extent of "jiggle-wiggle" vibration of brush head, causing tips of bristles to enter gingival sulci and facial embrasures (lingual embrasures when brush applied to lingual surfaces). After "jiggle-wiggling" for several seconds, move brush mesially (or distally) by one tooth (maintaining same bristle direction) and repeat the vibrating motion at each successive position until all facial and lingual surfaces are brushed. **C,** Brush applied as depicted in **(A)** and **(B).**

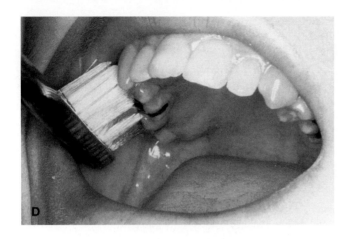

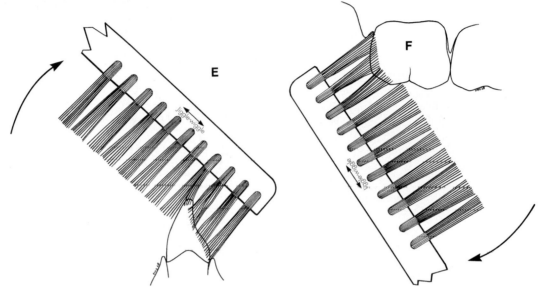

Fig. 3-47—cont'd. D, Sulcular vibrating the bristles on facial surfaces of maxillary posterior teeth. **E** and **F,** Sulcular-vibrating technique for lingual surfaces of mandibular anterior teeth (**E**) and a most posterior distal surface (**F**).

twice-a-month cleaning group had almost one-tenth the number of new lesions (0.34 surfaces/student) as the control group. This study demonstrated that professional plaque removal on grade school students, even as infrequent as once every 2 weeks, dramatically reduces the development of new carious lesions. Equal or greater reductions can be expected in patients who practice proper oral hygiene methods for plaque removal.

Pit and fissure sealants. Although fluoride treatments are most effective in preventing smooth surface caries, they are less effective in preventing pit and fissure caries. While occlusal surfaces account for only 12.5% of all tooth surfaces, they account for 50% of all caries in school-age children.[72] Thus, there is a great need for a preventive measure for pit and fissure caries. Pit and fissure sealants (Figs. 3-48 and 3-49) were specifically designed for this purpose and have been demonstrated to be effective.[27] Sealants have three important preventive effects. First, sealants mechanically fill pits and fissures with an acid-resistant resin. Second,

because the pits and fissures are filled, sealants deny *mutans streptococci* and other cariogenic organisms their preferred habitat. Third, sealants render the pits and fissures easier to clean by physical procedures including tooth brushing and mastication.

To date, acceptance of pit and fissure sealants by the dental profession has been slow and the procedure tends to be under-utilized (Table 3-21).[66] The reasons for this lack of professional acceptance have been concerns about the retention rate of sealants, fear of sealing caries under the sealant, and cost-effectiveness. These concerns have been addressed in various studies. For example, in a review of 15 independent clinical studies, Ripa[80] concluded that caries reductions of more than 80% after 1 year and 70% after 2 years are typical results that may be expected after a single application of sealant. One of these studies reported a 37% caries reduction after 5 years.[37] Ripa also found that all studies reported a progressive loss of sealants.[80] The typical retention rate was at least 80% at 1 year, 60% at 2 years,

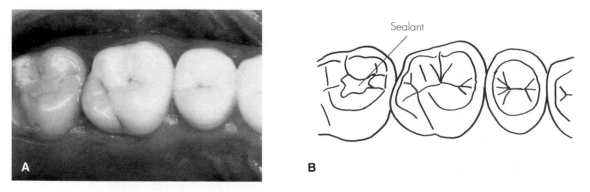

Fig. 3-48. A and **B,** Sealant applied to the central fossa of a maxillary second molar. This tooth was treated because of the appearance of chalky enamel and softening in the central fossa. A highly-filled composite was used (see Fig. 3-49).

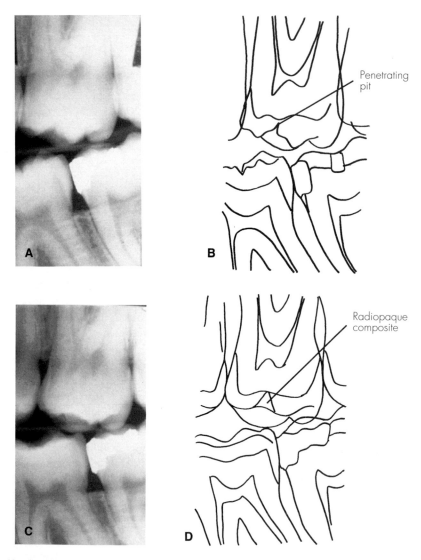

Fig. 3-49. A and **B,** Radiograph of a maxillary first molar with a deep central fossa pit that appears to penetrate to the dentin. **C** and **D,** The central pit was sealed with a highly-filled, radiopaque composite. The composite is readily visible on the radiograph.

Table 3-21. Indications for use of sealants

Criteria	Seal	Do not seal
Tooth age	Recently erupted teeth	Teeth that have remained caries-free for 4 years or longer, staining is usually present in pits/fissures
Tooth type	Molars	Premolars, except when patient is caries active
Occlusal morphology	Deep, retentive, narrow pits and fissures	Well-coalesced fossae and grooves; wide, easily cleaned grooves
Recent caries activity	Teeth showing signs of softening or opacity in pit or fissure	Teeth that have remained caries-free for 4 years or longer, staining is usually present in pits/fissures
General caries activity	Occlusal or smooth surface lesions on other teeth; no proximal cavitated lesions on tooth to be sealed	Proximal cavitated lesion on tooth to be sealed / Cavitation of occlusal (tooth will require restoration)
Availability of other preventive measures	Patient receiving appropriate systemic and/or topical fluoride therapy and still caries-active	Patient's water supply is fluoride-deficient / Patient is not cooperating in recommended caries-preventive program (restoration of pits and fissures is preferred)

and in one study, 42% at 5 years. In a 7-year-study involving 110 paired occlusal surfaces (one receiving a sealant and the other receiving an amalgam restoration), comparable effectiveness was found.[91] After the 7 years, only one sealed tooth was found to be carious while three amalgam restorations were found to have secondary caries. One half of the sealants were retained for the full 7 years, 30% required one reapplication, 10% required two reapplications, and 10% received three reapplications. The total average time required to apply the sealants was 10 minutes and 45 seconds while the average time for placement of the amalgams was 14 minutes and 26 seconds. This data demonstrates the equivalence of sealants and occlusal amalgam restorations. Sealants, therefore, have been shown to be effective, to have long-term retention, to cause regression of active lesions, and to be superior to amalgam restoration in terms of time requirements.

When a sealant is lost, it is most likely a result of a technical error in its application rather than a result of poor bond strength. Proper acid etch bonding of methacrylate and BIS-GMA* polymers to enamel produces a bond strong enough to retain restorations, orthodontic brackets, and even prosthetic bridges. This same bond, which is used for sealants, is unlikely to fail if the sealant is applied properly. Sealing partially erupted molar teeth is a demanding technical procedure. Saliva contamination of the etched enamel will result in precipitation of salivary glycoproteins that prevent the sealant polymers from bonding to the enamel. Re-drying the contaminated surface will not remove the precipitated salivary proteins even though the surface will still have an etched appearance. The contaminated surface must be re-etched to remove the precipitate and

properly recondition the enamel for effective bonding. Indeed, studies of sealant retention indicate the greatest loss of sealants occurs within the first 6 months of application, indicating bond failure most likely due to saliva contamination. Loss of the sealant's occlusal surface because of attrition is a less important problem. Whereas sealants lost because of bond failure leave the fissures exposed and caries-susceptible, loss of only the occlusal portion of sealants leave the depths of the fissures still filled with sealant and therefore caries-resistant.[81] It may be impossible to clinically distinguish between these two modes of sealant loss. Therefore sealant repair or replacement should be done in patients who remain in a high-risk category.

The concern about sealing active carious lesions has been reported by two other independent studies.[27,29] Both studies reported that *sealed lesions fail to progress* and the number of viable bacteria that could be recovered from the lesions was progressively reduced over the period of the studies. Both reports concluded that intentional sealing of carious lesions may be an acceptable treatment modality for pit and fissure caries. One of these studies by Going and others[27,66] reported an 89% reversal from caries-active to caries-inactive after 5 years. That study further states, "There is no doubt that sealing a suspected carious pit and fissure area is a better clinical service than watchful waiting for an interval of six months or more."

The cost-effectiveness of sealant treatment, including replacement of lost sealant versus amalgam treatment, has been studied by Leverett and others.[29,50] They concluded that, although the cost of sealant treatment in caries-inactive patients was not justified, *sealants were cost-effective in caries-active patients*. It is recommended, therefore, that sealants not be used on patients who do not have signs of caries activity. If caries activity is noted either clinically or radiographically, strong

*BIS-GMA, or Bowen resin, is the reaction product of glycidyl methacrylate and bisphenol A.

consideration for sealing all pits and fissures should be made.

The use of sealants is an effective preventive treatment for caries. Sealants (1) prevent caries in newly erupted teeth, (2) arrest incipient caries, (3) prevent odontopathogenic bacterial growth in sealed fissures, and (4) prevent infection of other sites. They should be used on the pits and fissures of patients at high risk for caries as an alternative to restorations. This includes the lingual pits on maxillary anterior teeth and facial pits on mandibular molars. Because caries primarily is a disease of childhood and adolescence, that time period should be when the patient receives frequent recalls and extra preventive treatment. Even though the occlusal portion of sealants may eventually wear off, *sealants offer essential caries protection during the time of high caries risk in childhood and adolescence.* Because of the well-established effectiveness of sealants, *it is not acceptable clinical practice to wait for caries to develop in pits and fissures and then restore these areas with amalgam.* Prompt sealing of the molar teeth after eruption should be a routine practice for most children.

Restorations. The status of a patient's existing restorations may have an important bearing on the outcome of preventive measures and caries treatment. Old, corroded metallic restorations that are rough and therefore plaque-retentive could be smoothed and polished or replaced. Restoration defects, such as overhangs, open proximal contacts, and defective contours, contribute to plaque formation and retention. These defects should be corrected, usually by replacement of the defective restoration. Detection of secondary caries can be difficult around old restorations. Discoloration of the enamel adjacent to a restoration is suggestive of secondary caries. This appears as a localized opalescent area next to the restoration margins. (Exception: A bluish color of facial or lingual enamel that directly overlies an old, other-

wise acceptable, amalgam restoration does not indicate replacement unless for improvement of esthetics. Such a discoloration may be due to the amalgam itself.) Since metallic restorations are radiopaque, the radiolucency of secondary caries may be masked. (See Chapter 5 for a discussion of diagnosis of caries.)

Tooth alignment. Tooth malalignment can also contribute to caries problems by providing sheltered areas for plaque retention. Correction of these problems by orthodontic or prosthetic treatment can contribute to the overall oral health of the patient.

Composition of the oral flora
Mutans streptococci. *Mutans streptococci* are prominently associated with the initiation of caries. Their presence usually is predictive of cavitation in the near future. Microbiological testing is useful for those patients in high-risk categories, especially those who do not yet have active, cavitated lesions. Detection of high *mutans streptococci* levels suggests the need for preventive measures including dietary analysis, oral hygiene instruction, sealants, and antimicrobial treatment (Table 3-22). Follow-up microbial assessments should be used to determine the effectiveness of the measures.

Lactobacilli. *Lactobacilli* are associated with active carious lesions and, thus, should be regarded as an indicator of active caries. *Lactobacilli* levels can be used to assess the effectiveness of caries control procedures.

Summary
Strict preventive measures for caries are not necessary for all patients. Some of those measures would result in expensive treatment with few benefits for low-risk patients. Only caries-active patients and those at high risk (who will most likely benefit from preventive measures) should be treated with comprehensive regimens (Fig. 3-50). Caries activity should be viewed as a problem of oral ecology in which there is an abnormal

Table 3-22. Antimicrobial agents

	Mechanism of action	Spectrum of antibacterial activity	Persistance in mouth	Side effects
Antibiotics				
Vancomycin	Blocks cell wall synthesis	Narrow	Short	Increases gram-negative flora
Kanamycin	Blocks protein synthesis	Broad	Short	Can increase caries activity
Actinobolin	Blocks protein synthesis	Streptococci	Long	Unknown
Bis Biguanides				
Alexidine	Antiseptic; prevents bacterial adherence	Broad	Long	Bitter taste; stains teeth and tongue brown; mucosal irritation
Chlorhexidine	Antiseptic; prevents bacterial adherence	Broad	Long	
Halogens				
Iodine	Bacteriocidal	Broad	Short	Metallic taste
Fluoride	1-10 ppm reduces acid production; 250 ppm bacteriostatic; 1000 ppm bacteriocidal	Broad	Long	Increases enamel resistance to caries attack; fluorosis in developing teeth with chronic high doses

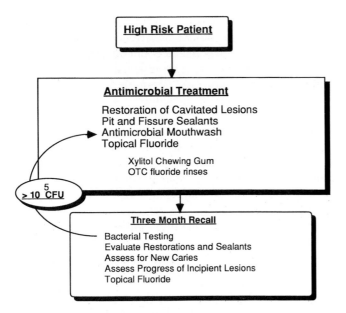

Fig. 3-50. A scheme for caries treatment based on the specific plaque hypothesis. Here caries is treated as an infectious bacteriologic disease. Signs of the disease, such as development of white spot lesions, indicate the need for antimicrobial treatment. Follow-up assessment is used to determine if the infection still persists and if new lesions are forming. Retreatment occurs if either is present. Restorative treatment in this model is an adjunct to the antimicrobial treatment, not the primary treatment.

abundance of cariogenic organisms. Preventive treatment is based on reducing the pathogen population size and increasing the resistance of the tooth to cariogenic attack. The cariogenicity of plaque can be controlled by denying the food supply, denying the habitat, using antimicrobial therapy, and stopping succession. The most successful preventive treatment combines all of these treatments in a specific program designed for an individual that considers both caries and periodontal disease.

CARIES CONTROL RESTORATIVE TREATMENT
Introduction

Much success has been obtained in decreasing the incidence of caries. Research activity has been intense in developing an understanding of the carious process and, consequently, in preventing caries. However, if the carious process cannot be prevented or reversed, it must be controlled. Currently there is no therapeutic medicament which will stop the progression of caries, and while the "arrested caries" phenomenon is recognized, it is not yet clearly understood so as to be universally applicable. Therefore, the recognized control of cavitated carious lesions occurs predominantly by the clinical removal of the infected area from the tooth and the subsequent restoration of the tooth to optimal form,

function, and esthetics. The specific clinical treatment depends on the extent of the destruction that has occurred, and subsequent chapters in this book relate to the definitive treatment of carious lesions.

Once caries has produced cavitation of the tooth surface, preventive measures are usually inadequate to prevent further progression of the lesion. Surgical removal of the lesion and restoration of the tooth then is required to eliminate the progression of the lesion. Currently, operative treatment constitutes the majority of all caries treatment. Restoration of carious lesions is the most effective method for control of the progression of active, cavitated lesions. The term *caries control* refers to an operative procedure in which multiple teeth with acute threatening caries are treated quickly by (1) removing the infected tooth structure, (2) medicating the teeth, and (3) restoring the defects with a temporary material. With this technique, most of the infecting organisms are removed, limiting further spread of caries throughout the mouth. The caries control procedure must be accompanied by other preventive measures which reduce the likelihood of continued buildup or presence of pathogenic organisms (Table 3-23). Teeth rapidly treated by caries control procedures are subsequently treated by using routine restorative techniques, if appropriate pulpal responses are obtained. Also, the intent of caries control procedures is to make immediate, corrective intervention in advanced carious lesions so as to both prevent and assess pulpal disease and avoid possible sequelae such as toothache, root canal therapy, or more complex ultimate restorations.

Table 3-23. Caries control restoration as a part of the medical model

Initial treatment	Thorough evaluation and documentation of lesions
	Temporization of all large cavitated lesions by caries control restorations
	Specific antimicrobial treatment, see Table 3-18, technique *B*
	Plaque control—Table 3-18, technique *C*
	Dietary control—Table 3-18, technique *A*
Preliminary assessment	Gingival response as a marker of plaque control effectiveness
	Pulpal response of teeth with caries control restorations
	Assess patient compliance with medications, oral hygiene, and dietary control measures
Follow-up care	Careful clinical evaluation of teeth
	Replacement of caries control restorations with permanent restorations
	Monitor plaque, *Mutans streptococci (MS)* levels
	New cavitations, incipient lesions, or high *MS* levels indicate need for further antimicrobial treatment, dietary reassessment

Caries control restoration

Objectives and indications. While caries has declined in the general population of the United States, there remains a significant segment of the population, including lower socioeconomic groups and minorities, that suffers from extensive caries. Victims of *acute caries* (lesions that have progressed at least half the distance from the DEJ to the pulp) typically have poor oral health care habits, minimal exposure to fluorides, deficient or highly cariogenic diet, and poor or limited access to dental care. The clinical situation often is complicated by missing teeth, retained roots, and periodontal and/or pulpal diseases (Fig. 3-51). Active, rapidly progressing caries urgently needs clinical treatment when dentin softening has progressed at least half the distance from the DEJ to the pulp. *Acute caries will progress rapidly without operative intervention.* Conventional restorative treatment techniques may not address acute problems with sufficient rapidity to prevent pulpal infection and/or death of the pulp. The treatment regimen for *caries control is to remove the decay from all of the advanced carious lesions, place appropriate pulpal medication, and restore the cavities in the most expedient manner.* Temporary restorative materials (Intermediate Restorative Material [IRM] or amalgam) are usually the treatment materials of choice. This treatment of acute lesions will quickly remove gross infectious lesions. This will not only buy some time while many of the other associated dental problems can be attended but also provide a time period for pulpal assessment of the more seriously compromised teeth. These temporary restorations usually should be replaced with more permanent restorations at a later date when the factors promoting caries formation have been controlled and the prognosis of the tooth pulp has been determined.

Caries control is an intermediate step in restorative treatment and has several other indications. Teeth with questionable pulpal prognosis should be treated with a caries control approach. In this way the progression of demineralization of the dentin is stopped, and the response of the pulp can be determined prior to making a commitment to permanent restoration. Another clinical situation where caries control is a useful approach occurs during an operative procedure when a tooth is unexpectedly found to have extensive caries. Caries control technique provides the busy practitioner the flexibility to respond rapidly to get the situation under control without causing major changes in the daily time schedule. The caries control procedure will allow quick removal of the caries, placement of a temporary restoration, and the rescheduling of the patient for a more time-consuming, permanent restoration. Before placement of a permanent restoration, a caries control procedure also provides a suitable delay that will give the pulp time to recover, allowing a better assessment of the pulpal status.

A caries control procedure is indicated when (1) the caries is extensive enough that adverse pulpal sequelae are soon likely to occur, (2) the goal of treatment is to remove the nidus of caries infection in the patient's mouth, or (3) a tooth has extensive carious involvement which cannot or should not be permanently restored because of inadequate available time or questionable pulpal prognosis.

Operative technique. When numerous acute lesions are present, the practitioner should treat these without delay in one or two appointments with the caries control procedure. Thus the rate of the carious process will be significantly reduced, potential pulpal irritation will be minimized, and the patient will be in a healthier and more comfortable state. The following description involves only a single tooth for the sake of simplicity. Temporization of multiple teeth in a single setting is a practical clinical procedure and is simply an extension of the procedure for a single tooth. Fig. 3-52 shows a schematic representation of the caries control procedure and Fig. 3-53 provides a preoperative radiograph of the tooth described in the following sections.

Anesthesia and isolation of the operating site. Anesthesia is indicated for the affected area unless a test cavity for pulpal vitality is to be performed. The indications and technique for a test cavity are presented in Chapter 5. Anesthesia is usually essential for providing patient comfort, reducing saliva flow, and promoting good patient cooperation during the procedure. Since pulpal death is a frequent occurrence when oral fluids

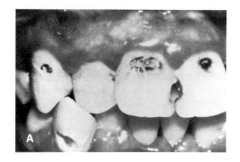
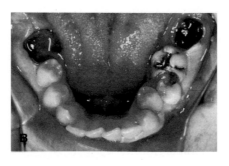

Fig. 3-51. Acute, rampant caries. **A,** Severe carious involvement in anterior teeth. **B,** Severe carious involvement in posterior teeth.

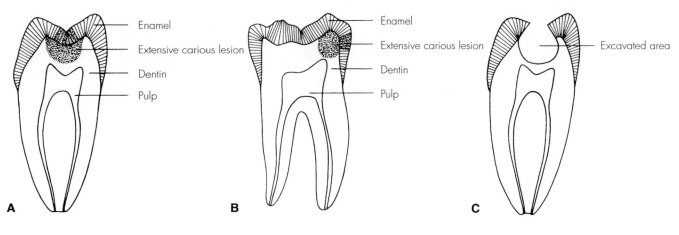

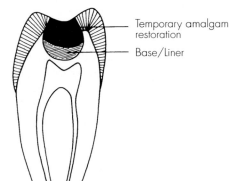

Fig. 3-52. Schematic representation of caries control procedure. Faciolingual (**A**) and mesiodistal (**B**) cross sections of mandibular first molar showing extensive preoperative occlusal and proximal carious lesions. **C**, Tooth after excavation of extensive caries. Note remaining unsupported enamel. **D**, Temporary amalgam restoration inserted after appropriate liner/base material is applied.

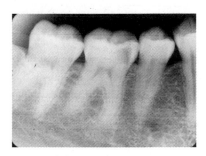

Fig. 3-53. Preoperative clinical radiograph illustrating extensive carious lesion in proximal and occlusal regions of mandibular right first molar.

contaminate exposure sites during excavation of advanced carious lesions, the operating site must be isolated. The ***rubber dam*** provides the best means of isolation and protection of the excavation site from contamination with oral fluids during the operative procedure, and therefore should be used routinely in caries control procedures.

Cavity preparation. The primary objective of the caries control cavity preparation is to provide adequate visual and mechanical *access* to the tooth to facilitate the

removal of the infected portion of the carious dentin. The initial opening of the tooth cavity is made with the largest carbide bur that can be used, such as a No. 4 or No. 6 round bur, or a No. 271 fissure bur. A high-speed handpiece with an air-water spray is the most practical instrument for this procedure (Fig. 3-54). Some steps of initial cavity preparation are modified for the caries control procedure. (See Chapter 7 for further considerations in cavity design.) Retaining unsupported enamel is permissible in cavity control procedures because this tooth structure, even though undermined, will assist in the retention of the temporary restorative material. Removal of the unsupported enamel will occur when the final restoration is placed at a later date. Retaining sound portions of old restorative material also may enhance the temporary restoration and reduce the risk of pulpal exposure. However, care must be exercised when deciding not to remove all old restorative material because it may mask residual infected dentin.

Once access has been gained, the identification and removal of caries depends primarily on the dentist's interpretation of tactile stimuli. Color differences cannot be used as a reliable index for complete caries removal. In rapidly advancing lesions, the softened dentin shows little or no color change while more slowly advancing lesions have more discoloration. *Dentin that appears leathery, peels off in small flakes, or can be penetrated by a sharp explorer should be removed.*

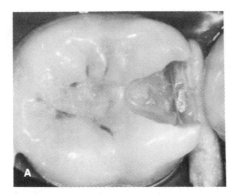 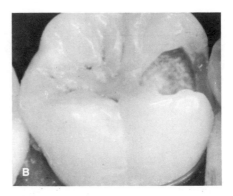

Fig. 3-54. Initial caries excavation of tooth in Fig. 3-53. **A,** Note remaining caries that requires further excavation. Also note wedge in place protecting rubber dam and soft tissue and that it has been lightly shaved by bur. **B,** Note remaining unsupported enamel under mesiolingual cusp.

Because fine tactile discrimination is required for complete removal of caries, the use of high-speed handpiece at full speed is contraindicated for the removal of deep caries. Effective caries removal can be accomplished with (1) hand instrumentation using spoon excavators, (2) slow-speed handpiece with a large round bur, or (3) high-speed handpiece using a round bur operated just above stalling speed (low speed). The use of spoon excavators may result in peeling off amounts of softened dentin larger than intended and therefore result in inadvertent pulp exposure. Thus, hand excavation requires great skill and sharp instruments. Rotary instruments provide good control and require less skill. The high-speed handpiece, when running just above stalling speed, provides good control. A simple technique is to run the handpiece slowly enough that the bur stalls shortly after contacting the dentin. Repeated applications of the bur will remove dentin in small increments and allow the operator to carefully monitor changes in both hardness and color. After removal of softened dentin, it is then helpful to evaluate the excavated area with a sharp explorer to determine if the remaining dentin is hard and sound. Extreme care must be used with the explorer to prevent penetration into the pulp. Penetration of the explorer into the pulp will cause pulpal infection, increasing the possibility of pulpal death.

Usually all soft, infected dentin is removed during caries control procedures. However, in asymptomatic teeth that have deep lesions (where complete excavation of softened dentin is anticipated to produce pulpal exposure), the softened dentin nearest the pulp may be left. The deliberate retention of softened dentin near the tooth pulp and medication of the remaining dentin with calcium hydroxide is termed an *indirect pulp cap.* The goals of this procedure are to prevent pulp exposure and aid pulpal recovery by medication. The portion of the remaining softened dentin is covered with a calcium hydroxide liner/base and the excavated area is restored with a temporary material. Calcium hydroxide promotes

reparative dentin bridges over any area of frank pulpal exposure. Such repair usually occurs in 6 to 8 weeks and may be evident radiographically in 10 to 12 weeks.

If the pulp is penetrated by an instrument during the operative procedure, then a decision must be made whether to proceed with root canal therapy or do a direct pulp cap. A *direct pulp cap* is a technique for treating a pulp exposure with calcium hydroxide to stimulate dentin bridge (reparative dentin) formation. If the exposure site is the consequence of infected dentin extending into the pulp, termed a *carious pulpal exposure,* it is likely that infection of the pulp has already occurred and removal of the tooth pulp is indicated. If, however, the pulp exposure occurs in an area of normal dentin (usually as a result of operator error or misjudgment), termed a *mechanical pulpal exposure,* and bacterial contamination from salivary exposure does not occur, the potential success of the direct pulp cap procedure is enhanced. With either type of exposure, a more favorable prognosis for the pulp following direct pulp capping may be expected if:

1. The tooth has been asymptomatic (no spontaneous pain, normal response to thermal testing, and is vital) prior to the operative procedure
2. The exposure is small, less than 0.5 mm in diameter
3. The hemorrhage from the exposure site is easily controlled
4. The exposure occurred in a clean, uncontaminated field (such as provided by rubber dam isolation)
5. The exposure was relatively atraumatic and little desiccation of the tooth occurred, with no evidence of aspiration of blood into the dentin (dentin blushing)

A deep caries excavation close to the pulp, which may result in either an undetected pulpal exposure or a visible pulpal exposure, should be covered with a calcium hydroxide liner that can stimulate formation of dentin bridges (reparative dentin) over the exposure. However, deep excavations not encroaching on the pulp should be covered with a zinc oxide and eugenol liner. Eugenol provides a sedative effect that decreases the potential for postoperative sensitivity. Calcium hydroxide and eugenol medications will contribute to thermal protection at thicknesses of 0.5 mm or greater as well as provide mechanical protection from amalgam condensation forces at thicknesses of 1 to 1.5 mm or greater.

Restoration. After the involved tooth has been prepared, excavated, and medicated, a suitable restorative material must be placed. The selection of a material depends on both the amount of missing tooth structure and the expected length of service anticipated for this temporary restoration. Amalgam and IRM are the most frequently used materials for caries control procedures.

If a long interval is anticipated between the caries control procedure and the permanent restoration, amalgam will ensure maintenance of tooth position and proper contour. If significant portions of the proximal or occlusal surfaces are missing, an amalgam temporary restoration will maintain the adjacent and occlusal tooth contact better than other temporary restorative materials, such as IRM. (See Chapter 2 for a discussion of problems due to loss of tooth position, such as drifting and pathological eruption.)

The extent of the access preparation and tooth structure loss will indicate the need for a matrix application before placement of the restorative material (Fig. 3-55). Matrix choice and application is described in Chapter 13. Condensation and carving should be accomplished in the conventional manner. Precise anatomical form is not necessary for temporary restorations. However, proper proximal contacts and contours should be established to maintain satisfactory dimension of the embrasures to foster inter-dental papilla health (Fig. 3-56). Teeth lacking interproximal contacts may drift, making subsequent restoration more difficult.

Controversies in caries control restorative treatment procedures

There are different opinions concerning various aspects of caries control technique. Some practitioners advocate removal of all caries in all teeth initially, regardless of the size of the lesion. This approach is undoubtedly the most effective for controlling the infection from dental caries. This approach, however, has disadvantages because it necessitates the excavation of all lesions, which is very laborious. Limiting caries control procedures to pulp-threatening, advanced, carious lesions is advocated in this text as a more practical procedure. The caries control restorations can be replaced after the remaining small-to-moderate-sized lesions are completely restored. The interval between the caries control restoration and its replacement with a permanent restoration provides time to complete the following: assessment of the pulpal response to excavation and medication, treatment of the cariogenic infection, assessment of the patient's ability to perform oral hygiene procedures, assessment of the patient's compliance with dietary changes, and assessment of caries activity elsewhere in the mouth. The outcome of these factors may have an important bearing on the choice of materials and techniques for the final restoration of the teeth. Regardless of the caries control concept endorsed, advanced carious lesions should be treated without delay to minimize the potential of adverse pulpal reaction and to provide time for assessment of the pulpal response to therapy.

There are also different opinions regarding the indication for indirect pulp capping procedures. Some practitioners routinely remove all softened dentin even if a pulpal exposure is likely. Other practitioners routinely leave a small amount of dentin in the area of a potential pulpal exposure, regardless of the status of such dentin. Finally, some practitioners use the indirect pulp capping technique only when the status of remaining dentin in

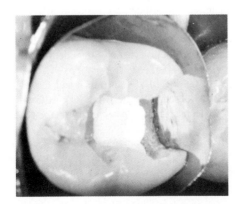

Fig. 3-55. Tooth ready for placement of temporary amalgam restoration. Carious involvement required further extension than in Fig. 3-54. Liner/base material has been applied to deepest excavated areas, and matrix, appropriately wedged, has been placed.

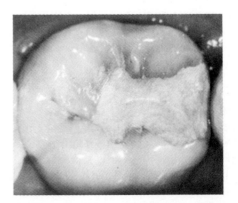

Fig. 3-56. Temporary amalgam restoration completed for caries control procedure. Carious process has been eliminated, the pulp adequately protected, and interarch and intraarch positions of tooth maintained by caries control procedure.

close proximity to the pulp is questionable. Data is not available to guide the final decision in this area.

Another controversial issue with the indirect pulp capping treatment is whether or not to reenter the treated tooth at a later time to determine if, in fact, the remaining dentin has remineralized, providing a sound bridge of tooth structure over the affected area. Some practitioners routinely reenter the affected area to verify this remineralization and/or to remove any caries left over the remineralized layer. Others believe that remineralization does occur and any remaining bacteria become inviable; consequently, reentry into the excavated area is not practical because such a procedure may cause additional pulpal irritation. Carefully controlled studies are lacking, but the consensus is shifting against reentry procedures.

There is also some controversy concerning the medication material to place over deeply excavated areas. Although most practitioners recognize the potential for stimulating reparative dentin formation with the use of calcium hydroxide materials, this is not universally accepted, and some practitioners subscribe to the use of zinc oxide–eugenol materials for this purpose. More importantly there is controversy regarding the mechanism of action for calcium hydroxide liners. One group of practitioners supports the concept that a calcium hydroxide liner must be in direct contact with pulpal tissue to cause reparative dentin formation. Therefore these practitioners believe that the use of calcium hydroxide bases in other than a direct pulpal exposure situation will not stimulate reparative dentin formation. However, other practitioners believe that the calcium hydroxide material is soluble and therefore is transmitted by the fluid in the dentinal tubules to the pulp and, consequently, causes reparative dentin formation.

Finally, there is minor controversy, or at least confusion, about the terminology related to this procedure. Although this section has termed the procedure *caries control restorative treatment*, other terms such as *interim restoration*, *treatment restoration*, or *temporary restoration* may be used. All of these descriptions have validity when applied to the technique of removing acute caries without delay and temporarily restoring the involved tooth or teeth.

SUMMARY

Prevention and control of dental caries must be the foremost objectives of operative dentistry. Research efforts in understanding the carious process, maximizing the benefits of fluoride use, and developing anticaries vaccines must be continued. Patient education and motivation in the prevention of dental caries must be stressed. Finally, the clinical treatment of cavitated, carious teeth must be accomplished expeditiously and judiciously.

REFERENCES

1. Alaluusua S et al: Salivary caries related tests as predictors of future caries increments in teenagers: a three-year longitudinal study, *Oral Microl Immunol* 5:77-81, 1990.
2. Alexander M: *Microbial ecology,* New York, 1971, John Wiley & Sons.
3. Antoku S et al: Effect of controllable parameters on oral radiographs. I. *Quintessence Int* 15:71-76, 1984.
4. Arnold RR et al: Antimicrobial activity of the seretory innate defense factors lactoferrin, lactoperoxidase, and lysozyme. In Guggenheim B, editor: *Cariology today,* Basel, 1984, Karger.
5. Backer Dirks O: Posteruptive changes in dental enamel, *J Dent Res* 45:503, 1966.
6. Baum LJ: Dentinal pulp conditions in relation to caries lesions, *Int Dent J* 20:309-337, 1970.
7. Bohannan HM et al: A summary of the results of the national preventive dentistry demonstration program, *Can Dent Assoc J* 51:435-41, 1985.
8. Bowden GH et al: The microflora associated with developing carious lesions of the distal surface on the upper first premolars in 13- to 14-year-old children. In Stiles HJ, Loesche WJ, O'Brien TC, editors: Microbial aspects of dental caries, *Microbiol Abstr Spec Suppl* 1:223, 1976.
9. Bowen WH: Nature of plaque. In Meleher AH, Zarb GA, editors: Preventive dentistry: nature, pathogenicity and clinical control of plaque, *Oral Sci Rev* 9:3, 1976.
10. Brannstom M, Gaberglio R: The dentinal tubules and the odontoblastic processes. A scanning electron microscopic study, *Acta Odontol Scand* 30:291-311, 1972.
11. Brannstrom M, Lind PO: Pulpal response to early dentinal caries, *J Dent Res* 44:1045-1050, 1965.
12. Brown LR, Dreizen S, Handler S: Effects of selected caries preventive regimens on microbial changes following radiation-induced xerostomia in cancer patients. In Stiles HM, Loesche WJ, O'Brien TC, editors: Microbial aspects of dental caries, *Microbiol Abstr Spec Suppl* 1:275, 1976.
13. Dawes C: The nature of dental plaque, films and calcarious deposits, *Ann NY Acad Sci* 153:102-119, 1968.
14. Dawes C: An analysis of factors influencing diffusion from dental plaque into a moving film of saliva and the implications for caries, *J Dent Res* 68:1483-1488, 1989.
15. Disney J et al: The University of North Carolina caries risk assessment study: further developments in caries risk prediction, *Community Dent Oral Epidemiol* 20:64-75, 1992.
16. Douglass CW, Gammon MD: The epidemiology of dental caries and its impact on the operative dentistry curriculum, *J Dent Ed* 48:547-555, 1984.
17. Dreizen S, Brown LR: Xerostomia and dental caries. In Stiles HM, Loesche WJ, O'Brien TC, editors: Microbial aspects of dental caries, *Microbiol Abstr Spec Suppl* 1:263, 1976.
18. Eggen KH, Rolla G: Information on the composition of the acquired pellicle. In Guggenheim B, editor: *Cariology today,* Basel, 1984, Karger.
19. Espelid I: Radiographic diagnosis and treatment decision on approximal caries, *Community Dent Oral Epidemiol* 14:265-270, 1986.
20. Fejerskov O et al: Plaque and caries development in experimental human fissures. Structural and microbiologic features (abstract), *J Dent Res* 56(Special Issue Abstract No. 457), 1977.

21. Frank RM, Voegel JC: Ultrastructure of the human odontoblast process and its mineralization during dental caries, *Caries Res* 19:367-380, 1980.

22. Fusayama T: *A simple pain-free adhesive restorative system by minimal reduction and total etching,* Tokyo, 1993, Ishiyaku EuroAmerica.

23. Fusayama T: Intratubular crystal deposition and remineralization of carious dentin, *J Biol Buccale* 19:255-262, 1991.

24. Fusayama T: *New concepts in operative dentistry,* Chicago, 1980, Quintessence Publishing.

25. Fusayama T: Two layers of carious dentin: diagnosis and treatment, *Oper Dent* 42:63, 1979.

26. Fusayama T, Okuse K, Hosoda H: Relationship between hardness, discoloration and microbial invasion in carious dentin, *J Dent Res* 45:1033, 1966.

27. Glass RL, editor: The first international conference on the declining prevalence of dental caries, *J Dent Res* 61:1301, 1982.

28. Going RE et al: The viability of microorganisms in carious lesions five years after covering with a fissure sealant, *J Am Dent Assoc* 97:455, 1978.

29. Govan JR: In vivo significance of bacterioicins and bacteriocin receptors, *Scand J Infect Dis Suppl* 49:31-37, 1986.

30. Handleman SL: Effect of sealant placement on occlusal caries progression, *Clin Prevent Dent* 4(5):11-16, 1982.

31. Hardie JM, Bowden GH: The normal microbial flora of the mouth. In Sykes G, Skinner FA, editors: *The normal microbial flora of man,* New York, 1974, Academic Press.

32. Hay DI: Specific functional salivary proteins. In Guggenheim B, editor: *Cariology today,* Basel, 1984, Karger.

33. Hay DI, Moreno EC: Macromolecular inhibitors of calcium phosphate precipitation in human saliva. Their roles in providing a protective environment for the teeth. In Kleinberg I, Ellison SA, Mandel ID, editors: *Saliva and dental caries* (supplement to *Microbiology Abstracts),* Washington, DC, 1979, Information Retrieval, Inc.

34. Hillman JD, Dzuback AL, Andrews SW: Colonization of the human oral cavity by a *Streptococcus mutans* mutant producing increased bacteriocin, *J Dent Res* 66(6):1092-1094, 1987.

35. Hillman JD, Yaphe BI, Johnson, KP: Colonization of the human oral cavity by a strain of *Streptococcus mutans, J Dent Res* 64(11):1272-1274, 1985.

36. Hodge HC: The concentration of fluoride in drinking water to give the point of minimum caries with maximum safety, *J Am Dent Assoc* 40:436, 1950.

37. Horowitz HS: The potential of fluorides and sealants to deal with problems of dental decay, *Pediatr Dent* 4:286, 1982.

38. Horowitz HS, Herfetz SB, Paulsen S: Retention and effectiveness of a single application of an adhesive sealant in preventing occlusal caries: final report after five years of study in Kalespel, Montana, *J Am Dent Assoc* 95:1133, 1977.

39. Jenkins GN: Salivary effects on plaque pH. In Kleinberg I, Ellison SA, Mandel ID, editors: *Saliva and dental caries* (supplement to *Microbiology Abstracts),* Washington, DC, 1979, Information Retrieval, Inc.

40. Jett BD, Gilmore MS: The growth inhibitory effect of the Enterococcus faecalis bacteriocin encoded by pAD1 extends to the oral streptococci, *J Dent Res* 69(10):1640-1645, 1990.

41. Juhl M: Three-dimensional replicas of pit and fissure morphology, *Scand J Dent Res* 91(2):90, 1983.

42. Kantor ML et al: Efficacy of dental radiographic practices: opinions or image receptors, examination selection, and patient selection, *J Am Dent Assoc* 119:259-268, 1989.

43. Kato S, Fusayama T: Recalcification of artificially decalcified dog dentin in vivo, *J Dent Res* 49:1061, 1970.

44. Kleinberg I, Kanapka JA, Craw D: Effect of saliva and salivary factors on the metabolism of the mixed oral flora. In Stiles HM, Loesche WJ, O'Brien TC, editors: *Proceedings: microbial aspects of dental caries* (supplement to *Microbiology Abstracts),* Washington, DC, 1976, Information Retrieval, Inc.

45. Klock B, Krasse B: Effect of caries preventive measures in children with high numbers of *S. mutans* and lactobacilli, *Scand J Dent Res* 86:221, 1978.

46. Koeur M, Bergen T, Mortensen N: DNA base composition of gram-positive cocci, *J Gen Microbiol* 69(pt. 2):167, 1971.

47. Koulourides T: Dynamics of biologic mineralization applied to dental caries. In Menker L, editor: *The biologic basis of dental caries,* New York, 1980, Harper & Row, Publishers.

48. Krasse B: *Caries risk,* Chicago, 1985, Quintessence Publishing.

49. Kuboki Y, Liu C-F, Fusayama T: Mechanism of differential staining in carious dentin, *J Dent Res* 62:713, 1983.

50. Lehner T, Challacombe SJ, Caldwell J: An immunological investigation in to the prevention of caries in deciduous teeth of rhesus monkeys, *Arch Oral Biol* 20:305, 1975.

51. Leverett JB et al: Cost effectiveness of sealants as an alternative to conventional restorations, *J Dent Res* 1143(57A):130, 1978 (abstract).

52. Listgarten MA, Mayo HE, Tremblay R: Development of dental plaque on epoxy resin crowns in man, *J Periodontol* 46(1):10, 1975.

53. Loe H: Human research model for the production and prevention of gingivitis, *J Dent Res* 50:256, 1971.

54. Loesche WJ: Role of *Streptococcus mutans* in human dental decay, *Microbiol Rev* 50:353-380, 1986.

55. Loesche WJ: Antimicrobials, can they be effective. In Guggenheim B, editor: *Cariology today,* Basel, 1984, Karger.

56. Loesche WJ: *Dental caries: a treatable infection,* Springfield, 1982, Charles C Thomas, Publisher.

57. Loesche WJ: Clinical and microbiological aspects of chemotherapeutic agents used according to the specific plaque hypothesis, *J Dent Res* 58:2404, 1979.

58. Reference deleted in proofs.

59. Loesche WJ: Chemotherapy of dental plaque infection, *Oral Sci Rev* 9:63-107, 1976.

60. Loesche WJ, Bradury DR, Woolfolk MP: Reduction of dental decay in rampant caries individuals following short term kanamycin treatment, *J Dent Res* 56:254-265, 1977.

61. Loyola-Rodriguiez JP et al: Purification and properties of extracellular mutacin, a bacteriocin from *Streptococcus sobrinus, J Gen Microbiol* 138(pt2):269-274, 1992.

62. Mandel ID: Caries prevention—a continuing need, *Int Dent J* 43:67-70, 1993.

dental schools for teaching the dental care of patients with bloodborne infectious diseases.[5] The guidelines specify a comprehensive array of basic and clinical topics including a description of transmissible infections, their epidemiology and mechanisms of transmission, principles and methods of infection control, use of barriers, instrument sterilization, and disinfection. The topics must necessarily be taught in keeping with the prevailing concept of universal precautions (i.e., treating all patients as infectious). The content was not intended to be presented in a separate course, but to be integrated into existing courses as appropriate. *This chapter integrates applicable topics on transmissible diseases, epidemiology, and infection control specified by the AADS curriculum guidelines into the teaching and practice of operative dentistry.* That content is also integrated with federal and other requirements related to infection control.

To meet clinical AADS guidelines, state and other requirements, dental schools also prepare and maintain a written *manual of infection control policies and procedures.*[6] The manual serves purposes of standardizing and documenting policies and procedures to protect patients and personnel, and for training students, faculty, and personnel in those regards. It is convenient to include required OSHA, state, and other regulations in sections of the same manual. Private dental offices develop an office infection control manual for the same reasons. Much of the content in this chapter can be adapted to such a manual.

FEDERAL AND STATE REGULATIONS TO REDUCE EXPOSURE RISKS FROM PATHOGENS IN BLOOD AND OTHER SOURCES OF INFECTION

The term, *"Infection Control Program"* (IC program), has a long tradition in hospital usage. *IC programs,* such as those recommended by the Centers for Disease Control (CDC) and the American Dental Association (ADA), *are designed to protect both patients and personnel.*

The federal Occupational Safety and Health Administration (OSHA) uses a different term, *"Exposure Control Plan,"* for a *required* office *program that is designed to protect personnel* against risks of exposure to infection. Guidelines and requirements of other agencies that pertain to areas of infection control not covered by OSHA will be discussed in the next section. State occupational safety and health agencies are now enforcing regulations finalized by the federal OSHA, whose *Final Rule* (or *The Standard*) on occupational exposure to bloodborne pathogens was published in December, 1991.[79]

The OSHA rule derives from the original *Occupational Safety and Health Act* passed by the U.S. Con-

gress in 1970.[99] This Act identified employers' obligations to protect employees from occupational risks. That Act has been the basis for all subsequent federal safety and health regulations. According to the Act, *each employer must furnish employees with a place and conditions of employment free from recognized hazards that presently cause, or are likely to cause, death or serious harm to them.* The Act created the Occupational Safety and Health Agency (OSHA) in the U.S. Department of Labor. In the late 1980s labor unions petitioned OSHA in federal courts to extend chemical hazards protection standards to employees in the health care professions. Shortly thereafter, concern about transmitting HIV to health care workers stimulated the unions to take similar action to obtain the OSHA regulation of blood and body-fluid exposure among health care personnel.

Thus the Act covers two regulated programs of compliance: (1) an OSHA Hazard Communications program concerning risks from environmental and chemical hazards in the workplace (see Chapter 6, section on safety and efficacy); and (2) an OSHA Bloodborne Pathogens program that addresses control of "occupational exposure to blood and other potentially infectious materials".[79,80]

The OSHA Hazard Communications program, which also must be implemented in every dental office, applies mainly to chemicals. Other requirements that fall between the two regulations and must not be overlooked include: maintenance of a complete first aid kit, full oxygen tank, and pocket resuscitation masks; a fire evacuation plan; fire extinguishers with annual inspection and actual personnel training updated; and general environmental safety, such as clear passageways without mechanical obstructions and with clearly marked exits, electrical safety (e.g., ground fault outlets near sinks), and adherence to radiation and nitrous oxide safety standards. An *occupational safety and health poster* stating the obligations of employers and employees to follow health and safety regulations, and workers rights and recourses, *must be displayed in a convenient place for employees to see.*

All aspects of the OSHA Bloodborne Pathogens program were required in every dental office by July 6, 1992.[79] Copies of the *OSHA Bloodborne Pathogens Standard of 1991* are available for $2 from the U.S. Government Printing Office, Superintendent of Documents, Washington, DC 20402 (specify GPO order no. 069-001- 0040-8). A federal translation of the standard (but not a substitute) for dentistry can be requested free by sending a return address label to the OSHA Publications Office, Room N-3101, 200 Constitution Ave. NW, Washington, DC 20210. Required copies of regulations, posters, and reporting forms, as well as other materials for training purposes are available from local state offices of the Division of Labor or of the Occupational Safety and Health Agency. Helpful brochures and manuals that provide copies of regulations, forms, and more detailed instruction are also available from some state health department divisions of dental health, or from state and national dental associations.

Written OSHA office exposure control plan (summary)

A written exposure control plan must be accessible to employees with exposure risks. The plan must be updated at least annually and when alterations in procedures create new occupational exposures.

The office exposure control plan applies to all operatory and laboratory personnel (such as the dentist, hygienist, dental assistant, and dental laboratory technicians, as well as dental equipment repair personnel, and laundry and custodial personnel who handle waste or laundry from operatories). These are persons who have regular, potential contact with blood/body fluids. This exposure determination shall be made without regard to use of personal protective equipment. *All such persons must be listed in the exposure control plan by name, job, and kind of exposure* (e.g., intraoral treatments, exposure to spatter of blood-contaminated oral fluids, and/or cleaning and sterilizing sharp instruments). Dentists who are employed by an office, corporation, or institution are also listed as personnel to whom all rules apply. Receptionists who never assist or work in the operatory and who do not have contact with body-fluid–contaminated charts would be exempt. If personnel do encounter blood/body fluid contamination on charts, etc., then they must be listed. Appropriate training, immunization, and protective materials must be provided. Clerical hospital personnel who handle blood-contaminated forms have shown elevated hepatitis B infection rates. Paper cuts have apparently been responsible.[83]

Dental students do not come under OSHA regulations unless they are employees of the school in capacities that involve blood-borne pathogen exposure. However, all dental schools have an infection control manual of standard operating procedures (SOPs) that apply to students based upon the school's OSHA exposure control plan for faculty and staff. As future employers or employees, dental students will have to become acquainted with OSHA's exposure control plan. A simple *implementation schedule* must be prepared to document how and when various aspects of compliance with the exposure control plan is provided for new and old employees. This can be done by notating a copy of the OSHA regulation.[79,100]

The OSHA exposure control plan uses terms that require definition. *Exposure* is defined in the OSHA regulation as, "specific eye, mouth, other mucous membrane, non-intact skin, or parenteral contact with blood or other potentially infectious materials that results from performance of an employee's duties."[79] *Universal pre-cautions* means that all patients and blood-contaminated body fluids are treated as infectious.

Means of compliance are expressed in the OSHA terminology of environmental safety engineers. *Work practice controls and engineering controls* are terms that describe precautions (e.g., careful handling of sharp instruments, and not putting hands into sharps containers) and use of devices to reduce contamination risks (e.g., using high-volume suction, rubber dam, and protective sharps containers). *Personal protective equipment (PPE)* is the term used for barriers, such as gloves, gown, or mask. *Housekeeping* is a term that relates to cleanup of treatment-soiled operatory equipment, instruments, counters, and floors, as well as to management of used gowns and waste. Housekeeping also relates to cautions for servicing contaminated equipment, and using only mechanical means to clean up contaminated broken glass.

Standard operating procedures (SOPs) is a term used in former OSHA regulations for step-by-step descriptions of tasks. Such task descriptions are preferred for training new personnel and comprise part of the training manual.

Following is a *summary of the current OSHA regulations* specifying what employers must furnish, directions employers must provide, and compliance required of employees (obtain and read a copy of the *Final OSHA Rule on Bloodborne Pathogens* to be apprised of complete and exact details[79]):

1. Provide hepatitis B immunization to employees without charge within 10 days of employment. A copy of the OSHA regulations on bloodborne pathogens from which this information is taken must also be provided by the employer to the health care professional responsible for providing the HB vaccine.
2. Require that universal precautions be observed to prevent contact with blood and other potentially infectious materials. Saliva is considered to be a blood-contaminated body fluid *in relation* to dental treatments.[23,33]
3. *Implement engineering controls* to reduce production of contaminated spatter, mists, and aerosols. Examples are use of rubber dam, high-volume suction, rubber prophy cup instead of brushes, scaling instruments for patients with respiratory infections instead of cavitron, and hard-wall containers to avoid contact with disposable and reusable sharps.[37,45,75]
4. *Implement work practice control* precautions to minimize splashing, spatter, or contact of bare hands with contaminated surfaces. For example, when using a brush to scrub instruments, hold the instruments well down in the sink, place the bristles on the upper surfaces of the instruments,

and brush away from yourself; never contact telephones, switches, door handles, or faucet handles with soiled gloves. *The subsequent items (5 to 18) are also work practice control regulations.*

5. Provide facilities and instruction for washing hands after removing gloves, and for washing other skin immediately or as soon as feasible after contact with blood or potentially infectious materials (see Figs. 4-2 and 4-3). Flush eye or mucosa immediately or as soon as feasible after any contact with blood or potentially infectious materials.

6. Prescribe safe handling of needles and other sharp items. Needles must not be bent or cut. When it can be shown necessary, needles may be re-sheathed with mechanical aids or other one-handed technique (see Chapter 10, Fig. 10-2).

7. Prescribe disposal of single-use needles, wires, carpules, and sharps as close to the place of use as possible, as soon as feasible, in hard-walled, leakproof containers that are closable, from which needles cannot be easily spilled. Containers must be red or bear a biohazard label, and must be kept upright and closed when moved (see Chapter 10, Fig. 10-1). Teeth must not be discarded into trash but can be given to the patient or discarded into sharps containers.

8. Contaminated reusable sharp instruments must not be stored or processed in a manner that requires employees to reach hands into containers to retrieve them. Use baskets or cassettes to place instruments into and retrieve them from soaking pans and ultrasonic cleaners. Use biohazard-labeled or red pans that are leakproof and puncture resistant.

9. Prohibit eating, drinking, handling contact lenses, and application (but not wearing) of facial cosmetics in contaminated environments such as operatories and cleanup areas. Ban storage of food and drinks in refrigerators or other spaces where blood or infectious materials are stored.

10. Place blood and contaminated specimens (e.g., impressions that have not been well cleaned and well disinfected, teeth, biopsy specimens, blood specimens, and culture specimens) to be shipped, transported, or stored into suitable closed containers that prevent leakage. An adequately strong plastic bag can be used for impressions. The surface of all containers must be clean or enclosed in another clean, red, or biohazard-labeled container.

11. At no cost to employees, provide them with necessary *personal protective equipment (PPE)* and clear directions for use of appropriate universal barrier protection in treating all patients and for all other contact with blood or other infectious materials (see Figs. 4-1 and 4-2). PPE must *not allow blood or other potentially infectious material to pass through to contaminate personal clothing, skin, or mucous membranes.* Namely, provide: protective gloves, or hypoallergenic gloves as needed; appropriate protective body clothing such as gowns, and "the type and characteristics will depend upon the task and degree of exposure anticipated" [79]; protective eyewear, chin-length face shields, goggles, or glasses with solid protective side shields; masks; pocket resuscitation masks for cardiopulmonary resuscitation (CPR); and surgical caps or shoe covers to be worn when required for surgery or whenever heavy contamination can be reasonably anticipated.

12. Ensure that employees correctly use and discard PPE or properly prepare it for reuse. Provide adequate facilities to discard gowns in the location where they are used. Note: *A face shield does not substitute for a mask.*

13. As soon as feasible after treatments, attend to *housekeeping* requirements including floors, countertops, sinks, and other environmental equipment that are subject to contamination. Also included are the use of protective covers that are changed after each appointment, or thoroughly clean and disinfect contaminated surfaces and operatory equipment items that cannot be covered, discarded, or removed and sterilized. (See Operatory Asepsis; and Procedures, Materials, and Devices for Cleaning Instruments Before Sterilization, for details.)

14. Provide a written schedule for cleaning and then using a decontaminating procedure for equipment, work surfaces, and contaminated floors. For contaminated spills, prescribe an appropriate method of cleaning and then applying disinfecting methods. Broken glassware that may be contaminated must be cleaned up with mechanical means, and never with gloved hands.

15. Contaminated equipment that requires service must first be decontaminated, or a biohazard label must be used to indicate contaminated parts.

16. Contaminated sharps are **regulated waste;** discard in hard-walled containers. For OSHA purposes in dentistry, *regulated waste* also means (1) liquid or semi-liquid blood or other potentially infectious materials, (2) contaminated

items that would release blood or other potentially infectious materials in a liquid or semi-liquid state if compressed, and (3) items that are caked with blood or other potentially infectious materials and are capable of releasing these materials during handling. Properly dispose of such regulated waste in biohazard-labeled or red closable bags or other labeled containers that prevent leakage. Containers contaminated on the outside must be placed in a secondary container. The secondary container must also be closable, prevent leakage, and be red or biohazard-labeled. Containers or bags must be closed when moved. If outsides of reusable containers are likely to become contaminated, they must be inspected, decontaminated, and cleaned on a regularly scheduled basis, and as soon as feasible if they become visibly contaminated.

Cabinets or other storage areas on the premises in which blood-contaminated waste is stored must be identified by a biohazard label.

17. Place reusable contaminated sharp instruments into a basket in a hard-walled container for transportation to the clean-up area. Personnel must not reach hands into containers of contaminated sharps.

18. Provide *laundering* of protective garments used for universal precautions at no cost to employees. Handle contaminated laundry as little as possible without sorting or rinsing. Bag all soiled linens where they are used in a color-coded bag recognized as requiring universal precautions. (See current American Dental Association [ADA] updates on their negotiations with OSHA on laundry management and other aspects of the plan.)

Emergency and exposure incident plan. An emergency and exposure incident plan must be developed *for employees*. A separate plan is needed for students if they use different medical care resources or methods for reporting exposure incidents.

A person must be identified who is the program coordinator and *contact person* when emergencies arise. That person may also become the trainer for office personnel. OSHA describes an exposure incident plan that emphasizes *documentation* of incidents and their follow up. During training sessions personnel must be told what to do in an emergency, but documenting a plan of medical emergency care is an equally important aspect of employee protection. Five *requirements* of an incident plan should be addressed.

1. Exposures to mucosa may not be associated with an injury; or an exposure incident may involve minor or severe injury (e.g., from a cutting instrument). Rapid and thorough cleaning of a wound or washing a splashed eye or mouth as quickly as possible is the most important first step to minimize infection risks. Blood tends to collect on the surface of puncture wounds created by solid pointed instruments, so washing puncture wounds is just as important.

Persons must be identified in the office to provide any help, direction, or transportation needed to obtain medical care. A brief written plan should be formulated of how to rapidly access medical attention. This content should comprise the first part of the exposure incident plan. Sufficient time will still be available for a designated responsible person to contact the patient and transmit medical records as well as other information to the attending physician, as presented next.

2. The source patients' written permission must be obtained to copy and convey their medical history to the attending physician, or to obtain other medical records regarding the patient. However, knowledge of risk behavior, blood test results, or other pertinent information can usually be conveyed verbally in confidence without permission in case of exposure. Consult local laws.

Some states only prescribe transmission of the name, address, and phone number of the patient and the name and phone number of the patient's physician to the physician attending the exposed person. The patient's physician is then contacted by the examining physician who deals with testing the patient.

3. As directed by OSHA regulations, employers must provide copies of the exposure incident plan and explain it to employees. Employers must document the route and circumstances of the exposure, identifying the source patient when possible. Employers must provide and pay for exposure incident evaluation and follow-up evaluations for an exposed employee unless paid for by workman's compensation.

4. If other local regulations do not prevail, employers must also (1) identify and contact the source patient if possible; (2) obtain the source person's permission to be tested, unless they are already known to be infected; (3) as soon as feasible have the source person's blood tested for evidence of current HIV and HBV infection (e.g., if blood is available, some states permit testing in exposure instances without permission); (4) provide results to the exposed employee in confidence (state laws often require counseling of the source patient for HIV testing as well as the exposed person); (5) with permission, test the employee's blood as

HIV is termed an *RNA retrovirus,* one that needs complementary DNA formed within the nucleus of a host cell (termed a provirus form) to reproduce the HIV. As HIV gains entry into the lymphocytes, reverse transcription of viral RNA begins resulting in formation of double stranded viral DNA in the infected cells. Once inserted into the cell's genetic structure (genome), this DNA becomes HIV provirus. HIV DNA may then divide and reproduce along with the cell's nuclear DNA for years. Antibody tests are now available to detect HIV provirus DNA fragments that regulate production of various parts of HIV structure (core proteins, gag; viral envelope, env; reverse transcriptase, pol).[61]

One drug found helpful in prolonging the health of HIV-infected persons is zidovudine (formerly azidothymidine ["AZT"]). This drug is one of a group of the dideoxy nucleoside drugs that interferes with reverse transcriptase action necessary to complete HIV infection of human cells.[61]

After remaining latent during the prolonged incubation period in infected helper lymphocyte cells, the HIV commences to replicate. The lymphocytes die, releasing virus into the blood, and thus the numbers of essential helper lymphocytes are drastically reduced. When helper cell counts fall to counts below 200 per mm^3 in the blood, many different opportunistic infections and tumors appear. These produce conditions that become increasingly more difficult to treat until *Pneumocystis* infection of the lungs is fatal, or until HIV or other infection of the brain causes death.[49] At the author's institution, patients with T-4 helper cell counts of 200 per mm^3 are considered to benefit from facilities, nursing care, and treatment expertise offered by the hospital dental service clinicians which are not available in the school.

Symptoms and oral manifestations

Within 3 months of infection, temporary flu-like symptoms of pharyngitis, myalgia, fatigue, fever, or diarrhea may occur when antibody to HIV becomes detectable. After prolonged incubation of about 1.5 to 12 years, any of several **early signs** of AIDS may be detected by the dentist, signaling gradual failure of the immune system.[8,62] (Refer to Chapter 5 for color illustrations of orofacial manifestations of AIDS.) Easily detected during examination are one or two *cervical lymph nodes*, especially below the mandible, that persist for more than 3 months. Nodes may be attached and painless, or movable, painful, and infected. Undifferentiated *non-Hodgkins lymphoma cancers* may arise in lymph nodes, or may appear in the mandible as well as in the central nervous system, eyes, bone marrow, and other vital organs.[8]

Persistent *oral candidiasis* is often seen with easily dislodged white curd-like patches scattered over the tongue. In AIDS such infection may not easily respond to treatment, and often recurs, developing into *atrophic candidiasis,* or *cheilitis* at the angles of the lips. Painful *herpes stomatitis* is also somewhat common. Untreated herpes or candidiasis may extend into *esophagitis* or *laryngitis,* impairing speech.[8]

Red, brownish to purple blotches that persist on the oral mucosa and skin of the individual typify a sarcoma of the capillaries, termed ***Kaposi's sarcoma.*** Oral lesions often develop into tumors that may require surgery and radiation therapy. Kaposi's sarcoma is often found on oral tissues of male homosexuals. Human papilloma virus can cause flat to cauliflower-like *oral warts* to develop.[8]

A persistent, severe, recurrent *gingivitis* and *periodontitis* typical of AIDS is a common finding that brings patients for dental care. The gingivitis may persist despite good plaque control.[62]

Early *systemic signs* of illness progressing toward AIDS are marked by *weight loss* of up to 50 pounds within a few months, and chronic *fever or night sweats* that persist for 3 months or more.[8,49] Early detection, and medical treatment of HIV infection is beneficial to the majority of patients. Current treatments are summarized in the annual JADA supplement update, *Facts about AIDS for the Dentist.*[8]

Serology of HIV infection

HIV infection is detected by blood tests (EIA or enzyme linked immunoassay, Western Blot, and fluorescent antibody tests) that detect antibodies formed against the virus. Tests for anti-HIV antibody are often positive within 3 months after infection; most are positive by 6 months; 1% take up to 12 months to become positive. A second positive test is necessary to confirm positive serologies.

Serological tests for the virus and provirus DNA have also been developed. Tests for T-4/T-8 (or CD4/CD8) lymphocyte ratios are used to indicate progress of the HIV infection. One criterion for starting zidovudine therapy is a T-4 helper cell count below 500 per mm^3 of blood.[8]

HIV risks for clinical personnel

Of all American health care workers injured by needles and sharp instruments used to treat HIV-infected persons, only 0.3% or less have become infected with HIV. This contrasts with 30% of workers who become infected with hepatitis B following parenteral exposure to infected blood.[24] Among all U.S. health care personnel, occupationally related HIV infections now total 101.[16] Negative base-line blood tests performed at the time of exposure were confirmed for only 32 of those personnel while initial negative tests were not confirmed for the remaining 69.

As was pointed out in the introduction, dental personnel have almost miraculously been spared infection with HIV. Thousands of unprotected dentists who unknowingly treated HIV-infected patients must have been exposed to HIV infection as the epidemic mounted during the 1980s before gloves and other barriers came into common use. Only six dentists who claim no other exposure risks appear to have acquired HIV infection by occupational exposure.[16] Testing for evidence of prior HIV infection at the time of exposure was not commonly performed in dentistry until the 1990s. Because none of the infected dentists had such baseline blood tests, their HIV infections cannot be firmly linked to time and circumstance of clinical exposure.

HIV infection has developed in a nurse and a technician spattered with HIV-infected blood. Five other medical personnel have acquired HIV infection related to spatter of infected blood to their non-intact skin. The serological status for HIV in these persons was apparently not known when they were exposed.[16,24] *Therefore personnel are required to protect eyes, mucosa, skin, and hands from spatter and direct contact with blood and blood-contaminated body fluids during dental treatments of all patients.*[100] *Precautions must also be made to minimize risks of injuries with sharp instrumentation.*

Patients seriously ill enough with AIDS to be seen in a hospital setting may also harbor transmissible respiratory infections, such as tuberculosis (TB) and cytomegalovirus infection (CMV).[17,53] As indicated in the section titled, Epidemiology of Other Infection Risks, transmission of drug-resistant TB from immunocompromised patients is a growing concern. Personnel without adequate barrier protection should avoid exposure to coughing, saliva-spatter, and heavy aerosols from HIV-infected persons with signs of respiratory infection. This applies especially to pregnant women, since CMV can be detrimental to the newborn infant of a mother recently infected with CMV. CMV is also bloodborne.

HIV infection risks for dental patients

With proper use of infection control measures in dental practice there should be no risk for a dental patient of contracting HIV or other transmissible infections from office personnel or other patients.

HIV has not been transmitted to dental patients from infected clinical personnel anywhere in the United States but in one unique outbreak.[20,32] In a situation that has stood by itself through mid-1993, a group of six patients were found to be infected with the same strain of HIV as infected a Florida dentist who treated them.[20,32] The patients had no other apparent risk factor

and the dentist with symptoms of well-developed AIDS had persisted in treating patients. Some kind of doctor-to-patient transmission seems likely. At this time there are no reports of other patients infected with HIV by infected dentists or physicians. One or more alleged HIV cross-infections between patients attributed to contaminated dental equipment have come under investigation.[16]

HIV data related to infection control

Data that provide a better understanding of disease agents, their survival qualities, and clinical transmission potentials help us institute effective infection control. HIV data are somewhat reassuring and explain the amazingly low occupational risk of HIV infection for dental personnel.[8,67]

1. Unlike hepatitis B virus, HIV has usually been found in very low levels in blood of infected persons. This is especially true of asymptomatic persons who are the most difficult to recognize and would be most likely to be treated in private offices.[3,25,68]

2. HIV was detected in only 28 of 50 samples of blood from infected persons. In saliva from infected persons, HIV was detectable in only 1 of 83 samples.[56]

3. In dried infected blood, 99% of HIV has been found by CDC investigators to be inactive in about 90 minutes.[25] Longer survival data on larger numbers of HIV grown in laboratory cell cultures have created false impressions about HIV survival in dried infected blood. However, *when kept wet* the virus may survive for 2 or more days.[93] Caution is required with containers of used needles in which the virus may remain wet.

4. HIV is killed by all methods of sterilization. When used properly all disinfectants except some quaternary ammonium compounds are said to inactivate HIV in less than 2 minutes.[8,25,91]

5. HIV has been transmitted by blood-contaminated fluids that have been heavily spattered or splashed.[25] However, aerosols, such as those produced during dental treatments, have not been found to transmit hepatitis B or HIV infection.[25,82]

6. *Barriers have proven successful in protecting dental personnel in hospital dentistry and in all other dental clinics against HIV and even more transmissible viral infections at the author's institution for over 10 years.*

A recent concern *for the immunocompromised person,* as well as for dental personnel, is airborne transmission of multi-drug−resistant *Mycobacterium tuberculosis.*[7,17,21]

VIRAL HEPATITIS (AGENTS, EPIDEMIOLOGY, INFECTION)

In the 8 years after AIDS was recognized, 38,000 persons developed AIDS. During that same period an estimated 38,400 persons died from hepatitis B, related cirrhosis, or liver carcinoma.[19,28,31]

Infective inflammation of the liver, termed *hepatitis,* can be caused by infection with five varieties of hepatitis viruses labeled A to E. The type of infection is specifically diagnosed by serological testing. A, B, and C types of hepatitis are roughly equally divided among viral hepatitis cases detected in population surveys, with type A being the most prevalent. Types B, C, and D are bloodborne infections. Types A and E are fecal-borne infections.[28,69]

Hepatitis B is found in 1/100 to 1/500 persons in the general population, including dental patients. *Incidence has peaked in areas in association with high rates of intravenous (IV) drug abuse and closely follows the incidence of HIV infection.* 1% to 3% of the U.S. population may carry type C.[23,38,69]

HBV infection, symptoms, and clinical findings

Hepatitis B virus (HBV) must enter the circulating blood in order to reach the liver where the viral DNA causes infected hepatic cells to reproduce the virus. Symptoms usually appear after 2 to 4 months of incubation. Extensive liver damage and illness occur rapidly in about 2 of 10 infected persons. *Symptoms and signs* include nausea, vomiting, chronic fatigue, mental depression, fever, joint aches, darkened urine, jaundice, elevated liver enzymes, and possibly diarrhea or rash. Mortality is 2% or less, but tends to be 2% or higher in persons over 30 years of age.[30,38] (Cytomegalovirus and Epstein-Barr virus infections may also produce jaundice and elevated liver enzymes.)

Since only 2 infected persons in 10 show symptoms, the remaining 8 persons usually are not aware of the infection. For this reason it is *impossible to detect many infected persons by medical history.* Whether infected persons are symptomatic or not, they can transmit hepatitis B. Usually within 1 year, 9 of the 10 persons develop immunity to hepatitis B and are no longer infectious. Unfortunately *1 out of each 10 infected persons remains infected and infectious,* often for the remainder of life. Acute cirrhosis may be fatal within a number of months. If illness was not severe and chronic infection persists, in 20 to over 30 years increased risks of cirrhosis or hepatocellular carcinoma may prove fatal. *The possibility of such an outcome produces an overall hepatitis mortality rate of 2%. There is no specific treatment against the virus after infection occurs.*

Other types of hepatitis produce symptoms somewhat similar to those of hepatitis B.[28,38,39,69] Type A has a shorter incubation of about 1 month, with lower mortality. Persons infected with type A do not remain infected or infectious beyond 8 weeks after symptoms subside. Type C hepatitis is often (75%) anicteric (without jaundice), being detected by an elevation of liver enzymes and serological tests. Type C hepatitis becomes chronic in about one half of persons infected, causing them to remain infectious.

Type D, or delta hepatitis virus, has a curious makeup. It has no outer coating and relies upon cells infected with HBV to provide the required outer layer. Once types B and D infect a person together, usually by the same route and source, the infection becomes much more severe and many times more fatal than infection with hepatitis B alone. Protection against hepatitis B also protects against type D, but not type A, C, or E.[28,69]

Transmission of viral hepatitis

The transmission of viral hepatitis types B, C, and D is mainly by *blood, IV drug abuse, and sexual contact.* Up to billions of hepatitis B virus may occur per milliliter of infectious blood.[24] Hepatitis B (HB) virus is also found in saliva at lower concentrations. HB can be transmitted by contamination of broken skin, the mouth, or eyes with blood-contaminated saliva. One in three exposed persons may be infected with HB. In studies performed *during dental treatments of HBV-infected persons, aerosolization of HBV could not be detected by tests for HB surface antigen.*[82]

Hepatitis B is transmitted in the population by the same routes as HIV infection. *Unlike HIV, however, HBV has been transmitted to family members* by prolonged associations that may involve repeated saliva or blood contamination (e.g., by shared shaving utensils, traces of blood left on bathroom towels, or perhaps extensive sharing of unwashed tooth brushes, or by drinking after one another). *In public, however, neither HIV nor HBV are transmitted by casual contact.*[28,54] Persons with risks for HIV infection are also more likely to be carriers of HBV. Up to 90% of HIV-infected persons have been infected with HBV. Mothers infected with HBV have nearly a 50% chance of infecting their infants at birth. If a mother's infection is recognized, *infants can be easily and safely protected with antiserum at birth.* If not, up to 90% of infected infants remain carriers for life and have the same increased risk of fatal liver cancer or cirrhosis in 20 to 30 years as adult carriers.

Hepatitis A is excreted from the infected liver into the bile. Both hepatitis A and E are transmitted by the fecal-oral route. Poor hygiene and contaminated food and water are common routes of infection. These types are not a major concern in dentistry.

Blood transfusions were a major source of type B

hepatitis until 1985, and of type C hepatitis until 1991. A test for type C hepatitis was developed in 1990. Testing instituted in hospitals since 1986 for type B and since 1991 for hepatitis C has virtually eliminated transfusions as a source of infections. *A remaining problem is to detect infectious donors during incubation.*[69]

Infection risks for personnel from HBV, HCV and HDV

Personnel can be infected by parenteral exposure, mucosal exposure to infected blood, blood-contaminated saliva, and by spatter of blood contamination to eyes, mouth, or broken skin. Plain saliva also can be weakly infectious. *Aerosolized, blood-contaminated saliva and respiratory secretions that can transmit many respiratory viruses and tuberculosis have not been shown to transmit hepatitis B.*[21,28,37,82]

In contrast to HIV infection, one in three parenteral exposures of personnel to HB-infected blood has caused hepatitis B infection.[38] Therefore, of 300 persons parenterally exposed to HBV, 100 will be infected, instead of the 1 person in 250 to 300 infected when exposed to HIV. With a 2% death probability, 2 of the 100 HBV-exposed persons may die compared with the 1 HIV-exposed person. Thus, a parenteral blood exposure of a nonimmune person to *HBV carries at least 2 times the mortality risk of a similar HIV exposure.* This mortality risk from HB infection could be 6.6 times that of HIV exposure when studies are considered that resulted in only 1/1000 HIV infections per exposure. This latter figure may more closely relate to exposures in dentistry.

Fortunately a vaccine is readily available against HBV. Mortality rates for personnel from HB exposure could approach zero.[28]

Hepatitis C virus (HCV) exposure risks for personnel are now being documented. Early data indicate that infection rates from parenteral exposure with HCV-infected blood are rather low, somewhere between rates for HBV and HIV.[69]

Serological tests related to hepatitis B

Serological tests are available for several *antigens* of hepatitis B virus and for the *serum antibodies* individuals produce against them.[28,38] Testing a blood sample for HBsAg (hepatitis B surface antigen) is used to determine the presence of infection by detecting the protein associated with the surface of the HB virus in the blood. The test is used to detect persons who are infected, whether they are symptomatic or not. Testing for HbeAg (hepatitis B, e antigen) determines presence of an HB antigen that is found in blood when HB virus concentrations are high and relate to the person's ability to infect others.

Testing for anti-HBc (antibody against HB core antigen) can detect antibody against a virus core protein that becomes positive in virtually all persons a few

months after infection and remains positive for years thereafter. *The antibody is used as a marker for previous HB infection, but this antibody is not protective.*

A test for anti-HBs (anti-hepatitis B surface antigen) is performed to determine the presence of *antibodies that can protect against future HB infection.* Detection of anti-HBs means that the person has been infected and has recovered or has been immunized with a vaccine.

Hepatitis A is detected by a test for anti-HAV antibody. Recent infection is indicated by an immunoglobulin M class of anti-HAV antibody.[69] An EIA screening test for type C hepatitis is now used to screen transfused blood; confirmatory tests are also available. Testing of patients and clinical persons is also available.[69] A test for anti-HDV can detect suprainfection with hepatitis D in HBV infection.[38]

Data related to control of hepatitis B

HBV is a relatively stable DNA hydrophilic virus that can withstand drying on surfaces, and presumably upon equipment and clothing, for over 7 days.[15] Up to 1 billion virus particles of HBV can be found per milliliter of infected blood. Disinfectants selected for their ability to inactivate TB and hydrophilic viruses appear able to inactivate HBV. All forms of sterilization destroy the virus.[26,51]

Immunization against hepatitis A and B

A vaccine against type A hepatitis has been developed and found effective in clinical trials. It should be available by 1994.[86]

Type B hepatitis is effectively prevented by either of two new, genetically engineered vaccines now derived from bread yeast, Engerix-B (Smith Kline and French Laboratories) and Recombivax B (Merck Sharp and Dohme).[38] The antigenic protein of these genetically engineered vaccines is identical to the purified viral surface protein antigen used in the original "killed" vaccine derived from the serum of HB-infected persons.

Vaccination requires one dose followed with another, 1 month later, and a third dose 6 months after the first. Hepatitis vaccines must be given in the arm, not the hip. Both vaccines (yeast and human derived) have as few or fewer side effects compared to other injected vaccines. Protection of those who form antibodies is virtually 100%.

Tests for HB antibody; boosters

Persons with a history of exposure to HB and those who have worked in dentistry for several years may prefer to be tested for anti-HBs before being immunized to see if they need the vaccine. A test for antigen (HBsAg) is useful to detect an asymptomatic carrier (chronically infected) state. Persons who are carriers (HBsAg positive) cannot produce antibody, and they would want to test family contacts and immunize those not already exposed.

One to 6 months after vaccination against hepatitis B is completed, it is important that dental personnel (as high risk persons) obtain a test to determine if protective anti-hepatitis B surface antigen antibodies (anti-HBs) were formed.[23,28] One or more in 30 vaccinated adults under 40 years of age may not respond to three vaccine injections. Still higher percentages of persons over 40 years do not respond since the immune response gradually lessens with age.[28]

Three or more years after they were vaccinated, many dental personnel realize that they have never had a follow-up antibody test. In the author's experience their antibody level is often undetectable by then and their ability to respond cannot be evaluated without a booster. Many prefer to save the cost of an initial test by getting a booster dose and a test a month later.

Boosters are not recommended for the general health care profession during the first 6 years after immunization.[28] A booster effect is usually experienced upon infection in a person who has produced antibodies. Because of the crisis situation that can surround an exposure, the time it takes to obtain test results after an exposure, and *the problem in dentistry of often never knowing when a small exposure has occurred,* dental personnel often prefer to have their blood tested with a radioimmunoassay test for anti-HBs to check immunity after 3 years. If test results are below 10 serum ratio units, in the author's opinion they should take a booster dose of HB antigen. This is in keeping with the recommendation for having a booster dose when a known exposure occurs and antibody in a previously immunized person is deficient.[28]

EPIDEMIOLOGY OF OTHER INFECTION RISKS

Agencies are concerned that dental personnel and patients are protected against risks of all infections borne by blood, saliva, and respiratory secretions. Routine medical histories are important, but cannot be relied upon for detecting infected patients or for limiting the use of specified "universal precautions" for all patients. In addition to HIV and hepatitis B, C, and D (discussed previously), other transmissible infections of concern include *infectious mononucleosis* (Epstein-Barr virus infection), *cytomegalovirus, herpes simplex I and II,* and *tuberculosis.* Agents of *measles, mumps,* other childhood infections, and some other *respiratory infections* are also transmissible, especially in indistinguishable early stages of infection. Measles and mumps can be severe in adults. (See Chapter 5, Patient Assessment, Plate 1, showing oral manifestations associated with communicable diseases.)

In 1990, 23% of measles infections occurred in persons over 19 years of age. The mortality rate was 0.3%; one third of fatal cases involved non-immunized adults.[22] Measles outbreaks among college students have been severe.[27]

Multi-drug–resistant tuberculosis bacteria (MDR-TB) are an increasing concern.[17] They are resistant to two or more of the more common therapeutic drugs and *are highly transmissible by aerosols produced by productive coughing.* Infections seldom become active in healthy adults, but an active infection can remove a clinical person from practice for months until the infection is controlled and is no longer transmissible. Infection with MDR-TB can be rapidly fatal for immunocompromised persons.[17]

The least familiar disease is cytomegalovirus infection, a sexually and blood-transmitted disease that often resembles infectious mononucleosis. Especially during pregnancy a newly infected woman is faced with possible intrauterine or perinatal infection of her infant. Developmental defects can occur in 5% to 10% of infected infants resulting in neuromuscular, auditory, and visual impairments.[53] This is just another infection to which operatory personnel are vulnerable and can be *prevented by universal use of barrier protection.*

Personnel should avail themselves to **immunizations** against measles, polio, and tetanus. Annual or semi-annual skin tests for tuberculosis (PPD) are urged and may soon be required for dental personnel. *Hepatitis B immunization is a Federal OSHA requirement unless an employee documents his or her understanding of the risks and his or her refusal.* Current regulations require employers to pay for hepatitis B immunization, but not for confirmatory testing a month after immunization is complete. Employers or workmen's compensation must pay for serological testing of employees following exposure incidents related to HIV and HBV. Measles vaccination is required for persons born after 1956, or they must show proof of immunity for admission to most colleges.[29] This is also an excellent requirement for dental personnel.

Immunization against viral influenza and pneumococcal pneumonia may be elected and are advisable. Mumps immunization is highly desirable for male and female personnel who lack a history of immunization or childhood infection. Diphtheria and pertussis immunizations are usually obtained during infancy. Vaccines to prevent HIV, hepatitis C virus, and other common infections are anticipated in years to come.

EXPOSURE ASSESSMENT PROTOCOL (see OSHA regulation)

OSHA does not regulate students. However, dental students are required to follow the same *exposure protocol incident plan* as dental employees, but with any appropriate differences for students such as source of medical care. This requires that if blood-contaminated body fluid from a patient is spattered to mucous membranes or broken skin of a clinical person, or if exposure is produced by cut or puncture with a contaminated sharp instrument, the protocol must be followed immediately before the patient leaves. If possible, the patient's potential to transmit hepatitis B and HIV infection is determined and the student's susceptibility to hepatitis B is determined. The attending physician who helps with these determinations then provides, if indicated, hepatitis B immunoglobulin, hepatitis booster, anti-HIV testing, and counseling.

MEDICAL HISTORY

The medical history serves several purposes: (1) to detect any unrecognized illness that requires medical diagnosis and care; (2) to identify any infection or high risk that may be important to a clinical person exposed during examination, treatment, or cleanup procedures; (3) to assist in managing and caring for infected patients; and (4) to reinforce use of adequate infection control procedures, bearing in mind that general history taking is not capable of detecting all infectious persons. *Only conscientious use of universal precautions provides safety.* Symptoms of persistent respiratory illness, night sweats, chronic fatigue, and weight loss can be symptomatic of either tuberculosis or HIV infection. With increasing occurrence of multi-drug–resistant tuberculosis bacteria (MDR-TB), a dentist's medical history of HIV-infected dental patients and others at high risk should be kept abreast of the current medical care and surveillance under the patient's physician. Be aware of the relationship of all infections (and their characteristics) when taking a medical history and performing an initial general examination at each appointment. Refer to Chapter 5 for more detail.

PERSONAL BARRIER PROTECTION
Gloves

Persons with chronic HBV or HIV infection should curtail any treatment activities that would jeopardize the patient. *All persons with weeping or draining lesions that could infect patients should abstain from patient contact.*[18] Dry, non-draining lesions should be kept well protected from clinical contamination.

OSHA regulations specify that all clinical personnel must wear **treatment gloves** during all treatment procedures. *After each appointment, or if a leak is detected, remove gloves, wash hands, and put on fresh gloves* (Figs. 4-3 and 4-4). *Gloves must not be washed or used with more than one patient.* Inexpensive disposable well-fitting treatment gloves are available for chairside

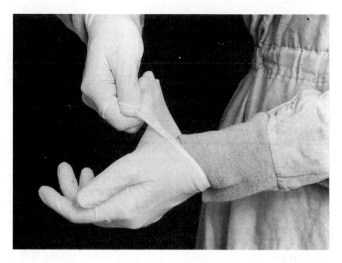

Fig 4-3. To remove a contaminated glove, pinch the palm side of outer cuff surface with gloved fingers of other hand. Pull off glove, inverting it. Both gloves can be removed simultaneously in this manner. Or, after removing one, *insert bare fingers under the cuff* to grasp and pull off remaining glove. *Discard gloves safely.*

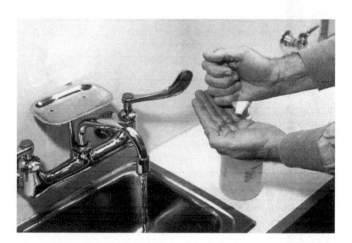

Fig. 4-4. To wash hands after removing treatment gloves, operate pump as shown with clean underside of a wrist. Also, operate faucet handles the same way to avoid contamination or use foot controls. Never touch handles with contaminated gloves.

use. They should be dispensed carefully to avoid contaminating others in the box. The value of gloves was emphasized by finding that occult blood persisted under dentists' fingernails for several days after patient contact.[4]

Treatment gloves cannot protect against punctures, so be cautious. Gloves that become penetrated or torn can imbibe patient fluids and must be removed. Instead of a barrier, gloves worn for more than one patient or for prolonged periods can harbor blood and saliva-borne microorganisms. Washing gloves with hand soaps can reduce glove integrity leaving personnel more vulnerable. Instead of attempting to wash the gloved hands prior to opening drawers or handling items adjacent to the operatory, use a paper towel or food handler's overglove to control contamination.

Increased marketing competition has reduced glove prices and improved quality of latex treatment gloves appreciably. *Viruses have been found to penetrate no more than 1 intact latex glove in 100.*[66] Gloves must meet new Food and Drug Administration (FDA) regulations; less than 4 per 100 can have a leak detectable by a water test.[52] Some companies set their standards at less than 2% to 3%. Store boxes of gloves out of sunlight and store multiple boxes in tightly closed, heavy plastic bags to minimize oxidation. If in doubt about a supplier's gloves, contact the distributor about FDA regulations and manufacturing standards of the product. Products that do not meet FDA standards and advertising claims are subject to removal from the market if consumers report lack of compliance.

While cleaning and sorting used sharp instruments, wear *puncture-resistant* **utility gloves.** Nitrile latex gloves are preferred; they can be washed inside and out, disinfected, or steam autoclaved, as needed. Wear treatment gloves inside the heavy gloves if they must be shared.

Instructions for handwashing

At the beginning of a routine treatment period, remove watches, jewelry, and rings, or at least those with enlarged projections or stones that can penetrate gloves; then **wash hands** with a suitable cleanser. Lather hands for at least 10 seconds, rubbing all surfaces, and rinse. Use a clean brush to scrub under and around nails. Repeat at least once to remove all soil. Wash hands well when changing gloves.[57] Even good quality surgical gloves develop minor pin holes or leaks during vigorous use. Prior to surgery use a prescribed surgical scrub, washing and rinsing from hands toward elbows. (Reserve a separate brush to clean instruments!)

Hand cleansers containing a mild antiseptic like 3% PCMX (p-chloro, meta-xylenole) or chlorhexidine are preferred to control transient pathogens and to suppress overgrowth of skin bacteria.[50] Hand cleansers with 4% chlorhexidine may have broader activity for special cleansing (e.g., for surgery, when a glove leaks, or when a clinical person experiences an injury), but can be hazardous to eyes.[65,94] PCMX cleansers have been found equally effective, non-irritating, and preferable for routine use.[94]

Protective eyewear; masks; hair protection

Protective eyewear may consist of goggles, or glasses with solid side-shields. Wear a **mask** to protect against aerosols. *Face shields* are appropriate for heavy spatter, but a mask is still required to protect against

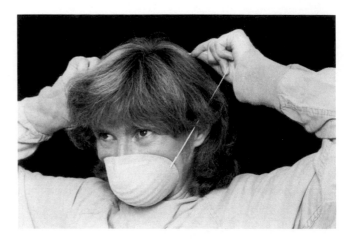

Fig. 4-5. Remove the mask as shown. Grasp the mask ties or elastic band behind the head instead of grasping the contaminated mask. Before treatments, put on mask and eyewear before washing and gloving hands. After treatments, first remove gloves, then eyewear (grasping only the temple pieces) and mask, and lastly wash hands.

aerosols that drift behind the shield.[11,79] Spatter can also pass under the edge of a short shield and strike the mouth. Anti-fog solution for eyewear can be obtained from opticians or product distributors.

Put on eyewear with clean hands before gloving and remove it with clean hands after gloves are removed. Grasp eyewear by the temple pieces. Grasp the mask only by the string or band at the sides or back of the head to remove it (Fig. 4-5). Change the mask every hour, or sooner if it becomes wet. Discard the mask when the patient is dismissed after a treatment instead of wearing it around the neck where contaminated edges can rub against the neck. Avoid touching facewear during treatments to avoid cross-contamination.

When eyewear or shields are removed they should be cleaned and disinfected. (To save time, have clean replacement eyewear available while disinfecting used eyewear.) Remove eyewear by grasping the temple pieces with clean fingers; place eyewear on a paper towel and spray with a water-based disinfectant that is allowed to stand for at least 5 minutes. Next, while wearing gloves (for protection against any contamination on lenses), wash eyewear well and reapply disinfectant for 10 minutes, or preferably allow it to soak in a 1:50 to 1:100 solution of 5% hypochlorite bleach, or other disinfectant solution that does not damage eyewear. (One-half ounce of bleach in a quart of water gives an acceptable 1:65 dilution.) Rinse well and dry. If preferred, goggles that can be autoclaved are available from dental distributors.

Masks with the highest filtration are rectangular, folded types used for surgeries.[35] *Dome-shaped masks* are adequate barriers against spatter and are considered to prevent hepatitis B and HIV infection.[82] They *are not adequate to hold back measles, influenza, and other aerosol-borne respiratory viruses or tuberculosis bacteria. To best protect against aerosols, press edges of the rectangular mask close around the bridge of the nose and face.* Masks have been rated according to porosity and effectiveness.[35]

Hair should be kept back out of the treatment field. Hair can trap heavy contamination that if not washed away can be rubbed back from a pillow onto the face at night. *Personnel must protect their hair with a surgical cap when encountering heavy spatter (e.g., from an ultrasonic scaling device).*

Protective overgarments

An *overgarment* must be protective of clothing and skin (see Fig. 4-2). Used overgarments should require a minimum of handling and should be easily laundered. Operatory clothing becomes highly spattered with invisible saliva and traces of blood throughout the day. Hepatitis B and many other microbes can live on dry materials for 1 or more days.[15,54,64,98] Spatter is heavy to the upper surface of the wrists and forearms.[11] Spatter remains on uncovered arms most of the day if not protected by long sleeves. Large cuffs of clinic coat sleeves drag across patient napkins and mouths, become grossly contaminated, and cross-contaminate patients.[104] Therefore, *sleeves with knit cuffs that tuck under gloves are preferred.* If not covered, arms must be washed after each patient if spatter was created. Most office sinks are not deep or wide enough for that purpose.

A simple, lightweight garment that covers the arms and chest up to the neck as well as the lap when seated appears to provide adequate protection. Cloth made of cotton or cotton/synthetic fiber like an isolation garment material appears to be thick enough to protect skin and street clothing from the spatter of most dental treatments. If surgeries or other treatments produce splashing that wets or penetrates a garment, change it as soon as possible and clean the skin. Wear impermeable cloth or plastic when needed to prevent penetration to skin or undergarments.

Wearing contaminated garments home or out of the clinical area is not permitted. Such garments can contaminate family members who sort, handle, and launder soiled clothing, or may infect young children who cling to or even mouth adults' clothing. Contamination with HBV, TB, and respiratory viruses (e.g., respiratory syncytial virus) are of most concern.

Used overgarments are removed and placed directly into a laundry bag with a minimum of handling or sorting before leaving the clinical area, or are left in the operatory if they are not heavily soiled or contaminated and are satisfactory to put back on the same day. *Guidelines call for managing used clinic garments to avoid handling or sorting* (e.g., searching pockets, removing name tags). Persons handling soiled clinical garments must wear protective gloves. Laundering must be provided by the employer. Bags that actually dissolve in the laundry water can eliminate handling.

Laundering with a regular cycle with regular laundry detergent is considered acceptable, following manufacturer's directions.[23] Hot water up to 70° C or cool water containing 50 to 150 ppm of chlorine provided by liquid laundry bleach would provide more antimicrobial action. Use of a hot air dryer and/or ironing is also beneficial.[23,57]

DISPOSAL OF CLINICAL WASTE

Infected blood and other *liquid clinical waste* can generally be poured down a sanitary sewer or drain designated for that purpose, but not mercury and certain chemicals. Aseptic precautions, cleaning, and disinfection must be applied to the basin around the drain. Adding 3 ounces of 5% hypochlorite in water (household bleach) to each 30 ounces of fluid collected in surgical aspiration bottles is recommended before disposing the fluid down the drain.

Contaminated materials such as used mask, gloves, blood/saliva-soaked sponges, cotton rolls, etc., must be discarded safely. OSHA regulations presented previously describe rules and labels required regarding *regulated sharps and soft waste disposal.* OSHA labeling requirements may differ from local protection agency requirements. As pathological waste, excised tissues require separate disposal and may not be discarded into the trash.

Federal Environmental Protection Agency (EPA) and local environmental protection or control agencies regulate the management and disposal of blood-contaminated waste. This usually applies to waste when it leaves the dental office or clinic. Local county and state regulations must be consulted.

As described, judgment is essential in bagging medical waste so injury or direct contact with liquids does not take place, since HIV and HBV can survive beyond a few days while wet. *Separating needles and sharps into hard-walled containers and out of soft trash has provided adequate safety.* Nevertheless, laws governing waste disposal range from the adequate recommendations of the Centers for Disease Control (CDC) to regulations requiring somewhat strict management and tracking of waste disposal at added expense.[23,25]

NEEDLE DISPOSAL

Goals for needle disposal are to (1) dispose of needles in a hard-walled leakproof container which has the OSHA biohazard label; (2) locate the needle-disposal container in the operatory close to where the needle will be used; and (3) avoid carrying unsheathed contaminated needles or containers in a manner that could endanger others or would allow the needles to be accidently spilled (see Chapter 10, Fig. 10-3).[79] If numbers of approved disposal containers are limited, move the well-closed container to where it is needed during cleanup. Follow local regulations for disposal of the container.

PRECAUTIONS TO AVOID INJURY EXPOSURE

Pointed instruments without a hollow lumen have minimal capacity to transmit infected blood into a puncture site. However, the same principles that apply to needles should be reasonably translated and applied to used burs, wires, and sharp instruments from the operatory. Use great care in passing instruments and syringes with unsheathed needles to another person. *Turn sharp and curved ends away from the recipient's hand.*

Two-handed resheathing of needles is not permitted. A needle sheath holder or other safety device or technique should be used for the operator to resheath the needle with only one hand (see Chapter 10, Fig. 10-1).[79]

Remove burs from handpieces when finished; or if left in the handpiece in a hanger, point the bur away from your hands and body. Hanging handpieces upside down in some types of hangers can angle the bur away from the operator. *Carefully and deliberately rehang a handpiece when a cutting instrument must be left in it.*

OVERVIEW OF ASEPTIC TECHNIQUES

Concept: What operatory personnel handle and contaminate has to be discarded or cleaned and properly prepared to prevent cross-contamination; what they do not contaminate, does not. A few simple rules help to avoid wasting costly time and effort between patient appointments:

During each appointment:
1. Directly touch only what has to be touched.
2. Remember, whatever is touched is contaminated.
3. Use one of the following to control contamination:
   A. Clean and sterilize it.
   B. Use a disposable device and discard it after use.
   C. Protect it with disposable, single-use covers.
   D. Scrub and disinfect it as well as possible.

Consistently practiced, these concepts of **asepsis** can reduce exposure risks, reduce cross-infection risks, and reduce cleaning and disinfecting numerous items in the operatory and even the reception office between appointments, where personnel may inappropriately wear contaminated gloves. Examples of items found needlessly contaminated in studies of dental offices include telephones, faucet handles, switches, cabinet and

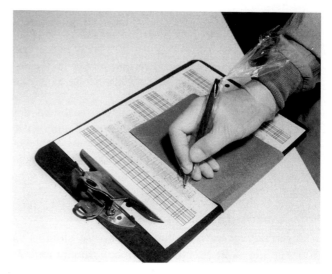

Fig. 4-6. Protect charts from contamination. When charting must be performed without help, rest writing hand on paper towel and use a pen covered (except tip) by plastic bag. Note that cuff of glove should overlap cloth overgarment. Surfaces of both glove and plastic bag must not contaminate chart and its contents.

drawer handles, radiography controls, lamp handles, door handles, charts, and pens.[64] A number of reports provide evidence of cross-contamination and cross-infection risks for patients and personnel related to contact with contaminated surfaces.*

With treatment-soiled gloves, avoid unnecessary contact with all switches, drawers, dispensers, or surfaces on the unit that need not be touched. Use the wrist, arm, or paper towel to operate faucet handles and soap handpump handles. Use a paper towel to handle the phone, drawer pulls, and charts, and a tongue blade to operate uncovered switches. Rest your gloved writing hand on a paper towel when it is necessary to record findings while charting a patient. Pull a slender clear bag over a pen, tip first, then pop the tip through the plastic end and tie the bag snugly in a knot at the other end; discard the bag between patients (Fig. 4-6).

Use single-use plastic bags on control unit and chair back, foil or plastic "baggies" on lamp handles, and adherent plastic sheets or a plastic bag on radiography cone (Fig. 4-7). Use a thin plastic overglove, or a gauze or paper towel to avoid contaminating other objects. Use foot controls for faucets, dental chair, and radiography button.

Once a day, or as needed, use any water-based tuberculocidal disinfectant licensed by the EPA to clean and disinfect other environmental surfaces in the operatory and laboratory.

*References 9,50,54,63,83,98,103.

OPERATORY ASEPSIS
Protection of operatory surfaces; principles

Operatory surfaces that will be repeatedly touched or soiled are best protected with *disposable covers* that can be discarded after each treatment (see Fig. 4-7).[33,43,102] Changing covers eliminates cleaning and disinfecting the surface, saves time, effort, and expense, and can be more protective. Paper ("white newsprint") is useful for work benches and operatory surfaces on which dry contaminated materials are placed. For dental unit trays, paper or plastic film or surgical pack towels should cover the entire tray, including edges. Use plastic or a small sheet of foil wrap on lamp handles, or use removable lamp handles that can be sterilized. (A plastic bag or foil wrap is less expensive and covers better than gauze sponges.) Inexpensive large *clear plastic bags* are used in numerous offices to cover chair back, control unit, and hose supports. Specially sized commercial bags offer various conveniences that are worth the extra price to a successful practice. For economy, clear plastic 15 gallon waste container bags fit many chair backs and control units; plastic, restaurant, silverware bags fit suction handles, air/water syringe handles, and motor ends of low-speed handpieces (see Fig. 4-7).

After each appointment, discard and replace these bags and covers without cleaning and disinfecting these equipment items if they remained covered and uncontaminated.

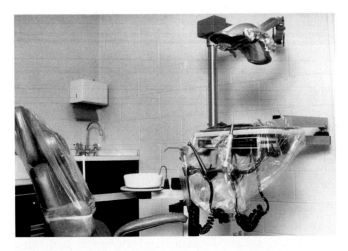

Fig. 4-7. Specially designed or generic plastic bags are used to cover chair, dental unit, and light handles. Changing bags after each patient is more effective and more rapid than disinfection. Damage to equipment from disinfectants is also avoided. Do not routinely disinfect surfaces that have been covered.

Preparation of semi-critical items (attached to the dental unit for reuse) and non-critical items (supporting or environmental)

Instruments that contact cut tissues or penetrate tissues are considered to be *critical items* that require thorough cleaning and sterilization for reuse.[13,33,51] A number of items are attached to the dental unit that are used intraorally, or are handled and touched interchangeably with mucosa by gloved hands coated with blood and saliva. New Centers for Disease Control guidelines consider these to be *semi-critical items*.[33,51] Items that are not ordinarily touched during treatments are termed *non-critical items*.

Semi-critical items. Semi-critical items that touch mucosa are the air/water syringe tip, suction tips, prophy angle, and handpieces. Others (air/water syringe handle, suction hose ends, lamp handle, and switches) are handled or touched interchangeably with treatment instruments that become contaminated with blood and saliva. *Semi-critical items must be removed for cleaning and sterilization unless they are disposable or can be protected from contamination with disposable plastic covers.* This applies especially to air/water syringe tips.

Semi-critical items should not be disinfected. As stated before, they should be covered, cleaned and sterilized, or discarded. Some bacteria often remain after use of the best disinfectant.[64] However, when a cover comes off, or when disinfection is the only recourse, semi-critical items must be scrubbed clean, preferably at the sink, disinfected, and then wiped again using a fresh, alcohol sponge. Surface disinfection is not adequate for items with a lumen such as air/water syringe tips.

Non-critical items. *Non-critical items are environmental surfaces* such as chairs, benches, floors, walls, *and supporting equipment of the dental unit that are not ordinarily touched during treatments.* Lengths of hoses that connect equipment to the control unit become spattered but need not be touched. Contaminated non-critical items require cleaning and disinfection.

Disinfection is always at least a two-step procedure: (1) the initial step involves vigorous scrubbing of the surfaces to be disinfected and wiping them clean; (2) the second step involves wetting the surface with a disinfectant and leaving it wet for the time prescribed by the manufacturer. Many water-based disinfectants contain detergents that make them effective cleaners. So, some products can be used in both steps. But there is no such thing as a "one-step disinfectant." The disinfectant step must always be preceded by cleaning.

Wear protective utility gloves to clean equipment that cannot be covered. For cleaning and disinfecting environmental surfaces, nitrile latex utility gloves are preferred. Disinfectants can penetrate treatment gloves to irritate covered skin, and these less sturdy gloves are prone to small tears. Use a water-based disinfectant cleaner (e.g., a synthetic phenolic complex disinfectant), a chlorhexidine antiseptic scrub, or other suitable cleaner to scrub equipment. Next, wipe items dry with a paper towel. Then wet them with an **EPA-registered disinfectant** and leave them wet for the time specified by the disinfectant manufacturer.

Although uncovered chair arms may become spattered and need to be covered or disinfected, *the chair itself is considered to be a non-critical item.* Areas of the chair not contaminated by spatter need not be disinfected, except for housekeeping purposes. Chair backs and control units are covered to protect control buttons from operator gloved finger contamination and spatter, as well as from the damaging effects of disinfectants; and time for disinfecting is saved.

Disinfectants. Preferred disinfectants are those that can inactivate polio or coxsackieviruses (because they are non-lipid viruses similar to hepatitis B in resistance).[7,13,14,51] Disinfectants must be active against *Mycobacterium* species, common respiratory viruses, and common bacterial hospital pathogens (*Staphylococcus, Pseudomonas* species, etc.). All such disinfectants readily inactivate HIV in 1 to 2 minutes.

Glutaraldehydes at concentrations used for instrument disinfection are far too toxic to be used on operatory surfaces and take 20 minutes at best to kill *Mycobacterium* species.

Unfortunately, the reliability of testing disinfectants against mycobacteria and hepatitis B is controversial and criteria for evaluating disinfectants are being revised.[89] Preferred disinfectants registered by the EPA include: 1:10 to 1:100 dilutions of 5% hypochlorite in water (household bleach); plain dilute iodine solutions; iodophor disinfectants containing phosphoric acid; water-based synthetic complex phenolic derivatives containing 9% o-phenyl-phenol and 1% o-benzyl-p-chlorophenol diluted 1 ounce to 1 quart of water to give O.3% final concentration of synthetic complex phenols; 79% ethyl alcohol sprays containing 0.1% phenylphenol, or other ethyl alcohol disinfectants containing 60% or more alcohol.[36] (Isopropyl alcohol may be used, but ethyl alcohol is preferred.) *Activity of all disinfectants is reduced by organic debris or blood.* Iodines are especially sensitive to blood.[36,97] While most disinfectants can be applied with paper towels or gauze pads, some types of cellulose paper or fiber react with iodine to produce an inactive greenish, black, or blue color reaction with iodine which usually indicates inactivation. Most water-based disinfectants are effective for removing dried blood. Alcohols harden whole blood dried on surfaces.[39,97] Remember, *disinfection cannot occur until fresh disinfectant is reapplied to the thoroughly cleaned surface.*[41,51]

Chlorine and iodine found in some disinfectants can react with or be absorbed by the plastic in some types of dispensing bottles which must be refilled with fresh solution daily. Consult and follow manufacturer's directions in this regard.

Manufacturers specify a time to leave items wet with disinfectant for disinfection. This is usually 10 minutes. Most disinfectants, except plain phenol, appear to be active in about 5 minutes according to manufacturer data. Equipment left wet until the next patient is seated has usually been wet for at least 5 minutes. But this should be taken into careful consideration. Data on kill times should be obtained from the manufacturer. After sufficient time, wet items can be wiped with a paper towel.

Step-by-step preparation of dental chair, dental unit, and instruments

As well as not being acceptable for semi-critical items, the disinfectants generally considered to be most active against microorganisms are unfortunately the most drying or destructive to plastic chair covers and equipment. That is the final argument for using covers wherever possible. Then the effectiveness of disinfectants used becomes less critical and choosing disinfectants in favor of protecting equipment is easier.

Following is an example of step-by-step standard operating procedures for preparation of the dental chair, dental unit, and instruments between appointments. (Remember, do not disinfect surfaces and items covered with plastic drape after each treatment unless the plastic cover was torn or came off during treatment.)

1. With hands still gloved after the last treatment, remove and invert chair back cover, discard cotton rolls and other disposable materials into the cover, and discard cover into the operatory trash bin. Remove and discard gloves aseptically.

2. Wash hands with antiseptic hand soap, rinse, and dry. Place three paper towels on the seat of the dental chair for later placement of air/water syringe and ends of suction hoses. *Put on nitrile latex utility gloves.*

3. With the used suction tip, clean saliva and debris from the cuspidor trap. Discard disposable suction tip into the operatory trash bin.

4. Remove (unscrew) from the anesthetic syringe the re-sheathed needle and discard it with all other sharp disposable items in a sharps container. Using a Stick-shield[R] is advised (see Chapter 10, Fig. 10-3, *C* to *F*).

   Note: Handling needles without using a protective one-handed capping device and gathering instruments without heavy protective gloves account for most injury exposure incidents.

5. Place any loose sharp instruments and instrument cassette into a perforated metal basket, and then lower the basket into disinfectant solution in a covered hard-walled pan. Return the air/water syringe tip, handpieces, and pan of instruments to the cleanup area. Using handles provided, remove the basket of instruments, rinse, and then place into the ultrasonic cleaner.

6. Before handling disinfectant-dispensing bottles, wash utility gloves (on hands) with antiseptic scrub, rinse, and dry.

7. Spray any used bottles, containers, tubes, and unused burs with disinfectant, and wipe with a paper towel. Spray again and leave damp with disinfectant as they are put away. (Spraying in this manner has been found to be effective.[97] However, if there is an objection to spraying a disinfectant, it may be applied with any disposable material that will not inactivate the disinfectant.)

8. Remove the air/water syringe (now minus its removable tip) and suction hoses from the hangers on the control unit. Remove the plastic covers from hose ends and discard. Lay the air/water syringe and suction hose ends on the paper towels previously placed on the dental chair.

9. Invert, remove, and discard plastic drapes from the control unit (Fig. 4-8); remove and discard protective covers from lamp handles, and surface covering from the side table. These disposables may be placed into the large bag removed from the control unit.

10. For any controls and switches that were not covered, wet a paper towel with disinfectant spray and wipe lamp switch and controls that were contaminated. (Do not spray control switches.) Wipe any *contaminated surfaces not previously covered:* side table, arms of dental chair, contaminated drawer handles, radiographic viewbox switch, and paper towel dispenser. Discard wet paper towels.

11. Use a second towel wet with disinfectant to re-wet these items and leave them wet. (Paper towels neutralize iodine disinfectants and should not be used to apply them.)

12. Spray the outside and inside of the cuspidor with disinfectant. Use two paper towels to prevent gloves from contacting the cuspidor while first wiping the outside and then the inside of the cuspidor. Discard towels. Wipe any overspray of disinfectant from the operatory floor. Discard towels into the trash bin.

13. Spray any *contaminated* faucet handles, sink counter top, and trash disposal openings with

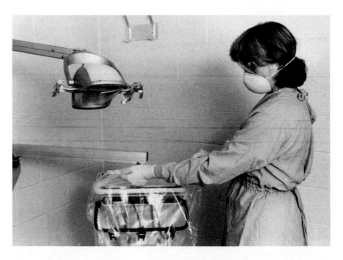

Fig. 4-8. Wear suitable protective gloves to undrape unit. Remove hoses from hangers and lay on paper towels on dental chair. Pull draping bag off control unit so it will invert. Pull clean bag over unit from the front with clean hands and tuck around the back and bottom. Cover equipment support arms as well.

disinfectant and wipe dry with paper towel. Discard towel and re-spray areas with disinfectant and leave damp.

14. Wash utility gloves (still on hands) with strong antiseptic hand scrub or disinfectant cleaner, rinse thoroughly, and dry them with paper towels. Discard towels into trash bin. *Remove utility gloves* and re-hang them in the operatory. Wash hands. Contaminated utility gloves can be cleaned and disinfected. Nitrile latex gloves can be autoclaved.

To prepare the unit for the next patient gloves need not be worn if only clean surfaces that have been protected with covers are touched. Use a paper towel or treatment glove to handle questionable surfaces such as hoses.

1. Pull a large clear plastic bag-cover over the dental control unit from the front and tuck excess up under the unit (see Fig. 4-8). Split the bag up one side to cover mobile delivery system units with large surfaces.

2. Pull another bag down over the chair back; also cover chair arms.

3. Install suction and air/water syringe tips. Place a slender bag over each tip, pushing the tip through the end of the bag and then sliding the bag down to cover all of the handle. For the suction tip, wrap autoclave tape at the tip/bag junction to secure the bag against creeping and to prevent contamination of the handle area of the hose (Fig. 4-9). It usually is not necessary to tape the bag onto the air/water syringe. Press handles into the

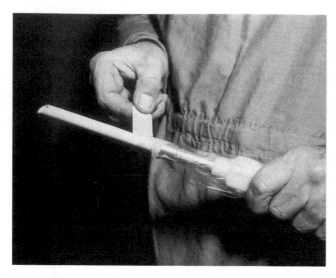

Fig. 4-9. Install suction tip and cover it with a slender plastic bag. Push tip through end of bag and continue sliding bag to cover handle area of hose. Wrap a piece of suitable tape at the bag/tip junction as shown to secure bag against creeping and prevent exposing handle to contamination. After use, bag will come off with plastic tip for easy removal and disposal.

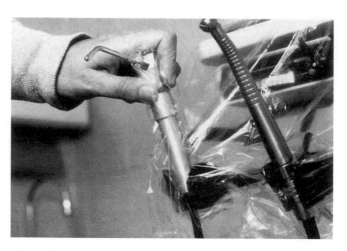

Fig. 4-10. Replace equipment attached to hoses by using the device to simply press loose plastic film into forked holder. Use tape or rubber band to hold plastic covers in place if indicated.

forked hangers on the unit that are covered by the plastic bag (Fig. 4-10).

4. Install sterilized handpieces. A plastic sleeve may be used to cover the motor-end of the low-speed handpiece that is not sterilized (see Fig. 4-7). Re-hang handpieces. If the plastic film obstructs the electric eye in the hanger, use a small finger to pull out the film when the handle is removed.

5. Set out materials and instrument packs; open packs being careful not to touch sterilized instruments with bare hands.

6. Seat the patient and put on a clean mask, eyewear, and gloves.

Protection of complex devices against contamination

Cameras and light-curing devices are examples of complex devices that must be protected against contamination. They are used in the operatory and *cannot be sterilized or even readily disinfected.* Clear plastic bags of suitable size obtained from plastics supply companies are effective single-use protective barriers. Tear a small hole to pull over the lens holder of the camera. A hole is usually not needed to expose the curing light lens or radiograph cones.

PROCEDURES, MATERIALS, AND DEVICES FOR CLEANING INSTRUMENTS BEFORE STERILIZATION

According to the American Dental Association guidelines and Centers for Disease Control specifications, instruments that touch mucosa or penetrate tissues must be *cleaned* and then sterilized before reuse (Box 4-1).[7,33]

Box 4-1. Do's and don'ts of instrument recycling

Do the following:

- Wear protective puncture-resistant gloves to handle used instruments
- Keep instruments wet in an antibacterial solution before cleaning
- Use an ultrasonic cleaning device
- Test and maintain the ultrasonic device periodically
- Use good quality sterilizer equipment
- Read the operator's manual and follow operation instructions for the sterilizer
- Have sterilizers annually inspected regarding gaskets, timer, valves, temperature and/or pressure gauges
- Use proper water or chemicals to operate, clean and maintain sterilizer
- Place only dry instruments in the sterilizer
- Use a wrap that will be penetrated by the steam or gas used
- Load the sterilizer loosely; leave air space between large packs
- Daily read sterilizer temperature and/or pressure gauges
- Use the complete sterilizer monitoring system outlined: use indicators daily; spore tests weekly
- Keep a record of daily indicators and spore tests

Don't do the following:

- Place wet instruments into any type of sterilizer unless so instructed
- Over-wrap cloth packs, or use impermeable wraps for steam or chemical vapor pressure sterilization
- Use closed, non-perforated trays, foil, canisters, or other sealed containers in gas or steam sterilizers
- Overload or cram packs together in the sterilizer
- Decrease the required time for sterilization
- Add instruments to a sterilizer without re-starting the cycle
- Sterilize viability control strips supplied with spore tests

Principles and procedures for handling and cleaning instruments after treatment

Instrument cleaning procedures should be designed to be effective while avoiding risks such as grasping and scrubbing groups of single- and double-ended sharp instruments. (Such hand grasping and scrubbing are the most exposure-prone tasks encountered after treatments, even when protective utility gloves are worn.)

*The safest and most efficient instrument cleaning procedures involve ultrasonic cleaning of used instruments kept in a perforated basket or cassette throughout the cleaning procedure. Wear **protective utility gloves at all times to handle contaminated containers and instruments.*** Transport to the cleanup area instrument cassettes and any loose instruments in a perforated metal basket lowered by handles into a disinfectant solution contained in a covered hard-walled pan. (Used instruments are commonly placed in an antimicrobial cleaning solution before cleaning them, as this softens and loosens debris.) Leave instruments in their basket or cassette while rinsing them well. Next, clean them in an ultrasonic cleaning device (Fig. 4-11), rinse them again, and then carefully inspect the instruments for debris. Use tongs to remove any instruments left uncleaned. Remove the debris from these instruments individually, keeping hands well protected with utility gloves. Dip instruments likely to rust into a rust inhibitor such as fresh rust-retarding cleaning solution (e.g., solution from Health Sonics Corp., Pleasanton, California). Drain and air-dry instruments in cassettes or carefully spill baskets of instruments onto an absorbent towel. Wet instruments can be patted with a thickly folded towel. Still wearing protective gloves, properly package the instruments together with internal and ex-ternal sterilization indicators suited to the sterilization process used.

Protective utility gloves made of nitrile latex are the most puncture resistant and are obtainable from dental suppliers. These gloves can be washed and wiped with disinfectant or autoclaved after use as needed. Household utility gloves are not suitable for handling and cleaning sharp instruments.

Instrument containers are used as specified by the OSHA regulations: (1) Immediately, or as soon as possible after use, place contaminated reusable sharps into appropriate containers until they are properly reprocessed. Containers must be puncture resistant, properly labeled or color coded, and leakproof on sides and bottom. Cover the container to transport the instruments to the cleanup area. (2) Reusable contaminated sharps shall not be stored or processed in a manner that requires employees (with or without protective gloves) to reach by hand into containers where these sharps have been placed.[79,100] If instruments can be securely enclosed in a cassette (Fig. 4-12), re-wrapping the cassette in its sturdy sterilization wrapping paper may be considered by OSHA authorities to provide sufficient protection against injury or contamination while transporting the instruments. This option should be verified with the cassette manufacturer or local OSHA authorities. Otherwise, the OSHA criteria are met by placing instruments into a basket or cassette with attachable handles, or by using other methods that avoid hand-reaching into the hard-walled containers to place, process, and remove used instruments.

Some OSHA consultants have prescribed that used instruments be placed in a hard-walled container of disinfectant soaking or holding solution before removing the instruments from the operatory. Although soaking is desirable to prevent debris from hardening on instruments, the OSHA regulation does not appear to address such holding solutions.

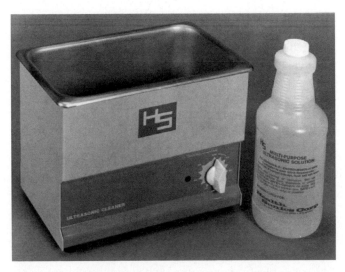

Fig. 4-11. Example of commercial ultrasonic cleaner with rust-inhibiting soaking and cleaning solution. (Courtesy of Health Sonics Corp., Pleasanton, California.)

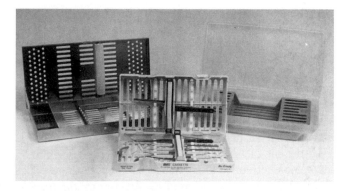

Fig. 4-12. Examples of three cassettes designed to hold instruments while they are cleaned and sterilized. (Supplied by Health Science Products, Birmingham, Alabama *(left)*, Hu-Friedy, Chicago, Illinois *(center)*, and Zirc Dental Products, Inc., Minneapolis, Minnesota *(right)*.

*A **disinfectant holding solution** for transporting and/or soaking used instruments* should contain a detergent, be economical so it can be discarded frequently, not corrode instruments in a reasonable time, be one of the least inactivated by organic debris, not give off toxic aldehyde vapors, and have 10 minute well-verified antimicrobial claims against TB and preferably against polio or coxsackievirus. Some concentrated phenolic-derivative products that must be diluted for use and a product recommended by an ultrasonic device manufacturer (Health Sonics Corp., Pleasanton, California) meet most of these criteria reasonably well. However, no product is currently considered able to completely disinfect soiled instruments, so protective gloves must still be worn until the instruments have been fully wrapped for sterilization.

When it is necessary to **clean instruments by hand,** *use a suitable brush along with a disinfectant cleaner.* Severe irritation, infection of unprotected eyes, or both can result from spatter of the disinfectant, detergents, or chlorhexidine gluconate hand cleansers often used to scrub instruments. Hand injury from double-ended instruments is the other main risk as indicated before.

Wear heavy gloves, eye protection, a mask or a face shield, and a protective garment or apron to protect against spatter. Use a long-handled pan-scrubbing brush. Grasp the mid-handle portion of only a few instruments at a time with fingers and thumb to protect the palm and to rotate the instruments. Brush away from yourself, down into the sink, using at least 5 strokes per end while rotating them. Pay attention to removing visible soil and debris. Rinse with an aerated stream of water to avoid spatter.

Scrape or use an appropriate solvent cleaner to remove coatings such as plaster, wax, cement, and impression material. When finished cleaning, use heavy gloves, disinfectant, and paper towels to clean up spattered or contaminated surfaces around the sink.

Ultrasonic cleaners and solutions

Ultrasonic cleaning is the safest and most efficient way to clean sharp instruments after instruments have been rinsed or soaked (see Fig. 4-11). *Burs* should be ultrasonically cleaned. To contain burs place them in a fine screen basket or kitchen type of metal tea ball. *Some hinged instruments* (e.g., some brands of orthodontics pliers) *should not be submerged in ultrasonic or disinfectant cleaning solutions if hinges will corrode or rust.* Consult their manufacturer.

Ultrasonic cleaning can be just as effective or up to 9 times more effective than hand cleaning if the device functions properly and is used as directed by the manufacturer.[96] An ultrasonic cleaning device should provide fast and thorough cleaning without damage to instruments, have a lid and well designed basket, have an audible timer, and be engineered to prevent electronic interference with other electronic equipment and office communication systems.

Observe operating precautions:

1. Operate the tank one-half to three-fourths full of cleaning solution at all times.
2. Use only cleaning solutions recommended by ultrasonic device manufacturers. Change solutions as directed. An antimicrobial cleaning solution is preferred. Studies sponsored by one company indicated that their antibacterial solution remained free of contamination for about 3 days of continued reuse (Health Sonics Corp., Pleasanton, California).
3. Operate the ultrasonic cleaner for 5 minutes or longer as directed by the manufacturer to give optimal cleaning.
4. Coatings such as plaster, wax, cement, and impression material can be removed with an appropriate solvent cleaner placed in a beaker in the ultrasonic device. Consult ultrasonic device manufacturers or dental product distributors.
5. Verify ultrasonic performance monthly and when poor performance is suspected by using a foil test. Devices that have less than two transducers do not pass the foil test and are not suitable for instrument cleaning. Performance of ultrasonic devices used without periodic testing and maintenance is often poor.[34]

To perform an **ultrasonic cleaner foil test,** remove the basket from the device. Add solution to the tank and operate the device for 5 minutes to expel dissolved gases as directed by the manufacturer. Measure the depth of the solution and the length (longest dimension) of the tank. From a roll of aluminum foil (regular weight at about 16 μm thickness), cut a sheet about 1 inch more than the depth of the solution in the metal tank. Cut the length 1 inch less than the length of the tank. Hold the foil like a curtain vertically submerged in the solution in the center of the tank about $\frac{1}{2}$ inch above the bottom. (Caution: do not immerse fingers.) Without allowing the edges of the curtain to touch the tank, operate the device for exactly 20 seconds. Upon close inspection, every square $\frac{1}{2}$ inch of the foil should show small visible indentations or perforations if the ultrasonic device functions properly. The foil test can be performed in the midline, front, and rear areas of the tank to determine uniformity. Labeled foil sheets can be filed to document test results. (This method was adapted from directions of Health Sonics Corp., Pleasanton, California.)

Instrument containment

Cloth **packs, wraps, tubes** of nylon film, or commercial paper/plastic **bags** are suitable for instrument containment if they are compatible with the method and temperature of sterilization. Various kinds of instrument *trays* and *cassettes* (see Fig. 4-12) are manufactured to contain instruments at chairside and they can be placed in an ultrasonic cleaner, rinsed, and packaged ready for sterilization. Cassettes provide convenience, safety in handling and cleaning batches of instruments, and maintenance of instrument organization for efficient use.

STERILIZATION

Infectious dental patients go undetected more often than they are recognized. Sterilization provides a method of instrument recycling that can be monitored and documented to show that conditions for control of disease transmission were indeed established. Since most instruments contact mucosa and/or penetrate oral tissues, it is essential that reused instruments be thoroughly cleaned and *sterilized* by accepted methods that can be routinely tested and monitored.[7,33,41] Heat sterilization takes less time than high-level sporicidal disinfection which is required when heat or gas sterilization cannot be used. It is important to recognize that sterilization practice was found unreliable in 15% to 31% of dental offices surveyed where routine **monitoring** *was not used* to evaluate and maintain correct sterilization performance.[81]

Accepted methods of sterilization

There are four accepted methods of sterilization:
1. Steam pressure sterilization (autoclave)
2. Chemical vapor pressure sterilization (chemiclave)
3. Dry heat sterilization (dryclave)
4. Ethylene oxide sterilization

Each method and each commercial modification has very specific requirements regarding timing, temperature, suitable packaging of materials, and kinds of items and materials that can be safely and effectively sterilized.[38,40,41] Ignoring any of these specifications can defeat sterilization or damage materials or instruments.

Selection of sterilization methods and equipment

It is best to evaluate office needs and examine various sterilizer capabilities; then carefully select one or two methods of sterilization. Kinds and sizes of sterilization equipment depend upon the treatment instrumentation used in the practice. Stainless steel instruments and mirrors used for operative, endodontic, periodontic or dental hygiene procedures can be sterilized by any accepted method. Both high- and low-speed handpieces are best autoclaved at the present time. Burs, discussed later, can be safely sterilized by dry heat or chemical vapor in a chemiclave or in a gas sterilizer, but, may rust or corrode if not protected from steam in the autoclave. Metal impression trays can be sterilized by any method, but dry heat above 345° F may remove sol-

dered handles. Orthodontic pliers of high quality stainless steel will resist corrosion in an autoclave; lower quality stainless steel found in some pliers must be sterilized by dry heat or chemical vapor. Towels and towelpacks of instruments needed for surgery are best sterilized by autoclaving; chemical vapor pressure sterilization does not penetrate cloth well. Perhaps the widest variety of instruments would be found in pediatric dentistry, and thus may require more than one sterilization method.

A sterilizer will be used every day of practice. Choose reliable sterilization equipment of proper size and cycle time compatible with needs of the practice. Patient load, turnaround time for instrument reuse, size of instrument inventory and instrument variety and instrument quality must all be balanced against the type and size of sterilizer selected and the number of auxiliary personnel employed. Some offices have personnel come in at night to clean and sterilize instruments. Careful planning toward a central goal is more practical, effective, and economical than adapting several sterilization methods to odds and ends of instrument varieties and qualities collected over a period of time. One complication in this systematic effort is that sterilizer modification and development is changing more rapidly now than ever before. *Choosing equipment that is well established still is the safest and most reliable approach.*

STEAM PRESSURE STERILIZATION (AUTOCLAVING)

Sterilization with steam under pressure is performed in a steam autoclave (Fig. 4-13). For a light load of instruments, the time required at 250° F (121° C) is a minimum of 15 minutes at 15 lbs pressure. Time for wrapped instruments can be reduced to 7 minutes if the

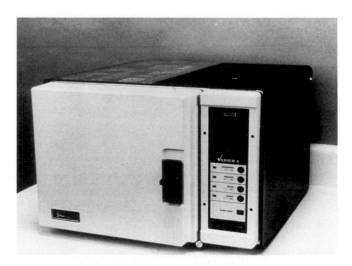

Fig. 4-13. Example of a steam pressure sterilizer (autoclave). (Courtesy of Pelton and Crane, Charlotte, North Carolina.)

temperature is raised to approximately 273° F (134° C) to give 30 lbs of pressure. Time required for the sterilizer to reach the correct temperature is not included. Bench models may be automatic or manually operated. Manual sterilizers should have both a temperature and pressure gauge so temperatures can be related to corresponding temperatures required for sterilization. Unlike hospital autoclaves, bench models depend upon gravity flow to distribute steam throughout the load rather than first evacuating air from the sterilizer and then refilling it with steam. Therefore, bench models require more caution against the use of large or tightly packed loads. Steam must enter and circulate around packs easily. Instrument pans or other impermeable instrument containers must be left open so steam can enter. Except for containers of solutions, all *metal items must be dry.* Moisture evaporating from instruments can slow the heating process. *Sterilization must be routinely tested* (see Monitors of Sterilization).[7,33]

Advantages of autoclaves

Autoclaving is the most rapid and effective method for sterilizing cloth surgical packs and towel packs. Other methods are not suitable for processing cloth packs. Autoclaves handle trays and paper-bagged instruments. Automated models are available, although they still can be misused or fail almost as often as nonautomated ones; they must be evaluated with a biological spore test monitoring system.

Disadvantages of autoclaves

Items sensitive to the elevated temperature cannot be autoclaved. Autoclaving tends to rust carbon steel instruments and burs. Steam appears to corrode the steel neck and shank portions of some diamond instruments and carbide burs.

Sterilization of burs in autoclaves

To avoid corrosion or rust, burs are most simply sterilized in a dry heat oven or ethylene oxide gas sterilizer. For **autoclave sterilization, burs** can be protected by keeping them submerged in a small amount of 2% sodium nitrite solution.[44] *Sodium nitrite crystals (not nitrate)* can be obtained from distributors of scientific products and chemicals, or a pharmacy. Add 20 g (⅔ oz) of nitrite to 1 L of pure water. Store tightly sealed. After ultrasonic cleaning, burs can be rinsed and placed into any small metal or glass beaker with a perforated lid (e.g., a metal salt shaker). Fill the beaker with sufficient fresh nitrite solution to have it above the burs about 1 cm. Leave the container uncovered or use a perforated cover. Place the container of burs and fluid into the sterilizer and operate a normal sterilization cycle. Discard the fluid from the container through the perforated lid. Use sterile forceps to place the burs into a

sterilized bur holder or tray. Store the burs dry. Before use, any nitrite residue can be wiped away, or rinsed off with clean or sterile water, if desired. Nitrites are commonly added to preserve processed meat (e.g., hot dogs).

CHEMICAL VAPOR PRESSURE STERILIZATION (CHEMICLAVING)

Sterilization by chemical vapor under pressure is performed in a Chemiclave (MDT Biologic Co., Rancho Dominguez, Calif.) (Fig. 4-14). Chemical vapor pressure sterilizers operate at 270° F (131° C) and 20 lbs pressure. They are similar to steam sterilizers and have a cycle time of about half an hour. Like ethylene oxide sterilizers, they must be used with a prescribed chemical. Newer models appear to handle aldehyde vapors well; vapors from older models must be safely vented. Loading cautions similar to those for autoclaving must be used. *Water left on instruments loaded into the chamber can defeat sterilization.*

Advantages of Chemiclaves

Carbon steel and other corrosion-sensitive burs, instruments, and pliers are said to be sterilized without rust or corrosion.

Disadvantages of Chemiclaves

Items sensitive to the elevated temperature will be damaged. Instruments must be lightly packaged in bags obtained from the sterilizer manufacturer. Towels and heavy cloth wrappings of surgical instruments may not be penetrated to provide sterilization. Routinely use biological spore test monitoring strips to confirm heat penetration of heavy packs before using them (see Mon-

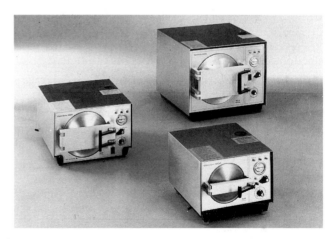

Fig. 4-14. Chemical vapor pressure sterilizer (Chemiclave). (Courtesy of MDT Biologic Co., Rancho Dominguez, California.)

itors of Sterilization). Only fluid purchased from the sterilizer manufacturer can be used. Load only dry instruments, and check the door gasket for leaks in order to avoid frequent sterilization monitoring failures.

DRY HEAT STERILIZATION
Conventional dry heat ovens

Dry heat sterilization is readily achieved at temperatures above 320° F (160° C). Conventional dry heat ovens are merely heated chambers that allow air to circulate by gravity flow (gravity convection). Packs of instruments must be placed at least 1 cm apart to allow heated air to circulate. Individual instruments must actually be at 320° F temperature for only 30 minutes to achieve sterilization.[45] However, a conventional oven may require an additional 0.5 to 1.5 hours to heat a lightly wrapped, properly spaced load of instrument packs to sterilization temperature. Time required in use will also depend upon the efficiency of the oven for its size, the size of the load, and how the load is packaged. Foil wrap or special nylon bags are used. Sixty to 90 minutes may be required to sterilize a medium load of lightly wrapped instruments in an oven set at a range of 335° F to 345° F. Temperatures vary at least 5 degrees above and below the setting, so a range rather than a specific temperature must be set.

Without careful calibration, more sterilization failures are obtained with ordinary gravity convection dry heat ovens than any other type of sterilizer. The only accurate way to calibrate a sterilization cycle in most relatively inexpensive industrial and professional dry heat ovens is by using an external temperature gauge (pyrometer) attached to a thermocouple wire. The other end of the wire is extended inside the oven and tied to an instrument in a centrally located pack to measure its exact temperature. Battery operated pyrometers are available from scientific supply companies for under $100. The pyrometer can continue to be used by fastening the wire to a control instrument left in the sterilizer.

Short-cycle high-temperature dry heat ovens

A rapid high-temperature process that uses a forced-draft oven (a *mechanical convection* oven that circulates air with a fan or blower) is now available that reduces total sterilization time to 6 minutes for unwrapped and 12 minutes for wrapped instruments (Fig. 4-15) (Cox Manufacturing Corp., and Dentronics Corp.). These short-cycle high-temperature dry heat ovens operate at approximately 370° F to 375° F. Chamber size of one brand is limited to processing about one set of instruments at a time, but is more effective for wrapped instruments, and also may be adapted for a shorter heat disinfection cycle (consult the Cox Manufacturing Corp.).

Ovens sold specifically for medical applications must first be examined by the U.S. Food and Drug Administration (FDA). This has not prevented clinicians from using their best efforts to adapt equipment for effective use in their offices. Legal professionals have also begun to anticipate how a jury may view use of home roasting ovens to sterilize professional treatment instruments. However, reasonably priced small ovens manufactured for industrial and scientific use by industrial manufacturers (e.g., Blue M Co., Blue Island, Illinois) can provide more accuracy and reliability for professional use than ovens designed for home use. Careful calibration is still imperative.

Proper, weekly monitoring of all sterilizers, including dry heat ovens, is imperative.

Advantages of dry heat

Carbon steel instruments and burs do not rust, corrode, or lose their temper or cutting edges if they are well dried before processing. Industrial forced-draft hot air ovens usually provide a larger capacity at a reasonable price. Rapid cycles are possible at high temperatures.

Disadvantages of dry heat

High temperatures may damage more heat-sensitive items, such as rubber or plastic goods. Sterilization cycles are prolonged at the lower temperatures. Heavy loads of instruments, crowding of packs, and heavy wrapping easily defeat sterilization. Cycles are not automatically timed on some models. Inaccurate calibration,

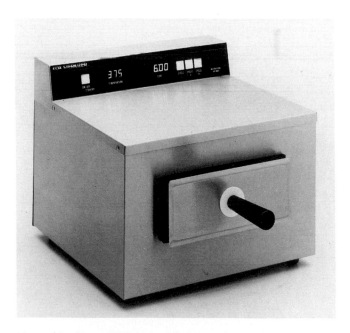

Fig. 4-15. Cox rapid heat transfer dry heat sterilizer. (Courtesy of E.T.M. Corp., Monrovia, California.)

lack of attention to proper settings, and adding instruments without re-starting the timing are other common sources of error.

ETHYLENE OXIDE STERILIZATION

Ethylene oxide sterilization is the most gentle method for sterilizing complex instruments and delicate materials. Automatic devices sterilize items in several hours and operate at elevated temperatures well below 100° C. Less expensive devices operate overnight to produce sterilization at room temperature (Fig. 4-16). Both types meet OSHA requirements. Porous and plastic materials absorb the gas and require aeration for 24 hours or more before it is safe for them to remain in contact with skin or tissues. Units with large chamber sizes hold more instruments or packs per cycle; however, the cost of large units is a significant consideration. Some chamber designs or sizes are better suited to accept stacks of instrument trays. Manufacturers should be consulted to obtain detailed information about these sterilizers. Consult infection control texts, or dental product distributors (Anderson Products Co., Haw River, North Carolina; 3M Co., Minneapolis).

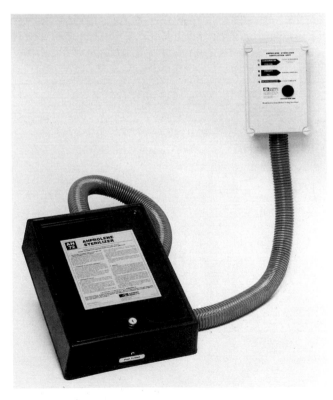

Fig. 4-16. Room temperature ethylene oxide sterilizer. (Courtesy of Anderson Products Co., Burlington, North Carolina.)

BOILING WATER

Boiling water does not kill spores and *cannot sterilize* instruments. However, heat can reach and kill bloodborne pathogens in places that liquid sterilants and disinfectants used at room temperature cannot reach. Boiling is a method of high-level disinfection that is useful when actual sterilization cannot be achieved (e.g., in case of a sterilizer breakdown).[13] Well-cleaned items must be completely submerged and allowed to boil at 98° C to 100° C (at sea level) for 10 minutes. Great care must be exercised that instruments do not boil dry. Simple steaming is not reliable. Pressure cooking, similar to steam autoclaving, is preferred and would be required at high altitudes.

NEW METHODS OF STERILIZATION

Various new methods of sterilization are under investigation and development. The microwave oven has major limitations for sterilizing metal items without damaging the machine and reaching all sides of the instruments. Research efforts to overcome such limitations are ongoing in industry. Use of peroxide vapor sterilization is under development (AMSCO, Erie, Pennsylvania). Ultraviolet light is not highly effective against RNA viruses such as HIV and is not very effective against bacterial spores.[91,95] Incomplete exposure of all surfaces and poor penetration of oil and debris are other limitations. Ultraviolet irradiation may be useful for sanitizing room air to help control tuberculosis bacteria.[21]

One valuable guide to whether a commercial device is an effective sterilizer rests upon whether the FDA can find it equivalent to other effective and proven devices now in common use. Before purchasing any medical device in question, require the manufacturer to provide documentation of FDA pre-marketing review.

MONITORS OF STERILIZATION

Sterilization assurance not only protects patients from cross-infections, but protects personnel from the infections of previous patients as well. Effective instrument sterilization is assured by routine monitoring of instrument sterilization.

In microbiology literature, *sterilization is defined as killing all forms of life including the most heat-resistant forms, bacterial spores.* For instruments that can penetrate tissues, this provides control of spore-forming tetanus and gas gangrene species, as well as all pathogens borne by blood and secretions. For instrumentation used in body cavities that routinely touches mucosa, using criteria for sterilization provides a margin of safety for assuring destruction of hepatitis B, mycobacteria and other pathogenic bacteria and viruses that can become involved in cross-infections.

Weekly sterilization monitoring of highly efficient automated sterilizers in hospitals has been mandated for many years by the Joint Commission of Accreditation of Hospitals (Chicago, Illinois), an organization formed by the profession to monitor and accredit its own performance. Many state examining or disciplinary boards have now provided that type of regulation. Defense against litigation has also become a concern of professional liability insurers. Sterilization must be tested weekly with biological spore tests using heat-resistant spores and tested daily with process indicators.[7,33] Routine monitoring and *documentation in a daily-entry sterilization notebook allows confirmation of sterilizer operator performance, as well as the proper functioning of the equipment.* Problems are caught and corrected. Evidence of sterilization assurance is also in hand when unavoidable localized or systemic post-treatment infections occur and instrument sterilization may be questioned. Sterilization monitoring has four components: (1) sterilization indicator on the bag and date of sterilization, (2) daily process indicator strips, (3) weekly biological spore test, and (4) documentation notebook.

Sterilization indicators and date

Sterilization indicators, both tapes and bags, are marked with heat-sensitive dyes that change color easily upon exposure to heat or sterilization chemicals. Such heat-sensitive markers are important to identify and *differentiate* those packs that have been in the sterilizer from those that have not. *Used alone, these indicators are not an adequate measure of sterilization conditions.* (On a hot day, test a strip of autoclave tape on the dashboard of your automobile parked in the sun!)

Date the packs to be sterilized. Ordinary paper-wrapped packs should be resterilized after 1 month; commercial pouches will preserve sterility for up to 1 year. Ask the manufacturer for product data.

Process indicator strips

Process indicator strips provide an inexpensive, qualitative, *daily monitor* of sterilizer function, operation, and heat penetration into packs. Place one of the inexpensive color-change process indicator strips into every surgical pack and in at least one operative instrument pack in the center of each load. Chemicals on the strip change color slowly, somewhat relative to the temperature reached in the pack. As soon as the pack is opened, the strip can immediately identify breakdowns and gross overloading. The strip is not an accurate measure of sterilization time and temperature exposure.

Biological monitoring strips

A biological monitoring spore test strip is the *accepted weekly monitor* of adequate time and temperature exposure. Spores dried on absorbent paper strips are calibrated to be killed when sterilization conditions are reached and maintained for the necessary time to kill all pathogenic microorganisms. An assistant processes a spore strip in a pack of instruments in an office sterilizer each week. Tests can be evaluated in the office. However, by sending the strip to a licensed reference laboratory for testing the dentist obtains independent documentation of monitoring frequency and sterilization effectiveness. In the event of failure, such laboratory personnel provide immediate expert consultation to help resolve the problem.

Documentation notebook

In a notebook affix a single dated, initialed, indicator strip to a sheet or calendar for each work day, followed by a weekly spore strip report. The *notebook* provides valuable sterilization documentation. Dated sterilized instrument packs, bags, and trays provide the final evidence of the sterilization program.

LIQUID STERILANTS/HIGH-LEVEL DISINFECTANTS

Liquid sterilants are those that can kill bacterial spores in 6 to 10 hours. These sterilants are high-level disinfectants and are registered by the Environmental Protection Agency. Sterilants used for high-level disinfection of items for reuse are glutaraldehydes at 2% to 3% concentrations. Greater dilutions are not encouraged for repeated use.

Organic matter and oxidation reduce activity of reused disinfectant baths. Placing wet items into disinfectant trays dilutes the solution. The level does not change because solution is carried out when the instruments are removed. Despite reuse claims of several weeks' duration, studies have shown that disinfectants in heavy use often lost activity during the second week.[88] Therefore, it is wise to place fresh disinfectant into trays on Monday and discard it at the end of Friday.

Glutaraldehydes are irritating, sensitizing to skin and respiratory passages, and can be toxic as indicated in manufacturers' safety data sheets.[51] Keep trays tightly covered in a well-vented area. *Do not use 2% glutaraldehyde solutions to wipe counters or equipment* (e.g., dental unit and chair). Most glutaraldehydes require 20 minutes to kill tuberculosis bacteria in contrast with some synthetic phenol complexes and alcohols that act in 10 minutes or less and are much less toxic.

USES OF HIGH-LEVEL DISINFECTION

Rule: according to the Centers for Disease Control, instruments that penetrate tissues or contact mucosa are termed critical or semi-critical and require cleaning and heat or gas sterilization before reuse.[26,33,51] *Few if any instruments now exist that cannot be heat sterilized.* High-level disinfection is used mainly for plastic items that enter the mouth and that cannot withstand heat sterilization. *Plastic cheek retractors, photographic mirrors, and similar heat-sensitive devices should be replaced with metal types that can be heat sterilized. Disinfection for 20 to 90 minutes in glutaraldehyde germicides is not appropriate for instruments used in the mouth.* Most require 6 or more hours for sterilization. Consult the label. Liquid sterilants cannot process prepackaged instruments or be completely monitored with biological indicators.

Prophy cups should be discarded and never disinfected for reuse. Some cups can be steam autoclave sterilized for reuse. Used anesthesia carpules and anesthesia needles must be discarded after a patient appointment and never be disinfected or heat sterilized for reuse.

TYPES OF INSTRUMENTS AND STERILIZATION METHODS

Periodontal, restorative, and endodontic instruments are readily processed by autoclave or chemical vapor pressure sterilization. Carbon steel instruments and burs, if dried well before sterilizing, are best sterilized by dry heat and chemical vapor pressure sterilizers with less risk of rust.

DENTAL CONTROL UNIT WATER SYSTEMS AND HANDPIECE ASEPSIS

The air-driven high-speed handpiece is one component of a complex system of instrumentation operated by the dental operatory master control unit. Within the head of the handpiece and supported by delicate bearings, an air-driven turbine assembly holds and rotates the cutting instrument at the speeds preferred for cavity preparation. The handpiece is attached by flexible plastic lines to the dental unit which controls air and water supplied to the handpiece. A small orifice located below the neck of the handpiece near the bur supplies either a jet of air to blow away cutting debris or an air-water spray emitted from the same orifice to lubricate and clean the cutting site; this spray cools the cutting bur as well.

These components comprise a complex system that is vulnerable to several unique kinds of **contamination by and through the handpiece.** Oral fluid contamination problems of rotary equipment and especially the high-speed handpiece involve (1) contamination of handpiece external surfaces and crevices, (2) turbine chamber contamination that enters the mouth, (3) water spray retraction and aspiration of oral fluids into the water line, growth of environmental aquatic bacteria in water lines, and (4) exposure of personnel to spatter and aerosols generated by intraoral use of rotary equipment.[1,11,45,47,70]

If not controlled, external and internal contamination of this equipment by oral fluids holds infection potentials for other healthy dental patients. Even sterilization of handpieces cannot control contamination related to water spray retraction and bacterial colonization of water lines that holds infection potentials for immunocompromised patients.

Handpiece surface contamination control

Blood and saliva contaminate the surfaces of handpieces during various dental treatments. Irregular surfaces and especially crevices around the bur chuck are difficult to clean and disinfect, especially by a brief wipe with a disinfectant-soaked sponge.

Submersion of a high-speed handpiece in a high-level disinfectant has not been an option accepted by manufacturers. In tests, thorough scrubbing and applying the best disinfectants to inoculated smooth handpiece surfaces reduced numbers of simple test bacteria but did not completely eliminate them.[85] *Only sterilization can approach complete infection control of handpiece surfaces.*

Turbine contamination control

Contaminated oral fluids may be drawn back into the turbine chamber by negative pressure created either by a Venturi effect during operation or when the turbine continues to spin whenever the drive air is stopped. Oral fluids may also enter around worn bearing seals, or be aspirated into the vent holes in the top of older handchuck operated handpieces or possibly into the air-water spray orifice which communicates with the turbine chamber in some makes. The question is whether debris that contains viable microbes in the turbine chamber may then be vented from holes in the top of the turbine chamber during the next treatment, as indicated by some investigators.[46,70,71]

While turbine contamination can be demonstrated experimentally under extreme conditions on a laboratory bench, it is not clear under what conditions this may occur during clinical treatments, *nor have air-driven high-speed handpieces been clearly implicated in this manner of cross-infection.* Cross-contamination potentials of water-driven handpieces that have been used in a hospital have been more easily demonstrated.[48]

Operating the handpiece between patients to flush the handpiece is prescribed to reduce this risk.[7,26] *Flushing* is most important if the handpiece has not been sterilized, or if water spray retraction has not been permanently corrected.

Water retraction system correction

Dental unit water control systems made before the mid- to late 1980s used water lines that easily expanded when air-water spray was used, and gradually contracted when water pressure was relieved. Handpieces had an annoying tendency to continue to drip immediately after having been used. To overcome the problem in those units, a device was installed that retracted water in the line whenever the spray was stopped. Unfortunately, more than just water could be retracted. Following treatments, oral bacteria have been readily recovered from water samples obtained from the handpieces and water lines of those older dental units.[10,46]

Most bacterial pathogens and viral agents are unable to grow in the water lines, although many may survive for several days. *The minimal recommendation is to operate the handpiece spray for 20 seconds between appointments to help expel any aspirated infectious microorganisms.*[26] If not completely expelled by this flushing, microbes could be expelled while the next patient is treated. Flushing for brief periods has been found helpful for reducing test bacteria.

Agencies recommend correcting water retraction by placing a one-way check valve in the water line.[26,40,42] Check valves clog and fail. *Systems should be tested monthly if not weekly to verify lack of water retraction.*[47] *A simple, inexpensive water retraction testing device is available* from major dental supply companies that takes only about 1 minute to use (Fig. 4-17).[46]

The industry has also responded to defeat the retraction problem. Since 1988 nearly all manufacturers have manufactured dental control units that simply cut off the water spray without retraction. The ultimate solution is to replace older dental control units with newer ones that do not retract.[33,46,47]

Inherent water system contamination

Bacterial growth in biofilms on the inner walls of dental unit water lines is a universal occurrence unless steps are taken to control it. Counts of bacteria that are shed from the biofilms into water of the dental unit range from thousands to hundreds of thousands of bacteria per milliliter.[1,12,73,92] This bioload could be compared with bacterial counts of some foods (e.g., juices, milk, and yogurt) except that the bacterial types present are not carefully controlled. The main inhabitants are opportunistic gram negative, aquaphilic bacteria, especially flavobacteria. Similar species are found in biofilms that form in swimming pools or wherever nonsterile water remains in prolonged contact with habitable surfaces. The bacteria may include atypical myco-

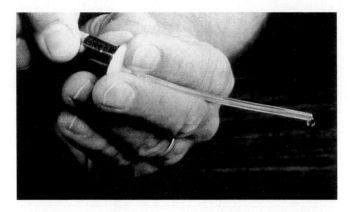

Fig. 4-17. Device used to detect retraction of water supplied to high-speed handpiece by older units when foot control is released. If water moves back into plastic tube, a new check valve is needed in handpiece water-line to prevent retraction of oral fluids during treatments. (Courtesy of A-DEC, Inc. Newberg, Oregon.)

bacteria and possibly *Legionella* bacteria which can present an infection risk to immunocompromised persons.[60,72,84,87] Flushing or sterilizing high-speed handpieces cannot be expected to overcome this source of contamination of patients and personnel that extends throughout the dental unit water system.

Clean water reservoir systems combined with disinfection or sterilization of equipment downstream have been developed by at least two companies. One has a large reservoir (ADEC, Portland, Oregon) (Fig. 4-18).[77,84] *Caution:* disinfectants, such as 0.5% hypochlorite solution, will damage the high-speed handpiece; therefore, *always remove the handpiece before disinfecting the system.*

Control of contamination from spatter and aerosol

Concerns regarding contamination from spatter and aerosol created by *rotary equipment* are valid. Operating this equipment in the mouths of patients necessarily *spatters oral fluids and microorganisms* onto the attending clinical personnel, and *aerosols* can readily be inhaled. Aerosolization of mycobacteria that cause pulmonary tuberculosis (*Mycobacterium tuberculosis*) has always been a concern. *Annual tuberculin testing of personnel has been a standard infection control recommendation in dentistry.* Concern is now being registered about nosocomial airborne transmission of multi-drug–resistant strains of mycobacteria that have exhibited an 85% infection rate and have been lethal for 75% of infected immunocompromised persons in 16 weeks.[21,17] This poses a new concern for health of dental personnel as well.

The rubber dam and high-volume evacuation (HVE) are very important and helpful methods to help reduce exposure to contamination.[37,75] (See Chapter 11 for

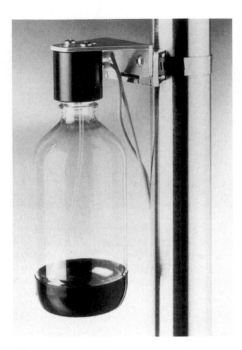

Fig. 4-18. Water reservoir shown can provide uncontaminated water to the syringe and to cool the high-speed bur. *After removing handpiece,* the reservoir and water lines downstream are disinfected weekly with 0.5% hypochlorite solution (handpiece is damaged by such solution). Uncontaminated water with 2 ppm hypochlorite solution is used routinely in the reservoir to discourage biofilm regrowth. (Courtesy of A-DEC, Inc., Newberg, Oregon.)

rubber dam isolation and HVE.) HVE can be up to 80% effective in reducing aerosol contamination. However, there is no way to eliminate airborne contamination, unless some method of continuous air purification can be used. Without the *universal use of personal barriers, drapes, and/or effective cleanup procedures,* personnel and subsequent patients can be subjected to oral fluid-borne contamination.

STERILIZATION OF HANDPIECES AND RELATED ROTARY EQUIPMENT

Prophy angles, latch angles, burs, and rotary stones used in the mouth must be cleaned and sterilized for reuse. All such items are readily sterilized by three or more methods of sterilization. Carbon steel burs require special protection in the autoclave (see Sterilization of Burs in Autoclave). Handpieces are semicritical instrumentation requiring sterilization.[7,33] Few brands now exist on the market that cannot be routinely autoclaved. *Such sterilization of handpieces can be monitored and documented.* In the armed forces, dental schools, and numerous private offices, handpieces have been sterilized for a number of years.

When handpiece surfaces were only disinfected, they still had to be removed to be scrubbed clean and thoroughly disinfected. When disinfected properly, even this process took time and necessitated having additional handpieces.

The more handpieces in inventory, the less each is used and the longer each should last until maintenance is needed. With proper care the cost of sterilizing and maintaining handpieces is between 1 and 2 dollars per patient, and this should be an added charge for infection control. Rapid turnaround time can be achieved between patients (i.e., the time needed to replace the handpiece between patients) if enough handpieces are available to replace a used one with a clean/sterile one for the next patient. A sufficient inventory of high-speed handpieces and at least the end sheaths of straight low-speed handpieces is needed per operatory in order to have as a minimum one of each at the unit, one of each on the shelf, and one of each in cleanup/sterilization. The investment is mainly the time for an assistant to keep this cycle going throughout the day. Another alternative is suggested under ethylene oxide sterilization of handpieces (see Other Methods of Handpiece Sterilization). The motor end of the attached low-speed handpiece can be covered by pulling a disposable, single use, slender plastic bag up over it and pushing (popping) the handpiece through the sealed end of the bag so the bag covers the motor end and part of the hose (see Fig. 4-7). Otherwise scrub and disinfect the motor-end for each reuse if it cannot be sterilized.

Steam sterilization of handpieces

Autoclave sterilization of handpieces is one of the most rapid methods. If proper cleaning and lubricating is performed as prescribed by the manufacturer, good utility is obtainable with regular autoclaving. Servicing is required about once a year, depending on patient load and number of handpieces. Fiber optics dim with repeated heat sterilization in a number of months to a year, apparently due to oil residue and debris baked on the ends of the optical fibers. Cleaning with detergent solution and wiping ends of optics with alcohol or other suitable organic solvents may prolong use before factory servicing. Manufacturers are improving methods of preparing handpieces for sterilization. *Consult the manufacturer's current advice and warnings.*

Procedure for handpieces with metal-bearing turbine. Scrub metal-bearing high-speed handpieces and the sheath or cone of the low-speed straight handpiece at the sink with running water and detergent. See manufacturer's directions for further cleaning and lubrication before and after sterilization. Bag the handpiece and sheath and autoclave them. *Note: when first operating a freshly lubricated handpiece, keep it in a plastic bag or the sterilization bag to avoid breathing the vaporized lubricant.*

Procedure for handpieces with "lube-free" ceramic-bearing turbine. Follow manufacturer's directions for cleaning high-speed handpieces with lubrication-free ceramic-bearing turbine (Den-Tal-Ez, Inc., Lancaster, Pennsylvania). For this type of handpiece, avoid using chemicals that will damage internal parts. Consult manufacturer's most current directions supplied with each handpiece for preparation of handpieces for sterilization. Attention to directions on cleaning fiber optics at both ends of the handpiece (e.g., with isopropyl alcohol) will prolong service life. Bag and autoclave handpiece.

Other methods of handpiece sterilization

Chemical vapor pressure sterilization recommended for some types of handpieces apparently works well with ceramic-bearing handpieces and may impair others. Always obtain the handpiece manufacturer's recommendations.

Ethylene oxide (ETOX) gas is the most gentle method of sterilization used for handpieces. Internal as well as external cleaning is important. Otherwise, preparation of handpieces before sterilization is not as critical since no heat is involved. Gas appears to penetrate high-speed handpieces. However, oil left in handpieces may impair sterilization.

ETOX processing takes the handpiece out of circulation for several hours or overnight. Some practitioners have purchased enough low-cost handpieces to treat their maximum number of patients seen per day, and use overnight ethylene oxide sterilization. This approach appears effective with adequate handpiece cleaning. Further research on the effectiveness and any limitations of ETOX handpiece sterilization is needed (consult Anderson Products, Haw River, North Carolina).

Dry heat sterilization of handpieces is generally not recommended. A rapid, high-temperature, dry heat disinfection has been developed for handpieces. Check with the handpiece manufacturer and the sterilizer manufacturer (Cox Sterilizer Co.) regarding use of this process.

INFECTION CONTROL FOR MAKING IMPRESSIONS AND ASSOCIATED REGISTRATIONS, AND TRANSPORTING TO A REMOTE LABORATORY
Infection control factors in making impressions and associated registrations

Precautions are required for infection control in making impressions and associated registrations, just as for other operative procedures. Universally apply barrier protection for personnel against contamination from mucosa, saliva, and blood by use of adequate personal protective equipment (PPE), such as gloves, mask, and appropriate overgarment.

To eliminate any chance of cross-contamination when sizing trays used for alginate or reversible hydrocolloid impressions, place the tray in a plastic baggy before it is tried in the mouth. After the appropriate size has been determined, remove the baggy and proceed with impression making. Indicate the tray size on the patient's chart to eliminate further try-ins.

For infection control, custom resin trays for impressions made with non-aqueous rubber impression materials are used once and then discarded. Likewise, stock trays are used only once and discarded.

Before making the impression and associated registrations, dispense using clean, gloved hands as many materials and disposable items as possible. This avoids contaminating their containers. Whenever possible use unit dose packaged materials, or use a paper towel or plastic film to handle tubes and other reused containers. Least satisfactory, but adequate, is wiping material's containers with a disinfectant *after* the procedures. A satisfactory disinfectant should be an EPA-approved tuberculocidal disinfectant.

Infection control concepts for transporting impressions and associated registrations to a remote laboratory

Transporting to a remote laboratory impressions and associated registrations is regulated by OSHA's specifications for handling and transporting specimens of blood or other potentially infectious materials (OPIM) such as blood-contaminated saliva: ". . . potentially infectious materials shall be placed in a container which prevents leakage during collection, handling, processing, storage, transport, or shipping (to the laboratory). Labeling or color coding is required when such specimens/containers leave the facility."[79]

There is controversy over two choices that may be used for preparing a potentially infectious item for transport: (1) *send it well-cleaned (rinsed) and un-disinfected in a biohazard-labeled, heat-sealed, plastic bag;* or (2) debride, clean (rinse), and adequately disinfect it, place it in a sealed transport bag labeled with the precautions taken, and assume responsibility for the aseptic condition of the item. In either choice most laboratories will disinfect the item (a second time in the second choice) to assure protection of laboratory personnel. Disinfecting twice is time wasted, and multiple exposures to disinfectant should be avoided.[74] The simplest and best approach may be the first. It avoids confusion over whether the item (e.g., an impression) is properly disinfected in the office, saves office time and materials for disinfection, and removes office liability. Special labeling of the item regarding potential contamination is not necessary (except for always having the OSHA biohazard label) if no item is disinfected and every item is assumed infected (thus satisfying the concept of universal precautions). This was the choice adopted in 1992 by the Washington State Department of Health, Dental Disciplinary Board.[101] This requires satisfactory labeling, including on the prescription the type of impression material. The National Association of Dental Laboratories recommends disinfecting all items received from the dental office and disinfecting all appliances before shipping them from the laboratory.[78]

Inexpensive, biohazard-labeled, heat-sealable bags are commercially available in various sizes made of sturdy clear plastic, and they are stamped with warnings to transporters and personnel (e.g., Seal-A-Case, Infection Control Services, Inc., P. O. Box 1389, Kent, WA 98035) (Fig. 4-19). The U.S. Postal Service also has specifications for double, leak-proof packaging and external labeling of such packaging if contaminated items must be sent by the U.S. Postal Service. (Mailing impressions would only apply to some non-aqueous impression materials which are relatively stable for a few days.)

Similar bags are also available for returning finished items to the office. They have no biohazard labels, but provide stamped instructions in green lettering advising office personnel that the contents are pre-cleaned and disinfected, and to handle the enclosed items appropriately for delivery to the patient (Fig. 4-20).

Generic, heat-sealable bags are available but must be appropriately labeled.

Infection control procedures for handling and transporting to a remote laboratory items from a non-aqueous polymer-based rubber impression technique and any associated registrations

Infection control procedures regarding the non-aqueous rubber impression and any associated registration are as follows:

1. Before the patient appointment, prepare one or more industrially clean, strong, clear, heat-sealable, *biohazard-labeled* plastic bag(s) of appropriate size, one for containing the scheduled impression and a separate one for any associated interocclusal registration. (Do *not* place any other item along with an impression in a bag to prevent the possibility of pressure-deformation of the impression caused by the additional item). Place each bag into an open canister of suitable size so that the bag's open end extends above the rim of the supporting canister, allowing a slight folding downward and outward of the bag's open edge. This helps to keep it open and also prevents contamination of the bag's outer surface during insertion of the item (in procedure 3).
2. Remove the impression, or interocclusal registration, or device from the mouth, and while still wearing barriers (gowns, gloves, etc.) remove

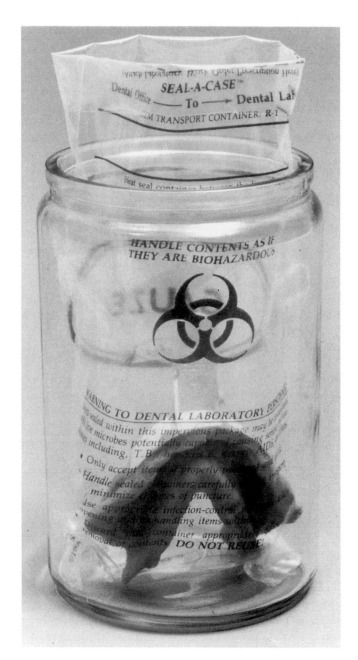

Fig. 4-19. Dentist or dental assistant prepares potentially infectious impression for transport (to remote laboratory or to on-site laboratory) by rinsing it and then placing in a biohazard-labeled plastic bag without contaminating bag's outer surface. Then with clean hands the bag is heat sealed.

any attached debris and rinse the item well with running tap water for 15 seconds to *remove saliva and blood.*
3. After rinsing, and while still wearing barriers, place the impression (or other item) into the designated, prepared bag without touching the bag's outer surface.
4. Now remove the gloves (because they are contaminated). With clean hands, close the bag while

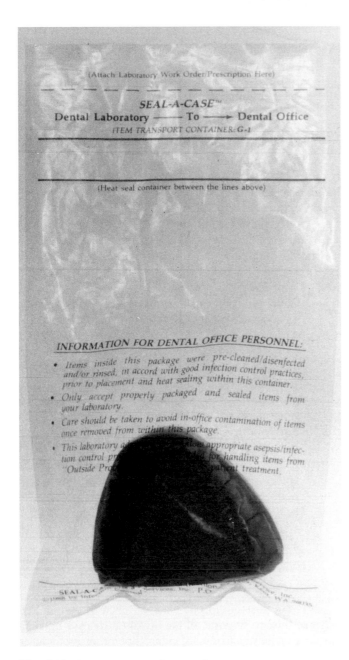

(Attach Laboratory Work Order/Prescription Here)

SEAL-A-CASE™
Dental Laboratory ——— To ——→ Dental Office
ITEM TRANSPORT CONTAINER: G-1

(Heat seal container between the lines above)

INFORMATION FOR DENTAL OFFICE PERSONNEL:

- *Items inside this package were pre-cleaned/disinfected and/or rinsed, in accord with good infection control practices, prior to placement and heat sealing within this container.*
- *Only accept properly packaged and sealed items from your laboratory.*
- *Care should be taken to avoid in-office contamination of items once removed from within this package.*
- *This laboratory ... appropriate asepsis/infection control pr... ...handling items from "Outside Pro... ...t treatment.*

Fig. 4-20. Laboratory disinfects appliance and then transports it in heat-sealed bag to dentist.

touching only the bag's clean outer surface, and heat-seal it.

5. Tape the prescription to the bag.

6. Attach a note or use a bag appropriately lettered to alert the laboratory that the item(s) in the bag was/were debrided and rinsed, but not disinfected. Communication with laboratory personnel can state also that this is how any item will be sent unless the laboratory has different require-

ments. Place the bag(s) into a suitable box and send to the remote laboratory. Laboratory personnel will proceed with disinfecting the items sent. Treat all potentially infectious items alike. Laboratory precautions and disinfection should be the same whether a patient has an infection or not. Only if a laboratory person has an exposure incident should the patient's history become important.

7. If the non-aqueous rubber impression is to be poured in the dental office, the impression must be disinfected before the cast is formed (see Infection Control for Handling Impressions and Associated Registrations to/in the On-site Laboratory).

Infection control procedures for handling and transporting to a remote laboratory items from an aqueous impression material technique (using alginate [irreversible hydrocolloid] or reversible hydrocolloid) and any associated registrations

If the aqueous impression is to be poured in-office and the resultant cast and associated items transported to a remote laboratory, infection control procedures are as follows:

1. Thoroughly rinse the impression under tap water (15 seconds recommended) to remove any saliva or blood.

2. Disinfect the impression by submerging it for 10 minutes in a fresh (prepared daily), 0.5% solution of commercial bleach (add 1 part of 5.25% sodium hypochlorite to 9 parts of water). An acceptable alternative is to follow the manufacturer's recommendation for a particular disinfectant. Do not exceed 30 minutes submersion time for reversible hydrocolloid.

3. With clean hands thoroughly rinse the disinfected impression under tap water to avoid prolonged exposure to the disinfectant and because any residual disinfectant can adversely affect surface hardness of the stone cast.

4. Shake-off excess water from the impression and pour the cast immediately. One reversible hydrocolloid manufacturer (Van R, 600 E. Hueneme Rd., Oxnard, CA 93033) offers two alternatives to immediate pouring of the impression after disinfection: option 1, submerge the impression into a 2% potassium sulfate solution for (up to) 20 minutes, and then remove, shake off excess, and pour the impression; option 2, place the impression into a humidor (for up to 4 hours with no temperature change), remove, submerge into the 2% potassium sulfate solution for 20 minutes, remove, shake-off excess, and pour the impression. (To make the potassium sulfate solution, Van R

supplies the crystals and instructs the user to dissolve 1 capfull of crystals to 1 pint of water.)

5. The cast from a disinfected impression does not need disinfecting.
6. *Carefully package the cast* for shipment to the remote laboratory; associated items (such as an interocclusal registration) which are from the mouth must be rinsed, disinfected, and then rinsed again. These may then be shipped along with the cast, but packaged to avoid harming it. Include also a *written note* stating that the impression and associated registration were disinfected and that the cast should not be subjected to a disinfection procedure which might compromise accuracy.

If the dentist desires to utilize a nearby commercial laboratory (having expeditious courier service) for pick-up of the aqueous impression and associated items, and for the disinfection and subsequent handling of these, the infection control procedures described in the previous section for handling a non-aqueous rubber impression to be transported to a remote laboratory should be followed.

INFECTION CONTROL FOR HANDLING IMPRESSIONS AND ASSOCIATED REGISTRATIONS TO/IN THE ON-SITE LABORATORY

Laboratory personnel are required to wear a clean uniform or laboratory jacket, coat, or gown, and these are supplied by the dentist. Disposable mask, protective eyewear, and protective gloves are also supplied, and their use is required when there is potential for exposure to dust or spatter.

Convey impressions and associated items removed from the mouth to the on-site laboratory technician using the same procedures described in the previous section (for transport to a remote laboratory). These procedures should maintain the outside surfaces of the bag in an uncontaminated condition, as well as protect the contents from accidental spillage.

Additional *infection control measures* for handling these items in the on-site laboratory are listed as follows:

1. A designated area *must* be available to receive the items. Personnel receiving them must wear disposable treatment gloves.
2. All incoming items to the dental laboratory must be properly labeled. With gloved hands, disinfect impressions (and associated registrations) by submerging (for 10 minutes) in 1:10 dilution (0.5%) of household liquid chlorine bleach (5.25% sodium hypochlorite) prepared fresh daily, or other accepted tuberculocidal disinfectant. As long as blood is not visible, containers can then be discarded in regular trash.
3. With gloved hands, spray articulators and any related equipment that have been contaminated, and which cannot be sterilized, with an alcohol disinfectant (see Operatory Asepsis) since chlorine in the hypochlorite-type disinfectant may damage the metal.
4. With clean hands, thoroughly rinse the impression under tap water (15 seconds) to remove any residual disinfectant, and follow manufacturer's directions for any additional procedures for treating the impression and forming the cast.
5. All outgoing items must be properly cleaned and placed in a leakproof bag or appropriate container prior to leaving the laboratory.
6. Contaminated countertops and work surfaces must be cleaned of debris and disinfected daily. After cleaning, spray surfaces with disinfectant, wipe dry with paper towels, and re-spray with disinfectant. Leave surfaces wet.
7. Do not use the same pumice for new work and repair work.* For repairs, pre-measure pumice in small amounts and discard it daily after use. Discard pumice used for new work weekly. Wet pumice with a mixture of green soap and a disinfectant. *Do not use water only!* Soak brush wheels and rag wheels in a disinfectant for 10 minutes after use. Air dry them overnight. After using pumice in a repair, disinfect the appliance again for 10 minutes. Disinfect model trimmers and pumice pans at the end of the day.[90]†

CONCLUSIONS; OTHER INFORMATION SOURCES

It is not possible in one chapter, even as comprehensive as this, to provide all the detail on disease updates, tests, vaccines, barriers, standard operating procedures, sterilization methods, and equipment. Infection control and auxiliary persons are referred to other more detailed literature and texts in the reference list, and are advised to attend continuing education programs to expand and update their infection control information.[7,33,39,43,105]

*NADL Health and Safety Committee: Fabrication Procedure: HS-1, Infection control procedures in the dental laboratory, *Trends and Techniques.*
†Specific infection control and safety procedures for training dental laboratory technicians are available from the NADL, 3801 Mt. Vernon Ave., Alexandria, VA 22305.

REFERENCES

1. Abel LC et al: Studies on dental aerobiology. IV. Bacterial contamination of water delivered by dental units, *J Dent Res* 50:1567-1569, 1971.

2. Ahtone J, Goodman RA: Hepatitis B and dental personnel: transmission to patients and prevention issues, *J Am Dent Assoc* 106(2):219-222, 1983.

3. Allain J-P et al: Long-term evaluation of HIV antigen and antibodies to p24 and gp41 in patients with hemophilia, *N Engl J Med* 317:1114-1121, 1987.

4. Allen A, Bryan R: Occult blood accumulation under fingernails, *J Am Dent Assoc* 105:358-362 Sept 1982.

5. American Association of Dental Schools: Curriculum guidelines for the dental care management of patients with bloodborne infectious diseases, *J Dent Educ* 55:609-619, 1991.

6. American Association of Dental Schools: Recommended clinical guidelines for infection control in dental education institutions, *J Dent Educ* 55:6221-630, 1991.

7. American Dental Association: Infection control for the dental office and dental laboratory, *J Am Dent Assoc* 123(suppl):1-8, Aug 1992.

8. American Dental Association: Facts about AIDS for the dental team, ed 3, *J Am Dent Assoc* 119(suppl):1-9, July, 1991.

9. Autio KK et al: Studies on cross-contamination in the dental office, *J Am Dent Assoc* 100(3):358-361, 1980.

10. Bagga BSR et al: Contamination of dental unit cooling water with oral microorganisms and its prevention, *J Am Dent Assoc* 109:712-716, 1984.

11. Bentley C, Burkhart NW, Crawford JJ: Evaluation of spatter and contamination during dental procedures, *Transmissions (Soc Inf Cont Dent)* 7:2, 1992.

12. Blake GC: The incidence and control of bacterial infection in dental spray reservoirs, *Brit Dent J* 115:413-416, 1963.

13. Bond WW et al: Effective use of liquid chemical germicides on medical instruments: instrument design problems. In Block SS, editor: *Disinfection, sterilization, and preservation*, ed 4, Philadelphia, 1991, Lea & Febiger.

14. Bond WW et al: Inactivation of hepatitis B by intermediate to high-level disinfectant chemicals, *J Clin Microbiol* 18:535-538, 1983.

15. Bond WW et al: Survival of hepatitis B virus after drying and storage for one week, *Lancet* 7:550-551, March 1981.

16. Centers for Disease Control: Surveillance for occupationally acquired HIV infection, United States 1981-1982, *MMWR* 41(No.43):823-825, 1992.

17. Centers for Disease Control: Nosocomial transmission of multidrug-resistant tuberculosis among HIV-infected persons—Florida and New York, 1988-1991, *MMWR* 40:585-591, 1991.

18. Centers for Disease Control: Recommendations for preventing transmission of human immunodeficiency virus and hepatitis B virus to patients during exposure prone invasive procedures, *MMWR* 40(RR-8):1-9, 1991.

19. Centers for Disease Control: Update: acquired immunodeficiency syndrome, United States, 1981-1991, *MMWR* 40(No.22):358-368, 1991.

20. Centers for Disease Control: Update: transmission of HIV infection during invasive dental procedure—Florida, *MMWR* 40(No.2):21-28, 1991.

21. Centers for Disease Control: Guidelines for preventing transmission of tuberculosis in health-care settings, with special focus on HIV-related issues, *MMWR* 39(RR17):1-29, 1990.

22. Centers for Disease Control: Measles—United States, 1990, *MMWR* 40(No. 22):369-372, 1990.

23. Centers for Disease Control: Guidelines for prevention of transmission of HIV and HBV to health care and public safety workers, *MMWR* 38(No.S-6), 1989.

24. Centers for Disease Control: Update: universal precautions for prevention of transmission of human immunodeficiency virus, hepatitis B virus, and other bloodborne pathogens in health-care settings, *MMWR* 37:377-387, 1988.

25. Centers for Disease Control: Recommendations for prevention of HIV transmission in health-care settings, *MMWR* 36(suppl 2S):1S-18S, 1987.

26. Centers for Disease Control: Recommended infection-control practices for dentistry, *MMWR* 35(15):237-242, 1986.

27. Centers for Disease Control: Measles on a college campus—Ohio, *MMWR* 34(7):89-90, 1985.

28. Centers for Disease Control, Immunization Practices Advisory Committee: Recommendation of the Immunization Practices Advisory Committee: Protection against viral hepatitis, *MMWR* 39(No.S-2):1-26, 1990.

29. Centers for Disease Control, Immunization Practices Advisory Committee: Measles prevention: recommendations of the Immunologic Practices Committee, *MMWR* 38(No.S-9), 1989.

30. Centers for Disease Control, Immunization Practices Advisory Committee: Recommendations for protection against viral hepatitis. U.S. Dept. of Health and Human Services, Public Health Service, *MMWR* 34 (22):314, 1985.

31. Centers for Disease Control, Immunization Practices Advisory Committee: Inactivated hepatitis B virus vaccine, *MMWR* 31:317-328, 1982.

32. Centers for Disease Control and Prevention: Update: investigations of persons treated by HIV-infected health-care workers—United States, *MMWR* 42(No.17):329-337, 1993.

33. Centers for Disease Control and Prevention: Update: recommended infection-control practices for dentistry, *MMWR* 142(No.RR-8):1-12, 1993.

34. Christensen RP: Ultrasonic cleaning equipment, *Clin Res Assoc Newsletter* 13(8):1-3, Aug 1989.

35. Christensen RP et al: Efficiency of 42 brands of face masks and two face shields in preventing inhalation of airborne debris, *Gen Dentistry* 39:414-421, 1991.

36. Christensen RP et al: Antimicrobial activity of environmental surface disinfectants in the absence and presence of bioburden, *J Am Dent Assoc* 119:493-504, 1989.

37. Cochran MA, Miller CH, Sheldrake MA: The efficiency of the rubber dam as a barrier to the spread of microorganisms during dental treatment, *J Am Dent Assoc* 119:141-144, 1989.

38. Cottone JA: Recent developments in hepatitis: new virus, vaccine and dosage recommendations, *J Am Dent Assoc* 120:501-508, 1990.

39. Cottone JA, Terezhalmy GT, Molinari JA, editors: *Practical infection control in dentistry,* Philadelphia, 1991, Lea & Febiger.

40. Council on Dental Materials, Instruments and Devices, American Dental Association: Dental units and water retraction, *J Am Dent Assoc* 116:417-420, 1988.

41. Council on Dental Therapeutics, Council on Dental Materials Instruments and Equipment, American Dental Association: *Monograph series on dental materials and therapeutics: safety and infection control in the dental office,* Chicago, 1990, American Dental Association.

42. Council on Dental Therapeutics, Council on Dental Practice, Council on Dental Materials Instruments and Equipment, American Dental Association: Infection control recommendations for the dental office and dental laboratory, *J Am Dent Assoc* 116:241-248, 1988.

43. Crawford JJ: *Clinical asepsis in dentistry: regulations, infection control,* Chapel Hill, NC, 1992, CIC Publishing.

44. Crawford JJ: State of the art: practical infection control in dentistry. In Mitchell E, Cottone J, editors: Proceedings of the national symposium on hepatitis B and the dental profession, *J Am Dent Assoc* 110:629-633, 1985.

45. Crawford JJ: Sterilization, disinfection, and asepsis in dentistry. In Block SS, editor: *Disinfection, sterilization, and preservation,* Philadelphia, 1983, Lea & Febiger.

46. Crawford JJ, Broderius C: Evaluation of a dental unit designed to prevent retraction of oral fluids, *Quintessence International* 21:47-51, 1989.

47. Crawford JJ, Broderius C: Control of cross infection risks in the dental operatory: prevention of water retraction by bur cooling spray systems, *J Am Dent Assoc* 116:695-687, 1988.

48. Crawford JJ, Fine J: Infection control in hospital dentistry. In Hooley J, Daun L, editors: *Hospital dentistry,* St Louis, 1980, Mosby.

49. DeVita VT Jr, Hellman S, Rosenberg SA, editors: *AIDS etiology, diagnosis, treatment, and prevention,* Philadelphia, 1985, JB Lippincott.

50. Ehrenkranz NJ, Alfanso BC: Failure of bland soap handwash to prevent hand transfer of patient bacteria to urethral catheters, *Infect Control Hosp Epidemiol* 12:654-662, 1991.

51. Favero MS, Bond WW: Chemical disinfection of medical materials. In Block SS, editor: *Disinfection, sterilization, and preservation,* ed 4, Philadelphia, 1991, Lea & Febiger.

52. Food and Drug Administration: Medical devices: patient examination and surgeons' gloves; adulteration. Final Rule, 21CFR Part 800. *Federal Register* 55(239):51254-52158, 1990.

53. Forbes B: Acquisition of cytomegalovirus infection: an update, *Clin Microbiol Rev* 2:204-216, 1989.

54. Francis D, Favero MS, Maynard JE: Transmission of hepatitis B virus, *Semin Liver Dis* 1(1):27-32, 1981.

55. Francis D et al: Occurrence of hepatitis A, B, non-A/non-B in the United States, *Am J Med* 76:69, Jan 1984.

56. Friedland GH, Klein RS: Transmission of the human immunodeficiency virus, *N Engl J Med* 317:1125-1135, 1987.

57. Garner JS, Favero MS: *Guideline for handwashing and hospital environmental control,* Atlanta, Public Health Service, Centers for Disease Control, HHS pub. No. 99-1117, 1985.

58. Gayle HD et al: Prevalence of the human immunodeficiency virus among university students, *N Engl J Med* 323:1538-1541, 1990.

59. Glasel M: *High-risk sexual practices in the transmission of AIDS.* In DeVita VT Jr, Hellman S, Rosenberg SA, editors: *AIDS etiology, diagnosis, treatment, and prevention,* Philadelphia, 1985, JB Lippincott.

60. Gold J: Mycobacterial infections in immunosuppressed patients, *Semin Respir Infect* 13:160-165, 1986.

61. Greene WC: The molecular biology of human immunodeficiency virus type 1, *N Engl J Med* 324:308-317, 1991.

62. Greenspan D, Greenspan CA, Winkler JR: Diagnosis and management of oral manifestations of HIV infection and AIDS, *Infect Dis Clin North Am* 2:373-385, 1988.

63. Gwaltney JM Jr, Hendley JO: Transmission of experimental rhinovirus infection by contaminated surfaces, *Am J Epidemiol* 116:828-833, 1989.

64. Hackney RW: *Oral bacteria as biological indicators for dental asepsis.* Doctoral Dissertation, School of Public Health, 1989, University of North Carolina at Chapel Hill.

65. Hamed LM et al: Hibiclens keratitis, *Am J Ophthalmol* 104:50-56, 1987.

66. Klein RC, Party E, Gershey EL: Virus penetration of examination gloves, *Biotechniques* 9:196-199, 1990.

67. Klein RS et al: Low occupational risk of human immunodeficiency virus infection among dental professionals, *N Engl J Med* 318:86-90, 1988.

68. Lange J, Goudsmit J: Decline of antibody reactivity to HIV core protein secondary to increased production of HIV antigen, *Lancet* p 19, Feb 19, 1987.

69. Lettau LA: The A,B,C,D, and E of viral hepatitis: spelling out the risks for health care workers, *Infect Control Hosp Epidemiol* 13:77-81, 1992.

70. Lewis DL, Boe RK: Cross-infection risks associated with current procedures for using high-speed dental handpieces, *J Clin Microbiol* 30:401-406, 1992.

71. Lewis DL et al: Cross-contamination potential with dental equipment, *Lancet* 340:1252-1254, Nov 21, 1992.

72. Martin MV: The significance of the bacterial contamination of dental unit water systems, *Br Dent J* 163:152-154, 1987.

73. McEntegart MG, Clark A: Colonization of dental units with water bacteria, *Br Dent J* 134:140-142, 1973.

74. Merchant VA: Infection control in the dental laboratory: concerns for the dentist, *Compend Contin Educ Dent* 14:(3)382-391, 1993.

75. Miller RL, Micik RE: Air pollution and its control in the dental office, *Dent Clin North Am* 22:453 1978.

76. Mitchell E: ADA council recommends hepatitis vaccine for dentists, students, and auxiliary personnel, *ADA News* 13:1, Aug 8, 1982.

77. Moriarty JD, Crawford JJ: Evaluation of an independent sterile water reservoir system for highspeed instrumentation, *J Dent Res* 55:(abstract no. 855), 1976.

78. National Association of Dental Laboratories: *A complete program of infection control for dental laboratories,* Alexandria, Va, 1989, The Association.

79. Occupational Safety and Health Administration: Blood borne pathogens. Section 1910, 1030 (26 U.S.C. 635), *Federal Register* 56(235):64175-64181, 1991.

80. Occupational Safety and Health Administration: Hazard communications standard, *Federal Register,* August 24, 1987.

81. Palenik CJ et al: A survey of sterilization practices in selected endodontic offices, *J Endodontics* 12:206-209, 1986.

82. Paterson NJ, Bond WW, Favero MS: Air sampling for hepatitis B surface antigen in a dental operatory, *J Am Dent Assoc* 99:465-467, 1979.

83. Pattison CP et al: Epidemic hepatitis B in a clinical laboratory; Possible association with computer card handling, *JAMA* 230:854-857, 1974.

84. Polinsky B et al: Sterile dental unit water reservoir to control mycobacteria and aquaphilic bacteria, *Control* 5:5, 1990.

85. Poole P, Summers T, Crawford JJ: Comparison of ultrasonic versus swabbing methods to evaluate handpiece disinfection, *Control* 6:4, 1991.

86. Raloff J: Successful hepatitis A vaccine debuts, *Science News* 142:103, 1992.

87. Reinthaler FF, Ascher FM, Stunzer D: Serologic examination for antibodies against *Legionella* species in dental personnel, *J Dent Res* 67:942-943, 1988.

88. Robinson RAN et al: A suspension method to determine reuse life of chemical disinfectants during clinical use, *Appl Microbiol* 54:158-164, 1988.

89. Rutala WA, Cole EC: Ineffectiveness of hospital disinfectants against bacteria, a collaborative study, *Infect Control* 8:501-506, 1987.

90. Sabatini B: Keeping the laboratory clean and safe; how to prevent cross-contamination, ADA, *Dental Teamwork* 4(No. 6):23-24, 1991.

91. Satter SA, Springthorpe VS: Survival and disinfectant inactivation of the human immunodeficiency virus: a critical review, *Rev Infect Dis* 1(13):430-447, 1991.

92. Sawyer DR et al: Bacterial contamination of the highspeed dental handpiece and the water it delivers, *Virginia Dent J* 53:14-23, 1976.

93. Slade JS et al: The survival of human immunodeficiency virus in water, sewage, and sea water, *Water Science and Technology* 21:55-59, 1989.

94. Soulsby ME, Barnett JB, Maddox S: Brief report: the antiseptic efficiency of chlorxylenol-containing vs. chlorhexidine gluconate-containing surgical scrub preparations, *Infect Control* 7:223-226, 1986.

95. Spire B et al: Inactivation of lymphadenopathy-associated virus by heat, gamma rays, and ultraviolet light, *Lancet* pp 188-189, Jan 26, 1985.

96. Stubbs B et al: A quantitative biological assay to evaluate pre-sterilization cleaning methods, *Transmissions; Society for Infect Control in Dentistry* 7:4, 1992.

97. Summers T, Poole P, Crawford J: Statistical evaluation of cleaning methods and chemicals for disinfecting handpieces, *Transmissions; Society for Infect Control in Dentistry* 6:2, 1991.

98. Thomas LE et al: Survival of herpes simplex and other selected microorganisms on patient charts: potential source of infection, *J Am Dent Assoc* 111:462-464, 1985.

99. U.S. Congress: *Occupational Safety and Health Act of 1970,* Sections 6 and 8, (29 U. S. C. 655, 657), CFR Part 1911 and Sec. of Labor's Orders Nos. 9-83 (48 FR 35736), and 29 CFR Part 1910, 1970.

100. U.S. Department of Labor, OSHA, *Controlling occupational exposure to bloodborne pathogens in dentistry,* Washington DC, 1992, U.S. Government Printing Office.

101. Washington State Department of Health, Dental Disciplinary Board, Small business economic impact statement. *Infection Control,* Chapter 246-816-720, March 3, 1992.

102. Whitacre RJ, Robins SK, Crawford JJ: *Dental asepsis,* Seattle, 1979, Stoma Press.

103. White SC, Glaze S: Interpatient microbial cross-contamination after dental radiographic exam, *J Am Dent Assoc* 96:801-804, 1978.

104. Williams N, Shay DE, Hasler JF: Indications of the sanitation level in a dental clinic, *J Balt Coll of Dent Surg* 31:18-34, 1976.

105. Wood PR, editor: *Cross infection control in dentistry,* Aylesbury, England, 1992, Wolf Publishing.

CHAPTER 5

Patient assessment, examination and diagnosis, and treatment planning

Daniel A. Shugars

Diane C. Shugars

Pretreatment considerations consisting of patient assessment, examination and diagnosis, and treatment planning are the foundation of sound dental care. These considerations follow a *stepwise progression* as the diagnosis and treatment plan depend on thorough assessment and examination of the patient.

Planning of dental treatment is a challenging and rewarding undertaking for the dentist. This endeavor is no longer the sole province of the treating dentist, however. Heightened consumer awareness and interest in personal health has resulted in increased participation by the patient in decisions about treatment. The financing of over one third of dental care by private dental insurance[11] has prompted third-party payers' interest in treatment decisions. Growing attention to using only the most effective and appropriate treatment has spawned the development of professional consensus conferences and practice parameters that serve to assist dentists with their treatment planning decisions.

The first section of this chapter describes several aspects of patient assessment that includes a review of medical condition and history, sociological and psychological conditions, dental history, and an evaluation of the patient's risk for dental disease. The second section, devoted to examination and diagnosis, reviews the clinical examination of orofacial soft tissues, clinical and radiographic examinations of teeth and periodontium, and clinical examination of the occlusion. The second section also reviews special considerations for the examination of a patient in pain. The final section discusses types of treatment plans, indications for operative treatment, and sequencing of dental procedures with an emphasis on interdisciplinary aspects of treatment planning.

Three pretreatment considerations—medical review, examination, and diagnosis—are necessary during each of the initial, emergency, re-evaluation, and recall visits. The *routine initial visit* involves obtaining detailed information for treatment planning. An *emergency visit* requires collecting basic information and then focusing on the patient's chief complaint. A *re-evaluation appointment* requires updating patient information and evaluating previous treatment. In contrast, a *recall appointment* demands reviewing the patient assessment information and comparing the patient's current status with previous conditions. Regardless of the type of visit, however, the dentist must routinely evaluate the patient's systemic condition, along with the status of the teeth, periodontium, occlusion, and facial structures.

Pretreatment assessment must be thorough and systematic. The results of this assessment must be recorded accurately in the ***patient record.*** Accurate records are maintained for proper patient care and for medical/legal and forensic purposes.

PATIENT ASSESSMENT

Before the examination and diagnosis of teeth, periodontium, and orofacial soft tissues, attention is given to infection control, medical review, sociological and psychological review, dental history, and risk assessment.

Infection control

Before, during, and after any patient visit, appropriate *infection control measures must be instituted.* For this information the reader is referred to Chapter 4, Infection Control.

Medical review

The patient completes a standard, comprehensive ***medical history*** form (Fig. 5-1). This form is the focus of the pre-examination *patient interview* which helps to identify conditions that could alter, complicate, or contraindicate proposed dental procedures. For instance, the practitioner may identify: (1) *communicable diseases* that require special precautions, procedures, or referral; (2) *allergies or medications* that may contraindicate the use of certain drugs; (3) *systemic diseases and cardiac abnormalities* that demand less strenuous procedures or prophylactic antibiotic coverage; and (4) *physiological changes associated with aging* that may alter clinical presentation and influence treatment. The practitioner may also identify a need for medical consultation or referral before initiating dental care. All of this information is carefully detailed in the patient's permanent record and is used as needed to shape subsequent treatment.

Communicable diseases. During the medical interview, the dentist must recognize the clinical manifestations of common infectious diseases because their presence can affect patient management and may constitute potential transmission hazards within the dental practice. *The dentist is sometimes the first health professional to identify a patient with a contagious disease.* Moreover, many communicable diseases are transmissible through the dental setting unless appropriate infection control measures are taken (see Chapter 4).

Of particular concern is the detection and prompt treatment of oral infections in ***immunocompromised patients.*** These individuals are at high risk of developing life-threatening illnesses due to the suppression of appropriate immune responses to infectious agents. This immunosuppression may be caused directly by diseases of the immune cells (e.g., leukemia, lymphomas, infection with the human immunodeficiency virus) or indirectly by the use of immunosuppressive drugs and therapies (e.g., drug administration to prevent rejection of transplanted tissues and irradiation therapy for some cancers). The oral manifestations of bacterial, fungal, and viral infections in these immunocompromised individuals frequently involve extensive, aggressive, and painful lesions that may occur in characteristic or uncharacteristic locations and too often result in lethal dissemination to vital organs. Therefore, careful examination, detection, and aggressive treatment of oral and perioral lesions in this population are critical steps in maintaining the health of immunocompromised patients.

A comprehensive treatise of the numerous oral and perioral manifestations associated with communicable diseases is beyond the scope of this book. The reader is referred to texts on oral medicine, oral microbiology, and oral pathology for additional information. A list of recommended readings is included at the end of this chapter. The more common infectious diseases and associated orofacial lesions are reviewed in this section.

Medical History Form

Date _____

Name _____   Home Phone (_____) _____
     Last   First   Middle

Address _____   Business Phone (_____) _____
      Number, Street

City _____ State _____ Zip Code _____

Occupation _____ Social Security No. _____

Date of Birth ___ / ___ / ___ Sex M F Height _____ Weight _____ Single _____ Married _____
           mo. day yr.

Name of Spouse _____ Closest Relative _____ Phone (_____) _____

If you are completing this form for another person, what is your relationship to that person? _____

Referred by _____

For the following questions, *circle yes or no*, whichever applies. Your answers are for our records only and will be considered confidential. Please note that during your initial visit you will be asked some questions about your responses to this questionnaire and there may be additional questions concerning your health.

1. Are you in good health? . . . . Yes   No
2. Has there been any change in your general health within the past year? . . . . Yes   No
3. My last physical examination was on _____
4. Are you now under the care of a physician? . . . . Yes   No
   If so, what is the condition being treated? _____
5. The name and address of my physician(s) is _____
   _____
   _____
   _____
6. Have you had any serious illness, operation, or been hospitalized in the past 5 years? . . . . Yes   No
   If so, what was the illness or problem? _____
7. Are you taking any medicine(s) including non-prescription medicine?. . . . . Yes   No
   If so, what medicine(s) are you taking? _____
8. Do you have or have you had any of the following diseases or problems?
   a. Damaged heart valves or artificial heart valves, including heart murmur or rheumatic heart disease . . . . Yes   No
   b. Cardiovascular disease (heart trouble, heart attack, angina, coronary insufficiency, coronary occlusion, high blood pressure, arteriosclerosis, stroke) . . . . Yes   No
      1. Do you have chest pain upon exertion? . . . . Yes   No
      2. Are you ever short of breath after mild exercise or when lying down? . . . . . . Yes   No
      3. Do your ankles swell? . . . . Yes   No
      4. Do you have inborn heart defects? . . . . Yes   No
      5. Do you have a cardiac pacemaker? . . . . Yes   No
   c. Allergy . . . . Yes   No
   d. Sinus trouble . . . . Yes   No
   e. Asthma or hay fever . . . . Yes   No
   f. Fainting spells or seizures . . . . Yes   No
   g. Persistent diarrhea or recent weight loss . . . . Yes   No
   h. Diabetes . . . . Yes   No
   i. Hepatitis, jaundice or liver disease . . . . Yes   No
   j. AIDS or HIV infection . . . . Yes   No
   k. Thyroid problems . . . . Yes   No
   l. Respiratory problems, emphysema, bronchitis, etc. . . . . Yes   No
   m. Arthritis or painful swollen joints . . . . Yes   No
   n. Stomach ulcer or hyperacidity . . . . Yes   No
   o. Kidney trouble . . . . Yes   No
   p. Tuberculosis . . . . Yes   No
   q. Persistent cough or cough that produces blood . . . . Yes   No
   r. Persistent swollen glands in neck . . . . Yes   No
   s. Low blood pressure . . . . Yes   No
   t. Sexually transmitted disease . . . . Yes   No
   u. Epilepsy or other neurological disease . . . . Yes   No
   v. Problems with mental health . . . . Yes   No
   w. Cancer . . . . Yes   No
   x. Problems of the immune system . . . . Yes   No

Fig. 5-1. A comprehensive medical review form is the focus of the patient interview (Form continued on next page). This form helps the practitioner identify conditions that may affect dental treatment or require referral to a physician. (Copyright by the American Dental Association. Reprinted by permission.)

9. Have you had abnormal bleeding?. . . . .   Yes   No
    a. Have you ever required a blood transfusion? . . . .   Yes   No

10. Do you have any blood disorder such as anemia? . . . .   Yes   No

11. Have you ever had any treatment for a tumor or growth? . . . . .   Yes   No

12. Are you allergic or have you had a reaction to:
    a. Local anesthetics . . . .   Yes   No
    b. Penicillin or other antibiotics . . . .   Yes   No
    c. Sulfa drugs . . . .   Yes   No
    d. Barbiturates, sedatives, or sleeping pills . . . .   Yes   No
    e. Aspirin . . . .   Yes   No
    f. Iodine . . . .   Yes   No
    g. Codeine or other narcotics . . . .   Yes   No
    h. Other _____

13. Have you had any serious trouble associated with any previous dental treatment? . . . .   Yes   No
    If so, explain _____
_____

14. Do you have any disease, condition, or problem not listed above that you think I should know about? . . . .   Yes   No
    If so, explain _____
_____

15. Are you wearing contact lenses? . . . .   Yes   No

16. Are you wearing removable dental appliances? . . . .   Yes   No

Women

17. Are you pregnant? . . . .   Yes   No

18. Do you have any problems associated with your menstrual period? . . . .   Yes   No

19. Are you nursing? . . . .   Yes   No

20. Are you taking birth control pills? . . . .   Yes   No

Chief Dental Complaint _____
_____

I certify that I have read and understand the above. I acknowledge that my questions, if any, about the inquiries set forth above have been answered to my satisfaction. I will not hold my dentist, or any other member of his/her staff, responsible for any errors or omissions that I may have made in the completion of this form.

_____
Signature of Patient

For completion by the dentist.
Comments on patient interview concerning medical history: _____
_____
_____

Significant findings from questionnaire or oral interview: _____
_____
_____

Dental management considerations: _____
_____
_____

_____   _____
(Date)   Signature of Dentist

Medical history update:

Date	Comments	Signature
_____	_____	_____
_____	_____	_____
_____	_____	_____
_____	_____	_____

Fig. 5-1 — cont'd.

Table 5-1. Communicable diseases of concern in dentistry

Infectious agent	Route of transmission	Disease
Herpes simplex viruses, types 1 and 2 (HSV types 1 and 2)	Congenital, oral (saliva), sexual, direct contact with lesions	Oral/genital herpes Primary herpetic gingivostomatitis Herpes labialis Herpetic whitlow (finger) Keratoconjunctivitis (eye)
Varicella zoster virus (VZV)	Aerosols, respiratory droplets, direct contact with lesions	Chickenpox, or varicella (primary infection) Shingles, or zoster (reactivated infection)
Papillomaviruses	Direct oral or sexual contact with lesions	Venereal warts, or condylomata acuminatum
Respiratory viruses		
Viruses such as rhinoviruses, respiratory syncytial virus, and influenza viruses	Direct contact with respiratory droplets, aerosols	Respiratory infections such as cold and flue
Paramyxoviruses	Direct contact with respiratory droplets, aerosols	Rubeola, or measles Mumps
Togavirus	Direct contact with respiratory droplets, aerosols	Rubella, or German measles
Epstein-Barr virus (EBV)	Direct contact with saliva	Infectious mononucleosis
Hepatitis B virus (HBV)	Bloodborne, sexual, perinatal, present in all body fluids, including saliva	Hepatitis, cirrhosis of the liver, hepatocellular carcinoma
Human immunodeficiency virus (HIV)	Blood, sexual, perinatal	Opportunistic infections Neoplastic lesions such as Kaposi's sarcoma Wasting syndrome AIDS
Mycobacterium tuberculosis	Respiratory droplets, aerosols, saliva, ingestion, direct contact	Pulmonary tuberculosis (TB), dissemination to the intestines, kidney, bones, meninges, lymph nodes, oral structures
Neisseria gonorrhoeae	Sexual contact	Gonorrhea, oral lesions, gonococcal arthritis, infections of the skin, eye, heart, meninges
Treponema pallidum	Sexual contact, congenital	Syphilis, oral lesions, disseminated infections to other organs, including the CNS, heart

Some of the clinical symptoms associated with contagious diseases that should be familiar to the dentist are listed in Table 5-1, and the intraoral and extraoral manifestations are shown in Plate 5-1. The dentist must be capable of detecting and identifying these manifestations either during the medical interview or during the subsequent examination of soft tissues of the head (intraoral and extraoral) and neck (see Examination of Orofacial Soft Tissues).

Herpes simplex virus (HSV). This infectious disease is probably the most common non-respiratory viral disease affecting humans. Transmitted primarily through saliva, the herpes simplex virus (HSV) preferentially infects the skin, mucous membranes, eyes, and nervous tissues. Generally, the two HSV types affect different regions of the body; type 1 involves the oral and perioral tissues ("above the waist") whereas type 2 involves the genital and surrounding areas ("below the waist").

Clinical characteristics	Treatment	Comment

Vesicles that rupture to form multiple shallow ulcers; inflamed gingiva may be present; lesions frequently recur when reactivated by various stimuli (e.g., stress)	Acyclovir
	  Topical ointment
	  Systemic use for severe cases
		Lesions of HSV type 1 are usually found above the waist, while those of HSV type 2 usually occur below the waist; herpetic infections may be severe and potentially life-threatening in newborns and immunosuppressed individuals

Vesicular lesions associated with chickenpox appear initially on the trunk and scalp and spread laterally; lesions associated with shingles follow a unilateral dermatome distribution	Acyclovir and vidarabine Topical and systemic use	VZV infections may have serious, fatal consequences in the neonate and immunocompromised individual
Flat or raised nodules that may coalesce into "cauliflower-like" clusters; typically asymptomatic; lesions frequently recur	Surgical or chemical removal	Certain lesions may progress to precancerous and cancerous growths
Sneezing, sore throat, fever, headache, malaise	Prophylactic prevention for flu by vaccination or amantadine treatment; palliative treatment for colds	Probably the most frequently transmitted diseases within dental practices
Rubeola—cough, conjunctivitis, fever, maculopapular rash, Koplik's spots	Childhood vaccination, palliative treatment	Serious infections may lead to life-threatening pneumonia
Mumps—salivary gland enlargement, headache, fever, malaise		
Low-grade fever, sore throat, mild exanthematous rash of short duration	Childhood vaccination, palliative treatment	May cause congenital defects in the neonate, including mental retardation, heart defects, deafness, and retarded growth
Lymphadenopathy, fever, petechiae	None	Infection is rarely serious
Fever, malaise, anorexia, gastrointestinal distress, chills, icteric symptoms of liver damage (jaundice, dark urine, pale stools)	Vaccination, palliative treatment	HBV infection is a serious occupational hazard to unprotected dentists and dental personnel
Acute, early illness—flu-like symptoms, fever, weight loss, chills, lymphadenopathy; chronic illness—extreme weight loss, chronic lymphadenopathy, intraoral lesions such as herpes labialis, hairy leukoplakia, candidiasis, HIV-associated gingivitis and periodontitis	No curative treatment is available; therapy with zidovudine (formerly azidothymidine or AZT) and/or similar medications may slow disease progression	HIV infection is a progressively debilitating and ultimately fatal illness which spans the clinical spectrum of no symptoms (asymptomatic period) to frank AIDS
Persistent cough, night sweats, loss of energy and appetite	Multi-drug chemotherapy such as isoniazid (INH) and rifampin, rest, proper nutrition	The incidence of TB is rising due largely to poor sanitary and living conditions, growing numbers of persons with AIDS, and reactivated disease
Urethral or vaginal discharge, pharyngitis; oral lesions are rare	Penicillin	One of the most prevalent sexually transmitted diseases
Primary syphilis—lymphadenopathy, chancre; secondary syphilis—generalized rash, bone lesions, red patches on mucosal membranes; tertiary syphilis—gummas, involvement of the CNS and circulatory system	Penicillin	Syphilis has been nicknamed "the great imitator" due to the varied clinical manifestations accompanying the infection

However, oral infections with *HSV type 2* and genital infections with *HSV type 1* are becoming more common and their disease manifestations are clinically indistinguishable. In relatively healthy patients, infections are localized to the skin and mucous membranes. However, virus dissemination within the immunosuppressed individual or newborn may lead to serious sequelae such as esophagitis, pneumonitis, hepatitis, meningitis, or viral encephalitis.[10]

Primary infection with HSV type 1 usually occurs in children and is typically subclinical, but may be preceded by malaise, headache, irritability, fever, lymphadenopathy, and pharyngitis. Oral manifestations of primary HSV infection present as **primary herpetic gingivostomatitis,** an intraoral condition characterized by intensely red gingiva and small, painful vesicles (fluid-filled lesions) on the lips, facial mucosa, palate, pharynx, tonsils, or gingiva (Plate 5-1, *A*). After the lesions rupture, they appear as shallow ulcers with irregular red borders ("halo") and are covered by a gray pseudomembranous covering (Plate 5-1, *B, left*). Symptoms may last from 10 to 14 days before resolving. It is important to note that infectious virus is present during this period and can be easily transmitted to others via contact with lesions and infected saliva.

During *primary infection,* the virus gains access to the nerve endings adjacent to the point of entry. HSV then retreats along the nerve to the sensory ganglia (trigeminal ganglion for oral lesions) where it lies dormant until reactivated by one of several factors (e.g., stress, sunlight, trauma, fatigue, or allergy). Upon reactivation, the virus travels down the nerve to the epithelium, where it produces secondary herpetic lesions on the lips (*"herpes labialis,"* commonly known as fever blisters or cold sores) (Plate 5-1, *C*) or, less frequently, within the oral cavity. These *secondary herpetic lesions,* usually seen in adults, are frequently preceded by a burning or tingling sensation at the site where a single vesicle or cluster of vesicles subsequently develops.

Intraoral herpetic lesions can be differentiated from *aphthous ulcers* (lesions usually of unknown origin, but often associated with trauma and subsequent infection) in that the former are confined to the attached tissues of the palate, gingiva, and alveolar ridges (Plate 5-1, *B, left*) whereas the latter usually present on movable mucosa (e.g., facial mucosa, alveolar mucosa, floor of mouth) (Plate 5-1, *B, right*). In addition, intraoral HSV lesions occur in clusters with well-defined borders; aphthous ulcers appear as solitary lesions with irregular borders. Topical or systemic administration of the antiviral drug acyclovir reduces the duration and severity of symptoms if given prior to the onset of skin lesions. However, the extensive lesions seen in immunosuppressed patients infected with HSV require lengthy systemic therapy for complete resolution.[2]

HSV infections are also of particular concern to those delivering patient care. **Herpetic whitlow,** HSV infection of the finger, has been documented in dental professionals (Plate 5-1, *D*). This painful lesion arises from contact of infected oral secretions with broken skin of the finger. In addition, *ocular infection* with HSV may occur following auto-inoculation from an oral infection, with potentially serious consequences of scarring and blindness. *The routine use of gloves and protective eyewear during patient treatment significantly reduces the occupational exposure to HSV.*

Chickenpox (varicella) and shingles (zoster). Infection with the *varicella zoster virus* presents as chickenpox (varicella) during initial exposure and as shingles (zoster) in reactivated (or recurrent) disease. Chickenpox, a common and relatively mild childhood disease, is easily transmitted by airborne droplets and direct contact. Following an incubation period of 2 to 3 weeks, infected individuals frequently complain of malaise and fever. A rash typically appears on the trunk and spreads centrifugally to the head and extremities (Plate 5-1, *E*). The rash is later replaced by crops of vesicles which rupture and crust. Lesions frequently appear on the oral mucosa as non-painful, blister-like ulcers that resemble aphthous ulcers (Plate 5-1, *F*).

After acute infection, the virus remains dormant indefinitely in the dorsal root ganglia of the affected sensory nerves. Reactivation in the form of shingles or zoster may occur decades later in the immunocompetent adult over the age of 50 or at any age in the immunosuppressed individual. *Reactivation of virus replication occurs along the sensory distribution of the affected nerve (dermatome)* and is frequently accompanied by itching and neuralgia. Skin lesions also occur characteristically along the unilateral dermatome distribution and appear as vesicles which erupt and ulcerate (Plate 5-1, *G*). In the relatively healthy adult, the active disease is brought under control within a few days. However, in the elderly or severely immunocompromised, the lesions may resolve slowly and neural pain may persist for several months. Treatment includes palliative agents to decrease itching and pain and the antiviral drug acyclovir to limit the duration and intensity of symptoms.

An infected patient with chickenpox may transmit virus via the respiratory route for 1 to 5 days following the appearance of the rash. Treating an infected patient in the dental office during that period may disseminate the infection to other susceptible patients and to dental personnel. Therefore, *routine dental care should be postponed in patients with chickenpox until all lesions have crusted.*

Condyloma acuminatum (venereal warts). Condyloma acuminatum, more commonly referred to as the venereal wart, is caused by the human papillomavirus. This transmissible and auto-inoculable disease affects the anogenital skin and mucosa. Oral lesions initially present as soft pink nodules on the gingiva or other mucosal surface. These nodules may remain flat with well-defined margins or may coalesce to form raised, papillomatous ("cauliflower-like") clusters (Plate 5-1, *H*). Typically asymptomatic, lesions may be localized or scattered throughout the mouth and frequently recur. Because some lesions have premalignant potential, removal by surgical excision, cryosurgery, or laser therapy is recommended.

Respiratory viruses. Arguably the most frequently transmitted diseases within the dental environment are those caused by respiratory viruses. This group of viruses includes both viruses whose primary disease manifestations directly affect the respiratory tract (e.g., rhinoviruses, respiratory syncytial viruses, and influenza viruses) and viruses that are transmitted via respiratory secretions but manifest themselves through other organ systems (e.g., rubeola and rubella). Transmission occurs through inhalation of or direct contact with droplets and aerosols. Depending on the etiological agent, symptoms may include sneezing, cough, low-grade fever, headache, malaise, conjunctivitis, and rash. In the immunocompetent individual, these respiratory infections are usually self-limiting and have few serious sequelae. However, in the immunocompromised or medically compromised patient, serious morbidity and mortality may result. The anti-viral agent amantadine may provide relief in these severe situations. Annual vaccination for influenza viruses is recommended, especially in the elderly and other highly susceptible populations. Vaccines are not currently available for the other respiratory viruses.

Rubeola (measles). Rubeola, also known as measles, is a highly contagious viral childhood disease that spreads via respiratory secretions. Following an incubation period of 10 to 12 days, virus multiplication in the upper respiratory tract and conjunctivae causes prodromal symptoms of dry cough, sore throat, headache, low-grade fever, and conjunctivitis. During this prodromal stage, characteristic intraoral lesions known as **Koplik spots** may appear on the facial mucosa opposite the first and second maxillary molars. These lesions resemble white grains of sand set within red, inflamed patches. Following the prodromal period, a red maculopapular rash appears on the head and face and quickly extends to the extremities. Pharyngitis is commonly present. Because virus shedding occurs during the prodromal period and for about 2 days after the appearance of the rash (before the disease can be recognized), measles is spread rapidly throughout populated regions and can quickly escalate to epidemic proportions. However, since widespread vaccination began in 1973, the number and geographical extent of measles outbreaks have been limited. Although this infection is usually self-limiting, secondary infection of the lesions with staphylococci or other bacteria may result.

Rubella (German measles). Rubella, commonly called German measles, results from infection with a togavirus, a virus distinct from the causative agent of rubeola. Rubella is an extremely mild disease characterized by fever, transient rash, and vesicular eruption, features that closely resemble rubeola but are of shorter duration. Like rubeola, rubella is transmitted by droplets from the mouth, nose, and throat, and is communicable before symptoms appear. Although rare, oral lesions appear as rose-colored lesions of the palatal mucosa and the posterior region of the oral cavity. The disease is usually benign and self-limiting; however, secondary staphylococcal infections may develop and infection during the first trimester of pregnancy can cause *serious congenital defects in the fetus. Therefore, female dental professionals and the spouses of male dental professionals should be protected by vaccination and by adherence to proper infection control measures.*

Mumps. Bilateral or unilateral enlargement of the parotid, submandibular, and/or sublingual glands is the hallmark of mumps, a childhood disease. The paramyxovirus, the etiological agent of mumps, is transmitted via respiratory droplets and saliva. Following an incubation period of 2 to 5 weeks, symptoms include headache, malaise, weight loss, fever, and swollen, tender salivary glands. Infected individuals are considered infectious approximately 2 days before swelling is noted, and remain infectious until approximately 9 days after swelling subsides. Although mumps can be an uncomfortable illness, it has few serious sequelae and an effective vaccine is available. Since this viral infection is spread by saliva via droplet dissemination and direct contact, *care must be taken to limit transmission in the dental practice.*

Infectious mononucleosis (IM). Primary infection with the **Epstein-Barr virus (EBV)** results in infectious mononucleosis (IM), an acute illness characterized by generalized lymphadenopathy, mild fever, and *petechiae (pin-point sub-surface hemorrhages) typically at the border of the hard and soft palates.* Although the virus is present in saliva and exudates, IM is not very contagious and is transmitted mainly by direct contact with infected saliva (hence the nickname, "kissing disease"). IM typically lasts from 1 to 4 weeks but may linger for several months or longer. No specific treatment is available for IM and serious complications rarely develop.

Hepatitis B virus (HBV). The hepatitis B virus (HBV) is readily transmitted through body fluids such as blood and saliva, and represents a *significant occupational hazard for the dental professional.* Fortunately, an effective vaccine is readily available for protection against HBV. Follow-up evaluation of immunization is also important to ensure that an appropriate immune response is generated. However, up to two thirds of acutely infected individuals report no symptoms and are unaware that they harbor the virus.[7] *Because both symptomatic and asymptomatic infected patients can transmit the virus, universal precautions must be taken with all patients to prevent disease transmission.* During the acute stage of infection, individuals may exhibit vague symptoms of nausea, gastrointestinal distress, muscular aches, low-grade fever, chronic fatigue, or *jaundice* (yellowing of the skin and sclera). No distinct oral changes are associated with HBV infection. Other aspects of HBV infection are detailed in Chapter 4.

Human immunodeficiency virus (HIV). The majority of individuals infected with the human immunodeficiency virus (HIV) present with some type of intraoral manifestation, many of which may be detected early in the disease course.[12] Lesions associated with HIV may arise from either newly-acquired infections or from re-activation of opportunistic infections, asymptomatic infections that are usually held in check by a competent immune system. However, during the course of HIV disease, the immune response slowly and progressively deteriorates, allowing these opportunistic infections to reappear and cause significant morbidity and mortality. HIV-associated lesions arise from a variety of sources: *fungal infections* (candidiasis), *viral infections* (herpetic lesions, hairy leukoplakia, warts), *bacterial infections* (HIV-gingivitis, HIV-periodontitis) and *neoplastic origin* (Kaposi's sarcoma), in addition to those of *generalized or undetermined origin* (lymphadenopathy, aphthous-like ulcers, HIV-associated salivary gland disease). Clinical manifestations not previously discussed in this section will be briefly addressed.

Oral candidiasis. The most prevalent oral infection in HIV-infected individuals, oral candidiasis, a fungal infection, often presents as the initial manifestation and frequently predicts the likelihood of other opportunistic infections.[5,13] Although occasionally observed in elderly patients, the detection of these lesions is strongly suggestive of HIV infection in a young person without a known cause such as xerostomia ("dry mouth") or therapy with antibiotics, corticosteroids, or other immunosuppressive drugs.

Candidiasis appears on oral mucosa as one of four distinct forms: (1) pseudomembranous, (2) hyperplastic, (3) atrophic or erythematous, or (4) angular cheilitis. *Pseudomembranous candidiasis,* or *thrush,* is characterized by white or yellow plaques that can be easily wiped off to reveal erythematous surfaces which easily bleed (Plate 5-1, *I*). The *hyperplastic form* also appears as light-colored plaques but cannot be removed by scraping. The *atrophic form* occurs as smooth, red patches, more commonly on palatal tissues, facial mucosa, or the dorsal surface of the tongue. *Angular cheilitis* appears as fissures or ulcers radiating from the corners of the mouth and are frequently associated with white plaques. Candidiasis is generally diagnosed by its clinical appearance and confirmed by staining with potassium hydroxide. If left untreated, oral candidiasis can extend into the esophagus and develop into a potentially life-threatening illness. In most cases, oral candidiasis can be treated effectively with antifungal agents such as nystatin, chlotrimazole, or ketoconazole; however, refractory cases may require systemic antifungal chemotherapy.

Hairy leukoplakia (HL). First reported by Greenspan et al.[6] in 1984, oral hairy leukoplakia (HL) describes an adherent, filamentous white plaque which exhibits a characteristic corrugated or "hairy" appearance (Plate 5-1, *J*). The lesion is typically observed on parakeratinized mucosa on the lateral border of the tongue, and may occur unilaterally or bilaterally. However, HL may

extend to cover the dorsal surface of the tongue and can also appear on facial mucosa. This lesion is caused by the Epstein-Barr virus, is usually asymptomatic, and has no known premalignant potential.

Kaposi's sarcoma (KS). HIV-infected patients may present with Kaposi's sarcoma (KS), a malignancy involving the endothelial covering of blood vessel walls. This lesion is often an initial manifestation of the severe stage of HIV disease known as **acquired immune deficiency syndrome (AIDS).** Over half of patients with mucocutaneous KS exhibit oral and perioral lesions.[3] The clinical appearance of oral KS is variable, but typically presents as blue, purple, or brown raised areas on the palate (Plate 5-1, *K),* and may also be present on the tongue, gingiva or other oral structures. Nearly two thirds of patients with oral KS have associated symptoms of pain or difficulty in swallowing.[14]

HIV-gingivitis. HIV-gingivitis is characterized by a marginal gingivitis associated with distinct linear marginal erythema or diffuse, punctate lesions involving the attached and alveolar mucosal surfaces (Plate 5-1, *L*). Petechiae are frequently an associated finding. Spontaneous bleeding or bleeding upon probing of the involved gingiva may be present even in patients with meticulous home care. Treatment consists of local debridement, with scaling and root planing, irrigation with an antimicrobial agent such as povidone-iodine, and rinses with chlorhexidine.

HIV-periodontitis. HIV-periodontitis presents all the features of HIV-gingivitis but includes severe soft tissue ulceration, gingival necrosis, and rapid destruction of the periodontal attachment and alveolar bone. These rapidly progressive lesions resemble acute necrotizing ulcerative gingivitis (ANUG) but are not confined to the soft tissues and do not recur episodically. *The intense pain and spontaneous bleeding associated with HIV-periodontitis often drive patients to seek dental care.* Patients usually respond to an aggressive course of debridement involving scaling and root planing, irrigation with the antimicrobial agent povidone-iodine (which also has a topical anesthetic effect), and rinses with chlorhexidine. However, refractory lesions may require further treatment by a specialist.

Lymphadenopathy. Lymphadenopathy, or swollen lymph glands, is an almost invariant feature of HIV infection. Lymphadenopathy may be present at any time throughout the course of infection. Manual palpation of the superficial lymph nodes of the neck will reveal the presence of cervical lymphadenopathy during the extraoral clinical examination.

Aphthous ulcers. Aphthous-like ulcerations may appear during the course of HIV infection (Plate 5-1, *B, right*). These ulcers usually persist and may be associated with ulcers of the esophagus and pharynx. The application of topical corticosteroids can hasten healing in many instances; however, systemic corticosteroid therapy may be required for lesions resistant to topical treatment.

Salivary-gland disease. Some HIV-infected individuals complain of xerostomia with or without enlargement of parotid and minor salivary glands during the early stage of infection. Although the cause of this salivary-gland disease is unclear, the xerostomia and glandular swelling both may be managed by conventional means and zidovudine (formerly azidothymidine [AZT]) therapy.

Tuberculosis (TB). Tuberculosis (TB) is a highly contagious granulomatous disease caused by the slow-growing, rod-shaped, acid-fast bacillus *Mycobacterium tuberculosis*. This bacillus is transmitted via inhalation of respiratory droplets and aerosols (e.g., sputum and saliva), ingestion, or direct inoculation. Initial infection usually occurs in the lungs or intestines, depending on the route of transmission. However, dissemination to other regions such as the bones, meninges, kidneys, skin, lymph nodes, and oral structures may occur. Unless aggressively treated with multi-drug chemotherapy, the unhealed bacterial lesions *(tubercles)* persist indefinitely within walled-off regions of the lungs and body tissues. *Caseation* (cheese-like) *necrosis* results as dead cells accumulate in the center of the tubercles. These caseous lesions may eventually heal by fibrosis and calcification to form radiodense *Ghon complexes* detectable upon radiographic evaluation of the lungs. However, in a small percentage of infected individuals, the lesions do not heal and release infectious particles that disseminate throughout the body to seed other organs *(miliary tuberculosis)*.

The accurate diagnosis of TB is a common and serious problem because the infection may not be suspected or recognized. Furthermore, symptoms resemble those of other infectious diseases such as HIV: fatigue, cough, excessive weight loss, low-grade fever, and recurrent night sweats. *Oral lesions,* which occur rarely and are usually secondary to pulmonary involvement, include tuberculosis gingivitis, tuberculosis of the lips, and persistent exudative ulcers of the tongue. Because these oral lesions may mimic squamous cell carcinoma, differential diagnosis should include one of several tests for TB: the skin test (PPD), sputum culture, and chest x-ray.

TB remains one of the most widespread and persistent human transmissible infections worldwide. Historically, the incidence of TB in developed countries has decreased due to effective chemotherapeutic agents and isolation procedures; however, TB remains a major cause of disease and death in underdeveloped and developing third-world countries. Unfortunately, the recent emergence of drug-resistant strains of *Mycobacterium tuberculosis* coupled with increasing poverty,

homelessness, crowding, and rising numbers of persons with AIDS have led to the *resurgence of TB as a significant public health problem in this country.* An important and growing source of TB is the elderly who were infected in the 1920s and 1930s and continued to harbor persistent bacillus. These individuals may experience a reactivation of their disease with deterioration of their immune response with aging.

The TB-infected patient represents a significant occupational hazard for dental personnel. Open lesions and infected sputum and saliva are highly contagious. Moreover, the outer lipid coating ("spore") of the bacillus allows the organism to survive in dried fluids for extended periods of time and renders it resistant to many germicidal agents. Therefore, *dental personnel must adhere to proper infection control measures which include personal protective barriers (e.g., eyewear, mask, and gloves) during patient treatment and the appropriate use of tuberculocidal disinfectants and sterilants (see Chapter 4).*

Gonorrhea. The bacterium *Neisseria gonorrhoeae,* a gram-negative diplococci, is the etiological agent for gonorrhea, one of the most prevalent sexually transmitted diseases today. This organism is spread by direct contact with infected mucosal lesions of the urogenital tract, eyes, and oral cavity. Following an incubation period of 2 to 21 days, infected individuals may experience purulent urethral or vaginal discharge and pharyngitis. Rare oral lesions appear as patchy edema and erythema of the tonsillar regions and uvula, and as vesicles at the site of primary contact. Diagnosis is made by culture of the organism or microscopic examination of the discharge. Although this infection is effectively treated with penicillin, the emergence of penicillin-resistant strains of gonorrhea has heightened the awareness of gonorrhea as a serious public health threat.

Syphilis. Caused by the bacteria *Treponema pallidum,* syphilis may be acquired congenitally or through direct contact with infected mucous membranes of the oral, genital, and anorectal regions. Syphilis is characterized by three stages. *Primary syphilis* of the oral cavity appears as a hard ulcer (chancre) of the lip, tongue, gingiva, or palate. Unless treated with an antibiotic such as penicillin, primary syphilis may progress to secondary syphilis. A red maculopapular rash on the body, highly infectious erythematous patches on mucous membranes, bone defects, and recurrences characterize the secondary form. Continued progression can lead to *tertiary syphilis* with neurological or cardiovascular involvement. Lesions may present intraorally as *gummas,* granulomatous lesions on the palate or tongue which may erode and/or affect the central nervous system. Although individuals in the tertiary stage are not infectious, untreated individuals in the primary and secondary stages are highly contagious.

In summary, dental professionals must be aware of the signs and symptoms of infectious diseases and their routes of transmission for the proper evaluation, diagnosis, and management of patients. *Since these contagious diseases may be spread from the infected patient to the dental team and to other patients, meticulous attention to infection control practices is essential.*

Allergies or medications. The patient interview should include a discussion of any allergies or medications noted on the medical history form. Sometimes patients report that they are "sensitive" or allergic to local anesthetic. They often refer to having had a reaction after the injection of "Novocaine." These alleged reactions are often attributable to excessive anesthetic deposited over too short a time, or, more likely, to an intravascular deposition. Nevertheless, when any patient relays *a history of "sensitivity" from injected dental anesthetic, the dentist must believe the patient until further investigation* (be it verbal questions and answers, or allergic testing in a sophisticated life support environment) disproves the patient's belief of an allergy. These precautions are necessary because *anaphylactic shock following an allergic reaction can be immediate and life-threatening.*

Medications used by the patient can also affect diagnosis and treatment. Certain medications can modify normal salivary flow and composition, alter normal appearance of oral soft tissues, or affect the metabolism and/or therapeutic effect of other pharmacologic agents. For example, *tricyclic antidepressants* may render patients extremely sensitive to epinephrine, anti-epileptic agents may cause gingival enlargement, and antibiotics may reduce the efficacy of oral contraceptives.

Systemic diseases and cardiac abnormalities. The presence of systemic diseases or cardiac abnormalities may require that treatment be altered. The reader is referred to Patient Physical Factors; Relationship to Anesthetic and Epinephrine, Chapter 10. Of special note are patients with certain heart disorders. The manipulation of mucosal surfaces during dental procedures may release bloodborne bacteria that lodge on abnormal or damaged heart valves or in the filial tissues, resulting in bacterial endocarditis. Patients with cardiac conditions such as valvular defects or heart murmurs are at an increased risk of acquiring bacterial endocarditis following surgical and dental procedures. Therefore, these patients should be treated prophylactically with an appropriate antibiotic prior to and following dental treatment. The reader is referred to the latest recommendations by the American Heart Association for information regarding antibiotic-dosing regimen, specific cardiac conditions for which endocarditis prophylaxis is recommended, and the dental procedures requiring coverage.[4]

As a screening test for underlying diseases such as hypertension, the patient's pulse and blood pressure are taken and recorded. This information provides a baseline for monitoring changes in the patient's health over time and for managing medical emergencies. If any patient presents with a systolic blood pressure >200 and/or diastolic blood pressure >115, *routine dental treatment should be deferred until acceptable levels are achieved.*

Physiological changes associated with aging. With the lengthening life span and increased retention of teeth by older patients, dentists are treating more *geriatric patients.* It is important to thoroughly understand the medical and dental background of older adult patients. The geriatric population can experience significant changes in behavior and diet, as well as in oral and systemic health. Certain medications and illnesses may alter oral physiology, oral hygiene, and dental health, necessitating changes in treatment. For example, *xerostomia,* or reduced salivary flow, may be a side effect of anticholinergic and antihypertensive medications and may result in increased caries incidence, mucosal alterations, and plaque retention. The use of salivary stimulants such as sugar-free candy drops, artificial saliva or pilocarpine in more serious cases, along with lowering drug dosage, may lessen or relieve this symptom. Additional considerations include the limited use of vasoconstrictors in patients with advanced cardiovascular disease, reduced dosages of diazepam to prevent over-sedation due to poor renal/hepatic clearance with aging, and interactions between drugs prescribed for dental purposes and the patient's other medications (e.g., epinephrine and antidepressants).

A number of *normal physiological changes* may occur in older patients and should not be mistaken for pathological conditions. For example, the skin and blood vessels lose their elasticity due to degeneration of the elastic connective tissue and delayed healing following surgical procedures may result. Bones become more brittle and easily broken with advancing age. Sensory impairment may lead to hearing loss, visual changes, and alterations in taste and smell.

Dental and mucosal changes may also be associated with the aging process. A tooth can change shape due to many years of attrition, abrasion, and wear of proximal surfaces. Variations in pulpal anatomy, physiology, and color changes due to extrinsic staining can occur with age and may lead to increased brittleness of the teeth. A continuous thickening of the cementum is frequently noted and is most pronounced in the apical regions. The gingivae can become edematous, friable with a loss of stippling, and recede. The diminished salivary flow results in loss of elasticity of the oral mucosa as well as increased caries rate. An understanding that these physiological or metabolical changes are not pathological is essential for proper operative treatment planning for the geriatric patient.

Table 5-2. Guidelines for prescribing dental radiographs for dentulous adults

New patients	Recall patients		
All new patients to assess dental diseases	Clinical caries or high-risk factors for caries*	No clinical caries and no high-risk factors for caries*	Periodontal disease or a history of periodontal treatment
Individualized radiographic examination consisting of posterior bitewings and selected periapicals; a full-mouth intraoral radiographic examination is appropriate when the patient has clinical evidence of generalized dental disease or a history of extensive dental treatment	Posterior bitewing examination at 12-18 month intervals	Posterior bitewing examination at 24-36 month intervals	Individualized radiographic examination consisting of selected periapical and/or bitewing radiographs for areas where periodontal disease (other than nonspecific gingivitis) can be demonstrated clinically

*See Table 5-3 for caries risk factors

Of primary importance in planning dental therapy is the biological or physiological age of the older patient, not the chronological age. Factors such as genetic predisposition, physical or mental capabilities, and the presence of chronic disease may make an individual's biological age older or younger than his or her chronological age. Consideration of these factors in the treatment plan is crucial for the long-term success of any dental treatment of the older patient.

Sociological and psychological review

During initial visits the clinician should ascertain the patient's attitudes, priorities, expectations, and motivations toward dental care. Attitudinal information combined with assessment of the patient's dental appreciation, educability, habits, parental history, occupation, and financial situation can indicate the patient's commitment to dental care. This commitment contributes to the overall success of dental treatment. As with every facet of patient assessment and examination, it is essential to maintain and update records of discussions and clinical findings.

During this portion of the pretreatment assessment, the dentist must begin to explore patient's preferences for dental care. The results of this exploration will affect the dentist's treatment recommendations.

Dental history and chief complaint

The dental history consists of reviewing previous dental experiences and current dental problems. Review of the dental history reveals information about past dental problems and treatment. Frequency of dental care and perceptions of that care may be indications of the patient's future behavior. Obviously if a patient has difficulty tolerating certain types of procedures or has encountered problems with previous dental care, an alteration of the treatment or environment may help to avoid future complications. Also, this discussion may lead to

identification of other problems such as areas of food impaction, inability to floss, areas of pain, and broken restorations and/or tooth structure. It is important to understand past experiences to provide optimal care in the future.

After review of the dental history, attention should be directed to the patient's present problem, with the chief complaint recorded verbatim in the chart. The patient should be encouraged and guided to discuss all aspects of the current problem, including onset, duration, and related factors. This information is vital to establish the need for additional diagnostic tests and to determine the cause and treatment of the complaint.

Finally, it is important to know the date and type of available radiographs to ascertain the need for additional radiographs and minimize the patient's exposure to unnecessary ionizing radiation. The Food and Drug Administration (FDA) guidelines[9] help direct the type and frequency of radiographs needed according to patient condition and risk factors (Table 5-2).

Risk assessment

Few diseases known to man are caused by a single factor. Instead most diseases have been shown to be associated with numerous behavioral/socio-demographic, physical/environmental, microbiological, or host factors. In addition, every patient possesses a different set of *risk factors* and as such presents a challenge to determine the likelihood that disease is present or will occur in the future. For example, patients who possess a number of the risk factors shown in Table 5-3 should be considered at high risk for dental caries. This assessment will then be used to guide treatment. A patient at high risk for dental caries should receive aggressive intervention to remove or alter as many risk factors as possible. Alternatively, watchful waiting or periodic reassessment of the condition may be appropriate for a patient at low risk for dental caries.

Table 5-3. Risk factors for caries

Factors	High-risk characteristics
Non-oral	
Age	Younger, <18 yr; older, >65 yr
Social-economic status (SES)	Lower SES
Medical condition	Reduced salivation
Medications	Reduced salivation
Fluoride history	Lack of fluoride during tooth development
Dietary habits	High intake of refined carbohydrates; tobacco and alcohol use
Genetic predisposition	Family history of disease
General health	Debilitation and decreased ability to give self-care
Oral	
Tooth anatomy/composition	Development fissures and low fluoride content
Oral flora/plaque	High levels of *mutans streptococcus* (see Chapter 3)
Previous infection/restorations	History of extensive restoration
Restorations	Defective restorations
Oral hygiene—skills, knowledge, motivation	Poor oral hygiene

Risk assessment is a relatively young science in the health care professions. Historically dentists have relied on their knowledge of the disease process in combination with their experiences and intuition to estimate the risk levels for their patients. To properly prescribe and determine appropriate preventive and therapeutic strategies, the dentist must consider the patient's overall risk status in the context of the current level of understanding disease progression. Though such understanding is not yet perfected, we do know that certain conditions place patients at a higher risk for dental disease. Knowing this, dentists try to identify and measure risk factors for dental disease during the initial oral examination and subsequent patient appointments.

EXAMINATION AND DIAGNOSIS

This section describes the examination and diagnosis of problems with orofacial soft tissues, teeth, restorations, periodontium, and occlusion. Special considerations for evaluating the patient presenting with pain are also reviewed. In practice each tooth is evaluated individually by using a combination of clinical and radiographic examinations and appropriate adjunctive tests. However, for the purpose of presentation, the clinical examination, radiographic survey, and use of adjunctive diagnostic aids are discussed separately.

General considerations

Clinical *examination* is the "hands-on" process of observing both normal and abnormal conditions. *Diagnosis* is a determination and judgment of variations from normal. During the clinical examination the dentist must be keenly sensitive to subtle signs, symptoms, and variations from normal to detect pathological conditions and etiological factors. Meticulous attention to detail generates a base of information for diagnosing the patient's general physical health and dental problems.

As alluded to in the previous section on infection control, *universal infection control* measures should be adhered to throughout the medical interview. Certainly before any "hands-on" examination, standard precautions must be taken to avoid the transmission of disease. These precautions include the *sterilization/disinfection* of all instruments, supplies, and operatory surfaces, as well as *barrier techniques* such as gloves, masks, protective eyewear, and gowns, consistent with prevailing standards (see Chapter 4).

While following accepted barrier techniques, the initial step in the clinical examination includes an observation of the patient's general physical health and oral condition to determine the presence of potentially harmful *communicable diseases* (see Plate 5-1 and Table 5-1). However, as emphasized in Chapter 4, some individual disease carriers such as those infected with HIV or HBV may not be identified during medical review and clinical examination. This underscores the necessity for routine and universal infection control for all dental patients.

An additional preliminary consideration is a cursory examination of the general tooth alignment and occlusal relationship since this information is helpful in the subsequent detailed examination.

Charting and records. Normal and abnormal clinical and radiographic findings are noted on a detailed chart as a permanent part of the patient's records (Fig. 5-2, pp. 182-183). The exact location and condition of all teeth, restorations, defects, and caries, and soft/hard tissues are necessary for many reasons: (1) *proper care*—a thorough charting of existing conditions provides basic information for an accurate, comprehensive treatment plan; (2) *third-party communication*—accurate records of the patient's conditions are useful in communicating with third-party payment agencies; (3) *practice audits/quality assessment*—dental charts and records are the foundation of many quality assurance programs because the content, completeness, and accuracy of records are used as measures of the care provided; (4) *legal proceedings*—the dental record is considered legal, admissible evidence in arbitration of contended negligence or malpractice; and (5) *forensic uses*—in many instances, the dental record is the only means of identifying the deceased person. In addition, there is growing use of *intraoral photographs* to supplement routine dental charting.

Although various formats are available for recording a patient's dental condition, an acceptable **charting system** should conform to certain standards. The chart should be (1) *uncomplicated*—should be easily understood by the dentist and staff and be an effective and accurate means of recording dental conditions; (2) *comprehensive*—should note all dental conditions, both normal and abnormal, and a detailed representation of location, nature, and size of all restorations; (3) *accessible*—should be part of the permanent patient record, which is easily accessible for referencing during treatment or recall appointments; and (4) *current*—should allow for continual updating as treatment is rendered and as dental or medical conditions change. If these guidelines are followed, the findings of a thorough and systematic examination can be maintained for each patient.

Denotation. To expedite the designation of teeth during examination and charting, a denotation system is used. There are several denotation systems in use, but the one used in this text is the *universal system*. In this system the teeth are numbered from 1 to 32 starting with the maxillary right third molar and continuing around the arch to the left third molar, then continuing with the mandibular left third molar as No. 17 and ending with the right third molar as No. 32.

Preparation for clinical examination. A chairside assistant familiar with the terminology, denotation system, and charting procedure can survey and record the teeth and existing restorations to save chair time for the dentist. Subsequently, the dentist will perform the examination, confirm the charting, make a diagnosis, and develop the treatment plan. The clinical examination is performed systematically in a clean, dry, well-illuminated mouth. Proper instruments including a mirror, explorer, and periodontal probe are required. A routine for charting should be established such as starting in the upper right quadrant with the most posterior tooth and progressing around the maxillary and mandibular arches. An accurate examination can occur only when the teeth are clean and dry. This may require initial scaling, flossing, and a toothbrushing prophylaxis before final clinical examination of the teeth. A cotton roll in the vestibular space and another under the tongue will maintain dryness and improve vision (Fig. 5-3). Dental floss is useful in determining overhanging restorations, improper contours, and open contacts.

Interpretation and use of diagnostic tests. The diagnostic effort of health professionals has been enhanced by the use of principles adopted from the discipline of **clinical epidemiology.** This analytical approach is a means of increasing the certainty in the interpretation of diagnostic tests. It relies on a "two by two" contingency table (Box 5-1). These tables are created from data de-

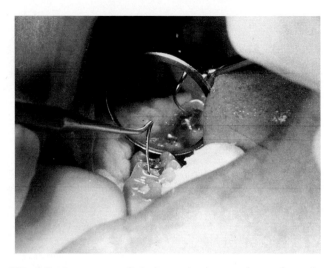

Fig. 5-3. An accurate clinical examination requires a clean, dry, well-illuminated mouth. Cotton rolls are placed in the vestibular space and under the tongue to maintain dryness and enhance visibility.

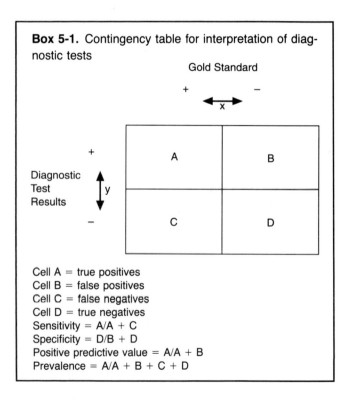

Box 5-1. Contingency table for interpretation of diagnostic tests

Gold Standard

Cell A = true positives
Cell B = false positives
Cell C = false negatives
Cell D = true negatives
Sensitivity = A/A + C
Specificity = D/B + D
Positive predictive value = A/A + B
Prevalence = A/A + B + C + D

rived from controlled clinical studies. Such studies compare the results of a diagnostic test with those obtained from a "gold standard" (knowledge of the actual condition) to determine how well the test diagnoses the "true" condition. The results of the diagnostic tests, positive or negative, are plotted on the y axis of the table, and the results of a gold standard or the "truth" are plotted on the x axis. Cell A of the table contains those

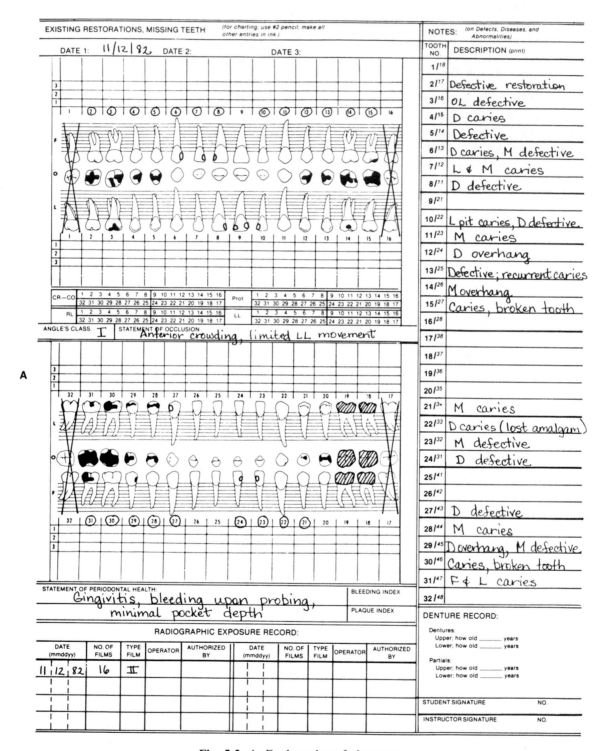

Fig. 5-2, A. For legend see facing page.

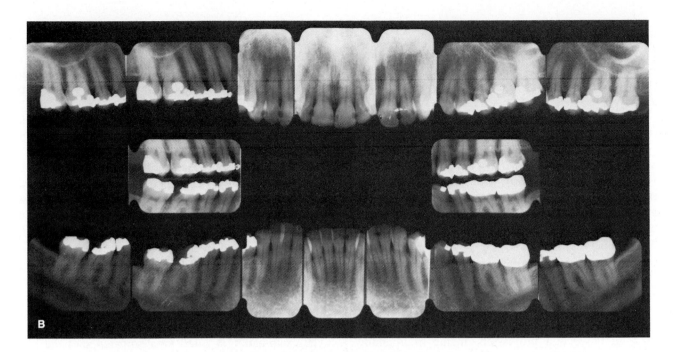

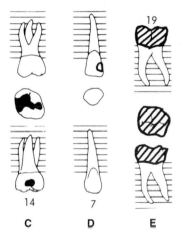

Fig. 5-2. **A,** An appropriate charting system designates location, type, and extent of existing restorations and presence of disease and defects, all of which become part of the permanent patient record. **B,** Radiographic findings obtained from this full-mouth series are correlated with the findings of the clinical examination and noted in the patient's record. The following may be used as keys to charting **A:** (1) *amalgam restorations* **(C)** are depicted by an outline drawing, blocked in solidly, showing the size, shape, and location of the restoration; (2) *tooth-colored restorations* **(D)** are depicted by an outline drawing of the size, shape, and location of the restoration; (3) *gold restorations* **(E)** are depicted by an outline drawing inscribed with diagonal lines of the size, shape, and location of the restoration; (4) *missing teeth* are depicted by a large **X** on the facial, occlusal, and lingual diagram of each tooth that is not visible in the mouth or on radiographs; (5) *caries* is recorded by circling the tooth number that is located at the apex of the involved tooth and by noting the presence and location of caries in the description column in the section corresponding to the tooth number on the right column; and (6) *defective restorations* are recorded by circling the tooth number and noting the defect in the description column.

cases that the test identifies as being both positive (or diseased) and confirmed by the gold standard. These cases are termed *true positives*. Cell B contains all cases for which there is a positive finding from the diagnostic test but a negative finding with the gold standard. This cell denotes *false positives*. Cell C includes those cases identified by the diagnostic test as being negative but found by the gold standard to be positive. Findings in this cell are termed *false negatives*. The final cell, cell D, includes *true negatives*. In cell D the diagnostic test accurately identifies the negative cases that are truly negative as confirmed by the gold standard. Thus, an ideal diagnostic test would result in most cases being assigned to cells A or D with few or no false positives (cell B) and false negatives (cell C).

Once the basics of this table are understood, there are several additional features that can be put to good use by the diagnostician. The first concept is *test sensitivity*. The sensitivity of a test is calculated as the number of true positives (A) divided by the number of total positive cases (A + C). This term indicates the proportion of positive cases in a population that are identified positively by the test. In contrast, *test specificity* is the proportion of negative cases properly classified by the diagnostic test and is the ratio of true negatives (D) to all negatives (B + D). Therefore, sensitivity and specificity relate to the proportion of cases in a population, positive or negative, that are predicted accurately by the diagnostic test. In contrast, the *positive predictive value* of a test is calculated by dividing the true positives (cell

A) by all cases tested as positive by the diagnostic test (cells A + B). The positive predictive value denotes the proportion of cases that test positive and are in fact positive.

Using these concepts, a clinician knows that if a diagnostic test has a high positive predictive value, there is a greater likelihood that a patient with a positive test does have the disease. Thus, if there is a positive result using a test with a high positive predictive value, the clinician has greater assurance that the diagnosed condition does actually exist. A test with low sensitivity indicates that there is a high probability that many of the cases with negative results will possess the disease and go undiagnosed (cell C—false negatives). Finally, tests with high specificity suggest that patients without the disease are highly likely to test negative.

These concepts are widely used in medical practice. While the necessary studies have not been conducted to develop these probabilities for dental conditions, there has been a growing interest in the use of clinical epidemiology in the dental profession. In the future more studies will be conducted that will provide this information for clinicians, and one should be prepared to take advantage of their use.

Examination of orofacial soft tissues

The reader is again referred to Plate 5-1 for a review of oral manifestations of contagious diseases and to Table 5-1 for clinical symptoms.

As with the other aspects of the clinical examination, *soft tissue evaluation* requires a systematic approach. Begin by examining the submandibular glands and cervical nodes for abnormalities in size, texture, mobility, and sensitivity to palpation. Then, palpate the masticatory muscles for pain or tenderness. Next, start in one area of the mouth and follow a routine pattern of visual examination and palpation of the cheeks, vestibules, mucosa, lips, lingual and facial alveolar mucosa, palate, tonsillar areas, tongue, and floor of the mouth. A thorough evaluation of all these structures is necessary before operative care is initiated. It is ill-advised to plan restorative procedures for a patient while a life-threatening disease process goes undiagnosed because a thorough examination was not conducted.

Examination of teeth and restorations

Clinical examination for caries. *Dental caries* is diagnosed by one or all of the following: (1) visual changes in tooth surface texture or color, (2) tactile sensation when an explorer is used, and (3) radiographs. The examination is aided by a knowledge of the likelihood of overall caries risk (Table 5-3), and patterns of susceptibility. For example, the patient's dental history, oral hygiene, diet, and age may suggest a certain pattern of caries activity. Caries also tends to occur bilaterally and on adjacent proximal surfaces (Fig. 5-4, *A* and *B*). If caries is found on the occlusal surface and a proximal surface in one tooth on one side of the arch, then the chances are increased that it will occur in the same locations on the opposite side. If caries is found on the

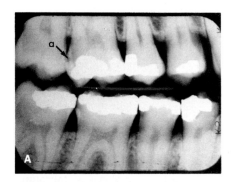
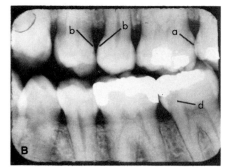
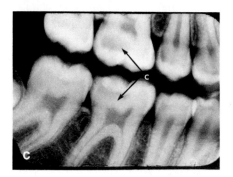
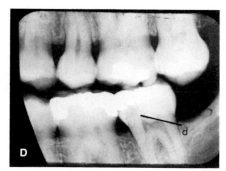

Fig. 5-4. Caries can be diagnosed radiographically as translucencies in the enamel or dentin. **A** and **B,** Proximal caries tends to occur bilaterally *(a)* and on adjacent surfaces *(b).* **C,** Occlusal caries *(c).* **D,** Recurrent caries gingival to an existing restoration *(d).* This same recurrent caries *(d)* is also shown in **B.**

proximal surface of one tooth, then the adjacent surface is suspect. In the clinical examination for caries, every questionable accessible surface of each tooth not only must be examined with an explorer to determine if cavitation is present but also must be inspected visually for localized changes in color, texture, and translucency.

Caries is most prevalent in the *faulty pits and fissures of the occlusal surfaces* where the developmental lobes of the posterior teeth failed to coalesce, partially or completely (Fig. 5-5, *B*). It is important to remember the distinction between primary occlusal grooves/fossae and occlusal fissures/pits. *Primary occlusal grooves/fossae* are smooth "valley/saucer" landmarks indicating the region of complete coalescence of developmental lobes. Normally, such *grooves/fossae are not susceptible to caries* because they are not niches for plaque (and bacteria), and furthermore are frequently cleansed by the rubbing action of food during mastication. Conversely, *occlusal fissure/pits* are deep, tight, crevices/holes in enamel where the lobes failed to coalesce, par-

tially or completely (see Fig. 2-12, in Chapter 2). Fissures/pits are detected visually and when a sharp explorer placed into the defect provides tug-back or resistance to removal. Generally this "catch" or resistance indicates that the developmental fault either has become carious or is likely to become carious. Sometimes it may be difficult to distinguish a wedging action of the explorer tip in a deep noncarious fissure/pit from the resistance felt when the explorer wedges into such a defect having walls affected by incipient caries. Clinical experience and judgment regarding the patient's susceptibility to caries help to differentiate the two conditions. In summary, *an occlusal surface is diagnosed as diseased* if any one of the following clinical/radiographic findings is present: (1) chalkiness or softening of the tooth structure forming the fissure/pit, (2) brown-gray discoloration radiating peripherally from the fissure/pit, or (3) radiolucency beneath the occlusal enamel surface. In contrast, *a non-diseased occlusal surface* will either have grooves/fossae or have shallow, very tight fis-

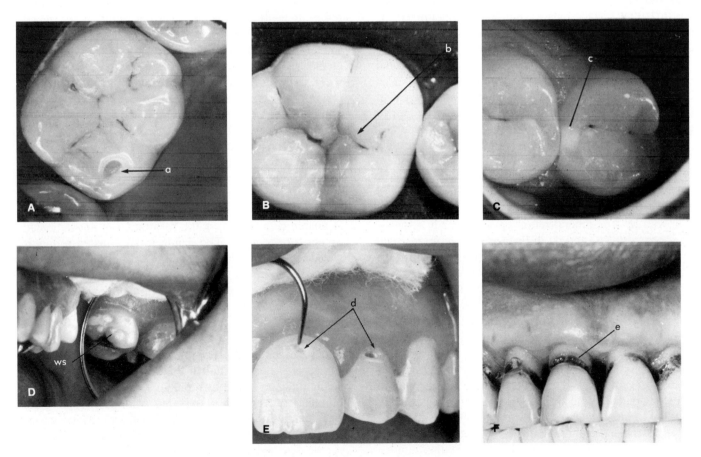

Fig. 5-5. Caries can be diagnosed clinically by careful inspection. **A,** Carious pit on cusp tip *(a)*. **B,** Loss of translucency and change in color of occlusal enamel *(b)* due to a carious fissure. **C,** White chalky appearance or shadow under marginal ridge *(c)*. **D,** Incipient smooth surface carious lesion, a white spot *(ws)*, has intact surface. **E,** Smooth surface caries can appear white or dark, depending on the degree of extrinsic staining *(d)*. **F,** Root surface caries *(e)*.

sures/pits which exhibit superficial staining and/or may cause a slight mechanical binding of an explorer but *has no radiographic evidence of caries*. This superficial staining is extrinsic and occurs over several years of oral exposure in a person with a low caries risk.

Precarious or carious pits are occasionally present on *cusp tips* (Figs. 5-5, *A* and 17-50). Typically these are the result of developmental enamel defects. *Carious pits and fissures* also occur on the *occlusal two-thirds of the facial or lingual surface of the posterior teeth* and on the *lingual surface of maxillary incisors* (see Caries Diagnosis, Chapter 3, for the U.S. Public Service criteria for the diagnosis of caries in pits and fissures.) As a supplement to tactile examination, occlusal enamel can be evaluated for loss of translucency and change in color, which are characteristic of caries (Fig. 5-5, *B*). This change in color can be dark gray and should not be confused with the noncarious fissures/pits that often become merely stained over time.

Proximal surface caries, one form of *smooth surface caries,* is usually diagnosed radiographically (Fig. 5-4, *A*). However, it may also be detected by careful visual and tactile examination. When caries has invaded the proximal surface enamel and has demineralized the dentin, a white chalky appearance or a shadow under the marginal ridge may become evident (Fig. 5-5, *C*). Careful probing with a sharp explorer on the proximal surface may detect cavitation, which is defined as a break in the surface contour of enamel. The use of all three examination methods is helpful in arriving at a final diagnosis.

Brown spots on intact, hard proximal surface enamel adjacent to and usually gingival to the contact area are often seen in older patients whose caries activity is low (Fig. 5-14, *C*). These discolored areas are a result of extrinsic staining during earlier caries episodes, each followed by a remineralization episode. Such a spot is no longer carious, and is, in fact, usually more resistant to caries due to fluorhydroxyapatite formation. *Restorative treatment is not indicated*. These arrested lesions sometimes challenge the diagnosis because of faint radiographic evidence of the remineralized lesion.

Proximal surface caries in anterior teeth may be identified by radiographic examination, visual inspection (trans-illumination optional), and/or probing with a sharp explorer. *Trans-illumination* is accomplished by placing the mirror or light source on the lingual side of the anterior teeth and directing light through the teeth. Proximal surface caries, if other than incipient, shows up as a dark area along the marginal ridge when light is directed through the tooth. In addition to trans-illumination, tactile exploration of the anterior teeth is appropriate to detect cavitation because the proximal surfaces generally are more visible and accessible than in the posterior regions. Small *incipient lesions* may be detectable only on the radiograph.

Another form of *smooth surface caries* often occurs on the *facial and lingual surfaces* of the teeth, particularly in gingival areas that are less accessible for cleaning. The earliest clinical evidence of *incipient caries* on these surfaces is a *white spot* that is visually different from the adjacent translucent enamel and will partially or totally disappear from vision by wetting. Drying again will cause it to reappear (Fig. 5-5, *D*). This disappearing-reappearing phenomenon distinguishes the smooth surface incipient carious lesion from the white spot resulting from non-hereditary enamel hypocalcification (see Clinical Examination for Additional Defects). Both types of white spots are undetectable tactilely because the surface is intact, smooth, and hard. For the carious white spot, preventive treatment discussed in Chapter 3 should be instituted to promote *remineralization* of the lesion.

The presence of several facial (or lingual) smooth surface carious lesions within a patient's dentition suggests a high caries rate. In a caries-susceptible patient, the gingival one third of the facial surfaces of maxillary posterior teeth and the gingival one third of the facial and lingual surfaces of the mandibular posterior teeth should be carefully evaluated as these teeth are at a greater risk for caries. Advanced smooth surface caries will exhibit discoloration and demineralization and will feel soft to penetration by the explorer. The discoloration can range from white to dark brown, with rapidly progressing caries being light in color (Fig. 5-5, *E*). With slowly progressing caries in a patient with low caries activity, darkening occurs over time because of extrinsic staining, and remineralization of decalcified tooth structure occasionally may harden the lesion. Such an *arrested lesion* may at times be rough though cleanable (Fig. 5-19), and a restoration is not indicated except for esthetics. The dentin in an arrested remineralized lesion is termed *eburnated* or *sclerotic.*

For the *geriatric patient,* extra care must be taken to inspect for *root surface caries,* carious lesions that occur on the cemental surfaces of teeth. A combination of cemental exposure, dietary changes, systemic diseases, and medications that affect the amount and character of saliva can predispose an older patient to root surface caries. It is not unusual to find caries at the cementoenamel junction (CEJ) or more apically on the cementum in older patients or in patients who have undergone periodontal surgery (Fig. 5-5, *F*). Root surface caries may be undetectable on radiographic examination but can be detected with a careful, thorough clinical examination. Active root caries is detected by the presence of softening and cavitation.

Regardless of the location or type of carious lesions,

a careful, thorough clinical examination is critical in the diagnosis of caries and *for confirmation of radiographic evidence of the disease.*

Clinical examination of amalgam restorations. Evaluation of all restorations must be done systematically in a clean, dry, well-lighted field. Clinical evaluation of **amalgam restorations** requires visual observation, application of tactile sense with the explorer, use of dental floss, interpretation of radiographs, and knowledge of the probabilities that a given condition is sound or at risk for further breakdown.

At least ten distinct conditions may be encountered when amalgam restorations are evaluated: (1) amalgam "blues," (2) proximal overhangs, (3) marginal ditching, (4) voids, (5) fracture lines, (6) lines indicating the interface between abutted restorations, (7) improper anatomical contours, (8) marginal ridge incompatibility, (9) improper proximal contacts, and (10) recurrent caries.

Discolored areas or **amalgam blues** are often seen through the enamel in teeth that have amalgam restorations (Fig. 5-6). This bluish hue results either from the leaching of corrosion products of amalgam into the dentinal tubules or from the color of underlying amalgam as seen through translucent enamel. The latter occurs when the enamel has no dentin support, such as in undermined cusps, marginal ridges, and regions adjacent to proximal margins. When other aspects of the restoration are sound, amalgam blues are not indicative of caries, do not warrant classifying the restoration as defective, and require no further treatment. However, replacement of the restoration may be considered for elective improvement of esthetics or for areas under heavy functional stress that may require a cusp capping restoration to prevent possible tooth fracture.

Proximal overhangs are diagnosed visually, tactilely, and radiographically (Fig. 5-7). The amalgam-tooth junction is evaluated by moving the explorer back and forth across it. If the explorer stops at the junction and then moves outwardly onto the amalgam, an overhang is present. Overhangs can also be confirmed by catching or tearing of dental floss. Such an overhang is

a plaque trap, provides an obstacle to good oral hygiene, and usually results in inflammation of the adjacent soft tissue. An overhang should be corrected, and this often indicates replacement of the defective restoration.

Marginal gap or **ditching** is the deterioration of the amalgam-tooth interface on the occlusal surfaces as a result of wear, fracture, or improper cavity preparation (Fig. 5-8, *A*). It can be diagnosed visually or by the explorer dropping into an opening as it crosses the margin. Shallow ditching less than 0.5 mm deep is not usually a reason for restoration replacement, for such a restoration usually looks worse than it really is. The self-sealing property of amalgam allows the restoration to continue serving adequately if it can be satisfactorily cleaned and maintained. However, if the ditch is too deep to be cleaned or jeopardizes the integrity of the remaining restoration or tooth structure, the restoration should be replaced.

Voids other than ditching also occur at the margins of amalgam restorations. If the void is at least 0.3 mm deep and is located in the gingival one third of the tooth crown, then the restoration is judged as defective and should be repaired or replaced. Accessible small voids in other marginal areas where the enamel is thicker may be corrected by recontouring or repairing with a small restoration.

A careful clinical examination will detect any **fracture line** across the occlusal portion of an amalgam restoration. A line that occurs in the isthmus region generally indicates fractured amalgam and thus a defective restoration that needs replacing (Fig. 5-9, *A*). However, care must be taken to evaluate correctly any such line, especially if it is in the mid-occlusal area because this may be an **interface line,** a manifestation of two abutted restorations, each accomplished at a separate appointment (Fig. 5-9, *B*). If other aspects of the abutted restorations are satisfactory, replacement is not necessary.

Amalgam restorations should duplicate the **normal anatomical contours** of the teeth. Restorations that impinge on the soft tissue, have inadequate embrasure

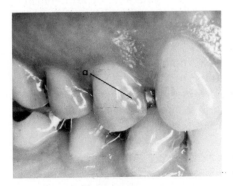

Fig. 5-6

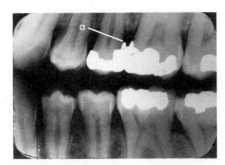

Fig. 5-7

Fig. 5-6. Discoloration *(a)* by amalgam is a bluish hue (amalgam blues) seen through a thin shell of enamel of a tooth. In the absence of any other problems this condition does not indicate replacement.

Fig. 5-7. Proximal overhang *(a)* can be diagnosed radiographically.

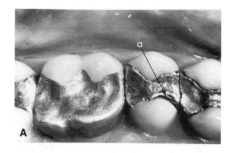

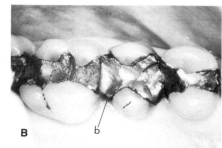

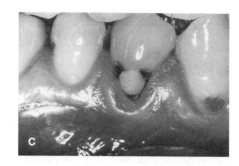

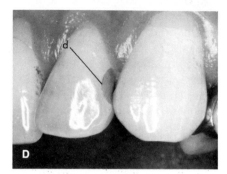

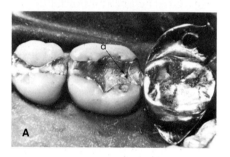

Fig. 5-8. Restorations can be diagnosed clinically as being defective by observing the following. **A,** Significant marginal ditching *(a)*. **B,** Improper contour *(b)*. **C,** Recurrent caries. **D,** Esthetically displeasing dark staining *(d)*.

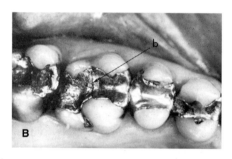

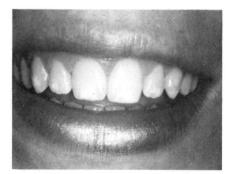

Fig. 5-9. Lines across the occlusal surface of an amalgam restoration may be **A,** fracture line *(a)* that indicates replacement, or **B,** interface line *(b)* that indicates two restorations placed at separate appointments, which by itself is not sufficient indication for replacement.

Fig. 5-10. Non-hereditary hypocalcified areas on facial surfaces. These areas may result from numerous factors but do not warrant restorative intervention unless they are esthetically offensive or if cavitation is present.

form or proximal contact, or prevent the use of dental floss should be classified as defective, indicating recontouring or replacement (Fig. 5-8, *B*).

The marginal ridge portion of the amalgam restoration should be ***compatible with the adjacent marginal ridge.*** Both ridges should be at approximately the same level and display correct occlusal embrasure form for passage of food to the facial and lingual and for proper proximal contact area. If the marginal ridges are not compatible and are associated with poor tissue health, food impaction, or the inability of the patient to floss, the restoration is defective and should be recontoured or replaced.

The ***proximal contact area*** of an amalgam restoration should touch (a "closed" contact) the adjacent tooth at the proper contact level and with correct embrasure

form. (Refer to Forming the Proximal Contour and Contact, Chapter 19.) If the contact of any restoration is suspected to be inadequate, it should be evaluated with dental floss and/or by trial angulations of a mouth mirror (held lingually when viewing from the facial aspect) to reflect light and actually see if there is a space at the contact ("open" contact). For this viewing, the contact must be free of saliva. Another evaluation method is to use a very slender strand of floss obtained by separating it into thin strands. If the contact is "open" and is associated with poor interproximal tissue health and/or food impaction, the restoration should be classified as defective and replaced. An "open" contact typically is annoying and even distressing to the patient; thus correcting the problem usually is a very appreciated service.

Recurrent caries at the marginal area of the restoration is detected visually, tactilely, or radiographically and is an indication for repair or replacement (Figs. 5-4, *D* and 5-8, *C*).

Clinical examination of cast restorations. Cast restorations should be evaluated clinically in the same manner as amalgam restorations. If any aspect of the restoration is not satisfactory or is causing tissue harm, it should be classified as defective and considered for recontouring, repair, or replacement.

Clinical examination of tooth-colored restorations. Tooth-colored restorations should be evaluated clinically in the same manner as amalgam and cast restorations. If there is an improper contour or proximal contact, an overhanging proximal margin, recurrent caries, or other condition that impairs cleaning, the restoration is considered defective. Corrective procedures include recontouring, polishing, repairing, or replacing.

One of the main concerns with anterior teeth is esthetics. If a tooth-colored restoration has dark marginal staining or is discolored to the extent that it is esthetically displeasing and the patient is unhappy with the appearance, the restoration should be judged defective (Fig. 5-8, *D*). Marginal staining that is judged non-carious may be corrected by a small repair restoration along the margin. Occasionally the staining is superficial and can be removed by resurfacing.

Clinical examination for additional defects. A thorough clinical examination will occasionally disclose localized intact, hard white areas on the facial (Fig. 5-10) or lingual surfaces, or on cusp tips of the teeth. Generally these are ***non-hereditary hypocalcified areas of enamel*** that may have resulted from factors such as childhood fever, trauma, or fluorosis that occurred dur-

ing the developmental stages of tooth formation. Another cause of hypocalcification is arrested and remineralized incipient caries, which leaves an opaque, discolored, and hard surface (Fig. 5-14, *C*). When smooth and cleanable, such areas do not warrant restorative intervention unless they are esthetically offensive to the patient. These areas remain visible regardless if the tooth is wet or dry. Recall that in contrast, the smooth surface incipient carious lesion also is opaque white when dried. Therefore, care must be exercised to distinguish the incipient carious lesion from non-hereditary developmental enamel hypocalcification.

Chemical erosion is the loss of surface tooth structure by chemical action in the continued presence of demineralizing agents (acids). The resulting defective surface is smooth. Though these agents are predominant causative factors, it is generally recognized that toothbrushing is a contributing factor. Exogenous acidic agents, such as lemon juice (by lemon sucking), cause crescent or dished defects (rounded as opposed to angular) on the surfaces of exposed teeth (Fig. 5-11, *A*), while endogenous acidic agents, such as gastric fluids, cause generalized erosion on the lingual, incisal, and occlusal surfaces (Fig. 5-11, *B*). The latter defective surfaces are associated with the binge-purge syndrome in ***bulimia,*** or with ***gastroesophogeal reflux.***

In contrast to chemical erosion, ***idiopathic erosion*** is thought by some to explain the cervical, wedge-shaped defect (angular as opposed to rounded) that is similar to the defect customarily associated with toothbrush abrasion (subsequently presented), but where the predominant causative factor (as proposed) is heavy force in eccentric occlusion shown in an associated wear facet, re-

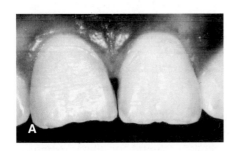

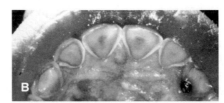

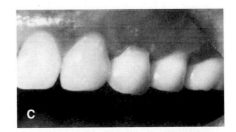

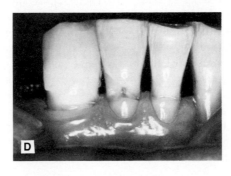

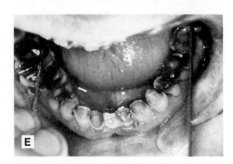

Fig. 5-11. Erosion. **A,** Crescent-shaped defects on enamel facial surfaces caused by exogenous demineralizing agent (from sucking lemons several years previous to time of photograph). **B,** Generalized erosion caused by endogenous fluids. **C,** Idiopathic erosion lesion at the DEJ is hypothesized to be associated with abnormal occlusal force. **D,** Wedge-shaped lesions caused by abrasion from toothbrush. **E,** Generalized attrition caused by excessive functional or parafunctional mandibular movements.

sulting in flexuring (elastic bending) of the tooth (Fig. 5-11, *C*). It is further hypothesized that the bending force produces tension stress in the affected wedge-shaped region on the tooth side away from the tooth bending direction, resulting in loss of surface tooth structure by microfractures (by abfractures). Proponents of this hypothesis also add that the microfractures can foster loss of tooth structure from toothbrush abrasion and from acids in the diet and/or plaque. The resulting defect has smooth surfaces.

Abrasion is abnormal tooth surface loss resulting from direct frictional forces between the teeth and external objects, or from frictional forces between contacting teeth in the presence of an abrasive medium.[8] Such wear is caused by improper brushing techniques or other habits such as holding a pipe stem between the teeth, tobacco chewing, and chewing on hard objects such as pens or pencils. Toothbrush abrasion is the most common example and is usually seen as a sharp wedge-shaped notch in the gingival portion of the facial aspects of the teeth (Fig. 5-11, *D*). The surface of the defect is smooth. The presence of such defects does not automatically warrant treatment. Rather, it is important to determine and eliminate the cause.

Attrition is mechanical wear of the incisal or occlusal tooth structure as a result of functional or para-functional movements of the mandible. Although a certain degree of attrition is expected with age, it is important to note abnormally advanced attrition (Fig. 5-11, *E*). If significant abnormal attrition is present, the patient's functional movements must be evaluated and inquiry made about any habits creating this problem such as tooth grinding, or *bruxism*, usually due to stress. In some older patients the enamel of the cusp tips (or incisal edges) is worn off resulting in cupped-out areas because the exposed, softer dentin wears faster than the surrounding enamel. Sometimes these areas are an annoyance because of food retention or the presence of peripheral, ragged, sharp enamel edges. Slowing such wear by appropriate restorative treatment is indicated. The sharp edges can result in tongue or cheek biting, and rounding these edges is a thoughtful and appreciated service.

Fracture or *craze lines* in a tooth are often visible, especially with advancing age, and should be considered as potential cleavage planes for possible future fractures. Appropriate dye materials or light reflected from a dental mirror aid in detecting fracture lines. Any tooth that has an extensive restoration and weakened cusps should be identified as being susceptible to future fracture (Fig. 5-12) and should be considered for a cusp-protecting restoration. *Deep developmental fissures across marginal or cusp ridges are cleavage planes, especially in the tooth weakened by caries or previous restoration.* A minor fracture of a tooth can of-

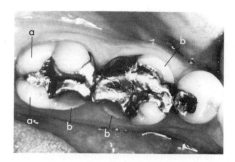

Fig. 5-12. Extensively restored teeth with weakened *(a)* and fractured *(b)* cusps. Note in second molar the distal developmental fissure, which further predisposes the distal cusps to fracture.

ten be treated by recontouring and polishing. If the fracture is more extensive, the tooth should be restored. The examination and diagnosis of the incomplete fracture of a posterior tooth is presented in a subsequent section titled, Examination of the Patient in Pain.

The dental examination may also reveal *dental anomalies* that include variations in size, shape, structure, or number of teeth such as *dens in dente* (see Lingual Pits of Maxillary Incisors, Chapter 12), *macrodontia, microdontia, gemination, concrescence, dilaceration, amelogenesis imperfecta,* and *dentinogenesis imperfecta.* Thorough discussion of these anomalies is beyond the scope of this text; the reader should refer to an oral pathology textbook for additional information.

Radiographic examination of teeth and restorations. Dental radiographs are an indispensable part of the contemporary dentist's diagnostic armamentarium. As with most things in life, however, the use of diagnostic *ionizing radiation* is not without risks. Exposure to any amount of ionizing radiation can potentially result in a range of adverse affects. Therefore, the diagnostic yield or potential benefit that could be gained from a radiograph must be weighed carefully against the financial costs and the potential adverse affects of exposure to radiation.

To assist the clinician with assessing the risks and benefits, the FDA sponsored a panel of dental experts to develop radiograph selection criteria for dental patients. Their report specifies guidelines based on patient age and risk of dental disease for prescribing dental radiographs.[9] As a general rule, patients at higher risk for caries or periodontal disease should receive more frequent and more extensive radiographic surveys. Table 5-2, adapted from the FDA guidelines, lists the preferred types of radiographs and the intervals at which they should be used for the dentulous adult patient. Specific clinical situations for which radiographs may be indicated are also shown in Box 5-2.

For diagnosis of *proximal surface caries, restoration*

overhangs, or *poorly contoured restorations,* posterior bitewing and anterior periapical radiographs are most helpful. When interpreting the radiographic presentation of proximal tooth surfaces, it is necessary to know the normal anatomical picture presented in a radiograph before any abnormalities can be diagnosed. In a radiograph, proximal caries appears as a dark area or a radiolucency in the proximal enamel at or gingival to the contact of the teeth (Fig. 5-4, *A*). This radiolucency is triangular and has its apex toward the dentoenamel junction (DEJ). Moderate-to-deep occlusal caries can be seen as a radiolucency extending into dentin (Fig. 5-4, *C*). Some defective aspects of restorations may also be

identified radiographically. These include improper contour, overhangs (Fig. 5-7), and *recurrent caries* gingival to restorations (Fig. 5-4, *D*). Pulpal abnormalities such as **pulp stones** and **internal resorption** may be identified in the anterior periapical radiographs (Fig. 5-13, *A* and *B*). The height and integrity of the *marginal periodontium* may be evaluated from the bitewing radiographs. Periapical radiographs are helpful in diagnosing changes in the periapical periodontium such as **periapical abscesses, dental granulomas,** or **cysts** (Fig. 5-13, *C*). Impacted third molars, supernumerary teeth, and other congenital or acquired abnormalities may also be discovered upon periapical radiographic examination. However, it should be kept in mind that the sensitivity and specificity of dental radiographs will vary according to the diagnostic task.

Always interpret dental radiographs cautiously. Remember the limitations imposed by interpreting a dental film that is a two-dimensional representation of three dimensions. In addition, the dentist should realize that the interpretation of dental radiographs will produce a certain number of false positive and false negative diagnoses. For instance, misdiagnosis can occur when **cervical burnout** (the radiographic picture of the normal structure and contour of the cervical third of the crown) mimics caries (Fig. 5-14, *A* to *C*). Furthermore, a Class V lesion or a radiolucent tooth-colored restoration may be radiographically superimposed on the proximal area, mimicking proximal caries (Fig. 5-14, *D* and *E*). *Finally, always assume caries is more extensive clinically than it appears radiographically.* Although radiographs are excellent diagnostic media, they do have limitations. The only way to guard against these limitations is to continually correlate clinical and radiographic findings.

Box 5-2. Clinical situations for which radiographs may be indicated

1. Previous periodontal or root canal therapy
2. History of pain or trauma
3. Familial history of dental anomalies
4. Clinical evidence of periodontal disease
5. Large or deep restorations
6. Deep carious lesions
7. Malposed or clinically impacted teeth
8. Swellling
9. Mobility of teeth
10. Fistula or sinus tract infection
11. Growth abnormalities
12. Oral involvement in known or suspected systemic disease
13. Evidence of foreign objects
14. Abutment teeth for fixed or removable partial prosthesis
15. Unexplained bleeding
16. Unexplained sensitivity of teeth
17. Unusual tooth morphology, calcification, or color
18. Missing teeth with unknown reason

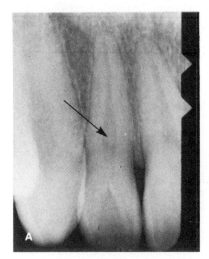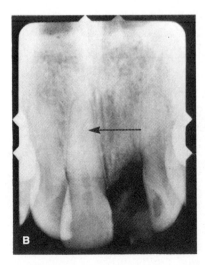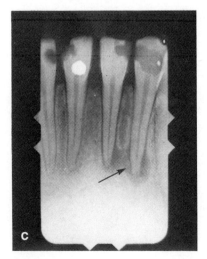

Fig. 5-13. Pulpal abnormalities. **A,** Pulp stone. **B,** Internal resorption. **C,** Periapical abscess, granuloma, or cyst.

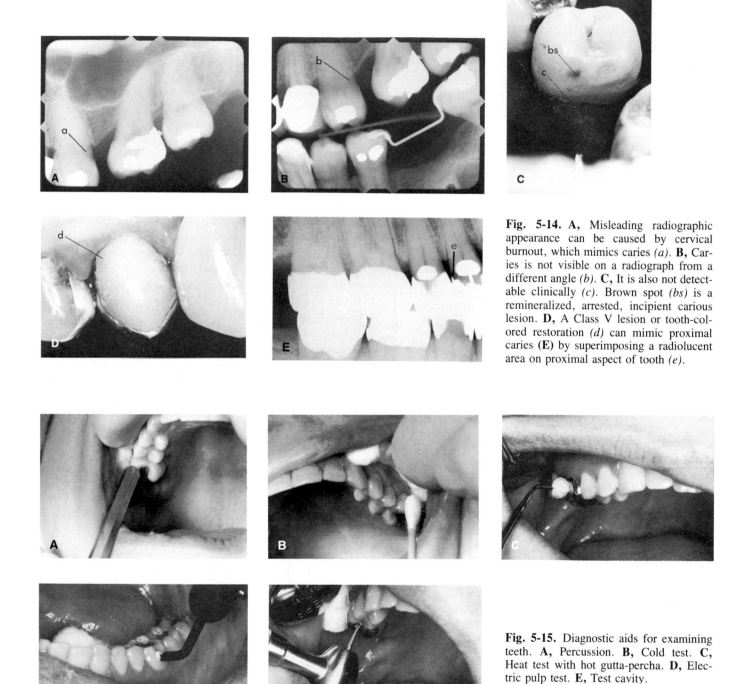

Fig. 5-14. A, Misleading radiographic appearance can be caused by cervical burnout, which mimics caries *(a)*. **B,** Caries is not visible on a radiograph from a different angle *(b)*. **C,** It is also not detectable clinically *(c)*. Brown spot *(bs)* is a remineralized, arrested, incipient carious lesion. **D,** A Class V lesion or tooth-colored restoration *(d)* can mimic proximal caries (**E**) by superimposing a radiolucent area on proximal aspect of tooth *(e)*.

Fig. 5-15. Diagnostic aids for examining teeth. **A,** Percussion. **B,** Cold test. **C,** Heat test with hot gutta-percha. **D,** Electric pulp test. **E,** Test cavity.

Adjunctive aids for examining teeth and restorations. Adjunctive aids or tests, such as the *percussion test, palpation, thermal tests, electric pulp test,* and *test cavity,* are useful when further information is needed to discern the health of the teeth and supporting structures. Remember, however, that these are only aids in arriving at a diagnosis. Positive results on only one test should not be considered conclusive, as a test is seldom 100% accurate. Rather, all available information, including history, examination, radiographs, and other test results, and comparable findings on adjacent and contralateral teeth should be used in concert to confirm the diagnosis.

A *percussion test* is performed by gently tapping the occlusal or incisal surfaces of the suspected tooth and adjacent teeth with the end of the mirror handle to determine the presence of tenderness (Fig. 5-15, *A*). Pain on percussion suggests possible injury to the periodontal membrane from pulpal or periodontal inflammation. Care must be taken when interpreting a positive response on maxillary teeth, since teeth in close proximity to the maxillary sinuses may also exhibit pain on percussion when the patient is suffering from maxillary sinusitis.

Palpation is performed by rubbing the index finger along the facial and lingual mucosa overlying the apical region of the tooth. An alveolar abscess in an advanced stage or other periapical pathosis may cause tenderness to palpation. Palpation can also reveal nontender swellings which may be otherwise overlooked.

An indication of pulp vitality can be obtained through the results of thermal tests, an electric pulp test, and a test cavity. In addition, before any tooth is restored with a casting, pulpal evaluation should be performed. To conduct a *thermal test,* a cotton applicator tip sprayed with a freezing agent (HistoFreeze®*) or hot gutta-percha is applied directly to the tooth (Fig. 5-15, *B* and *C*). Hot and cold testing should elicit from the healthy pulp a response that will subside within a few seconds following removal of the stimulus. Pain lasting 10 to 15 seconds or less after stimulation by heat or cold suggests a *hyperemia,* an inflammation that may be reversed by timely removal of the irritant(s). Intense pain of longer duration from hot or cold usually suggests *irreversible pulpitis,* which can only be treated by root canal therapy or extraction. Pain that results from heat but is quickly relieved by cold also suggests irreversible pulpitis. Lack of response to thermal tests may indicate that the pulp is necrotic. Adjacent and/or contralateral unaffected teeth should be tested for baseline comparisons as the duration of pain may differ among individuals.

The *electric pulp tester* also has value in determining the vitality of the dental pulp (Fig. 5-15, *D*). The electric pulp tester is placed on the tooth and not on a restoration. A small electric current delivered to the tooth causes a tingling sensation when the pulp is vital and no response when the pulp is nonvital. It is important to obtain readings on adjacent and contralateral teeth so the tooth in question can be evaluated relative to the responses of the other teeth. Results of an electric pulp test should not be the sole basis for a pulpal diagnosis since false positives/negatives can occur. Instead, electric pulp test results provide additional information that, when combined with other findings, may lead to a diagnosis. Electric pulp testing is sometimes not possible in teeth with large or full-coverage restorations.

A *test cavity* can be performed to help in the evaluation of pulpal vitality when a large restoration in the tooth may be resulting in false negative responses with other evaluation methods. This test particularly is an option for diagnosing questionable pulpal vitality of a tooth contemplated for a replacement casting restoration. By using a round bur and no anesthetic, a test cavity is made through the existing restoration into the dentin (Fig. 5-15, *E*). Lack of sensitivity (response) when the dentin is cut may indicate a nonvital pulp. However, sclerosed dentin can result in a false negative. Moreover, on a multiple-rooted tooth, one region of the dentin may respond, whereas there may be no response at another site, possibly indicating a degeneration of a portion of the pulp. Furthermore, heat generated by the bur might cause a response, but the pulp may not be healthy. Though there are indications for the test cavity, its use and diagnostic information attained are limited.

When extensive restorative therapy is contemplated, *study casts* are helpful in providing an understanding of occlusal relationships, developing the treatment plan, and educating the patient. Accurately mounted study casts provide an opportunity for a thorough evaluation of the tooth interdigitation, the functional occlusion, and any occlusal abnormalities that may need treatment. For example, study casts provide for further evaluation of the plane of occlusion, tilted or extruded teeth, crossbites, plunger cusps, wear facets and defective restorations, coronal contours, proximal contacts, and embrasure spaces between the teeth. Combined with clinical and radiographic findings, study casts allow the practitioner to develop a treatment plan without the patient present, thus saving valuable chair time. When a proposed plan of treatment is discussed with the patient, study casts can be valuable educational media in helping the patient to understand and visualize existing conditions and the need for proposed treatment.

Additional aids for diagnosis of additional problems are discussed in later sections of this chapter, and these include transillumination, the rubber wheel biting test, mobility testing, the anesthetic test, and occlusal analysis.

*HistoFreeze®, Fisher brand, Fisher Scientific, Pittsburgh, PA 15219.

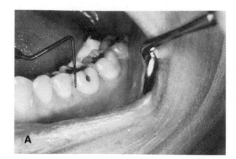 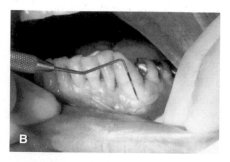 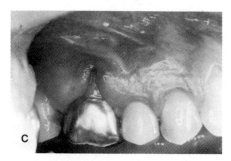

Fig. 5-16. Periodontal examination. **A,** Probing to measure sulcus depth. **B,** Lack of attached gingiva next to a tooth requiring restoration with a subgingival margin. **C,** Gingival recession.

Review of periodontium

Determination of operative treatment should occur only after the status of the ***periodontium*** has been evaluated. Because the periodontium and the teeth must exist in a mutually beneficial physiological environment, an accurate diagnosis of the periodontal condition is critical to the planning of operative treatment.

Clinical examination. The periodontium is evaluated clinically through a series of steps. The gingival color and texture are important indices of periodontal health. Healthy gingiva is light pink in color, firm, knife-edged, and stippled; unhealthy gingiva is often red, soft, edematous, and has a glazed, smooth surface. The depth of the gingival sulcus around each tooth is determined by systematic probing using a specialized instrument (periodontal probe) having a round-ended, thin shaft with millimeter indications (Fig. 5-16, *A*). Sulcus depth is assessed at six locations around each tooth, three facially (mesiofacial, mid-facial, distofacial), and three lingually (mesiolingual, mid-lingual, and distolingual). A sulcus depth greater than 3 mm and sites that bleed upon probing should be recorded in the patient's chart. The presence of a pocket (a sulcus depth greater than 3 mm) or the presence of hemorrhage or exudate may indicate periodontal disease.

The next step in probing is to evaluate the presence of bifurcation or trifurcation involvement. These regions should be explored with a furcation probe and classified according to the amount of penetration. The presence of furcation involvement reduces the long-term prognosis of the tooth and affects the restorative treatment plan.

After probing is completed, it is imperative to note areas of ***gingival recession*** and areas with a minimal or lack of attached gingiva, especially if these areas are near a tooth surface that requires a subgingival restorative margin (Fig. 5-16, *B*). With a lack of attached gingiva in these areas, restorative manipulations such as margination, temporization, and impressions can further aggravate the gingival problem (Fig. 5-16, *C*).

Teeth should be evaluated for ***mobility*** and noted with appropriate classification (1, 2, 3). Class 1 mobility is barely distinguishable mobility (physiological) in a faciolingual direction of only a few tenths of a millimeter (total); class 2 is mobility (non-physiological) in any transverse direction greater than a few tenths up to 1 mm; and class 3 mobility (non-physiological) is greater than 1 mm in any transverse direction. Teeth that can be depressed or rotated are also scored as class 3. Mobility signifies loss of bone support or the result of improper occlusal forces, either of which could affect subsequent operative treatment. The occlusal relationship of the teeth should be closely evaluated. Well-positioned occlusal contacts are necessary to prevent occlusal trauma to the periodontium. Non-physiological mobility observed during functional contacts should be recorded since this information is useful in treatment planning.

The presence of ***plaque,*** debris, and inflammation, and the general level of home care must be noted for two reasons. First, the teeth cannot be properly restored when they are covered by debris and surrounded by unhealthy tissues that bleed easily. The gingiva should be firm and healthy so that restorative procedures can be performed in a clean, dry field. Second, the long-term prognosis of any operative treatment is highly dependent on the long-term periodontal health and the patient's ability to keep the restoration and tooth surfaces clean.

Restorations should be ***correctly contoured*** to maintain proper periodontal health. Proximal, facial, and lingual surfaces should not be overcontoured because such contouring can impinge on the soft tissue or act as a plaque trap. Physiological proximal contacts should be achieved to prevent interproximal food impaction and tooth movement, as well as foster during mastication proper movement of food facially and lingually due to correct lingual, occlusal, and facial embrasures.

Radiographic examination. ***Radiographs*** are another valuable aid in assessing periodontal health. Bitewing

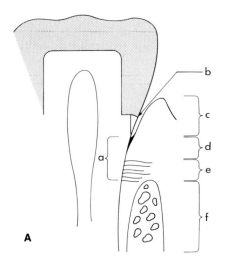

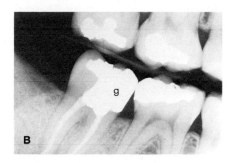

Fig. 5-17. A, Biological width *(a)* is the physiological dimension needed for the junctional epithelium *(d)* and the connective tissue attachment *(e)*, which is measured from the base of the sulcus *(c)* to the level of the bone crest *(f)*. The margin of the restoration *(b)* must not violate this dimension. **B,** Tooth with an existing restoration *(g)* that encroaches on the biological width requires crown-lengthening procedures before placement of a new restoration.

radiographs, exposed at the proper angulation, are the best means of radiographically assessing bone levels. Vertical bitewing radiographs are recommended for patients with periodontitis involving substantial bone loss. Localized or generalized bone loss, vertical or horizontal, should be noted.

Radiographs aid in determining the relationship between the margins of existing or proposed restorations and the bone. A ***biological width*** of at least 2 mm is required for the junctional epithelium and connective tissue attachments located between the base of the sulcus and the alveolar bone crest (Fig. 5-17, *A*). In addition to this physiological dimension, the restoration margin should be placed as far away as possible from the base of the sulcus to foster gingival health. Encroachment on this biological width may cause breakdown and apical migration of the attachment apparatus. The attachment breakdown and apical migration are in response to the inflammatory process caused by bacterial plaque which accumulates at the inaccessible restoration margins. The final position of a proposed gingival margin, which is dictated by the existing restoration, caries, or retention features, must be estimated to determine if *crown-lengthening* procedures are indicated before restoration (Fig. 5-17, *B*). These procedures involve the surgical removal of the gingiva and/or bone to create a longer clinical crown, and thus provide more tooth structure for placing the restoration margin in a cleansable area and for increasing retention form.

Because of the obvious importance of the periodontium, operative procedures must continually be performed with respect, understanding, and concern for the periodontium. Therefore, the relationship of the periodontium and operative procedures must always be considered.

Examination of occlusion

There are several reasons for completing a thorough occlusal examination for developing an analysis and understanding of the patient's occlusion before initiating restorative care. First, the patient's presenting condition can be established prior to any alterations by the operator. This documentation includes the identification of signs of occlusal trauma, such as enamel cracks or tooth mobility, and notation of occlusal abnormalities that contribute to pathological conditions, such as bone loss. Second, the potential effect of proposed restorative treatment on the occlusion can be assessed. For example, the potential of proposed restorations to provide a beneficial and harmonious occlusion must be determined. Third, the effect of the current occlusal scheme on proposed restorative treatment can be identified, and the existing occlusion altered if needed prior to placement of restorations.

The static and dynamic occlusion must be carefully examined. Although not all occlusal abnormalities require treatment, the clinician must always be able to identify deviations from normal and be prepared to treat, refer, or make allowances for these problems in any planned therapy. A description of the patient's static anatomical occlusion in maximum intercuspation, or the ***intercuspal position*** (IP), including the relationship of the molars and canines (Angle's Class I, II, or III), and the amount of ***vertical overlap*** (overbite) and ***horizontal overlap*** (overjet) of the anterior teeth should be recorded. The presence of missing teeth and the relationship of the maxillary and mandibular midlines should be evaluated. The appropriateness of the occlusal plane and the positions of malposed teeth should be identified. Super-erupted teeth, spacing, fractured teeth and marginal ridge discrepancies should be noted. The dynamic functional occlusion in all movements of the mandible (right, left, forward, and all excursions in-between) should be evaluated. This evaluation also includes assessing the most retruded (unforced) contact position (RCP) of the teeth when the condyle head is in *centric relation,* the most anterior-superior physiological position in the glenoid fossa with the disc interposed, and then relating this RCP position to the IP, noting any differences between these two positions. There is a small, physiological slide (a few tenths of a millimeter) of the condyle head upward and rearward from the IP to the RCP. Functional movements of the mandible are evaluated to determine if *canine guidance* or *group function* exists. The presence and amount of *anterior guidance* is evaluated to note the degree of potential posterior disclusion. *Nonfunctional contacts* are recorded so that they may be eliminated and any planned restorative care for involved teeth will not perpetuate these contacts. Any mobility of teeth during function is identified. Movement of the mandible from maximum intercuspation to maximum opening is observed; any clicking of the joint(s) during such movement may be an indication of a pathological condition.

Teeth are examined for abnormal wear patterns. If signs of abnormal wear are present, the patient is queried as to the presence of any contributing habits such as nocturnal bruxism or parafunctional habits. The examination should also disclose possible unfavorable occlusal relationships, such as a *plunger cusp,* which is a pointed cusp "plunging" deep into the occlusal plane of the opposing arch. A plunger cusp may be contacting the lower of two adjacent marginal ridges of different levels, or contacting directly between two adjacent marginal ridges in maximum intercuspation, or positioned in a deep fossa. These may result in food impaction or tooth/restoration fracture.

The results of the occlusal analysis should be included in the dental record and considered in the restorative treatment plan. Acceptable aspects of the occlusion must be preserved and not altered during treatment. When possible, improvement of the occlusal relationship is desirable; assuredly, abnormalities must not be perpetuated in the restorative treatment.

Examination of the patient in pain

One of the most perplexing yet challenging problems a dentist encounters is the treatment of patients who have pain in the jaws or teeth. Such problems often can test the dentist's diagnostic skills. The cause of discomfort must be determined before relief can be provided. The problem can be identified and treated by carefully piecing together subjective information from the patient and objective information from the clinical examination supplemented with appropriate diagnostic tests.

Regardless of whether the patient is new to the practice or is a patient of record, the medical history must be reviewed to uncover potential health-related problems. The patient is then asked to describe various characteristics of the pain, particularly: (1) the onset and duration, (2) stimuli, (3) spontaneity, (4) intensity, and (5) factors that relieve it (Box 5-3). After carefully listening to a thorough description of the characteristics, the practitioner guides the discussion to obtain more information. During this discussion the dentist begins to formulate an idea about the potential cause of the pain and a means for verifying it. Care should be taken, however, not to focus too quickly; instead, all possible sources of pain must be considered: systemic, pulpal, periapical, periodontal, restorative, degenerative, and neoplastic.

After assessing the subjective symptoms described by the patient and developing a preliminary diagnosis, the dentist should apply *objective tests* to confirm the diagnosis. These include a *percussion test* to determine possible inflammation in the periodontal ligament (PDL), *palpation* to examine for any tenderness in the apical region, and *transillumination* to check for cracks or caries in the tooth as well as for tooth color changes which may indicate loss of vitality. If a tooth is suspected of having a pulpal problem, *electric pulp testing* combined with *thermal testing* may assist in the diagnosis. *Periodontal probing* helps rule out periodontal abscess. The *integrity of restorations is evaluated* by examining them for fractures, recurrent caries, wear marks, shiny spots, or mobility (looseness).

One of the more challenging diagnostic problems is to locate the offending, posterior tooth that has an *incomplete fracture* not directly involving the pulp chamber/canal(s) of a vital pulp. If the chief complaint is, "When I chew on this side it hurts," the examiner must be especially alert for an *incomplete fracture of a vital posterior tooth.* Frequently the patient gives a history of seeking relief from the dentist over an extended period. Sensitivity to cold usually is an additional complaint. All fracture lines in the enamel of the teeth on the affected side of the arches, maxillary and mandibular, should be noted. Such lines usually are found in the remaining enamel of teeth weakened by extensive caries or restorations. Particularly suspect are those fracture lines emanating from enamel developmental fissures (natural cleavage planes), extending through marginal or cusp ridges, and then extending gingivally in axial surface enamel, thus leaving the included cusps liable to this incomplete fracture under occlusal load (Fig. 5-18). The incompletely fractured cusp causes *sharp pain when masticatory pressure is released* resulting in the fractured dentinal surfaces rubbing together creating hydrodynamic pressures in the dentinal tubules to thus elicit pulpal pain; also the fractured dentinal surfaces become hypersensitive because of salivary contamina-

Box 5-3. For the diagnosis of dental pain an inventory of information should be obtained from the patient interview and from the clinical and radiographic examinations

1. Questions asked of the patient
   a. Can you point to the tooth or area that bothers you?   _____
      top right   top left   top front
      bottom right   bottom left   bottom front
   b. When did you first notice the pain or discomfort?   _____
   c. How long has it hurt?   _____
   d. Circle any of the following that describe(s) character of your pain.
      pulsating   dull   sudden   constant
      nagging   sharp   off and on
   e. Does the tooth start hurting by itself or on its own?   yes   no
   f. Does the pain wake you up at night?   yes   no
   g. What makes it hurt? Please circle the correct response(s).
      (1) hot   yes   no   don't know
      (2) cold   yes   no   don't know
      (3) sweets   yes   no   don't know
      (4) chewing/biting   yes   no   don't know
      (5) air   yes   no   don't know
      (6) other   _____
   h. Does the pain linger?   yes   no
   i. What relieves the pain?   _____
2. Clinical examination
   a. Caries   yes   no
   b. Extensive restoration   yes   no
   c. Sensitive to percussion   yes   no
   d. Sensitive to palpation   yes   no
   e. Response to cold test   normal   no response   pain lingers
   f. Response to heat test   normal   no response   pain lingers
   g. Periodontal pocket depths   ML _____ L _____ DL _____ MF _____ F _____ DF _____
   h. Mobility   yes   no
   i. Wear facets or signs of occlusal trauma   yes   no
   j. Rubber wheel test   yes   no
   k. Craze lines emanating from developmental fissures   yes   no
   l. Exposed root surface   yes   no
   m. Presence of sinus tract   yes   no
   n. Tooth discoloration   yes   no
   o. Other   _____
3. Radiographic examination
   a. Caries   yes   no
   b. Extensive restoration   yes   no
   c. Periapical pathology
      widened PDL   yes   no
      radiolucent lesion   yes   no
   d. Root fracture   yes   no
   e. Bone levels
      furcation   _____
      interproximally   _____

tion. Often it is difficult to determine which tooth is affected; however, a differential diagnosis frequently can be made with a *rubber wheel test*. This is accomplished by applying a small rubber disc over each suspect cusp and asking the patient to bite on and then release the disk (Fig. 5-18, *A* and *B*). Sharp pain on release of pressure helps to identify the offending tooth and its partially fractured component. A properly designed cast restoration (with extracoronal resistance features) often provides relief, since the fractured part is either re-

moved during preparation or is encompassed by the restoration.

An *incomplete fracture that exposes the vital pulp of a posterior tooth* is characterized by symptoms different from those given for an incomplete fracture without pulpal exposure; in a short time the former will result in severe, almost constant, throbbing pain from irreversible pulpitis. Sometimes temporary relief follows pulpal death, but intervention therapies of root canal treatment or tooth extraction are indicated for long-term

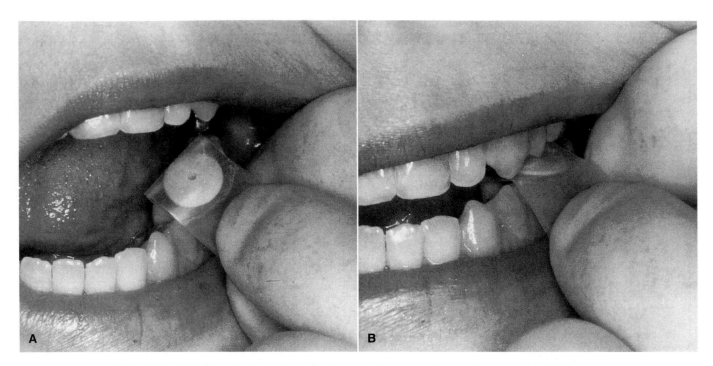

Fig. 5-18. A, Rubber wheel test is used to detect an incomplete fracture in a posterior vital tooth. Wheel (Sulci* miniature polishing disc) is held in loop of clear Scotch† tape, adhesive side inward, and positioned over each suspect cusp for patient to apply biting pressure, **B.** (Loops, each with wheel, are made up by freshly-gloved office personnel during non-appointment hours; this item is discarded as waste after one-patient use.) **C,** Tooth that yielded a positive response to the rubber wheel test, indicating a possible incomplete fracture. **D,** Removal of existing restoration confirms diagnosis of an incomplete fracture.

success. The choice of these therapies depends on several factors, including restorability, usefulness, supporting tissue, and patient preferences.

If the patient is unable to localize the arch in which the offending tooth is located, an ***anesthetic test*** may be used. The suspected tooth is anesthetized to determine if the patient gains any relief. If the symptoms subside, the offending tooth likely has been identified.

Exposed root surfaces can result in sharp annoying pain. For treatment refer to a later section titled, Treatment of Root Surface Sensitivity.

Along with a discussion of the patient's symptoms and a thorough clinical examination and the use of adjunctive tests, a radiograph of the involved region may provide additional information. Radiographs are useful in identifying significant interdental or periradicular bone loss associated with pulpal pathosis. Also, deep restorations and pulpal abnormalities can be detected through radiographic evaluation.

After diagnosis of the probable cause of pain, appropriate treatment should be instituted. Occasionally, examination findings may be so inconclusive that the patient may need to be advised that no definitive treatment is indicated at the moment and that it is best to wait for the symptoms to change or localize. Finally, treatment should be as conservative as possible. This means that unless otherwise indicated, the most palliative form of treatment should be initiated first.

Summary

A thorough and exacting examination of the orofacial soft tissue, teeth, periodontium, and occlusion provides adequate information on which to base a diagnosis. Only after abnormalities of these structures are diagnosed and recorded should the treatment planning process begin. A treatment plan and subsequent treatment are only as effective as the quality of information obtained during the examination.

*Jelenko, New York, NY.
†3M Consumer Products Group, St. Paul, Minn.

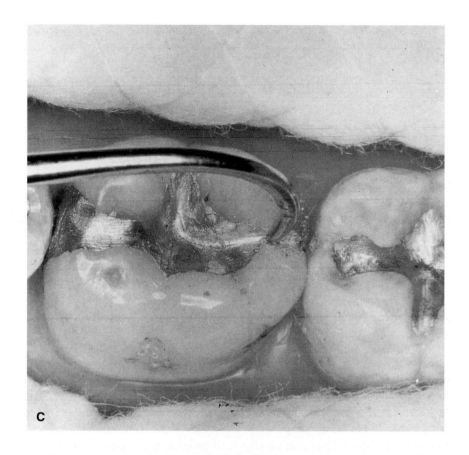

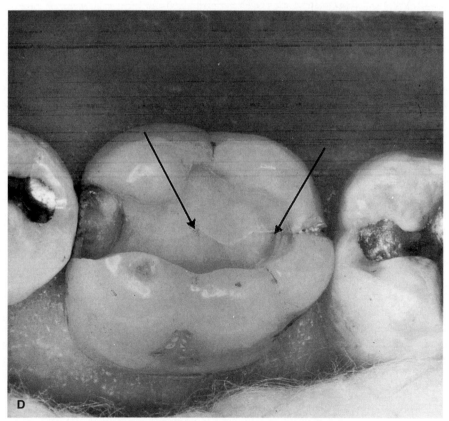

Fig. 5-18, C and **D.** For legend see opposite page.

TREATMENT PLANNING
General considerations

A *treatment plan* is a carefully sequenced series of services designed to eliminate or control etiological factors, repair existing damage, and create a functional, maintainable environment. A sound treatment plan depends on thorough patient evaluation, dentist expertise, understanding of indications and contraindications, and a prediction of the patient's response to treatment. An accurate *prognosis* for each tooth and for the patient's overall dental health is central to a successful treatment plan. To establish a prognosis, the practitioner must be able to forecast possible results given the patient's current condition and the possible outcomes of contemplated treatment.

The development of a dental treatment plan for a patient consists of four steps: (1) examination and problem identification, (2) decision to recommend intervention, (3) identification of treatment alternatives, and (4) selection of the treatment with the patient's involvement. *Step one,* examination and diagnosis, discussed in detail in the second part of this chapter, results in a list of dental problems. *Step two,* deciding to intervene, is dependent upon a determination that a tooth is diseased, restoration is defective, or that either tooth or restoration is at some increased risk of further deterioration. If any of these conditions exist, then intervention is recommended to the patient. *Step three,* identification of treatment alternatives, involves establishing the list of one or more reasonable interventions from the set of possible alternatives. Treatment alternatives for a specific condition can include: "watchful waiting" (periodic re-evaluation to monitor the condition); chemotherapeutics (e.g., fluoride applications to promote remineralization); recontouring defective restorations or irregular tooth surfaces; repair (patching a defective restoration); and restoration. This list of reasonable treatment alternatives is based upon the current knowledge of the effectiveness of the treatment, the prevailing standards of care, and both clinical and non-clinical patient factors. *Step four,* selection of the treatment, is conducted in consultation with the patient. The patient is advised of the reasonable treatment alternatives and their related risks and benefits. After the patient is fully informed, the doctor and patient can select a course of action that is most appropriate for that patient.

Treatment plans are influenced by patient preferences, motivation, systemic health, emotional status, and financial capabilities. The dentist's knowledge, experience, and training; laboratory support; dentist-patient compatibility; and the availability of specialists; as well as functional, esthetic, and technical demands also can modify a treatment plan. Even when modification is necessary, the practitioner is ethically and profession-ally responsible for providing the best level of care possible. For instance, if a tooth ideally should be treated with a cast restoration but the patient is unable to afford this care, then optimal treatment would consist of a large, multi-surface, amalgam restoration. Although this is optimal rather than ideal treatment, it does not give the dentist license to perform an inadequate amalgam restoration. The best amalgam restoration possible should be done under the circumstances.

Finally, a treatment plan is not a static list of services. Rather, it is a multiphase and dynamic series of events. Its success is determined by its suitableness to meet the patient's initial and long-term needs. A treatment plan should allow for reevaluation and be adaptable to meet the changing needs, preferences, and health conditions of the patient. Therefore the patient must realize that the plan may have to be altered as conditions change.

Treatment plan sequencing

Treatment plan sequencing is the process of scheduling the needed procedures into a time frame. Proper sequencing is a critical component of a successful treatment plan. Certain treatments must naturally follow others in a logical order, while other treatments can or must occur concurrently and thus require coordination. Complex treatment plans often should be sequenced in phases, including a *control phase,* a *holding phase,* a *definitive phase,* and a *maintenance phase.* However, for most patients, the first three phases are accomplished in a single phase.

Generally, the concept of "greatest need" dictates the order in which treatment is sequenced. *This concept dictates that what the patient needs most is performed first.*

Control phase. The control phase of treatment is meant to (1) eliminate pain, (2) eliminate active disease such as caries and inflammation, (3) remove conditions preventing maintenance, (4) eliminate potential causes of disease, and (5) begin preventive dentistry activities. The goals of this phase are to remove etiological factors, and stabilize the patient's dental health. Examples of control phase treatment include extractions, endodontics, periodontal debridement and scaling, occlusal adjustment as needed, caries removal, and the replacement or repair of defective restorations, such as those with gingival overhangs.

As part of the control phase, the dentist should develop a plan for the management and prevention of dental caries. After the patient's caries status and caries risk have been determined, chemical, surgical, behavioral, mechanical, and dietary techniques (Box 5-4) can be used to improve host resistance and alter the oral flora. Chapter 3 presents a detailed discussion of caries etiology, prevention, and control.

Box 5-4. Preventinon and management of caries

Chemical—The use of antimicrobial agents to alter the oral
flora and topical fluoride administration to stimulate remineralization
Surgical—Removal of diseased tooth structure and replacement of missing tooth structure with restorative material
Behavioral—Applying appropriate techniques to help patient
develop the skills, knowledge, and attitudes to alter deleterious dietary intake and improve oral hygiene
Mechanical—Mechanical alteration of tooth surfaces at high
risk (sealants), remove overhangs, reestablish proximal
contacts, restore defective contours
Dietary—Change character of diet
Other—Stimulate salivary flow by increasing chewing, altering medications; using artificial saliva

Holding phase. The holding phase is a time between the control and definitive phases that allows for resolution of inflammation and time for healing. Home care habits are reinforced, motivation for further treatment is assessed, and initial treatment is re-evaluated before definitive care is begun.

Definitive phase. After the dentist reassesses initial treatment and determines the need for further care, the patient enters a more definitive phase of treatment. This includes some forms of endodontics, periodontics, orthodontics, oral surgery, and operative procedures prior to fixed or removable prosthodontic treatment. This phase is discussed in detail in a following section titled, Interdisciplinary Considerations in Operative Treatment Planning.

Maintenance phase. This phase includes regular recall examinations that (1) may reveal the need for adjustments to prevent future breakdown and (2) provide an opportunity to reinforce home care. The frequency of re-evaluation examinations during the maintenance phase depends in large part on the patient's risk for dental disease. A patient who has stable periodontal health and a recent history of no caries should have longer intervals (such as 9 to 12 months or longer) between recall visits. In contrast, those at high risk for dental caries and periodontal breakdown should be examined much more frequently (i.e., 3 to 4 months).

Interdisciplinary considerations in operative treatment planning

When an operative procedure is performed during the control or definitive phases, there are general guidelines for when operative treatment should occur relative to other forms of care. Following is a discussion of how to *sequence operative care with endodontic, periodontal, orthodontic, oral surgical, and prosthodontic treatments.*

Endodontics. All teeth to be restored with large or cast restorations should have a pulpal/periapical evaluation. If indicated, they should have root canal treatment before restoration is completed. Also, a tooth previously root canal–treated that shows no evidence of healing, or has an inadequate fill, or a fill exposed to oral fluids should be evaluated for retreatment before restorative therapy is initiated.

Periodontics. Generally, periodontal treatment should precede operative care, especially when improved oral hygiene, initial scaling, and root planing procedures can create a more desirable environment for performing operative treatment. Obviously a tooth with a questionable periodontal prognosis should not receive an extensive restoration until the time when periodontal treatment provides a more favorable prognosis. However, if a tooth has a good periodontal prognosis, operative treatment can occur before or after periodontal treatment as long as the operative treatment is not compromised by the existing tissue condition. Treatment of deep carious lesions often requires caries control, amalgam foundations, temporization and/or root canal therapy prior to periodontal treatment. The correction of gross restorative defects in restoration contours (such as open contacts, gingival overhangs, and poor embrasure form) is considered a part of initial periodontal therapy, and such corrections enhance a favorable tissue response. If periodontal surgical procedures are required, permanent restorations such as inlays/onlays, crowns, and prosthesis should be delayed until the surgical phase is completed.

Patients with gingivitis and early periodontitis generally respond favorably to improved oral hygiene and scaling/root planing procedures. More advanced periodontitis patients may require surgical pocket elimination/reduction procedures or various regenerative procedures. An increase in the zones of attached gingiva and the elimination of abnormal frenal tension should be provided by corrective periodontal surgical procedures around teeth receiving restorations with subgingival margins. In addition, any teeth requiring restorations that may encroach on the biological width of periodontium should have appropriate crown-lengthening surgical procedures performed before restoration is started. Usually a minimum of 4 to 5 weeks is required following the surgery prior to final restorative procedures.

Orthodontics. Orthodontic therapy may include extrusion or realignment of teeth to provide favorable interdental spacing, stress distribution, function, and esthetics. All teeth should be free of caries before orthodontic banding. Treatment of caries may include the placement of amalgam and composite resin restorations. There are few indications for cast restorations before orthodontic treatment is completed.

Oral surgery. In most instances impacted, unerupted,

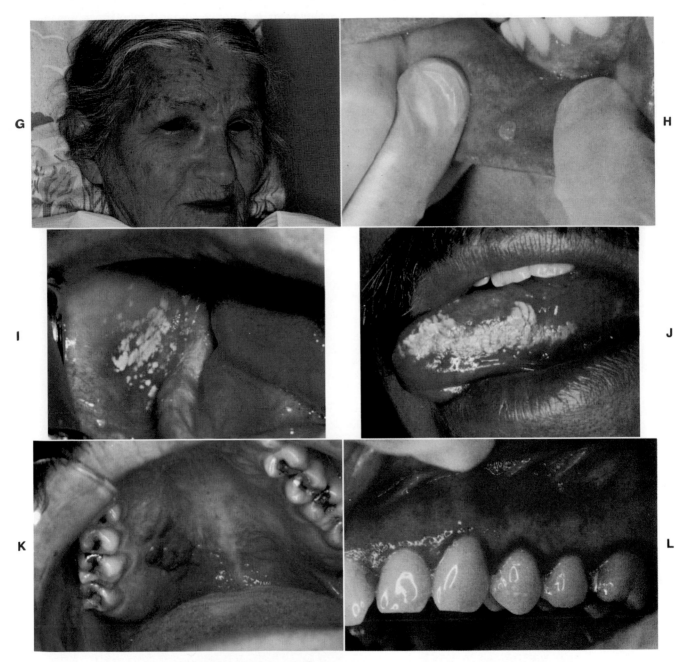

Plate 5-1, continued from previous page. G, Herpes zoster (shingles), supra-orbital dermatome distribution. **H,** Condylomata acuminatum, or venereal wart. **I,** Pseudomembranous candidiasis, facial mucosa. **J,** Hairy leukoplakia, lateral border of the tongue. **K,** Kaposi's sarcoma, maxillary palate. **L,** HIV-gingivitis. (**A,** courtesy Dr. William F. Vann, University of North Carolina, Chapel Hill; **B,** courtesy Dr. Diane C. Shugars, University of North Carolina, Chapel Hill; **C,** courtesy Dr. Lauren Patton, University of North Carolina, Chapel Hill; **D,** courtesy Dr. James Crawford, University of North Carolina, Chapel Hill; **E and F,** courtesy Dr. William F. Vann, University of North Carolina, Chapel Hill; **G,** courtesy Dr. Diane C. Shugars, University of North Carolina, Chapel Hill; **H to K,** courtesy Centers for Disease Control, Atlanta; **L,** courtesy Dr. James R. Winkler, University of California, San Francisco.)

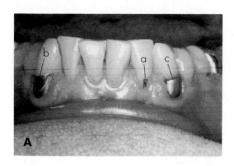 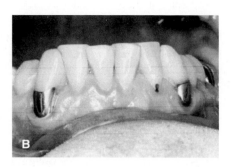 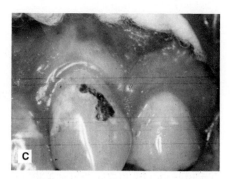

Fig. 5-19. A, Forty-year-old, arrested, root surface carious lesion *(a)* showing darkened, eburnated (sclerotic) dentin. Lesion should not be restored unless esthetically objectionable. Twenty-year-old gold inlay restoration *(b)* and 36-year-old amalgam restoration *(c)*. **B,** Same patient as shown in **A** 12 years later (lesion 52 years old, gold inlay 32 years old, amalgam restoration 48 years old). **C,** Arrested carious lesions on facial surface of canine. Both lesions feel hard to explorer, are cleanable, and should not be restored except to improve esthetics.

the patient population and tooth retention have emphasized this growing problem. Areas with root surface caries usually should be restored when there is clinical or radiographic evidence of cavitation. However, care must be exercised to distinguish the *active* root surface carious lesion from the root surface lesion that once was active but has become *inactive* (arrested) (Fig. 5-19, *A* and *B*). The latter lesion shows **eburnated dentin (sclerotic dentin)** that has darkened from extrinsic staining, is firm to the touch of an explorer, may be rough but is cleanable, and is seen in patients (usually older) whose oral hygiene and diet in recent years are good. Generally these lesions should not be restored except when elected by the patient.

If it is determined that the lesion needs restoration, the lesion can be restored with amalgam or tooth-colored materials. Restorative treatment of root surface caries may be enhanced by future refinement of dentinal adhesive restorative materials.

Obviously prevention is preferred over restoration. It is recommended that appropriate preventive steps such as improvements in diet and oral hygiene, as well as fluoride treatment, be taken in hopes of avoiding carious breakdown and the need for restoration.

Treatment of root surface sensitivity. It is not unusual for patients to complain of root surface sensitivity, which is annoying sharp pain usually associated with gingival recession and exposed root surfaces. Several theories have been advanced to explain the unusual sensitivity and response of such exposed dentin to a stimulus or irritation. The most accepted theory is the **hydrodynamic theory,** which postulates that the pain results from indirect innervation caused by dentinal fluid movement in the tubules which stimulates mechanoreceptors near the predentin. (See The Pulp-dentin Complex, Chapter 2.) Some of the causes of such fluid shifts are temperature change, air-drying, and osmotic pressure (e.g., by sucrose). *Any treatment that can reduce these fluid shifts by partially or totally occluding the tubules helps to reduce the sensitivity.*

Dentinal hypersensitivity is a particular problem in patients immediately after periodontal surgery that results in the clinical exposure of root surfaces. Numerous forms of treatment have been used to provide relief, such as topical fluoride, fluoride rinses, oxalate solutions, dentinal bonding agents, sealants, iontophoresis, and desensitizing toothpastes. All of these methods have met with varying degrees of success, and none has been totally effective. When these conservative methods fail to provide relief, restorative treatment is indicated.

Replacement of existing restorations. Generally a restoration should not be replaced unless (1) it has significant discrepancies, (2) the tooth is at risk for caries or fracture, or (3) the restoration is an etiological factor to adjacent teeth or tissue.[1] In many instances recontouring or resurfacing the existing restoration can delay replacement.

Some indications for replacing restorations are as follows: (1) marginal void, especially in the gingival one third, that cannot be repaired; (2) poor proximal contour or a gingival overhang, since these conditions contribute to periodontal breakdown; (3) a marginal ridge discrepancy that contributes to food impaction; (4) over-contour of facial or lingual surface resulting in plaque gingival to the height of contour and resultant inflammation of gingiva overprotected from rubbing-cleansing action of food bolus or toothbrush; (5) poor proximal contact that is either open, resulting in interproximal food impaction and inflammation of impacted gingival papilla, or improper in location or size (see Forming Proximal Contour and Contact, Chapter 19); (6) recurrent caries that cannot be adequately treated by a repair restoration; and (7) ditching deeper than 0.5 mm of the occlusal amalgam margin that is judged carious or caries-prone. By itself, the presence of shallow ditching around an amalgam restoration is not an indication for replacement.

Some indications for replacing tooth-colored restorations are (1) improper contours that cannot be repaired, (2) large voids, (3) dark marginal staining, (4) recurrent caries, or (5) unacceptable esthetics. Restorations that have only light marginal staining and are judged noncarious can be corrected by a shallow, narrow, marginal repair restoration.

As with every aspect of treatment planning, all factors must be considered before making a decision to replace a restoration.

Indications for amalgam restorations. Dental amalgam has evolved into an excellent restorative material. It is generally indicated for small cavitated lesions or for the replacement of small restorations on the distal surface of canines and posterior tooth surfaces. Amalgam also may be used on the lingual surface of the anterior teeth and when esthetics will not be affected. Consideration is given to capping cusps with amalgam or treating the tooth with a gold onlay when the width of the isthmus of an amalgam restoration approaches half of the distance between the cusp tips.

The use of amalgam in dentistry has been the source of controversy. This is due to the perceived adverse effects on the environment by mercury and amalgam waste resulting as amalgam is removed from the teeth. The reader is referred to Chapter 6, Dental Materials, for a more complete discussion of the issue.

Indications for direct-fill tooth-colored restorations. The direct application of composite is indicated for the treatment of cavities in the anterior teeth and is often indicated for cavities of the posterior teeth. There has been a great deal of research on the use of composite restorations for Classes I and II cavities in posterior teeth. Currently their use in these areas is acceptable if at least one centric-holding contact remains on tooth structure and isolation is satisfactory for bonding. Their routine use will depend on further improvements in dentinal bonding systems, verification from long-term clinical studies, and full acceptance by the American Dental Association (ADA) Council on Dental Materials and Devices. The reader is referred to Chapters 6, 16, and 17 for further details on the direct use of composites and glass ionomers.

Indications for indirectly fabricated tooth-colored restorations. Tooth-colored restorations that are indirectly fabricated out of the mouth often are indicated for Classes I and II preparations primarily when esthetics is of significant concern. Moreover, because of the potential of bonded restorations to strengthen remaining tooth structure, indirectly fabricated tooth-colored restorations also occasionally are *selected for the conservative restoration of weakened posterior teeth in esthetically critical areas.*

Indirectly fabricated tooth-colored restorations include (1) processed composite, (2) feldspathic porcelain, (3) cast ceramic, and (4) computer-generated (CAD/CAM) inlays and onlays. While all types offer superior physical characteristics when compared to direct-fill tooth-colored restorations, they also are more costly owing to the indirect process required for fabrication or due to the expense of CAD/CAM equipment.

Although *processed composite* restorations possess improved wear resistance over direct-fill posterior composites, they still should be reserved primarily for conservative Classes I and II preparations in low-to-moderate stress areas to ensure optimal performance. *Feldspathic porcelain* inlays and onlays for Classes I and II restorations are highly esthetic but suffer from a relatively high incidence of fracture, especially if subjected to heavy occlusal forces. Porcelain restorations also have the potential to wear opposing tooth structure.

Cast ceramic inlays and onlays (Dicor™) for Classes I and II preparations offer excellent marginal fit, low abrasion to opposing tooth structure, and superior strength compared to processed composite or feldspathic porcelain. However, the material is highly translucent and unesthetic unless used in conjunction with feldspathic porcelain surface stains, which increase the abrasiveness of the final restoration. Nonetheless, cast ceramic inlays and onlays offer an excellent esthetic alternative to cast metal restorations.

Computer-generated ceramic restorations (Dicor MGC™) for Classes I and II preparations possess high strength, low abrasiveness and are highly esthetic owing to the intrinsic coloration and highly polishable nature of the material. Although onlays can be generated, inlays are best fabricated with this system because of the difficulty in establishing occlusal morphology. Because these restorations are fabricated chairside (CEREC System™), only one appointment is required for placement as compared to the two appointments required for the other types of indirectly fabricated tooth-colored restorations.

Since all indirectly fabricated tooth-colored restorations depend largely on the establishment of an adhesive bond with enamel, *restoration of deeply subgingival preparations is not recommended.* Moreover, it must be noted that even though the physical characteristics of all types of indirectly fabricated tooth-colored restorations are superior to those of direct-fill types, the bonding medium used to cement these restorations often is inferior to the restoration itself and is the primary source of failure in large, stress-bearing restorations.

Indications for cast metal restorations. Although there are very few indications for intracoronal castings, a gold onlay that includes the occlusal surface of the tooth and preferably also *skirts at least three of the axial tooth line angles* (see Chapter 19) is an excellent restoration. Cast metal restorations are generally the treatment of choice for patients undergoing occlusal rehabilitation. Teeth with deep subgingival margins are best treated with cast restorations since, compared to amalgams, they provide a better opportunity for control of proximal contours and for restoration of the difficult subgingival margin. Teeth with facial and lingual surfaces unaffected by caries or restorations but whose cusps are fractured or weak may be restored by the above-mentioned "brace onlays" that skirt the line angles to improve both the resistance form as well as the retention form.

CONCLUSION

Proper diagnosis and treatment planning play a critical role in the quality of dental care. Each patient must be evaluated individually in a thorough and systematic fashion. After the patient's condition is understood and recorded, a treatment plan can be developed and rendered.

A successful treatment plan carefully integrates and sequences all necessary procedures indicated for the patient. There are few absolutes in treatment planning; the available information must be considered carefully and incorporated into a plan to fit the needs of the individual. Patients should have an active role in the process; they should be made aware of the findings, be advised of the risks and benefits of the proposed treatment, and be given the opportunity to help decide the course of treatment.

Examination, diagnosis, and treatment planning are extremely challenging and rewarding for both the patient and the dentist if done thoroughly and properly with the patient's best interest in mind.

REFERENCES

1. Anusavice KJ, editor: *Quality evaluation of dental restorations: criteria for placement and replacement,* Chicago, 1989, Quintessence Publishing.
2. Barr C: *Dental management of HIV-associated oral mucosal lesions: current and experimental techniques.* In Robertson PB, Greenspan JS, editors: *Oral manifestations of AIDS,* Littleton, Massachusetts, 1988, PSG Publishing.
3. Barr CE, Marder MZ: *Aids: a guide for dental practice,* Chicago, 1987, Quintessence Publishing.
4. Dajani AS et al: Prevention of bacterial endocarditis: recommendations by the American Heart Association, *JAMA* 264:2919-2922, 1990.
5. Greenspan D et al: *AIDS and the mouth,* Copenhagen, 1990, Munksgaard.
6. Greenspan D et al: Oral "hairy" leukoplakia in male homosexuals: evidence of association with both papillomavirus and a herpes-group virus, *Lancet* 2:831-834, 1984.
7. Hoofnagle JH: Type B hepatitis: virology, serology and clinical course, *Semin Liver Dis* 1:7-14, 1981.
8. Marzouk MA et al: *Operative dentistry,* ed 1, St Louis, 1985, Ishiyaku EuroAmerica.
9. Matteson SR et al: The report of the panel to develop radiographic selection criteria for dental patients, *Gen Dent* 39:264, July/August 1991.
10. Merchant VA: Herpes viruses and other microorganisms of concern in dentistry, *Dent Clin North Am* 35:283-298, 1991.
11. National Center for Health Statistics, Jack SS and Bloom B: Use of dental services and dental health, United States, 1986. Vital and Health Statistics. Series 10, No. 165. DHEW Pub No. (PHS) 88-1593. Public Health Service. Hyattsville, MD, 1988, U.S. Government Printing Office.
12. Reichart PA et al: The HIV-infection: virology, etiology, origin, immunology, precautions and clinical observations in 110 patients, *Int J Oral Maxillofac Surg* 16:129-153, 1987.
13. Samaranayake LP, Scully C: Oral candidiasis in HIV infection, *Lancet* 2:1491-1492, 1989.
14. Silverman S et al: Oral findings in people with or at high risk for AIDS: a study of 375 homosexual males, *J Am Dent Assoc* 112:187-192, 1986.

RECOMMENDED READINGS

Cottone JA: Hepatitis B: current status in dentistry, *Dent Clin North Am* 35:269-282, 1991.
Dolan MM, Yankell SL: *Transmissible infections in dentistry.* In Slots J, Taubman MA, editors: *Contemporary oral microbiology and immunology,* St Louis, 1991, Mosby.
Greenspan D et al: *AIDS and the mouth,* Copenhagen, 1990, Munksgaard.
Merchant VA: Herpes viruses and other microorganisms of concern in dentistry, *Dent Clin North Am* 35:283-298, 1991.
Schuster GS, editor: *Oral microbiology & infectious disease,* ed 3, Philadelphia, 1990, BC Decker.
Scully C et al: Oral manifestations of HIV infection and their management. I. More common lesions, *Oral Surg Oral Med Oral Pathol* 71:158-166, 1991.
Scully C et al: Oral manifestations of HIV infection and their management. II. Less common lesions, *Oral Surg Oral Med Oral Pathol* 71:167-171, 1991.
Silverman S: *Color atlas of oral manifestations of AIDS,* Toronto, 1989, Decker.
Syrjänen S: Viral infections in oral mucosa, *Scand J Dent Res* 100:17-31, 1992.

CHAPTER 6

Dental Materials

Stephen C. Bayne

Duane F. Taylor

INTRODUCTION

Dental materials science for restorative dentistry is derived from materials science. The field of materials science can be organized in terms of four categories of materials, with four categories of structural considerations governing their properties, and with four categories of general properties. For each of these there is a rich basis of materials science definitions. This information is presented in depth in textbooks of dental materials* but is reviewed here for reference during discussions in other parts of this book.

Review of materials science definitions

Materials categories. The four categories of materials are metals, ceramics, polymers, and composites. Each one of these has characteristic structures and resulting properties. It is paramount in every situation in restorative dentistry that the structures and properties involved be known.

Formal engineering definitions of each category are not practically useful. The following definitions are most often substituted instead.

Metals. A metal is based on an element which diffusely shares valence electrons amongst all of the atoms in the solid, instead of forming local ionic or covalent bonds. A **metal alloy** is an intentional mixture of metallic elements which occurs in a chemically intimate manner. As a result of mixing, the elements may be completely soluble (e.g., Au-Cu) or may be only partially soluble (e.g., Ag-Sn), producing more than one phase. Different **phases** represent locally different chemical compositions. The distribution of phases is influenced by the thermal and mechanical history of the solid, allowing a wide range of properties to be developed from a single overall composition. The periodic table consists mostly of metallic elements. Thus, there are a wide range of metallurgical systems which are possible.

Ceramics. Ceramics are chemically intimate mixtures of metallic and nonmetallic elements, that allow ionic (K_2O) and/or covalent bonding (SiO_2) to occur. In the periodic table, there are only a few nonmetallic elements, such as oxygen, nitrogen, hydrogen, and chlorine. The most common ceramics in dentistry are alloys of three main metallic oxides (SiO_2, Al_2O_3, K_2O). Ceramics also may result from corrosion of metals (Fe_2O_3, SnO, Ag_2S).

The corrosion behavior of metallic elements is classified as **active, passive,** or **immune** with respect to chemical or electrochemical reactions with other elements in their environment. Active metals corrode to

*References 6,7,17,30,33,35,36,52,59,76,93,114,120,122, 123,127,129,159,168.

form solid ceramic products or soluble products. For example, iron reacts with oxygen to form iron oxide. Passive metals corrode to form thin films of ceramic products that remain adherent to their surfaces and prevent further corrosion *(passivation)*. Titanium reacts with oxygen to form a titanium dioxide coating (TiO_2) that prevents further reaction and thus protects the surface. Immune metals, such as gold, are not reactive under normal environmental conditions. Most metals are active, and thus ceramics are much more common than metals in the world. Many of the key ceramics used for dentistry are oxides.

Polymers. Polymers are long molecules composed principally of nonmetallic elements (e.g., C, O, N, H) that are chemically bonded by covalent bonds. Their principal distinction from other common organic materials is their large size, and thus molecular weight. The process of forming a polymer from identifiable subunits, **monomers,** is called **polymerization.** The word *monomer* means "one unit." The word *polymer* means "many units."

A common commercial and dental example is the polymerization of methyl methacrylate monomer (100 gm/mole) into methyl methacrylate polymer (typically 300,000 gm/mole). Most polymers are named by adding *poly* as a prefix to the word for the major monomer in the polymer chain (polymethyl methacrylate) or by adding poly to the description of the chemical links formed between monomer units (polyamide, polysaccharide, polyester, polyether, polyurethane). In other cases, the original commercial brand name has become the common name (Nylon, Teflon, Dacron, Plexiglas).

Polymers may be classified in terms of the kinetics of the polymerization reaction. *Chain reaction polymerization* involves rapid monomer addition to growing chains. *Stepwise reaction polymerization* occurs slowly by random addition of monomers to any growing chain ends.

Composites. Composites are physical mixtures (or blends) of metals, ceramics, and/or polymers. The goal is to average the properties of the parts to obtain intermediate properties or to take advantage of good properties of each part. The classic mixture for dental restorations involves ceramic particles mixed with a polymer matrix. This is commonly called **dental composite.**

The properties of dental composites can be explained readily in terms of the volume fraction of the phases being physically mixed. This principle is called the *rule-of-mixtures* and actually has wide application for all materials. By knowing the phases present in the structure of any material and the interfacial interactions, it is possible to predict the overall properties fairly well.

Composites can be described as a **dispersed (filler) phase** mixed into a **continuous (matrix) phase.** The matrix phase is generally the phase which is transiently fluid during manipulation or placement of the materials. It is also the phase which tends to have the least desirable properties in the mixture. As a general rule, *minimizing the matrix of any system produces materials with more desirable clinical properties*. For a composite to distribute energy within the system to all of the phases, *it is important that the dispersed phase be bonded effectively to the continuous phase*.

Materials structure. Traditionally, a material is defined in terms of its composition. However, the composition of a material is only one of four important categories describing its structure, and hence properties. The four **structural categories** are **atomic arrangement, bonding, composition,** and **defects.** *Atomic arrangement* may be crystalline (ordered) or noncrystalline (disordered, glassy, amorphous). *Primary bonding* may include metallic, ionic, and/or covalent chemical bonds. *Secondary bonding* is much weaker and may include van der Waals or hydrogen bonds. *Composition* includes the elemental components and the resulting phases which form. The *defects* encompass a wide range of imperfections from those on the atomic scale to voids or pores. The thermal and mechanical histories strongly influence these structural categories, producing a wide range of possible properties for the same overall chemical composition. Gold alloys will have different mechanical properties if their defect concentrations are changed. SiO_2 can be produced as a noncrystalline solid or as any of three equilibrium crystalline solids (crystobalite, trydimite, or quartz).

Materials properties. Properties are descriptions of a material's interactions with the energy in its environment. *The four common **material's property categories** are physical, mechanical, chemical, and biological properties.* **Physical properties** include mass properties, thermal properties, electrical properties, optical properties, and surface properties. **Mechanical properties** include descriptions of stresses and strains within a material as a result of an external force. **Chemical properties** include chemical and electrochemical interactions. **Biological properties** include characterization of toxicity or sensitivity reactions during clinical use.

Physical properties. Physical properties involve reversible interactions of a material with its environment. A few of the more common physical properties are reviewed here with respect to important dental situations.

Metals, ceramics, polymers, and composites have different types and numbers of bonds. During temperature changes, therefore, they respond differently. During temperature increases, more rapid atomic motions stretch bonds and produce net expansion. During temperature decreases, solids undergo contraction. The relative rate of change is called the **coefficient of thermal expansion (or contraction).** If it is referenced to a sin-

Table 6-1. Linear coefficients of thermal expansion (LCTE)

Dental materials and dental structures	LCTE (ppm/°C)
Aluminous dental porcelain	4
Titanium implants	8-9
Traditional dental cements	8-10
Tooth structure	9-11
Stainless steel	11
PFM ceramics	14
PFM alloys	14
Gold foil	14-15
Gold casting alloys	16-18
Co-Cr alloys	18-20
Hybrid glass ionomers	20-25
Dental amalgam	25
Highly filled posterior composites	28-35
Anterior composites	35-45
PMMA direct-filling resins	72-83
Dental wax	260-600

After Bayne SC, Taylor DF, Zardiackas LD: *Biomaterials science,* ed 6, Chapel Hill, NC, 1992, Brightstar Publishing.

gle dimension, it is called the **linear coefficient of thermal expansion** (LCTE) and is symbolized by the Greek letter, alpha (α). The LCTE is expressed in units of inch/inch/°F, cm/cm/°C, or ppm/°C. Because the rate of change is small, the actual value is typically a multiple of 10^{-6} cm/cm/°C and is reduced to ppm/°C. Ceramics have an LCTE from 1 to 15 ppm/°C. Metals have values from 10 to 30 ppm/°C. Polymers have values from 30 to 600 ppm/°C. Tooth structure's LCTE is approximately 9 to 11 ppm/°C. It is important that the LCTE of a restorative material be as near that of tooth structure as possible. Important examples of values for dental materials are reported in Table 6-1.

One of the consequences of thermal expansion and contraction differences between a restorative material and adjacent tooth structure is percolation. This process is typified by an intracoronal dental amalgam restoration. During cooling, the amalgam contracts faster than tooth structure and recedes from the cavity wall, allowing the ingress of oral fluids. During subsequent expansion, the fluid is expressed. Cyclic ingress and egress of fluids at the restoration margin is called **percolation**. This is schematically presented in Fig. 6-1.

Other important physical properties involve **heat flow** through materials. Enamel and dentin are primarily composed of ceramic crystals (i.e., hydroxyapatite, $Ca_{10}(PO_4)_6(OH)_2$) that make those structures act as thermal insulators. If tooth structure is replaced with metallic restorations, which tend to be thermal conductors, then it is important to place additional thermal insulation to protect the dental pulp from rapid increases or decreases in temperature in the mouth. Generally, dental cements which are used as bases act as insula-

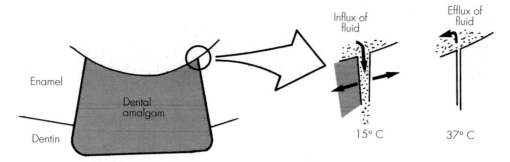

Fig. 6-1. Percolation along margins of dental amalgam restoration due to its difference in linear coefficient of thermal expansion from tooth structure during intraoral temperature changes. Fluid influx occurs during cooling (contraction). Fluid efflux occures during heating (expansion).

tors. One of the advantages of dental composites is low thermal conductivity, and therefore these materials do not need liners/bases to provide thermal insulation. Heat flow through a material is measured in terms of either the relative rate of heat conduction *(thermal conductivity)* or the amount of heat conduction per unit time *(thermal diffusivity)*. Thermal diffusivity is the more important property because it determines the amount of heat flow per unit time toward the pulp through a restoration. The dental pulp can withstand small temperature changes (from 37°C up to 42°C) for relatively short periods (30 to 60 seconds) without any permanent damage. Under most circumstances, the microcirculation of the pulp transports the heat entering the pulp away to other parts of the body where it is dissipated easily. However, extreme temperature changes or extended times of exposure to high temperatures will cause pulpal changes.

Electrical conductivity is a measure of the relative rate of electron transport through a material. This is important for metallic restorations which easily conduct electricity. If a galvanic cell (electrochemical cell) is present, then electrical current may flow and that process would stimulate nerves in the pulp. This may occur accidentally, such as when a tinfoil chewing gum wrapper contacts a cast gold restoration and produces a minor electrical shock.

Mass properties of materials involve density or specific gravity. *Density* is a material's weight (or mass) per unit volume. Most metallic materials have relatively high densities in the range of 6 to 19 gm/cm³. Ceramics are typically 2 to 6 gm/cm³. Polymers are in the range of 0.8 to 1.2 gm/cm³. The density is an important consideration for certain dental processing methods such as casting. Dense metal alloys are much easier to cast by centrifugal casting methods. Density must be considered in estimating the properties of mixtures of different materials (composites) because the final properties of the mixture are proportional to the volume of mixed materials (and not the weight). On occasion, the relative

density (or *specific gravity)* may be reported. Relative density is the density of the material of interest compared with the density of water under a standard set of conditions. At 25°C at 1 atmosphere of pressure, the density of water is 1.00 gm/cm³. Therefore, a specific gravity of 1.2 translates into a density of 1.2 gm/cm³ under the same conditions.

Optical properties of bulk materials include interactions with electromagnetic radiation (e.g., visible light) that involve *reflection, refraction, absorption (and fluorescence),* and/or *transmission* (Fig. 6-2). The radiation typically involves different intensities for different wavelengths (or energies) over the range of interest (spectrum).

Any of these interactive events can be measured using a relative scale or an absolute scale. When the electromagnetic radiation is visible light, the amount of reflection can be measured in relative terms as *gloss,* or in absolute terms as *percent reflection.* Visible light absorption can be measured in absolute terms as *percent absorption* (or *transmission)* for every wavelength (in the visible spectrum). *Color* is a perception by an observer of the distribution of wavelengths. The same color sensation may be produced by different absorption spectra *(metamerism).* An individual's eye is capable of sensing dominant wavelength, luminous reflectance (intensity), and excitation purity. Variations among individuals' abilities to sense these characteristics gives rise to varying perceptions of color.

Color measurement techniques do not measure these quantities directly. Color has traditionally been measured using the *Munsell color system* in terms of *hue, value,* and *chroma.* These terms correspond approximately to wavelength, intensity, and purity. The relationships of these quantities are represented schematically in Fig. 6-3. Shade guides for matching restorative dental materials to tooth structure are based on this system of describing color (see Chapter 16). The quality of color also is measured by the *CIE* (Commision Internationale de l'Eclairage) *system* as tristimulus values and

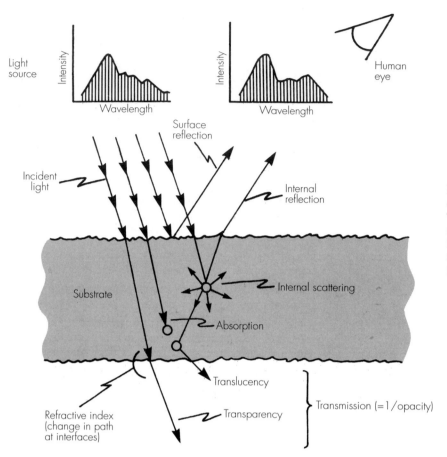

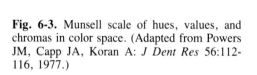

Fig. 6-2. Schematic summary of interactions of electromagnetic radiation with materials. The color perceived by observer is the result of a number of interactions between substrate and incoming radiation producing reflection, internal scattering, absorption, fluorescence, and transmission.

Fig. 6-3. Munsell scale of hues, values, and chromas in color space. (Adapted from Powers JM, Capp JA, Koran A: *J Dent Res* 56:112-116, 1977.)

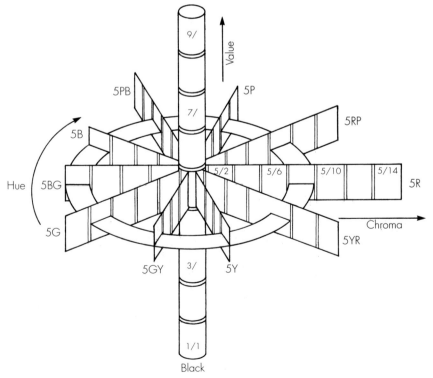

reported as color differences (L*, a*, and b*) in comparison to standard conditions.

One should always remember that *color is more than a property of a material. It is coupled to the electromagnetic spectrum involved* (and the relative intensity of every wavelength in the spectrum) *and the perceptive abilities of the observer.* A practical example of the importance of the spectrum and the observer would be the appearance of anterior dental porcelain crowns in a nightclub in which the lighting involves low-level fluorescent lamps. The crowns fluoresce differently in that light and appear different from adjacent natural teeth, as compared with a very natural appearance in full spectrum visible daylight.

Radiation of still another wavelength may be preferentially absorbed (e.g., x-rays). Dental composites that contain lithium, barium, strontium, or other good x-ray absorbers may appear *radiopaque* (radio-dense) in dental x-rays. Materials that are good absorbers (for whatever form of radiation) are described as *opaque.*

The appearance of a dental restoration is a combination of events of surface reflection, absorption, and internal scattering. The scattering may simply deflect the path of the radiation during transmission *(refraction),* or it may internally reflect the radiation from varying depths back out of a solid to the observer *(translucency).* Enamel naturally displays a high degree of translucency, therefore that is a desirable characteristic for restorative materials attempting to mimic enamel.

A wet tooth that is isolated from the wetting by saliva soon has a transient whiter appearance (see Chapter 11, Isolation of the Operating Field). Most of this shade change is due to the effect of loosely-bound water which is lost from subsurface enamel (by dehydration) between hydroxyapatite crystals. *This increases internal scattering of light* with much of it

reflected back to the observer (see internal reflection in Fig. 6-2). This probably explains why it takes 15 to 20 minutes for the isolated tooth to develop the whiter appearance, and 30 minutes or more for it to regain its original appearance after isolation is terminated. Larmas *et al.* showed that 0.8% to 1% by weight of pulverized moist enamel is exchangeable water, and that it can be removed at 4% relative humidity and 20°C.[72] Loosely-bound water also provides channels for *diffusion through enamel* of ions and molecules (see Histology of Enamel, in Chapter 3).

The direction of radiation may be perturbed as it crosses an interface from a medium of one type of optical character to another. *Refractive index* is the angle of change of the path for a standard wavelength of light energy under standard conditions.

Another group of physical properties of great interest is *surface properties.* Surfaces are important because all restorative dental materials meet and interact with tooth structure at a surface. Also, all dental surfaces interact with intraoral constituents such as saliva and bacteria. The extent of that interaction can be mitigated by changing a material's surface properties. The type of interaction between two materials at an interface is defined as the energy of interaction, and this is conveniently measured for a liquid interacting with a solid under a standard set of conditions as the *contact angle* (θ). The contact angle is measured as the angle which a drop of liquid makes with the surface on which it rests, as shown in Fig. 6-4, *A.* This angle is the result of an equilibrium between the surface tensions of the liquid-gas interface (γ_{LG}), solid-gas interface (γ_{SG}), and solid-liquid interface (γ_{SL}). These relationships can be expressed as an equation as shown in Fig. 6-4, *A.* If the energy difference of the two materials in contact is large, then they will have a large contact angle. If the

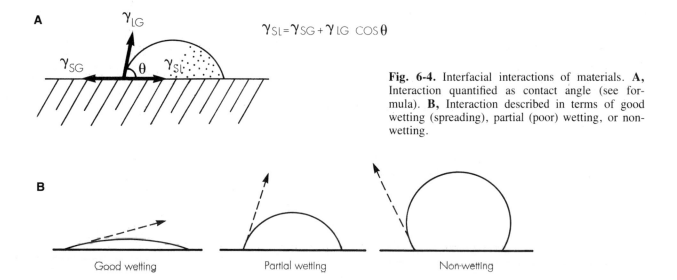

$$\gamma_{SL} = \gamma_{SG} + \gamma_{LG} \cos\theta$$

Fig. 6-4. Interfacial interactions of materials. **A,** Interaction quantified as contact angle (see formula). **B,** Interaction described in terms of good wetting (spreading), partial (poor) wetting, or non-wetting.

energy difference is very small, then the contact angle will be low and the liquid will appear to wet the solid by spreading. *Wetting* is a qualitative description of the contact angle. Good wetting, or spreading, represents a low contact angle. Partial (poor) wetting describes a contact angle approaching 90 degrees. Non-wetting is a contact angle approaching 180 degrees (Fig. 6-4, *B*).

It is very important that film formers such as varnishes, liners, cements, and bonding agents (all of which are discussed later in this chapter) have good wetting on cavity preparation surfaces on which these materials may be placed, so that they adapt to the microscopic interstices of the surfaces. However, in other instances, poor wetting may be an advantage. For example, experimental posterior dental composites have been formulated to have high contact angles to retard water and/or bacterial interactions. In most cases, wetting can be anticipated on the basis of the *hydrophilicity* (water-loving) or *hydrophobicity* (water-hating) of materials. Hydrophilic surfaces are not wet well by hydrophobic liquids.

Mechanical properties. The mechanical properties of a material describe its response to *loading*. Although most clinical situations involve complicated three-dimensional loading situations, it is common to simply describe the external load in terms of a single dimension (direction) as *compression, tension,* or *shear.* Combinations of these can produce *torsion* (twisting) or *flexion* (transverse bending). These modes of loading are represented schematically in Fig. 6-5 with respect to a simple cylinder and a mesio-occlusal (MO) amalgam restoration. For testing purposes, often it is impossible to grip and pull a specimen in tension without introducing other more complicated stresses at the same time. To circumvent problems for tensile testing of cylinders, it is possible to compress the sides of a cylinder and introduce stresses equivalent to tension. This variation of tension is called *diametral tension* (or diametral compression).

When a load is applied, the structure undergoes deformation as its bonds are compressed, stretched, or sheared. The load-deformation characteristics are only useful information if the absolute size and geometry of the structure involved are known. Therefore, it is typical to normalize load and deformation (in one dimension) as stress and strain. *Stress* (abbreviated, σ) is load per unit of cross-sectional area (within the material). It is expressed in units of load/area (pounds/in^2 = psi, or N/mm^2 = MPa). *Strain* (abbreviated, ϵ) is deformation (ΔL) per unit of length (L). It is expressed in units of length/length (inch/inch, or cm/cm), which is a dimensionless number. A schematic summary is presented in Fig. 6-6. During loading, bonds are generally not compressed as easily as they are stretched. Therefore, materials resist compression more readily and are said to be

stronger in compression than in tension. Materials have different properties under different directions of loading. *It is important to determine what the clinical direction of loading is before assessing the mechanical property of interest.*

As loading continues, the structure is deformed. At first this deformation (or strain) is completely reversible *(elastic strain).* However, increased loading finally produces some irreversible strain as well *(plastic*

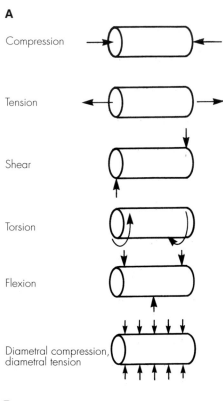

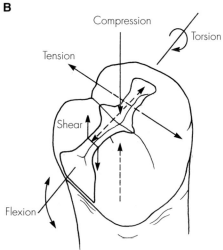

Fig. 6-5. Examples of directions of loading. **A,** Uniaxial loading of cylinder. **B,** Uniaxial loading of an MO amalgam restoration.

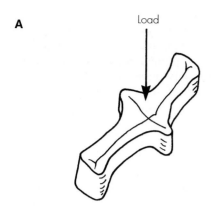

A

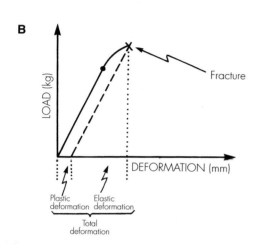

B

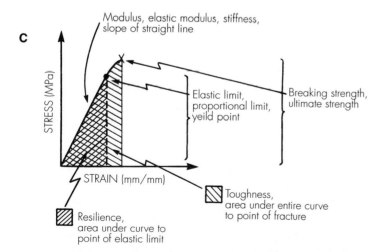

C

Fig. 6-6. Schematic summary of mechanical properties with respect to dental amalgam restoration in function. **A,** Occlusal loading of Class I amalgam restoration. **B,** Load/deformation curve describing behavior of amalgam. **C,** Normalization of load/deformation curve to stress/strain curve with important characteristics of curve indicated. (Mechanical responses depend on temperature and strain rate involved.)

strain), which causes permanent deformation. The point of onset of plastic strain is called the *elastic limit (proportional limit, yield point)*. This is indicated on the stress-strain diagram (Fig. 6-6) as the point at which the straight line starts to become curved. Continuing plastic strain ultimately leads to failure by fracture. The highest stress before fracture is the *ultimate strength* (Fig. 6-6, *C*). The total plastic tensile strain at fracture is called the *elongation*. This may also be expressed as the percent elongation. Materials that undergo extensive plastic deformation prior to fracture are called *ductile* (in tension) or *malleable* (in compression). Those which undergo very little plastic deformation are called *brittle*.

The slope of the linear portion (constant slope) of the stress-strain curve (from no stress up to the elastic limit) is called the *modulus, modulus of elasticity, Young's modulus,* or the *stiffness* of the material, and is abbreviated as E. It represents the amount of strain produced in response to each amount of stress. Ceramics typically have much higher modulus values (high stiffness) than polymeric materials (low stiffness). Because the slope of the line is calculated as the stress divided by the strain ($E = \sigma/\epsilon$), modulus values have the same units as stress (e.g., psi or MPa).

Two of the most useful mechanical properties are the modulus of elasticity and the elastic limit. A restorative material generally should be very stiff so that under load, its elastic deformation will be extremely small. An exception is Class V composites, which should be less stiff to accommodate tooth flexure (see Microfill Composites, in Chapter 16). If at all possible, a material should be selected for an application so that the stress level during function usually will not exceed the elastic limit. If the stress exceeds the elastic limit a small amount, the associated plastic deformation will tend to be very small. If the stress is well beyond the elastic limit, then the resulting deformation is primarily plastic strain and at some point ultimately results in failure.

Often it is convenient to determine the elastic limit in a relative manner by comparing the onset of plastic deformation of different materials using scratch or indentation tests, called *hardness tests*. The Mohs hardness scale ranks scratch resistance of a material in comparison to a range of standard materials. The Mohs scale is presented in Table 6-2. *Rockwell, Brinell,* and *Knoop* hardness tests employ indentors instead.

The energy that a material can absorb before the onset of any plastic deformation is called its *resilience* (Fig. 6-6, *C*), and is described as the area under the stress-strain curve up to the elastic limit. The total energy absorbed to the point of fracture is called the *toughness* and is related to the entire area under the stress-strain curve (Fig. 6-6, *C*).

Table 6-2. Mohs hardness scale

Mohs hardness	Reference material	Materials examples
10	Diamond	
—		(Silicon carbide, Tungsten carbide)
9	Corundum	
—		
8	Topaz	
—		(Tool steels)
7	Quartz	
—		
6	Orthoclase	
—		Dental enamel
5	Apatite	
—		(Low carbon steels)
4	Fluorite	
—		
3	Calcite	
—		
2	Gypsum	
—		
1	Talc	

After Greener EH, Harcourt JK, Lautenschlager EP: *Materials science in dentistry,* Baltimore, 1972, Williams & Wilkins.

Mechanical events are both temperature dependent and time dependent. Those conditions must be carefully described for any reported mechanical property. Generally, as the temperature increases, the mechanical property values decrease. The stress-strain curve appears to move to the right and downward. The opposite occurs during cooling. As the rate of loading decreases, the mechanical properties decrease. This is described as *strain rate sensitivity* and has important clinical implications. To momentarily make a material's behavior stiffer and/or more elastic, strain it quickly. *For recording undercut areas in an elastic intraoral impression, remove it rapidly so that it will be more elastic and more accurately record the absolute dimensions of the structures.* This is an excellent example of applied materials science.

Other time-dependent responses to stress or strain also occur. Deformation with time in response to a constant stress is called *creep* (or *strain relaxation*). Materials which are relatively weak or which are relatively close to their melting temperature are more susceptible to creep. Dental wax deforms (creeps) under its own weight over short periods of time. Traditional dental amalgam restorations are involved in intraoral creep. Deformation over time in response to a constant strain is called *stress relaxation.*

During loading, for all practical purposes, the strain below the elastic limit is all elastic strain. There is an infinitesimal amount of plastic strain, but it is so small that it is ignored. However, during multiple cycles, these very small amounts of plastic strain begin to accrue. After millions of cycles, the total plastic strain accumulated at low stress levels may be sufficient to represent the strain required to produce fracture. This process of multiple cycling at low stresses is called *fatigue* (Fig. 6-7, *A*). A standard engineering design limit for dental restorative materials is about 10 million cycles (or about 10 years of intraoral service). A rule-of-thumb is that materials on working surfaces of teeth are mechanically cycled about 1 million times per year on the average. The curve correlating cyclic stress levels (S) to the number of cycles to failure (N) is called a fatigue curve (S-N curve). These curves have only been determined for a few dental materials, because conducting the tests requires such a long period of time.[172] The compressive fatigue curves for Tytin and Dispersalloy dental amalgams are shown as part of Fig. 6-7, *B*.

Chemical properties. Chemical properties of a material are those which involve changes in primary or secondary bonding. *Primary bonding* changes occur during chemical reactions and electrochemical reactions. *Secondary bonding* changes occur during processes such as adsorption and absorption.

For metallic materials in the oral environment, the principal changes in primary bonding occur as a result of *chemical corrosion (tarnish)* or *electrochemical corrosion.* Chemical corrosion involves direct reaction of species by contact in solution or at an interface. An example of this process is the sulfide tarnishing of silver in dental amalgams to produce a black surface film. Another example is the oxidation of very high-copper-containing casting alloys to produce a green patina.

For any material, a number of electrochemical corrosion processes may happen as well. Electrochemical corrosion involves two coupled chemical reactions (half cells) at separate sites. These sites are connected by two paths, one (a circuit) is capable of transporting electrons, and the other (an electrolyte) is capable of transferring metallic ions.[155] Therefore, the basic components required for any *electrochemical cell* are (1) an anode (site of corrosion), (2) a cathode, (3) a circuit, and (4) an electrolyte (Fig. 6-8).

Electrochemical corrosion occurs intraorally any time these four components are present. The conditions define which of the metallic sites acts as an anode. A number of types of electrochemical cells are possible. Examples are shown schematically in Fig. 6-9.

A number of these electrochemical cells are possible in a simple restorative dentistry situation, such as that pictured in Fig. 6-22. When a dental amalgam is in contact with a gold alloy restoration, there are possibilities for galvanic corrosion, local galvanic corrosion, crevice corrosion, and stress corrosion. *Galvanic corrosion* is associated with the presence of macroscopically different electrode sites (amalgam and gold alloy). *Local galvanic corrosion (structure-selective corrosion)* is due to the electrochemical differences of different phases in a

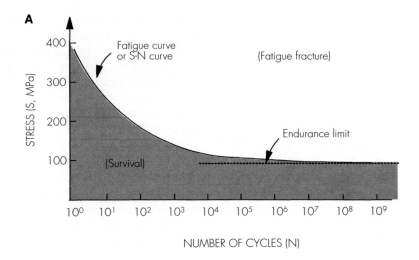

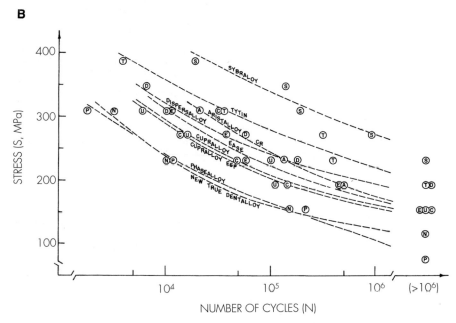

Fig. 6-7. Fatigue curves. **A,** Typical fatigue curve and characteristic regions (survival; fracture). **B,** Fatigue curves in compression for several commercial dental amalgams. (Courtesy Zardiackas LD, Bayne SC: *Biomat* 6:49-54, 1985.)

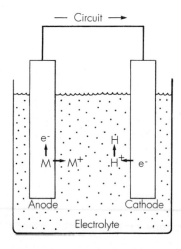

Fig. 6-8. Schematic representation of electrochemical cell. (Courtesy Bayne SC, Taylor DF, Zardiackas LD: *Biomaterials Science,* ed 6, Chapel Hill, NC, 1992, Brightstar Publishing.)

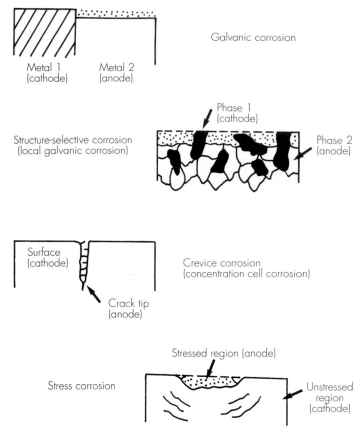

Fig. 6-9. Types of electrochemical cells. (After Tomashov ND: *Theory of corrosion and protection of metals*, ed 1, New York, 1966, Macmillan Publishing.) Dotted areas indicate material being lost during corrosion.

single material (such as dental amalgam). Electrochemical cells may arise whenever a portion of the amalgam is covered by plaque or soft tissue. The covered area has a locally lowered oxygen and/or increased hydrogen ion concentration, making it behave more anodically and corrode *(concentration cell corrosion)*. Cracks and crevices produce similar conditions and encourage concentration cell corrosion. Both corrosion processes are commonly termed **crevice corrosion.** When the restoration is under stress, the distribution of mechanical energy is not uniform and this produces different corrosion potentials. This process is called **stress corrosion.**

Ceramics and polymers do not undergo chemical or electrochemical corrosion in the same sense. Most of their changes are related to either chemical dissolution, absorption, or adsorption. **Chemical dissolution** normally occurs due to the solubilization created by hydrogen bonding effects of water and locally high acidity. Tooth structure is dissolved by high concentrations of lactic acid under dental plaque (see Chapter 3). Dental porcelains may be dissolved by very acidic fluoride solutions (acidulated phosphate fluoride, APF) used for protecting outer layers of dental enamel against dental caries.

Sorption events include both **adsorption** (adding molecules to a surface by secondary bonding) or **absorption** (penetration of molecules into a solid by diffusion). Protein adsorption alters the behavior and reactivity of dental materials' surfaces. Water absorption into dental polymers affects their mechanical properties.

Biological properties. Biological properties of dental materials are concerned with **toxicity** and **sensitivity** reactions that occur both locally within the associated tissue and systemically. Most dental materials interface locally with a variety of tissues (enamel, dentin/pulp, periodontium, cheek, tongue) and so local reactions may vary. It is possible to evaluate local toxic effects on cells by clinical pulp studies or by tissue culture tests. Unset materials may release components which are cytotoxic. However, in clinical situations there is rarely evidence of this problem. Two important clinical factors determining toxicity are the *exposure time* and the *concentration* of the potentially toxic substance. Generally, restorative materials set quickly and/or are not readily soluble in tissue fluids. Therefore, potentially toxic products do not have time to diffuse into tissues. Even more importantly, *the concentration makes the poison!* Some authorities believe that if the amount of material involved is small, then the pulp or other tissues can transport and excrete it without significant biochemical damage. Others believe that there is no threshold. A **threshold level** for toxicity is one below which no effect can be detected.

Systemic changes due to biomaterials' interactions have been very difficult if not impossible to monitor. Most evidence of biocompatibility has come from long-term usage and indirect monitoring. *This is an area of increasing concern for understanding potential risks of new or alternative restorative dental materials.*

Finally, toxicology is undergoing rapid evolution. In the 1970s most toxicological screening involved the use of the Ames test for determining mutagenicity. The inventor of that test has now withdrawn support for the conclusions derived from that screening procedure.[5,51] Therefore, results from earlier screening tests of dental materials may have to be reconsidered.

Biomechanics for restorative dentistry

Teeth are subjected to many forces during normal use. The interactions between the applied forces, the shape and structure of teeth, the supporting structures, and the mechanical properties of tooth components and restorative materials are all included in the subject of **biomechanics.** Biomechanics is the study of loads (or stresses) and deformations (or strains) occurring in biological systems.

The biomechanical behavior of restored teeth can be studied at any level from gross to microscopic. Examples of situations of interest include the calculation of stress transfer to the margin of an amalgam restoration, from the amalgam to tooth structure, from tooth structure to the periodontal ligament, from several teeth to bone, and throughout bone. The most common analysis focuses on stress transfer at the interface between a restoration and tooth structure.

Biomechanical unit. The standard biomechanical unit involves the (1) restorative material, (2) tooth structure, and (3) interface (interfacial zone) between the restoration and tooth. Different restorative procedures can involve very different interfaces. Composite/enamel interfaces are micro-mechanically bonded. Amalgam/enamel interfaces are weak and discontinuous unless a bonding system is used. Cemented crown/enamel interfaces are weak but are continuous. The importance of considering three structures in the biomechanical unit is to detect stresses that may cause unwanted fractures or debonding. The restorative material may be strong enough to resist fracture, but the interface or tooth structure may not be.

Stress transfer. Normal tooth structure transfers external biting loads through enamel into dentin as compression (Fig. 6-10). The concentrated external loads are distributed over a large internal volume of tooth structure and thus local stresses are lower. During this process a small amount of dentin deformation may occur which results in tooth flexure. These deformations will be discussed more carefully subsequently (see the following section in this chapter).

A restored tooth tends to transfer stress differently than an intact tooth. Any force on the restoration produces compression, tension, or shear along the tooth/restoration interface.[87,88] Once enamel is no longer continuous, its resistance is much lower. Therefore, most restorations are designed to distribute stresses onto sound dentin, rather than to enamel (Fig. 6-11).[100] Once in dentin the stresses are resolved in a manner similar to a normal tooth. The process of stress transfer

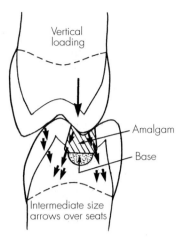

Fig. 6-11. Stress in tooth restored with dental amalgam is transferred to dentin (and not enamel) whenever possible. Note the facial and lingual seats at initial cavity preparation pulpal wall level (before removal of remaining infected dentin and placement of base).

to dentin becomes more complicated when the amount of remaining dentin is thin and the restoration must bridge a significant distance to seat onto thicker dentin (see Liners and Bases).

For an amalgam restoration in a pulpally deep cavity preparation, a total of 1 to 2 mm of underlying dentin and/or other insulating material is preferred pulpal of the amalgam to provide adequate *thermal and mechanical protection of the pulp.*[123] If inadequate thickness of dentin remains, the insertion of an insulating liner or base is recommended. *However, it is still wise to ensure that the amalgam restoration is "seated" on sound dentin at three or more widely separated areas at the level of the initial cavity preparation pulpal wall.* **This provides optimal stress transfer.** For a nonmetallic restoration, which has better insulating properties than a metallic one, 0.5 to 1 mm of dentin and/or liner or base is sufficient for thermal and mechanical protection.

Strain within tooth structure (tooth flexure). Teeth are not rigid structures. They undergo deformation (strain) during normal loading.[135] Intraoral loads (forces) vary widely and have been reported to range from 10 to 431 N (1 N = 0.225 lb of force), with a functional load of 70 N considered clinically normal.[58] Obviously, the number of teeth, type of occlusion, and occlusal habits of patients, such as bruxism, affect the load per tooth.

The amount of strain will be roughly proportional to the amount of stress. However, because tooth structure is heterogeneous and asymmetrical and its properties change with time, there is no simple description of the state of stress or amount of strain. To date, there is increasing evidence that the amount of strain and its effect on tooth structure may be very important in fatigue.

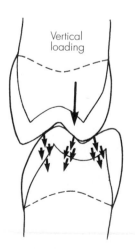

Fig. 6-10. Stress transfer in unrestored tooth occurs through dental enamel into dentin.

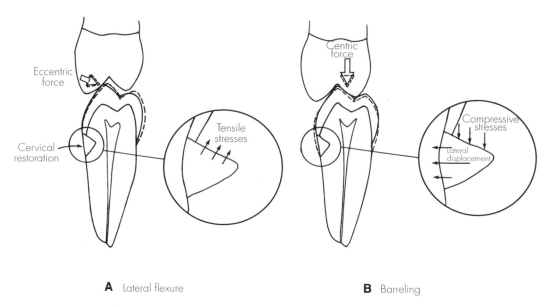

A Lateral flexure   **B** Barreling

Fig. 6-12. Schematic diagram of tooth flexure creating cervical stresses. **A,** Lateral flexure results from eccentric forces which produce tensile stresses at marginal interface with cervical restoration placed in facial CEJ region. **B,** Barreling results from heavy centric forces which produce compressive stresses along marginal interface with cervical restoration in entire CEJ region, resulting in lateral displacement (loss) of the restoration. (Courtesy Heymann HO et al: *J Am Dent Assoc* 122:41-47, 1991.)

Tooth flexure has been described as either a lateral bending or an axial bending of a tooth during occlusal loading.[61] This flexure produces the maximal strain in the cervical region, and the strain appears to be resolved in tension or compression within local regions, causing the loss of bonded Class V restorations in preparations with no retention grooves (Fig. 6-12). Moreover, *one current hypothesis is that tensile or compressive strains gradually produce micro-fractures*[53,56,73] (called **ab-fractions** by some authors) in the thinnest region of enamel at the cementoenamel junction (CEJ) (Fig. 6-13). Such fractures predispose enamel to loss when

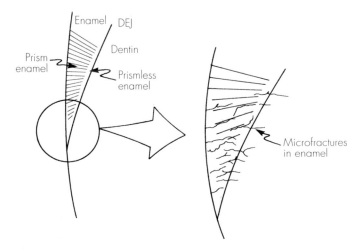

Fig. 6-13. Schematic view of micro-fractures developing between enamel rods in cervical enamel. The enamel near the junction of the CEJ and DEJ is prismless. (After Lee WC, Eakle WS: *J Prosthet Dent* 52:374-380, 1984.)

subjected to toothbrush abrasion and/or chemical erosion. This process may be key in the formation of Class V defects (Fig. 6-14). Additionally, in unbonded or leaking restorations, this flexure of the dentin may also produce changes in fluid flow and microleakage leading to sensitivity and pulpal inflammation, respectively (see Pulp-Dentin Complex, in Chapter 2). These events are just beginning to be carefully documented.

Effects of aging. As a tooth becomes older it undergoes changes in structural mass and in the character of the remaining tissue. Older teeth have lost most prismless enamel along the outer surface and may have encountered numerous microfractures in cervical portions, as just discussed. In response to disease assaults, such as caries or other external stimuli, odontoblastic processes may have laid down more peritubular dentin occluding the outer zones of dentinal tubules.[50] Peritubular dentin is mostly hydroxyapatite and would tend to stiffen dentin. Secondary and reparative dentin also may have been produced, replacing some of the pulp chamber and canals. There is also strong evidence that with aging, all type I collagen in the human body becomes more crosslinked.[171] A strong suspicion is that this process of crosslinking makes the intertubular dentin more brittle. Therefore, it is logical that the modulus of teeth is observed to increase with aging (50% increase from 20 to 29 years of age, to 40 to 49 years of age) and that teeth behave in a more brittle fashion.[46,170] This alteration, coupled with microcracks that may have developed with fatigue, may produce large cracks or fractures in the tooth over time.

These changes produce a substrate that may not

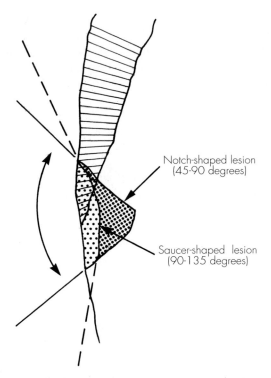

Fig. 6-14. Schematic view of Class V cervical defects comparing shallow saucer-shaped lesions to deep notch-shaped lesions. Angulation is determined by average slope of walls and not walls at perimeter of the lesion. (Courtesy Bayne SC et al: *J Dent Res* 71A:314, 1992 (abstract 1669.)

Notch-shaped lesion (45-90 degrees)

Saucer-shaped lesion (90-135 degrees)

transfer stress as readily and which may no longer be well-matched to the properties of a restorative material which has survived for a long time. The complete implication of these changes is not yet fully understood.

Principles of biomechanics. Stress transfer and the resulting deformations of structures are principally governed by (1) the elastic limit of the materials, (2) the ratio of the elastic moduli involved, and (3) the thickness of the structures. Materials with a high elastic modulus transfer stresses without much strain. Lower modulus materials undergo dangerous strains where stresses are concentrated, unless there is adequate thickness. The resistance to strain increases approximately as the fourth power of the thickness of the material involved. Doubling the thickness increases the resistance to elastic strain by sixteen-fold. If the local stress does exceed the material's elastic limit, then the capacity for plastic deformation before fracture will determine when fracture actually occurs.

These principles can be demonstrated easily using the case of a mesioocclusodistal (MOD) restoration in a first molar. A low modulus material, such as amalgam, must have sufficient thickness to resist flexural deformation that would produce fracture in this brittle material. Increased amalgam thickness improves its resistance to

flexure but compromises the resistance of the remaining dentin and base floor for the restoration. However, properly prepared and condensed amalgam in a proper cavity preparation that provides the recommended occlusopulpal restoration thickness serves for many years without fracture.

DIRECT RESTORATIVE DENTAL MATERIALS
Introduction

Loss of tooth structure to dental caries or other processes usually proceeds in a gradual way. Therefore, a patient's initial encounter with a dentist often involves the restoration of a small portion of tooth structure that is cavitated. This can be accomplished relatively easily by designing a cavity preparation with retention features and restoring it with a pliable material that is capable of hardening in situ. While in a moldable stage, the material can be adapted to the tooth structure and shaped to re-create normal anatomic contours. This process is called *direct restorative dentistry,* because it is accomplished directly in the intraoral environment. The development or selection of materials for direct application may require compromise of mechanical properties or other desired characteristics. *If there is extensive loss of tooth structure, then the restorative materials must provide better stress distribution characteristics and be more carefully bonded to remaining tooth structure.* In most cases, this requires the use of materials that cannot be made fluid for direct use. These materials must be fabricated into a restoration outside of the mouth and cemented or bonded in place. The procedures involved with this approach are categorized as *indirect restorative dentistry.*

Dental amalgam

Terminology. *Amalgam* technically means an alloy of mercury with any other metal. *Dental amalgam* is an alloy made by mixing mercury (Hg) with a silver-tin dental amalgam alloy (Ag-Sn). In dentistry, it is common to use the term *amalgam* to mean dental amalgam.

Dental amalgam alloy is a silver-tin alloy to which varying amounts of copper and small amounts of zinc have been added. *Low-copper dental amalgam* alloys contain 2% to 5% copper. The earliest successful dental amalgams were made by combining filings of such alloys with mercury. A typical modern low-copper dental amalgam alloy may contain 69.4% Ag, 26.2% Sn, 3.6% Cu, and 0.8% Zn. Amalgams made from such low-copper alloy filings are often referred to as *conventional dental amalgams*. *High-copper dental amalgam* alloys contain 12% to 30% copper and, due to their higher copper content, display significantly better corrosion resistance than low-copper dental amalgams. A typical high-copper dental amalgam alloy may contain

60% Ag, 27% Sn, 13% Cu, and 0% Zn. The particles of these alloys which are mixed with mercury may be filings but are often small spheres.

Dental amalgam is mixed for use by combining dental amalgam alloy particles with mercury, vigorously mixing the components for a few seconds during the initial reaction, placing the plastic mass into a cavity preparation, compressing the mixture (*condensation*) to remove the excess mercury-rich phase, and then carving and finishing the hardening mass.

Because of a concern about the possible toxicity of mercury in dental amalgams, a number of materials have been developed as *dental amalgam substitutes*. Most are compositions which contain some of the components of dental amalgam (such as Ag-Sn alloy particles) but which do not contain mercury. *Gallium alloys* are an example of such a substitute that is made with Ag-Sn particles in Ga-In.[116,146] Gallium melts at 28°C and can be used to produce liquid alloys at room temperature by the addition of small amounts of other elements such as indium. In this case, Ga-In has been substituted for Hg in dental amalgam. Other systems are being explored which use Au mixed with other noble metals to form the restoration matrix.[161]

The American Dental Association, in combination with the National Institute on Standards Technology (ADA-NIST), has patented a *mercury-free direct filling alloy* based on Ag coated Ag-Sn particles that can be self-welded by compaction to create a restoration. This approach is being proposed as an alternative to dental amalgam.

Other transitional approaches include redesigning amalgam to have much less initial mercury. If alloy particle sizes are judiciously chosen to pack together well, it is possible to minimize the mercury required for mixing to the 15% to 25% range. The actual clinical properties of these *low-mercury amalgams* are not yet known.

Classification. The major approaches to classification of dental amalgams and the dental amalgam alloys on which they are based are in terms of (1) *dental amalgam alloy particle geometry and size,* (2) *copper content,* and (3) *zinc content.* Each of these is discussed subsequently in an historical context.

In the 1830s, dental amalgam alloy was obtained by filing or grinding silver coins into coarse particles to mix with mercury. The compositions were inconsistent at best and the reaction conditions were quite variable. This process could not reliably produce a final amalgam with uniform properties. During the 1860s and 1870s, Townsend, Flagg, and others contributed immensely to investigations of composition versus properties. However, true dental amalgam science began with investigations by G.V. Black during the 1890s. *Traditional (or conventional) dental amalgam alloys* were produced by early dental manufacturers, such as S.S. White, and predominated from 1900 until 1970. The basic compo-

sition was 65% Ag, 30% Sn, 5% Cu, and <1% Zn.

Traditional dental amalgam was mixed initially by proportioning alloy and mercury components into a mortar and then grinding the mixture with a pestle. The process of manual mixing is known as *trituration.* Alloy was manufactured in bricks that were ground with a file into *filings* and mixed with mercury. A more efficient process was grinding up the ingot of alloy, typically on a lathe. For that reason, those particles became known as *lathe-cut particles* (Fig. 6-15). Filings were irregular in shape and gradually were produced in finer and finer sizes by manufacturers to control the reaction, produce smoother mixtures, and enhance final properties. Lathe-cut particles could be purchased in regular cut, fine cut, and micro-fine cut versions. *Conventional amalgam alloys were commonly classified on this basis of particle size.*

Irregular powder particles pack together relatively

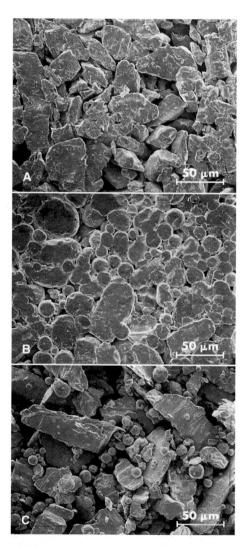

Fig. 6-15. Examples of amalgam alloy particles. **A,** Filings (New True Dentalloy). **B,** Spheres (Cupralloy). **C,** Mixed geometries (Dispersalloy). (Courtesy SC Bayne, School of Dentistry, University of North Carolina, Chapel Hill, NC.)

poorly (Fig. 6-15, *A*) and require a relatively large amount of mercury (50% to 60% by weight in the mixture) to fill in the spaces. After transfer of the mixture to the cavity preparation, it is possible to compact the mass and extrude some of the mercury-rich matrix. By eliminating the mercury-rich matrix as much as possible, the amount of reaction product matrix which forms is limited, thereby improving the overall properties of the set dental amalgam. Mercury-rich mixtures, after trituration but before placement into the cavity, historically could be partially condensed by wringing the mass in a squeeze cloth. In the 1960s, Eames was the first to promote a low mercury-to-alloy mixing ratio (*Eames technique* or no squeeze cloth technique).[41] Later, it was demonstrated that by spherodizing the alloy particles,[39] the particles packed more efficiently (Fig. 6-15, *B*) and required much less mercury to make a practical mixture. *Spherical particles* also increased the fluidity of the mixture by presenting less resistance to particle sliding. Using some or all spherical alloy particles, it is possible to reduce the mercury portion of the mixture to less than 50% by weight. The distinction between irregular (lathe-cut) and spherical particle geometries became the next major basis for classification of dental amalgam alloys. Most modern pre-capsulated dental amalgams are formulated with only 42% to 45% mercury by weight.

During the early part of the twentieth century, alloy powder and mercury were proportioned crudely and mixed manually (Fig. 6-16, *A*). To proportion and mix dental amalgam more carefully, manufacturers later recommended the use of alloy pellets, mercury dispensers, reusable mixing *capsules* and *pestles,* and *amalgamators* (Fig. 6-16, *B*). A typical reusable capsule (Fig. 6-17, *A*) was a hollow tube with rounded ends constructed as two pieces that could be friction-fit or screwed together. Amalgam alloy was dispensed into the capsule as a pellet of pressed powder of standard weight. Mercury was dispensed into the capsule as a standard-sized droplet from an automatic dropper bottle. A small metal or plastic pestle (Fig. 6-17, *B*) was added to the capsule and it was closed. The capsule and its contents were then automatically mixed using an amalgamator. The typical amalgamator has been designed to grasp the ends of the capsule in a claw that is oscillated in a figure-eight like pattern. This accelerates the mixture toward each end of the capsule during each throw and impacts the mixture with the pestle.

To guarantee that amalgam alloy and mercury are mixed both efficiently and consistently, it is very impor-

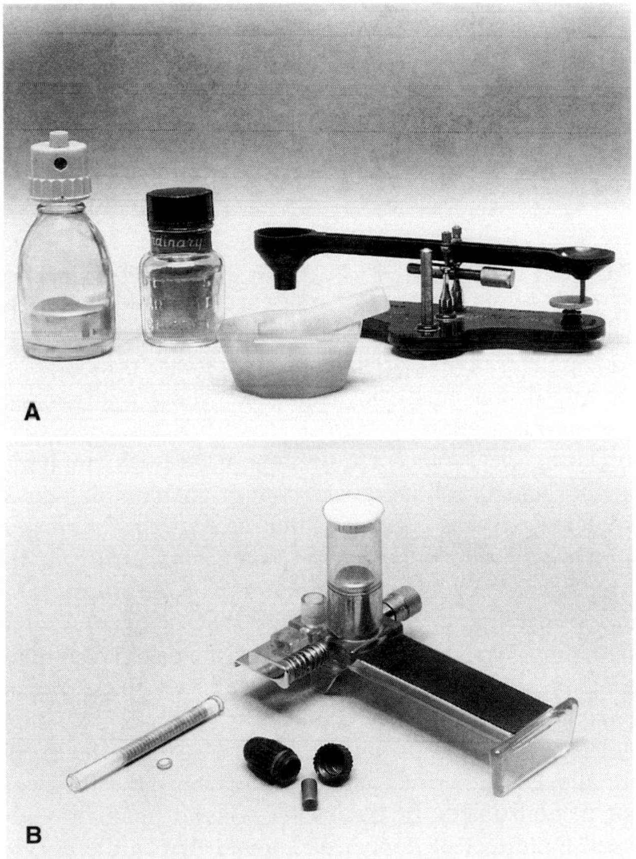

Fig. 6-16. Earlier methods of dental amalgam trituration. **A,** Equipment for hand mixing of alloy powder and mercury in mortar and pestle using excess mercury (circa 1900 to 1940 AD). **B,** Equipment for mixing of alloy pellets and controlled mercury in reusable capsules with mechanical mixing in amalgamator (circa 1940 to 1970 AD).

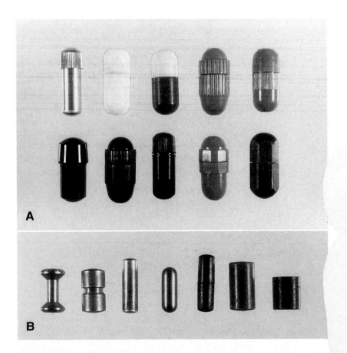

Fig. 6-17. Pestles and capsules for automatically mixing dental amalgam constituents using amalgamator. **A,** Reusable capsules. **B,** Magnified view of pestles.

tant to periodically calibrate dental amalgamators. After several years of use, the bearings become worn and the mixes no longer are sufficiently triturated. On standard electric amalgamators (Fig. 6-18, *A*), the trituration speed and trituration time are manually set on the front of the equipment. Settings vary for different products. Electronic amalgamators (Fig. 6-18, *B*) have digital controls and permit programming of settings.

Modern dental amalgams are produced from pre-capsulated alloy and mercury. The components are separated in the capsule by a special diaphragm that is broken when the capsule is "activated" just before mixing (Fig. 6-19). Precapsulated *(preproportioned) dental*

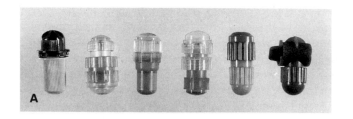

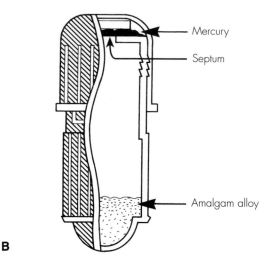

Fig. 6-19. Preproportioned capsules for mixing dental amalgam constituents using amalgamator. **A,** Examples of preproportioned capsule designs. **B,** Schematic of preproportioned capsule showing mercury and powder separated by septum that must be perforated before mixing. (After Rinne VW: *J Dent Res* 62:116-117, 1983.)

amalgam (Fig. 6-19, *A*) provides convenience but also provides some degree of assurance that the materials will not be contaminated before use or spilled prior to mixing. *Mercury hygiene* is an important consideration for safe dental amalgam management and is discussed later in this section.

During the 1960s there was major research emphasis on the benefits of increased copper contents in dental amalgams. It was confirmed that *increasing the copper content above 12% by weight in the dental amalgam alloy effectively suppressed formation of the phase (Sn-Hg) which was prone to intraoral corrosion.* A dramatic improvement in corrosion resistance led to a doubling or tripling of clinical longevity of these dental amalgams. The effect of copper was originally explored by Flagg in the 1860s but the copper was not effectively pre-alloyed with silver and/or tin. Thus, the effect was not demonstrated. In the 1930s, Gayler again investigated the effect of copper and found that in the coarse filing alloys of that time, copper contents above 6% produced excessive expansion and the corrosion-reducing effect at higher copper contents was not realized. Also in the 1930s, early pioneers were admixing copper amalgams with dental amalgams to produce very corro-

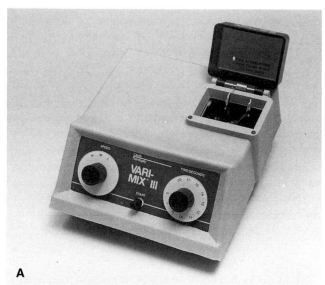

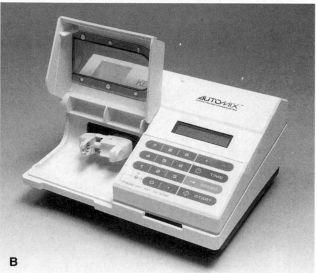

Fig. 6-18. Examples of dental amalgamators for automatically mixing dental amalgam in capsules (shown with protective cover open on equipment). **A,** Amalgamator with manually set trituration speeds and times. **B,** Amalgamator with digital controls and programming for trituration speeds and times.

sion-resistant compositions. However, the setting times of the mixtures were slow and the compositions were quite variable. It was not until Innes and Youdelis[64] added Ag-Cu spheres to conventional amalgam alloy with the intent of producing dispersion-hardened amalgams, that the advantageous effect of copper on corrosion resistance was clearly observed.

Classification of dental amalgams based on copper contents is the main system in use today (Table 6-3). High-copper dental amalgams can be produced from dental amalgam alloy particles that are irregular and/or spherical.

Another important additive to amalgam alloy was **zinc**. Originally zinc was added to conventional dental amalgams as a processing aid to suppress oxidation of the key elements in the alloy. Zinc tends to oxidize preferentially forming a zinc oxide film that covers the surface of liquid alloy during manufacture and suppresses oxidation of other elements. Generally, 1% or more is added to accomplish this end. However, some (0.2% to 1%) is left in the dental amalgam alloy at the end. A detrimental side effect of this residual zinc was that moisture contamination prior to setting converted the zinc to zinc oxide and produced hydrogen gas that could expand the amalgam excessively, resulting in patient pain. Once the mechanism of **delayed expansion** was understood, care during dental amalgam manipulation prevented this problem. Some manufacturers also produced **non-zinc amalgams** as an alternative. These alloys were often favored where isolation was difficult. *It now seems as though zinc may have some beneficial effect on amalgam longevity.* There is clinical research evidence[80,81,117] that zinc-containing low-copper and high-copper amalgams may last 20% to 50% longer than zinc-free ones. On the basis of this new evidence, **amalgams** continue to be produced and designated as **zinc** (zinc-containing) or **non-zinc** (zinc-free), although improved manufacturing techniques have largely eliminated the original need for it as a manufacturing aid.

Composition, structure, and properties. Examples of *compositions and structure* of dental amalgams of all types are summarized in Table 6-3. *The principal considerations for any dental amalgam are the amount of mercury in the final restoration and the types of reaction products which are formed.*

Conventional dental amalgam sets by the reaction of Ag and Sn from Ag-Sn particles with mercury to produce two reaction product phases, a Ag-Hg phase and a Sn-Hg phase. These form solids and cause the mass to harden. The reaction is very complicated metallurgically and is influenced by a number of variables. Schematically, the reaction is summarized in a simple way in Fig. 6-20. Because the original mixture contains a large excess of Ag-Sn alloy particles, only a minor portion of the outside of the particles is consumed during the reaction with mercury. The unreacted portion of the original dental amalgam alloy particles remains as residual alloy particles, reinforcing the final structure. Reaction products form a matrix surrounding the residual alloy particles. Because the residual alloy particles have physical, chemical, and mechanical properties that are significantly better than those of the reaction products, *it is key to minimize the amount of matrix which forms during the reaction.* Depending on the geometry and packing of the dental amalgam alloy particles, different amounts of mercury will be required to initially create a condensable mixture. After the reaction begins and the amalgam has been placed in the cavity preparation, it is important to compress (condense) the mixture to reduce voids in the material, adapt it closely to the cavity preparation walls, and to express excess mercury-rich matrix. The mercury-rich matrix is removed from the surfaces of condensed material increments. *This process ensures that the final structure is composed predominantly of reinforcing residual alloy within a minimum of reaction product matrix.*

Table 6-3. Compositions and structure of dental amalgam alloys*

Amalgam alloys	Classification	Particle type	Ag	Sn	Cu	Zn	Hg	Other
New true dentalloy	Low copper	Lathe-cut	70.8	25.8	2.4	1.0	0.0	—
Micro II	Low copper	Lathe-cut	70.1	21.0	8.6	0.3	0.0	—
Dispersalloy	High copper	Mixed	69.5	17.7	11.9	0.9	0.0	—
Tytin	High copper	Spherical	59.2	27.8	13.0	0.0	0.0	—
Sybraloy	High copper	Spherical	41.5	30.2	28.3	0.0	0.0	—
Cupralloy	High copper	Mixed	62.2	15.1	22.7	0.0	0.0	—
Aristalloy CR	High copper	Spherical	58.7	28.4	12.9	0.0	0.0	—
Indiloy	High copper	Lathe-cut	60.5	24.0	12.1	0.0	0.0	3.4 In
Valiant	High copper	Lathe-cut	49.5	30.0	20.0	0.0	0.0	0.5 Pd
Valiant PhD	High copper	Mixed	52.7	29.7	17.4	0.0	0.0	0.5 Pd

After Osborne JW et al: *J Dent Res* 57:983-988, 1978; Vrijhoef MMA, Vermeersch AG, Spanauf AJ: *Dental amalgam*, Chicago, 1980, Quintessence Publishing.
*Elements in the composition are reported in weight percent.

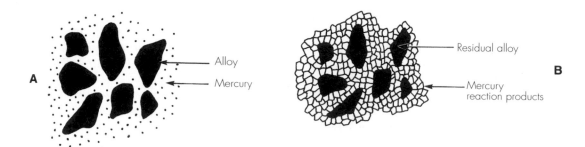

Fig. 6-20. Schematic summary of setting reaction of dental amalgam and its associated micro-structure. **A,** Before reaction, alloy particles are dispersed in mercury. **B,** After reaction, residual alloy particles are embedded in matrix of reaction products. Only small amount of the powder particles is required to completely react with mercury. (Courtesy Bayne SC, Barton RE. In Richardson RE, Barton RE, editors: *The dental assistant,* ed 6, Philadelphia, 1988, Lea & Febiger.)

The major reaction product phases of Ag-Hg and Sn-Hg are approximately Ag_2Hg_3 and $Sn_{7-8}Hg$, and are non-stoichiometric. In metallurgical terminology, the original alloy is designated as *gamma phase* (γ) and the reaction product phases are called *gamma-one* (γ_1) and *gamma-two* (γ_2), respectively.

Ag-Hg (gamma-one) crystals are generally small and equiaxed. Most of the matrix is Ag-Hg. That phase has intermediate corrosion resistance. *Sn-Hg (gamma-two)* reaction product crystals are long and blade-like, penetrating throughout the matrix. Although they constitute less than 10% of the final composition, they form a penetrating matrix because of inter-crystalline contacts between the blades. That image is reinforced by the scanning electron microscopy (SEM) picture of Sn-Hg crystals in Fig. 6-21. This phase is prone to corrosion in clinical restorations, a process which proceeds from the outside of the amalgam, along the crystals, connecting to new crystals at inter-crystalline contacts. This produces *penetrating corrosion* that generates a porous and spongy amalgam with minimal mechanical resistance.

Two key features of this degradation process are the corrosion-prone character of the Sn-Hg phase and the connecting path formed by the blade-like geometry of the crystals. Both of these are eliminated by the use of more copper in the initial composition.

High-copper dental amalgams set in a manner similar to low-copper amalgams except that Sn-Hg reactions are suppressed by the preferential formation of Cu-Sn phases instead. *Cu-Sn phases which are part of the set dental amalgam matrix are much less corrosion-prone than the Sn-Hg phase they replace.* The Cu-Sn phases are still the most corrosion-prone ones in the amalgam. However, when they corrode, penetrating corrosion does not occur because individual crystals generally are not connected.

Both low-copper and high-copper dental amalgams undergo two kinds of corrosion, *chemical corrosion*

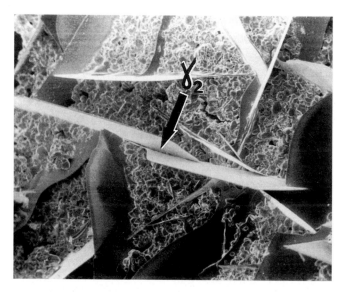

Fig. 6-21. SEM view of Sn-Hg (γ_2) crystals that occur in matrix of set low-copper dental amalgams. (Note blade-like crystals that penetrate amalgam and touch each other to create continuous matrix.)

and *electrochemical corrosion* (Fig. 6-22). Chemical corrosion occurs most notably on the occlusal surface and produces a black Ag-S tarnish film. This reaction is limited to the surface and does not compromise any properties, except for esthetics. Those amalgams with very high levels of copper also are capable of producing a copper oxide patina, but that is relatively uncommon. Electrochemical corrosion is an important mechanism of amalgam corrosion and has the potential to occur virtually anywhere on or within a set dental amalgam. Electrochemical corrosion occurs whenever chemically different sites act as an anode and cathode (see Chemical Properties). This requires that the sites be connected by an electrical circuit in the presence of an electrolyte,

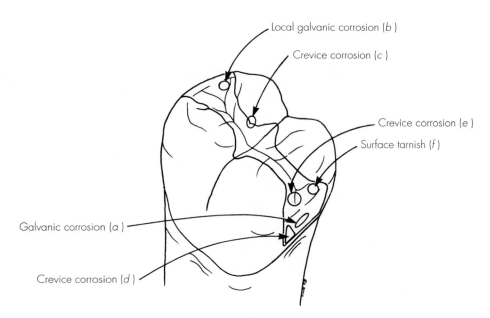

Local galvanic corrosion (b)

Crevice corrosion (c)

Crevice corrosion (e)

Surface tarnish (f)

Galvanic corrosion (a)

Crevice corrosion (d)

Fig. 6-22. Examples of sites susceptible to electrochemical and chemical corrosion on dental amalgams. Galvanic corrosion *(a)* at interproximal contact with metallic restoration such as gold casting alloy. Local galvanic *(b)* corrosion on occlusal surface at grain boundaries between different metallic phases. Crevice corrosion *(c)* at margin due to lower pH and oxygen concentration of saliva. Crevice corrosion *(d)* under retained interproximal plaque due to lower local pH. Crevice corrosion *(e)* within unpolished scratches or detailed secondary anatomy. Chemical corrosion *(f)* of occlusal surface with sulfide ions in saliva producing surface tarnish.

typically saliva. The anode corrodes, producing soluble and insoluble reaction products.

If a dental amalgam is in direct contact with an adjacent metallic restoration such as a gold crown, the dental amalgam is the anode in the circuit. This type of electrochemical corrosion is called **galvanic corrosion** and is associated with the presence of macroscopically different electrode sites. *The same process may occur microscopically* **(local galvanic corrosion or structure selective corrosion)** *due to the electrochemical differences of different phases.* Residual dental amalgam alloy particles act as the strongest cathodes. Sn-Hg or Cu-Sn reaction product phases are the strongest anodes in low-copper and high-copper dental amalgams, respectively. Local electrochemical cells may also arise whenever a portion of the amalgam is covered by plaque or soft tissue. The covered area has a locally lowered oxygen and/or higher hydrogen ion concentration, making it behave more anodically and corrode. Cracks and crevices produce similar conditions and preferentially corrode (concentration cell corrosion or **crevice corrosion**). Regions within a dental amalgam that are under stress also display a greater propensity for corrosion **(stress corrosion)**.

For an occlusal dental amalgam, *the greatest combination of corrosion and mechanical stresses occurs along margins.* Therefore, most visible changes are associated with margins. These are discussed subsequently in detail.

During electrochemical corrosion of low-copper dental amalgams, the Sn-Hg phase is oxidized to Sn-O and/or Sn-O-Cl.[91,92] The oxychloride species is soluble. The oxide precipitates as crystals and tends to fill up the spaces occupied by the original Sn-Hg phase. Along the margins of the amalgam, Sn-O helps to seal the space against microleakage (Fig. 6-23). Dental amalgam has a linear coefficient of thermal expansion that is 2.5 times greater than tooth structure, and it has not been bonded to tooth structure (until recently with the increasing use of amalgam bonding agents). Therefore, during expansion and contraction, percolation could otherwise occur along the external walls (see Fig. 6-1) if corrosion products did not impede fluid flow.

Electrochemical corrosion of Sn-Hg does not release free mercury into the oral environment. Rather, mercury immediately reacts with locally available Ag and Sn from residual amalgam alloy particles and is re-consumed to form more reaction products. Electrochemical corrosion of Cu-Sn in high-copper amalgams produces both copper and tin oxides and oxychlorides, but no mercury is involved in the process. *Electrochemical corrosion is not a mechanism of mercury liberation from set dental amalgams!*

Principal mechanical properties of dental amalgam are reported in Table 6-4 and include values for compressive strength, tensile strength, and creep. The compressive strengths of high-copper dental amalgams are greater than those of low-copper amalgams due to the

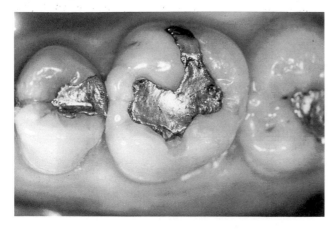

Fig. 6-26. Occlusal dental amalgam restoration with extensive marginal deterioration (Courtesy AD Wilder, School of Dentistry, University of North Carolina, Chapel Hill, NC).

that is below (No. 1), intermediate (No. 3, No. 5, No. 7, and No. 9), or greater (No. 11) than the main scale images.

Unfortunately, the impression of extensive (progressive) marginal fracture (to Mahler values of 6-11) for low-copper amalgams has been translated as a reason to clinically intervene and replace high-copper amalgams. High-copper dental amalgams also undergo marginal fracture. However, despite early ditching, they do not progress to levels of extensive ditching that would place them at high risk for secondary caries. Instead, *high-copper dental amalgams display only modest marginal fracture (Mahler values of 3-5) over long periods of time*. There is excellent clinical research evidence that substantiates clinical half-lives for well-placed high-copper dental amalgam restorations of 24 to 25 years (which will be addressed later in Clinical Considerations).

High-copper dental amalgams which are left in place

may eventually fail due to bulk fracture. It is hypothesized that such bulk fracture is the result of *mechanical fatigue*. A rule-of-thumb for clinical service is that occlusal restorations are stressed an average of 1 million times per year. A 25-year service life would correspond to 25 million cycles of mechanical stress. Typically, materials fail in the 10 to 100 million cycle range during laboratory testing. The events contributing to mechanical fatigue affect both the restoration and the tooth structure. The stresses and strains in both must be considered together, particularly in the case of restorations bonded to tooth structure.

Mercury management. Like all other materials in the world, *mercury* (Hg) has the potential to be hazardous if not managed properly. Therefore, it is very important that the alloying reaction of mercury with the Ag-Sn alloy go to completion to ensure that mercury does not diffuse into the oral environment. *Once the reaction is complete, only extremely minute levels of mercury can be released and those are far below the current health standard.* Mercury is ubiquitous in the environment and is taken into the body in one form or another via water, air, and food on a daily basis.

The contribution of mercury derived from dental amalgam to the overall body burden has been the source of much controversy but appears to be relatively low. The important perspective is that mercury enters the body everyday no matter what restorative filling materials are present in the mouth. Under normal circumstances, that mercury is biochemically processed and excreted. As long as the levels are low, there is no threat for mercury toxicity. Although poorly understood, *mercury hypersensitivity* has also at times been claimed as a potential hazard. This is an immune system response to very low levels of mercury. However, the number of individuals identified as potentially hypersensitive is extremely low, and the sensitivity reac-

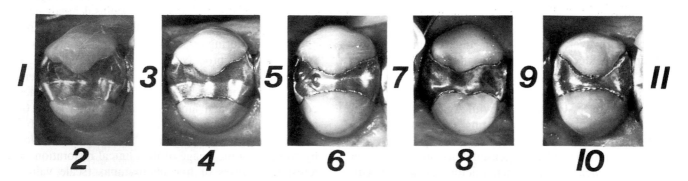

Fig. 6-27. Mahler scale showing levels of marginal deterioration (No. 1 = none; No. 11 = extensive). The numbers on scale indicate ratings assigned to restoration's appearance based on comparison to scale. (Courtesy DB Mahler, School of Dentistry, Oregon Health Sciences Center, Portland OR).

tion is very mild. It is not life-threatening. Mackert[84,85] and Mandel[90] have reviewed these issues in detail and scientifically refuted the hypothesized problems.

Early claims of mercury problems appeared as soon as dental amalgams were first used in the United States. The original amalgamation process was demonstrated by a chemist in France.[27] In 1833 two English entrepreneurs, the Crawcour brothers, realized the practical importance for dentistry, carried the idea to New York, and promoted the material as an inexpensive and convenient restoration.[99] However, there was no attention to the proper mercury-alloy ratios or the type of alloy being used. For the most part, the alloy mixed with the mercury was prepared by filing silver coins whose composition was considerably variable. In many cases, the inconsistency in materials and techniques led to slow-setting amalgams that released mercury from the unset mass into unprotected dentinal tubules. Although there are no reported cases of patient deaths, there were several cases of pulp death.

A complex battle ensued *(the so-called First Amalgam War)* between dentists using traditional restorative techniques based on gold foil and those using amalgam. The dispute was based on philosophical choices as to dental standards and differences in points of view about the safety of dental amalgam. Periodically, there were calls for eliminating dental amalgam use because of potentially harmful mercury release. In the 1920s another series of challenges to dental amalgam use occurred when there were inferences that mercury was not tightly bound in dental amalgams.[150] The next serious controversy arose in 1980 when Dr. Hal Huggins publicly condemned dental amalgam. Dr. Huggins, a practicing dentist in Colorado, was convinced that mercury released from dental amalgam was responsible for a plethora of human diseases affecting the cardiovascular and nervous systems. Patients claimed recoveries from multiple sclerosis, Alzheimer's disease, and other afflictions as a result of removing their dental amalgam fillings. For almost a decade, a loyal following of patients and dentists expanded the call to ban dental amalgam. Research in the United States and other first world countries has since demonstrated clearly that there was no basis for any of these claims.

In 1991, the general American public was widely exposed to the controversy when it was reported by a major television program *(60 Minutes)*. In response to numerous public questions, the profession, the National Institute of Health-National Institute for Dental Research (NIH-NIDR), the Food and Drug Administration (FDA), and several other groups held forums involving world-famous scientists and clinicians to reexamine the issue. Although these experts agreed dental amalgam research was needed and should continue, they concluded that there was *no basis for claims that dental amalgam was a signif-*

icant health hazard.[109] They strictly recommended that dental amalgams not be removed for that reason. However, the controversy is far from being resolved. There continue to be claims of hazards published in both local papers and nonscientific journals, and occasionally as well in scientific journals.[55,158] However, all published research demonstrates clearly that there is no cause-and-effect relationship between dental amalgam restorations and other health problems. This controversy will probably never be resolved because there will always be a certain percentage of patients seeking a miracle cure for their problems. However, fears of dental amalgam are not a basis for amalgam removal.[115]

Understanding the issues related to dental amalgam use has been a challenging problem for dental patients. The issues are complex and dealing with them requires some knowledge of physical chemistry and biochemical processes. It is not realistic to think that a general dentist has the time to effectively communicate this information. In addition, most dentists are perceived by patients as having a vested interest in the decision to use dental amalgam. Yet, clearly the public wants to know. Fortunately, very clear and concise reviews of the controversy have been published by reputable consumer affairs groups (Fig. 6-28).[95] *Reprints of these reviews*

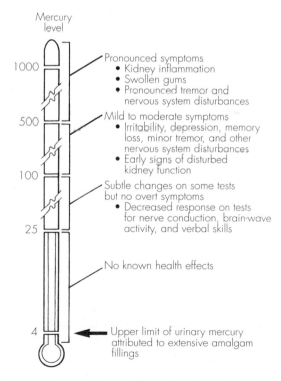

Fig. 6-28. Mercury thermometer portraying different levels of mercury toxicity. Chronic exposure can be assessed by urinary mercury concentration (as micrograms of mercury per gram of creatinine. (Courtesy *Consumer Reports,* pp 316-319, May 1991.)

have provided the best means of patient education.

The health risk from dental amalgam use is clearly greater for members of the dental office team than for a patient. Historically a major, though rare, source of mercury contamination in dental offices was the accidental spillage of quantities of liquid mercury. Mercury was commonly purchased in bottles containing a pound or more. This was then transferred to dispensers and eventually to individual capsules for mixing. Mishandling at any stage could result in mercury splashing on the bench or floor and being widely scattered as small droplets. Fortunately the current use of pre-capsulated amalgam has eliminated most opportunities for a major spill, but care must be maintained to avoid hazards in routine use of amalgam. Careful review of dental amalgam handling procedures reveals that the critical times are when metallic mercury exists in liquid or vapor form, rather than bound in a set dental amalgam. *As a vapor, metallic mercury can be inhaled and absorbed through the alveoli in the lungs at 80% efficiency.* This is clearly the major route of entry into the human body. Metallic mercury is poorly absorbed through the skin or via the gastrointestinal tract. A summary of absorption routes is presented in Table 6-5.

In addition to metallic mercury, both inorganic and organic mercury compounds are potentially toxic. Mercury is normally mined as an inorganic sulfide (cinnabar) ore which is heated in air to oxidize and drive off the sulfur.[126] The mercury is then collected as a liquid. *Mercury can exist in a wide variety of **inorganic compounds*** in addition to the sulfide. Many of them are water-soluble and release mercury ions into solution. Some of these compounds have been used in the past as medicaments. Such materials are poorly absorbed through the lungs but are easily absorbed in the gastrointestinal tract.

Mercury can also form organic compounds such as methyl mercury. Such mercury compounds are readily absorbed by many organisms and concentrated as they are passed up the food chain. *The concentration of naturally derived mercury in food is at times aggravated by the use of fungicides and pesticides containing methyl mercury. For most people **organically bound mercury** in food is the primary source of mercury exposure.* Humans absorb methyl mercury from food readily but excrete it less effectively than other forms of mercury. Once absorbed it has a tendency to concentrate in certain organs such as the liver, kidney, and brain. It is eventually all excreted, but the rate is dependent upon the body's ability to convert it to other forms.

It has been suggested that metallic mercury can be changed into methyl mercury by microorganisms in either the mouth or gastrointestinal tract. However, careful examination of blood mercury concentrations indicates that no biotransformation seems to occur.[26]

In the dental office, the sources of mercury exposure related to dental amalgam include (1) dental amalgam raw materials being stored for use (usually as pre-capsulated packages), (2) mixed but unhardened dental amalgam during trituration, insertion, and intraoral setting, (3) dental amalgam scrap that has insufficient alloy to completely consume the mercury present, (4) dental amalgam undergoing finishing and polishing operations, and (5) dental amalgam restorations being removed. Each of these is more carefully reviewed in the following paragraphs. Specific recommendations by the American Dental Association[4] are summarized in Box 6-1.

It is difficult if not impossible to totally contain liquid or gaseous mercury because it is very mobile, has a high diffusion rate, and penetrates through extremely fine spaces. Even in packages that include plastic blister wrapping and layers of cardboard, mercury vapor leakage is possible. Therefore, mercury-containing products should not be stored in the open, but rather in closets or cabinets, to minimize local concentrations in the rest of the offices. *Storage locations should be near a vent that exhausts air out of the building.*

*During dental **amalgam trituration,** small amounts of material may escape from capsules.* Both reusable capsules and pre-capsulated designs have some leakage. Small local spills or spatters of triturated materials are best dealt with by collection with a vacuum aspirator (not a vacuum cleaner). During trituration, the high frequency of agitation can force some mercury-rich material out of the capsule and create both an aerosol of liquid droplets and a vapor that may extend 6 to 12 feet away from the triturator. To minimize this risk, small covers are mounted on mechanical triturators to contain the aerosol to the region of the triturator. This does not eliminate the hazard. These materials persist as air contaminants or as particles which may drop onto the floor and contaminate carpeting or cracks between tiles. *Air contamination is managed by ensuring that air flow is reasonably high and that fresh air is brought into the office in a path from the waiting room, through the outer office, and then into the operatories, before being expelled to the outside of the building without contaminating other building areas.*

Once small droplets of mercury-rich material contaminate the *floor coverings,* the only practical approach to decontaminating the area is to replace those cover-

Table 6-5. Absorption efficiencies for different forms of mercury

	Skin	Lungs	Gastrointestinal tract
Elemental	—	80%	0.01%
Inorganic	—	80%	7%
Organic	—	—	95%-98%

No information is reported for some routes because the values are suspected to be very low and are not yet well-established.[162]

ings. *There is no effective treatment for removing liquid mercury from carpeting.* Mercury will react with sulfur to form a stable sulfide *(cinnabar)* but the reaction is slow and inefficient. Therefore, sprinkling sulfur powder onto sites of mercury spills will not adequately control the problem.

Box 6-1. Dental mercury hygiene recommendations

1. SYMPTOMS: Know the potential hazards and symptoms of mercury exposure such as the development of sensitivity and neuropathy.
2. HAZARDS: Know the potential sources of mercury vapor such as: (a) spills, (b) leaky dispensers or capsules, (c) polishing amalgams, (d) removing amalgams, and (e) heating of amalgam-contaminated instruments.
3. VENTILATION: Provide proper ventilation in the workplace by having fresh air exchanges and periodic replacement of filters which may act as traps for mercury.
4. MONITOR OFFICE: Monitor the mercury vapor level in the office periodically. (This may be done by using dosimeter badges.) The current OSHA limit for mercury vapor is 50 microgram/cubic meter (time weighted average) in any 8-hour work shift over a 40-hour work week.
5. MONITOR PERSONNEL: Monitor office personnel by periodic analysis. (The average mercury level in urine is 6.1 µg/liter for dental office personnel.)
6. OFFICE DESIGN: Use proper work area design to facilitate spill containment and cleanup.
7. PRECAPSULATED ALLOYS: Use precapsulated alloys to eliminate the possibility of a bulk mercury spill. Otherwise store bulk mercury properly in unbreakable containers on stable surfaces.
8. AMALGAMATOR COVER: Use an amalgamator fitted with a cover.
9. HANDLING CARE: Use care in handling amalgam. Avoid skin contact with mercury or freshly mixed amalgam.
10. EVACUATION SYSTEMS: Use high-volume evacuation when finishing or removing amalgam. Evacuation systems should have traps or filters. Check, clean, or replace traps and filters periodically.
11. MASKS: Change mask as necessary when removing amalgam restorations. (The mask will trap airborne particles and may discourage vapor transport but will not stop vapor passage.)
12. RECYCLING: Store amalgam scrap under radiographic fixer solution in a covered container. Recycle amalgam scraps through refiners who are properly licensed by the EPA. Find out how long the company has been in business and what are its assets.
13. CONTAMINATED ITEMS: Dispose of mercury-contaminated items in sealed bags according to applicable regulations.
14. SPILLS: Clean up spilled mercury properly by using trap bottles, tapes, or fresh mixes of amalgam to pick-up droplets; or use commercial cleanup kits. Do not use household vacuum cleaner.
15. CLOTHING: Wear professional clothing only in the dental operatory.

Quoted in part from American Dental Association CDMIE: *J Am Dent Assoc* 122(9):112, 1991.

During insertion of dental amalgam into cavity preparations, the mixture is not yet fully reacted and the *high vapor pressure of mercury* causes contamination of the air above the material. While the unhardened material sits in a Dappen dish for loading an amalgam carrier, some vapor is released. This should be cleared by the air flow system for the room. During the intraoral placement and condensation procedures some mercury vapor is released. To control the vapor, a *rubber dam* should be used to isolate the patient and *high-volume evacuation* should be used to prevent intraoral vapor from diffusing. After initial setting, the material has hardened to a solid and the vapor pressure drops several orders of magnitude.

Scrap dental amalgam from condensation procedures should be collected and stored under water, glycerine, or spent x-ray fixer in a tightly capped jar. The jar should be nearly filled with liquid to minimize the gas space where mercury vapor can collect. The unused dental amalgam will set but the mercury-rich material in the scrap does not have sufficient alloy present to become completely reacted. Spent x-ray fixer has an advantage for controlling mercury because it is a source of both silver and sulfide ions for reaction to a solid product. Periodically, this material should be recycled for profit for the office and to minimize the amount of material being stored. *No more than a small jar of material should be present in the office at any time.* Recycling mercury, silver, and other elements is a professional job. The only known case of human death related to mercury management was due to a misinformed dental technician trying to distill mercury out of amalgam scrap in the basement of his home.

Once dental amalgam has solidified, the mercury is tightly bound. However, one of the reaction products, Ag_2Hg_3, has a very low melting point (127°C). *It can be easily liquefied during finishing or polishing procedures that generate heat* and then it has a much higher vapor pressure. This situation routinely arises when *amalgams are polished* by dentists or dental hygienists without using adequate cooling water and slow polishing. This process is very deceptive. *The Ag-Hg phase is melted producing a mercury-rich liquid phase that is easily smeared over the dental amalgam surface making it look bright and shiny.* The operator can misinterpret this appearance as a highly polished surface.

Melting of the Ag-Hg phase also occurs during *amalgam removal.* It is common where high-speed burs contact tooth structure for surface temperatures to increase a couple of hundred degrees centigrade.[70] This is well above the temperatures for melting the Ag-Hg phase and vaporizing mercury. *Rubber dam, high volume evacuation, and water cooling should be used to control this situation.*

Instruments which are used for inserting, finishing, polishing, or removing dental amalgam restorations do contain some amalgam material on their surfaces. During instrument sterilization techniques this material may be heated and can release mercury liquid or vapor. Therefore, it is advisable to properly isolate or specially vent the air from sterilization areas.

Historically, capsules and other contaminated surfaces have not been managed very well in the opera-*ory. **Spent capsules and mercury-contaminated cotton *lls or paper napkins** should not be thrown out with *gular trash.* They should be stored in a tightly capped *lastic container for separate disposal. In most loca-*cions, that material can be placed into a sanitary landfill but those regulations may change in the near future.

A summary of all of the potential mercury management problems is presented in Fig. 6-29. In addition to materials storage and materials recycling, there are routine cautions for exposure. By using a rubber dam and high-volume evacuation, the patient is well protected from even minor, transient exposure to mercury vapor. These cautions are easy to provide and effectively protect the dentist, assistant, and hygienist from the same vapor. *Mercury vapor which may escape into the room air is not removed by infection control masks.* Masks may catch particulate debris above 1 μm in size and catch droplets or sprays in the air, but they will not filter mercury vapor from the air. *Routine exposures can be monitored with* **exposure badges** *worn by individuals in the office.*[48]

In the dental office, the dentist, assistant, hygienist, and other staff are at more risk of mercury toxicity than patients because of their long-term contact with mercury vapor. American Dental Association (ADA) monitoring of mercury levels in dentists has shown that they are in safe ranges despite the fact that the levels are almost twice the national average for non-dentists. As a group, dentists actually show better-than-average survival rates. The inference is that if dentists are exposed and survive better than most individuals, then there does not seem to be any basis for the perceived problem.

Much of the confusion about mercury effects is related to inadequate understanding of **mercury processing by the human body.** Mercury that is absorbed into the circulatory system may be deposited in any tissue. Higher-than-average accumulations occur in the brain, liver, and kidneys. Mercury ions (Hg^{+2}) circulate readily in the blood but pass the membrane barriers of the brain and placenta only with difficulty. In contrast, nonionized mercury (Hg^0) is capable of crossing

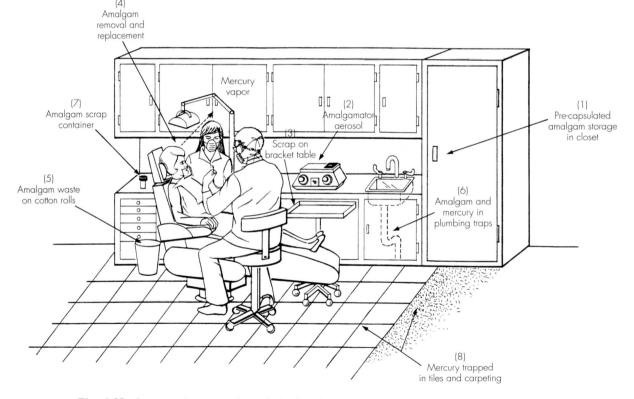

Fig. 6-29. Sources of mercury hazards in dental operatory include (1) some mercury vapor released from stored materials; (2) small losses from capsules during trituration; (3) spillage during manipulation for cavity restorations; (4) some vapor exposures to dentist, assistant, and patient during removal, placement, or finishing and/or polishing of dental amalgam; (5) contamination of cotton rolls; (6) collection of debris via vacuum suction into plumbing system and sewer system; (7) collection of remnants in jar for recycling; and (8) mercury that is trapped in small cracks between floor tiles and/or in carpet fibers.

through lipid layers at these barriers and, if subsequently oxidized within these tissues, is only slowly removed. This fact has become the basis for many claims of neuromuscular problems in patients with dental amalgams. However, this mercury is not uniquely from dental amalgam, the levels are low, and removing dental amalgam restorations does not eliminate exposure to mercury. Mercury does not collect irreversibly in human tissues. There is an *average half-life of 55 days for transport through the body to the point of excretion.* *Thus, mercury that came into the body years ago, is no longer present in the body.*

There are a variety of events which mitigate the conversion of mercury into ions and affect the conversion of the ions to other compounds. For example, ethyl alcohol is known to interrupt some of the biochemical steps required for blood-brain transport, thereby facilitating its rapid excretion.

The placental barrier is less effective than the blood-brain barrier, and some mercury ions are capable of placental transfer, as is about anything else in the circulatory system. Fetal mercury contents, while elevated, are lower than brain concentrations in the mother. *Effects on fetal development* are not fully known. All of the contemporary evidence from surveys and post-hoc surveys indicates that *female dentists, assistants, and hygienists who are pregnant are at no higher risk to miscarriage or fetal mis-development.* Even so, it seems to be judicious to minimize any exposure of these individuals to any potential hazard such as mercury during pregnancy.

In philosophical terms, the threat that may some day eliminate dental amalgam use as a restorative material is not a question of human toxicity, but rather of environmental protection.[12] It is now well known that improper disposal of contaminated waste greatly affects the environment. There are federal regulations to control large-scale industries which pollute. However, there has not yet been a focus on small-scale polluters, which could include local hospitals and dental offices. Although the relative contributions are small, the local community problems may mandate that *either dental offices control all mercury effluent or cease using dental amalgam.*

This important consideration, combined with evidence that (1) current dental amalgams last 3 to 5 times longer than low-copper dental amalgams, (2) dental caries rates are lower due to fluoridation effects, and (3) anterior restorations are now exclusively made from tooth-colored materials, has resulted in a *dramatic reduction overall in dental amalgam use.* Recent ADA surveys indicate that dental amalgam use decreased 45% from 1979 to 1990 alone.[108] If this trend continues, the amount of dental amalgam used for new restorations by the year 2010 may be almost insignificant. This pattern, however, does not eliminate the *profes-sion's problem of mercury containment during dental amalgam removal.*

Clinical considerations. Clinical longevity is a primary concern for selecting any restorative dental material. *Clinical longevity is the median age for a "group" of related or similar restorations at which 50% of the restorations have been replaced due to clinical failure.* Clinical longevity is determined by monitoring many restorations for clinical failure over a long period of time (longitudinal clinical research study) or by collecting information on random failures over a short period of time (cross-sectional clinical study).

Clinical failure is the point at which the restoration is no longer serviceable or at which time the restoration poses other severe risks if it is not replaced. Amalgam restoration-related failures include (1) *bulk fracture of the restoration* per se, (2) *corrosion and excessive marginal fracture,* (3) *sensitivity or pain,* (4) *secondary caries,* and (5) *fracture of tooth structure* forming the restorative cavity preparation wall(s). The incidence of different failure modes depends on a large number of factors. Restorations in caries-prone individuals may fail more often due to *secondary caries.* Restorations in caries-free individuals generally survive much longer, to the point that either fatigue may result in *bulk fracture of the restoration* or that *remaining tooth structure fractures* from masticatory force because the resistance form of the cavity preparation is inadequate.

In many cases, amalgam restorations are not permitted to reach the point of clinical failure. They are replaced before that time in anticipation of failure *(clinical replacement).* An example would be the replacement of a functionally sound restoration because of unacceptable esthetics. *Therefore, the clinical failure time is often longer than the clinical replacement time* (Fig. 6-30).[8] For any single restoration, clinical failure or replacement may be shorter or longer than the clinical longevity value describing a group of restorations.

Failure or replacement times may vary from a few months to as many as 45 to 50 years. This distribution is typified by the curve in Fig. 6-31. This average has been designated the CL_{50} (clinical longevity for 50% of the restorations) value.[19]

Many clinical failures of dental amalgam restorations occur because of some combination of electrochemical corrosion and mechanical stress. The combination produces *continual marginal breakdown* that creates conditions for more frequent failure due to secondary dental caries. In anticipation of this failure, amalgams with advanced marginal breakdown are often replaced. The average replacement age of conventional (low-copper) amalgams in clinical practice is in the range of 5 to 8 years (Table 6-6). *There is much less corrosion and marginal fracture in high-copper dental amalgams.* They more commonly fail due to *bulk fracture,* presum-

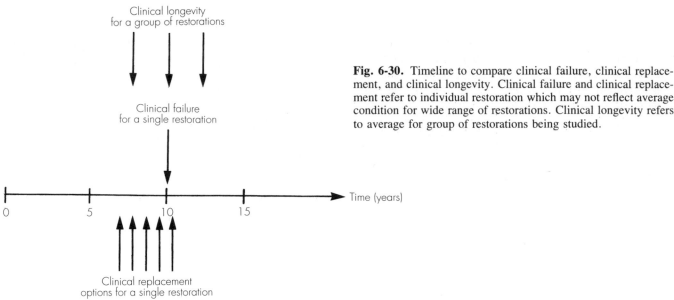

Fig. 6-30. Timeline to compare clinical failure, clinical replacement, and clinical longevity. Clinical failure and clinical replacement refer to individual restoration which may not reflect average condition for wide range of restorations. Clinical longevity refers to average for group of restorations being studied.

Fig. 6-31. Distribution of clinical failures of dental restorations. (Courtesy SC Bayne, School of Dentistry, University of North Carolina, Chapel Hill, NC.)

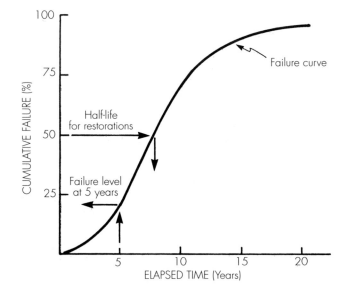

Table 6-6. Lifetimes reported for dental amalgams in use in general clinical practices*

Citation, year	Study type	Amalgam type	Restorations	Survival level	50% Longevity
Robinson, 1971	(Cross-sectional)	Low copper	145	25% at 20 yrs	10 yr
Allan, 1977	(Cross-sectional)	Low copper	241	10% at 15-20 yr	5-8 yr
Crabb, 1981	(Cross-sectional)	(Low copper)	1081		7-8 yr
Elderton, 1983	(Cross-sectional)	(Low copper)	1206	52% at 4.5 yr	
Patterson, 1984	(Cross-sectional)	(Low copper)	2344		7.5 yr
Bentley and Drake, 1986	(Longitudinal)	(Low and high copper)	433	71%-92% at 10 yr	
Mjor, 1981	(Cross-sectional)	Low and high copper	3527	40% at >10 yr	
Smales, 1991	Longitudinal	Low and high copper	1042	>70% at 10 yr	
Smales et al., 1991	Longitudinal	Low and high copper	1801	75% at 10.9 yr	
Smales et al., 1992	Longitudinal	Low and high copper	1813	70% at 20 yr	20-24 yr (est.)
Dawson and Smales, 1992	(Longitudinal)	Low and high copper	1345	75% at 6.6 yr	14.4 yr
Letzel et al., 1982	Longitudinal	Low and high copper	360	73.6% at 7 yr	
Letzel et al., 1990	Longitudinal	High copper		83%-91% at 10 yr	24 yr (est.)

*Parentheses indicate that information not stated definitively in reference.

ably related to fatigue. In recent years there has been mounting evidence that high-copper dental amalgams, regardless of initial compositional differences, have a CL_{50} of 24 to 25 years. High-copper dental amalgams not containing zinc do not last quite as long.

There is normally very little early failure of amalgams, but when it does occur it is related to either bulk fracture, improper design factors, or postoperative sensitivity. Conventional dental amalgams have very low tensile strength at first due to slow overall reaction. Therefore, they must be protected from high stresses during the first few hours after placement. Spherical high-copper dental amalgams develop strength more rapidly and are relatively immune to early fracture from loading. However, if the final dental amalgam does not have adequate depth and/or width at the narrowest portion of its bulk, then it is possible for intraoral loads to produce high resolved stresses causing fracture in the isthmus of the restoration. This is true of all amalgams.

During setting, most amalgams undergo very little dimensional change. Improperly manipulated and/or improperly condensed amalgams, however, might undergo increased expansion. This could produce stresses on tooth structure and create unusual postoperative sensitivity or pain. However, it should not be confused with slight sensitivity due to the fact that a dental amalgam is a metallic restoration that may conduct heat or become electrochemically coupled and produce a minor current that may induce pulpal sensitivity for a few hours. After that time, corrosion products eliminate the problem. Until initial corrosion occurs, some oral fluid penetration may occur along the walls of the cavity preparation. If the dentin is not adequately sealed with a solution liner or bonding agent, then fluid flow in the tubules may be induced and sensitivity could result. This should not occur with adequately sealed dentin surfaces. The normal resolution of the problem of persistent sensitivity is replacement of the restoration.

There are occasional reports of high incidences of dental amalgam sensitivity with some spherical alloys, but there is no careful documentation of any cause and effect. Complaints arise only sporadically and are certainly not universal. No investigation has been able to identify the causes or solutions to this problem. The prevalence of this type of sensitivity is presumed to be very low.

External surfaces on dental amalgams should be relatively smooth. This discourages the formation of crevice sites for electrochemical corrosion or for stress concentration during mechanical loading. The rule-of-thumb for carving a dental amalgam is to produce only surfaces and grooves that can be made smooth. Detailed secondary tooth anatomy, which can be carved into amalgam surfaces, is usually more of a liability to longevity than an esthetic advantage.

For many years there has been concern over the smoothness of the restoration surface as a means of reducing corrosion sites. Until 1985, it was standard procedure to wait for more than 24 hours and then to polish the dental amalgam at a subsequent visit. *Polishing has been replaced by burnishing the surface at the time of placement* (see Chapter 12) and only polishing surfaces on amalgams later that were not smooth when inspected. Clinical studies have shown no detectable clinical advantage for polished restorations compared with initially smooth restorations.[29,78]

Dental amalgam repair is possible to a limited extent. If secondary caries or fracture involves only a portion of an amalgam restoration, it is possible to leave the unaffected portion and prepare a cavity preparation that includes the old restoration as one of its external walls. Differences in dental amalgam compositions and corrosion behaviors will contribute to corrosion, but the effect appears to be insignificant.

At sites in which there is inadequate support for remaining tooth structure, amalgam bonding systems have been proposed to provide retention and strengthen weak tooth structure. These procedures are inadequate for stress distribution except in situations with the lowest stresses and should be considered as only temporary measures prior to more conventional restorative procedures. Cuspal elements that have been significantly weakened by previous cavity preparation or caries should be protected from subsequent fracture by cusp capping procedures along with circumferential restoration design for bracing (see Chapters 13 and 19). However, amalgam bonding agents (see Bonding Systems) can be used to seal cavity preparations, bond new to old amalgam, and/or repair marginal defects.

Liners and bases

Introduction. Many restorative dental materials that provide excellent properties for the bulk of a dental restoration may not protect the dental pulp during setting or during cyclic thermal or mechanical stressing. ***Pulpal protection*** requires consideration of (1) *chemical protection*, (2) *electrical protection*, (3) *thermal protection*, (4) *pulpal medication*, and (5) *mechanical protection* (Fig. 6-32). These concerns become more important as the cavity preparation extends closer to the pulp. ***Liners*** and ***bases*** are materials placed between dentin and the restoration to provide pulpal protection. Protective needs for a restoration vary depending upon the extent and location of the preparation as well as the restorative material to be used. The characteristics of the liner or base selected are largely determined by the purposes it is expected to serve. Because they share similar objectives, liners and bases are not fully distinguishable in all cases, but some generalizations can be made.

Terminology and classification. *Liners* are relatively

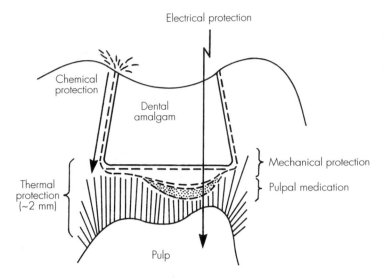

Fig. 6-32. Schematic view of needs for pulpal protection below metallic restoration. Varnishes, liners, and/or bases are added to cavity preparation under dental amalgam for purposes of chemical protection, electrical protection, thermal protection, mechanical protection, and/or pulpal medication. (Courtesy Bayne SC, Barton RE. In Richardson RE, Barton RE, editors: *The dental assistant,* ed 6, Philadelphia, 1988, Lea & Febiger.)

thin layers of material used primarily to provide a barrier to protect the dentin from residual reactants diffusing out of a restoration and/or oral fluids which may penetrate leaky tooth-restoration interfaces. They also contribute initial electrical insulation, generate some thermal protection, and, in some formulations, provide pulpal treatment as well (Fig. 6-33). The need for liners is greatest with metallic restorations that are not well-bonded to tooth structure and which are not

insulating, such as amalgam and cast gold, or with other indirect restorations. Direct composite restorations, indirect composite or ceramic restorations, and resin-modified glass ionomer restorations routinely are bonded to tooth structure. *The insulating nature of these tooth-colored materials and the sealing effects of the bonding agents preclude the need for traditional liners and bases unless the cavity preparation is extremely close to the pulp and pulpal medication becomes a concern.* This situation is described in more depth later in discussions of bonding agents (see Bonding Agents). Thin film liners (1 to 50 μm) can be divided into *solution liners* (varnishes, 2 to 5 μm) and *suspension liners* (typically 20 to 25 μm). Thicker liners (200 to 1000 μm = 0.2 to 1 mm), selected primarily for pulpal medication and thermal protection, are sometimes identified as *cement liners.*

Bases (cement bases, typically 1 to 2 mm), are used to provide thermal protection for the pulp and to supplement mechanical support for the restoration by distributing local stresses from the restoration across the underlying dentin surface. This mechanical support provides resistance against disruption of thin dentin over the pulp during amalgam condensation procedures or cementation procedures of indirect restorations. Metallic restorations should seat (rest) on sound dentin peripheral to the lined and/or based regions that result from excavating infected dentin (Fig. 6-33). Various liners and bases may be combined in a single preparation, and the total *cavity preparation base may be described as the combination of natural dentin, liner, and base.*

Objectives of pulpal protection. To understand the actions of these agents, it is extremely important to recall the anatomy and physiology of dentin that were

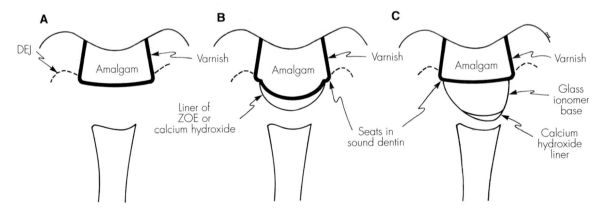

Fig. 6-33. Schematic examples of use of liners and bases for amalgam restorations. **A,** For shallow amalgam cavity preparations, varnish is applied to walls of preparation before insertion of restoration. **B,** For moderate depth cavity preparations, liners may be placed for thermal protection and pulpal medication. (Note seats in sound dentin for amalgam restoration.) **C,** In very deep preparation, light-cured calcium hydroxide in placed in deepest region in which infected dentin was excavated, and then base of glass ionomer is inserted. Amalgam bonding systems are being advocated as a substitute for liner and varnish, except for calcium hydroxide liner in the deepest region (judged to be within 0.5 mm of pulp).

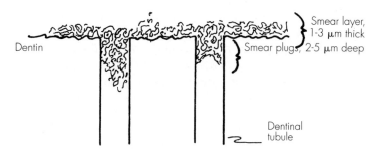

Fig. 6-34. Schematic view of dentin smear layer.

presented in Chapter 2. Normal coronal dentin includes dentinal tubules that contain cellular extensions (odontoblastic processes) of the cells (odontoblasts) which originally laid down dentin during dentinogenesis. These columnar cells remain as a layer along the periphery of the dental pulp, partially embedded in poorly mineralized dentin (pre-dentin), and with processes extending outward into dentinal tubules. The processes are surrounded by dentinal fluid when they do not contact the walls of the tubules. In response to mild, long-term chemical or mechanical insults, the processes slowly recede toward the pulp while occluding the tubules with peritubular dentin by depositing hydroxyapatite crystals (see Chapter 2). If the insult is strong and/or near to the pulp, the processes are retracted more rapidly from that region and a thin local bridge of hydroxyapatite is created across the affected tubules. Both of these are natural defense mechanisms to insulate the pulp from chemical, thermal, mechanical, or biological challenges.

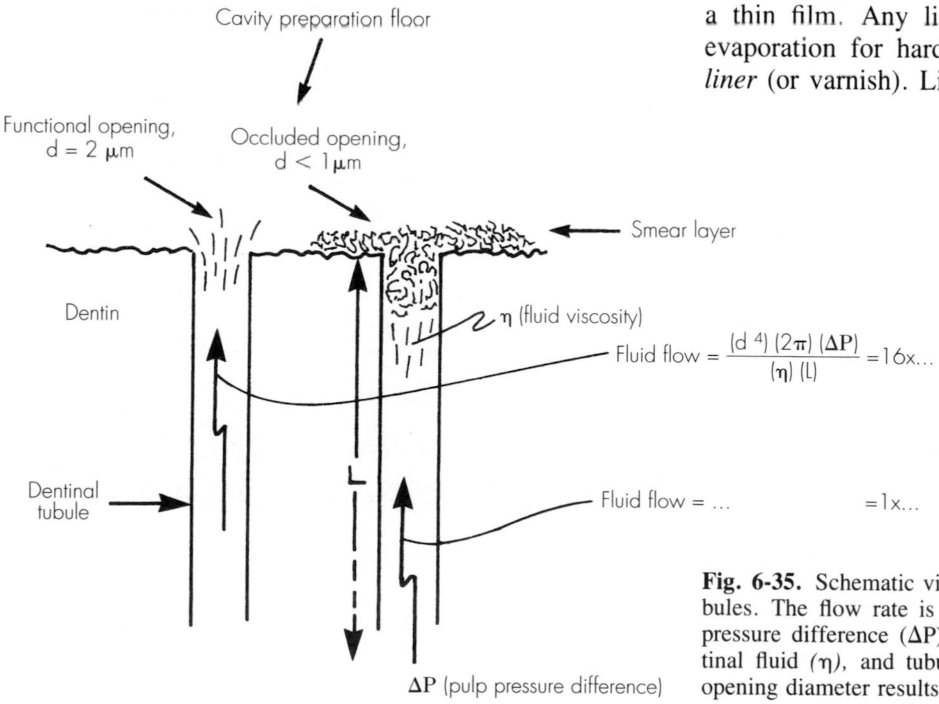

If the insult produces conditions allowing fluid flow in or out of the dentinal tubules, the pressure change is sensed by mechanoreceptors within the pulp, and the patient experiences sensitivity. If leakage of chemical irritants from dental materials or bacteria occurs, then the pulp complex can become inflamed. To protect against these events, it is paramount to seal the outer ends of the tubules along the dentinal cavity preparation wall.

Cavity preparation with rotary instruments generates cutting debris, some of which is compacted unavoidably into a layer on the cut surface. That layer of material is called a **smear layer** and is typical of any cut surface, dental or otherwise. Enamel and dentin smear layers are left in place for unbonded dental amalgam restorations. The dentin smear layer (Fig. 6-34) produces some degree of dentinal tubule sealing, although it is 25% to 30% porous. Flow or microleakage in or out of tubules is proportional to the fourth power of the diameter of the opening (Fig. 6-35). Halving the diameter of the opening produces a 16-fold reduction in flow. Therefore, the smear layer is a very effective barrier. However, because it is partially porous, it can not prevent slow long-term diffusion. Therefore, for dental amalgam restorations which can leak along their enamel margins, the smear layer should be sealed with an overlying layer of a *liner*. This produces chemical protection. *Dentin and amalgam bonding systems, which are discussed later in this chapter, can produce the same effect and are becoming substitutes for liners.*

To produce a very thin film liner, liner ingredients are dissolved in a volatile nonaqueous solvent. The solution is applied to tooth structure and dries to generate a thin film. Any liner based on nonaqueous solvent evaporation for hardening is designated as a *solution liner* (or varnish). Liners based on water have many of

Cavity preparation floor

Functional opening, d = 2 μm

Occluded opening, d < 1 μm

Smear layer

Dentin

η (fluid viscosity)

$$\text{Fluid flow} = \frac{(d^4)(2\pi)(\Delta P)}{(\eta)(L)} = 16x...$$

Dentinal tubule

Fluid flow = ...   = 1x...

ΔP (pulp pressure difference)

Fig. 6-35. Schematic view of fluid flow physics for dentinal tubules. The flow rate is function of tubule diameter *(d)*, pulpal pressure difference (ΔP) to ambient pressure, viscosity of dentinal fluid *(η)*, and tubule length *(L)*. A two-fold reduction in opening diameter results in 16-fold reduction in fluid flow.

the constituents suspended instead of dissolved and are called *suspension liners*. Liners that are intended to provide thermal protection as well need to be thicker in dimension.

Most varnish coatings are produced by drying solutions of copal or other resin dissolved in a volatile solvent. Copalite (H.J. Bosworth) has been used more widely than most other varnishes and contains 10% copal resin in a combination of ether, alcohol, and acetone. The resin content is kept intentionally low to produce a thin film on drying. Thin films work the best because they are flexible and dry rapidly. Thick films tend to trap solvent during rapid superficial drying and become brittle when they finally dry. Most solvent loss occurs in 8 to 10 seconds and does not require forced air assistance. A thin film of 2 to 5 μm is formed over smear layers along the cavity preparation wall. Because there is some moisture in the smear layer and varnishes are hydrophobic, the film does not wet the surfaces well. A single coat effectively covers only 55% of the surface (Fig. 6-36). *A second thin layer is recommended to produce sealing of 80% to 85% of the surface.*

Suspension liners can produce the same effect, but dry more slowly and produce thicker films. The typical film thickness is 20 to 25 microns in contrast to the 2 to 5 micron film produced by solution liners (varnishes). Both types of liner are often extended out over the cavosurface margins of the preparation. Excess material on external surfaces is not necessary but is difficult to avoid. It is easily abraded off. The primary purpose of the liners is to provide a protective seal on the exposed dentin surface. The liner layer at the restoration enamel interface also *provides a means of electrically isolating metallic restorations from external electrical circuits with restorations in adjacent teeth.* Otherwise amalgam restorations may produce small electrical currents during the first few days that cause patient pain or discomfort. This sensitivity rapidly disappears as electrochemical corrosion and/or tarnish modify the surfaces of the dental amalgam.

A key function of enamel and dentin is *thermal insulation of the pulp.* Most restorative materials are not as insulating as dentin and therefore thermal insults may occur during intraoral temperature changes. The need for insulation is greatest for metallic restorations. Thermal insulation is proportional to the thickness of the insulating materials. Ideally 2 mm of dentin or an equally insulating material should exist to protect the pulp (Fig. 6-32). This thickness is not always possible, but 1 to 1.5 mm of insulation is accepted as a practical thickness. As the cavity preparation extends closer to the pulp, a thick liner or a base is used to augment dentin to this thickness range. Such a liner or base cannot harden by evaporation of solvent or water because it would not

dry effectively. Material used for this purpose hardens by a chemical reaction or is light-cured.

In addition to thermal protection, *liners are formulated to provide pulpal medication whenever possible.* Two important aspects of pulpal medication are the relief of pulpal inflammation and facilitation of dentinal bridging for physiological protection. The materials which are most commonly used to provide these two functions are not compatible and cannot be used in the same formulation.

Eugenol is used to alleviate discomfort resulting from mild-to-moderate pulpal inflammation. Eugenol is a para-substituted phenolic compound that is slightly acidic and produces palliative or obtundent actions on the pulp when used in very low concentrations. High concentrations can be chemically irritating. Several eugenol-containing dental materials are based on the reaction of eugenol with zinc oxide (ZOE) to produce lin-

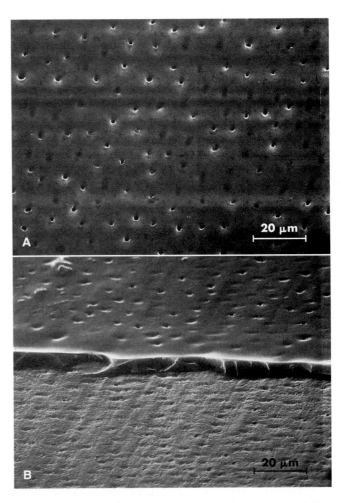

Fig. 6-36. Copalite varnish partially occluding dentinal tubules. **A,** SEM of one layer of Copalite varnish over smear layer that seals about 55% of the tubules. **B,** SEM of two layers of Copalite varnish adjacent to region protected only by smear layer. (SEM micrographs courtesy SC Bayne, School of Dentistry, University of North Carolina, Chapel Hill, NC.)

ers, bases, or cements. In the liner compositions, small amounts of eugenol are released during setting and over several days. For this reason, these liners have been widely used *in those sites where cavity preparations are moderately deep.*

In the deepest portions of the preparation or when a microscopic pulp exposure is suspected, it is more important to encourage dentinal bridging by using *calcium hydroxide* compositions. Calcium hydroxide in saturated solutions (suspensions) is extremely caustic (pH>11) but when ionized in low concentrations it stimulates the formation of reparative dentin. Traditionally *calcium hydroxide liners* are formulated to undergo a chemical setting reaction but do allow minor amounts of calcium hydroxide to be released from the liner surface to produce the desired effect. Calcium hydroxide liners generally are based on the reaction of calcium ions from calcium hydroxide particles with phenolic moieties on mono- or multi-functional molecules. There is excess calcium hydroxide in the composition, so that some is always available as a source of calcium and hydroxyl ions. Unfortunately these liners may become degraded to a great degree over long periods of time, to an extent that they no longer provide mechanical support for the overlying restoration.

Water is an important component for the chemical setting of both eugenol- and calcium-based liners. The setting reaction of ZOE is accelerated by moisture. Most formulations contain reaction modifiers to produce setting in a reliable way, but moisture does not interfere with the reaction. For calcium hydroxide–based liners, the setting reaction involves calcium ions. To start the reaction, some calcium hydroxide must be dissociated by moisture from air or from moist dental surfaces. If the site has been dried excessively, a moist cotton pledget may have to be introduced to make the liner set correctly.

Eugenol and calcium hydroxide cannot be incorporated into the same formulation because eugenol rapidly chelates calcium ions in a strongly exothermic reaction. Therefore, the choice of eugenol-based versus calcium hydroxide–based liners is connected to the relative depth of the cavity preparation.

New liners place less emphasis on pulpal medication and focus more on chemical protection by sealing, adhesion, and mechanical protection. Sealing may prove to be the most important property overall. As long as the compositions are based primarily on ceramic and/or polymer materials, they will provide excellent thermal insulation as well. These newer compositions rely on mechanically strong acrylic resin matrices that partially or totally replace traditional matrices. This choice makes the release of eugenol or calcium hydroxide ions from the composition much more difficult or impossible.

Historically, restorative materials bases have been generated by mixing dental cements at higher-than-normal powder-to-liquid ratios to increase the final compressive strength and reduce the concentration of potentially irritating liquids. (The thick mixes of some materials are sticky and at times lead to problems with adaptation and with control of the amount and contour of base material. For this reason the flow technique described in Chapter 19 was developed.)

Zinc phosphate cement and resin-reinforced ZOE cement were widely used for bases before the 1960s. Polycarboxylate cement gained popularity for this application starting in 1970. Glass ionomer cement has become more popular during the period from 1985 to 1994. Highly modified forms of glass ionomer cement (light-cured resin-modified glass ionomers) provide chemical adhesion, good mechanical strength, potential fluoride release, well-controlled setting, and rapid achievement of strength.

Before the development of modified glass ionomers, the functions of liners and bases were relatively distinct, but have since begun to converge. Previously, in a deep preparation, a calcium hydroxide liner would be placed first. Then a base would be added to provide mechanical support and stress distribution. The base would be covered with varnish at the same time the tooth structure walls were varnished (except that when using zinc phosphate cement the varnish would be applied prior to the cement), and the amalgam would be placed. Currently, light-cured calcium hydroxide and glass ionomer materials are being used to both line and base relatively deep preparations (see Fig. 6-33, *C*).

For indirect restorations, provisions must be made to prevent dislodgment of the base during impression taking or removal of a temporary restoration. Mechanical undercuts or bonding of the base material to prepared dentin are used depending on the type of base material (see Fig. 19-11).

Composition, structure, and properties. Representative examples of the composition, structure, and important properties of solution liners (varnishes), liners, and bases are reported in Tables 6-7, 6-8, and 6-9, respectively.

Clinical considerations. Clinical judgments about the need for specific liners and bases are linked to the amount of remaining dentin, considerations of adhesive materials, and the type of restorative material being used.

In a *shallow cavity preparation,* which includes 1.5 to 2 mm or more of remaining dentin, there is no need for pulpal protection other than in terms of chemical protection. For a dental amalgam restoration, the cavity is coated with two thin coats of a varnish and restored. For a composite restoration, the cavity is etched, primed, coated with a single coat of a bonding agent,

Table 6-7. Composition, structure, and properties of a typical solution liner (varnish).*

	Copal resin varnish (Copalite)
Components	
Solid	10% copal resin
Solvent	90% ether, acetone, alcohol
Setting reaction	Physical (by solvent evaporation)
Structure	
Arrangement	Amorphous film
Bonding	Covalently bonded organic material
Composition (phases)	Single phase
Defects	Pores and cracks
Physical properties	
Thermal	[Insulator]
Electrical	[Insulator]
LCTE (ppm/°C)	[High]
Wetting	[Poor on hydrophilic surfaces]
Chemical properties	
Solubility (% in water)	[Low]
Mechanical properties	
Tensile strength (MPa)	<<1
Elongation (%)	<<0.1% [Brittle]
Biological properties	
Toxicity	[None, if solvent eliminated safely]

*Relative properties are reported in brackets.

and then restored. Both the varnish for dental amalgams and the bonding system for dental composites provide chemical protection. To provide adhesion of amalgams to the surfaces of the cavity preparation, amalgam bonding systems are being substituted for cavity varnishes.

In a dental amalgam cavity preparation that includes *some extension of the preparation toward the pulp so that a region includes less-than-ideal dentin protection*, it is judicious to apply a liner only at that site of zinc oxide eugenol or calcium hydroxide. Either one will provide pulpal medication but the effects will be different. Zinc oxide–eugenol cement will release minor quantities of eugenol to act as an obtundent to the pulp. It will also provide thermal insulation. In a composite cavity preparation, *eugenol has the potential to inhibit polymerization* of layers of bonding agent or composite in contact with it. Therefore, calcium hydroxide is normally used. If the remaining dentin thickness is very small or if there is the potential problem of a pulp expo-

Table 6-8. Composition, structure, and properties of typical liners.*

	Calcium hydroxide (VLC Dycal)	Traditional glass ionomer (Fuji Lining LC)	Reinforced ZOE (IRM)
Components			
Components 1 and 2	Paste (with Ca(OH)₂; LC resin, and polyphenolics)	Powder (Al-silicate glass); liquid (polyalkenoate acid, LC resin)	Paste (with ZnO); paste (with Eugenol)
P/L or paste/paste ratio	(1 component)	1.4/1.0 by weight	6.0/1.0 by weight
Setting reaction	Acid-base reaction	Acid-base reaction	Acid-base reaction
Structure			
Arrangement	Amorphous matrix Crystalline fillers	Amorphous matrix Crystalline fillers	Crystalline matrix Crystalline fillers
Bonding	Covalent; ionic	Covalent; ionic	Covalent; ionic
Composition (phases)	Multiphase	Multiphase	Multiphase
Defects	Pores; cracks	Pores; cracks	Pores; cracks
Physical properties			
LCTE (ppm/°C)	[Low]	[Low]	[Low]
Thermal conductivity	[Insulator]	[Insulator]	[Insulator]
Electrical conductivity	[Insulator]	[Insulator]	[Insulator]
Radiopacity (mm Al)	—	4	—
Chemical properties			
Solubility (% in water)	0.3-0.5 [high]	0.08 [low]	[Modest]
Shrinkage on setting (μm/mm)	—	24 [low]	—
Mechanical properties			
Elastic modulus (MPa)	588	1820	—
Hardness (KHN₁₀₀)	—	—	—
Elongation (%)	—	—	—
Compressive strength, >24 hr (MPa)	138	128	71
Diametral tensile strength (MPa)	—	24	—
Flexural strength (MPa)	—	46	—
Shear bond strength to dentin (MPa)	—	5.8	—
Biological properties			
Biocompatibility	[Acceptable]	[Acceptable]	[Acceptable]

*Relative properties are shown in brackets. The values reported are from a variety of published sources from 1988-1993, including manufacturer's product bulletins. Comparisions should be made only in terms of the overall application requirements and not in terms of any single property.

Table 6-9. Composition, structure, and properties of typical bases*

	Zinc phosphate cement (Modern Tenacin)	Polycarboxylate cement (Durelon)	Glass ionomer cement (Ketac-Cem)
Components			
Component 1	ZnO powder	ZnO powder H_2O	F-Al-Si glass powder
Component 2	H_3PO_4/H_2O liquid	Polyacrylic acid/H_2O liquid	Polyacrylic acid/H_2O liquid
P/L ratio	[High]	[High]	[High]
Setting reaction	Acid-base reaction	Acid-base reaction	Acid-base reaction
Structure			
Arrangement	Crystalline matrix	Amorphous matrix	Amorphous matrix
	Crystalline fillers	Crystalline fillers	Crystalline fillers
Bonding	Ionic	Covalent; ionic	Covalent; ionic
Composition (phases)	Multiphase	Multiphase	Multiphase
Defects	Pores and cracks	Pores and cracks	Pores and cracks
Physical properties			
Thermal	[Insulator]	[Insulator]	[Insulator]
Electrical	[Insulator]	[Insulator]	[Insulator]
LCTE (ppm/°C)	[Low]	[Low]	10 [Low]
Chemical properties			
Solubility (% in water)	0.10 [Low]	[Low]	0.10 [Low]
Mechanical properties			
Modulus (MPa)	—	—	—
Hardness (KHN$_{100}$)	—	—	—
Percent elongation (%)	—	—	—
Compressive strength (MPa)	77	[100]	120
Diametral tensile strength (MPa)	—	[17]	—
Biological properties			
Safety	[Acceptable]	[Acceptable]	[Acceptable]

*Relative or estimated properties are shown in brackets.

sure, then calcium hydroxide is used to stimulate reparative dentin. A thickness of 0.5 to 1 mm of set calcium hydroxide liner is sufficient to treat a near or actual pulp exposure and provide adequate resistance for dental amalgam condensation forces. Under these circumstances, when a minimum thickness of material is protecting the pulp, a spherical dental amalgam is recommended for use because less condensation pressure is required. A solution liner (varnish) or dental amalgam bonding system is then applied before placing a final dental amalgam restoration. In the case of a dental composite procedure, a bonding system is applied.

If extensive dentin is lost during the caries process or the cavity preparation, then a dental cement base should be applied. If an adhesive cement base is chosen (i.e., polycarboxylate cement or glass ionomer cement) for amalgam or composite situations, then the adhesive base should be applied over the liner and tooth structure to permit chemical adhesion to occur. Varnish or bonding agent is not applied until after the base is in place.

In indirect restorative procedures requiring multiple appointments, a base must be placed with its own retentive features. This guarantees that it will not be displaced during impression procedures or during the removal of temporary restorations.

Survival of liners and bases below restorations has never been well understood. Even during restoration removal, it is difficult to completely remove the restorative materials and to assess the acceptability of the liners and bases. Solution liners (varnishes) are relatively brittle and thin and may only provide chemical protection for a matter of days to weeks. However, that should be sufficient for their purpose. Bonding agents may survive years. Liners and bases may be sufficiently intact to limit the extent of cavity re-preparation to the outline for the bulk restorative material. There are suspicions that traditional calcium hydroxide liners continue to dissolve and may lose 10% to 30% of their volume over 10 or more years.[128] Radiolucent lines are often observed in dental radiographs at the border of liners. Thus, liners may need to be replaced or augmented if such changes are obvious when the restoration is replaced. Long-term changes in both cement liners and cement bases are not well characterized.

Dental adhesion

Terminology. *Adhesion* is a process of solid and/or liquid interaction of one material (*adhesive* or *adherent*) with another (*adherend*) at a single interface.[25] Most instances of **dental adhesion** also are called **dental bonding.** Adhesive bond strength is evaluated by debonding the system.

Most situations involving dental adhesion really involve adhesive joints. An ***adhesive joint*** is the result of interactions of a layer of intermediate material ***(adhesive*** or ***adherent)*** with two surfaces ***(adherends)*** producing two adhesive interfaces (Fig. 6-37). Examples of the classification of different dental situations are presented in Fig. 6-38. A pit and fissure sealant bonded to etched enamel is a case of dental adhesion. An enamel bonding agent which bonds together etched enamel with dental composite is a classic dental adhesive joint.

Bond strength (or bond stress) is reported as the initial mechanical load to fracture divided by the simple, geometrically defined, cross-sectional area of the bond. In most cases, the true contact area between the materials involved may be much greater because of a mechan-

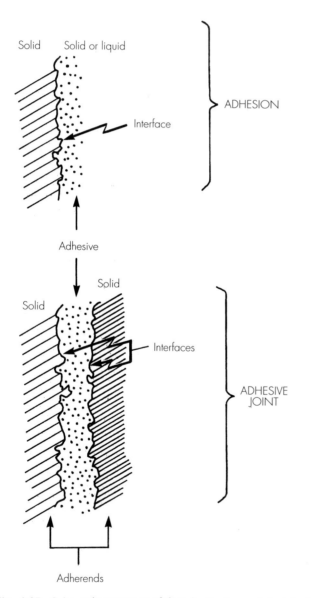

Fig. 6-37. Schematic summary of dental adhesion and dental adhesive joint.

ically rough interface. However, the roughness is not considered in the calculation. The type of bond strength test is categorized in terms of the initial mechanical loading direction, and not the resolved loading direction. Almost all bond strength tests are categorized as ***tensile*** or ***shear bond strengths.*** In a practical sense, most tensile bond strengths are only about half of the value of shear bond strengths. Any comparison of bond strengths should be in terms of equivalent testing conditions.[147]

Classification. The interactions which occur at the interface are classified generally in terms of types of atomic interactions which may be involved. Adhesion is classified as physical, chemical, and/or mechanical bonding. ***Physical bonding*** involves van der Waals or other electrostatic interactions that are relatively weak (Fig. 6-39). It may be the only type of bonding if surfaces are smooth and chemically dissimilar. ***Chemical bonding*** involves bonds between atoms formed across the interface from the adhesive to the adherend. Because the materials are often dissimilar, the extent to which this bonding is possible is limited and the overall contribution to bond strength is normally quite low. ***Mechanical bonding*** is the result of an interface that involves undercuts and other irregularities that produce interlocking of the materials. The microscopic degree to which this occurs dictates the magnitude of the bonding. Almost every case of *dental adhesion* is based primarily on mechanical bonding. Chemical bonding may occur as well, but generally makes only a small contribution to the overall bond strength.

The common method for producing surface roughness for better mechanical bonding is to grind or etch the surface. *Grinding produces gross mechanical roughness but leaves a **smear layer*** of hydroxyapatite crystals and denatured collagen that is approximately 1 to 3 microns thick. ***Acid etching or conditioning*** dissolves this layer and produces microscopic relief with undercuts on the surface to create an opportunity for mechanical bonding.[24] If the mechanical roughness produces microscopically interlocked adhesive and adherend with dimensions of less than about 10 microns, then the situation is described as ***micro-mechanical bonding (micro-mechanical retention or micro-retention).***

Requirements for adhesion. To develop good adhesion (good bonding) it is necessary to form a microscopically intimate interface. The adhesive must be able to approach the molecules of the substrate within a few nanometers. Forming the interface is described in terms of the adhesive ***wetting*** the adherend.

To produce good bonding, there must be good wetting. Wetting is a measure of the energy of interaction of the materials (see Fig. 6-4, *B*). Materials which interact significantly, producing chemical bonds and reducing their total energy, are said to wet one another. A

Fig. 6-38. Examples of classification of dental adhesion (**A** to **C**) and dental adhesive joints (**D** to **F**). **A,** Fissure sealant. **B,** Varnished wall of amalgam preparation. **C,** Surface sealer on composite restoration. **D,** Orthodontic bracket bonding resin. **E.** Enamel bonding system for a composite restoration. **F,** Bonded porcelain veneer.

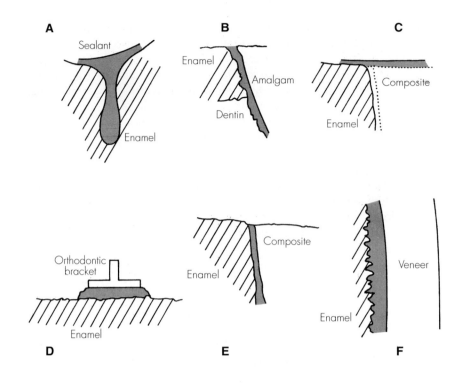

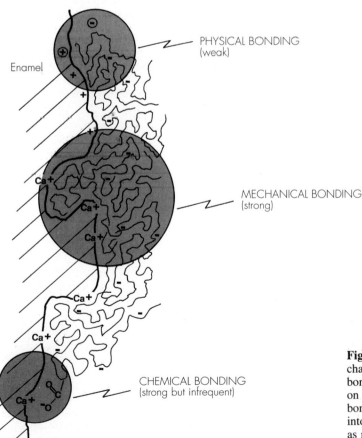

Fig. 6-39. Schematic summary of contribution of physical, mechanical, and chemical bonding to interfacial adhesion. Physical bonding occurs when negative and positive sites on polymer and on tooth structure are attracted electrostatically. Mechanical bonding occurs when bonding agent is mechanically interlocked into micro-undercuts on tooth surfaces. Chemical bonding occurs as reactive sites on polymer form primary bonds with surfaces of tooth structure.

liquid which wets a solid spreads readily onto the solid surface. If a state of complete wetting occurs, the contact angle approaches zero degrees.

A second requirement for adhesion is that the surfaces being joined are clean. Quite often this is a difficult situation to produce and maintain. Clean surfaces are at a high energy state and rapidly absorb contaminants from the air, such as moisture or dust. If contaminants are not excluded, then the adhesive interface will be weak. A standard process for cleaning any surface is the application of solvents or acids to dissolve or dislodge contaminants.

Bonding strengths. Most often the bond strengths of materials are measured by shearing the adhesive or adhesive joint to produce fracture. Bond strength is measured as a single cycle stress to fracture. In the clinical situation, however, fatigue may be much more important than single-cycle loading. Fatigue is too complex to be simulated in laboratory bond strength tests at the moment. The fracture strength that is measured depends on the path of the fracture. For an adhesive joint, such as composite bonded to dentin with a dentin bonding agent, the bulk materials' strengths control the fracture path. Dentin is stronger than composite, which is stronger than the dentin bonding agent. If the interfaces are well-bonded, then the fracture occurs within the dentin bonding agent or is driven into the adherends. If one or both of the interfaces is not well-bonded, then the fracture occurs along the weakest interface.

If the dentin bonding agent is chemically matched to the composite, it will be wet well by the composite, chemically intermix with it, and produce true chemical bonding that will create a very strong interface. Bond strengths for the interface of bonding systems with dentin depend on the degree to which wetting occurs. Cut dentin contains a smear layer, is moist, and is not necessarily micro-mechanically rough. Selective etching removes some or all of the smear layer, locally controls the wetness, and produces a micro-mechanically rough surface. However, dentin is still **hydrophilic** (water loving). Therefore, the dentin bonding agent must be designed to be hydrophilic. This quality produces a chemically intimate and micro-mechanically well-bonded interface. Most current dentin bonding systems are designed with conditioning, priming, and bonding steps to accomplish this end.

As the interfacial bond strengths of an adhesive joint become stronger, the bulk strength of the adhesive becomes the limiting factor to adhesive joint strength. One way of improving the bond strength is to decrease the adhesive thickness to the point that a fracture cannot propagate through it in a practical sense. If the adhesive is thin and/or tortuous in geometry, then any crack is constantly driven into one or the other adherends. Thus the joint begins to behave more like the simple adhesion

of the two materials on either side of the adhesive. This is the situation for the current dentin bonding agents. By impregnating a finely etched or conditioned dentin surface, the final thickness of the dentin bonding agent approaches 1 micron. Fractures are now diverted into dentin, and bond strengths of 25 to 40 MPa are recorded.

The problem for dentistry is that different situations require different chemical characteristics for an adhesive to produce good wetting and/or a thin film. Materials which are good dentin or enamel bonding agents are not necessarily good porcelain-bonded-to-metal repair bonding agents or amalgam bonding agents.

A number of dental adhesion or adhesive joint situations are tabulated in Table 6-10 with examples of bond strengths. These situations are described in the following paragraphs.

Bonding systems. In dentistry, the agents producing adhesive dental joints are referred to as bonding systems and classified on the basis of the primary adherend.

Enamel bonding systems. Enamel bonding systems most often consist of an unfilled liquid acrylic monomer mixture placed onto acid-etched or conditioned enamel. The monomer flows into interstices between and within enamel rods.

Enamel bonding depends on **resin tags** becoming interlocked with the surface irregularities created by etching. Resin tags which form between enamel rod periph-

Table 6-10. Summary and comparison of shear strengths for different materials and systems involved with dental adhesion.*

Adherend/(adhesive)/(adherend)	Shear strength (MPa)
Enamel	90-200
Dentin	170
Composite	30-120
Traditional glass ionomer	—
Resin-modified glass ionomer	—
Dental amalgam	[125]
Enamel/enamel SL	4-6
Dentin/dentin SL	4-6
Enamel/EBS/composite	18-22
Enamel/ABS/composite	10-12
Enamel/ABS/amalgam	2-22
Enamel/no SL/traditional glass ionomer	8-12
Enamel/EBS/orthodontic bracket	18-20
Enamel/composite cement/Maryland bridge	—
Dentin/DBS/composite	22-35
Dentin/SL/traditional glass ionomer	[6]
Dentin/no SL/light-cured hybrid glass ionomer	10-12
Composite/EBS/resurfacing composite	10-27

*Estimated values are shown in brackets. The combination of adherend, adhesive, and/or overlying adherend is indicated in the left-hand column.
†EBS = enamel bonding system; DBS = dentin bonding system; ABS = amalgam bonding system; SL = smear layer.

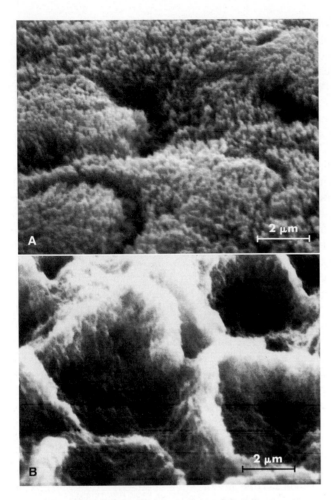

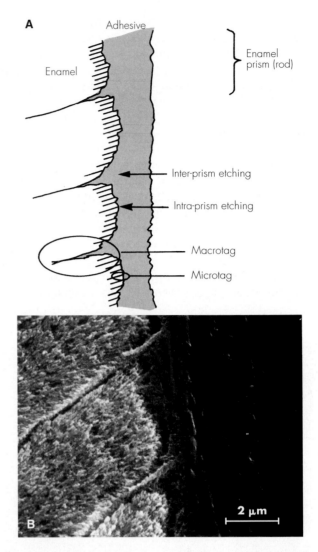

Fig. 6-40. Micro-mechanical retention of bonding systems to dental enamel. **A,** SEM view of etched enamel showing relief between enamel rods and within their ends. **B,** SEM view of enamel bonding agent, from which etched enamel has been removed, with cup-shaped macrotags and thousands of fine microtags on each one. (Courtesy SC Bayne, School of Dentistry, University of North Carolina, Chapel Hill, NC.)

Fig. 6-41. Cross-sectional views of micro-mechanical retention of enamel bonding systems. **A,** Schematic view of macrotags and microtags. **B,** SEM cross-sectional view of interface of enamel bonding agent with enamel revealing microtags between macrotags. (Courtesy SC Bayne, School of Dentistry, University of North Carolina, Chapel Hill, NC.)

eries are called *macrotags* (Figs. 6-40 and 6-41).[15] A much finer network of thousands of smaller tags form across the end of each rod where individual hydroxyapatite crystals have been dissolved leaving crypts outlined by residual organic material. These fine tags are called *microtags.* Macrotags and microtags are the basis for micro-mechanical bonding. Microtags are probably more important because of their large number and great surface of contact. During the 1970s and 1980s before these details were known, bonding studies concentrated more on the length of macrotags and the patterns of etching. However, macrotag length is unimportant because fracture occurs in the neck of the tag. Most macrotags are only 2 to 5 μm in length. Rod etching patterns also are generally not important to the resulting bond strength.

The bonding agent co-polymerizes on its other side with the matrix phase of dental composite, producing strong chemical bonding. The bond strength for the joint is 18 to 22 MPa and is limited by the film thickness of the bonding agent and then by the shear strength of adjacent enamel rods. The theoretical upper limit for joint strength is probably about 50 MPa. The current bond strengths of about 20 MPa appear to clinically be very acceptable. More than 20 years of clinical use has not detected any degradation of the mechanical bonds due to routine stress or fatigue.

Dentin bonding systems. Dentin bonding systems involve an unfilled, liquid acrylic monomer mixture which is placed onto an acid conditioned and primed dentin surface. The bonding primer is based on *hydro-*

philic monomers such as 2-hydroxyethyl methacrylate (*2-HEMA* or *HEMA*) to wet dentin surfaces that may contain some moisture. Although primer and/or bonding agent may flow into dentinal tubules, the bond strength is primarily related to micro-mechanical bonding to the *intertubular dentin* which occurs between tubules along the cut dentin surface. Despite the fact that many dentin bonding agents have been formulated to allow chemical reactions to take place with dentin, this has had little or no apparent contribution to the final bond strength.[149] Generally, 90% or more of dentin bond strengths are presumed to be due to mechanical bonding.

As noted earlier, mechanical preparation of dentin leaves behind a highly distorted debris layer (smear layer) that covers the surface and conceals the underlying structures (Fig. 6-42, *A*). Early dentin bonding agents were hydrophobic and were bonded directly to the dentin smear layer. Therefore, shear bond strengths

were less than 6 MPa because the smear layer had about that adhesive strength to sound dentin. Initial dentin conditioning processes removed the smear layer but tended to over-etch dentin (Fig. 6-42, *B*). Bond strengths of 10 to 12 MPa were produced but were not significantly greater until bonding systems were chemically modified to be more hydrophilic (18 to 20 MPa). Careful dentin conditioning produced micro-mechanical relief for bonding between tubules (intertubular dentin) without excessive demineralization of peritubular dentin. Coupled with hydrophilic primers, bond strengths increased to 22 to 35 MPa. The theoretical limit for dentin bonding agent strength may actually be higher than that for enamel, because dentin is more resistant to shear fracture. The clinically important limit for dentin bonding is not yet known. However, because of the presence of more water in dentin than enamel, *the clinical longevity of dentin bonding may not be as long.*

As portrayed in Fig. 6-43, the primer in dentin bonding systems is designed to penetrate through remnant smear layer and into the intertubular dentin to fill the spaces left by dissolved hydroxyapatite crystals. This allows the primer to form an interpenetrating network around dentin collagen. This layer is called the *hybrid zone (interdiffusion zone* or *interpenetration zone)* by Nakabayashi.[107] Depending on the particular chemistry of a bonding system, the hybrid layer may vary from 1 to 5 μm deep. Unfortunately, excessive etching may decalcify dentin from 1 to 10 μm deep. If this decalcified dentin zone is not filled (bonded) by the primer, it may act as a weakened layer or zone contributing to fracture. The extent of the etching effect on the strength of the collagen fibers is not yet known either. However, these systems demonstrate that stronger dentin bonding is possible and portend a bright future for bonding systems.

The key ingredient in primers in most dentin bonding systems is hydroxyethyl methacrylate (HEMA; Fig. 6-44, *A*). This molecule is an analog to methyl methacrylate, except that the pendant methyl ester is replaced by an ethoxy ester group to make it hydrophilic. Importantly, it is relatively volatile and has some tendency to produce mild sensitivity. Dentists and assistants should be aware that it is very mobile, can diffuse through rubber gloves[105] (see information in Fig. 6-72 in the MSDS [material safety data sheet] for a dentin bonding agent), and will cause skin dryness and cracking in many individuals. *Therefore, during the use of primers and bonding agents, high volume evacuation should be used to minimize HEMA vapor contact.*

Amalgam bonding systems. Amalgam bonding systems may be used to bond amalgam to tooth structure, amalgam to amalgam, or amalgam to other metal substrates. They require dual characteristics to achieve optimal wetting. Dental amalgam is strongly hydrophobic,

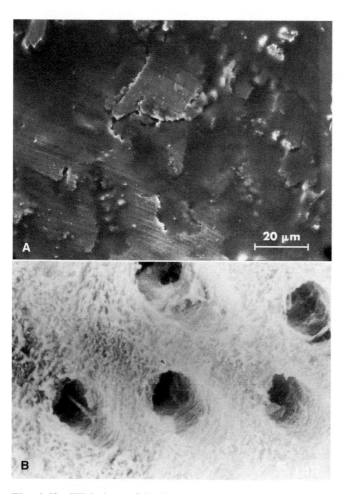

Fig. 6-42. SEM views of dentin in various stages of etching. **A,** Unetched dentin with smear layer. **B,** Over-etched dentin revealing intertubular spaces and enlarged dentin tubule openings. (**A,** courtesy SC Bayne, School of Dentistry, University of North Carolina, Chapel Hill, NC; **B,** courtesy K Bruggers, School of Dentistry, University of North Carolina, Chapel Hill, NC.)

while enamel is hydrophilic. Therefore, the bonding agent must be modified with a wetting agent (co-monomer) that has the capacity to wet both hydrophobic or hydrophilic surfaces. *4-META* (4-methyloxy ethyl trimellitic anhydride) is frequently used. This monomer molecule has hydrophobic and hydrophilic ends (Fig. 6-44, *B*).

Bonding system strengths for joining amalgam to dentin have been relatively low (2 to 6 MPa). Improved conditioning of tooth structure and better wetting seem to enhance bond strengths. Although there has been good bonding to tooth structure, there has been poor micro-mechanical bonding at the amalgam to bonding agent interface. Most debonding occurs by fractures along the interface of bonding agent with amalgam. These systems will continue to be modified to mimic the experience gained with dentin bonding systems for composites. *For the moment, **the primary advantage for amalgam bonding agents is sealing of dentin.*** Adhesion of tooth structure to amalgam may not be neces-

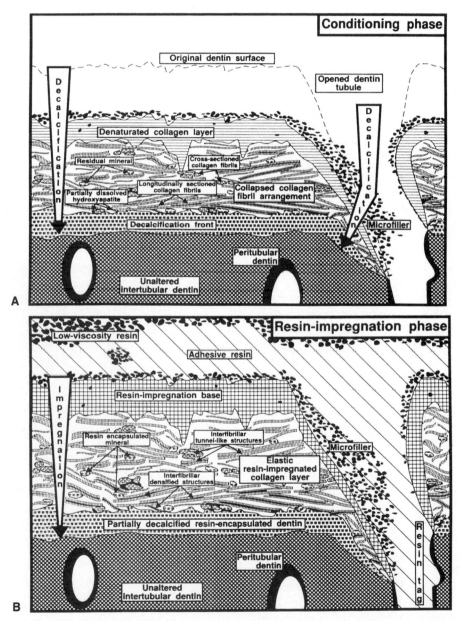

Fig. 6-43. Cross-sectional views of micro-mechanical retention of dentin bonding systems. **A,** Schematic view of conditioning phase for dentin bonding systems. **B,** Schematic view of resin-impregnation phase showing the development of macrotags in tubules and microtags within intertubular dentin between collagen bundles. (Courtesy Van Meerbeek B et al: *J Dent Res* 72:495-501, 1993.)

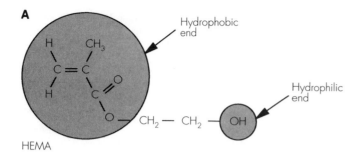

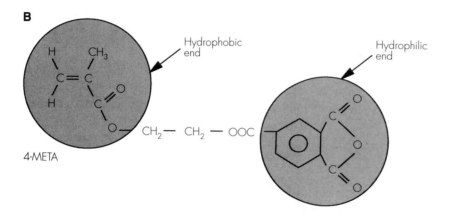

Fig. 6-44. Examples of acrylic monomers used in bonding systems because of their hydrophilicity. **A,** HEMA (hydroxyethyl methacrylate). **B,** 4-META (4-methyloxy ethyl trimellitic anyhydride).

sary in many clinical circumstances where satisfactory retention and resistance forms of cavity preparation already exist. However, much interest remains in micromechanical adhesion of amalgam to weakened tooth structure in order to improve the overall resistance form of the restored tooth. *Those bonding systems that produce a relatively thick (10 to 20 μm) bonding agent layer permit the interlocking of microstructural features of amalgam during condensation and create a strong interface* (see Fig. 6-45). The advantages and disadvantages of self-curing versus light-curing systems are not yet well researched and understood. *In any case, as these materials improve they should completely replace traditional liners and bases.*

For simplicity, most dental product manufacturers are combining their bonding agents into a single system which is either capable of bonding to all substrates or which can be varied to optimize the bonding to specific substrates. These systems are called ***multi-purpose bonding agents.*** They are presumed to be useful for enamel bonding, dentin bonding, amalgam bonding, and composite-to-metal bonding for fracture repairs. Bonding agents that are used below insulating restorations, such as dental composite, replace traditional liners and bases except when the cavity preparation is extremely close to the pulp (<0.5 mm). In that case a traditional liner is used for pulpal medication, either to mitigate pulpal inflammation or stimulate reparative dentin (see Fig. 6-33). When possible, a liner should be

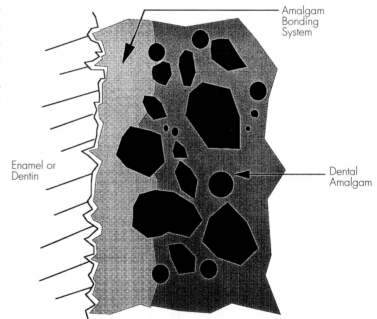

Fig. 6-45. Schematic view of the adhesive joint created with dental amalgam bonding agent. Micro-mechanical bonding holds bonding agent to the surface of conditioned tooth structure. Alloy particles and amalgam irregularities provide retentions to bonding agent where adhesive film is thick enough to allow micro-mechanical interlocking to occur. (Courtesy SC Bayne, School of Dentistry, University of North Carolina, Chapel Hill, NC).

chosen that can be bonded to tooth structure and to the overlying dental restorative materials.

Cast restoration bonding/luting systems. Cast restorations are retained to tooth structure by dental cements whose structure and properties will be detailed later in this chapter. The adhesion process involves cement adaptation to surface irregularities ***(dental luting cement)*** in a way that prevents the restoration's withdrawal along the original path of insertion. Cements may be chemically adhesive (polycarboxylate or glass ionomer), but most of the bond strength results from mechanical adhesion. The limits to bond strength in these situations relate to (1) the relatively poor wetting characteristics of viscous luting cements and (2) the relative thickness of luting cement. Both of these features contribute to low bond strength. If the cement does not wet the substrate well, then fractures propagate easily along the interface, typically with dentin. If the cement is more hydrophilic and wets dentin well, then fractures propagate within the weakest solid in the joint, which is the dental cement. *The adhesive joint bond strength is improved by using stronger cements (composite cements), roughening and etching the casting surfaces and dentin surfaces, using composite materials that contain wetting agents, and attempting to reduce the cement thickness in the adhesive joint.* All of these features are included in composite cements used for Maryland bridges (see Chapter 18).

These same principles are equally applicable to all other situations involving adhesion in dentistry, such as sealants, bonded orthodontic brackets, denture adhesives, porcelain-to-metal bonding, and osseointegration of implants.

Pit and fissure sealants

Terminology. Pit and fissure *sealants* were first proposed for dentistry in the late 1960s. They are an alternative to cavity preparation and restoration techniques for the elimination of caries-prone pits and fissures on occlusal surfaces of teeth. Pits and fissures that are not self-cleansing are considered caries-prone (see Figs. 3-21, 5-5, *B,* and 17-1, *A*). Normally, they accumulate organic debris and oral bacteria, providing an ideal site for the development of dental caries. The objective of pit and fissure sealants is simply to eliminate the geometry which harbors bacteria. Sealants are used to occlude portions of these sites that are not self-cleansing. Any material which is placed to seal these sites tends to overfill the area. Because sealant has only modest wear resistance, contact area wear and food abrasion quickly wear it away from naturally self-cleansing areas where it is not needed. However, key areas remain occluded, resulting in continued benefits.

The principal feature of a sealant that is required for success is *adequate retention*. Most pits and fissures have some degree of macro-retention but there may be debris in the fault, inadequate access, or insufficient fluidity of the sealant to allow its penetration to the deepest recesses of these sites. Therefore, micro-mechanical retention is required. Sealant is applied only after gross debridement and acid etching of the surfaces. Sealant cannot be applied so precisely that there is no excess extending onto self-cleansing areas of occlusal surfaces. Therefore, it is important that the material be adjusted as needed following placement (see Chapter 17 for technique) so that it does not interfere with normal occlusal contacts or disrupt occlusal paths. Once it has been removed from self-cleansing areas, the remaining sealant blocks bacterial accumulation occurring in otherwise non–self-cleansing locations (Fig. 6-46).

Classification. The division of sealants into classification categories is trivial. Sealants are categorized in terms of polymerization method, as ***self-curing*** or ***visible light-curing***. Early sealants were based on methyl methacrylate or cyanoacrylate cements but virtually all contemporary compositions are unfilled and based on difunctional monomers such as those used for the matrix of dental composites. The principal monomer (e.g., BIS-GMA, see the section in this chapter on dental composites—Historical Development) may be diluted with lower molecular weight species (e.g., TEGDMA) to reduce the viscosity. Small amounts of colorant, such as TiO_2, may be added to make the appearance slightly different from occlusal enamel. Otherwise the sealant is clear and difficult to locate during clinical inspection on recall. Self-curing compositions have the advantage of curing quickly enough that they are retained in sites whose orientation may encourage flow away from the area. Self-curing materials have to be applied so that they are fluid enough to penetrate the pit or fissure but so that they begin to cure before running away from the site. This combination of characteristics sometimes causes problems in obtaining adequate penetration. If occlusal surfaces are easily oriented during the procedure to control flow, then light-curing materials are actually simpler to use. They can be applied and allowed to flow for a convenient time before exposure to a visible light source for curing.

Composition, structure, and properties. Because the primary clinical property is flow into small access spaces, a ***penetration coefficient*** is normally calculated for comparison of products. It describes the relative rate of flow in a standard sized orifice. Penetration is a function of both capillary action and viscosity. If the site is well-cleaned, etched, rinsed, and dried, then acrylic monomers such as BIS-GMA tend to wet the surface reasonably well. Even if the opening in the pit or fissure is small, if there is good wetting, then capillary action will tend to draw the material into the orifice. The viscosity must be low enough for a long enough time for

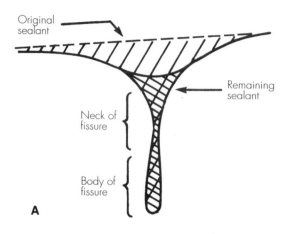

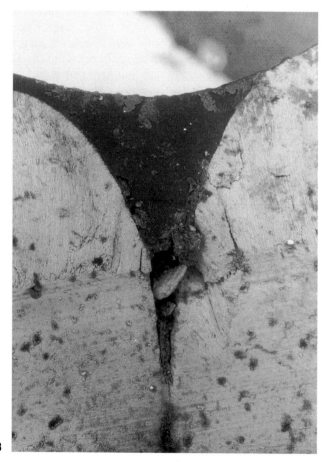

Fig. 6-46. Fissure sealants. **A,** Schematic view of idealized fissure after sealing and after loss of excess sealant. **B,** SEM cross section of sealed fissure. Sealant does not penetrate into entire fissure. Excess sealant on occlusal surface has been mostly worn away to boundary of self-cleansing zone. (**A,** After Bayne SC, Barton RE. In Richardson RE, Barton RE, editors: *The dental assistant,* ed 6, Philadelphia, 1988, Lea & Febiger; **B,** courtesy S Mitchell, School of Dentistry, University of North Carolina, Chapel Hill, NC.)

the material to penetrate into the defect site. Penetration coefficients for several sealants are reported in Table 6-11.

Complete penetration of sealant does not seem to be absolutely critical. It is possible to occlude only the neck region of a fissure and produce clinically acceptable results. An example of a fissure is shown in Fig. 6-46, *A*. An example of a typical cross-sectional view is shown in Fig. 6-46, *B*. Quite often, the local geometry creates a defect with a wide orifice.

When glass ionomer compositions were originally explored for dentistry, they were evaluated in pit and fissure applications. However, they were unsuccessful because they lacked abrasion resistance. In addition, they were brittle and were prone to fracture, exposing the underlying portions of unfilled pits or fissures to the intraoral environment.

Composites, by themselves, are not good sealants because they do not penetrate into pits and fissures readily due to their comparatively high viscosity. However, they may be involved in treating pit or fissure caries, especially when used with a bonding adhesive. *If a fissure is minimally carious, then excavation of the caries and restoration with a composite provides the same type of conservative management of the defective enamel region* (see Chapter 17).

The properties of sealants are essentially those of the resin matrix component of composite materials. However, there is no evidence that water absorption, chemical degradation, or other events which have been observed with composites detract from the longevity of these materials.

Clinical considerations. During the early 1970s a large number of clinical studies were initiated to determine the relative reduction in dental caries possible with sealant use and to determine the longevity of the materials. Simonsen[141] has reported excellent clinical suc-

Table 6-11. Penetration coefficients for typical pit-and-fissure sealants and surface sealers

Sealant system	Penetration coefficient
Adaptic bonding agent	12.8 cm/s
Delton pit and fissure sealant	7.22 cm/s
	10.0 cm/s
Concise enamel bond	6.40 cm/s
	4.80 cm/s
Nuva seal	3.0 cm/s
Concise white sealant	2.43 cm/s
Adaptic glaze	0.62 cm/s

Derived from Retief DH, Mallory WP: *Pediatr Dent* 3:12-16, 1981; O'Brien WJ, Fan PL, Apostolides A: *Oper Dent* 3:51-56, 1978; and Fan PL, O'Brien WJ, Craig RG: *Oper Dent* 4:100-103, 1979.

cess after 15 years with teeth sealed only with a single application of sealant. Prevention of occlusal dental caries at defects depends simply on the exclusion of bacteria (Fig. 6-47). Numerous clinical investigations have demonstrated that as long as pits and fissures remain completely sealed, there is 100% prevention of caries at those sites.[110,132] As long as the sealant is retained, it will achieve this end. There are differences among sealant types in both short-term and long-term retention.[96]

There is absolutely no evidence that sealant ever wears out. If the sealant is lost or leaks, then the site is once again at risk to caries. It may be lost due to failure of the acid etching or the micro-mechanical retention to the acid-etched surface. It is common for saliva or moist air contamination to interfere with the effects of acid etching. However, loss of sealant from areas that are not self-cleansing is minimal.

The ideal time to apply sealants is as soon as occlusal surfaces erupt in the oral environment. However, at that time, very little of the tooth has erupted and it is difficult or impossible to use a rubber dam for moisture control. Therefore, cotton rolls and/or absorbent wedges are used instead. Without special care it is common for some contamination of the acid-etched enamel to occur. This contamination prevents resin penetration into micro-mechanical spaces and leads to premature failure. During recalls, if the sealant has been lost, then it can be re-applied. With careful management and repair of sealed surfaces it is possible to achieve 100% reduction in occlusal caries.

Despite the enormous long-term benefit for patients with sealed pits and fissures, this prevention method was used routinely by only about 16% of dental practices in the United States in 1992. To some degree this poor use has been based on limited enthusiasm for prevention by dentists and by delayed commitments of insurance carriers to reimburse dental practices for these procedures. However, it is quite clear that *sealants provide outstanding service for very low costs. In societies committed to dental care, this is a core strategy for early management of dental caries.*

Sealants also have been applied to smooth surface tooth structure to try to eliminate caries. For smooth surfaces, fluoridated water is very effective in reducing caries prevalence. Sealants which have been applied to smooth surfaces are abraded by food and/or toothbrushes and are lost at relatively rapid rates. Because toothbrush bristles are large, they do not affect sealants in pits and fissures.

Recently, sealants containing fluoride have been investigated. *The contribution of fluoride in these circumstances may be very small at best.* Clinical studies in which sealants were used to seal fissures that were minimally carious produced complete inhibition of the caries process. Therefore, fluoride modification of the enamel would not seem to be very beneficial. Although not proven, there is strong suspicion that any retained sealants do not leak. Those which are poorly bonded are lost almost immediately. In those circumstances, the limited time for diffusion of fluoride from the sealant to the underlying tooth structure would probably not provide sufficient fluoride to completely discourage caries.

Another important consideration for sealant use is the degree to which children and adolescents are susceptible to caries. There is strong evidence that there are two categories of these patients, one with a much greater dental caries predisposition (see Chapter 3). This category of patients would benefit the most from the use of pit and fissure sealants. One sure indication of apparent caries susceptibility is a dental history of caries on the occlusal surfaces of primary teeth.[9,40,138] If all individuals were routinely being examined by a dentist, then their record would provide simple evidence for the choice whether to apply sealants to the permanent teeth.

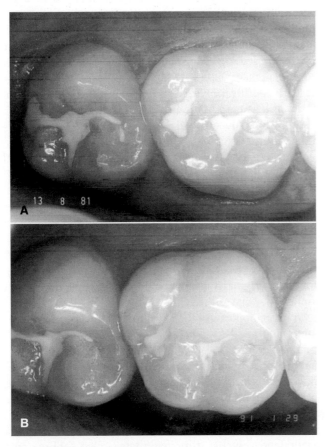

Fig. 6-47. Example of functioning of sealant on first molar after: **A,** 5 years, and **B,** 15 years of clinical service. Some abrasion of sealant has occurred in occlusal areas that appear self-cleansing. (Courtesy Simonsen RJ: *J Am Dent Assoc* 122(11):34-42, 1992.)

Dental composites

Terminology. A *composite* is a physical mixture of materials. The parts of the mixture generally are chosen with the purpose of averaging the properties of the parts to achieve intermediate properties. Quite often a single material does not have the appropriate properties for a specific dental application.

A schematic view of a generalized composite is presented in Fig. 6-48. Composites typically involve a *dispersed phase* of *filler particles* that are distributed within a *continuous phase (matrix phase)*. In most cases the matrix phase is fluid at some point during the manufacture or fabrication of a composite system.

A *dental composite* has traditionally indicated a mixture of silicate glass particles with an acrylic monomer that is polymerized during the application. The silicate particles provide mechanical reinforcement of the mixture (reinforcing fillers) and produce light transmission and light scattering that adds enamel-like translucency to the mixture. The acrylic monomers make the initial mixture fluid and moldable for placement into a cavity preparation. That matrix flows to adapt to cavity preparation walls and penetrate into micro-mechanical spaces on etched enamel or dentin surfaces.

Because the flow of uncured composite is quite limited, most composite manufacturers provide a *bonding system.* It is primarily an unfilled acrylic monomer mixture, similar to the matrix of the composite, that is pre-placed onto conditioned (etched) tooth surfaces to form a 1 to 5 micron film. It micro-mechanically interlocks with the etched surfaces, seals the walls of the preparation, and co-polymerizes with the composite restorative material that fills the cavity preparation. Dentin and/or enamel bonding systems, or universal bonding systems,

may be provided as part of the composite product package.

Although "dental composite" is the technically correct term for these materials, a variety of slang terms have been widely accepted as well. Dental composites have often been called *composites, composite restorative materials, filled resins, composite resins, resin composites,* or *filled composites.*

These alternative terms become more confusing as the field of dental polymers becomes more sophisticated and simultaneously more complex. Most dental materials are composites of some type. If these compositions are modified to include special polymer phases, then they may be called resin-containing composites. Glass ionomer cements have been modified with both polymer-containing fillers and monomer-containing matrices. They are classified as *hybrid* or *resin-modified glass ionomers* but could equally well be described as modified dental composites.

Historical development. Early attempts at esthetic filling materials which predated acrylic resins and composites were based on silicate cements. These cements resulted from reactions of phosphoric acid with acid-soluble glass particles to form a silica gel matrix containing residual glass particles. Solubility problems with these materials led to the introduction of unfilled acrylic systems based on polymethyl methacrylate (PMMA). Methyl methacrylate (MMA) monomer contracted excessively during polymerization, permitting subsequent marginal leakage. Also, PMMA was not strong enough to support occlusal loads. Therefore, reinforcing ceramic fillers, principally containing silica, were added to the composition. Retrospectively, the original PMMA materials now are called **unfilled acrylics.** (If the amount of filler or filler-like phase added to a resin matrix is small, the overall composition is considered as unfilled. Therefore, 1% to 2% filler-modified sealant compositions are still classified as unfilled.)

MMA-based matrices were supplanted by **BIS-GMA** (alternatively Bis-GMA). BIS-GMA is a difunctional monomer originally produced as the reaction product of bisphenol-A and glycidyl methacrylate (Fig. 6-49, *A*).[22] Several analogues of that structure have been investigated (modified BIS-GMA). Another very similar difunctional molecule also is used, *UDM* (urethane dimethacrylate, also abbreviated UDMA). UDM replaces the bisphenol-A backbone with a linear isocyanate one (Fig. 6-49, *B*). Both BIS-GMA and UDM are extremely viscous. For practical reasons, they are diluted with another difunctional monomer with an aliphatic backbone, *TEGDMA* (triethylene glycol dimethacrylate, also abbreviated TEGDM or TGDMA), of much lower viscosity (Fig. 6-49, *C*).

To gain the full advantage of a composite formulation, it is very important to provide interfacial bonding

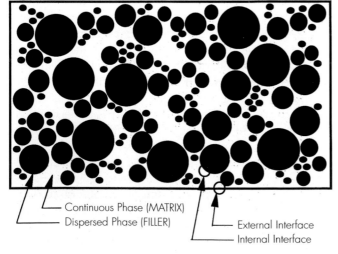

Continuous Phase (MATRIX)
Dispersed Phase (FILLER)
External Interface
Internal Interface

Fig. 6-48. Key components of composites. Schematic view of generalized composite showing continuous phase, dispersed phase, internal interfaces, and external interface.

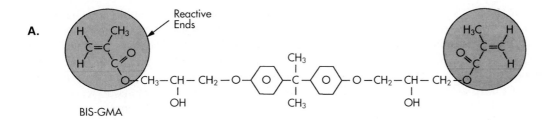

A.

BIS-GMA

B.

UDM

R₁ = Aliphatic Species
R₂ = Aromatic Species

C.

TEGDMA

Fig. 6-49. Chemical formulas of difunctional monomers commonly used in dental composites. **A,** BIS-GMA monomer. **B,** UDM monomer. **C,** TEGDMA monomer.

between the phases. In modern composites, silica particles are pre-coated with mono-molecular films of *silane coupling agents.* These molecules are difunctional. One end is capable of bonding to hydroxyl groups, which exist along the surface of the silica particles, and the other end is capable of co-polymerizing with double bonds of monomers in the matrix phase. Coupling agents work best with silica particles. Therefore, all dental composites have been based on silica-containing fillers.

Filler compositions are often modified with other ions to produce desirable changes in properties. Li (lithium) and Al (aluminum) ions make the glass easier to crush to generate small particles. Ba (barium), Zn (zinc), B (boron), Zr (zirconium), and Y (yttrium) ions have been used to produce *radiopacity* in the filler particles. Excessive modification (by replacement of the silicon in the structure) however, can reduce the efficacy of the coupling agent.

Pure silica occurs in several crystalline forms (such as crystobalite, tridymite, or quartz) and in a noncrystalline form (glass). Crystalline forms are stronger and harder, but make composites which are difficult to finish and polish (Fig. 6-50). Therefore, most composites are now produced using silicate glass. *Barium, zinc, and yttrium glasses are currently the most popular fillers.*

The *fluidity* of a mixture of filler and matrix monomer is affected by the fluidity of the monomer and the amount of filler. The friction between the filler particle surfaces and the monomer is a principal factor controlling the fluidity. As the filler surface area increases, the fluidity decreases. Large filler particles have a relatively small amount of particle surface area per unit of filler particle volume. As an equivalent volume of smaller filler particles is used to replace larger ones, the surface area increases rapidly. For example, when filler particles with diameters that are one-tenth as large are substituted, the surface area increases 10 times. The situation is further exacerbated for microfiller particles made from SiO_2 which tend to agglomerate into chains and clusters.

Placement of dental composites cannot be accomplished so precisely that there will not be a need for adjustments to anatomical contours after curing. Typically, the restoration is produced by intentionally overfilling the cavity preparation a small amount. The anatomical contours are accomplished by gross cutting *(grinding),* fine cutting *(finishing),* and then smoothing *(polishing)* the material after polymerization.

Particle sizes in dental composites affect other properties as well as fluidity. For example, filler particle size has a direct effect on the surface roughness of the ground, finished, or polished dental composite. Filler particles are harder than the matrix. Therefore, during finishing some particles may be left protruding from the surface, while others are stripped out of the surface leaving holes. If the particles are very small, then the resulting surface roughness is of little concern. This effect is illustrated schematically in Fig. 6-50. Otherwise, the rough areas may contribute to light scattering and collection of organic debris or stain.

Classification. Dental composites generally are classified with respect to the components, amounts, or properties of their filler or matrix phases. The most common classification method is based on filler content (weight or volume percent), filler particle size, and method of filler addition. Composites could be defined, as well, on the basis of the matrix composition (*BIS-GMA or UDM*) or polymerization method *(self-curing, ultraviolet light-curing, visible light-curing, dual curing, or staged curing),* but these do not communicate as much information about the properties.

Almost all important properties of composites are

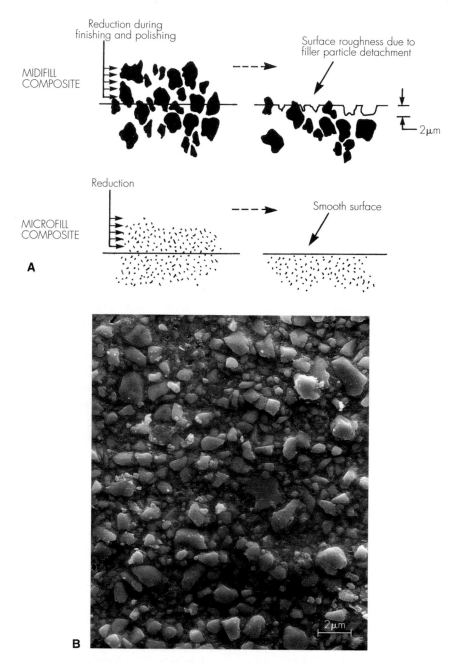

Fig. 6-50. Effect of particle size on surface finish of dental composite. **A,** Schematic illustration of finishing midifill versus microfill composite surfaces. **B,** SEM view of finished midifill composite surface. (Courtesy SC Bayne, School of Dentistry, University of North Carolina, Chapel Hill, NC.)

improved by using higher filler levels. The only practical problem is that as the filler level is increased, the fluidity decreases. Highly filled compositions typically contain large filler particles, but as previously stated, this composition results in a rough finished surface. Smaller filler particles are used to guarantee that composites have a relatively smooth finished surface, but this choice compromises the filler level that is possible.

The degree of filler addition is represented in terms of the weight percent or volume percent of filler. Because silica fillers are about three times as dense as acrylic monomer (or polymer), 75 weight percent filler is equivalent to approximately 50 volume percent filler. Properties of composites are proportional to the volume percent of the phases involved. But, it is much easier to both measure and formulate composites using weight percentages rather than volume percentages and, in dentistry, the weight percent is much more commonly reported. A conversion of *filler levels* is presented in Table 6-12.

Filler particle sizes for the earliest dental composites averaged 10 to 20 microns (μm) in diameter with many of the larger particles as large as 50 microns (Figs. 6-51 and 6-52). At first there was no need to distinguish the

Table 6-12. Examples of filler level ranges for typical dental composites in terms of the weight and volume percent.*

Weight % filler	Volume % filler	Composites
0	0	[Unfilled resins; bonding agents; pit and fissure sealants; surface sealers]
	10	[Sealants filled with colorants]
	20	
50	30	Homogeneous microfills
	40	
75	50	Macrofills, midifills
	60	Hybrid midifills, heterogeneous microfills
85	70	Hybrid minifills
	80	[ENAMEL]
	90	
100	100	

*The composites are reported using a classification system based on filler particle sizes. Systems which are not dental composites are reported in brackets.

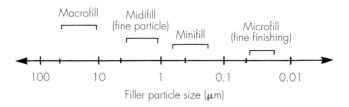

Fig. 6-52. Composite filler ranges versus particle size (shown on logarithmic scale).

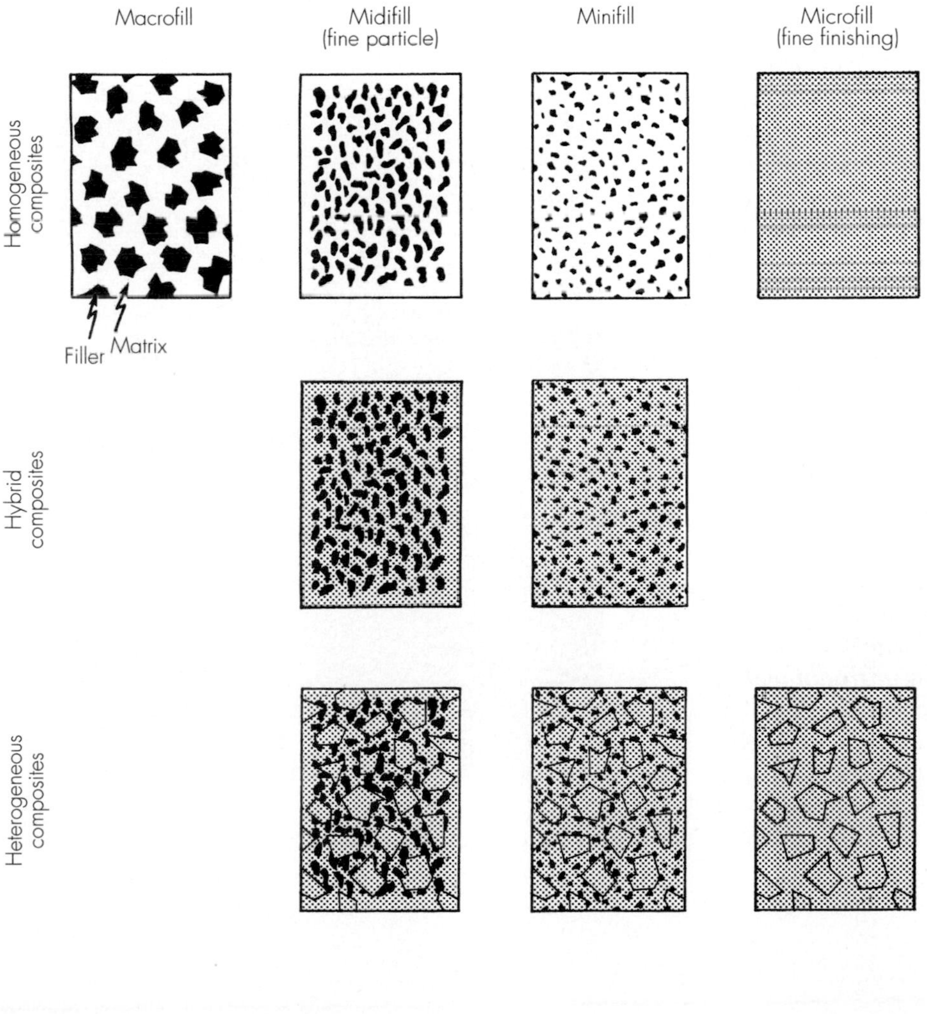

Fig. 6-51. Summary of filler particle size-based classification system for dental composites. Composites are grouped on basis of (1) range of average particle size, (2) whether or not they are hybrid due to particle size mixing, and (3) whether composite is homogeneous mixture of filler and resin or includes precured composite (heterogeneous).

particle size range or ranges of composites because all commercial products were in about the same range. During the evolution of the formulations for better finishing characteristics and greater resistance to wear, smaller and smaller filler particles were used. Because the early filler particles were relatively large, dental composites based on those large fillers became known as *macrofill* materials. The terms macrofill or macrofiller are preferred to macrofilled because they properly describe the filler particle size and not the method of producing the mixture. During the course of composite evolution, nomenclatures and classification systems have been neither consistent nor uniform.* In the following sections, composites will be classified either in terms of their (1) particle size range or (2) comparative finishing characteristics. Both classifications are presented here.

Classification of composites based on the range of filler particle size range has been partially developed by several authors.† That system is extended here to include the particle size by order of magnitude, acknowledging mixed ranges of particle sizes, and distinguishing pre-cured composite pieces as special filler. Composite filler particles are called *macrofillers* in the range of 10 to 100 microns, *midifillers* from 1 to 10 microns, *minifillers* from 0.1 to 1 micron, and *microfillers* from 0.01 to 0.1 micron. Very large individual filler particles, called *megafillers,* have also been used in special circumstances. New ultra-small fillers are being investigated that are from 0.005 to 0.01 micron in diameter and are called *nanofillers.* Accordingly, composites are classified by particle size as *megafill, macrofill, midifill, minifill, microfill,* and *nanofill.* Composites with mixed ranges of particle sizes are called *hybrids,* and the largest particle size range is used to define the hybrid type (e.g., minifill hybrid) because microfillers are normally the second part of the mixture. If the composite simply consists of filler and uncured matrix material, it is classified as *homogeneous.* If it includes pre-cured composite or other unusual filler, it is called *heterogeneous.*

After the early macrofill composites, the next generation had fillers that were 8 to 10 microns in average size (midifillers) and were originally designated *fine particle* composites to imply their improved finishing characteristics. These new materials quickly became popular and were used primarily for anterior restorations in place of silicate cements and direct filling resins. The category soon became known as *traditional* or *conventional* composites, but that designation has become confusing as newer composites continue to evolve with even smaller particle size ranges. The next step

was to utilize 0.02 to 0.04 micron diameter particles to produce *microfill* composites. The term microfiller was already in common use for these particles in non-dental applications. Microfill composites were also called *fine finishing* composites. The small filler particle size produced high viscosities in the uncured mixes of BIS-GMA with TEGDMA and required the addition of greater amounts of monomer diluents along with a reduced overall filler content to maintain workable consistencies.

To circumvent part of the viscosity problem, two strategies were developed. The first was to blend precured microfill composite with uncured material. Precured particles were generated by grinding cured composites to a 1 to 20 micron size. The pre-cured particles become chemically bonded to the new material, provide islands that have better properties, and are fine finishing. These variants are known as *heterogeneous microfills* (or *organic filler* composites). An example is shown schematically in Fig. 6-51 (and later a scanning electron micrograph of the same is illustrated in Fig. 6-53). Unmodified microfills are called *homogeneous microfills.* A second approach has been to sinter small filler particles into large but porous filler particles, impregnate them with monomer, and add the new particles to a microfill composite. Within the local region of the sintered filler particle, the material is highly filled and yet capable of being polished.

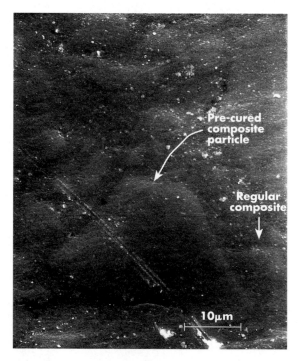

Fig. 6-53. SEM cross-sectional view of heterogeneous microfill composite. (Courtesy SC Bayne and DF Taylor, School of Dentistry, University of North Carolina, Chapel Hill, NC.)

*References 34,71,82,136,156,165,166.
†References 65,67,71,82,136,156.

After it was realized that highly filled microfills were difficult to use, dental composites were formulated with mixtures of particles in the microfiller range and 2 to 5 micron range. These bimodal distributions allowed higher filler levels and still permitted good finishing. All types of mixtures are known collectively as *hybrid* composites. Currently, the principal particle size for newer materials is in the 0.1 to 1 micron range.

New composites are being contemplated with nanofillers that range in size from 0.005 to 0.01 micron, which is below the wavelength range for visible light (0.02 to 2 micron).[43] Since these particles do not interact with visible light, they do not produce scattering or significant absorption. Non-silicate–based compositions can be used for nanofillers because they are effectively invisible. Non-silicate fillers do not tend to agglomerate or cluster like typical silica-based fillers. Nanofillers are so small that they fit between several polymer chains. These characteristics permit the opportunity to achieve very high filler loading levels in composites while still maintaining workable consistencies. Consideration of nanofillers, particularly of compositions other than silica, complicate the classification system for composites even further. Potentially the composition will have to be stated along with the particle size range.

For the purposes of examining the properties of composites in this section, the classification based on particle size range will be used. However, in other sections of the text, some of the historic terms may be substituted.

Examples of the filled composite designations are shown in Fig. 6-51. Mean filler particle sizes of those designations are shown in Fig. 6-52. Mean filler particle sizes may often not correspond to any actual particle size due to polydisperse distributions. Fig. 6-54 shows examples of the particle size distributions for several composites. There is no practical limitation on the complexity of filler particle compositions or particle size distributions. New composites may be better described simply as polydisperse.

In addition to inorganic or composite fillers, it is possible to add *crystalline polymer fillers.* Some newer composites include crystalline polymer to supplement traditional fillers. Crystalline polymer is not nearly as strong as inorganic filler, but it is stronger than simply amorphous polymer matrix.

Microfill and hybrid dental composites utilize microfillers of SiO_2 that can be produced in a variety of ways and, therefore, are designated with different names. Two forms are primarily used in dental compositions. *Colloidal silica* is chemically precipitated from a liquid solution as amorphous silica particles. *Pyrogenic silica* is precipitated from a gaseous phase as amorphous particles.[63] The actual properties of each form are slightly different but the differences have not yet been shown to

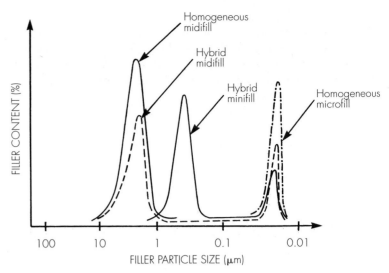

Fig. 6-54. Schematic of particle size distributions for homogeneous midifill, hybrid midifill, hybrid minifill, and homogeneous microfill composites.

produce different clinical properties for dental composites.

For posterior composite applications, it is also possible to place one or two large glass inserts (0.5 to 2 mm particles) into composites at points of occlusal contact or high wear. These pieces of glass are referred to as *inserts* (or *megafillers*). Although they have demonstrated improved wear resistance to contact area wear, the techniques are more complicated and do not totally eliminate wear of regular composite in contact-free areas. Furthermore, the bonding of the composite to the insert is questionable.

Matrix monomers for dental composites used in the United States traditionally have been based on BIS-GMA as the primary monomer. UDM has been more popular in European dental composites. Initially, better adhesion and/or resistance to color change was predicted for the UDM formulations, but clinical studies have not been able to document these advantages.

Matrix monomers can be polymerized in a variety of ways. The original dental composites adopted self-curing chemistry that was typical of dental denture base compositions. These composites have been called *self-cured, chemically cured,* or *two component systems.* Amine accelerators which were used to increase polymerization rates, however, contributed to discoloration after 3 to 5 years of intraoral service. An alternative system then was introduced that used *ultraviolet light (UV light-cured)* to initiate polymerization. The curing units which were required were of limited reliability and presented some safety problems. They, in turn, were replaced with *visible light-cured (VLC,* or *light-cured, LC)* systems.

VLC composites are the most popular today, but their success depends on the access of high-intensity light to cure the matrix material (Fig. 6-55). If the composite thickness exceeds 1.5 to 2 mm, then the light intensity can be inadequate to produce complete curing, especially with darker shades of composite. Filler particles and coloring agents tend to scatter or absorb the curing light in the first 1 to 2 mm of material. Darker shades and microfills are more difficult to cure. Access to interproximal areas is limited and requires special approaches to guarantee adequate light-curing energy. Because of these problems, more and more composite compositions are **dual cured,** combining self-curing and light-curing. The self-curing rate is slow and is designed to cure only those portions that are not adequately light-cured. Another approach is to provide **staged curing.** Often composite finishing is complicated by the relatively hard, fully cured material. By filtering the light from the curing unit during an initial cure, it is possible to produce a soft, partially cured material that can be easily finished. Afterwards, the filter is removed and the dental composite curing is completed with full spectrum visible light.

Composites were originally designed for restoration of Classes III, IV, and V cavity preparations, but are now used in modified forms for many other restorative dentistry applications. Based on their intended application, they can be used in all Classes (I to VI) of restorations, cements, bases, cores, veneers, or repair materials.

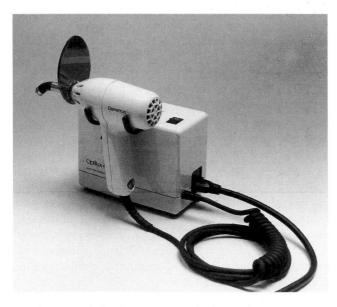

Fig. 6-55. Example of visible light-curing unit for use with dental composites, bonding agents, and other light-curing materials. The main power supply is connected to pistol-grip light gun that generates beam that is passed through fiber optic tube. A shield is supplied to protect against direct observation of high-intensity light at tip.

Composition, structure, and properties. A summary of the composition, structure, and properties of five composite compositions is provided in Table 6-13 as examples of commercially available materials. Note that *as the overall filler content increases, the physical, chemical, and mechanical properties generally improve.*

The physical property of principal concern is the LCTE. As previously stated in the properties section, tooth structure expands and contracts at a linear rate of about 9 to 11 ppm/°C. Unfilled acrylics (such as PMMA) have linear rates of 72 ppm/°C. The LCTE for composites (28 to 45 ppm/°C) may be almost twice as much as the value for dental amalgam (25 ppm/°C) and three to four times greater than that for tooth structure. Thus, during extreme intraoral temperature changes, significant stresses may be generated at the tooth/restoration interfaces where composites are micro-mechanically bonded. If the interfacial bond fails, microleakage may produce unesthetic staining, pulpal sensitivity due to dentinal fluid flow, pulpal irritation due to diffusion of bacterial endotoxins, and/or predisposition toward recurrent caries.

Well-cured dental composites are very resistant to chemical change. However, *most compositions only can be practically cured to levels of 55% to 65% conversion of the reactive monomer sites.* This is partly due to steric hindrance problems during polymerization, and partly due to inadequate energy for forcing the reaction to completion. Both problems can be circumvented in some cases by heating the dental composite (indirect composite inlays) and thus facilitating polymer chain mobility and increasing contacts between unreacted double bonds and growing polymer chain ends. However, this approach is not practical for intraorally-cured composites. In many cases, the poor degree of conversion is due to inadequate curing energy from the VLC unit or from improper positioning of the curing light (Fig. 6-56). Therefore, additional light-curing after the original curing step, termed **post-curing,** improves the degree of conversion.

The composite material which is not reacted may be in the form of partially polymerized or unpolymerized monomer. *Unreacted monomer is capable of diffusing out of the polymer* either into dentin or onto external tooth surfaces. However, most of the unreacted double bonds are pendant groups on partially reacted monomer units and are not diffusable.

Water absorption swells the polymer portion of the dental composite and promotes diffusion and desorption of any unbound monomer. Water with other small molecules potentially plasticize the composite, as well as chemically degrade the matrix into monomer or other derivatives.[119] Beef esterase has been shown to produce chemical decomposition of polymer matrices into formaldehyde and/or low molecular monomer species.[49,106]

Table 6-13. Physical, chemical, and mechanical properties of typical dental composites from 1983-1993*

	Traditional macrofill (Adaptic)	Midifill (Concise)	Heterogeneous microfill: (Silux Plus)	Hybrid minifill (Herculite XR)	Hybrid minifill (TPH)
Components					
Matrix monomer	BIS-GMA	BIS-GMA	BIS-GMA	BIS-GMA	BIS-GMA
Diluent monomer	TEGDMA	TEGDMA	TEGDMA	TEGDMA	TEDGMA
Filler	Quartz	Quartz	Colloidal silica	Colloidal silica, Ba-Al-B-F-Si glass	Ba glass, fumed silica
Filler level (wt%)	78	81	56	76-78	—
Filler level (vol%)	64	68	40	58	—
Average filler diameter (μm)	25-35	8	0.04	0.6	<1.0
Setting reaction	Self-cured	Self-cured	Light-cured	Light-cured	Light-cured
Physical properties					
LCTE (ppm/°C)	31	37	—	26	—
Thermal conductivity	[Insulator]	[Insulator]	[Insulator]	[Insulator]	[Insulator]
Opacity	—	—	—	—	35
Radiopacity (mm Al)	[Poor]	[Fair]	[Poor]	—	3
Chemical properties					
Polymerization shrinkage (%)	—	—	—	—	—
Solubility (% in water)	—	—	—	—	—
Water absorption (%)	—	—	—	—	[Low]
Mechanical properties					
Modulus (MPa)	—	—	—	13,800	—
Knoop hardness (KHN_{100})	—	76	—	—	—
Elongation (percent)	—	—	—	—	—
Compressive strength (MPa)	236	262	355	455	381
Diametral tensile strength (MPa)	—	63	52	60	71
Flexural strength (MPa)	100	111		130	145
Fracture toughness	[Poor]	[Poor]	[Fair]	[Good]	[Good]
Wear resistance	[Poor]	[Poor]	[Excellent]	[Very good]	[Very good]
Biological properties					
Biocompatibility (set materials)	[Acceptable]	[Acceptable]	[Acceptable]	[Acceptable]	[Acceptable]

*Relative properties are shown in brackets. The values reported are from a variety of published sources from 1983-1993, including manufacturer's product bulletins. Comparisons should be made only in terms of the overall application requirements and not in terms of any single property.

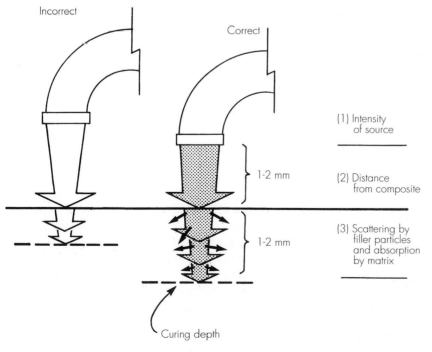

Fig. 6-56. Light intensity variables affecting depth of curing of composite restorations.

The consequences for the properties of the composite are obvious. The biological consequences of small releases of these materials are not known.

Curing efficiency is strongly related to the effectiveness of light energy penetration into the composite (Fig. 6-56). *Visible light-curing* involves light energy in the range of 410 to 500 nm with a peak intensity of about 470 nm. The intensity of light striking the composite depends on the output of the curing light itself and its distance from the composite. The intensity of light striking the composite is inversely proportional to the distance from the tip of the fiber-optic bundle of the curing light to the dental composite surface. Ideally, *the tip should be within 2 mm of the dental composite* to be effective.

All visible light-curing generators should be periodically monitored with a radiometer to ensure that adequate curing output energy is present. The output energy should be about 300 mW/cm² to be assured of adequate composite curing. Primary causes of output failure relate to reduced bulb output and deterioration of internal filters, due to cumulative damage from excess heat.

Composite filler particles tend to scatter the light, and darker colorants tend to absorb the light. Therefore, it is generally *recommended that no more than 1.5 to 2 mm increments be light-cured at a time.*[31,94] Smaller filler particles, in the range of 0.1 to 1 micron, interfere with the light the most which maximizes scattering, because those particle sizes are within the spectrum of wavelengths of the light being used for curing.

To permit closer approximation of the curing light to the composite, **light transmitting wedges** have been promoted for interproximal curing, and **light focusing tips** have become available for access into proximal boxes.[45]

The degree of conversion of monomer-to-polymer is strongly related not only to the intensity of light exposure, but also the duration of exposure. Most light-curing requires a minimum of 20 seconds for adequate curing under optimal conditions of access. To guarantee adequate curing has occurred, it has become common practice to post-cure for 20 to 60 seconds. There is some evidence that this may slightly improve the surface layer properties such as *wear resistance* as well.

There is no clear relationship of clinical performance to any single mechanical property. However, most investigators agree that stronger composites should resist intraoral occlusal stresses better in most situations. Therefore, there is a general consensus that filler contents should be maximized. The material's elastic *modulus* is of concern as well. There is now evidence that teeth deform more than previously suspected.[61] Dental composites with high elastic moduli may not be able to accommodate to some changes in tooth shape associated

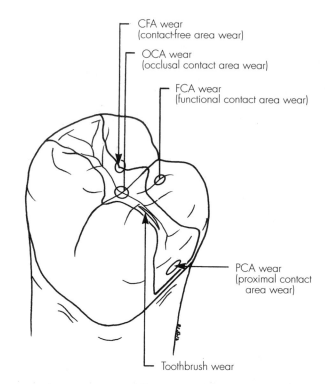

Fig. 6-57. Locations of different types of wear on posterior composite restorations.

with flexural forces. This limitation could result in debonding of the composite restoration from enamel or dentin. This situation is more critical for cervical restorations on facial surfaces where flexural stresses may produce large deformations (see Fig. 6-12). *Flexible restorations (low elastic modulus) would be clinically more retentive because of improved accommodation to flexural forces. The opposite requirement would be true for large MOD restorations. Composites in those cases should be very rigid and thus minimize tooth flexure of remaining cusps.*

Wear resistance of composites on posterior occlusal surfaces has received considerable attention in clinical studies.* There are at least five types (Fig. 6-57) of composite wear events: (1) wear by food (*contact-free area,* or CFA wear), (2) impact by tooth contact in centric (*occlusal contact area,* or OCA wear), (3) sliding by tooth contact in function (*functional contact area,* or FCA wear), (4) rubbing by tooth contact interproximally (*proximal contact area,* or PCA wear), and (5) wear from oral prophylaxis methods (*toothbrush or dentifrice abrasion*). The relative contributions of these processes are poorly understood.

Several mechanisms of wear have been hypothesized based on clinical information collected for contact-free area wear on relatively small posterior occlusal restora-

*References 23,62,74,81,112,164.

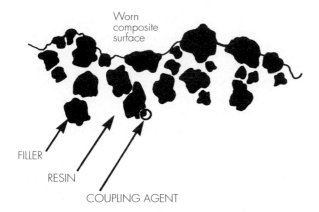

Fig. 6-58. Schematic view of wear of composite restoration. (Courtesy Bayne SC, Taylor DF, Heymann HO: *Dent Mater* 8:305-309, 1992.)

tions. In general, the process of wear is envisioned with respect to failures of the key components shown in Fig. 6-58. The **microfracture theory** proposes that high modulus filler particles are compressed onto the adjacent matrix during occlusal loading and this creates microfractures in the weaker matrix.[75] With the passage of time, these microfractures become connected and surface layers of the composite are exfoliated. The **hydrolysis theory**[148] purports that the silane bond between the resin matrix and filler particle is hydrolytically unstable and becomes debonded. This bond failure allows surface filler particles to be lost. The **chemical degradation theory**[169] supposes that materials from food and saliva are absorbed into the matrix, causing matrix degradation and sloughing from the surface. Finally, the **protection theory**[16,68] proposes that the weak matrix is eroded between the particles.

If a posterior occlusal restoration is narrow enough, occlusal contact wear is significantly reduced or eliminated, and wear is due almost entirely to food bolus contact (CFA wear, Fig. 6-59, *A*). It now appears that CFA wear resistance is not related to composite mechanical strength, but rather to filler spacing. Filler particles are much harder than the polymer matrix, and thus resist wear very well. If filler particles are closely spaced, then they shelter the intervening matrix polymer. This is called **micro-protection** (Fig. 6-59, *B*). In microfilled composites the particles are very small and therefore the inter-particle spacing is very small.[16] As a result, microfills, even with their low filler contents, show very good contact-free wear resistance. However, if their strengths are low, then they do not resist direct tooth contact wear forces very well. Composite restorations with relatively narrow cavity preparations minimize food bolus contact and provide sheltering of the restoration. This process is called **macro-protection** (Fig. 6-59, *A*). The size of the anticipated restoration is a good indication for the discretionary use of posterior composite materials. *If the cavity preparation is narrow, then composites can be used with little concern about wear. If the cavity preparation is wide, and/or is located in a molar tooth (which are most frequently involved in masticating the food bolus), then the restoration will be more susceptible to wear.*

Large, extensive posterior composites that include total occlusal contact coverage are more prone to failure due to both impact (OCA wear) and fatigue (FCA wear).[83,136] If the opponent teeth contact only the dental composite restoration, then undesirable composite

Fig. 6-59. Protection theory of CFA wear. **A,** Macro-protection of composite by sheltering effect of narrow cavity preparation. **B,** Micro-protection of matrix resin by close inter-particle spacing of filler particles. (Courtesy Bayne SC, Taylor DF, Heymann HO: *Dent Mater* 8:305-309, 1992.)

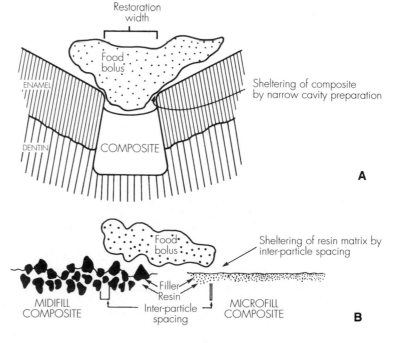

wear usually occurs at those contacts. *However, this process is restricted if there remain centric contacts on enamel elsewhere in the restored tooth.*

Wear resistance of posterior composites has been extensively evaluated in longitudinal clinical studies at the University of North Carolina* and the University of Alabama[74] over 15 years. Results of this research have demonstrated that *microfill composites are the most wear-resistant formulations.* Numerous in vitro wear simulators have been investigated over more than 30 years to try to duplicate the complicated combination of intraoral wear events. Only one device[77] has demonstrated excellent correlation with current clinical results.

Toothbrush (and toothpaste) abrasion of composites is poorly understood. There is no direct evidence from anterior composites that this process occurs other than at very low rates. Still, there exists some intuitive thinking that aggressive tooth brushing may produce significant abrasion.

Clinical considerations. Dental composites are monitored in clinical studies in terms of USPHS (United States Public Health Service) categories[37,137] of interest: color matching, interfacial staining, secondary caries, anatomical form (wear), and marginal integrity.

Color matching depends on not only proper initial color match, but also on the relative changes which occur with time. Both the restoration and tooth structure are known to change in color with age. The assessment is made with the tooth structure properly hydrated. Temporarily drying the tooth structure makes it appear lighter and whiter in color due to dehydration of enamel (refer to the discussion of optical properties in the section, Materials Properties). With time, chemical changes in the matrix polymer cause the dental composite to appear more yellow. This process is accelerated by UV light, oxidation, and moisture. Anterior restorative materials with high matrix contents that are self-cured are more likely to undergo yellowing.[163] Newer systems that are visible light-cured, that contain higher filler contents, and are modified with UV absorbers and anti-oxidants, are more resistant to color change. Even if the composite is relatively color stable, tooth structure undergoes a change in its appearance with time due to dentin darkening from aging. Aged tooth structure appears more opaque and darker yellow. The challenge is to match the rate and type of color change of the restoration with the tooth structure. A color mismatch that appears after several years is difficult to avoid. Dentin is likely to change color most rapidly during middle age (35 to 60 years old).

Another important consideration for esthetics is a gradual transition in color and translucency between the restoration and tooth structure. This goal is accomplished in two ways. *Beveling* the enamel tends to blend any color difference associated with the margin over about 0.5 to 1 mm (depending on the preparation size and requirements for bevel width) rather than making it abrupt. This step is particularly important for anterior restorations. It also produces more surface area for a well-bonded margin that does not leak. Marginal leakage leads to the accumulation of subsurface *interfacial staining* that is difficult or impossible to remove and which creates a marked boundary for the restoration appearance. Restorations which have been properly acid-etched should be well bonded for years. The longevity of micro-mechanical enamel retention is unknown. Likewise the effects of fatigue stresses or other intraoral events are unknown. However, clinical studies as long as 14 years indicate relatively good resistance to interfacial staining.

As long as margins are well bonded and no marginal fractures occur, there should be good resistance to secondary caries. Although not well documented, *most secondary caries seems to occur along proximal or cervical margins* where enamel is thin, less well-oriented for bonding, difficult to access during the restorative procedure, and potentially subject to flexural stresses as well. Only rarely is secondary caries observed along margins on occlusal surfaces or non-cervical aspects of other surfaces. The incidence of caries is quite variable depending on the degree of technical excellence during composite placement. *Clinical research studies indicate that for well-controlled insertion techniques the incidence of secondary caries after 10 years can be as low as 3%.*[20] Under these circumstances, the primary reason for composite failure is poor esthetics or excessive wear. Cross-sectional studies of dental practices that did not strictly conform to recommended techniques indicate that caries levels as high as 25% to 30% have been observed after 10 years for composites placed during the 1970s and early 1980s.

The principal concern for posterior composites has been that occlusal *wear* could occur at a high rate and continue over long periods of time, exposing underlying dentin and leading to secondary caries or sensitivity. There is now excellent evidence from clinical research studies for small- to medium-width restorations that indicates the rate of occlusal wear tends to decrease over time, with total wear approaching an average limiting value of about 250 microns over about 5 years (Fig. 6-60). Wear-resistant composites still wear but take longer to achieve that level of wear. There is only rare evidence that composites actually wear to the point of exposing underlying dentin. Morever, after many years of clinical service, worn restorations can be repaired by rebonding a new surface onto the old composite to replace a worn or discolored surface.

Wear of posterior composite restorations has been

*References 19,62,133,151,153,164.

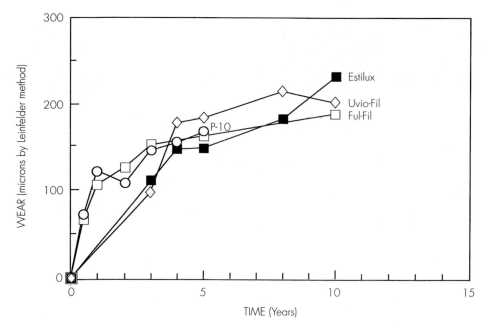

Fig. 6-60. Wear curves for several dental composite materials over 10 years demonstrating decreasing wear due to sheltering from occlusal cavity margins of small restorations. (Derived from Sturdevant et al: *J Dent Res* 71A:204, 1992 (abstract 794); Wilder et al: *J Dent* 19:214-220, 1991.)

compared in references to that for amalgams, but this comparison may be misleading. Occlusal dental amalgams do wear but the wear is gradually compensated by continuing expansion of the restoration. Therefore, the dental amalgam restoration appears to have the same occlusal contour. While this expansion may be a functional advantage, the biological effects of the wear of the dental amalgam are not known.

Marginal integrity of composites is very good under most circumstances. Clinical appearance is affected by the nature of the margin. Butt joint margins emphasize composite wear more than beveled margins. Butt joint margins of well-bonded restorations wear more slowly and create a meniscus appearance against the enamel. As beveled composite margins wear, thinner ledges of material are produced that are prone to fracture.

Bulk fracture of posterior composite restorations is very rare. Although there has been a persistent rumor that microfilled composites are more subject to fracture at OCAs, there is no published evidence of that fact except for a few restorations.[62] While bulk fracture may be the most prevalent failure mechanism for high-copper dental amalgam restorations, it is only rarely observed for intracoronal composite restorations.

Another clinical concern for all filling material procedures has been the onset of *postoperative sensitivity*. Actual causes of this event are poorly researched but are hypothesized to be due either to (1) marginal diffusion of species which induce fluid flow within dentin or (2) dimensional changes of the restoration itself. Contrac-

tion resulting from polymerization shrinkage and/or expansion from water sorption can cause flexure of bonded cusps and produce pain. The incidence of postoperative sensitivity for posterior composite restorations is less than 1%. In most cases, it occurs within the first 6 months to 1 year of the procedure and subsides within 6 months of initial onset. Only rarely must a posterior composite be removed to manage the problem.[11]

There are only limited problems of *biocompatibility* for most composites with respect to the dental pulp. Although the unpolymerized materials are potentially cytotoxic and may even have been classified as carcinogenic, they are very poorly soluble in water and are polymerized into a bound state before there is significant time for dissolution and diffusion. Monomers which do not polymerize may diffuse slowly out of the restoration, but the concentration at any given time is so low that the materials do not appear to represent any practical risk. As noted with mercury migration from dental amalgam restorations, concentration and time are the key factors in assessing biohazards. However, these events still need to be examined more closely. *From long-term clinical studies there is no evidence of any clinical problems resulting in pulp death or soft tissue changes.*

Glass ionomer cements

Terminology and classification. Glass ionomers are materials consisting of ion-crosslinked polymer matrices surrounding glass-reinforcing filler particles. The earliest glass ionomer materials for restorations were based on a solution of polyacrylic acid liquid that was mixed with a complex alumino-silicate powder containing calcium and fluoride. The acidic liquid solution (pH $\leq$ 1.0) dissolved portions of the periphery of the silicate glass particle releasing calcium, aluminum, fluoride, silicon, and other ions. Divalent calcium ions were quickly chelated by ionized carboxyl side groups on polyacrylic acid polymer chains, crosslinking the chains and producing an amorphous polymer gel. During the next 24 to 72 hours, the calcium ions were replaced by more slowly reacting aluminum ions to produce a more highly crosslinked matrix that was stronger.[167] It is now suspected that during the maturation involving aluminum ion crosslinking, silicon ions and unbound water participate in producing an inorganic co-matrix best described as a hydrated silicate.[111]

The same carboxylic acid side groups are also capable of chelating surface ions on the glass particles or calcium ions from tooth structure. *This process generates true chemical bonds at all internal and external interfaces when the reaction conditions are correct.* Set materials have modest properties compared with composites but have relatively good adhesion and the *ability to release fluoride ions* from the matrix for incorporation into neighboring tooth structure to suppress dental caries. The perceived *advantages of adhesion and fluoride release* have driven more than 20 years of intense research to improve glass ionomer products to the point of being competitive with other restorative materials options.

Historical development. The design of the original glass ionomer cements was a hybrid formulation of silicate and polycarboxylate cements. Glass ionomers used the aluminosilicate powder from silicates and the polyacrylic acid liquid of polycarboxylates. The earliest commercial product was named using the acronym for this hybrid formulation and was called ASPA (aluminosilicate polyacrylic acid). The different types of compositions and variables which have been explored subsequently are summarized in Box 6-2. A schematic of the variety of chemical reactions involved in the setting and adhesion of glass ionomer compositions is shown in Fig. 6-61.

A significant number of liquid and powder modifications were soon made to improve the physical, chemical, and mechanical properties. Despite these changes, however, these *early materials were very technique sensitive.* Mixing, placement, and early intraoral conditions were critical to the properties achieved.[103,104]

The original polyacrylic acid in the liquid component was modified by co-polymerization with different amounts of maleic acid, itaconic acid, and/or tartaric acid to increase the stability of the liquid and modify its reactivity. Powder particles were reduced in size. At the

---

Box 6-2. Variety of compositions and changes in the evolution of glass ionomer materials

1. Traditional glass ionomers: (liners, bases, cements)
   a. Modifications by adding co-monomers to polyacrylic acid
   b. Smaller powder particle size
   c. Experimentation with dehydrated liquid component
2. Metal-modified glass ionomers: (filling materials, bases, cores)
   a. Miracle mixtures (with amalgam alloy admixed with cement)
   b. Cermet particle reinforcement
3. Light-cured glass ionomers: (liners, bases)
   a. HEMA added to liquid component
      Polymers in liquid modified with acrylic functional groups
   b. Other powder particles mixed with alumino-silicate glass
4. Hybrid (resin-modified) glass ionomers: (cements, restorative filling materials, cores)
   a. HEMA and other polymers added to liquid component
   b. Polymers and other phases added to powder component
   c. Silicate glass of composites substitued for some of powder
   d. Pre-cured glass ionomer blended into composites

---

same time, the powder was modified by incorporating additional types of powder particles for reinforcement. Ag-Sn particles (amalgam alloy particles) were admixed in some formulations to produce an amalgam substitute. This combination[140] became known as the *"miracle mixture,"* because it was initially introduced during the early 1980s at the time when the mercury controversy was increasing dentists' questions about the safety of dental amalgams. However, the properties of miracle mixtures were far inferior to dental amalgam, and it has not been well-received as a restorative material. In part, the problem with the admixture was that the matrix would not strongly adhere to the Ag-Sn alloy particles.

To circumvent this difficulty, Ag-Pd was substituted. Ag-Pd generates a passivating oxide film of PdO which is chemically reactive by chelation with polyacrylic acid. These mixtures, termed ceramic-metal *(cermets)* mixtures (Fig. 6-61, *B*), were much stronger than unmodified glass ionomer cements, but had poor esthetics and could not be highly modified or else they would not set as well.

In the face of limited success with these modifications, glass ionomer compositions were promoted for less demanding applications, such as *liners, bases, cements, cores, and root canal filling materials* rather than as restoration materials. During the 1980s the utilization of glass ionomers for such applications increased. However, glass ionomers were plagued by

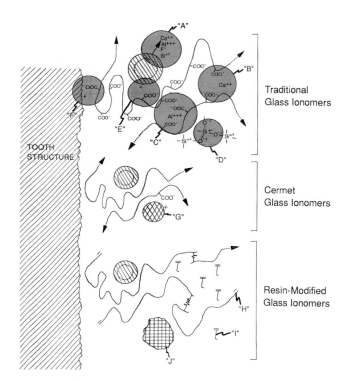

Traditional
Glass Ionomers

Cermet
Glass Ionomers

Resin-Modified
Glass Ionomers

Fig. 6-61. Schematic view of setting and adhesion reactions for a variety of glass ionomer compositions. Traditional glass ionomers: *(A)* Ions released from periphery of alumino-silicate glass particle by acid liquid. *(B)* Divalent Ca ions initially crosslink adjacent carboxyl ions on polymer chains to cause setting. *(C)* Trivalent Al ions gradually replace divalent Ca ions and form tighter network of crosslinks between polymer chains. *(D)* Si ions react with available water and form covalent silicate network. *(E)* Pendant carboxyl groups on polymer chains chelate surface ions on powder particles to produce internal bonding. *(F)* Pendant carboxyl groups on polymer chains chelate surface ions on tooth structure to produce chemical bonding. Glass ionomers that are metal-modified for mechanical reinforcement: *(G)* Cermet filler particles with ceramic coatings are bonded to pendant carboxyl groups on polymer chains. Hybrid or resin-modified glass ionomers: *(H)* Acrylic functional modifications of polymer allow light curing to cause initial crosslinking. *(I)* Water soluble monomers added for polymerization during light-curing reactions. *(J)* Resin, silica, or composite filler particles added as modifiers.

technique sensitivities due to mixing requirements, potential problems with postoperative sensitivity, and the need for moisture protection to prevent surface degradation before the secondary setting reaction was completed. With careful attention to procedural details, glass ionomers were proven clinically successful in many applications.[103] However, in restorative filling applications, glass ionomers were not as esthetic as dental composites.

There have been recent modifications that replace part or most of the original formulation with alternative filler particles and/or matrix setting reactions to make

these materials *more composite-like* (Fig. 6-61, *H-J*).[97] These materials are categorized as **hybrid** or **resin-modified glass ionomers.** *They are light-cured, less technique sensitive, and may be finished at the time of placement.* As these modifications were made, the new formulations came to look very much like composite formulations. Because resin-modified glass ionomers are significantly stronger than the original glass ionomers, they are recommended for Class V restorations and Classes I and II restorations in primary teeth.

Composition, structure, and properties. Examples of some glass ionomer cements, glass ionomer cermets, and resin-modified glass ionomers are listed in Table 6-14 along with key properties.

Clinical considerations. The mainstay arguments for glass ionomer use are *chemical adhesion* and *fluoride release.* Despite intuitive belief in benefits due to these properties, there is little or no clinical evidence that these products produce better restorations than systems based on composites. Relative advantages of these two factors and other considerations are discussed in this section.

Adhesion of conventional glass ionomers (not resin-modified) to enamel and/or dentin only produces bond strengths in the range of 6 to 12 MPa. By comparison, dentin bonding agents now can produce bond strengths of 22 to 35 MPa. Most glass ionomers are aqueous systems (before setting) that wet tooth structure very well because they are hydrophilic. However, glass ionomers tend to have relatively high viscosities and therefore do not flow and adapt to micro-mechanical spaces very readily. In contrast, bonding agents are hydrophobic but have been formulated for use with hydrophilic primers to facilitate wetting, flow, and bonding. Bonding by glass ionomers is achieved in part by mechanical retention and in part by chemical chelation. Although there always has been enchantment with chemical bonding for dental systems, the bond density per unit area of retentive interface is actually higher for mechanical bonding than for chemical bonding. Excellent bonding cannot be achieved by chemical bonding alone. In most cases, *good mechanical bonding is much more important than chemical bonding. Thus, the potential of glass ionomers for chemical bonding* is only an advantage in situations where it is difficult or impossible to produce micro-mechanical retention.

Historically, there was widespread evidence that there was little or no secondary caries associated with fluoride-containing silicate cement restorations despite significant marginal disintegration during restoration solubilization. That same success is expected with glass ionomers, but the pattern has never been directly demonstrated. There are two points which limit the influence of fluoride ion release. First, fluoride ion release is proportional to the concentration which can diffuse

way for more than a century, the process is tedious, demanding, and relatively expensive for the patient. These reasons, in addition to the fact that the restoration is not entirely trouble free, has resulted in disuse of this technique by most general practitioners.

Terminology and classification. Gold for direct filling restorations may be classified on the basis of (1) the geometric form in which it is supplied, (2) the surface condition of the piece, and (3) the microstructure of the piece. It may be supplied as *ropes, sheets, strips,* or *pellets* (Chapter 20). The surface condition is described as **cohesive** (clean) or **non-cohesive** (containing adsorbed gas). To prevent unwanted adsorption of hard-to-remove gases, the piece may be intentionally protected by ammonia gas adsorption. At the time of use, the ammonia layer is removed easily by properly heating the piece, making it cohesive once again. Different microstructural conditions are possible in forms referred to as **gold foil, mat gold,** or **powdered gold.**

Composition, structure, and properties. Direct gold is essentially 100% gold. Pre-alloying with other elements would reduce the weldability and malleability at room temperature. However, other elements may be incorporated (platinum or calcium) indirectly into the final structure by layering them onto the gold in forms such as gold foils.

During cold welding, much greater compaction pressures are required to remove pores or spaces in mat gold and powdered golds than in gold foil. However, these other forms are often used because they reduce the time required to build up a restoration. Restorations of mat or powdered golds are never quite as dense as those made from gold foil, and therefore, the former have lower flexural strengths. The theoretical density for defect-free pure gold is 19.3 gm/cm^3, but as can be seen by reference to Fig. 6-64, final restorations range from 14.3 to 15.9 gm/cm^3.

Clinical considerations. The LCTE of gold is 16.2 ppm/°C, which is closer to tooth structure (9 to 11 ppm/°C) than all other currently available direct filling materials except for traditional glass ionomer cement. There is very little differential expansion at the margins of the restoration and percolation is not a problem.

Placing a liner or base may result in compaction and welding problems. Gold foil is not indicated for restoring extensive lesions. Sometimes there is pulpal sensitivity to a thermal stimulus because of gold's high conductivity. However, usually this ceases after several months.

Direct filling gold restorations have transverse strength that is significantly lower than that for cast alloys (five to six times lower) and less than that for tooth structure (two times lower). Because direct gold has a low elastic limit, large restorations cannot adequately distribute occlusal stresses without plastic deformation.

Another major disadvantage is that direct filling gold

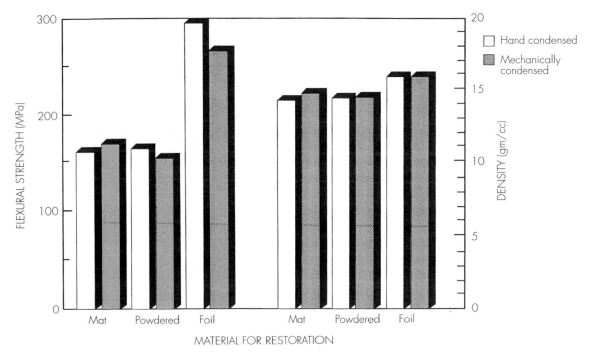

Fig. 6-64. Bar graph comparing the flexural strengths and densities of differenct direct filling golds for conditions of hand condensing versus mechanical condensing for cold welding. (Derived from Skinner EW, Phillips RW. In *Science of dental materials,* ed 6, Philadelphia, 1967, WB Saunders.)

restorations are not adhesive to tooth structure. Therefore, they cannot function to reinforce tooth structure in a manner similar to that for strong, properly bonded composites or bonded ceramic restorations.

Finally, gold foil is not an esthetic restorative material. Most patients are less than pleased by its appearance.

INDIRECT RESTORATIVE DENTAL MATERIALS
Introduction

Traditional stages of fabricating dental restorations by indirect restorative techniques involve impressions, dies, wax patterns, investing, casting or molding, finishing and polishing, and cementing. CAD/CAM approaches are possible as well and are discussed in a later section, Machined Restorations. Because of the multiple stages of these techniques, errors that enter into the procedures at any point tend to be compounded and carried into the next stage. It is important to faithfully adhere to the procedural details of all of the stages, or else the final restoration will not fit. Those clinical procedures that involve impression materials, choice of restorative materials, and cementing of restorations are discussed in Chapters 17, 18, and 19. The rationale for these procedural choices are discussed in this section in a limited way.

Impression materials

Terminology and classification. Impression materials are used to record the surface topography and detail of hard and soft tissues, and thereby produce a mold for making a replica (cast) of those structures. There are nine types of impression materials that have been used historically in dentistry. Their generic compositions, common names, and key clinical properties are summarized in Table 6-15.

Plaster, compound, and *ZOE* are rigid solids that are incapable of being removed directly from undercut areas of hard or soft tissues. Therefore, they have limited use for dentulous patients. *Alginate (irreversible hydrocolloid)* and *reversible hydrocolloid (agar-agar)* are elastic and have the advantage of wetting intraoral surfaces well, but have very limited dimensional stability because they include as much as 85% water in their composition. *Polysulfide (rubber base, Thiokol rubber), silicone (condensation silicone, conventional silicone), polyether,* and *polyvinyl siloxane (vinyl polysiloxane, addition silicone, addition polydimethyl siloxane)* are non-aqueous polymer-based rubber impression materials that have good elasticity (see Table 6-15). They are listed in order of development. Polyvinyl siloxane is now the most widely used.

Composition, structure, and properties. To be totally effective, an impression material must be fluid before setting, be hydrophilic to wet intraoral surfaces, undergo complete conversion to an elastic solid, be highly elastic to prevent permanent distortion during removal, be sterilizable, be dimensionally stable, and be compatible with the cast material. To meet these mechanical requirements, the most common approach to formulating an impression material is as a composite with a flexible matrix.

Elastomeric polymer matrices are produced by polymerizing fluid monomer and/or oligomer mixtures by either stepwise polymerization or chain reaction polymerization reactions. Polysulfide, condensation silicones, and polyether impression materials involve *stepwise polymerization.*

Stepwise reactions are relatively slow and do not go to completion for several hours. About 65% to 85% conversion occurs within 6 to 8 minutes during initial setting before a dental impression is removed from the mouth. As long as the impression is in the mouth, the shrinkage is confined to noncritical areas because the intraoral surfaces restrain the impression material. After removal, the impression experiences more shrinkage as the polymerization continues. Although these materials are elastic, the elastic recovery is viscoelastic and requires 20 to 30 minutes to reach a point of accurately returning to the intraoral dimensions that are being duplicated. During this pause for elastic recovery, continued polymerization can distort the impression size and shape. To minimize these effects, high levels of fillers

---

Table 6-15. Classification of dental impression materials

Type (and synonyms)	Mechanical behavior	Setting reaction
Impression plaster	Rigid	Chemical (Irreversible)
Impression compound	Rigid	Physical (Reversible)
Zinc oxide–Eugenol (ZOE)	Rigid	Chemical (Irreversible)
Alginate (irreversible hydrocolloid)	Flexible	Chemical (Irreversible)
Agar-Agar (reversible hydrocolloid)	Flexible	Physical (Reversible)
Polysulfide (rubber base, thiokol rubber)	Flexible	Chemical (Irreversible)
Silicone (conventional silicone, condensation silicone)	Flexible	Chemical (Irreversible)
Polyether	Flexible	Chemical (Irreversible)
Polyvinyl siloxane (vinyl polysiloxane, addition silicone)	Flexible	Chemical (Irreversible)

are incorporated in the matrix. Filler levels vary between 15 and 60 weight percent and are chosen on the basis of being compatible with the matrix material and inexpensive.

Portions of the impression that must record fine details of the tooth structure are normally impressed with the least-filled formulations (light-bodied material) so that there is maximal flow and adaptation to intraoral structure before curing. However, the bulk of the impression is the highly filled material (heavy bodied material) to minimize shrinkage contributions to inaccuracy. Examples of the relative degree of dimensional change versus filler content and material types are reported in Fig. 6-65.

Polyvinyl siloxane undergoes a chain reaction polymerization (which is also an addition reaction) during setting that is fast, goes almost to completion, and does not generate condensation by-products. This characteristic provides a major advantage for these materials compared with other elastic impression materials. Once the impression is removed, it is dimensionally stable, and the casts which will be fabricated from the impression can be produced at any time. In the case of the other rubber elastic impression materials, the impression should be poured immediately after pausing 20 to 30 minutes for viscoelastic recovery.

Polyvinyl siloxanes commonly use exotic curing systems based on chloroplatinic acid. During the reaction, the acid decomposes and generates small amounts of hydrogen gas as a by-product. Early versions of polyvinyl siloxane were plagued by gas bubble formation that ruined casts poured in the impressions unless 24 to 48 hours were permitted for out-gassing. However, newer materials contain hydrogen scavengers that react with and tie up the hydrogen by-products.

Clinical considerations. The most significant clinical consideration when using an elastic impression material is the ***rate of removal*** of the initially set impression. All polymer-based materials are *strain rate sensitive*. If they are stressed quickly, they behave as though they are stronger and more elastic than if stressed slowly. Therefore, elastic impression materials should be removed from intraoral surfaces with a relatively rapid motion. The objective is to minimize the time that the impression is distorted. This approach prevents conversion of mechanical energy into plastic rather than elastic deformation. Teasing or slowly deforming an impression produces unwanted plastic deformation and introduces inaccuracies into both the final impression and resulting cast.

Properties of impression materials influence not only clinical techniques, but also preparation of casts and dies. Hydrophobic impressions are not wet well by water-based cast and die materials. ***Wetting agents*** are used to avert air entrapment in detailed areas under these conditions. A final mechanical property of the impression material dictates ease of cast removal. The stiffness of impressions (e.g., polyether material) can cause breakage of thin "teeth" of the cast.

The impression must remain accurate while being

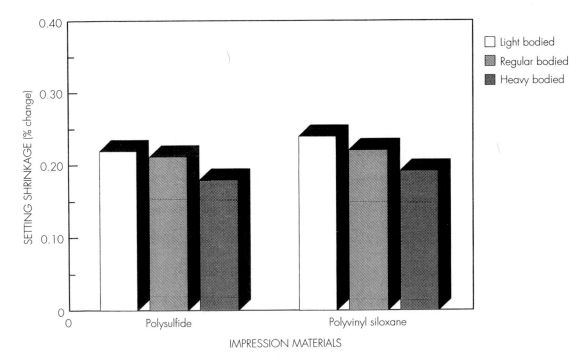

Fig. 6-65. Examples of setting shrinkage of polysulfide and polyviny siloxane impression materials for light, regular, and heavy bodied consistencies. (Derived from Eames et al: *J Prosthet Dent* 42:159-162, 1979.)

disinfected. See Chapter 4 for *infection control of the impression* and related items.

Cast metal restorations

Creation of a cast metal restoration involves a chain of stages from waxing on a die a pattern of the intended final restoration, investing the pattern to create a mold space for casting, casting the restoration, finishing and polishing the casting, and cementing the restoration intraorally. Because of the complexity of this sequence, properties desirable for a casting alloy are as much governed by technique limitations as by the final intraoral service considerations. Each of these is addressed in the following paragraphs.

Terminology. Cast metal may be used to form the entire restoration or may be designed as a substructure and veneered with porcelain to create a tooth-colored restoration. Those that are veneered with porcelain may be generically described as *porcelain-bonded-to-metal* (PBM), *ceramic-bonded-to-metal* (CBM) or *porcelain-fused-to-metal* (PFM) restorations. For successful porcelain application, the metal alloy must have a relatively high melting point in order to tolerate the high firing temperatures without sagging or melting. The melting temperature of restorations that are all metal (without porcelain) can be any temperature that can be conveniently processed.

Classification. *Corrosion resistance* is an essential characteristic of dental casting alloys. These alloys are categorized in terms of their (1) mechanism of corrosion resistance and (2) main elements in the composition affecting the corrosion resistance (see next section, Composition, Structure, and Properties). Corrosion resistance is achieved with either *immune* or *passivating* alloy systems. For dentistry, immune systems are divided into *gold systems* and *gold substitute systems*. Passivating systems are divided into *Ni-Cr, Co-Cr, Fe-Cr,* and *Ti* systems.

Many of the terms relating to corrosion resistance have very special meanings. *Noble metal alloys* are very resistant to both corrosion and electrochemical corrosion. These systems are based on gold, platinum, palladium, rhodium, iridium, ruthenium, and/or osmium. *Precious metal alloys* contain metals of high economic value and, as a group, traditionally include all of the noble metals and silver. *Low-gold alloys* contain only 3 to 50 weight percent gold or other noble metal elements. If less than half (75 weight percent) of the atoms in a gold alloy are corrosion-resistant ones (Au, Pt, or Pd), the overall corrosion resistance decreases dramatically. Low-gold alloys are attempts at producing lower cost alloys that still retain some of the qualities of premium-priced gold-based alloys. However, the actual quantity of gold may be deceptively low.

Gold substitute alloys are precious metal alloys that do not contain gold. The best examples are Ag-Pd systems and other Pd alloys.

Base metal alloys are based on active metallic elements that corrode but which develop corrosion resistance via surface oxidation that produces a thin, tightly adherent film which inhibits further corrosion. Alloys are formulated with 18% to 28% by weight Cr which produces films of Cr_2O_3 that passivate the surface. The films are brittle and may be ruptured but re-form immediately if sufficient Cr remains locally in the composition. Oxidation of other elements such as Ni and Co also produce superficial oxides, but Cr_2O_3 is principally responsible for the corrosion resistance. Ti (and Ti-6Al-4V) alloy is widely used in dentistry for implant systems, because it passivates by forming TiO_2, is biocompatible, and permits osseointegration with bone.

Composition, structure, and properties of gold castings. Cast restorations are constructed traditionally from gold alloys because of their potentially excellent corrosion resistance. In the nineteenth century, gold coins had been used as the source of alloy for casting restorations. Standardization of casting materials occurred in the 1930s. Dental gold casting alloys were defined in terms of their relative noble metal concentration, physical properties (fusion temperature), and mechanical properties (hardness, elongation, and yield point). The original *ADA classification system* defined Types A, B, and C gold alloys.[154] This specification was then revised and extended to include four types (I, II, III, IV) of alloys. Types I, II, and III corresponded to the original Types A, B, and C, while Type IV included higher strength alloys.[3] These four alloy types contain $\geq$ 83%, 78%, 78%, or 75% noble metal elements, respectively, of which gold is the principal one. Types I and II alloys are not capable of being heat treated, while Types III and IV alloys are. *Type I* compositions are intended for small inlays which do not involve significant occlusal loads. *Type II* alloys are for inlays and onlays. *Type III* alloys are for onlays and crowns. *Type IV* alloys are for crowns, bridges, and removable partial dentures.

The *major elemental components of gold casting alloys* are listed in Table 6-16 for several commercial products. Gold is primarily responsible for producing corrosion resistance but it also is relatively soft and requires other alloying element additions to *solution-harden* the composition. *Copper* is the primary alloying element which increases the hardness of the material. However, copper also tends to make the color less yellow and more orange. *Silver* is added to offset the color contributions of copper. *Palladium* is added to increase the hardness of the alloy and has a strong whitening effect on the color. Both palladium and *platinum* tend to raise the melting range for the alloy. Finally, *zinc* is added as a processing aid to scavenge oxygen at the surface of a melt and prevent oxidation and loss of other key elements during the casting procedure.

In recent years, the relatively high cost of gold has

Table 6-16. Objectives for alloying the components of gold casting alloys

Alloying element	(Chemical symbol)	Major contribution to casting alloy	Density, gm/cm³	Melting point (°C)	Corrosion behavior
Gold	(Au)	Corrosion resistance	19.28	1063	Immune
Copper	(Cu)	Solution hardening	8.93	1083	Active
Silver	(Ag)	Counteract orange color of copper	10.50	961	Active
Palladium	(Pd)	Increase hardness; elevate melting range	12.02	1552	Immune
Platinum	(Pt)	Elevate melting range	21.45	1769	Immune
Zinc	(Zn)	Scavenge oxygen during processing	7.14	420	Active

prompted increased use of low-gold, gold substitute, and **base metal alloys** for dental castings. Cast partial dentures are almost exclusively made of *base metal alloy*. Many full crowns and fixed bridges are made of palladium-based **gold substitute alloys,** but the mechanical properties of these materials make them difficult to fabricate into inlays and onlays. However, gradual improvement in the materials has made the **low-gold alloys** acceptable for selective use for these applications. *A number of products containing about 50 weight percent of gold have been introduced that exhibit acceptable tarnish resistance and adequate properties, if extensive marginal burnishing is not required.*

Key properties for casting alloys are reported in Table 6-17. A low melting range is desirable for simplified heating and casting procedures. Moderately high density is advantageous, because most dental alloys are normally cast by centrifugal force casting machines. High density helps to force the alloy quickly into the intricate details of the pattern within the casting mold before cooling solidifies the material. Gold-based alloys are much better in this regard than most other alloys. Finally, a low coefficient of thermal expansion helps to reduce the shrinkage which occurs from the solidus temperature down to room temperature. Because cooling produces shrinkage, there must be some expansion somewhere else in the technique sequence to compensate for dimensional changes upon cooling. Alloys with

Table 6-17. Properties of typical gold casting alloys*

Representative alloy (supplier)	Pentron I (Pentron)	Modulay (Jelenko)	Firmalay (Jelenko)	Sterngold 100 (Sterngold)
Composition (wt%)				
Au	84.0	77.0	74.5	60.0
Cu	Balance	Balance	Balance	Balance
Ag	12.0	14.0	11.0	19.0
Pt	—	—	—	—
Pd	1.0	1.0	3.5	4.0
Zn	<1	<1	<1	<1
Classification				
Gold content	High gold	High gold	High gold	High gold
ADA type	I	II	III	IV
Physical properties				
Color	Gold	Gold	Gold	Gold
LCTE (ppm/°C)	[14-18]	[14-18]	[14-18]	[14-18]
Density (gm/cm³)	16.60	15.90	15.50	13.90
Chemical properties				
Corrosion resistance	[Excellent]	[Excellent]	[Excellent]	[Excellent]
Tarnish resistance	[Good]	[Good]	[Good]	[Good]
Mechanical properties				
Modulus (MPa)	—	—	—	—
Elongation (%)	0-22	0-38	19-39	4-25
Hardness (BHN, soft/hard)	68/—	101/—	110/165	150/257
Compressive strength (MPa)	—	—	—	—
Tensile strength (MPa)	—	—	—	—
Biological properties				
Biocompatibility	[Acceptable]	[Acceptable]	[Acceptable]	[Acceptable]

*Relative properties are shown in brackets.

low coefficients of thermal contraction and which possess low melting temperatures can be controlled more easily.

Certainly the **primary chemical property** *of concern is the corrosion resistance*. To achieve this quality it is desirable that the entire alloy be a single phase composition. Two phase compositions will be prone to local galvanic (structure-selective) corrosion. Types I, II, and III compositions are **single phase** alloys. Type IV compositions may include **two phases.** There is a mechanical advantage with a second phase due to a hardening effect, but that benefit must be weighed against the loss of some corrosion resistance. Contamination or improper casting of gold-based alloys can produce unwanted phases that compromise both the mechanical properties and the corrosion resistance.

The **primary mechanical properties** *of interest for the final cast restoration are a high modulus of elasticity* **(stiffness)** *and a high elastic limit* **(hardness)** *to resist deformation in service*. However, these are not necessarily desirable properties during the fabrication of the restoration. Laboratory procedures such as finishing, polishing, and burnishing are more complicated if the restoration has a high resistance to plastic deformation (high hardness). During these processes, it is important for the casting metal near the margins to be adapted closely to the die (but without damaging the die) by minimal mechanical deformation **(burnishing).** Marginal gaps that exceed 0.1 mm should not be burnished. Rather the casting should be remade. Alloys with a high percentage elongation and a low yield point (low hardness) facilitate burnishing. After these procedures are complete, it is desirable to increase the overall hardness to high levels for clinical service. This goal can be accomplished with Types III and IV ADA gold alloys, which are heat-treatable. The *heat treatment* produces disorder-order and/or spinodal hardening processes.

Cast alloys should not produce toxic reaction products or release toxic elements from their surfaces. Immune and passive alloys appear to have excellent **biological properties.** However, there are some casting alloys that are active and which generate soluble corrosion products. Although the restorations look unchanged, soluble products which are toxic can be released.

Clinical considerations. The three principal clinical considerations for long-term success of cast restorations are *close fit, corrosion resistance, and retention*. Sturdevant *et al*[152] and Morris[102] have shown that gold-based alloys demonstrate excellent corrosion resistance for at least 10 years. *If the cemented restorations have a close fit* (within 20 μm) *and the cavity preparations are adequately designed, then the conventional dental cements resist degradation and provide excellent retention and service for 20 to 40 years.*

Retention and service life of cast restorations are produced by a combination of factors, such as the taper of the cavity preparation, stress distribution design of the cavity preparation to protect remaining tooth structure against fracture (see Enhancing Retention and Resistance Forms, in Chapter 19), the cement type, surface roughness on the internal aspects of the restoration, and potential micro-mechanical or chemical bonding of cement with the restoration and tooth structure. Under most circumstances the restoration surface for gold-based alloys is not well-suited to cement adhesion. The gold alloy surfaces are not wet well with cements and do not have the potential to be chemically bonded by existing formulations. However, *if the internal surfaces are sandblasted, then sufficient micro-mechanical irregularities are produced to permit excellent luting*. Tin or other metal plating also can be used as a surface modification which is chemically reactive toward some cements.

In some cases, such as Maryland bridges, the retention of the casting is dependent on well-developed micro-mechanical spaces along the bonded surfaces of enamel and the casting. The retentive surface of the casting is accomplished by choosing a two-phase dental casting alloy. The metal surface to be bonded is then relieved by chemical or electrolytic etching of one phase in preference to the other. The relieved surface is micro-mechanically interlocked with composite cement onto etched tooth structure.

Dental cements

Traditional dental cements are based on reactions between acidic liquids and basic powders to produce reaction product salts that form a solid matrix surrounding residual powder particles. Microscopically, these cements are classic examples of composite structures. Newer cements are formulated as modified versions of materials originally developed as dental composite restorative materials. In all cements, the properties of interest are governed by the extent to which the matrix is minimized in the final material.

Terminology and classification. Traditional dental cements are listed in Table 6-18 along with identification of the major powder and liquid components and the reaction products. *ZOE, reinforced ZOE, ZOE-EBA, silicate,* and *zinc silicophosphate cements* are no longer routinely used to permanently cement restorations. *Zinc phosphate* cement has been extensively replaced by *polycarboxylate* or *glass ionomer cements*.[28] The latter two are based on ion-crosslinked polyacrylic acid matrices that have the potential to react chemically with residual powder particles and the surface of tooth structure.

Polycarboxylate cement was developed in the 1960s by Dennis Smith in an effort to circumvent potential

Table 6-18. Summary of dental cement classifications, abbreviations, reactants, and reaction products

Classification by components	Abbreviation	Liquid components	Powder components	Reaction product matrix
1. Zinc oxide/eugenol				
a. Unmodified	ZOE	Eugenol	ZnO	Crystalline zinc eugenolate
b. Reinforced	ZOE-Reinf	Eugenol	ZnO, polymer, rosin	Crystalline zinc eugenolate
c. ZOE-EBA	EBA	Eugenol, EBA	ZnO, Al_2O_3, rosin	Crystalline zinc eugenolate; zinc ethoxybenzoate
2. Hexyl vanillate*	HV-EBA	HV, EBA	ZnO, Al_2O_3, rosin	Zinc hexyl vanillate; zinc ethoxybenzoate
3. Zinc phosphate	ZP	H_3PO_4, H_2O	ZnO	Tertiary zinc phosphate crystals
4. Silicate	SC	H_3PO_4, H_2O	F-Al-silicate glass	Amorphous silicophosphate
5. Zinc silico-phosphate	ZSP	H_3PO_4, H_2O	ZnO, F-Al-silicate glass	Amorphous zinc phosphate and silicophosphate
6. Polycarboxylate	PC	Polyacrylic acid, H_2O	ZnO	Zinc polyacrylate gel
7. Glass ionomer				
a. Conventional	GI	Polyacrylic acid, H_2O	F-Al-silicate glass	Aluminum polyacrylate gel; silicate gel
b. Light cured	LC-GI	Polyacrylic acid, H_2O, monomers	F-Al-silicate glass	Aluminum polyacrylate gel; silicate gel; crosslinked polymer
b. Resin modified (hybrid)	RGI	Polyacrylic acid, H_2O, monomers	F-Al-silicate glass; resin	Aluminum polyacrylate gel; silicate gel; crosslinked polymer
8. Calcium hydroxide	CH	Phenolic esters	$Ca(OH)_2$	Calcium chelates
9. Composite	COM	(monomers)	(Silica fillers)	Crosslinked polymer

*Experimental

pulpal problems associated with the low pH of traditional cements and biocompatibility problems related to the mobility of small acidic ions. By choosing an acid-functional polymer as a substitute for phosphoric acid in forming the matrix, it was also possible to produce cements that could adhere via chelation to dental surfaces. The original acid-functional polymer was polyacrylic acid. However, in most current commercial products there are several comonomers involved in the polymer and it is technically more correct to refer to the polymer as a *polyalkenoate.* Cements based on solutions of these polymers (i.e., polycarboxylate or glass ionomer cements) may be called *polyalkenoic cements.*

Glass ionomer cements are hybrids of silicate and polycarboxylate cements designed to combine the optical and fluoride-releasing properties of silicate particles with the chemically adhesive and more biocompatible characteristics of the polyacrylic acid matrix compared with the extremely acidic matrix of silicate cement.

Although dental cements are most often used for *luting* indirect restorations, they also may be used as bases. As *luting agents, the most important clinical requirements are flow, wetting, and film thickness.* To enhance flow, the materials are mixed at relatively low powder-to-liquid ratios. To guarantee that a film thickness of less than 25 microns can be produced, cement particles of 5 microns or less in diameter should be used. The actual film thickness that is achieved ranges from 20 to 100 microns and depends on (1) the viscos-

ity of the mixture and (2) the availability of space for displacement of the cement (as discussed in the next section). Although low powder-to-liquid ratios produce low viscosities for luting agents, cements used for *bases* should be mechanically stronger and are mixed with the maximum powder content that is manageable.

Composition, structure, and properties. Final properties of dental cements depend on the powder-to-liquid ratios used during mixing. Higher powder-to-liquid ratios not only increase the mechanical strength, but also increase the viscosity and reduce wetting and flow. The final matrices of the set cement are indicated in Table 6-18. Details of the cementing procedures are presented in Chapters 17, 18, and 19. A brief summary of dental cement properties is reported in Table 6-19.

Cements are routinely evaluated for their solubility and disintegration in laboratory tests. No laboratory tests or pseudo-clinical tests of restorations have ever been correlated with clinical performance categories, such as retention. A unique clinical research study was performed at the University of Michigan by Silvey and Myers[139] to compare zinc phosphate, reinforced zinc oxide–eugenol, and polycarboxylate cements for retention of crowns and bridges over 7 years. There was practically no difference in failure rates (ZP = 2%, ZOE-EBA = 8%, PC = 5%) and no differences were statistically significant. Mechanisms of failure for these materials are not well-understood.

Clinical considerations. Zinc phosphate cements

Table 6-19. Characteristic properties of categories of luting dental cements*

	ZOE-Rein	EBA	ZP	ZSP	PC	GI	COM
Working characteristics							
P/L ratio	[Low]	[Low]	[Low]	[Low]	[Low]	[Low]	[Low]
Film thickness (μm, ADA flow test)	32	25	18	25	21	24	10-60
Setting time range (minutes)	6-8	—	5-7	—	2-3	3-5	—
Physical properties							
LCTE (ppm/°C)	[Low]	[Low]	[Low]	[Low]	—	—	50
Thermal conductivity	[Low]	[Low]	[Low]	[Low]	[Low]	[Low]	[Low]
Chemical properties							
Solubility/disintegration (%, ADA test)	0.08	0.05	0.06	0.40	0.60	1.25	0-0.01
Mechanical properties							
Compressive strength (MPa)	48	55	100	145	55	86	66
Diametral tensile strength (MPa)	4	4	5	8	6	6	—
Biological properties							
Pulpal response	[Mild]	[Mild]	[Moderate]	[Moderate]	[Mild]	[Mild]	—

*Relative values are shown in brackets. See Table 6-18 for abbreviations for cements. These values are representative of a wide range of possible values.

have the potential during setting to release components from the acid-rich matrix into dentin and irritate the pulp. Therefore, when using zinc phosphate cement, dentin is routinely protected with cavity varnish. However, other cements that can chemically bond to dentin must be allowed to come into direct contact with that surface. *Thus, varnishes should not be used to coat dentin if a polycarboxylate or glass ionomer cement is to be used.* When bonding composite or ceramic restorations, the dentin should not be varnished because bonding requires conditioning of all cavity walls (see Chapter 17).

Cement displacement is a key factor for successfully cementing restorations. The process is an *hydraulic* (liquid in motion) one, dependent on *rapid flow* and escape of excess cement from between the restoration and cavity preparation during cementation. To produce cement flow, *loading* must be applied rapidly, at sufficiently high levels, and steadily maintained until the cement has initially set. The *seating* of the restoration must be completed within a few seconds while the cement is sufficiently fluid. One way to increase the potential of maximum seating is to make multiple channels large enough (larger if they are longer) to permit rapid escape of cement that otherwise would be entrapped. For metal castings, the channels could be created internally in the wax pattern or cut in the casting, extending gingivally from the occlusal (pulpal wall) aspect of the preparation (casting) to a point approximately 0.5 mm short of the restoration margins. The final result ideally is a restoration so well-seated that its cavity-side surface is in intimate contact with the tooth preparation, particularly along the margins, so that practically, the cement film thickness is no greater than 25 μm. *Inlay and onlay preparations have short enough external walls so that the castings do not require escape*

channels (see Chapter 19), but crowns often require them if considerable axial length is present. Channels allow seating with 330 N load (75 lb), the recognized possible masticatory pressure achievable in the molar region (see Chapter 17, Cementation).

Machined restorations

Until 1988, indirect ceramic dental restorations were fabricated by casting and/or sintering techniques, and neither were pore-free. Cooling shrinkage distortions and residual stresses could initiate fractures at residual pores in ceramics. However, pore-free restorations now can be produced by machining blocks of pore-free ceramic.

Terminology and classification. There are two principal *machining approaches* for dental restorations: (1) copy milling and (2) CAD/CAM milling. Examples of commercial systems are indicated in Box 6-3.

Copy milling uses a replica (e.g., wax, plastic, stone, or metal) of the desired form as a guide for a milling machine. The surface of the replica is traced by turning the pattern and touching the surface with a finger guide. The positions of the pattern and finger guide are used to adjust the positions of a block of restorative material and a milling tool cutting the block, respectively. This procedure is schematically represented in Fig. 6-66.

Because titanium has a very high melting temperature, it is difficult to conveniently cast. However, it can be copy milled easily and inexpensively. Composite and ceramic materials are being used more commonly for copy milling. The choice of material depends in large part on the type of margin required for the restoration. Virtually any geometry and size can be copy milled as long as there is direct access of the finger guide and cutting tool to the surfaces involved.

Box 6-3. Examples of commercial CAD/CAM and copy milling systems in dentistry (circa 1993)

1. CEREC (Ceramic Reconstruction) system:
   Applications: inlays, onlays, veneers
   Inventors: Martin Brandestini, Werner Moermann
   Corporate developer: Siemens
2. SOPHA system:
   Applications: inlays, onlays, veneers, crowns
   Inventor: Francois Duret
   Corporate developer: Bioconcept Inc.
3. DentiCAD system:
   Applications: inlays, onlays, crowns, (bridges)
   Inventor: E. Dianne Rekow
   Corporate developer: Digital Dental Systems (US);
      BEGO (Europe)
4. CICERO (Computer Integrated Crown Reconstruction) system:
   Applications: PFM Crowns
   Corporate developer: Elephant (Holland)
5. ProCera system:
   Applications: Copy-milled crowns and bridges as metal
      or PFM restorations
   Corporate developer: Nobelpharma
6. CELAY:
   Applications: Copy-milled composite or ceramic inlays,
      onlays, and veneers
   Corporate Developer: Mikrona Technologie AG (Europe) and Vident (US)

CAD/CAM milling uses digital information about the cavity preparation or a pattern of the restoration to provide a *c*omputer-*a*ided *d*esign (CAD) on the video monitor for inspection and modification. The image is the reference for designing a restoration on the video monitor. Once the three-dimensional image for the restoration design is accepted, the computer translates the image into a set of instructions to guide a milling tool (*c*omputer-*a*ssisted *m*anufacturing, [CAM]) in cutting the restoration from a block of material (Fig. 6-67).

Stages of fabrication. A number of approaches to CAD/CAM for restorative dentistry have evolved, but all systems ideally involve five basic stages: (1) computerized surface digitization, (2) computer-aided design, (3) computer-assisted manufacturing, (4) computer-aided esthetics, and (5) computer-aided finishing.[10,13] The last two stages are very difficult and have not yet been included in commercial systems. Various computerized surface digitization techniques have been explored. Examples of different approaches are listed in Box 6-4. Laser techniques and contact digitization are the most promising approaches from the point of view of cost and accuracy.

The *CEREC* (*Ce*ramic *Re*construction) *System* (Siemens) was the first commercially available CAD/CAM system used in dentistry. An intraoral video camera images the cavity preparation and the adjacent tooth surfaces. Elevations of the imaged surfaces are calculated by Moire fringe displacement. Features of the cavity

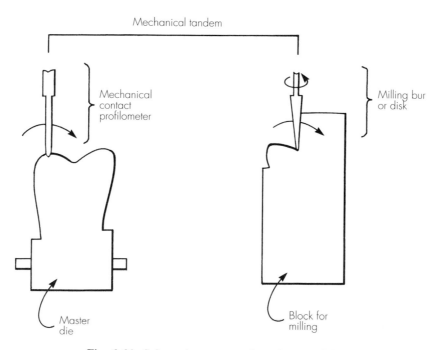

Fig. 6-66. Schematic representation of copy milling.

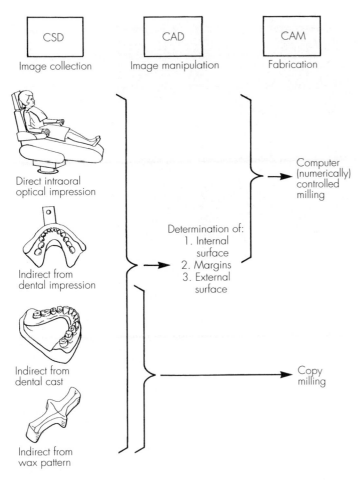

Fig. 6-67. Schematic summary of CAD/CAM and copy milling operations.

Box 6-4. List of computerized surface digitization techniques

1. Photogrammetry
2. Moire
3. Laser scanning
4. Computerized tomography scanning
5. Magnetic resonance imaging
6. Ultrasound
7. Contact profilometry

---

preparation are used to define the limits of the restoration. External surfaces of the restoration are estimated as distances to adjacent tooth structure in the computer view. Occlusal surfaces are much more highly refined later by the operator intraorally after cementing the CEREC restoration.

Composition, structure, and properties of machined materials. Restorations are machined from either *modified feldspathic porcelain* or *special fluoro alumino silicate compositions* with excellent **fracture and wear resistance**. The materials being machined are **pore-free**

and generally have both crystalline and noncrystalline phases. A two-phase composition permits differential etching of internal restoration walls for micro-mechanical retention using bonding agents and/or luting cements. Table 6-20 summarizes the typical properties of machinable ceramic materials in clinical use. Fig. 6-68 shows an example of the phases revealed by etching for bonding of Dicor MGC.

CAD/CAM restorations are fabricated primarily from ceramic materials. They are bonded to tooth structure by (1) etching for a bond to enamel; (2) conditioning, priming, and applying the bonding agent to dentin (when appropriate); (3) etching (by **HF acid**) and then priming *(silanating)* the inlay; and (4) cementing the inlay with composite cement. This situation is schematically summarized in Fig. 6-69.

CAD/CAM systems for fabricating restorations are not currently designed to produce esthetics comparable to the characterization possible in a dental laboratory. Most CAD/CAM systems utilize uniform color (monolithic) materials for the entire restoration. Despite the fact that increased shades of ceramic are becoming available for use with the CEREC system, the final *esthetics* rely on a combination of color match to adjacent tooth structure and light scattering from adjacent tooth structure into the restoration. Small restorations display color that is governed more by scattered light and look very esthetic. Larger restorations appear to be duller and less esthetic. While this situation cannot be totally

Table 6-20. Properties of a typical machinable ceramic material in clinical use with CAD/CAM systems

	Dicor MGC
Physical properties	
Density	2.8 gm/cm^2
Crystal size	2 μm
Refractive index	1.52
Translucency	0.41
Thermal conductivity	1.6 W/m-K
Thermal diffusivity	0.79 mm^2/sec
Specific heat	74.1 J/kg-K
LCTE	6.4 ppm/C
Chemical properties	
Solubility at pH=6	0.007 mg/cm^2
Solubility at pH=7	0.006 mg/cm^2
Mechanical properties	
Elastic modulus	680,000 MPa
Modulus of rupture	138 MPa
Biaxial flexure strength	147 MPa
Fracture toughness	1.5 MPa-m$^{1/2}$
Microhardness	330 KHN$_{100}$
Biological properties	
Biocompatibility	[Non-toxic (tissue culture test)]

After Grossman DG: *Proceedings of the International Symposium on Computer Restorations,* Chicago, 1991, Quintessence Publishing.

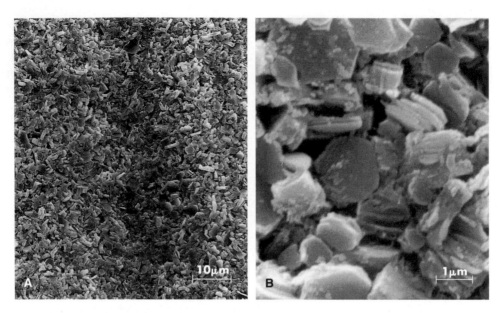

Fig. 6-68. Ammonium bifluoride acid-etched Dicor MGC inlay in preparation for cementation. Approximately 65% of ceramic is fluoromica crystals that are embedded in amorphous matrix. The matrix at surface is partially dissolved by etching. **A,** Etching partially reveals crystals that are 1 to 5 microns in size. **B,** Higher magnification view of crystals that provide micromechanical interlocking for bonding. (Courtesy SC Bayne, School of Dentistry, University of North Carolina, Chapel Hill, NC.)

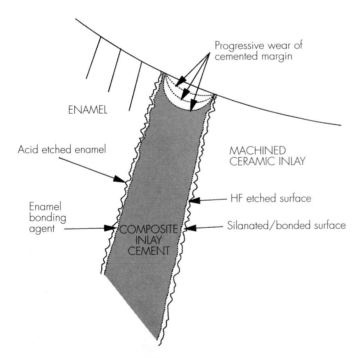

Fig. 6-69. Schematic summary of attaching ceramic CAD/CAM inlays to tooth structure. Enamel is etched for retention of bonding agents. Inlays are etched (HF acid) and primed (silanated). The restoration is cemented with composite cement.

remedied, some color variation can be introduced by cutting troughs into the internal (tooth side) surface of the CAD/CAM inlay. The troughs are then filled with varying shades of composite. This technique produces an optical effect of different dentin colors and enhances the overall esthetic appearance.

Composition, structure, and properties of composite cements. The weak link with these systems is the *cement gap* along occlusal surfaces that may be wider than desired. Normal food abrasion produces cement loss and ditching. This wear permits stain accumulation in marginal gaps and leaves exposed enamel and ceramic margins. Minimizing this gap depends on the computer digitization, design, and manufacturing steps being sufficiently accurate.

CAD/CAM restorations are routinely cemented with moderately filled composites (homogeneous microfills or hybrids). *The composite cements are not as mechanically strong as composite restorative materials but do provide the best abrasion resistance due to the microprotection effect of closely spaced filler particles.*

Clinical considerations. The clinical longevity of these restorations is difficult to project, because only relatively short-term clinical research information is available.[60,66,101] However, review of the earliest restorations indicates that while cement margins may degrade, the restorations themselves survive equally as well as amalgam or composite restorations of the same type. There is no evidence of postoperative sensitivity or secondary caries.

Major advantages of milled ceramics are excellent flexural strength and the ability to rigidly bond remaining tooth structure together. Occasional restoration fractures have been reported, but in most cases they are associated with onlay designs that are too thin and subject to stress concentration during flexure or fatigue fracture. It is still important to *use adequate thickness in the restoration design to resist flexure.*

Additionally, restorations from these systems are ***repairable,*** since they are etchable and defects can be restored using bonded composites. There should be no reason to completely replace the restoration unless it has undergone bulk fracture.

SAFETY AND EFFICACY

The availability of dental materials of high quality and dependability is due in large part to the existence of standards for the safety and efficacy of such products. Yet, very few clinicians are aware of or understand the intricate system of voluntary and mandatory controls that are currently in place to accomplish this purpose.

Standards programs

The large number of organizations involved in standards programs and their acronyms are summarized in Box 6-5.

Standards programs can be broadly divided into dental *professional organizations,* larger *interest groups* that include all professional organizations, and *government agencies.* These hierarchies exist both within the *United States* and throughout the *world* as a whole. Fig. 6-70 attempts to interrelate these groups. In the discussion which follows, individual group activities are addressed. Most professional organizations attempt to coordinate their standards with other organizations so that there is a rational system of tests that involve evaluating similar events.

Box 6-5. Acronyms for national and international groups interested in dental standards

NDA	National Dental Association
ADA	American Dental Association
	CDMIE = Council on Dental Materials, Instruments, and Equipment
	CDT = Council on Dental Therapeutics
ANSI	American National Standards Institute
	ASC MD156 = Accredited Standards Committee, Medical Devices
FDA	Food and Drug Administration
ASTM	American Society for Testing and Materials
FDI	Federation Dentaire Internationale
ISO	International Organizations for Standards
	ISO TC106 = ISO Technical Committee

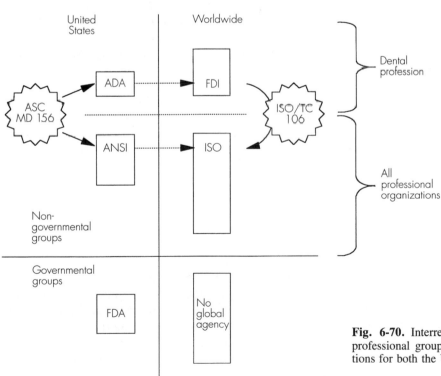

Fig. 6-70. Interrelationships of dental professional and other professional group standards versus government agency regulations for both the United States and the whole world.

Professional organizations develop *voluntary standards* which are often the basis for governmental *regulatory standards* whenever governments become involved. In many cases, the good faith standards and self-regulation of industry obviates the need for government involvement.

American Dental Association. Within the American Dental Association (ADA) there have been two councils, the *Council on Dental Materials, Instruments, and Equipment* (CDMIE) and the *Council on Dental Therapeutics* (CDT), which review products voluntarily submitted to them by manufacturers.[2,3] These councils were responsible for developing standards for testing. They manage the acceptance program and the certification program which evaluate and identify suitable products. Based on clinical information about safety and efficacy, products which were submitted for the *acceptance program* were awarded a classification of (1) *full acceptance* or (2) *conditional acceptance*. Accepted products displayed the *ADA seal of acceptance* (Fig. 6-71) in all advertising as evidence of compliance with ADA standards. Products for which laboratory test information has been demonstrated to predict safety and efficacy in lieu of clinical research may be submitted under the ADA's *certification* program on the basis of those laboratory tests. Certified products displayed the ADA seal of certification (Fig. 6-71). Dental amalgam and impression material products, for example, were reviewed by certification programs. However, posterior composite materials and dentin bonding products were considered through the acceptance program. Now both programs have been merged. Approved products may display the ADA seal of acceptance. This simplifies the information being conveyed to a practitioner.

American National Standards Institute. The American National Standards Institute (ANSI) is a clearinghouse for national standards.

The Accredited Standards Committee (ASC) MD156 is a liaison group between the ADA and ANSI. It is an independent committee of both organizations that is sponsored by the ADA and accredited by ANSI for dentistry in the United States. ADA standards that are developed are submitted to ANSI for approval as national standards.

Food and Drug Administration. Since 1976, the Food and Drug Administration (FDA) has been charged with regulating dental devices (including materials). In this role, they classify individual *materials as Class I, II, or III*. Class I materials are simply required to be produced under conditions of good manufacturing practices to assure reproducibility and continuing safety. Class II materials are required to present evidence of meeting standards as well, such as the ADA standards for acceptance or certification. Class III materials are required, in addition, to submit evidence of safety and efficacy using biocompatibility and clinical data to show satisfactory performance in tissue culture tests, implantation tests, and/or usage tests. Tests for the relative safety of dental materials (biocompatibility) are described as part of ANSI/ADA document No. 41. These tests are in large part controversial, because they are continually evolving and may be reinterpreted in light of new or more sophisticated understandings of *biocompatibility*.

American Society for Testing and Materials. The American Society for Testing and Materials (ASTM) is a non-governmental group that is involved widely in the development of standards for test methods for use in industry. It has recently become interested in standards for dentistry (dental materials and devices) as well as the development of appropriate terminology, nomenclature, and test methods. ASTM's F-4 subcommittee has developed specifications for surgical implants. ASTM's F-8 subcommittee governs sports devices such as mouth guards. ASTM's D-2 committee is concerned with rubber products, such as rubber gloves.

Federation Dentaire Internationale. The worldwide voluntary federation of national dental organizations is known as the Federation Dentaire Internationale (FDI).

International Organization for Standards. An International Organization for Standards (ISO) exists for the purpose of developing international standards for all activities, not only dentistry. ISO is a non-treaty organization. ANSI is the United States member of ISO.

FDI maintains a permanent liaison with ISO through its ISO/TC 106-Dentistry group. To the extent that each group coordinates its activities with each other, the ADA role has been a major one in initiating standards for a range of current standards organizations.

Safety for dental professionals

While there are numerous organizations and standards for regulating the safety of dental materials with regard to the patient, there are quite different ones concerned with the health of dental professionals. In many situations the scope and regulations of different groups are overlapping and inconsistent.

Occupational Safety and Health Administration. The *Occupational Safety and Health Administration*

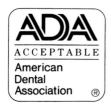
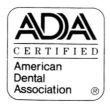

Fig. 6-71. ADA Seals of Acceptance and of Certification. (Courtesy ADA CDMIE, Chicago Ill.)

(OSHA) is the U.S. federal agency charged with responsibility for maintaining safety in the workplace. It differs from the organizations discussed previously in that OSHA has the legal authority to enforce compliance. During 1970, the United States adopted a wide range of OSHA regulations with the goal of reducing the potential for illness or injury to employees from chemical exposures. Many of these regulations were enforced only sparingly during the 1980s, and usually only for large businesses. *Since 1992, there has been stricter enforcement of these standards for dental offices and dental laboratories.* OSHA has issued regulations involved with a wide range of issues such as (1) hazard communications, (2) blood-borne pathogens, and (3) waste disposal.

Hazard communications include public posting of OSHA regulations, office record keeping, office emergency planning, office employee training, and office planning for workman's compensation. These processes involve *seven categories of responsibilities* which are described in the following paragraphs. Detailed information is provided by the ADA to dental professionals in this regard.

First Category of Responsibility. To ensure that all employees are aware of the processes that are required to guarantee the safety and health of the employees, an **OSHA poster** *must be continuously displayed within the office* (at one or more sites) *so as to be seen by all personnel.* This location is most often a kitchen, apparel changing location, or employee lounge area. The poster is titled "Job Health and Safety Protection."

Second Category of Responsibility. For many years, large businesses and laboratories have had to meet OSHA requirements involving hazardous chemicals to protect the health of their employees. The enforcement of these requirements has been extended recently to cover dental offices. While modifications of office routines are required, dentistry can benefit from the prior experience of industry in refining the application of these safety principles. *Hazardous chemical materials are routinely managed by proper labeling and storage as well as by certifying that all office personnel are fully informed of possible risks and the necessary precautions in those regards.* The requirement for hazardous chemical labeling is waived for FDA-regulated items such as most products in dental offices. However, the information about the nature of the chemical hazard and its management is still a responsibility of the office. This information is published on *material safety data sheets (MSDSs)* and is available from individual manufacturers. Manufacturers have the primary responsibility to determine whether an MSDS is required and to supply that information. Commercial chemicals generally are packaged with MSDSs. However, often dental products cannot conveniently include the MSDS, because the sheet is too big for the package in which materials are sold. Only some dental products include MSDSs, and therefore, absent MSDS information must be collected after the fact. The ADA maintains a list of available MSDSs by company (and code). Therefore, it is relatively easy to check off the MSDSs that are required. Some manufacturers have not supplied this information to the ADA and will not be listed. In that case, it is the responsibility of the dental office to contact the manufacturer directly and obtain the MSDSs if they are available.

Most personnel in a dental office are not familiar with key information they need on materials to be able to make an informed judgment about relative risks or hazards. Therefore, *the best approach is to inventory everything in the office* (by company or supplier) *and then check a published list for the presence or absence of an MSDS.*

These sheets must be available for review by all potentially exposed office personnel and should be stored in a central location with bold labeling or identification of the site. Most sheets are 3-hole punched for convenient insertion into an *MSDS notebook.* A common recommendation is to label the notebook "MSDS" on the spine and on the front. *The notebook should be of a color that is distinct from any other notebooks or books that might be in the same area. All MSDSs should be organized within the notebook* in a logical fashion for easy locating.

MSDSs are typically a two- to four-page summary of the material's names, chemical reactivity, potential risks in storage or biological contact, methods of managing emergencies, and summaries of key biological information. A sample MSDS is shown in Fig. 6-72, with categorical sections indicated.

Third Category of Responsibility. The information, once collected, *must be communicated to all employees on a regular basis. In the same notebook with the MSDSs, records should be kept on procedures and times for* **annual employee hazard communications training.** This record should include information about non-routine tasks such as cleaning the dental unit suction reservoirs, training new employees, training service personnel for the office (e.g., janitorial personnel), and inventorying new materials, equipment, or devices that might require updating the MSDSs. This process is rigorously defined and the appropriate details can be obtained from OSHA and the ADA. Some of the details are emphasized in the following discussions.

Fourth Category of Responsibility. For safety in the general office enviroment *and during servicing, sterilization, and maintenance of equipment and instruments,* it is mandatory that precautionary measures (e.g., ventilation), personal protective equipment (e.g., protective gloves, apron, and goggles), and emergency equipment

3M General Offices
3M Center
St. Paul, Minnesota 55144-1000
612/733-1110
    Duns No.: 00-617-3082

00-78
745

MATERIAL SAFETY
DATA SHEET

3M

DIVISION: DENTAL PRODUCTS
TRADE NAME:
SCOTCHBOND MULTIPURPOSE ADHESIVE

3M I.D. NUMBER: 70-2010-0402-8

ISSUED: MAY 11, 1992
SUPERSEDES: APRIL 16, 1992
DOCUMENT: 05-4869-3

1. INGREDIENT

INGREDIENT	C.A.S. NO.	PERCENT	
BISPHENOL A DIGLYCIDYL ETHER			
DIMETHACRYLATE	1565-94-2	60.0	70.0
2-HYDROXYETHYL METHACRYLATE	868-77-9	30.0	40.0
DL-CAMPHORQUINONE	10373-78-1	<	1.0
N,N-DIMETHYLBENZOCAINE	10287-53-3	<	1.0
DIPHENYLIODONIUM			
HEXAFLUOROPHOSPHATE	58109-40-3	<	1.0

2. PHYSICAL DATA

BOILING POINT: .... > 95 F
VAPOR PRESSURE: .... < 16 psi
VAPOR DENSITY: .... N/A
EVAPORATION RATE: .... N/A
SOLUBILITY IN WATER: .... N/A
SP. GRAVITY: .... 1.15 Water = 1
PERCENT VOLATILE: .... N/A
VOLATILE ORGANICS: .... N/A
VOC LESS H2O & EXEMPT SOLVENT N/A
pH: .... N/A
VISCOSITY: .... 250 CPS Brkfld
MELTING POINT: .... N/A
APPEARANCE AND ODOR: Liquid, CLEAR, SLIGHTLY YELLOW, SLIGHT ACRYLATE ODOR

3. FIRE AND EXPLOSION HAZARD DATA

FLASH POINT: .... 214 F
FLAMMABLE LIMITS - LEL: ..... N/A
FLAMMABLE LIMITS - UEL: ..... N/A
AUTOIGNITION TEMPERATURE: ... N/A
EXTINGUISHING MEDIA:
    Carbon dioxide, Dry chemical
SPECIAL FIRE FIGHTING PROCEDURES:
    Not applicable
UNUSUAL FIRE AND EXPLOSION HAZARDS:
    Not applicable.
NFPA-HAZARD-CODES: HEALTH 1 FIRE 1 REACTIVITY 0
        UNUSUAL REACTION HAZARD: none
OSHA FIRE HAZARD CLASS: Not applicable

4. REACTIVITY DATA

STABILITY: Stable
INCOMPATIBILITY - MATERIALS TO AVOID:
N/A

HAZARDOUS POLYMERIZATION: Will Not Occur
HAZARDOUS DECOMPOSITION PRODUCTS:
N/A

5. ENVIRONMENTAL INFORMATION

SPILL RESPONSE:
    Observe precautions from other sections. Ventilate area. Cover with
    absorbent material. Place in metal container.

    USE PROTECTIVE GLOVES

RECOMMENDED DISPOSAL:
    Dispose of completely cured (or polymerized) material in a sanitary
    landfill.

    SINCE REGULATIONS VARY, CONSULT APPLICABLE REGULATIONS OR
    AUTHORITIES BEFORE DISPOSAL.

ENVIRONMENTAL DATA:
    Not applicable.

    NOT A MARINE POLLUTANT

REGULATORY INFORMATION:
    U.S. EPA Hazardous Waste Number = None (Not U.S. EPA Hazardous).
    Since regulations vary, consult applicable regulations or authorities
    before disposal.

SARA HAZARD CLASS:
    FIRE HAZARD: No PRESSURE: No REACTIVITY: No ACUTE: Yes CHRONIC: No

6. SUGGESTED FIRST AID

EYE CONTACT:
    Immediately flush eyes with large amounts of water for at least 15
    minutes. Get immediate medical attention.

SKIN CONTACT:
    Flush skin with large amounts of water. If irritation persists, call
    a physician. Wash contaminated clothing before reuse.

INHALATION:
    No need for first aid is anticipated.

IF SWALLOWED:
    Do not induce vomiting. Drink two glasses of water. Call a physician.

OTHER FIRST AID:
    MUCOSAL CONTACT: FLUSH WITH PLENTY OF WATER

7. PRECAUTIONARY INFORMATION

EYE PROTECTION:
    Avoid eye contact.

SKIN PROTECTION:
    Wear appropriate gloves when handling this material. A pair of
    gloves made from the following material(s) are recommended: nitrile
    rubber.

VENTILATION PROTECTION:
    Not applicable.

RESPIRATORY PROTECTION:
    Not applicable.

PREVENTION OF ACCIDENTAL INGESTION:
    Do not ingest.

RECOMMENDED STORAGE:
    Store at room temperature.

FIRE AND EXPLOSION AVOIDANCE:
    Not applicable.

OTHER PRECAUTIONARY INFORMATION:
    N/A

EXPOSURE LIMITS

INGREDIENTS	VALUE	UNIT	TYPE AUTH SKIN*
BISPHENOL A DIGLYCIDYL ETHER			
DIMETHACRYLATE	NONE	NONE	NONE NONE
2-HYDROXYETHYL METHACRYLATE	NONE	NONE	NONE NONE
DL-CAMPHORQUINONE	NONE	NONE	NONE NONE
N,N-DIMETHYLBENZOCAINE	NONE	NONE	NONE NONE
DIPHENYLIODONIUM			
HEXAFLUOROPHOSPHATE	NONE	NONE	NONE NONE

* SKIN NOTATION: Listed substances indicated with "Y" under SKIN refer to
the potential contribution to the overall exposure by the cutaneous route
including mucous membrane and eye, either by airborne or, more particularly,
by direct contact with the substance. Vehicles can alter skin absorption.

SOURCE OF EXPOSURE LIMIT DATA:
- NONE: None Established

8. HEALTH HAZARD DATA

EYE CONTACT:
    Severe Eye Irritation: signs/symptoms can include redness, swelling,
    pain, tearing, cloudy appearance of the cornea, impaired vision and
    possible permanently impaired vision.

SKIN CONTACT:
    Allergic Skin Reaction: signs/symptoms can include redness, swelling,
    blistering, and itching.

    Mild Skin Irritation: signs/symptoms can include redness, swelling,
    and itching.

INHALATION:
    No adverse health effects are expected from inhalation exposure

IF SWALLOWED:
    No adverse health effects are expected from swallowing.

SECTION CHANGE DATES

INGREDIENTS   SECTION CHANGED SINCE APRIL 16, 1992 ISSUE

Abbreviations: N/D - Not Determined N/A - Not Applicable

The information on this Data Sheet represents our current data and best
opinion as to the proper use in handling of this material under normal
conditions. Any use of the material which is not in conformance with this
Data Sheet or which involves using the material in combination with any
other material or any other process is the responsibility of the user.

Fig. 6-72. Example of a Material Safety Data Sheet (MSDS) for dentin bonding agent containing information on the material's (1) ingredients and identity, (2) physical (and chemical) characteristics, (3) fire and explosion hazard data, (4) reactivity data, (5) environmental precautions, (6) suggested first aid, (7) precautions for safe handling and use, and (8) health hazard data.

(e.g., eyewash fountain, fire extinguisher, and resuscitator mask) be available and appropriately used. *These precautions should be reviewed at least annually.* Review of the *emergency equipment should be checked at least monthly.* A complete review of emergency preparedness for a small office for health and safety can generally be conducted in a matter of 10 to 15 minutes. This review is an infinitesimal investment for minimizing employee and patient risks.

Fifth Category of Responsibility. *Any incidents that require medical attention* or involve loss of work should be documented. *A range of forms are needed to* (1) maintain permanent records of incidents, follow-ups, and new preventive measures, (2) summarize incidents and dates for periodic review, and (3) file workman's compensation reports.

Sixth Category of Responsibility. In addition to OSHA's initial concern with *hazard communications,* there have been relatively recent emphases on **universal precautions against exposure to bloodborne pathogens** and **waste disposal** for dental offices. Infection control practices for blood-borne pathogens have become much more sophisticated because of concern about the increase in hepatitis and human immunodeficiency virus (HIV) transmissions. These problems and related procedures for offices are discussed in detail in Chapter 4.

Waste disposal currently is not regulated by OSHA. It really involves collection, transport, and management operations. Within the dental office, the collection systems must necessarily be more sophisticated than in many businesses because of infection control regulations. *Trash must be separated* on the basis of being (1) **biohazard waste (hazardous),** (2) **chemical waste (hazardous),** or (3) **regular (nonhazardous) waste.** *Nonhazardous waste can be placed in sanitary landfills. The other materials must be incinerated or buried in continuously managed waste disposal sites.*

At the moment, most communities have focused only on medical waste. Containers, such as dentin bonding agent vials or pre-capsulated amalgam capsules, although considered chemical waste, can be disposed in the nonhazardous waste. Waste transport may occur within a building and/or from the building to an approved disposal facility or site. *The owner of the office generating the waste is responsible for guaranteeing appropriate and safe transport for disposal.* At the moment there are numerous careless or unscrupulous transporters and managers of waste disposal who are inadequately informed or unconvinced about the care needed. For the most part, there is some responsibility for the dental office personnel to ensure the reliability of individuals providing these services.

Seventh Category of Responsibility. *Finally there must be employee training and education programs at least annually with respect to hazards, management of* blood-borne pathogens, and waste disposal. *All **new** employees must be trained immediately. Records must be kept of the training procedures and training times. All individual records should be kept either in the MSDS notebook and/or in personnel records.*

Environmental Protection Agency. All by-products of dental procedures end up as solid, liquid, or gaseous waste, and their disposal can be regulated by the **Environmental Protection Agency (EPA).** At the present time, most waste disposal is regulated by local authorities.

Hazardous gases or vapors, such as nitrous oxide, should be vented directly to the outside air or should be collected from the air using scrubbing devices, both to protect intraoffice individuals and to prevent inadvertent contamination of other local air systems.

Liquid wastes that are emptied into the sewer or drainage systems have some potential to contaminate the waste treatment plant or ground water supplies. Therefore, it is becoming increasingly important to separate hazardous liquids such as waste solvents for controlled disposal. Small amounts of water-based chemicals can be diluted and flushed into the sewer system. However, water-immiscible materials are best disposed of in alternative ways. Waste disposal of blood and body fluids into sanitary sewers is a commonly accepted practice.

Solid wastes include the trash from an office and the effluent disposed into the sewer system. Collected amalgam scrap should be recycled (see Mercury Management and Box 6-1). Amalgam scrap in waste water is becoming an important issue in European countries and separating devices are becoming required to separate suspended solid. Special filters are available for this purpose. The situation in the United States is not yet defined.

REFERENCES

1. Allan DN: A longitudinal study of dental restorations, *Brit Dent J* 143:87-89, 1977.
2. American Dental Association: *Accepted dental therapeutics,* ed 40, Chicago, 1984, American Dental Association.
3. American Dental Association: *Dentist's desk reference: materials, instruments, and equipment,* ed 1, Chicago, 1981, American Dental Association.
4. American Dental Association CDMIE: Dental mercury hygiene: summary of recommendations in 1990, *J Am Dent Assoc* 122(9):112, 1991.
5. Ames BN, Gold LS: Too many rodent carcinogens: mitogenesis versus mutagenesis, *Science* 249:970-971, 1990.
6. Anderson JN: *Applied dental materials,* ed 6, London, 1976, Blackwell Scientific Publications.
7. Anusavice KJ: *Dental biomaterials III: dental materials for clinical practice,* ed 1, Gainesville, 1992, University of Florida.

8. Bader JD, Shugars DA: Agreement among dentists' recommendations for restorative treatment, *J Dent Res* 72:891-896, 1993.

9. Bader JD et al: Identifying children who will experience high caries increments, *Community Dent Oral Epidemiol* 14:198-201, 1986.

10. Bayne SC: What is the future of CAD/CAM materials and techniques? In *Symposium on esthetic restorative materials,* 117-125, Chicago, 1993, American Dental Association CDMIE.

11. Bayne SC: Dental composites/glass ionomers: clinical reports. In Effects and side effects of dental restorative materials proceedings, *Adv Dent Res* 6:65-77, 1992.

12. Bayne SC: The mercury controversy, *Quint Int* 22(4):247-248, 1991 (editorial).

13. Bayne SC: CAD/CAM: science and technology, *Trans Acad Dent Mater* 2(1):3-7, 1989.

14. Bayne SC, Barton RE: Dental materials for direct restorations. In Richardson RE, Barton RE, editors: *The dental assistant,* ed 6, Philadelphia, 1988, Lea & Febiger.

15. Bayne SC, Fleming JE, Faison S: SEM-EDS analysis of macro and micro resin tags of laminates, *J Dent Res* 61A:304, 1982 (abstract 1128).

16. Bayne SC, Taylor DF, Heymann HO: Protection hypothesis for composite wear, *Dent Mater* 8:305-309, 1992.

17. Bayne SC, Taylor DF, Zardiackas LD: *Biomaterials science,* ed 6, Chapel Hill, NC, 1992, Brightstar Publishing.

18. Bayne SC et al: Class V angulation, size, and depth effects on composite retention, *J Dent Res* 71A:314, 1992 (abstract 1669).

19. Bayne SC et al: Clinical longevity of ten posterior composite materials based on wear, *J Dent Res* 70A:344, 1991 (abstract 630).

20. Bayne SC et al: Long term clinical failures in posterior composites, *J Dent Res* 68A:185, 1989 (abstract 32).

21. Bentley C, Drake CW: Longevity of restorations in a dental school clinic, *J Dent Educ* 50:594-600, 1986.

22. Bowen RL: Dental filling material comprising vinyl silane treated fused silica and a binder consisting of the reaction product of BIS phenol and glycidyl acrylate. *US Patent 3,066,112,* 1962.

23. Braem M et al: In vivo evaluation of four posterior composites: quantitative wear measurements and clinical behavior, *Dent Mater* 2:106-113, 1986.

24. Buonocore MG: Simple method of increasing the adhesion of acrylic filling materials to enamel surfaces, *J Dent Res* 34:849-853, 1955.

25. Cagle CV: *Handbook of adhesive bonding,* ed 1, New York, 1973, McGraw-Hill.

26. Chang SB, Siew C, Gruninger SE: Factors affecting blood mercury concentrations in practicing dentists, *J Dent Res* 71:66-74, 1992.

27. Charles AD: The story of dental amalgam, *Bull Hist Dent* 30:2-6, 1982.

28. Christensen G: Use survey—1990, *CRA Newsletter* 14(12):1, 1990.

29. Collins CJ, Bryant RW: Finishing of amalgam restorations: a three-year clinical trial, *J Dent Res* 20:202-206, 1992.

30. Combe EC: *Notes on dental materials,* ed 4, Edinburgh, 1981, Churchill Livingstone.

31. Cook WD: Factors affecting the depth of cure of UV-polymerized composites, *J Dent Res* 59:800-808, 1980.

32. Crabb HSM: The survival of dental restorations in a teaching hospital, *Brit Dent J* 150:315-318, 1981.

33. Craig RG: *Restorative dental materials,* ed 9, 1993, St Louis, Mosby.

34. Craig RG: Overview of posterior composite resins for use in clinical practice. In Vanherle G, Smith DC, editors: *Posterior composite resin dental restorative materials,* Netherlands, 1985, Peter Szulc Publishing.

35. Craig RG: *Dental materials—a problem oriented approach,* ed 1, St Louis, 1978, Mosby.

36. Craig RG, O'Brien WJ, Powers JM: *Dental materials—properties and manipulation,* ed 3, St Louis, 1983, Mosby.

37. Cvar JF, Ryge G: Criteria for the clinical evaluation of dental restorative materials, *US Dept HEW PHS,* Dental Health Center, San Francisco, 1973, US Government Printing Office, Publ No 7902244.

38. Dawson AS, Smales RJ: Restoration longevity in an Australian defense force population, *Aust Dent J* 37:196-200, 1992.

39. Demaree NC, Taylor DF: Properties of dental amalgams made from spherical alloy powders, *J Dent Res* 41:890-906, 1962.

40. Disney JA et al: The University of North Carolina caries risk assessment study: further developments in caries risk assessment, *Community Dent Oral Epidemiol* 20:64-75, 1992.

41. Eames WB: Preparation and condensation of amalgam with low mercury-alloy ratio, *J Am Dent Assoc* 58(4):78-83, 1959.

42. Eames WB et al: Accuracy and dimensional stability of elastomeric impression materials, *J Prosthet Dent* 42:159-162, 1979.

43. Eastman J, Siegel RW: Nanophase synthesis assembles materials from atomic clusters, *Res & Devel* Jan:56-60, 1989.

44. Elderton RJ: Longitudinal study of dental treatment in the general dental service in Scotland, *Brit Dent J* 155:91-96, 1983.

45. Ericson D, Derand T: Increase of in vitro curing depth of class II composite resin restorations, *J Prosthet Dent* 70:219-223, 1993.

46. Evans FG: *Mechanical properties of bone,* ed 1, Springfield, Ill, 1973, Charles C Thomas Publisher.

47. Fan PL, O'Brien WJ, Craig RG: Wetting properties of sealants and glazes, *Oper Dent* 4:100-103, 1979.

48. Fisher Scientific: 3M vapor monitors, 1991, p 727, *Laboratory Supplies Catalogue.*

49. Freund M, Munksgaard EC: Enzymatic degradation of Bis-GMA/TEGDMA-polymers causing decreased microhardness and greater wear in vitro, *Scand J Dent Res* 98:351-355, 1990.

50. Fried K: Changes in innervation of dentine and pulp with age. In Ferguson DF, editor: *The aging mouth,* Basel, 1987, Karger.

51. Gold LS et al: Rodent carcinogens: setting priorities, *Science* 258:261-265, 1992.

52. Greener EH, Harcourt JK, Lautenschlager EP: *Materials science in dentistry,* Baltimore, 1972, Williams & Wilkins.

53. Grippo JO, Masi JV: Role of biodental engineering factors (BEF) in the etiology of root caries, *J Esthet Dent* 3:71-76, 1991.

54. Grossman DG: Structure and physical properties of Dicor/MGC glass-ceramic. *Proceedings of the International Symposium on Computer Restorations,* pp 103-115, Chicago, 1991, Quintessence Publishing.

55. Hahn LJ et al: Dental "silver" tooth fillings: a source of mercury exposure revealed by whole-body image scan and tissue analysis, *FASEB* 3:2641-2646, 1989.

56. Haines D, Berry DC, Poole DFG: Behavior of tooth enamel under load, *J Dent Res* 42:885-888, 1963.

57. Hasegawa J: Dental casting materials, *Trans Acad Dent Mater* 2(3):190-201, 1989.

58. Helkimo E, Carlsson GE, Helkimo M: Bite force and state of dentition, *Acta Odont Scand* 35:297-303, 1977.

59. Hench LL, Ethridge EC: *Biomaterials, an interfacial approach,* ed 1, New York, 1982, Academic Press.

60. Heymann HO et al: Two-year clinical performance of CEREC CAD/CAM-generated MGC inlays, *J Dent Res* 71A:207, 1992 (abstract 814).

61. Heymann HO et al: Tooth flexure effects on cervical restorations: a two-year study, *J Am Dent Assoc* 122:41-47, 1991.

62. Heymann HO et al: Two-year clinical study of composite resins in posterior teeth, *Dent Mater* 2:37-41, 1986.

63. Iler RK: *The chemistry of silica. Solubility, polymerization, colloid, and surface properties, and biochemistry,* New York, 1979, John Wiley & Sons.

64. Innes DBK, Youdelis WV: Dispersion strengthened amalgams, *J Can Dent Assoc* 29:587-593, 1963.

65. Inokoshi S et al: Dual-cure luting composites. I. Filler particle distribution, *J Oral Rehabil* 20:133-146, 1993.

66. Isenberg BP, Essig ME, Leinfelder KF: Three-year clinical evaluation of CAD/CAM restorations, *J Esthet Dent* 4:173-175, 1992.

67. Jaarda MJ et al: Measurement of composite resin filler particles by using scanning electron microscopy and digital imaging, *J Prosthet Dent* 69:416-424, 1993.

68. Jorgensen KD: Occlusal abrasion of a composite resin with ultra-fine filler—an initial study, *Quint Int* 6:73-78, 1978.

69. Jorgensen KD: The mechanism of marginal fracture of amalgam fillings, *Acta Odont Scand* 23:347-389, 1965.

70. Lammie GA: A comparison of the cutting efficiency and heat production of tungsten carbide and steel burs, *Brit Dent J* 90:251-259, 1951.

71. Lang BR, Jaarda M, Wang RF: Filler particle size and composite resin classification systems, *J Oral Rehabil* 19:569-684, 1992.

72. Larmas MA, Hayrynen H, Lajunen LHJ: Thermogravimetric studies on sound and carious human enamel and dentin as well as hydroxyapatite, *Scand J Dent Res* 101:185-191, 1993.

73. Lee WC, Eakle WS: Possible role of tensile stress in the etiology of cervical erosive lesions of teeth, *J Prosthet Dent* 52:374-380, 1984.

74. Leinfelder KF: Wear patterns and rates of posterior composite resins, *Int Dent J* 37:152-157, 1987.

75. Leinfelder KF: Composites: current status and future developments. In *International state-of-the-art conference on restorative dental materials,* Bethesda Md, 1986, National Institute of Dental Research.

76. Leinfelder KF, Lemons JF: *Clinical restorative materials and techniques,* ed 1, Philadelphia, 1988, Lea & Febiger.

77. Leinfelder KF et al: An in vitro device for determining wear of posterior composites, *J Dent Res* 70A:345, 1991 (abstract 636).

78. Leinfelder KF et al: Burnished amalgam restorations: a two-year clinical evaluation, *Oper Dent* 3:2-8, 1978.

79. Letzel H: Four-year survival and failures of posterior composite restorations in a multicentre controlled clinical trial, *J Dent Res* 68A:206, 1989 (abstract 197).

80. Letzel H, Vrijhoef MMA: Survival rates of dental amalgam restorations, *J Dent Res* 61A:269, 1982 (abstract 820).

81. Letzel H et al: Materials influences on the survival of amalgam and composite restorations, *J Dent Res* 69A:287, 1990 (abstract 1426).

82. Lutz F, Phillips RW: A classification and evaluation of composite resin systems, *J Prosthet Dent* 50:480-488, 1983.

83. Lutz F et al: In vivo and in vitro wear of potential posterior composites, *J Dent Res* 63:914-920, 1984.

84. Mackert JR: Dental amalgam and mercury, *J Am Dent Assoc* 122(8):54-61, 1991.

85. Mackert JR et al: Lymphocyte levels in subjects with and without amalgam restorations, *J Am Dent Assoc* 122(3):49-53, 1991.

86. Mahler DB: Standardizing amalgam marginal fracture evaluation, *J Dent Res* 65:219, 1986 (abstract 445).

87. Mahler DB, Peyton FA: Photoelasticity as a research technique for analyzing stress in dental structures, *J Dent Res* 34:831-838, 1955.

88. Mahler DB, Terkla LC: Analysis of stress in dental structures. In *Dental Clinics of North America: Symposium on dental materials,* Philadelphia, 1958, WB Saunders.

89. Mahler DB, Terkla LG, Eysden JV: Marginal fracture of amalgam restorations, *J Dent Res* 52:823-827, 1973.

90. Mandel ID: Amalgam hazards. An assessment of research, *J Am Dent Assoc* 122(8):62-65, 1991.

91. Marshall SJ, Marshall GW, Jr: $Sn_4(OH)_6Cl_2$ and SnO corrosion products on amalgams, *J Dent Res* 59:820-823, 1980.

92. Marshall GW, Sarkar NK, Greener EH: Detection of oxygen in corrosion products of dental amalgam, *J Dent Res* 54:904, 1975.

93. McCabe JF: *Applied dental materials,* ed 2, London, 1990, Blackwell Scientific Publications.

94. McCabe JF, Carrick TE: Output from visible-light activation units and depth of cure of light-activated composites, *J Dent Res* 68:1534-1539, 1989.

95. The mercury in your mouth, *Consumer Reports* 316-319, May 1991.

96. Mertz-Fairhurst EJ et al: A comparative clinical study of two pit and fissure sealants: 7-year results in Augusta, Ga, *J Am Dent Assoc* 109:252-255, 1984.

97. Mitra SB, Li MY, Culler SR: Setting reaction of Vitrebond light cure glass ionomer liner/base. In Setting mechanisms of dental materials, *Trans Acad Dent Mater* 5(2):1-22, 1992.

98. Mjor IA: Placement and replacement of restorations, *Oper Dent* 6:49-54, 1981.

99. Molin C: Amalgam—fact and fiction, *Scand J Dent Res* 100:66-73, 1992.

100. Morin DL et al: Biophysical stress analysis of restored teeth: modeling and analysis, *Dent Mater* 4:77-84, 1988.

101. Mormann W, Krejci I: Computer-designed inlays after 5 years in situ: clinical performance and scanning electron microscope evaluation, *Quint Int* 23:109-115, 1992.

102. Morris HF: Veterans Administration Cooperative Studies Project No. 147. Part VIII. Plaque accumulation on metal ceramic restorations cast from noble and nickel-based alloys. A five-year report, *J Prosthet Dent* 61:543-9, 1989.

103. Mount GJ: Glass ionomer cements: clinical considerations, In *Clinical dentistry*, New York, 1984, Harper & Row, Publishers.

104. Mount GJ: Restoration with glass-ionomer cement: requirements for clinical success, *Oper Dent* 6:59-65, 1981.

105. Munksgaard EC: Permeability of protective gloves to (di)methacrylates in resinous dental materials, *Scand J Dent Res* 100:189-192, 1992.

106. Munksgaard EC, Freund M: Enzymatic hydrolysis of (di)methacrylates and their polymers, *Scand J Dent Res* 98:261-267, 1990.

107. Nakabayashi N, Ashizawa M, Nakamura M: Identification of a resin-dentin hybrid layer in vital human dentin created in vivo: durable bonding to vital dentin, *Quint Int* 23:135-141, 1992.

108. Nash KD, Bentley JE: Is restorative dentistry on its way out? *J Am Dent Assoc* 122(9):79-80, 1991.

109. National Institutes of Health: Effects and side effects of dental restorative materials—NIH Technology Assessment Conference Statement, *Natl Lib Med* 1-18, 1991.

110. National Institutes of Health: Consensus development conference statement on dental sealants in the prevention of tooth decay, *J Am Dent Assoc* 108:233-236, 1984.

111. Nicholson JW, Wasson EA: The setting of glass-polyalkenoate ("glass-ionomer") cements. In: Setting mechanisms of dental materials, *Trans Acad Dent Mater* 5(2):1-14, 1992.

112. Norman RD, Wilson NHF: Three-year findings of a multicentre trial for a posterior composite, *J Prosthet Dent* 59:577-583, 1986.

113. O'Brien WJ, Fan PL, Apostolides A: Penetrativity of sealants and glazes, *Oper Dent* 3:51-56, 1978.

114. O'Brien WJ, Ryge G: *An outline of dental materials and their selection*, ed 1, Philadelphia, 1990, WB Saunders.

115. Odom JG: Ethics and dental amalgam removal, *J Am Dent Assoc* 122(7):69-71, 1991.

116. Okamoto Y, Horibe T: Liquid gallium alloys for metallic plastic fillings, *Brit Dent J* 170:23-26, 1991.

117. Osborne JW, Berry TG: Zinc-containing high-copper amalgams: a 3-year clinical evaluation, *Am J Dent* 5:43-45, 1992.

118. Osborne JW et al: Clinical performance and physical properties of twelve amalgam alloys, *J Dent Res* 57:983-988, 1978.

119. Oysaed H, Ruyter IE, Sjovik-Kleven IJ: Release of formaldehyde from dental composites, *J Dent Res* 67:1289-1294, 1988.

120. Park JB: *Biomaterials: an introduction,* ed 1, New York, 1979, Plenum Publishing.

121. Patterson N: The longevity of restorations: a study of 200 regular attenders in a general dental practice, *Brit Dent J* 157:23-25, 1984.

122. Peyton FA: *Restorative dental materials,* ed 3, St Louis, 1968, Mosby.

123. Phillips RW: *Skinner's science of dental materials,* ed 9, Philadelphia, 1991, WB Saunders.

124. Port RM, Marshall GW: Characteristics of amalgam restorations with variable clinical appearance, *J Am Dent Assoc* 110:491-495, 1985.

125. Powers JM, Capp JA, Koran A: Color of gingival tissues of blacks and whites, *J Dent Res* 56:112-116, 1977.

126. Putnam JJ: Quicksilver and slow death, *National Geographic* 142(4):507-527, 1972.

127. Reese JA, Valega TM: *Restorative dental materials: an overview, vol* 1, Guildford, Surrey, 1985, FDI, Biddles Ltd.

128. Rehfeld RL et al: Evolution of various forms of calcium hydroxide in the monitoring of microleakage, *Dent Mater* 7:202-205, 1991.

129. Reisbick MH: *Dental materials in clinical dentistry,* ed 1, Boston, 1982, John Wright PSG Inc.

130. Retief DH, Mallory WP: Evaluation of two pit and fissure sealants: an in vitro study, *Pediatr Dent* 3:12-16, 1981.

131. Rinne VW: Aluminum foil pouch packaging in pre-measured amalgam capsules, *J Dent Res* 62:116-117, 1983.

132. Ripa LW: Occlusal sealing: rationale of the technique and historical review, *J Am Soc Prev Dent* 3:32-39, 1973.

133. Roberson TM et al: Five-year clinical wear analysis of 19 posterior composites, *J Dent Res* 67A:120, 1988 (abstract 63).

134. Robinson AD: The life of a filling, *Br Dent J* 130:206-208, 1971.

135. Ross GK et al: Measurement of deformation of teeth in vivo, *J Dent Res* 71A:569, 1992 (abstract 432).

136. Roulet JF: *Degradation of dental polymers,* Basel, 1987, Karger.

137. Ryge G: Clinical criteria, *Int Dent J* 30:347-358, 1980.

138. Scheinin A et al: Multifactorial modeling for root caries predictions, *Community Dent Oral Epidemiol* 20:35-37, 1992.

139. Silvey RG, Myers GE: Clinical study of dental cements. VII. A study of bridge retainers luted with three different dental cements, *J Dent Res* 57:703-707, 1978.

140. Simmons JJ: The miracle mixture: glass ionomer and alloy powder, *Tex Dent J* 100:10-12, 1983.

141. Simonsen RJ: Retention and effectiveness of dental sealant after 15 years, *J Am Dent Assoc* 122(11):34-42, 1992.

142. Skinner EW, Phillips RW: Direct filling gold and its manipulation. In *Science of dental materials,* ed 6, Philadelphia, 1967, WB Saunders.

143. Smales RJ: Long-term deterioration of composite resin and amalgam restorations, *Oper Dent* 16:202-209, 1991.

144. Smales RJ, Webster DA, Leppard PI: Predictions of restoration deterioration, *J Dent* 20:215-220, 1992.

145. Smales RJ et al: Prediction of amalgam restoration longevity, *J Dent* 19:18-23, 1991.

146. Smith DL, Caul HJ: Alloys of gallium with powdered metals as possible replacement for dental amalgam, *J Am Dent Assoc* 53:315-324, 1956.

147. Soderholm KJ: Correlation of in vivo and in vitro performance of adhesive restorative materials: a report of the ASC MD156 task group for the adhesion of restorative materials, *Dent Mater* 7:74-83, 1991.

148. Soderholm KJ: Degradation of glass filler in experimental composites, *J Dent Res* 60:1867-1875, 1981.

149. Spencer P et al: Chemical characterization of the dentin/adhesive interface by Fourier transform photoacoustic spectroscopy, *Dent Mater* 8:8-10, 1992.

150. Stock A: Die Gefahrlichkeit des Quecksilberdampfes und der Amalgame, *Med Klin* 22:1209-1212, 1250-1252, 1926.

151. Sturdevant JR et al: Ten-year clinical analysis of 3 barium glass filled posterior composites, *J Dent Res* 71A:204, 1992 (abstract 794).

152. Sturdevant JR et al: The 8-year clinical performance of 15 low-gold casting alloys, *Dent Mater* 3:347-352, 1987.

153. Taylor DF et al: Pooling of long term clinical wear data for posterior composites, *Am J Dentistry* 7(3):(in press), 1994.

154. Taylor NO, Paffenbarger GC, Sweeney WT: Inlay casting golds: physical properties and specification, *J Am Dent Assoc* 19:36-53, 1932.

155. Tomashov ND: *Theory of corrosion and protection of metals,* Ed 1, New York, 1966, Macmillan Publishing.

156. Vanherle G, Lambrechts P, Braem M: Overview of the clinical requirements for posterior composites. In Vanherle G, Smith DC, editors: *Posterior composite resin dental restorative materials,* Netherlands, 1985, Peter Szulc Publishing.

157. Van Meerbeek B et al: Comparative SEM and TEM examination of the ultrastructure of the resin-dentin interdiffusion zone, *J Dent Res* 72:495-501, 1993.

158. Vimy MF, Takahashi Y, Lorscheider FL: Maternal-fetal distribution of mercury (^{203}Hg) released from dental amalgam fillings, *Am J Physiol* 258(4-Pt2):R939-945, 1990.

159. Von Fraunhofer JA: *Scientific aspects of dental materials,* ed 1, London, 1975, Butterworth Publishers.

160. Vrijhoef MMA, Vermeersch AG, Spanauf AJ: *Dental amalgam,* Chicago, 1980, Quintessence Publishing.

161. Waterstrat RM: New alloys show extraordinary resistance to fracture and wear, *J Am Dent Assoc* 123(12):33-36, 1992.

162. WHO: *Environmental health criteria 118: inorganic mercury,* Geneva, 1991, World Health Organization.

163. Wilder AD et al: Long term clinical color-matching analysis for 30 dental composites, *J Dent Res* 71A:206, 1992 (abstract 801).

164. Wilder AD et al: Five-year clinical study of UV polymerized posterior composites, *J Dent* 19:214-220, 1991.

165. Willems G et al: Composite resins in the twenty-first century, *Quint Int* 24:641-658, 1993.

166. Willems G et al: A classification of dental composites according to their morphological and mechanical characteristics. *Dent Mater* 8:310-319, 1992.

167. Wilson AD, Kent BE: A new translucent cement for dentistry—the glass ionomer cement, *Brit Dent J* 132:133-135, 1972.

168. Wilson HJ, McLean JW, Brown D: *Dental materials and their clinical applications,* ed 1, London, 1988, British Dental Association, William Clowes Ltd.

169. Wu W, Cobb EN: A silver staining technique for investigating wear of restorative dental composites, *J Biomed Mater Res* 15:343-348, 1981.

170. Yamada H: *Strength of biological materials,* ed 1, Huntington NY, 1973, RE Krieger Publishing.

171. Yamauchi M, Woodley DT, Mechanic GT: Aging and cross-linking of skin collagen, *Biochem Biophys Res Commun* 158:898-903, 1988.

172. Zardiackas LD, Bayne SC: Fatigue characterization of nine dental amalgams, *Biomat* 6:49-54, 1985.

CHAPTER 7

Fundamentals in cavity preparation

Theodore M. Roberson

Clifford M. Sturdevant

Roger E. Barton*

Joe T. Wall*

*These authors are inactive this edition; see Preface.

INTRODUCTION

Cavity preparation is defined as the mechanical alteration of a defective, injured, or diseased tooth in order to best receive a restorative material which will reestablish a healthy state for the tooth including esthetic corrections where indicated, along with normal form and function. This textbook covers such preparations except the preparation for either a three-quarter crown or full crown. *Nomenclature* associated with cavity preparation, particularly the classification of cavities, is presented in this chapter.

The discipline of operative dentistry harbors the essential knowledge of basic cavity preparation, which is of utmost importance to the dental student and dental practitioner. This basic knowledge must not be construed as simply the treatment of a tooth, but in the context of treating a person. The physiological and psychological aspects of the patient must be given proper consideration (see sections, Patient Physical Factors and Patient Psychological Factors, in Chapter 10). In the sense of local treatment, biological and mechanical factors regarding care of tooth tissues and contiguous oral tissues are paramount. Procedural organization is also emphasized in this chapter.

Need for restorations

Teeth need restorative intervention for a variety of reasons. Foremost is the need to repair a tooth after destruction from a *carious lesion*. A large, extensive restoration may be required in treating a large carious lesion, or a smaller, more conservative restoration may restore the tooth to proper form and function when the lesion is small. Another often-occurring need is the *replacement or repair* of restorations with serious defects, such as improper proximal contact, gingival excess, caries-risk margins, and poor esthetics. Restorations are also indicated to restore proper form and function to *fractured teeth*. Such teeth present with minor to major tooth structure missing or with an incomplete fracture ("greenstick fracture"), resulting in a tooth that has compromised function and, many times, pain or sensitivity. A tooth may require a restoration to simply *restore form or function* absent as a result of congenital malformation. A careful assessment of other diagnostic factors must be undertaken prior to restoration of such teeth to avoid unnecessary restorative intervention. With an increasing number of older persons who are retaining their natural teeth, the prevalence of incomplete tooth fracture is expected to increase. The proper restoration of such fractured teeth will require early diagnosis and knowledgeable, skillful treatment (see Chapters 5, 15, and 19).

As previously mentioned, *esthetic* demands of patients are a reason for placing (and replacing) restorations. An increasing percentage of practitioners' operative treatments are solely as a result of patient desires to improve appearance (see Chapter 18). These may or may not involve complex cavity preparations. Restorations are also required for teeth simply as part of fulfilling *other restorative needs*. For example, when replacing a missing tooth with a fixed or removable bridge, the teeth adjacent to the space usually require some type of restorative procedure to allow for adequate function of the prosthesis. Lastly, a tooth may be restored in a *preventive* sense. Since caries is an infectious disease, the removal of the caries during the restoration of a tooth reduces the microorganisms involved in the disease and thereby may reduce the potential spread. However, it should be completely understood that *restorative intervention primarily repairs damage caused by caries and by itself does not rid the patient of the factors that caused the disease initially.* To accomplish an effective preventive program that places the patient into a low-risk status for developing future carious or periodontal disease, a complete assessment must be made of (1) the type and number of microorganisms present; (2) the patient's homecare ability, effectiveness, and motivation; (3) the need for antimicrobial therapy; and (4) nutritional factors (see Caries Prevention, in Chapter 3).

Objectives of cavity preparation

In general terms the objectives of cavity preparation are to (1) remove all defects and give the necessary protection to the pulp, (2) locate the margins of the restoration as conservatively as possible, (3) form the cavity so that under the force of mastication the tooth or the restoration or both will not fracture and the restoration will not be displaced, and (4) allow for the esthetic and functional placement of a restorative material.

Much of the scientific foundation on which these objectives are executed was presented by Black.[3] For many years the Black cavity preparations, with few modifications, formed the basis for most operative cavity preparation procedures. Modifications of Black's principles of cavity preparation have resulted from the influence of Bronner,[4] Ireland,[16] Markley,[20] R. Sturdevant,[36] Sockwell,[31] and C. Sturdevant,[34] as well as from improvements in restorative materials, instruments, and techniques, and the increased knowledge and application of preventive measures for caries and periodontal disease.

Definition of cavity preparation

As previously stated, *cavity preparation* is the mechanical alteration of a tooth to receive a restorative material which will return the tooth and area to proper form, function, and esthetics. Included in the procedure of preparing the tooth is the removal of all defective or friable tooth structure. Any remaining infected or friable tooth structure may result in further carious progression, sensitivity or pain, or fracture of the tooth and/or restoration.

Stages and steps of cavity preparation

For efficiency in cavity preparation, the procedure is divided into two stages, with each stage having several steps. These stages and steps of cavity preparation are discussed comprehensively in this chapter in the section, Stages and Steps in Cavity Preparation. At this time it is important to realize that the stages do exist for specific reasons. The first stage of cavity preparation is referred to as the ***initial cavity preparation stage.*** In this stage the mechanical alterations of the tooth are *extended to sound tooth structure* (enamel supported by non-carious dentin) in *all* directions (facially, lingually, gingivally, incisally or occlusally, mesially, and distally) *while adhering to a specific, limited pulpal depth* (Fig. 7-1; see also Figs. 19-22, *B* and *C,* and 19-25). In this way the final dimensions of the restoration can be anticipated (minus bevels). The cavity walls are designed in the initial stage of cavity preparation to both retain the restorative material in the tooth and resist potential fracture of the tooth or restoration from masticatory forces delivered principally in the long axis of the tooth. Additional features for retaining the restorative material and protecting against fracture may be deemed necessary as part of the final stage of cavity preparation.

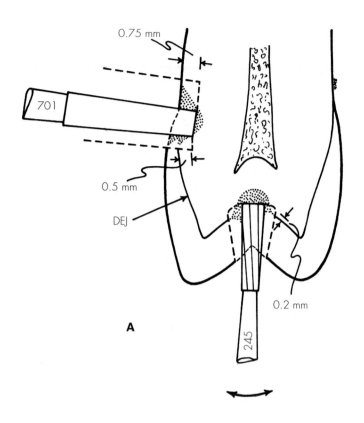

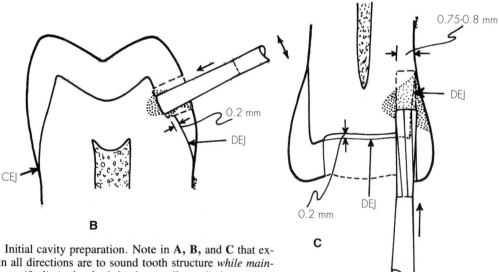

Fig. 7-1. Initial cavity preparation. Note in **A, B,** and **C** that extensions in all directions are to sound tooth structure *while maintaining a specific limited pulpal depth* regardless whether end (or side) of bur is in dentin, caries, old restorative material, or air. Dentinoenamel junction (DEJ); cementoenamel junction (CEJ) indicated in **B.** Note in **A** that initial depth is approximately two thirds of 3 mm bur head length, or 2 mm, as related to prepared facial and lingual walls, but is half the bur head length, or 1.5 mm, as related to central fissure location.

Guidelines for appropriate extensions during initial cavity preparation are discussed in detail later.

Final cavity preparation, the second stage of cavity preparation, is the completion of the cavity preparation. It includes excavating any remaining, infected carious dentin; removing old restorative material if indicated; protecting the pulp; incorporating additional cavity design features that both minimize the chance of tooth or restoration fracture against oblique forces and maximize the retention of the material in the tooth; finishing preparation walls (particularly regarding the margins); and performing the final procedures of cleaning, inspecting, and varnishing (varnishing of preparations for amalgam) the cavity preparation to receive the restorative material. Specific final cavity preparation steps and features which relate to completing the preparation procedure are discussed in subsequent sections. (Conditioning the preparation walls for adhesive bonding of restorative materials is the first procedure in the insertion of the restoration.)

FACTORS AFFECTING CAVITY PREPARATION

Preparing a tooth to receive a restorative material is a comprehensive endeavor. As routine or mundane as it may seem, there are many factors that affect the appropriate cavity preparation design for a given tooth. These factors must be considered for each restorative procedure contemplated, the end result being that no two cavity preparations will be the same. This section will present many of the factors that must be considered prior to any mechanical alteration of a tooth.

General factors

Diagnosis. Prior to any restorative procedure, a complete and thorough diagnosis must be made. There must be a reason to place a restoration in the tooth. The reasons, as presented earlier, may include caries, fractured teeth, esthetic needs, or needs for improved form or function. A careful examination as described in Chapter 5 must be made in order to determine a diagnosis and subsequent treatment recommendation. An assessment of both pulpal and periodontal status will influence the potential treatment of the tooth, especially in terms of the choice of restorative material as well as the design of the cavity preparation.

Likewise, an assessment of the *occlusal relationships* must be made. Such knowledge often affects the design of the cavity preparation and the choice of material. The patient's concern for *esthetics* should be considered when planning the restorative procedure and will influence the restorative material selected. Esthetic considerations will also influence the cavity preparation by altering, in some situations, the extension or design.

The relationship of a specific restorative procedure with *other treatment* planned for the patient must be considered. For example, if the tooth is an abutment for a fixed or removable partial denture, the design of the restoration may need to be altered to accommodate maximum effectiveness of that prosthesis.

Lastly, the *risk potential* of the patient to further dental disease should be assessed. If appropriate, tests should be performed which may indicate the risk the patient has for further dental caries. A high-risk patient may require altered treatment planning initially, until the risk factors are controlled better. This may mean that caries control procedures should be instituted followed by more definitive treatment once the patient's homecare, nutritional habits, and microbiologic assays are improved. Also, more conservative, less expensive restorative procedures may be planned initially until caries factors are controlled.

Knowledge of dental anatomy. Proper cavity preparation is accomplished through systematic procedures based on definite physical and mechanical principles. A prerequisite for understanding cavity preparation is knowledge of the anatomy of each tooth and its related parts. A gross picture, both internal and external, of the individual tooth being operated must be visualized. The direction of the enamel rods, the thickness of the enamel, the dentin body, the size and position of the pulp, the relationship of the tooth to investing tissues, and other factors must all be known to facilitate accurate judgment in cavity preparation.

Patient factors. Patient factors must play an important role in determining the appropriate restorative treatment rendered. The *patient's knowledge and appreciation of good dental health* will influence his or her desire for restorative care and may influence his or her choice of restorative materials. Certainly the patient's *economic status* will be a factor in selecting the type of restorative care selected, but the patient's input in this regard must be obtained. Too often dentists predetermine what they believe is the patient's best economic alternatives and realize later that their assessment was incorrect and other, more suitable, treatment alternatives should have been pursued.

The patient's *age* may be a factor in determining the restorative material and, consequently, the cavity preparation to be used. With more elderly in the population, the treatment of the elderly may pose restorative considerations. Elderly who have physical or medical complications may require special positioning for restorative treatment as well as shorter, less stressful appointments. Such considerations may influence the type of procedure that is planned. Because many elderly will have new or replacement restorative needs that are completely or partially on the root surfaces, the treatment of many of these areas will be more complex. The prevalence of root surface restorative needs is increasing significantly. Whether or not adequate *isolation of the operating site* can be obtained may affect the restorative material selection.

Conservation of tooth structure

Although one of the chief aims of operative dentistry is to arrest the damage from dental caries, the preservation of the vitality of the tooth is paramount. Although pulp tolerance to insult is usually favorable, it should not be subjected to unnecessary abuse by the application of poor or careless operative procedures on the tooth. The less tooth structure removed, the less potential damage that may occur to the pulp.

Every effort should be made to make restorations as small as possible. The smaller the cavity preparation, the easier it is to retain the restorative material in the tooth. Small cavity preparations will result in restorations that have less effect on both intraarch and interarch relationships, as well as esthetics. Naturally, the smaller the cavity preparation, the stronger is the remaining unprepared tooth structure.

Examples of conservative cavity preparation features will be discussed later in this chapter as well as in the technique chapters of this textbook. Included in those features will be concepts relating to (1) *minimal extensions* of the cavity preparations, especially faciolingually and pulpally, (2) *supragingival margins,* and (3) *rounded internal line angles.*

NOMENCLATURE

Nomenclature refers to a set of terms used in communication by persons in the same profession that enables them to better understand one another. The prudent student will master these terms early in the study of dentistry, since their comprehension will aid in diagnosing and treating disease and defects of the teeth.

Caries terminology

As stated in Chapter 3, dental caries is an infectious microbiological disease that results in localized dissolution and destruction of the calcified tissues of the teeth; moreover, caries is episodic with alternating phases of demineralization and remineralization, and these processes may be occurring simultaneously in the same lesion.

Location of caries. Caries can be described according to location, extent, and rate.[12] The latter two descriptive determinants are presented subsequent to this location determinant.

Primary caries. Primary caries is the original carious lesion of the tooth. The etiology, morphology, control, and prevention of caries are presented in Chapter 3. Associated with certain areas of the teeth, there are variations of this pathological condition that fundamentally

influence cavity preparation and, therefore, should be emphasized. Accordingly three *morphological types of primary caries* are evident in clinical observation, namely, carious lesions originating in enamel pits and fissures, or on enamel smooth surfaces, or on root surfaces. Also described in the following sections are backward caries, forward caries, and residual caries.

Caries of pit and fissure origin. Pit and fissure caries can form in the regions of pits and fissures that result from the imperfect coalescence of the developmental enamel lobes as long as other oral conditions conducive to caries are present (Fig. 7-2, *A*). As caries progresses in these areas, sometimes very little evidence is clinically noticeable until the forces of mastication fracture unsupported enamel. The caries forms a small area of penetration in the enamel at the bottom of a pit or fissure and does not spread laterally to a great extent until the *dentinoenamel junction* (*DEJ*) is reached. At this time the disintegration spreads along the junction and begins to penetrate the dentin toward the pulp via the dentinal tubules. In diagrammatic terms the pit and fissure caries may be represented as two cones, base to base, with the apex of the enamel cone at the point of origin and the apex of the dentin cone directed toward the pulp.

Perfect coalescence of the enamel developmental lobes is indicated by faultless enamel areas termed *grooves and fossae.* Usually these areas are not susceptible to caries because they are cleansed by the rubbing of food during mastication. However, in areas of no masticatory action in neglected mouths, caries may develop in a groove or fossa.

Caries of enamel smooth surface origin. Smooth surface caries does not begin in an enamel defect, but rather in a smooth area of the enamel surface that is habitually unclean, and is thereby continually, or usually, covered by plaque (Fig. 7-2, *B* and *C*). It is emphasized in Chapter 3 that plaque is necessary for caries, and that additional oral conditions also must be present for caries to ensue. The disintegration in smooth surface caries in the enamel may also be pictured as a cone, but with its base on the enamel surface and the apex at, or directed to, the dentinoenamel junction. The caries again spreads at this junction in the same manner as in pit and fissure caries. Thus the apex of the cone of caries in the enamel contacts the base of the cone of caries in the dentin.

Backward caries. When the spread of caries along the dentinoenamel junction exceeds the caries in the contiguous enamel, caries extends into this enamel from the junction and is termed backward caries (Fig. 7-3).

Forward caries. Forward caries is wherever the caries cone in enamel is larger or at least the same size as that in dentin[21] (see Fig. 7-2, *A*).

Residual caries. Residual caries is caries that remains in a completed cavity preparation, whether by operator intention or by accident. Such caries is not ac-

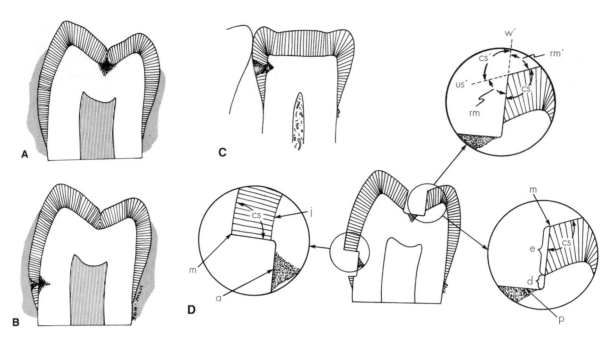

Fig. 7-2. Graphic example of cones of caries (decay) in pit and fissure of tooth (**A**) and on facial (**B**) and proximal (**C**) surfaces when caries has penetrated approximately same depth into dentin. Note differences in loss of enamel on external surfaces. **D,** Sectional view of initial stage of cavity preparations for lesions in **A** and **B** showing cavosurface angle *(cs);* axial wall *(a);* pulpal wall *(p);* enamel wall *(e);* dentinal wall *(d);* margin *(m);* and dentinoenamel junction *(j).* Note in upper exploded view that cavosurface angle *(cs)* can be visualized by imaginary projections *(w')* of the preparation wall and *(us')* of the unprepared surface contiguous with margin, forming angle *cs.'* Angles *(cs)* and *(cs')* are equal because opposite angles formed at the intersection of two straight lines are equal. Likewise, minimal restorative material angle *(rm)* is equal to angle *(rm').*

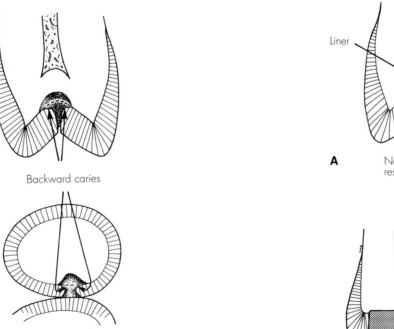

Fig. 7-3. Backward caries extends *from* dentinoenamel junction into enamel.

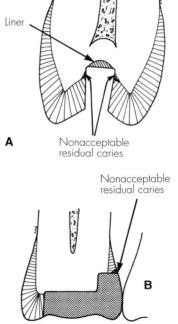

Fig. 7-4. Nonacceptable types of residual caries remaining after cavity preparation: **A,** at dentinoenamel junction and, **B,** on enamel wall of cavity preparation. In postoperative radiograph, **B** appears similar to secondary (recurrent) caries.

ceptable if at the dentinoenamel junction or on the prepared enamel cavity wall (Fig. 7-4, *A* and *B;* see also Fig. 13-11). It is acceptable, however, when it is *affected dentin,* especially near the pulp (see Affected and Infected Dentin).

Root surface caries (senile caries). Root surface caries, sometimes referred to as *senile caries,* may occur on the tooth root that has been both exposed to the oral environment and habitually covered with plaque (Fig. 7-5; see also Fig. 5-5, *F*). Additional oral conditions (discussed in Chapter 3) conducive for caries must also be present, and these are often prevailing in the older population. *Root caries is usually more rapid than other forms of caries, and thus should be detected and treated early.* Root caries is becoming more prevalent because there is an increasing number of elderly who are retaining more of their teeth and experiencing gingival recession, both of which increase the likelihood of root caries development.

Secondary (recurrent) caries. Secondary caries occurs at the borders of a restoration, and then under it. It is often termed *recurrent caries.* This condition usually indicates that microleakage is present, along with other conditions conducive to caries (Fig. 7-6; see also Figs. 5-4, *D* and 5-8, *C*).

Extent of caries

Incipient caries (reversible). Incipient caries is the first evidence of caries activity in the enamel. On smooth surface enamel the lesion will appear opaque white when air-dried, and will seem to disappear (not be distinguishable from contiguous unaffected enamel) if wetted. (See *white spot, ws,* in Fig. 5-5, *D*.) This lesion of demineralized enamel has not extended to the dentinoenamel junction, and the enamel surface is fairly hard and still intact (smooth to the touch). The lesion can be *remineralized* if immediate corrective measures alter the oral environment, including plaque removal and control. This lesion, then, may be stated as *reversible.* A remineralized lesion is either opaque white, or a

shade of brown-to-black from extrinsic coloration, has a hard surface, and appears the same whether wet or dry. (See *brown spot, bs,* in Fig. 5-14, *C*.)

Cavitated caries (nonreversible). In cavitated caries the lesion has advanced into dentin, the enamel surface is broken (not intact), and remineralization is not possible (see Fig. 5-5, *E*). Treatment by cavity preparation and restoration is indicated.

Rate (speed) of caries

Acute (rampant) caries. Acute caries, often termed *rampant caries,* is when the disease is rapid in damaging the tooth; is usually in the form of many, soft-to-the-touch, light-colored lesions in a mouth; and is infectious (see Fig. 5-5, *E*). Less time for extrinsic pigmentation explains the lighter coloration.

Chronic (slow, or arrested) caries. Chronic caries is *slow,* or it may be *arrested* following several active phases. The slow rate results from periods when demineralized tooth structure is almost remineralized (the disease is episodic over time due to changes in the oral environment). The condition may be in only a few locations in a mouth, and the lesion is discolored and fairly hard (see Fig. 5-19, *C*). The slow rate of caries allows time for extrinsic pigmentation. An arrested, enamel lesion is brown-to-black, hard, and due to fluoride may be more caries-resistant than contiguous, unaffected enamel (see Fig. 5-14, *C [bs]*). An arrested, dentinal lesion typically is "open" (allowing debridement from toothbrushing), dark and hard, and this dentin is termed ***eburnated*** (or ***sclerotic***) ***dentin*** (see Fig. 5-19, *A [a]* and *B*).

Grooves and fissures; fossae and pits. On the enamel surface, grooves or fissures mark the location of the union of developmental enamel lobes (see Fig. 2-2). Where such union is complete, this "landmark" is only slightly involuted, smooth, hard, shallow, accessible to cleansing, and is termed a *groove.* (Note in Fig. 2-2 on the upper left illustration the good coalescence of the facial cusps to form an occlusofacial groove.) Where such

Secondary caries

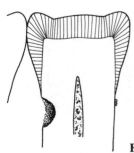

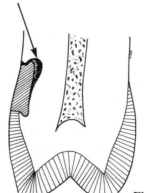

Fig. 7-5. Root surface caries (senile caries).

Root caries

Fig. 7-6. Secondary (recurrent) caries.

union is incomplete, the landmark is sharply involuted to form a narrow, inaccessible canal of varying depths in the enamel and is termed a *fissure* (note in Fig. 2-2 on the upper left illustration the mesial portion of the central fissure). It is a trap for plaque and other oral elements that together can cause caries unless the surface enamel of the canal is fluoride-rich (Fig. 2-12). Caries-preventive treatment of fissured enamel is presented in Chapter 3; and corrective treatments are discussed in this chapter and subsequent chapters.

The distinction made between a groove and a fissure also applies between an enamel surface *fossa* that is nondefective and a *pit* that is defective.

Extension for prevention; enameloplasty; sealant; preventive resin restoration; and conservative composite restoration. Black[3] noted that in cavity preparations for smooth surface caries the restoration should be extended to areas that are normally self-cleansing to prevent recurrence of caries. This principle has come to be known as **extension for prevention.** However, this principle has been broadened to include the extension necessary to remove remaining enamel defects, such as pits and fissures.

The practice of extension for prevention on smooth surfaces has virtually been eliminated because of the relative caries immunity provided by preventive measures, such as fluoride, improved oral hygiene, and proper diet. This has fostered a conservative philosophy wherein the factors determining extension on smooth surfaces are the extent of caries or injury and the restorative material to be used.

Likewise, extension for prevention to include the full length of enamel fissures has been reduced by treatments that conserve tooth structure; thereby, restored teeth are stronger and more resistant to fracture. Such treatments are enameloplasty (see Fig. 12-6), application of pit and fissure sealant (see Fig. 17-1), the preventive resin restoration[30] (see Fig. 17-10), and the conservative composite restoration (see Fig. 17-9).

Enameloplasty is grinding away a shallow, enamel developmental fissure/pit to create a smooth, saucer-shaped surface which is self-cleansing or easily cleaned, as well as an area that enhances proper finishing of a restoration whose margin crosses it. Not only can this prophylactic procedure be applied to fissures/pits and deep supplemental grooves, but also to some shallow, smooth surface enamel defects. (For more details regarding enameloplasty, see later section, Enameloplasty, discussed under subject titled, Initial Cavity Preparation Stage, the Features of Step 1.)

Resin sealant application does not require any tooth preparation and is the preferred preventive method. An alternative to sealant application is the **preventive resin restoration,** whereby a small rotary cutting instrument is used to explore suspicious fissures/pits which are sub-sequently restored with composite and sealant. The **conservative composite restoration** restores a diagnosed, cavitated, small fissure/pit while sealing other suspicious or caries-prone occlusal areas. (See Class I Cavity Preparation, in Chapter 17.)

Prophylactic odontotomy. Prophylactic odontotomy[18] is minimally cutting open and filling with amalgam developmental, structural imperfections of the enamel, such as pits and fissures, to prevent caries originating in these sites. It is no longer advocated as a preventive measure.

Affected and infected dentin. Fusayama reported that carious dentin consists of two distinct layers, an **outer** and an **inner.**[10] This textbook refers to the outer layer as **infected dentin** (zones 4 and 5 discussed in Chapter 3) and the inner layer as **affected dentin** (zones 2 and 3 discussed in Chapter 3). *In cavity preparation, it is desirable that only infected dentin be removed, leaving the affected dentin which then may be remineralized in a vital tooth following the completion of restorative treatment.* This principle for the removal of dentinal caries is supported by Fusayama's observation that the softening front of the lesion always precedes the discoloration front which in turn always precedes the bacterial front[11] (Figs. 7-7 and 7-8).

Infected dentin (bacteria present) is irreversibly denatured (the collagen), not remineralizable, and must be removed. Affected dentin is reversibly denatured, not infected, remineralizable, and should be preserved. To distinguish (differentiate) clinically between these two

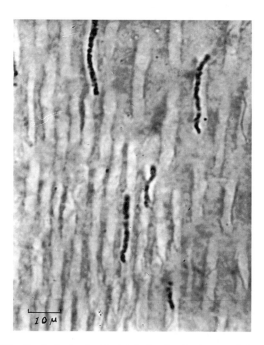

Fig. 7-7. Bacteria in dentinal tubules in the bacterial front of a carious lesion. (Courtesy of Takao Fusayama and the *Journal of Dental Research.*)

layers, the operator traditionally observes the degree of discoloration (extrinsic staining) and tests the area for hardness by the feel of an explorer tine or a slowly revolving bur. Some difficulties occur with this approach because (1) the discoloration may be very slight and gradually changeable in acute (rapid) caries, and (2) the hardness (softness) felt by the hand through an instrument may be an inexact guide. As an alternative method, Fusayama has suggested the application of a 1% solution of acid red (a food dye) in propylene glycol to disclose infected dentin.[10]

In **chronic caries** (rate is slow), infected dentin usually is discolored, and because the bacterial front is close to the discoloration front, it is advisable in caries removal to remove all discolored dentin unless judged to be within 0.5 mm of the pulp (Fig. 7-9). Since in **acute caries** (rate is rapid) the discoloration is very slight and the bacterial front is well behind the discoloration front, some discolored dentin may be left, although any "clinically remarkable" discoloration should be removed.[11]

Non-carious tooth defects terminology

Abrasion. Abrasion is abnormal tooth surface loss resulting from direct friction forces between the teeth and external objects, or from frictional forces between contacting teeth components in the presence of an abrasive medium.[22] Abrasion may occur from (1) improper brushing techniques, (2) habits such as holding a pipe stem by the teeth, (3) tobacco chewing, or (4) vigorous use of toothpicks between adjacent teeth. Toothbrush

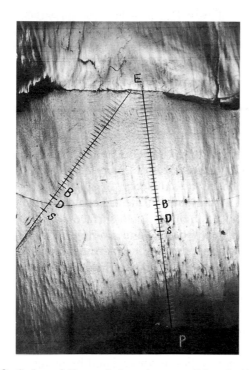

Fig. 7-8. Series of Knoop indentations parallel and oblique to dentinal tubules. *(E)*, Dentinoenamel junction; *(B)* bacterial invasion front; *(D)*, discoloration front; *(S)*, softening front; *(P)*, pulp chamber wall. (Courtesy of Takao Fusayama and the *Journal of Dental Research.*)

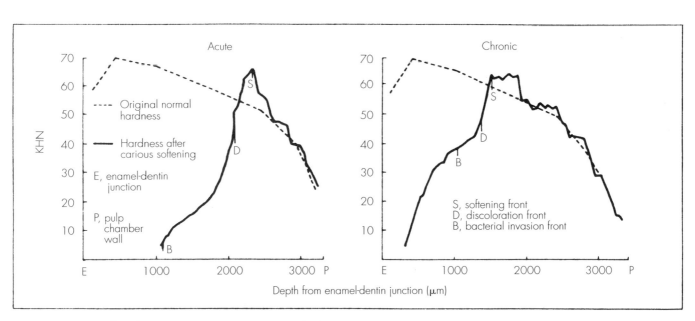

Fig. 7-9. Graphs comparing acute and chronic caries regarding closeness, hardness, and depth factors of the softening, discoloration, and bacterial invasion fronts. (Courtesy of Takao Fusayama.)

tum do not meet, thereby leaving a narrow region of exposed dentin.

Enamel margin strength. One of the more important principles in cavity preparation is the concept of the *strongest enamel margin*. This margin has two significant features: (1) it is formed by full-length enamel rods whose inner ends are on sound dentin; and (2) these enamel rods are buttressed cavity-side by progressively shorter rods whose outer ends have been cut off but whose inner ends are on sound dentin (see Figs. 7-1, *D*, and 12-4). Because enamel rods usually are perpendicular to the enamel surface, the strongest enamel margin will result in cavosurface angle greater than 90 degrees.

An enamel margin composed of full-length rods that are on sound dentin but are *not* buttressed cavity-side by shorter rods also on sound dentin is termed *strong* (but not the strongest). Generally, this margin will result in a 90-degree cavosurface angle (see Fig. 13-7).

An enamel margin composed of rods that do not run uninterrupted from the surface to sound dentin is termed *weak* and this marginal enamel will tend to split off, leaving a V-shaped ditch along the margin of a restoration (see Fig. 2-4, *A*). Usually, this weak enamel margin will have a cavosurface angle less than 90 degrees.

Longitudinal (vertical) and transverse (horizontal) terminology. It is customary through habitual use to describe cavity preparation features or sections (of teeth) which are parallel (or nearly so) to the long axis of the tooth crown as *vertical,* such as vertical height of cusps, or vertical walls. However, for greater correctness this textbook uses the term *longitudinal* in lieu of vertical. Likewise, cavity preparation features which are perpendicular (or nearly so) to the long axis of the tooth are termed *transverse* instead of *horizontal.* When longitudinal (vertical) or transverse (horizontal) are first used in a chapter, the parenthetical alternate will be included, but not thereafter.

Intracoronal and extracoronal cavity preparations. An intracoronal cavity preparation is "box-like," having both internal and external cavity walls (see Fig. 7-10). With conservative cavity preparation for treatment of a small lesion, much of the tooth crown, as well as crown surface, is not involved. Nevertheless, the remaining tooth usually is weakened, and the resto ration may or may not restore the tooth strength.

Conversely, the extracoronal cavity preparation is usually "stump-like," having walls or surfaces that result from removal of most to all of the enamel. The extracoronal restoration, termed a *crown* or *cap,* envelopes the remaining tooth crown and thereby usually restores some of its strength. This textbook does not include extracoronal cavity preparation for crown restorations. However, included in Chapter 19 are *cast metal onlay restorations* which by design encompass the transitional longitudinal tooth corners and thereby strengthen the tooth against post-restorative fracture.

Anatomical tooth crown and clinical tooth crown. The anatomical tooth crown is that portion of the tooth which is covered by enamel. The clinical tooth crown is that portion of the tooth which is exposed to the oral cavity.

Cavity classification

Classification of cavities according to anatomical areas involved as well as by the associated type of treatment was presented by Black and is designated as Class I, Class II, Class III, Class IV, and Class V.[3] Since then an additional class has been added, Class VI. Class I cavities are pit and fissure cavities, whereas the remaining classes are smooth surface cavities. Classification of cavities was originally based on the observed frequency of carious lesions on certain aspects of the tooth. Even though the relative frequency of caries locations may have changed over the years, the original cavity classification is still used, and the various *classes are also used to identify restorations* (i.e., a Class I amalgam restoration). This method of classification is used throughout this textbook.

Class I cavities/restorations. All pit and fissure cavities/restorations are *Class I,* and there are three groupings, as follows:

Cavities/restorations on occlusal surface of premolars and molars. The names of the walls, line angles, and point angles of an occlusal cavity preparation are identified by the labels and legends in Figs. 7-12, 7-13, and 7-14, noting again that a preparation will take the name of the tooth surface (or aspect) that the wall is toward.

Cavities/restorations on occlusal two-thirds of the facial and lingual surfaces of molars. The names of the walls, line angles, and point angles of these cavity preparations (see Fig. 12-28) are the same as those depicted for the preparations for Class V cavities (see Class V Cavities/Restorations).

Cavities/restorations on lingual surface of maxillary incisors. The names of the walls, line angles, and point angles of these cavity preparations (see Fig. 12-29) are the same as those depicted for the preparations for Class V cavities (see Class V Cavities/Restorations).

Class II cavities/restorations. Cavities/restorations on the proximal surfaces of posterior teeth are *Class II.* A proximoocclusal (mesioocclusal, or MO) preparation illustrates and designates walls, line angles, and point angles (Figs. 7-15, 7-16, and 7-17). A distoocclusal preparation has the same walls, line angles, and point angles, except the distal wall (in the MO) will be a mesial wall (in the DO); and the line angles and point angles relating to a distal wall (in the MO) will be relating to a mesial wall (in the DO). A mesioocclusodistal (MOD) preparation will have similar walls, line angles, and point angles, but there is neither a mesial wall nor a distal wall, and therefore line angles and point angles

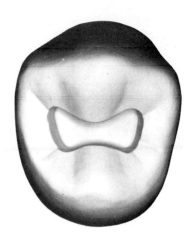

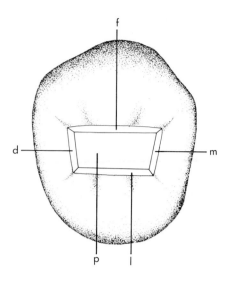

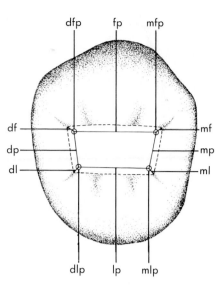

Fig. 7-12. Typical Class I cavity preparation for amalgam on maxillary premolar.

Fig. 7-13. Schematic representation (for descriptive purpose) of Fig. 7-12 illustrating cavity preparation *walls:* facial *(f)*, distal *(d)*, lingual *(l)*, mesial *(m)*, and pulpal *(p)*.

Fig. 7-14. Schematic representation (for descriptive purpose) of Fig. 7-12 illustrating cavity preparation line angles and point angles. *Line angles* are: faciopulpal *(fp)*, distofacial *(df)*, distopulpal *(dp)*, distolingual *(dl)*, linguopulpal *(lp)*, mesiolingual *(ml)*, mesiopulpal *(mp)*, and mesiofacial *(mf)*. *Point angles* are: distofaciopulpal *(dfp)*, distolinguopulpal *(dlp)*, mesiolinguopulpal *(mlp)*, and mesiofaciopulpal *(mfp)*.

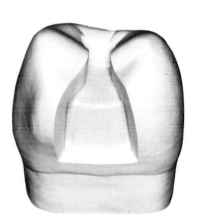

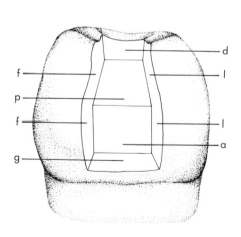

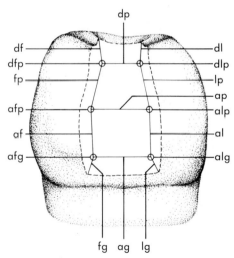

Fig. 7-15. Typical Class II mesioocclusal cavity preparation for amalgam on maxillary premolar.

Fig. 7-16. Schematic representation (for descriptive purpose) of Fig. 7-15 illustrating cavity preparation *walls:* facial *(f)* of proximal and occlusal portions, gingival *(g)*, lingual *(l)* of proximal and occlusal portions, distal *(d)*, pulpal *(p)*, and axial *(a)*.

Fig. 7-17. Schematic representation (for descriptive purpose) of Fig. 7-15 illustrating cavity preparation line angles and point angles. *Line angles* are: distofacial *(df)*, faciopulpal *(fp)*, axiofacial *(af)*, faciogingival *(fg)*, axiogingival *(ag)*, linguogingival *(lg)*, axiolingual *(al)*, axiopulpal *(ap)*, linguopulpal *(lp)*, distolingual *(dl)*, and distopulpal *(dp)*. *Point angles* are: distofaciopulpal *(dfp)*, axiofaciopulpal *(afp)*, axiofaciogingival *(afg)*, axiolinguogingival *(alg)*, axiolinguopulpal *(alp)*, and distolinguopulpal *(dlp)*.

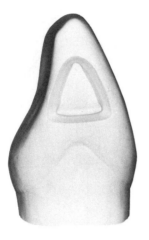

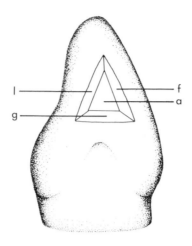

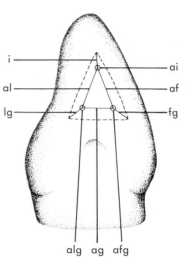

Fig. 7-18. Class III cavity preparation on maxillary central incisor.

Fig. 7-19. Schematic representation (for descriptive purpose) of Fig. 7-18 illustrating cavity preparation *walls*: facial *(f)*, lingual *(l)*, gingival *(g)*, and axial *(a)*.

Fig. 7-20. Schematic representation (for descriptive purpose) of Fig. 7-18 illustrating cavity preparation line angles and point angles. *Line angles* are: axiolingual *(al)*, linguogingival *(lg)*, axiogingival *(ag)*, faciogingival *(fg)*, axiofacial *(af)*, and incisal *(i)*. *Point angles* are: axiolinguogingival *(alg)*, axiofaciogingival *(afg)*, and axioincisal *(ai)*. (Note that names for incisal line angle and point angle are exceptions to the general naming rule.)

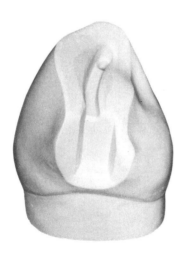

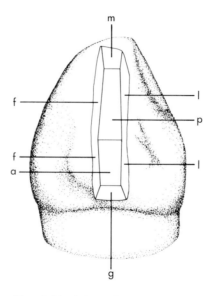

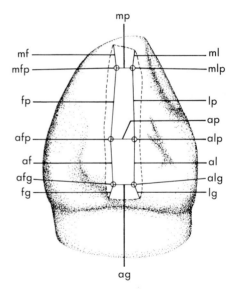

Fig. 7-21. Class IV cavity preparation for inlay on maxillary canine.

Fig. 7-22. Schematic representation (for descriptive purpose) of Fig. 7-21 illustrating cavity preparation *walls*: facial *(f)* of proximal and incisal portions, gingival *(g)*, lingual *(l)* of proximal and incisal portions, axial *(a)*, and mesial *(m)*.

Fig. 7-23. Schematic representation (for descriptive purpose) of Fig. 7-21 illustrating cavity preparation line and point angles. *Line angles* are: mesiofacial *(mf)*, faciopulpal *(fp)*, axiofacial *(af)*, faciogingival *(fg)*, axiogingival *(ag)*, linguogingival *(lg)*, axiolingual *(al)*, axiopulpal *(ap)*, linguopulpal *(lp)*, mesiolingual *(ml)*, and mesiopulpal *(mp)*. *Point angles* are: mesiofaciopulpal *(mfp)*, axiofaciopulpal *(afp)*, axiofaciogingival *(afg)*, axiolinguogingival *(alg)*, axiolinguopulpal *(alp)*, and mesiolinguopulpal *(mlp)*.

associated with mesial and distal walls are not present.

Class III cavities/restorations. Cavities/restorations on the proximal surfaces of anterior teeth that do *not* involve the incisal angle are *Class III*. Walls, line angles, and point angles of a representative cavity preparation are identified in Figs. 7-18, 7-19, and 7-20. Note that the faciolingual line angle at the incisal is termed the *incisal line angle;* likewise, the faciolinguoincisal point angle is termed the *axioincisal point angle.*

Class IV cavities/restorations. Cavities/restorations on the proximal surfaces of anterior teeth that *do* involve the incisal edge are *Class IV*. Walls, line angles, and point angles of a representative cavity preparation are designated in Figs. 7-21, 7-22, and 7-23.

Class V cavities/restorations. Cavities/restorations on the gingival third of the facial or lingual surfaces of all teeth (not pit and fissure cavities) are *Class V*. Walls, line angles, and point angles of a representative cavity preparation on an anterior tooth are designated in Figs. 7-24, 7-25, and 7-26. For posterior teeth the incisal *(i)* becomes occlusal *(o)*.

Class VI cavities/restorations. Cavities/restorations on the incisal edge of anterior teeth or the occlusal cusp heights of posterior teeth are *Class VI*. Walls, line an-

gles, and point angles of these cavity preparations are the same as those depicted for the preparations of occlusal pit and fissure cavities (see Cavities/Restorations on Occlusal Surfaces of Premolars and Molars).

STAGES AND STEPS IN CAVITY PREPARATION

Proper cavity preparation is accomplished through systematic procedures based on definite physical and mechanical principles. Also, the differences between clinically manifested physiological and pathological processes of teeth and investing tissues must be recognized. Moreover, the physical properties and capabilities of the different restorative materials must be appreciated. All these things are determining factors in understanding proper cavity preparation. Without this background knowledge, plus additional information concerning the mechanics of cutting and patient management, the exercise of proper judgment for efficient and proper cavity preparation cannot be achieved.

As stated earlier, the cavity preparation procedure is divided into two stages, each with several steps. The reasoning behind each stage must be thoroughly understood, and each step must be accomplished as perfectly

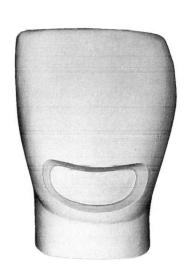

Fig. 7-24. Class V cavity preparation.

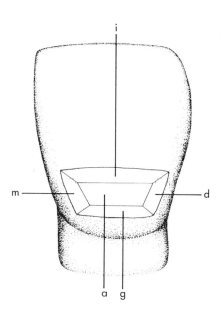

Fig. 7-25. Schematic representation (for descriptive purpose) of Fig. 7-24 illustrating cavity preparation *walls*: mesial *(m)*, gingival *(g)*, distal *(d)*, incisal *(i)* (or occlusal *[o]* if preparation on posterior tooth), and axial *(a)*.

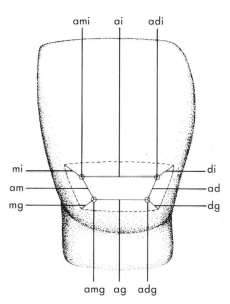

Fig. 7-26. Schematic representation (for descriptive purpose) of Fig. 7-24 illustrating cavity preparation line angles and point angles. *Line angles* are: mesioincisal *(mi)* (or mesioocclusal *[mo]*), axiomesial *(am)*, mesiogingival *(mg)*, axiogingival *(ag)*, distogingival *(dg)*, axiodistal *(ad)*, distoincisal *(di)* (or distoocclusal *[do]*), and axioincisal *(ai)* (or axioocclusal *[ao]*). *Point angles* are: axiomesioincisal *(ami)*, (or axiomesioocclusal *[amo]*), axiomesiogingival *(amg)*, axiodistogingival *(adg)*, and axiodistoincisal *(adi)* (or axiodistoocclusal *[ado]*).

as possible before proceeding to the next. There are occasions, however, where the sequence is altered, but this is the exception and not the general rule (see Caries Control Restoration, in Chapter 3). The stages as they are presented are in the sequence in which they should be followed if consistent, ideal results are to be obtained. Much attention should be given to this area of study of operative dentistry to ensure that operators possess proper habits in cavity preparation that will result in optimal operation and attention to detail without undue strain and lost motion.

The stages and steps in cavity preparation follow:
Initial cavity preparation stage
Step 1.   Outline form and initial depth
Step 2.   Primary resistance form
Step 3.   Primary retention form
Step 4.   Convenience form
Final cavity preparation stage
Step 5.   Removal of any remaining enamel pit/fissure, and/or infected dentin, and/or old restorative material if indicated
Step 6.   Pulp protection
Step 7.   Secondary resistance and retention forms
Step 8.   Procedures for finishing external walls
Step 9.   Final procedures: cleaning; inspecting; varnishing; conditioning

As stated earlier, under certain circumstances this sequence is changed, such as extensive caries that may involve the pulp. Then it may be advisable to place the removal of infected dentin earlier in the procedure. When this becomes necessary, it is also important to place the desired liner and/or base in the preparation at this time, especially if a pulp capping procedure is necessary (see Chapter 3). Normally, however, much of the caries is removed in completing the initial cavity preparation and any remaining infected dentin is removed later.

Specific procedures and instrumentation are discussed in detail in areas of the text concerned with preparation of the various classes of cavities in conjunction with specific restorative materials. *The discussion in this section is concerned with what should be accomplished and why,* and not specifically how it should be accomplished.

Operating site

Before any restorative procedure can be undertaken, the environment in which the procedure will be done must be readied. *Most restorative materials require a moisture-free environment, otherwise the physical properties of the material are compromised.* Chapter 11 of this textbook presents the methods of field isolation, assuring maximum effectiveness of the restorative material. In most cases, the use of the **rubber dam** best assures the correct isolation. Some operators prefer to

place the rubber dam after the initial stage of cavity preparation but prior to excavating infected dentin and placement of secondary retentive features.

Also, the treatment and management of the remainder of the oral environment must be considered. *Protecting the contiguous soft tissues in the operating site must be a primary objective.* Oral mucosa, lips, cheek, and tongue should be protected against deleterious effects from substances placed in the mouth during a restorative procedure as well as from possible mechanical injury caused by the procedure. Likewise, these tissues must be treated carefully so as not to cause any lasting harm. This requires specific actions which will provide appropriate soft tissue response. Proper manipulation of the gingiva requires appropriate use of retraction cord, protection by wedge placement, and development of restoration contours that engender postoperative gingival health. (Placement of retraction cord and wedge[s] is presented in Chapter 11.) For years it was thought to be best to place restoration margins into the gingival sulcus, a region thought to be immune to recurrent caries. It is now accepted that the gingival sulcus is not immune to recurrent caries. Moreover, soft tissue responds negatively to margins placed in the crevice. Therefore *margins should be limited to supragingival locations whenever possible.* Obviously, the less the gingival tissue is affected by the restoration, the less likelihood of future gingival harm caused by either the operative procedure or the restoration contour. Also, and just as important, less extension gingivally is more conservative of tooth structure, leaving the tooth stronger. Specific factors that best assure proper soft tissue health both during and after a restorative procedure will be presented in the chapters describing the various operative restorative techniques.

Initial cavity preparation stage

The initial stage of cavity preparation is the development of the initial cavity preparation. As stated earlier, **initial cavity preparation** *is the extension and initial design of the external walls of the preparation at a specified, limited depth so as to provide access to the cavity or defect, reach sound tooth structure (except for later removal of infected dentin on the pulpal or axial walls), resist fracture of the tooth or restorative material from masticatory forces principally directed with the long axis of the tooth, and retain the restorative material in the tooth* (except for the Class V preparation). The preparation is extended internally no deeper than 0.2 mm (0.5 mm when restoring with direct gold) into dentin for pit and fissure cavities and 0.2 to 0.8 mm into dentin for smooth surface cavities (the greater at a level on the root surface; see Fig. 7-1). This necessitates during the final stage of cavity preparation the need for additional deepening of the preparation in the areas of excavation of any remaining faulty tooth structure, faulty old restorative material, or infected dentin. In this way, the operator can maximize the use of the preparation instrumentation before making changes and can perform the final preparation techniques with better access and visibility. However, when the carious lesion is very extensive, the sequence of these steps is altered in order to determine the pulpal involvement and protect the pulpal tissue as early in the procedure as possible. The *steps in initial cavity preparation* are: (1) develop the outline form and initial depth, (2) establish primary resistance form, (3) establish primary retention form, and (4) provide convenience form. These steps are discussed in detail in the following sections.

Step 1—outline form and initial depth. The first step in initial cavity preparation is determining and developing the outline form while establishing the initial depth.

Definition. Establishing the **outline form** means (1) placing the *cavity margins* in the positions they will occupy in the final preparation, except for finishing enamel walls and margins, and (2) preparing an **initial depth** of 0.2 to 0.8 mm pulpally of the dentinoenamel junction position or normal root surface position (*never deeper no matter whether in tooth structure, air, old restorative material, or caries* unless the occlusal enamel thickness is minimal and greater dimension is necessary for strength of the restorative material!). The deeper depth is for extensions onto the root surface. Otherwise the depth into dentin is not to exceed 0.2 to 0.5 mm (see Fig. 7-1). The outline form must be visualized before any mechanical alteration to the tooth is begun. Occasionally, extensive caries, fractured enamel, and other conditions may prevent an accurate preoperative mental visualization at the onset of cavity preparation; although a dentist with sufficient clinical experience usually can do this. With the principles governing the outline form as a background, this preoperative visualization of the outline form will act as a deterrent to overcutting and overextension, which very often causes weak remaining tooth structure and an unesthetic restoration. Thus, it is very important to preoperatively assess the proposed cavity preparation extensions prior to mechanical removal of any tooth structure, chiefly enamel.

Principles. There are three general principles, not without exception, on which outline form is established regardless of the type of cavity being prepared: (1) all friable and/or weakened enamel should be removed (recall previous Nomenclature section, Enamel Margin Strength), (2) all faults should be included, and (3) all margins should be placed in a position to afford good finishing of the margins of the restoration. The third principle has ramifications that differ for pit and fissure cavities as compared with smooth surface cavities.

Factors. In determining the outline form of a pro-

posed cavity preparation, certain conditions or factors must first be assessed. These conditions will affect the outline form and often will dictate the extensions. Obviously the *extent of the carious lesion, defect, or faulty old restoration* will affect the outline form of the proposed cavity preparation since *the objective is to extend to sound tooth structure, except in a pulpal direction.* There is one extension exception: not uncommonly, a cavity preparation outline for a new restoration will contact or extend slightly into a sound, existing restoration (e.g., a new MO abutting a sound DO; see Fig. 13-26, *A* and *B*). *This is an acceptable practice (i.e, to have a margin of a new restoration placed into an existing, sound restoration).* In addition to these factors, esthetic and occlusal conditions will affect the proposed preparation. *Esthetic considerations* will not only affect the choice of restorative material but also the design of the cavity preparation in an effort to maximize the esthetic result of the restoration. Correcting or improving *occlusal relationships* may also necessitate altering the cavity preparation to accommodate such changes, even when the involved tooth structure is not faulty (i.e., perhaps a cuspal form must be altered to effect better occlusal relationships). Another example is the attempt to avoid including in the outline form an area of heavy occlusal contact, such as centric holding, in a composite restoration for a tooth with no other enamel centric holding area. Likewise, the *adjacent tooth contour* may dictate specific cavity preparation extensions which both secure appropriate proximal relationships and provide the restored tooth with optimal form and strength. Lastly, the desired *cavosurface marginal configuration* of the proposed restoration will affect the outline form. Restorative materials which are more effective when having beveled margins will require cavity preparation outline form extensions that must anticipate the final cavosurface position and form. All of these factors will be discussed in subsequent chapters which present the clinical techniques for the various operative restorations.

Features. Generally there are six specific, typical features of establishing proper outline form and initial depth. These are (1) preserving cuspal strength, (2) preserving marginal ridge strength, (3) minimizing faciolingual extensions, (4) using enameloplasty, (5) connecting two close (less than 0.5 mm apart) faults or cavity preparations, and (6) restricting the depth of the preparation into dentin to a maximum of 0.2 mm for pit and fissure caries and 0.2 to 0.8 mm for the axial wall of smooth surface caries (the greater depth indicated only for an extension gingivally onto the root surface). These features will be discussed as they relate to both pit and fissure cavities and smooth surface cavities.

Outline form and initial depth for pit and fissure cavities. Outline form and initial depth in pit and fissure cavities are controlled by three factors: (1) the extent to which the enamel has been involved by the carious process, (2) the extensions that must be made along the fissures to achieve sound and smooth margins, and (3) the steady (unchanging) limited bur depth related to the tooth's original surface (real, or "visualized" if missing due to disease or defect) while extending the preparation to sound external walls that have a pulpal depth of approximately 2 mm and usually a maximum depth into dentin of 0.2 mm (see Fig. 7-1, *A* and *B*). It should be noted in Fig. 7-1, *A*, that this depth measured in relation to the location of the fissure itself is 1.5 mm.

Certain conditions are involved in establishing sound procedures as a result of these three factors. These considerations may be interpreted as **rules to follow in establishing outline form for pit and fissure cavities:**

1. Extend the cavity margin until sound tooth structure is obtained and no unsupported and/or weakened enamel remains (see Fig. 12-4). Avoid terminating the margin on extreme eminences such as cusp heights or ridge crests. If the extension from a primary groove includes one half or more of the cusp incline, consideration should be given to **capping the cusp.** If the extension is two thirds, the cusp capping procedure is most often the proper procedure (Fig. 7-27). This will remove the margination from the area of masticatory stresses.

2. Extend the cavity margin to include all the fissure that cannot be eliminated by appropriate **enameloplasty** (Fig. 7-28; see also Figs. 12-6 and 19-5) (see Extension for Prevention; Enameloplasty; Sealant; Preventive Resin Restoration; and Conservative Composite Restoration).

3. Restrict the depth of the preparation to a maximum of 0.2 mm into dentin (except when preparing a tooth for a gold foil restoration, in which case the initial depth is 0.5 mm into dentin as described in Chapter 20). *To be as conservative as possible, the preparation for an occlusal surface pit and fissure cavity is first prepared to a depth of 1.5 mm, as measured at the central fissure* (see Figs. 12-1, *G* and 13-1, *C*). Depending on the cuspal steepness angles, the facial and lingual prepared walls usually will be greater than 1.5 mm. It should be noted in Fig. 7-1, *A*, that the initial depth is two thirds of a 3 mm long bur blade, or 2 mm, as related to the prepared facial and lingual walls, but is only half the blade length, or 1.5 mm, as related to the preoperative central fissure location. However, once this depth is established, if remaining enamel pit/fissure is present on less than 50% of the pulpal floor, it is removed during the final stage of cavity preparation (see Step 5—Removal of any Remaining Enamel Pit/Fissure and/or Infected Dentin and/or Old Restorative Material if Indicated). (See Figs. 12-9 and 12-10.) However, if the amount of pit/fissure remaining is greater than 50% of the pulpal floor, the entire pulpal floor is deepened (at this time of preparing outline form) to a maximum initial depth of 0.2 mm into dentin (see Fig. 12-8). This will mean 0.2 mm into dentin when extension is to sound tooth structure (i.e., a 0.2 mm dentinal wall, with the remainder of the wall formed in enamel). Thus, the actual depth of the preparation may vary from 1.5 mm depending on the thickness of the enamel and the steepness of the cuspal inclines. *During this cutting procedure, the end of the bur may be in air (over a hole or caries depression), in old restorative material, or in caries.*

4. When two pit and fissure cavities have less than 0.5 mm of sound tooth structure between them, they should be joined to eliminate a weak enamel wall between them.

5. Extend the outline form to provide sufficient ac-

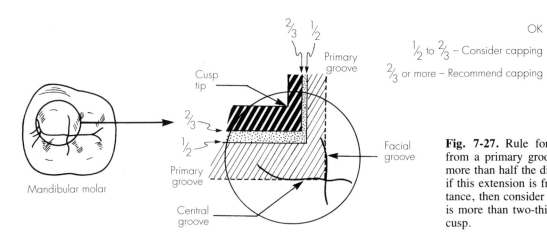

Fig. 7-27. Rule for cusp capping: If extension from a primary groove toward the cusp tip is no more than half the distance, then no cusp capping; if this extension is from half to two-thirds the distance, then consider cusp capping; if the extension is more than two-thirds the distance, then cap the cusp.

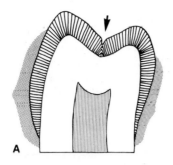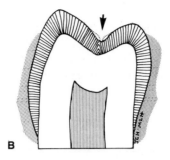

Fig. 7-28. A, Enameloplasty on area of imperfect coalescence of enamel. **B,** No more than one third of the enamel thickness should be removed.

cess for proper cavity preparation, restoration placement, and finishing procedures (see Step 4—Convenience Form).

In the application of these rules, adequate extension of the outline form cannot be overemphasized; however, the improvement of restorative materials and increased knowledge about caries have permitted a more conservative approach to preparation extension than was originally expressed by Black. Therefore conservative, minimal cavity preparation extension should be pursued while conforming to the sound principles of outline form.

Naturally the typical outline form varies with the anatomical form of the particular tooth being operated on. In extending fissures or connecting pits and fissures on the occlusal surfaces of teeth the margins usually do not assume a straight line from one point to another (see Fig. 7-32); rather, they are in *smooth curves* which preserve as much strong cusp structure as possible. Another example of this circumventing of cusps is the Class I preparation on maxillary premolars when cavity extension includes an occlusal fissure, mesial and distal pits, and facial and lingual radiating fissures (see Fig. 12-1, *A*). The outline form resulting from proper preparation of this cavity somewhat resembles a butterfly in flight and is often referred to as "butterfly"-type preparation. The most narrow portion of the preparation, faciolingually, is between the cusp heights. *As much of the cusp incline as possible should be preserved in any preparation involving the occlusal surface,* provided that other principles are maintained at the same time. It is emphasized that the outline will vary from tooth to tooth and that it is *not* extended except as dictated by these rules.

On the occlusal surfaces of molars all developmental grooves should be included to the extent of their being fissured, with appropriate consideration first being given to utilization of enameloplasty, or the preventive resin restoration, or the conservative composite restoration (see Extension for Prevention; Enameloplasty; Sealant; Preventive Resin Restoration; Conservative Composite

Restoration). At times this may necessitate extending onto the facial or lingual surfaces (particularly the facial surface of the mandibular molar and the lingual surface of the maxillary molar) in the form of a small step (see Fig. 12-19). The methods of including the facial or lingual fissures and pits are discussed under amalgam (Chapter 12), composite (Chapter 17), and gold restorations (Chapter 19).

For faulty pits on the lingual surfaces of maxillary anterior teeth and occlusal two thirds of the lingual and facial surfaces of molars the extent of caries or defect and provision of minimal manipulative access are the chief criteria for cavity extension (see Figs. 12-28 and 12-29).

Outline form and initial depth for smooth surface cavities. Smooth surface cavities are in two very different locations: (1) proximal surfaces or (2) the gingival portion of the facial and lingual surfaces (see Fig. 7-2, *B* and *C*). For discussion of outline features and initial depth in initial cavity preparation, each location must be considered separately.

Proximal surfaces (Classes II, III, and IV). The proximal surface presents another controlling factor in establishing outline form, namely, the location of the contact area in relation to the adjacent tooth.

The following fundamental considerations are *rules for establishing outline forms for proximal surface cavities:*

1. Extend the cavity margins until sound tooth structure is obtained and no unsupported and/or weakened enamel remains. (Sometimes unsupported but not friable enamel may remain in cavity preparations for esthetic restorations.)
2. Avoid terminating the margin on extreme eminences such as cusp heights or ridge crests.
3. Extend the margins to allow sufficient access for proper manipulative procedures.
4. Restrict the axial wall pulpal depth of the proximal preparation to a maximum of 0.2 to 0.8 mm into dentin (the greater depth when the extension is onto the root surface; the lesser depth when no

retention grooves will be placed) (see Figs. 7-1, C; 13-3, C; and 14-8). Typically, in this stage of cavity preparation for Class II amalgam restorations the cutting instrument (bur) is positioned by being held parallel to the dentinoenamel junction and thereby creating a cut approximately 0.3 mm into enamel with the remainder of the instrument diameter (approximately 0.5 mm) into dentin (see Fig. 7-1, C). During initial cutting, portions of the instrument may be in air (from a void caused by deeper caries) but it must not remove dentin caries that is deeper pulpally than 0.5 mm from the "dentinoenamel junction position."

5. Extend gingival margins of cavities apically of the contact to provide a minimum clearance of 0.5 mm between the gingival margin and the adjacent tooth (see Fig. 13-3, F). Otherwise this gingival extension is to sound tooth structure and no farther.

6. Extend the facial and lingual margins in proximal cavity preparations into the respective embrasures to provide specified clearance between the prepared margins and the adjacent tooth. The purpose of this clearance is to place the margins away from close contact with the adjacent tooth so that the margins can be visualized, instrumented, and better cleaned (see Figs. 13-21, A and B; 13-24, A and B; 14-5; and 14-19).

In the Class II preparation involving two surfaces, the occlusal outline is governed by the factors that determine the placement of margins of pit and fissure cavities and for inlays the preparation of a dovetail on the occlusal surface in the area of the occlusal pit opposite the involved proximal surface (see Chapter 19).

When extending the proximal surface incisally *in Class III preparations, it is acceptable to position the incisal margin in the area of contact,* especially when an esthetic restorative material is used or when the incisal embrasure is not large enough to allow extension incisal of contact and still have a strong incisal angle of the tooth (see Figs. 14-17 and 16-28, A and B). An incisal margin of sound enamel in the contact area should not be extended incisally to clear the contact unless necessary for instrumentation in cavity preparation or restoration, such as may be required in gold foil.

Gingival portion of facial and lingual surfaces (Class V). The **outline form of Class V cavities** is governed ordinarily *only* by the extent of the lesion, except pulpally. Therefore, extension mesially, gingivally, distally, and occlusally (incisally) is limited to that when sound tooth structure is reached; and during this initial cavity preparation, the bur depth is usually no deeper than 0.8 to 1.25 mm pulpally from the original (when unaffected) tooth surface. The lesser axial wall depth (0.8 mm) is at a gingival wall without an enamel portion (i.e., the margin is on the root surface; see Fig 7-1, A). The axial wall pulpal depth at the occlusal (incisal) wall is that which provides a 0.5 mm extension into dentin (the remainder being enamel). It is to be understood that infected caries deeper than these described depths is *not* removed by the cutting instrument during this preparation stage.

Restricted and increased extensions. Conditions that may warrant consideration of restricted or reduced extensions for smooth surface cavity preparations are (1) proximal contours and root proximity, (2) esthetic requirements, and (3) the use of modified cavity preparations for composite restorations.

Some conditions that may necessitate increased extensions for smooth surface cavity preparations are (1) mental or physical handicaps, (2) advanced age of the patient, (3) restoration of teeth as partial denture abutments or as units of a splint, (4) need for additional measures for retention and resistance form, and (5) need to adjust tooth contours.

Enameloplasty. Sometimes a pit or groove (fissured or not) does not penetrate to any great depth into the enamel and does not, except by undesirable extension, allow proper preparation of cavity margins. This is always true of the end of a fissure. If such a shallow feature is removed and the convolution of the enamel is rounded or "saucered," the area becomes cleanable, finishable, and allows conservative placement of cavity margins. This procedure of reshaping the enamel surface with suitable rotary cutting instruments is termed **enameloplasty** (Fig. 7-28). Specific applications of this procedure are covered and illustrated in detail in chapters pertaining to cavity preparations for inlay and amalgam restorations (see Figs. 12-6 and 19-5, A and B). *Enameloplasty does not extend the outline form.* The restorative material is not placed into the recontoured area, and thus the thickness of the restorative material at the enameloplastied margin (or pulpal depth of the external wall) is decreased.

The operator must be selective in the choice of areas on which this operation is performed. A fissure should be eliminated by normal preparation procedures if it penetrates to more than one-third the thickness of the enamel in the area. If one third or less of the enamel depth is involved, the fissure may be removed without preparing or extending a cavity preparation. This procedure is applicable also to supplemental grooves (fissured or not) extending up cusp inclines. If the ends of these grooves had to be included by extending the cavity preparation, the cusp could be weakened to the extent that it would need to be reduced for capping. Provided these areas are "saucered," the cusp strength can be retained and a smooth union effected between the restorative material and the enamel margin, because the grooved enamel is eliminated.

Another instance where enameloplasty is indicated is on a shallow fissure that approaches or crosses a lingual or facial ridge (see Fig. 19-20). This fissure, if extended under cavity extension principles, would involve two surfaces of the tooth. Use of the enameloplasty procedure can often confine the cavity preparation to one surface and realize a smooth union of the tooth surface and restorative material. An example would be the lingual fissure of a mandibular first molar that terminates on the occlusolingual ridge. Conventional extension should terminate when approximately 2 mm of tooth structure remains between the bur and the lingual surface, and the remainder of the fissure then reshaped provided the terminal portion of the fissure is no more than one third of the enamel in depth. Otherwise the cavity preparation must be extended onto the lingual surface (see Fig. 19-20).

As specific cavity preparations are detailed, several additional applications of this principle will be cited. Enameloplasty may also be applied to teeth in which no preparation is anticipated. However, extreme prudence must be used in the selection of these areas and the depth of which the enamel is removed. This procedure should not be used unless the fissure can be made into a groove with a saucer base by a minimal reduction of enamel and unless centric contacts can be maintained.

Step 2—primary resistance form. While extending the external cavity walls to sound tooth structure, the shape and form of the cavity walls must be initiated. Depending on the restorative material to be used, and in Classes I, II, and IV cavities, the cavity wall design at this initial stage must provide for both protection against fracture from forces delivered in the tooth's long axis (primary resistance form) and retention of the material in the tooth against forces in reverse.

Definition. Primary resistance form may be defined as that shape and placement of the cavity walls that best enable both the restoration and the tooth to withstand, without fracture, masticatory forces delivered princi-pally in the long axis of the tooth. (For protection principally against oblique forces, see Step 7—Secondary Resistance and Retention Forms, in a later section, Final Cavity Preparation Stage.) The relatively flat pulpal and gingival walls prepared perpendicular to the tooth's long axis *resist* forces in the long axis of the tooth and prevent tooth fracture from wedging effects (Fig. 7-29).

Principles. The fundamental principles involved in obtaining primary resistance form follow: (1) to utilize the box shape with a relatively *flat floor,* which helps the tooth to resist occlusal loading by virtue of being at right angles to those forces of mastication that are directed in the long axis of the tooth; (2) to *restrict the extension* of the external walls (keep as small as possible) to allow strong cusp and ridge areas to remain with sufficient dentin support; (3) to have a *slight rounding* (coving) *of internal line angles* to reduce stress concentrations in tooth structure; (4) in extensive cavity preparations, to *cap weak cusps and envelope or include enough of a weakened tooth* within the restoration to prevent or resist fracture of the tooth by forces both in the long axis and obliquely (laterally) directed (most resistance to oblique or lateral forces is attained later in the final cavity preparation stage); and (5) to provide enough *thickness of restorative material* to prevent its fracture under load.

During extension of external walls to sound tooth in developing outline form in Classes I and II cavities, the end of the cutting instrument prepares a relatively flat pulpal wall of uniform depth into the tooth (1.5 to 2 mm overall depth or 0.2 mm into dentin) (see Fig. 7-1, *A* and *C*). *The pulpal wall, therefore, is as flat as the original occlusal surface and the dentinoenamel junction (these roughly paralleling each other).* This semblance of flatness (see Fig. 7-29) is perpendicular to those masticatory forces directed nearly in the long axis of the tooth, and thus is ideal for the stable seating of a restoration which can best *resist* such forces without fracture of the tooth (both wedging forces on the tooth

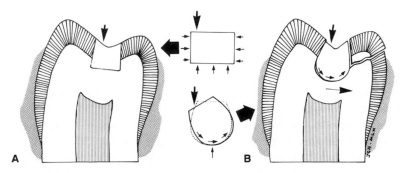

Fig. 7-29. Resistance forms must consider resistance of tooth to fracture from forces exerted on restoration. Flat floor (**A**) will prevent restoration movement, whereas rounded pulpal floor (**B**) is conducive to restoration rocking action producing a wedging force, resulting in shearing of tooth structure.

or tilting forces on the restoration are unlikely). Following the same principle, in Class II cavities, the end of the cutting instrument prepares a *gingival wall (floor) that is flat* and relatively perpendicular to these forces.

Minimally extended facial and lingual walls conserve dentin supporting the cusps as well as facial and lingual ridges, thereby maintaining as much strength of the remaining tooth structure as possible. This *resistance* is against obliquely delivered forces, as well as those in the tooth's long axis.

Internal and external faced angles within the cavity preparation are slightly rounded (coved) so that stresses in the tooth and restoration from masticatory forces will not be as concentrated at these line angles.[23] Rounding internal faced line angles (those with apices directed internally) reduces the stress on the tooth, thus *resistance* to fracture of the tooth is increased. Rounding external faced angles (those with apices directed externally [e.g., axiopulpal line angles]) reduces the stress on some restorative materials (amalgam and porcelain), thus *resistance* to fracture of the restorative material is increased. Details regarding these cavity preparation modifications are described in Chapters 12 to 15, 17, and 19 (also see Fig. 7-32).

A tooth weakened by extensive caries deserves consideration of the fourth principle (capping weakened cusp[s] and/or extending to include cusp[s] entirely) in obtaining primary resistance form during cavity preparation. In extensive caries, extension facially or lingually of the pulpal or gingival walls indicates: (1) reduction of weak cusps for capping by the restorative material (see rules for cusp reduction in the Features section of Step 2—Primary Resistance Form; see Figs. 7-27, 15-2, and 19-22), and/or (2) extension of gingival floors around axial tooth corners onto facial or lingual surfaces (see Figs. 13-31 and 19-24, *J* to *P)*. Either of these features provides some *resistance* both to forces in the long axis and to those obliquely (laterally) directed.

Restorative material thickness affects the ability of a material to resist fracture. The minimal occlusal thickness for amalgam for appropriate resistance to fracture is 1.5 mm, cast metal 1 to 2 mm (depending on the region), and porcelain 2 mm.

When considering the resistance form in anterior proximoincisal preparations (Class IV), one must recognize the narrowness faciolingually of the anterior teeth (and therefore the lesser dentinal support) in applying the principles of obtaining resistance form.

In pulpless teeth special consideration is applied in obtaining resistance form because of the brittle nature of the remaining structure.[9] The weakened cusps are reduced, enveloped, and covered with restorative material to prevent the cracking or splitting of the remaining tooth structure in accord with the fourth principle mentioned previously. Methods of cusp protection are discussed in Chapters 13, 15, and 19.

Factors. The need to develop resistance form in a cavity preparation is a result of several factors. Certain conditions must be assessed to plan for the reduction of the potential fracture of either the restoration or the tooth. Foremost is the assessment of the *occlusal contact* potential on both the restoration and the remaining tooth structure. Obviously, the greater the occlusal force and contacts, the greater is the potential for future fracture (e.g., the further posterior the tooth, the greater is the effective masticatory force since the tooth is closer to the condyle head).

The amount of *remaining tooth structure* also impacts the need and type of resistance form. Very large teeth, even though extensively involved with caries or defects, may require less resistance form consideration, especially in regard to capping cusps, because the remaining tooth structure is still bulky and strong enough to resist fracture. Weakened, friable tooth structure should always be removed in the cavity preparation, but sometimes unsupported, but not friable, enamel may be left. This is usually for esthetic reasons in anterior teeth, especially on the facial surfaces of maxillary teeth where stresses are minimal.

The type of *restorative material* also dictates resistance form needs. Amalgam requires a minimum thickness of 1.5 mm for adequate strength and longevity in relation to wear. Cast metal requires less thickness to resist fracture but should still have a dimension of at least 1 mm in areas of wear, even though the marginal dimensions of cast metal restorations are thinner. Porcelain requires a minimum dimension of 2 mm to resist bulk fracture. The dimensional needs of composite are more dependent on the occlusal wear potential of the restored area. In posterior teeth, the thickness requirement is greater than for anterior teeth. Composite can be used in thinner applications such as veneers or minor esthetic enhancements as long as the wear potential is considered.

Features. The design features of cavity preparation that enhance primary resistance form are:
1. Relatively flat floors
2. Box shape
3. Inclusion of weakened tooth structure
4. Preservation of cusps and marginal ridges
5. Rounded internal line angles
6. Adequate thickness of restorative material
7. Seats on sound dentin peripheral to excavations of infected dentin
8. Reduction of cusps for capping when indicated

These special features will be discussed in more detail in the technique chapters. However, the need for peripheral seats in dentin requires further coverage at this time. A major principle of primary resistance form is that *the restoration should rest on flat sound tooth structure preferably perpendicular to occlusal forces directed parallel to the tooth's long axis* (see Fig. 12-10,

C). If a restoration has the potential to rotate while having forces exerted on it, the chance of fracture or microleakage is greatly increased. By incorporating at least three seats on sound dentin peripheral to an excavation of infected dentin, even in a very large cavity preparation, the restorative material will have a stable contact with the tooth (see Fig. 12-13 and note flat seats peripheral to the excavation). Four seats are even better. Then, when the described forces are applied to the tooth or restoration, they do not cause potential rocking of the restoration.

Reduction of cusps, when indicated, occurs as early as possible in the cavity preparation in order to improve access and visibility. Obviously the decision to reduce a cusp (for capping) is a very important one, and careful consideration should be applied. Although the cusp size and occlusal considerations may affect the decision, there is a basic rule to guide the reduction of cusps during initial cavity preparation. This *rule* is: (1) cusp reduction should be *considered* when the outline form has extended *half the distance from a primary groove to a cusp tip,* and (2) cusp reduction usually is *mandatory* when the outline form has extended *two-thirds the distance from a primary groove to a cusp tip* (see Chapters 15 and 19 and Figs. 7-27, 15-2, and 19-22). The exception to capping a cusp where extension has been two-thirds from a primary groove toward the cusp tip is where the cusp is unusually large and the operator judges that adequate cuspal strength remains.

Step 3—primary retention form. During initial cavity preparation, not only does the form and shape of the preparation need to provide resistance against fracture, but also the design of the preparation must provide for the retention of the restorative material in the tooth (Fig. 7-30). Often, features which enhance the retention form of a cavity preparation also enhance the resistance form (e.g., *pins placed in a manner so that one portion of a tooth supports another portion of the tooth;* see Fig. 15-1).

Definition. *Primary retention form is that shape or form of the prepared cavity that resists displacement or removal of the restoration from tipping or lifting forces.*

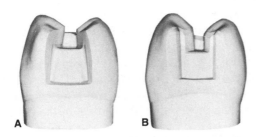

Fig. 7-30. Basic primary retention form in Class II cavity preparations for amalgam **(A)** with longitudinal external walls of proximal and occlusal portions converging occlusally and for inlay **(B)** with similar walls slightly diverging occlusally.

In many respects retention form and resistance form are accomplished in the same cutting procedure and are sometimes discussed together. Although they are separate entities, the same prepared form may contribute to both the resistance and retention qualities of the preparation.

The retention form developed during initial cavity preparation may be adequate to retain the restorative material in the tooth. Often, however, additional retention features must be incorporated in the final stage of cavity preparation.

Principles. Since retention needs are related to the restorative material used, the principles of primary retention form vary depending on the material.

For **amalgam** restorations in most Class I and all Class II cavity preparations, the material is retained in the tooth by developing external cavity **walls that converge occlusally** (see Fig. 7-30, *A)*. In this way, once the amalgam is placed in the cavity and hardens, it cannot come out without some type of fracture occurring. In these preparations the facial and lingual walls of the occlusal portion of the preparation, as well as the proximal portion, converge toward the occlusal surface. This convergence should not be overdone for fear of leaving unsupported enamel rods on the cavosurface margin of the occlusal surface. The occlusal convergence of the proximal portion has several advantages in addition to producing retention. It allows slight facial and/or lingual extension of the proximal portion of the preparation in the gingival area while conserving the marginal ridge, thus reducing the forces of mastication on critical areas of the restoration. The cavosurface angle where the proximal facial and lingual walls meet the marginal ridge is a desirable 90 degrees because of the occlusal convergence of the preparation.

In other preparations for amalgam (such as Classes III and V) the external walls diverge outwardly to provide strong enamel margins, and therefore **retention coves or grooves** are prepared in the dentinal walls to provide the retention form (see Step 7—Secondary Resistance and Retention Forms.)

Adhesive systems are showing promise not only for providing some retention by micro-mechanically **bonding amalgam to tooth structure** but also for **reducing/eliminating microleakage.**[1] However, until longevity studies demonstrate that bonding systems provide complete retention form, traditional retention features should be provided, especially for root surface restorations.

Composite restorations primarily are retained in the tooth by a **mechanical bond** that develops between the material and **conditioned, prepared tooth structure.** In such restorations, the enamel is etched by an acid and the dentin may be conditioned for a dentin bonding agent. These procedures are discussed in a subsequent section, Final Cavity Preparation Stage, and in Chapters

16 to 18. Sometimes the cavity preparation for composite restorations requires the use of mechanical retention form, which also is considered to be part of the final stage of cavity preparation and will be presented in Chapters 16 to 18. As an example, in a Class V cavity preparation (or any portion thereof) on the root surface, groove retention is usually recommended in addition to the use of a bonding system. Because of the strong bond that is developed between etched enamel and composite, the initial cavity preparation of many composite restorations results in a beveled enamel marginal configuration that is ready to be etched. These would be considered the modified composite cavity preparations. Other conventional-type composite restorations require a separate enamel beveling procedure which would be done in final cavity preparation.

Cast metal (usually a gold alloy) *intracoronal restorations* rely primarily on almost parallel longitudinal (vertical) walls to provide retention of the casting in the tooth. During initial cavity preparation, the cavity walls must be designed not only to provide for draw or draft (in order for the casting to be placed into the tooth) but also to provide for an appropriate *small angle of divergence* (2 to 5 degrees per wall) from the line of draw which will enhance *retention form*. The degree of divergence needed is dependent primarily on the length of the prepared cavity walls; the greater the longitudinal height of the walls, the more the divergence permitted and recommended, but within the range described.

In inlay and onlay preparations for cast metal restorations the side walls diverge outwardly by only a few degrees to each other and to a draw path that is usually perpendicular to the floor of the preparation (see Fig. 7-30, *B*). Having sufficient length of these almost parallel walls allows enough frictional resistance and mechanical locking of the cement into minute irregularities of both the casting and the cavity walls to counteract the pull of sticky foods. Close "parallelism" is the principal retention form for cast metal restorations.

In proximoocclusal preparations (Class II) where only one of the two proximal surfaces is involved, an *occlusal dovetail* may aid in preventing the tipping of the restoration by occlusal forces. This occlusal dovetail is placed, when necessary, whether or not there is caries on the occlusal surface. The dovetail simulates a Class I occlusal preparation in the area opposite the proximal involvement (see Fig. 19-6).

One form of *retention* that is inherent in *gold foil* restorations is the elastic compression developed in the dentin as a result of condensation of the foil. This is not a form established in cavity preparation, but it does occur when gold foil restorations are properly condensed. The specific cavity preparation features of a gold foil restoration are presented in Chapter 20.

There is more than one consideration in obtaining retention form. In addition to compensating for the forces of mastication, the pull of sticky foods also must be considered. In all cases, the cavity preparation design must provide for the retention of the restorative material in the tooth. While features of primary retention form are very important, usually additional, secondary retentive features are necessary in the final stage of cavity preparation for most restorations, although the introduction of bonding systems may modify this principle.

Factors. The factors that affect primary retention form have already been presented in the preceding section.

Features. Likewise, the features of primary retention form were presented in a preceding section.

Step 4—convenience form. *Convenience form is that shape or form of the cavity that provides for adequate observation, accessibility, and ease of operation in preparing and restoring the cavity.* On occasion obtaining this form may necessitate extension of mesial, facial, or lingual walls to gain adequate access to the deeper portion of the cavity. An example of this is the cavity preparation and restoration of a mesial (or distal) root surface carious lesion (see Fig. 13-23). The extension of facial margins on anterior teeth is contraindicated for esthetic reasons.

In preparations for gold foil, convenience form assumes an additional purpose other than accessibility for instrumentation (see Chapter 20). It includes establishing convenience points for the starting of foil condensation. These are prepared by deepening, or making more acute, one or more point angles of the preparation. Usually proper refinement of the line and point angles of Class I and Class V preparations is sufficient to produce the necessary convenience form, but additional accentuation may be practiced if desired. The most common application of convenience points is in the gingival area of proximal cavities and is for the convenience of the operator in starting the condensation of the foil. These angles or points are placed with small instruments and should not be "sunk" into the gingival floor.

The occlusal divergence of longitudinal (vertical) walls of cavity preparations for Class II cast restorations may also be considered as convenience form. Extending proximal preparations beyond proximal contacts is another convenience form procedure. Although exceptions may be made to such an extension, preparing the proximal walls to obtain clearance with an adjacent proximal surface affords better access to finish the cavity walls and the restorative material. For cast restorations, clearance with the adjacent proximal surface is mandatory in order to finish the cavity walls, make an accurate impression of the prepared tooth, and try-in the casting.

Final cavity preparation stage

Once the extensions and wall designs have fulfilled the objectives of initial cavity preparation, the preparation should be inspected carefully for other needs. With conservative amalgam or composite restorations the preparation may be complete after initial cavity preparation except for (1) varnishing the cavity walls for amalgam or (2) conditioning the walls for the bonding agent(s) for amalgam or composite. Often, however, there is need for the additional steps (steps 5 through 9) in the final cavity preparation stage. These steps are discussed in the next sections.

Step 5—removal of any remaining enamel pit/fissure and/or infected dentin and/or old restorative material if indicated. In teeth in which the carious lesion is minimal, the carious material is probably removed in completing the initial cavity preparation. If, however, carious infected dentin remains after completion of the previous steps, it should be removed now.

Definition. Removal of any remaining enamel pit/fissure and/or infected dentin and/or old restorative material is the elimination of any infected carious tooth structure or faulty restorative material left in the tooth after initial cavity preparation. The exception to the removal of infected carious tooth structure is when it is decided to perform an indirect pulp cap as described in Caries Control Restoration, in Chapter 3. Removal of remaining enamel pit/fissure typically occurs as small, minimally extended excavations on isolated faulty areas of the pulpal floor. Removal of defective old restorative material is addressed later in this section.

However, in dentin, as caries progresses, an area of decalcification precedes the penetration of microorganisms. This area of decalcification often appears discolored in comparison with undisturbed dentin, yet it does not exhibit the soft texture of caries. This dentin condition may be termed **affected dentin** and differs from **infected dentin** in that it has *not* been significantly invaded by microorganisms. It is accepted and appropriate practice to allow affected dentin to remain in a prepared tooth (see Affected and Infected Dentin).

The use of color alone to determine how much dentin to remove is unreliable. One risks the commitment to overcut on the one hand and to leave infected dentin on the other hand. Often soft, acute (rapid) caries manifests itself entirely within the normal range of color for dentin; thus the eye may not differentiate among infected, affected, or unaffected, normal dentin. On the other hand, distinctly discolored dentin, certainly affected, is often sound and comparable in firmness to surrounding unaffected, normal dentin.

A clinical description of exactly where infected dentin stops and affected dentin begins is practically impossible. It is an empirical decision that is enhanced by practical knowledge and experience, although there are some chemical dyes that may aid that decision. Fortunately the decision does not require exactness, for it is not necessary that all dentin invaded by microorganisms be removed. In shallow or moderately deep cavities, the removal of the masses of microorganisms and the subsequent sealing of the cavity by a restoration at best destroy those comparatively few remaining microorganisms and at worst reduce them to inactivity or dormancy.[27] Even in deep caries where actual invasion of the pulp may have occurred, the recovery of the pulp requires only that, between virulence of the organisms and resistance of the host, a favorable balance be established for the pulp. This is often accomplished by removing all soft caries with its numerous organisms.[32] *It is not acceptable to leave carious dentin at the dentinoenamel junction area* (see Fig. 7-4, *A;* see also Residual Caries).

After initial cavity preparation, the initial depths may result in old restorative material remaining on the pulpal or axial walls. *Any remaining old restorative material should be removed if any of the following conditions are present:* (1) the old material may affect negatively the esthetic result of the new restoration (i.e., old amalgam material left under a new composite restoration), (2) the old material may compromise the amount of anticipated needed retention (i.e., old glass ionomer material having a weaker bond to the tooth than the new composite restoration using enamel and dentin conditioning), (3) there is radiographic evidence of caries under the old material, (4) the tooth pulp was symptomatic preoperatively, or (5) the periphery of the remaining old restorative material is not intact (i.e., there is some breach in the junction of the material with the adjacent tooth structure which may indicate caries under the old material). *If none of these conditions is present, the operator may elect to leave the remaining old restorative material to serve as a liner/base, rather than risk unnecessary excavation nearer to the pulp, which may result in pulpal irritation or exposure.*

Technique. When a pulpal or axial wall has been established at the proper initial cavity preparation position and a small amount of infected carious material remains, only this material should be removed, leaving a rounded, concave area in the wall. The level or position of the wall peripheral to the caries removal depression should not be altered.

In large cavities with extensive soft caries, the removal of infected dentin may be accomplished early in the initial cavity preparation. When the extensive caries is removed, the condition of both the pulp and the remaining tooth structure has a definite bearing on the type of restoration placed. For this reason it is more expedient to remove extensive caries early in the cavity preparation before time and effort are spent in preparing a cavity for a certain restorative material which is then deemed inadequate for satisfactory restoration of the tooth.

Another instance in which the removal of caries is indicated early in cavity preparation is when a patient has numerous teeth with extensive caries. In one seating or appointment infected dentin is removed from several teeth and temporary restorations are placed. After all the teeth containing extensive caries are so treated, then individual teeth are restored as definitively planned. This procedure stops the progress of caries and is often referred to as the ***caries control technique*** (see Chapter 3). It should be obvious that this practice will allow many more teeth to remain serviceable than if a single, seriously involved tooth were treated to completion at the expense of others in the same condition in the same mouth.

It is generally agreed that *large areas of soft caries are best removed with* **spoon excavators** by flaking up the caries around the periphery of the infected mass and peeling it off in layers. The bulk of this material is thus easily removed in a few large pieces.

Regarding the removal of the harder, heavily discolored dentin, opinions vary between the use of spoon excavators, round steel burs at very low speed, and round carbide burs rotating at high speeds. There are several considerations in the removal of this type of caries in deep-seated cavities, although basically the primary concern is for the pulp. Pulpal damage may result from the creation of frictional heat with the use of a bur. The pulp may become infected by forcing microorganisms into the dentinal tubules through excessive pressure with a spoon excavator, or it may be exposed when either instrument is used. The ideal method of removing this material would be one in which minimal pressure is exerted, frictional heat is minimized, and complete control of the instrument is available. *Consideration of these factors usually favors the use of a round carbide bur, with air coolant and slow speed (just above stall-out).* This technique will give the operator complete control of the instrument, minimize pressure and heat generation, and permit adequate vision of the area being operated on. *Examination of the area with an explorer following the removal of infected dentin is advisable, but should be done judiciously to avoid perforation into the pulp.* Caries that rapidly develops sometimes is relatively unstained, and unless the sense of touch is relied on to detect softness the operator may unintentionally leave infected dentin. Ideally, removal of infected dentin should continue until the remaining dentin feels as hard as normal dentin. However, heavy pressure should not be applied with an explorer, or any other instrument, on what is believed to be a thin layer of reasonably firm dentin next to a healthy pulp, for fear of creating an unnecessary pulpal exposure.

Removal of remaining old restorative material, when indicated, is accomplished with use of a round carbide bur, at slow speed (just above stall-out) with air or (better) air-water coolant. The water spray (along with high-volume evacuation) is used when removing old amalgam material to reduce the amount of ***mercury vapor.***

Step 6—pulp protection. Although the placement of cavity liners and bases is not a step in cavity preparation in the strict sense of the word, it is a step in adapting the preparation for receiving the final restorative material. Therefore a basic discussion of this subject follows.

The reason for using traditional liners or bases is to either protect the pulp or to aid pulpal recovery or both. When the thickness of the remaining dentin is less than 2 mm, *heat generated by injudicious cutting can result in a pulpal burn lesion, an abscess formation, or the death of the pulp.* Thus a water or air-water spray coolant must be used with the high-speed rotary instrument. *Cutting the dentinal odontoblastic fibrils* that previously have not been exposed to any irritating episode such as caries or tooth wear will result in degeneration and death of the affected primary odontoblasts and their extensions. The involved tubules become open, ***dead tracts.*** Worse still, if the remaining dentin thickness is 1.5 mm or more and the cutting was done atraumatically using high speed with water or air-water spray, the pulp is not irritated enough to form replacement odontoblasts and therefore no reparative dentin is formed to seal the pulpal side of the dead tracts. Thus it is all the more important to place a liner or base to protect the pulp.[32] (See next paragraph regarding dentin bonding agents for sealing.) ***Other pulpal irritants*** that affect operative procedures are (1) some ingredients of various materials, (2) thermal changes conducted through restorative materials, (3) forces transmitted through materials to the dentin, (4) galvanic shock, and (5) the ingress of noxious products and bacteria through microleakage.

Because the ingress of bacteria is most commonly associated with various pulpal responses, more emphasis should be given to the complete sealing of the prepared dentinal tubules. Effective tubular sealing will prevent penetration of bacteria or their toxins. ***Dentin bonding agents are being recognized as beneficial for dentinal sealing under any type of restorative material.*** As this technology and technique are developed further, more information will become available. If such technology is deemed appropriate, the presented use of liners, bases, and varnishes will be significantly altered if not eliminated. *In spite of that likelihood, the following information is presented about traditional use of liners, bases, and varnishes.*

There are certain physical, chemical, and biological factors to be considered in the selection of a traditional liner or base. The material used should be one that under the circumstances more nearly satisfies the needs of the individual tooth. The attainment of generic status by popularization is insufficient basis for selecting a particular material. Rather, selection should be based on an assessment of the anatomical, physiological, and biological response characteristics of the pulp, as well as the physical and chemical properties of the considered material.

In the following discussion of traditional liners and bases, the use of the term *liners is reserved for those volatile or aqueous suspensions or dispersions of zinc oxide or calcium hydroxide that can be applied to a cavity surface in a relatively thin film*[13] *and are used to effect a particular pulpal response.* Liners may also provide (1) a barrier which protects the dentin from noxious agents from either the restorative material or oral fluids, (2) initial electrical insulation, and/or (3) some thermal protection. *Bases are considered to be those cements commonly used in thicker dimensions beneath permanent restorations to provide for mechanical, chemical, and thermal protection of the pulp.* Examples of bases include zinc phosphate, zinc oxide–eugenol, calcium hydroxide, polycarboxylate, and glass ionomer. For purposes of discussion *varnishes* are also included.

A traditional liner is used to medicate the pulp when suspected trauma has occurred. The desired pulpal effects include both sedation and stimulation, the latter resulting in reparative dentin formation. The choice of liner dictates the specific pulpal response. If the removal of infected dentin does not extend deeper than 1 mm from the initially prepared pulpal or axial wall, usually no liner is indicated. *If the excavation extends into or very close to the pulpal tissue, a calcium hydroxide liner is selected in order to stimulate reparative dentin.* If the excavation depth is between the above examples, a *zinc oxide–eugenol liner is selected (except for composite restorations,* where it may impede the polymerization process) *to provide a palliative, sedative pulpal response,* thus decreasing the potential for postoperative sensitivity.

Both zinc oxide–eugenol and calcium hydroxide liners (chemosetting types which harden) in thicknesses of 0.5 mm or greater have adequate strength to support (resist) condensation forces of amalgam[7] and provide protection against short-term thermal changes. However, when a very deep excavation occurs, it may be necessary to overlay the liner with a stronger base material. As a general rule, it is desirable to have at least a 2 mm dimension of bulk between the pulp and a metallic restorative material. This bulk may include remaining dentin, liner, or base. The base materials offer greater pulpal protection from mechanical, thermal, and chemical irritants. However, *for composite restorative materials,* which are thermal insulators and passively inserted, *a liner of calcium hydroxide is indicated only when there is a pulpal exposure or the excavation is judged to be within 0.5 mm of the pulp.*

The ability of calcium hydroxide to stimulate the formation of reparative dentin when it is in contact with pulpal tissue makes it the material of choice for application to very deep excavations and known pulpal exposures. Very deep excavations may contain **microscopic pulpal exposures** that are not visible to the naked eye. Hemorrhage is the usual evidence of a vital pulp exposure, but with microscopic exposures, such evidence may be lacking. Nevertheless, these exposures are large enough to allow direct pulpal access for bacteria and fluids. *Liners and bases in exposure areas should be applied without pressure.* It is recommended to have at least a 1 mm thickness of calcium hydroxide (chemoset) over near or actual exposures, which then may be overlaid with a base.

When zinc phosphate, glass ionomer, or polycarboxylate cement bases are used, cavity depth and the properties of prior liners determine the technique of placement. When there is known or suspected exposure to the pulp, care must be exercised against forcing material into the pulp chamber. Therefore it is essential to either first use a calcium hydroxide cement in adequate thickness or a nonpressure technique for placing an overlay base.

In instances when either an adequate thickness of calcium hydroxide liner has been placed over an exposure or the excavation is not deep enough to provide danger of forcing cement into the pulp chamber by pressure, a base material may be packed (condensed) into place. In these instances the cement base is used in a putty-like consistency and may be conveyed to the preparation with a hand instrument. The cement base may then be shaped with appropriate hand instruments. A base of zinc phosphate placed in this manner has advantages of less free acid and often the elimination of the use of rotary instruments in forming the surface of the base. *Deep excavations where no exposure or suspicion of exposure exists are appropriately lined with zinc oxide–eugenol material for its mildly anesthetic effect on the pulp.* Under amalgam restorations, a thin layer (0.5 mm) of zinc oxide–eugenol cement may be placed in such excavations with no overlaying of other base material.

In cavity preparations for castings, deeply excavated areas must be covered with positively retained liner/base material that will withstand the subsequent procedural forces. Zinc phosphate, glass ionomer, and polycarboxylate cements fulfill the requirements for such overlay base material. *Bases for cast restorations need to be positively retained against possible displacement in subsequent procedures.* Often undercuts resulting from removal of infected dentin provide retention for the cement base. However, there may be cavity preparations in which prepared undercuts must be provided to retain the cement base. If this is the case, a small round bur is used to place small indentations in the excavation in dentin in areas away from the pulp. Usually two such undercuts opposing each other will be sufficient to hold the cement base. The prepared undercuts need not be deeper than the diameter of the bur (see Figs. 19-10 and 19-11).

The protective qualities of zinc phosphate, polycarboxylate, and glass ionomer cements are somewhat in proportion to the bulk of material used. Thus a thin layer will not afford the protection of a thicker layer. However, *the level to which a base is built should never compromise the desired cavity preparation depth resulting in inadequate restorative material thickness.*

No liner or base exhibits the crushing strength of amalgam. Therefore in the placement of these materials, *ideally there should be at the least three seats, tripodally distributed, for the amalgam on sound dentin at the prescribed level of the pulpal wall in initial cavity preparation* (see Figs. 12-10, *C* and 13-9). This will allow the restoration and the tooth structure, rather than the liner or base, to bear the load after the amalgam has set.

Cavity varnish is a solution liner which seals most of the dentinal tubules and is placed on all cavity preparation walls for amalgam and on dentinal walls of cavity preparations for cast gold, but not used for composites. The application of cavity varnish usually occurs just prior to the insertion of an amalgam or cementation of a cast gold restoration, but will be discussed at this time as it relates to pulpal protection.

Two coats of cavity varnish should be applied to the prepared surfaces for amalgams. Cavity varnish is the only material necessary for shallow excavations in such preparations. The varnish prevents penetration of materials into the dentin[14] and helps to prevent microleakage.[37] Varnishes also may *reduce postoperative sensitivity* by reducing the infiltration of fluids and salivary components at the margins of newly placed restorations.[13]

Two coats of cavity varnish are applied to dentin surfaces (not on enamel walls) of cavity preparations for cast gold restorations. The varnish barrier helps reduce pulpal irritation from the luting cement.

Although varnishes are valuable in reducing postoperative sensitivity, their thin film thickness is insufficient to provide thermal insulation even when applied in two coats.[40] However, their presence significantly *reduces the diffusion of acid* from cements into dentin. Consequently, their use is recommended routinely, especially in deep cavities, with any restorative or cementing material containing acid.[13]

Cavity varnishes should not be used under composites because the solvent in the varnish may react with or soften the resin component in the composite, adversely affecting polymerization. Furthermore, the free monomer of the resin may dissolve the varnish film, rendering it ineffective.[13] Obviously, varnish is not to be ap-

plied to any prepared cavity walls that will be, or are, conditioned for bonding (see Cavity Wall Conditioning Features).

Darkening of tooth structure adjacent to amalgam restoration is observed on occasion. This may be caused by the gradual diffusion of metallic ions into the dentin or by light passing through the translucent enamel that is reflected from the underlying amalgam.[23] Placement of a cement liner or base when replacing such a restoration will decrease this unnatural appearance. This use of liner or base is for esthetic purposes rather than strictly for pulp protection.

Again it should be mentioned that the preceding information about traditional liners, bases, and varnishes may become obsolete as more knowledge is obtained about **bonding agents' effects on sealing dentinal tubules.** As evidence increases regarding the benefits of such materials, the use of liners, bases, and varnishes may be limited to clinical situations where pulpal exposure has occurred; and yet, it furthermore may be shown that reparative dentin formation may not be stimulated by calcium hydroxide. Therefore there may be no indications for traditional liner/base use. Regardless of the materials used, protecting the pulp appropriately is mandatory for the successful restoration of teeth.

Step 7—secondary resistance and retention forms. After removal of any remaining enamel pit/fissure, infected dentin, and/or old restorative material (if indicated) and pulpal protection provided by appropriate liners or bases, additional resistance and retention features may be deemed necessary for the cavity preparation. Most compound and complex cavity preparations require these additional features, the exception being those preparations that are very conservative. When a tooth preparation includes both occlusal and proximal surfaces, each of those areas must have independent retention and resistance features.

Since many preparation features that improve retention form also improve resistance form, and the reverse is true, they will be presented together. *The secondary retention and resistance forms are of two types: (1) mechanical features and (2) cavity wall conditioning features.* However, the second type (cavity wall conditioning features) is not really considered as a part of cavity preparation but, rather, as the first step for the insertion of the restorative material. Regardless, some general comments are presented about such conditioning features.

Mechanical features. There are a variety of mechanical alterations to the preparation that will enhance retention form. These alterations require additional removal of tooth structure. These are discussed fully in the respective technique chapters but are briefly identified in the next five sections.

Retention locks, grooves, and coves. Longitudinally

oriented retention locks and retention grooves are used to provide additional retention for proximal portions of cavity preparations; the locks are for amalgams (see Fig. 13-14) and the grooves are for cast metal restorations (see Fig. 19-8). Transversely oriented retention grooves are prepared in Classes III and V cavity preparations for amalgam (see Figs. 14-7 and 14-33) and in root surface cavity preparations for composite (see Fig. 16-44). Retention coves are appropriately placed undercuts for the incisal retention of Class III amalgams (see Fig. 14-9), occlusal portion of some amalgam restorations (see Fig. 12-26, *C* and *D),* some Class V amalgams (see Fig. 14-34), and occasionally for facilitating the start of insertion of certain gold foil restorations.

Retention locks in Class II preparations for amalgam restorations are generally thought to increase retention of the proximal portion against movement proximally due to creep; also, they are believed to increase the resistance form of the restoration against fracture at the junction of the proximal and occlusal portions. In vivo studies do not substantiate the necessity of these locks in proximoocclusal preparations with occlusal dovetail outline forms or in MOD preparations.[35,39] However, they are recommended for extensive cavity preparations for amalgam involving, for example, wide proximal boxes faciolingually and/or cusp capping.

Groove extensions. Additional retention of the restorative material may be obtained by arbitrarily extending the cavity preparation for molars onto the facial or lingual surface to include a facial or lingual groove. Such an extension is usually performed for cast metal restorations, and results in additional longitudinal (vertical), almost-parallel walls for retention. This feature also enhances resistance for the remaining tooth due to envelopment. (See Figs. 19-26, *I* and 19-29, *I.)*

Skirts. Skirts are preparation features used in cast gold restorations that extend the preparation around some, if not all, of the transitional longitudinal angles of the tooth (see Figs. 19-28 and 19-29). When properly prepared, skirts provide additional, opposed longitudinal walls for added retention. The placement of skirts also significantly increases resistance form by enveloping the tooth, thereby resisting fracture of the remaining tooth from occlusal forces.

Beveled enamel margins. Both cast gold/metal and composite restorations utilize beveled marginal configurations. The bevels for cast metal may slightly improve retention form when there are opposing bevels, but are used primarily to afford a better junctional relationship between the metal and the tooth. Most enamel margins of composite restorations are beveled to increase both the surface area of etchable enamel as well as to maximize the effectiveness of the bond by etching more enamel rod ends.

Pins, slots, steps, and amalgapins. When there is an unusually large need for increased retention form, especially for amalgam restorations, there are several other features that may be incorporated into the cavity preparation. The use of pins and slots increases both retention and resistance forms (see Figs. 15-1 and 15-4). Amalgapins and properly positioned steps also improve retention form, but not to the extent of pins or slots (see Fig. 15-8). All of these procedures are described in Chapter 15.

Cavity wall conditioning features. In addition to mechanical alterations to the cavity preparation, certain alterations to the cavity walls by actions of various materials also afford increased retention, as well as resistance to fracture. Both enamel and dentin surfaces may be conditioned for certain restorative procedures. While such conditioning is considered to be the first step in the insertion of the restorative material, some general comments are presented here.

Enamel wall conditioning. Enamel walls are conditioned for bonded restorations which utilize porcelain, composite, amalgam, or glass ionomer restorative materials. The conditioning consists of etching the enamel by an appropriate acid, resulting in microscopic undercuts in which the bonding material is mechanically bound.

Dentin conditioning. Dentinal surfaces may require conditioning when using bonded porcelain, composite, amalgam, or glass ionomer restorations. The actual conditioner varies with the restorative material utilized, but for most composite restorations, a dentin bonding agent is recommended. Sometimes a glass ionomer material is utilized as a dentin conditioner prior to the restoration of the tooth with another restorative material, and the advantages and disadvantages of this technique are presented in Chapters 16 and 17.

Lastly, it should be noted that retention of indirect restorations (fabricated extraorally) is enhanced by the luting agent used. Although not considered to be part of the cavity preparation, the cementation procedure does affect the retention of these restorations, and some cementing materials do require pretreatment of the dentin.

Step 8—procedures for finishing the external walls of the cavity preparation. Finishing the external walls of the cavity preparation entails consideration of both degree of smoothness and cavosurface design, since each restorative material has its maximum effectiveness when these conditions are developed for that specific material. All cavity preparations do not require special finishing of the external walls at this stage because the walls may already have been finished during earlier steps in the cavity preparation. This is particularly true for small, conservative composite cavity preparations and most amalgam cavity preparations.

Since most cavity preparations have external walls in enamel, most of the following discussion relates to the appropriate finishing of enamel walls. Nevertheless, when a cavity preparation has extended onto the root surface (no enamel present), the root surface cavosurface angle should be either 90 degrees (for amalgam, composite, or porcelain restorations) or beveled (for intracoronal cast metal restorations). The 90-degree root surface margin provides a butt joint relationship between the restorative material and the cementum/dentin preparation wall, a configuration that provides appropriate strength to both. The beveled root surface margin provides the benefits addressed in later paragraphs of this section.

Definition. Finishing the cavity walls is the further development, when indicated, of a specific cavosurface design and degree of smoothness that produces the maximum effectiveness of the restorative material being used.

Objectives. The objectives of finishing the cavity walls are to: (1) create the best marginal seal possible between the restorative material and the tooth structure, (2) afford a smooth marginal junction, and (3) provide maximum strength of both the tooth and the restorative material at and near the margin. Several *factors* must be considered in the finishing of enamel walls and margins: (1) the direction of the enamel rods, (2) the support of the enamel rods both at the dentinoenamel junction and laterally (cavity side), (3) the type of restorative material to be placed in the preparation, (4) the location of the margin, and (5) the degree of smoothness desired.

Theoretically the enamel rods radiate from the dentinoenamel junction to the external surface of the enamel and are perpendicular to the tooth surface. All rods extend full length from the dentin to the enamel surface. The rods converge from the dentinoenamel junction toward concave enamel surfaces and diverge outwardly toward convex surfaces. In general then, the rods converge toward the center of developmental grooves and diverge toward the height of cusps and ridges (see Fig. 7-2, *B* and *C*). In the gingival third of enamel of the smooth surfaces in the permanent dentition the rods incline slightly apically (see Fig. 7-33).

In some instances the rods of occlusal enamel appear to be harder than those of axial (mesial, facial, distal, lingual) enamel. This can be attributed to the amount of interlacing or twisting of the rods in the former as compared with the straight rods of the latter. Enamel with such interlacing of the rods is termed **gnarled enamel** (see Fig. 2-7).

Having a thorough knowledge of the direction of the enamel rods on various tooth surfaces, the operator should finish all enamel walls so that all rods forming the prepared enamel wall have their inner ends resting on sound dentin. Enamel rods that do not run uninterrupted from the cavity margin to dentin tend to split off, leaving a V-shaped ditch along the cavosurface margin

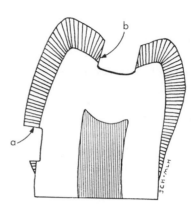

Fig. 7-31. All enamel walls must consist of either full-length enamel rods on sound dentin *(a)* or full-length enamel rods on sound dentin supported on cavity side by shortened rods also on sound dentin *(b)*.

area of the restoration (see Fig. 13-7, *A)*. This should not be interpreted that all enamel walls should consist of full-length rods. *The strongest enamel margin is that margin which is composed of full-length enamel rods that are supported on the cavity (preparation) side by shorter enamel rods, all of which extend to sound dentin* (Fig. 7-31). The shorter enamel rods buttress the full length enamel rods which form the margin, thus increasing the strength of the enamel margin (see Fig. 12-4).

An acute, abrupt change in an enamel wall outline form results in fracture potential, even though the enamel may have dentin support. This indicates that the cavity outline and walls should have *smooth curves or straight lines*. When two enamel walls join, the resulting line angle may be "sharp." If so, it should be slightly curved ("softened"). This slight rounding usually results in a similar curve at the margin. It is to be understood that this discussion is *not* about cavosurface (marginal) bevels. In other words, *line angles formed by the junction of enamel walls should be slightly rounded whether they are obtuse or acute* (Fig. 7-32).

Features. As already stated, there are two primary features related to the finishing of external walls: (1) the design of the cavosurface angle, and (2) the degree of smoothness of the wall.

The *design of the cavosurface angle* is dependent on the restorative material being used. Because of the low edge strength or friability of amalgam, a cavity preparation cavosurface angle of 90 degrees produces maximal strength for both the amalgam and the tooth. This junctional relationship should be obtained by an extension of the entire enamel wall (when in enamel) and not by the use of a short bevel at the cavosurface margin. In Class I cavities for amalgam, the incline planes of the cusp and the converging walls (for retentive purposes) of the cavity preparation approximate the desirable 90-degree butt joint junction, and very little additional,

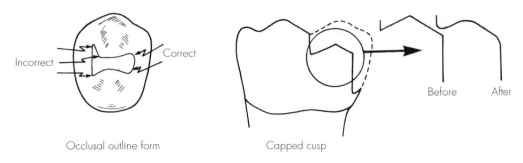

Fig. 7-32. The junctions of enamel walls (and respective margins) should be slightly rounded, whether obtuse or acute.

special cavity preparation is necessary, provided there is sound underlying dentin. However, as can be noted in Fig. 12-13, *A*, when extending the facial and lingual walls *in treating extensive occlusal caries, tilting the bur is often indicated to conservatively extend the margins and provide a 90- to 100-degree cavosurface angle. The extent of this alteration in bur orientation is dictated by the inclination of the contiguous unprepared enamel surfaces.*

Beveling the external walls is a preparation technique employed when using some materials such as intracoronal cast gold/metal and composite restorations. Occasionally some margins in preparations for gold foil are beveled, but these bevels form a cavosurface angle much less obtuse than for gold/metal castings and composites.

Beveling can serve four useful purposes in the cavity preparation for a casting: (1) it produces a stronger enamel margin, (2) it permits a marginal seal in slightly undersized castings, (3) it provides marginal metal that is more easily burnished and adapted, and (4) it assists in adaptation of gingival margins of castings that fail to seat by a very slight amount. The bevel of the cavity margin in a preparation for castings should produce a cavosurface angle that will result in 30- to 40-degree marginal metal (see Figs. 19-12 to 19-14). The marginal gold alloy will be too thin and weak if the angle of the gold bevel is less than 30 degrees. If the angle is greater than 40 degrees, the marginal gold will be too thick and therefore too difficult to burnish satisfactorily. The steepness of cuspal inclines is a factor when beveling *occlusal margins,* even eliminating the need for a bevel when inclines are very steep. (See Fig. 19-14 for developing 140-degree occlusal cavosurface margins.) The *gingival margin* of a casting is a very critical one; an improper beveling of this area may lead to early failure of the restoration. Providing 30-degree beveled metal in this area will result in a sliding, lap fit that definitely improves adaptation of metal to tooth at this margin (see Fig. 19-12).

When amalgam is used, beveling is contraindicated except on the gingival floor of a Class II cavity preparation when enamel is still present. In these instances, it is usually necessary to place a slight *bevel (approximately 15 to 20 degrees) only on the enamel portion of the wall in order to remove unsupported enamel rods.* This is necessary because of the gingival orientation of enamel rods in the cervical area of the tooth crown. This minimal bevel is placed with an appropriate gingival margin trimmer hand instrument and, once placed, still results in a 90-degree amalgam marginal angle (Fig. 7-33).

If the angle of marginal amalgam is less than 80 to 90 degrees (90 degrees is best), it is likely to fracture because it has low edge strength. Such a fracture will leave a crevice at the interface. Thus, the external walls of amalgam preparations need to be designed to result in 80 degrees or greater amalgam marginal angle.

Tooth-colored materials such as porcelain and silicate cement have traditionally belonged to that category of materials which contraindicated beveling the cavosurface margins. However, the use of bevels with most composite cavity preparations is advocated because of the advantages of the acid etch technique. When bevels can be employed with preparations for composites, the potential for retention is increased by increasing the surface area of enamel available for etch plus having a more effective area of etch obtained by etching the cut ends of the enamel rods. Other advantages of beveling composites are that adjacent, minor defects can be included with a bevel and the esthetic quality may be enhanced by a bevel creating an area of gradual increase in composite thickness from the margin to the bulk of the restoration.

The *degree of smoothness* is the second consideration in finishing external walls. Although both the selection of finishing instruments and the methods of finishing enamel walls are reserved for sections describing specific types of preparations, the reasoning for finishing procedures is reviewed in this section. The advent of high-speed cutting procedures has produced two pertinent factors related to finishing enamel walls: (1) the

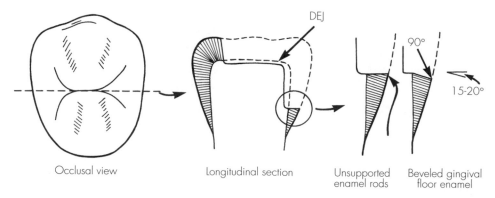

Occlusal view   Longitudinal section   Unsupported   Beveled gingival
                                          enamel rods   floor enamel

Fig. 7-33. Longitudinal section of Class II cavity preparation. Gingival floor enamel (and margin) is unsupported on dentin and friable unless beveled by gingival margin trimmer hand instrument having appropriately angled cutting edge to form 90- to 100-degree cavosurface angle.

lessening of tactile sense and (2) the rapid removal of tooth structure. Performing enamel finishing with high speed can be and is accomplished by the highly skilled and experienced operator; however, in the hands of inexperienced operators, high speed can lead to overextension of margins, grooved walls, and/or rounded cavosurface angles, especially on proximal margins. If this method is used, *plain cut fissure burs produce the finest surface*.[17] These burs produce a smoother surface than crosscut burs, diamonds, or carborundum stones.[5] In fact, at stall-out speeds with an air turbine handpiece, an excellent finish is achieved with this type of bur.

In instances when proximal margins are left at minimal extension for esthetic reasons, rotating instruments (burs, stones, wheels, or discs) cannot be used because of lack of proper access. In such locations, *hand instruments* must be used. The planing action of a razor-sharp hand instrument can result in a smooth enamel wall, although it may not be as smooth as that achieved with other instruments.[33] Hand instruments such as enamel hatchets and margin trimmers may be used in planing enamel walls, cleaving enamel, and establishing enamel bevels. Their usefulness in this capacity should not be overlooked.

The desired fineness or smoothness of an enamel wall is dictated primarily by the restorative material being used. The prepared walls of inlay or onlay preparations require a very smooth surface to permit undistorted impressions and close adaptation of the casting to the enamel margins.[6] In areas of sufficient access fine sandpaper discs can create a very smooth surface; however, proper use of hand instruments, plain fissure burs, or fine diamond stones also will create satisfactory enamel margins for cast preparations.

*When using **gold foil, amalgam, and composite** restorative materials, a very smooth preparation wall is not as desirable as for cast restorations.* When the

above-mentioned materials are used,[24] it has been demonstrated that a rough surface-prepared wall markedly improves resistance to marginal leakage. This does not mean, however, that finishing of the enamel wall should be ignored, but it does indicate that no strict rule for the selection of the finishing instrument can be applied in all instances.

Step 9—final procedures: cleaning; inspecting; varnishing; conditioning. Final procedures in cavity preparation include the cleaning of the cavity, inspecting the cavity preparation, and applying varnish when indicated. Conditioning the cavity walls, when appropriate, is reviewed but is considered the first step in material insertion. The first procedure includes removing all chips and loose debris that have accumulated, drying the cavity (do not desiccate), and making a final complete inspection of the preparation for any remaining infected dentin, unsound enamel margins, or any condition that renders the cavity unacceptable to receive the restorative material. Naturally most of the gross debris has been removed during the preparation steps, but there is usually some fine debris remaining on the cavity walls after all cutting is completed.

The usual procedure in cleaning the cavity is to free the preparation of visible debris with warm water from the syringe and then to remove the visible moisture with a few light surges of air from the air syringe. (Regarding moisture on the dentinal surface, be mindful that dentin bonding systems have specific requirements for conditioning, priming, and applying the bonding agent, which usually is hydrophilic). In some instances debris will cling to the walls and angles despite the above efforts, and it may be necessary to loosen this material with an explorer or small cotton pellet. After all the visible debris has been removed, the cavity is dried free of visible moisture. It is important that the *tooth not be dehydrated by overuse of air* or by the application of alcohol. Once the cavity has been cleaned adequately, the preparation is *visually inspected* to confirm the appropriateness of the cavity preparation.

If a cavity liner or base material has been used, it should be determined that coverage extends only to desired surfaces. *Varnish-type cavity liners* should extend to cover enamel margins for amalgam and should be limited in cast restorations to covering dentinal surfaces. Two coats of copal varnish are recommended in each of these situations. Microleakage in the early days of a newly inserted amalgam restoration is significantly decreased due to the ability of the varnish to seal the tubules.

Composite restorations, which are bonded to the tooth, *require some conditioning of the cavity preparation* prior to insertion of the restorative material. Also, *bonding systems for amalgam restorations have conditioning and bonding agents.* This conditioning may include etching the enamel, placing a dentin bonding agent, or applying a glass ionomer liner. Some of the conditioning steps are presented earlier in this chapter (see Step 7—Secondary Resistance and Retention Forms) and are discussed in detail in Chapters 16 to 18. In all cases, the **smear layer** is either altered or removed and a hybrid layer is formed which is characterized by an intermingling of the resin adhesive (bonding agent) with collagen fibrils of the intertubular dentin. This creates a strong mechanical bond between the composite and the dentin. Additional strong mechanical bonding may occur between the composite and the etched enamel, when enamel is present.

In accomplishing the final procedures before insertion of the restorative material, *sterilization of the cavity preparation* will be considered. The act of sterilizing a cavity preparation before inserting a restoration may be a logical procedure. Some operators do place medicaments in cavities for sterilization purposes, based on empirical factors. Others who have studied this procedure find the literature controversial on the subject of cavity sterilization.

The dentin tubule lumen, varying from 1 to 4 μm in diameter at varying distances between the dentinoenamel junction and the pulp, certainly presents sufficient size for the entrance of microorganisms. Investigators have verified the presence of microorganisms in dentin tubules beneath cavity walls. However, this fact in no way indicates that caries is progressing or that failures will automatically result. Besic,[2] as early as 1943, contended that caries in dentin stops or gradually ceases as soon as the carious lesion is closed to the oral environment, even if microorganisms remain in dentin. Investigators have noted that the number of bacteria in the dentin tubules is relatively small compared with the numerous microorganisms found in the superficial carious lesion. The question is whether these remaining organisms are capable of extending caries under the environmental circumstances of a restored tooth.[32]

Of course, the possible infection of the pulp is always a consideration when bacteria remain in a channel that terminates in the pulp chamber. In this respect the resistance of vital tissue to the ingress of bacteria must be considered. In many instances the presence of reparative dentin deposited as a result of pulpal insult constitutes a significant deterrent to bacterial progress. Another possible answer as to why all teeth with carious involvement do not eventually have pulpal infection is that bacteria may be in a dormant condition as the result of the altered environment of a restored tooth.

The basic considerations in cavity sterilization follow: (1) Is the agent used effective? (2) Is it capable of maintaining a sterile field? and (3) Is it harmful to the pulp?

Early investigators[25] indicated that the common antiseptics once used routinely for cavity sterilization were effective only as a surface disinfectant when applied for a limited amount of time. Therefore simply swabbing the cavity preparation with such agents as silver nitrate, phenol, or ethyl alcohol only leads to a false sense of security. If some of these agents are allowed to remain for a longer period of time, to permit penetration of the tubules, irreparable pulpal damage would result.[8] In deep cavities, microscopic pulp exposures are not always visible to the naked eye and the placement of harmful sterilization agents in such cavities would likely produce pulpal damage.

Assuming that a surface disinfectant is successful, it is doubtful that the sterilization can exist for any appreciable length of time because of the difference between the thermal coefficients of expansion of the tooth and filling materials.[14,15] Although differing in amounts, marginal leakage has been demonstrated for many restorative materials.[26,37,38] However, a large percentage of unsterilized restorations exhibit no caries on the internal wall as a result of this oral fluid penetration; therefore it is possible that the natural defense mechanism of the tooth or the germicidal action of the restorative material destroys any invading bacteria. The germicidal or protective effect ranges from the fluoride content of some materials to the deposition of corrosive products at the interface of the cavity wall and an amalgam. Zinc oxide—eugenol cement has marked germicidal properties over an extended period of time. Therefore some protection from further carious action is afforded by some restorative materials.[29]

The objective of the previous discussion is not to determine whether cavity sterilization via medicaments is essential or nonessential in the practice of sound dentistry but to ascertain if it is justified in routine procedures. *The routine use of specific sterilization medicaments should no longer be a strong consideration.*

However, as stated previously, the use of dentin bonding agents to effect a dentin tubular seal is recognized. *Eliminating bacterial penetration is so important that the use of dentin bonding agents will likely become universal (under all restorations) rather than remain only for composite materials.*

ADDITIONAL CONCEPTS IN CAVITY PREPARATION

A thorough understanding of the principles and concepts of cavity preparation must be obtained by an effective operative dentist. Applying those to a specific restorative procedure, combined with appropriate operating skills and proper handling of the restorative materials will result in successful treatment. Because many new techniques are being advocated for the restoration of teeth, the operator must assess each such proposed method of treatment on the basis of the fundamentals of cavity preparation presented in this chapter. Understanding these fundamental principles makes the assessment of new approaches easier and wiser.

Because amalgam and composite restorations are done more often than other operative procedures, most of the proposed new ways to restore teeth relate to these types of restorations.

Amalgam restorations

Several *new restorative techniques* have been advocated for use with amalgam restorations. In assessing these and future proposals, *the operator must remember the fundamental requirements for a successful amalgam cavity preparation.* These prerequisites for success are: (1) 90-degree junctions of amalgam with tooth structure, (2) mechanical retention form, and (3) adequate thickness for the amalgam material.

Box-only cavity preparations. Box-only cavity preparations for amalgam are advocated for those posterior teeth in which a proximal surface requires restoration but the occlusal surface is not faulty (see Fig. 13-22). A proximal box is prepared and specific retention form is provided, but no occlusal step is included. Such restorations obviously are more conservative, in that less tooth structure is removed. That conservation of tooth structure must be weighed against possible loss of retention form provided by the occlusal step of a typical Class II amalgam cavity preparation.

Tunnel cavity preparations. In an effort to be conservative of tooth structure removal, others advocate a tunnel cavity preparation. This preparation joins an occlusal lesion with a proximal lesion by means of a prepared tunnel under the involved marginal ridge. In this way, the marginal ridge remains essentially intact. In assessing this technique, the adequacy of preparation access may be controversial. Developing appropriately formed

cavity walls and excavating caries may be compromised by lack of access and visibility. Whether or not the marginal ridge is preserved in a strong state is also controversial.

Bonded amalgams. Another new technique advocated for amalgam restorations is the use of various materials which bond the amalgam material to tooth structure. Although the proposed techniques vary, the essential procedure is to prepare the tooth similar to typical amalgam cavity preparations except that more weakened, remaining tooth structure may be retained. Next, the cavity preparation walls are treated or covered with specific adhesive lining materials which bond to both the tooth and the amalgam. The amalgam is condensed onto or into this lining material and a bond develops between the amalgam and liner. Such a technique, if proven to work, will become a significant alternative to cast restorations for severely broken down teeth.

Composite restorations

Likewise there are *new concepts* relating to the use of composite to restore teeth. Some of the newer concepts relating to cavity preparations for composite restorations are presented in Chapters 16 to 18. In these chapters modified cavity preparations are presented as well as cavity preparations relating to expanded uses of composite such as composite inlays, esthetic enhancements, the conservative composite restoration of posterior occlusal surfaces, the preventive resin restoration, veneers, and porcelain inlays cemented with composite materials. In addition to those newer concepts, there are several others that should be addressed.

Again, it is *imperative that the operator understand the requirements of successful composite restorations* when assessing any proposed modifications. For a composite restoration to be successful: (1) most marginal enamel should be beveled and all should be etched; (2) dentin bonding agents should be used, when appropriate; and (3) non-enamel (root surface) external walls should provide butt joint shapes and have appropriately placed mechanical retention form.

Box-only cavity preparations. The box-only cavity preparations for composite restorations are similar to those for amalgam restorations except the box form is less distinct, having "roughed out" marginal configurations rather than refined, 90-degree butt joints. The enamel walls are etched, which provides the retention form of the material in the tooth.

Tunnel cavity preparations. The tunnel cavity preparation, as described above, is also advocated for composite restorations. Usually it is also advocated to use a glass ionomer liner under the composite and some suggest this preparation design be completely restored with a glass ionomer material.

"Sandwich" technique. Another proposed treatment is the use of a *glass ionomer material as a liner* under most, if not all, composite restorations. The advantages of this technique are purported to be the following: (1) the glass ionomer material bonds both to the tooth structure and the composite, thereby increasing retention form, (2) fluoride contained in the glass ionomer material reduces the potential of recurrent caries, and (3) the glass ionomer material, because of its bond to tooth structure, provides a better seal when used at non-enamel margins. There is controversy about these suggested advantages.

Some considerations an operator must make about the "sandwich" technique are the following: (1) Is the retention increased or decreased? (2) Is the resistance form of the restoration compromised because the composite does not rest on tooth structure? (3) Does the cavity preparation need to be deeper into the tooth to provide enough space for both materials? and (4) Is the esthetic result sometimes compromised?

When it is necessary to use an esthetic restorative material in a preparation that has some non-enamel margins, the use of a glass ionomer material to restore that portion of the tooth may have benefits because of both its fluoride content and bond to tooth structure.

"Bonded" restorations strengthen weakened tooth structure. Another controversial issue is whether or not the placement of a bonded composite restoration will bind remaining portions of weakened tooth structure together. The bond created between etched enamel and composite is very strong and may not only be adequate to hold the composite in the tooth but also strengthen remaining unprepared tooth structure. If additional research endorses this concept, the use of large composite restorations may be a valid alternative to more complex and expensive cast restorations for badly broken-down posterior teeth. A factor in utilizing this concept must still be the occlusal relationship of the involved tooth. If some centric contact remains on a nonrestored portion of the occlusal surface, a large composite restoration may withstand the loss of surface integrity caused by wear. If, however, all the occlusal contact is on the restorative material, the wear rate of the composite will be greater.

Some of these new concepts in restoring teeth will become accepted methods of treatment. If the bonded amalgam and large bonded composite restorations are found to be successful and even improve the strength of the tooth, there will be substantial need for their use. Because of the aging population, there will be increased need for the restoration of teeth having large existing, but failing restorations, and these treatment modalities (if endorsed) will provide a technique that is relatively fast, inexpensive, stress-free, and reliable.

SUMMARY

This chapter has addressed the principles of cavity preparations. Specific cavity preparation techniques are presented in various chapters later in the textbook. What should be apparent at this time is that a cavity preparation is determined by many factors and each time a tooth is to be restored, each of these factors must be assessed. If the principles of cavity preparation are adhered to, the success of the restoration is greatly increased. No two cavity preparations are the same.

To summarize, the factors that should be considered before initiating a cavity preparation are many. While the following is a list of many of those factors, it is not all-inclusive:

Extent of caries	Extent of old restorative material
Occlusion	
Pulpal involvement	Extent of defect
Esthetics	Pulpal protection
Patient's age	Contours
Patient's homecare	Economics
Gingival status	Patient's risk status
Anesthesia	Bur design
Bone support	Radiographic assessment
Patient's desires	Other treatment factors
Material limitations	Patient cooperation
Operator skill	Fracture lines
Enamel rod direction	Tooth anatomy
	Ability to isolate area

The increasing bond strengths of enamel and dentin bonding are likely to result in significant emphasis on *bonded restorations.* Likewise, *the improved ability to bond to tooth structure will likely alter significantly the entire cavity preparation procedure.* When materials can be effectively bonded to a tooth while restoring the inherent strength of the tooth, the need for refined cavity preparations will be reduced or eliminated. The only factors necessary then for successful tooth restoration will be the ability and knowledge to (1) completely remove infected dentin and friable enamel, (2) appropriately condition/prime the enamel and dentin, (3) properly manipulate the to-be-bonded restorative material, and (4) contour the restoration to provide proper form and function. *Thus emphasis will shift away from cavity preparation to knowledge of restorative materials and dental anatomy.*

REFERENCES

1. Ben-Amar A: Reduction of microleakage around new amalgam restorations, *J Am Dent Assoc* 119:725, Dec 1989.
2. Besic FC: The fate of bacteria sealed in dental cavities, *J Dent Res* 22:349, 1943.
3. Black GV: *Operative dentistry,* ed 8, 2 vols, Woodstock, Ill, 1947-1948, Medico-Dental Publishing.

4. Bronner FJ: Mechanical, physiological, and pathological aspects of operative procedures, *Dent Cosmos* 73:577, 1931.

5. Cantwell KR, Aplin AW, Mahler DB: Cavity finish with high-speed handpieces, *Dent Progr* 1:42, Oct 1960.

6. Charbeneau GT, Peyton FA: Some effects of cavity instrumentation on the adaptation of gold castings and amalgam, *J Prosthet Dent* 8:514, 1958.

7. Chong WF, Swartz ML, Phillips RW: Displacement of cement bases by amalgam condensation, *J Am Dent Assoc* 74(1):97, 1967.

8. Englander HR, James VE, Massler M: Histologic effects of silver nitrate on human dentin and pulp, *J Am Dent Assoc* 57:621, 1958.

9. Frank AL: Protective coronal coverage of the pulpless tooth, *J Am Dent Assoc* 59:895, 1959.

10. Fusayama T: Two layers of carious dentin: diagnosis and treatment, *Oper Dent* 4:63-70, 1979.

11. Fusayama T, Okuse K, Hosoda H: Relationship between hardness, discoloration, and microbial invasion in carious dentin, *J Dent Res* 45(4):1033-1046, 1966.

12. Gilmore HW et al: *Operative dentistry,* ed 4, St Louis, 1982, Mosby.

13. Going RE: Status report on cement bases, cavity liners, varnishes, primers, and cleaners, *J Am Dent Assoc* 85:654, 1972.

14. Going RE, Massler M: Influence of cavity liners under amalgam restorations on penetration by radioactive isotopes, *J Prosthet Dent* 11:298, 1961.

15. Going RE, Massler M, Dute HL: Marginal penetration of dental restorations by different radioactive isotopes, *J Dent Res* 39:273, 1960.

16. Guard WF, Haack DC, Ireland RL: Photoelastic stress analysis of buccolingual sections of Class II cavity restorations, *J Am Dent Assoc* 57:631, 1958.

17. Hartley JL, Hudson DC: *Clinical evaluation of devices and technics for the removal of tooth structure,* March 1959, Air University, Randolph Air Force Base, Texas.

18. Hyatt TP: Prophylactic odontotomy: the ideal procedure in dentistry for children, *Dent Cosmos* 78:353, 1936.

19. Lee WC, Eakle WS: Possible role of tensile stress in the etiology of cervical erosive lesions of teeth, *J Prosthet Dent* 52(3):374-380, 1984.

20. Markley MR: Restorations of silver amalgam, *J Am Dent Assoc* 43:133, Aug 1951.

21. Marzouk MA et al: *Operative dentistry,* ed 1, p 8, St Louis, 1985, Ishiyaku EuroAmerica.

22. Marzouk MA et al: *Operative dentistry,* ed 1, p 418, St Louis, 1985, Ishiyaku EuroAmerica.

23. Massler M, Barber TK: Action of amalgam on dentin, *J Am Dent Assoc* 47:415, 1953.

24. Menegale CM, Swartz ML, Phillips RW: Adaptation of restorative materials as influenced by the roughness of cavity walls, *J Dent Res* 39:825, 1960.

25. Muntz JA, Dorfman A, Stephan RM: In vitro studies on sterilization of carious dentin: evaluation of germicides, *J Am Dent Assoc* 30:1893, 1943.

26. Nelson RJ, Wolcott RB, Paffenbarger GC: Fluid exchange at the margins of dental restorations, *J Am Dent Assoc* 44:288, 1962.

27. Reeves R, Stanley HR: The relationship of bacterial penetration and pulpal pathosis in carious teeth, *Oral Surg* 22:59, July 1966.

28. Shafer WG, Hines MK, Levy BM: *Oral pathology,* ed 4, p 51, Philadelphia, 1983, WB Saunders.

29. Shay DE, Allen TJ, Mantz RF: Antibacterial effects of some dental restorative materials, *J Dent Res* 35:25, Feb 1956.

30. Simonsen RJ: Preventive resin restoration, *Quintessence Int* 9(1):69-76, 1978.

31. Sockwell CL: Dental handpieces and rotary cutting instruments, *Dent Clin North Am* 15:219, Jan 1971.

32. Stanley HR: *Human pulp response to operative dental procedures,* Gainesville, Fla, 1976, Storter Printing Co Inc.

33. Street EV: Effects of various instruments on enamel walls, *J Am Dent Assoc* 46:274, 1953.

34. Sturdevant CM et al: *The art and science of operative dentistry,* ed 1, New York, 1968, McGraw-Hill.

35. Sturdevant JR et al: Clinical study of conservative designs for Class II amalgams, *J Dent Res* 67:306, 1988 (abstract No. 1549).

36. Sturdevant RE: A further study of inlay problems, *J Am Dent Assoc* and *Dent Cosmos* 25:611, 1938.

37. Swartz ML, Phillips RW: In vitro studies on the marginal leakage of restorative materials, *J Am Dent Assoc* 62:141, Feb 1961.

38. Swartz ML et al: Role of cavity varnishes and bases in the penetration of cement constituents through tooth structure, *J Prosthet Dent* 16:963, 1966.

39. Terkla LG, Mahler DB, Eysden JV: Analysis of amalgam cavity design, *J Prosthet Dent* 29:204, Feb 1973.

40. Voth ED, Phillips RW, Swartz ML: Thermal diffusion through amalgam and various liners, *J Dent Res* 45:1184, 1966.

CHAPTER 8

Instruments and equipment for tooth preparation

Duane F. Taylor

Stephen C. Bayne

Clifford M. Sturdevant

HAND INSTRUMENTS FOR CUTTING

The removal and shaping of tooth structure is an essential part of restorative dentistry. Initially this was a difficult process accomplished entirely by the use of hand instruments. The introduction of rotary, powered cutting equipment was one of the truly major advances in dentistry. From the time of the first hand-powered dental drill to the present-day air-powered handpiece, tremendous strides have been made in the mechanical reduction of tooth structure and thus in the ease with which teeth can be restored. Modern high-speed equipment has eliminated the need for many hand instruments for cavity preparation. Nevertheless, hand instruments remain an essential part of the armamentarium for quality restorative dentistry.

The early hand-operating instruments, with their large, heavy handles (Fig. 8-1) and inferior (by present standards) metal alloys in the blades, were cumber-

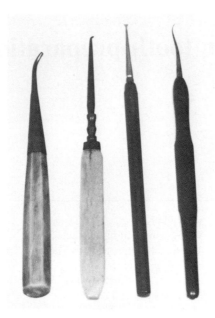

Fig. 8-1. Designs of some early hand instruments. These instruments were individually hand-made, variable in design, and cumbersome to use. Because of nature of the handles, effective sterilization was a problem.

some, awkward to use, and ineffective in many situations. Likewise, there was no uniformity of manufacture or nomenclature. Many dentists made their own hand instruments in an effort to find a suitable instrument for a specific need. As the commercial manufacture of hand instruments increased and dentists began to express ideas on cavity preparation, it became apparent that some scheme for identifying these instruments was necessary. G.V. Black,[4] among his many contributions to modern dentistry, is credited with the first acceptable *nomenclature for and classification of hand instruments.* His classification system enabled both dentists and manufacturers to communicate more clearly and effectively in regard to instrument design and function.

Modern hand instruments, when properly used, produce beneficial results for both the operator and the patient. It should be noted that some of these results can be satisfactorily achieved only with hand instruments and not with rotary instruments. Cavity form dictates some circumstances in which hand instruments are to be used, whereas accessibility dictates others.

Materials

Hand cutting instruments are manufactured from two main materials: *carbon steel* and *stainless steel.* In addition some instruments are made with *carbide* inserts to provide more durable cutting edges. Carbon steel is harder than stainless steel, but when unprotected, it will corrode. Stainless steel remains bright under most conditions but loses a keen edge during use much more quickly than does carbon steel. Carbide, while hard and

wear resistant, is brittle and cannot be used in all designs.

Other alloys of nickel, cobalt, or chromium are used in the manufacture of hand instruments, but they are usually restricted to instruments other than those used for the cutting of tooth structures.

Hardening and tempering heat treatments. To gain maximal benefits from carbon steel or stainless steel, the manufacturer must submit them to two heat treatments: hardening and tempering. The hardening heat treatment hardens the alloy, but it also makes it brittle, especially when the carbon content is high. The tempering heat treatment relieves strains and increases toughness. These properties are optimized by the manufacturer. Subsequent heating of hand instruments during dental use can alter the original properties of the alloy and render it unserviceable. Flaming or improper sterilizing procedures can easily ruin a well-manufactured instrument.

Effects of sterilization. Methods of sterilization are sporicidal cold disinfection, boiling water, steam under pressure (autoclave), chemical vapor, and hot air (dry heat). See Chapter 4 for details regarding acceptable methods of sterilization. Sterilizing carbon steel instruments by any of the first three methods causes *discoloration, rust, and corrosion.* However, several methods for protecting against or minimizing these problems are available. One method used by the manufacturer is to electroplate the instrument. This affords protection except on the blade, where use and sharpening remove the plating. The plating may also pit or peel on the handle and shank under certain circumstances. A second method of protection is by use of rust inhibitors, which are soluble alkaline compounds. These are usually incorporated into commercial sporicidal cold disinfectant solutions, and special preparations are available for use in boiling water and autoclaves. The third method of minimizing the effect of moisture is to remove the instruments promptly at the end of the recommended sterilizing period, dry them thoroughly, and place them in the instrument cabinet or on the tray setup. Leaving instruments exposed to moisture for extended periods or overnight is definitely contraindicated.

The boiling water or autoclave methods of sterilization do not produce discoloration, rust, or corrosion of stainless steel instruments. However, prolonged immersion in cold disinfectant solutions may cause rust. It is advisable to leave stainless steel instruments exposed to moisture only for the recommended time. Dry-heat sterilizers do not rust and corrode carbon steel instruments, but the high heat may reduce the hardness of the alloy. This effect would reduce the ability of the instruments to retain a sharp cutting edge.

The choice of alloy in the hand instrument is up to the operator, but whichever is selected to suit the immediate needs will soon prove unsatisfactory if proper manipulation and sterilization are not continually followed.

Terminology and classification

Instrument categories. The hand instruments used in the dental operatory may be categorized as: (1) cutting (excavators, chisels, and others) or (2) non-cutting (amalgam condensers, mirrors, explorers, probes).[4] *Excavators* may be further subdivided into *ordinary hatchets, hoes, angle formers, and spoons.* **Chisels** are primarily used for cutting enamel, and may be further subdivided into *straight chisels, curved chisels, bin-angle chisels, enamel hatchets, and gingival margin trimmers.* Other cutting instruments may be subdivided as *knives, files, scalers, and carvers.* In addition to the cutting instruments, there is also a very large group of non-cutting instruments (not illustrated in this chapter).

Instrument design. Most hand instruments, regardless of use, are composed of three parts: *handle, shank,* and *blade* (Fig. 8-2). For many non-cutting instruments, the part corresponding to the blade is termed the **nib.** The end of the nib, or working surface, is known as the **face.** The blade or nib is the working end of the instrument and is connected to the handle by the shank. Some instruments have a blade on both ends of the handle and are known as *double-ended instruments.* The blades are of many designs and sizes, depending on the function they are to perform.

Handles are available in various sizes and shapes. Early hand instruments had handles of quite large diameter and were grasped in the palm of the hand. A large, heavy handle is not always conducive to delicate manipulation. In North America, most instrument handles are small in diameter (5.5 mm) and light. They are commonly eight-sided and knurled to facilitate control. In Europe, the handles are often larger in diameter and tapered.

Shanks serve to connect the handles to the working ends of the instruments. They are normally smooth, round, and tapered. Shanks often have one or more

bends to avoid the instrument having a tendency to twist in use when force is applied.

Enamel and dentin are difficult substances to cut and require the generation of substantial forces at the tip of the instrument. Hand instruments must be balanced to allow for the concentration of force onto the blade without causing rotation of the instrument in the grasp. This *balance* is accomplished by designing the angles of the shank so that *the cutting edge of the blade lies within the projected diameter of the handle* and nearly coincides with the projected axis of the handle (Figs. 8-2 and 8-3). For optimal anti-rotational design the blade edge must not be off axis by more than 1 to 2 mm. All

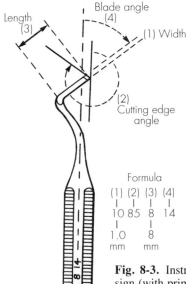

Fig. 8-3. Instrument shank and blade design (with primary cutting edge positioned close to handle axis to produce *balance*). The complete instrument formula (four numbers) is expressed as the *blade width* (1) in 0.1 mm increments, *cutting edge angle* (2) in centigrades, *blade length* (3) in mm, and *blade angle* (4) in centigrades.

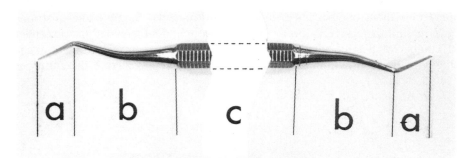

Fig. 8-2. Double-ended instrument illustrating three component parts of hand instruments: blade *(a)*, shank *(b)*, and handle *(c)*.

dental instruments and equipment need to satisfy this principle of balance.

Instrument shank angles. The functional orientation and length of the blade determines the number of angles necessary in the shank to balance the instrument. G.V. Black[3] classified instruments based on the number of shank angles, as: *mon-angle* (one), *bin-angle* (two), or *triple-angle* (three).

Instruments with small, short blades may be easily designed in mon-angle form, while confining the cutting edge within the required limit. Instruments with longer blades or more complex orientations may require two or three angles in the shank to bring the cutting edge near to the long axis of the handle. Such shanks are termed *contra-angled.*

Instrument name. Black classified all instruments by *name.* In addition, for hand cutting instruments, he developed a numeric *formula* to characterize the dimensions and angles of the working end (see the next section for details of the formula). Black's classification system[3] by instrument name categorized instruments by (1) function (e.g., scaler, excavator), (2) manner of use (e.g., hand condenser), (3) design of the working end (e.g., spoon excavator, sickle scaler), or (4) shape of the shank (e.g., mon-angle, bin-angle, contra-angle). These names were combined to form the complete description of the instrument (e.g., bin-angle spoon excavator).

Operative cutting instrument formulas. Cutting instruments have *formulas* describing the dimensions and angles of the working end. These are placed on the handle using a code of three or four numbers separated by dashes or spaces (e.g., 10-85-8-14) (Fig. 8-3). The first number indicates the *width of the blade* or primary cutting edge in tenths of a millimeter (0.1 mm) (e.g., 10 = 1.0 mm). The second number of a four number code indicates the *primary cutting edge angle* measured from a line parallel to the long axis of the instrument handle in clockwise centigrades (angle expressed as a percent of 360 degrees). The instrument is positioned so that this number always exceeds 50. If the edge is locally perpendicular to the blade, then this number is normally omitted resulting in a three number code. The third number (second number of a three number code) indicates the *blade length* in millimeters (1.0 mm). The fourth number (third number of a three number code) indicates the *blade angle* relative to the long axis of the

handle in clockwise centigrade. For these measurements, the instrument is positioned so that this number is always 50 or less. The most commonly used hand instruments, including those specified in this text, are shown in Figs. 8-5 through 8-9 *with their formulas indicated.*

In some instances there is an additional number on the handle that is the manufacturer's identification number. It should not be confused with the formula number. It is simply to assist the specific manufacturer in cataloging, ordering, and so on.

Cutting instrument bevels. Most hand cutting instruments have on the end of the blade a *single bevel* that forms the *primary cutting edge.* Two additional edges, called *secondary cutting* edges, extend from the primary edge for the length of the blade (Fig. 8-4). *Bibeveled* instruments, such as ordinary hatchets, have two bevels that form the cutting edge (Fig. 8-5, *A*).

Certain single-beveled instruments such as spoon excavators (Fig. 8-6) and gingival margin trimmers (Fig. 8-8, *B* and *C*) are used with a scraping or lateral cutting motion. Others such as enamel hatchets (Fig. 8-8, *A*) may be used with a planing or direct cutting motion, as well as a lateral cutting motion. For such single-beveled designs, the instruments must be made in pairs, having the bevels on opposite sides of the blade. Such instruments are designated as *right* or *left* beveled and are indicated by appending the letter R or L to the instrument formula. To determine whether the instrument has a *right* or *left bevel,* the primary cutting edge is held down and pointing away, and if the bevel appears on the right side of the blade it is the right instrument of the pair. This instrument, when used in a scraping motion, is moved from right to left. The opposite holds true for the left instrument of the pair. Thus one instrument is suited for work on one side of the cavity, and the other is suited for the opposite side of the cavity.

Most instruments are available with blades and shanks on both ends of the handle. Such instruments are termed *double-ended.* In many cases the right instrument of the pair is on one end of the handle, and the left instrument is on the other end. Sometimes similar blades of different widths are placed on double-ended instruments. Single-ended instruments may be safer to use, but double-ended instruments are more efficient because they reduce instrument exchange.

Instruments having the cutting edge perpendicular to

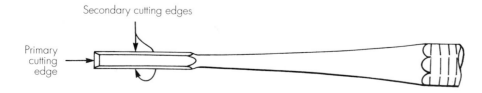

Fig. 8-4. Chisel blade design showing primary and secondary cutting edges.

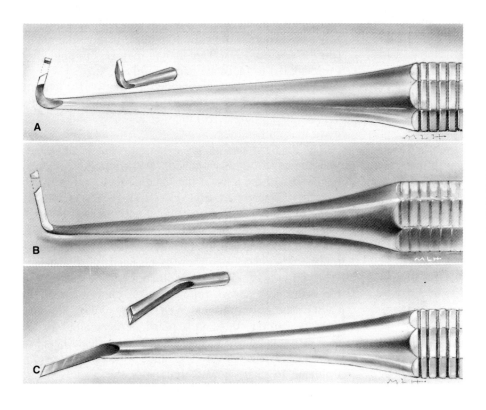

Fig. 8-5. Examples of hand instruments called excavators (with corresponding instrument formulas): **A,** Bibeveled ordinary hatchet (3-2-28). **B,** Hoe (4½-1½-22). **C,** Angle former (12-85-5-8).

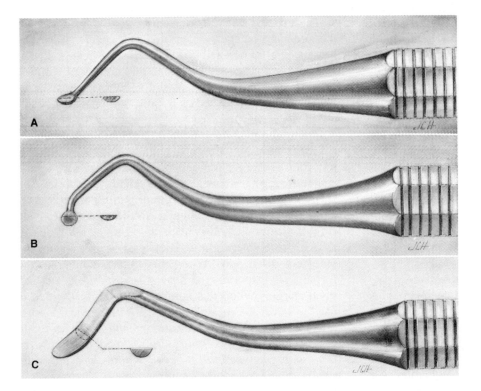

Fig. 8-6. Examples of hand instruments called spoon excavators (with corresponding instrument formulas): **A,** Bin-angle spoon (13-7-14). **B,** Triple-angle spoon (13-7-14). **C,** Spoon (15-8-14).

the axis of the handle, such as bin-angle chisels (Fig. 8-7, *C*), those with a slight blade curvature (Wedelstaedt chisels) (Fig. 8-7, *B)*, and hoes (Fig. 8-5, *B),* are single-beveled and not designated as rights or lefts, but as having a *mesial bevel* or a *distal bevel*. If when one observes the inside of the blade curvature (or the inside of the angle at the junction of the blade and shank) the primary bevel is not visible, the instrument has a *distal bevel*. Conversely, if the primary bevel can be seen (from the same viewpoint) the instrument has a *mesial* or *reverse bevel* (Fig. 8-7).

As previously described, instruments such as chisels and hatchets have three cutting edges, one primary and two secondary. These allow cutting in three directions as the occasion presents. The secondary edges permit more effective cutting than the primary edge in several instances. They are particularly effective in work on the facial and lingual walls of the proximal portion of a proximoocclusal cavity. The operator should not forget the usefulness of these secondary cutting edges because they enhance the use of the instrument.

Cutting instrument applications

The cutting instruments are used to cut hard or soft tissues of the mouth. Excavators are used for removal of caries and refinement of the internal parts of the cavity. Chisels are used primarily for cutting enamel.

Excavators. The four subdivisions of excavators are ordinary hatchets, hoes, angle formers, and spoons.

An *ordinary hatchet excavator* has the cutting edge of the blade directed in the same plane as that of the long axis of the handle and is bibeveled (Fig. 8-5, *A*). These instruments are used primarily on anterior teeth for preparing retentive areas and sharpening internal line angles, particularly in preparations for direct gold restorations.

The *hoe excavator* has the primary cutting edge of the blade perpendicular to the axis of the handle (Fig. 8-5, *B*). This type of instrument is used for planing cavity preparation walls and forming line angles. It is commonly used in Classes III and V preparations for direct gold restorations. Some sets of cutting instruments contain hoes with longer and heavier blades with the shanks contra-angled. These are intended for use on enamel or posterior teeth.

A special type of excavator is the *angle-former* (Fig. 8-5, *C*). It is used primarily for sharpening line angles and creating retentive features in dentin in preparation for gold restorations. It may also be used in placing a bevel on enamel margins. It is mon-angled and has the primary cutting edge at an angle (other than 90 degrees) to the blade. It may be described as a combination of a chisel and gingival margin trimmer. It is available in pairs (right and left).

Spoon excavators (Fig. 8-6) are used for removing caries and carving amalgam or direct wax patterns. The blades are slightly curved and the cutting edges are either circular or claw-like. The circular edge is known as a *discoid,* whereas the claw-like blade is termed a *cleoid* (Fig. 8-9, *C* and *D*). The shanks may be bin-angled or triple-angled to facilitate accessibility.

Chisels. Chisels are intended primarily for cutting enamel and may be grouped as: (a) straight, slightly curved, or bin-angle, (b) enamel hatchets, and (c) gingival margin trimmers.

The *straight chisel* has a straight shank and blade with the bevel on only one side. Its primary edge is perpendicular to the axis of the handle. It is similar in design to a carpenter's chisel (Fig. 8-7, *A*). The shank and blade of the chisel also may be slightly curved (Wedelstaedt design) (Fig. 8-7, *B*) or may be bin-angled (Fig. 8-7, *C*). The force used with all these chisels is essentially a straight thrust. There is no need for a right and left type in a straight chisel, since a 180-degree turn of the instrument allows for its use on either side of the cavity. The *bin-angle* and *Wedelstaedt chisels* have the primary cutting edges in a plane perpendicular to the axis of the handle and may have either a distal bevel or a mesial (reverse) bevel. The blade with a distal bevel is designed to plane a wall that faces the blade's inside surface (Fig. 8-5, *A* and *B*). The blade with a mesial bevel is designed to plane a wall that faces the blade's outside surface (Fig. 8-7, *B* and *C*).

The *enamel hatchet* is a chisel similar in design to the ordinary hatchet except that the blade is larger, heavier, and is beveled on only one side (Fig. 8-8, *A*). It has its cutting edges in a plane that is parallel with the axis of the handle. It is used for cutting enamel and comes as right or left types for use on opposite sides of the cavity.

The *gingival margin trimmer* is designed to produce a proper bevel on gingival enamel margins of proximoocclusal preparations. It is similar in design to the enamel hatchet, except the blade is curved (similar to a spoon excavator), and the primary cutting edge is at an angle (other than perpendicular) to the axis of the blade (Fig. 8-8, *B* and *C*). It is made as *right* and *left* types. It also is made so a right and left pair is either a mesial pair or a distal pair. When the second number in the formula is 90 to 100, the pair is used on the distal gingival margin. When this number is 85 to 75, the pair is used to bevel the mesial margin. *The 100 and 75 pairs are for inlay/onlay preparations with steep gingival bevels. The 90 and 85 pairs are for amalgam preparations with gingival enamel bevels that decline gingivally only slightly.* Among other uses for these instruments is the rounding or beveling of the axiopulpal line angle of two-surface preparations.

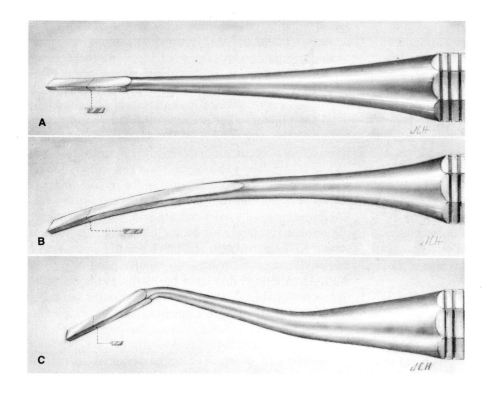

Fig. 8-7. Examples of hand instruments called chisels (with corresponding instrument formulas): **A,** Straight (12-7-0). **B,** Wedelstaedt (11½-15-3). **C,** Bin-angle (10-7-8).

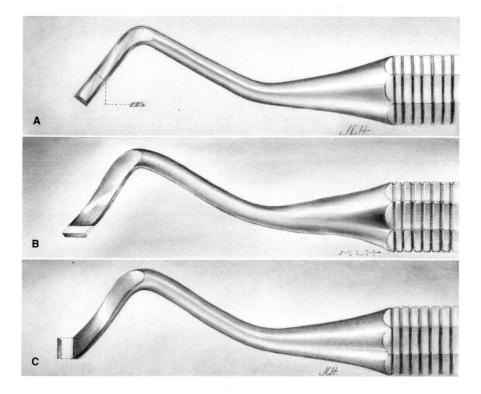

Fig. 8-8. Examples of hand instruments called chisels (with corresponding instrument formulas): **A,** Enamel hatchet (10-7-14). **B,** Gingival margin trimmer (12½-100-8-14). **C,** Gingival margin trimmer (12½-75-8-14).

Other cutting instruments. Other hand cutting instruments, such as the knife, file, and discoid-cleoid instrument, are used for trimming restorative material rather than for cutting tooth structure.

Knives, known as finishing knives, amalgam knives, or gold knives, are designed with a thin, knife-like blade that is made in various sizes and shapes (Fig. 8-9, *A* and *B*). Knives are used for trimming excess filling material on the gingival, facial, or lingual margins of a proximal restoration or trimming and contouring the surface of a class V restoration. Sharp secondary edges on the heel aspect of the blade are very useful in a scrape-pull mode.

Files (Fig. 8-9, *C*) also can be used to trim excess filling material. They are particularly useful at gingival margins. Blades of files are very thin, and teeth on the cutting surfaces are short. The teeth of the instrument are designed to make the file either a *push* or a *pull* instrument. Files are manufactured in various shapes and angles to allow access to restorations.

The *discoid-cleoid* (Fig. 8-9, *D* and *E*) instrument is used principally for carving occlusal anatomy in unset amalgam restorations. It also may be used to trim or burnish inlay-onlay margins. The working ends of this instrument are larger than the discoid or cleoid end of an excavator.

Hand instrument techniques

There are four grasps used with hand instruments: (1) modified pen, (2) inverted pen, (3) palm-and-thumb, and (4) modified palm-and-thumb. *The pen grasp is not an acceptable instrument grasp* (Fig. 8-10, *A*).

Modified pen grasp. The grasp that permits the greatest delicacy of touch is the modified pen grasp (Fig. 8-10, *B*). As the name implies, it is similar to that used in holding a pen, but not identical. Pads of the thumb, index, and middle fingers contact the instrument, while the tip of the ring finger, or tips of the ring and little fingers, is placed on a nearby tooth surface of the same arch as a *rest.* The palm of the hand generally is facing away from the operator. The pad of the middle finger is placed near the topside of the instrument; and by this finger working with wrist and forearm, cutting or cleaving pressure is generated on the blade. The instrument should not be allowed to rest on or near the first joint of the middle finger as in the conventional pen grasp (Fig. 8-10, *A*). Although this latter position may appear to be more comfortable, it limits the application of pressure. Recall that a balanced instrument design allows the application of suitable force without the instrument tending to rotate in the fingers (Fig. 8-3).

Inverted pen grasp. The finger positions of the inverted pen grasp are the same as for the modified pen

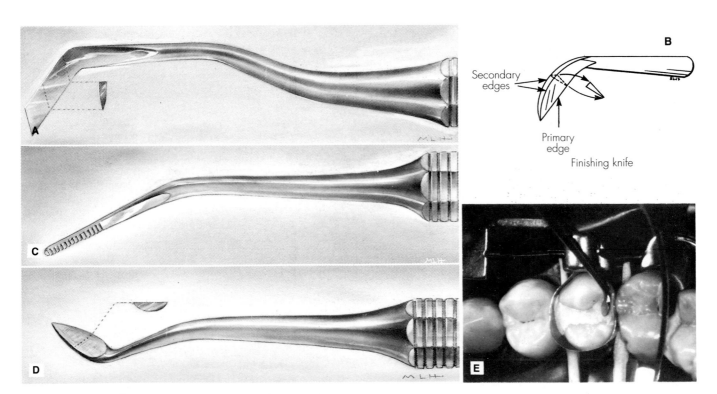

Fig. 8-9. Examples of other hand instruments for cutting: **A,** Finishing knife. **B,** Alternative knife design emphasizing secondary cutting edges. **C,** Dental file. **D,** Cleoid blade. **E,** Discoid blade carving dental amalgam.

Fig. 8-10   Fig. 8-11   Fig. 8-12

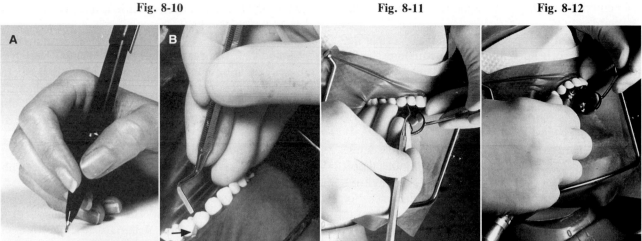

Fig. 8-13

Fig. 8-10. Pen grasps. **A,** Conventional pen grasp. Side of middle finger is on writing instrument. **B,** Modified pen grasp. Correct position of middle finger is near "topside" of instrument for good control and cutting pressure. The **rest** is tip(s) of ring finger (ring and little fingers) on tooth (teeth) of same arch. Note gingival wedge *(arrow)* serving as **guard.**

Fig. 8-11. Inverted pen grasp. Palm faces more toward operator. The **rest** is similar to that shown for modified pen grasp (Fig. 8-10, *B*).

Fig. 8-12. Palm-and-thumb grasp. This grasp has limited use, such as cutting incisal retention in a Class III preparation on maxillary incisor. The **rest** is tip of thumb on tooth in same arch.

Fig. 8-13. Modified palm-and-thumb grasp. This modification allows greater ease of instrument movement and more control against slippage during thrust stroke compared to palm-and-thumb grasp. The **rest** is tip of thumb on tooth being prepared or adjacent tooth. Note how instrument is braced against pad and end joint of thumb.

grasp. However, the hand is rotated so that the palm faces more toward the operator (Fig. 8-11). This grasp is used mostly for cavity preparations utilizing the lingual approach on anterior teeth.

Palm-and-thumb grasp. The palm-and-thumb grasp is similar to that used for holding a knife while paring the skin from an apple. The handle is placed in the palm of the hand and grasped by all the fingers, while the thumb is free of the instrument and the *rest* is provided by supporting the tip of the thumb on a nearby tooth of the same arch or on a firm, stable structure. For suitable control, this grasp requires careful utilization during cutting. An example of an appropriate use is holding a handpiece for cutting incisal retention for a Class III preparation on a maxillary incisor (Fig. 8-12).

Modified palm-and-thumb grasp. The modified palm-and-thumb grasp may be used when it is feasible to *rest the thumb on the tooth being prepared or the adjacent tooth* (Fig. 8-13). The handle of the instrument is held by all four fingers, whose pads press the handle against the distal area of the palm as well as the pad and first joint of the thumb. Grasping the handle under the first joint of the

ring and little fingers acts as a stabilizer. This grip fosters control against slippage.

The modified pen and inverted pen grasps are practically universal. The modified palm-and-thumb grasp is usually used in the area of the maxillary arch and is best adopted when the dentist is operating from a rear-chair position.

Rests. A proper instrument grasp must include a firm rest to steady the hand during operating procedures. When the modified pen and inverted pen grasps are used, rests are established by placing the ring or ring and little fingers on a tooth (or teeth) of the same arch and as close to the operating site as possible (Figs. 8-10 and 8-11). The closer the rest areas are to the operating area, the more reliable they are. When the palm-and-thumb grasps are used, rests are created by placing the tip of the thumb on the tooth being operated on, on an adjacent tooth, or on a convenient area of the same arch (Figs. 8-12 and 8-13).

In some instances it is impossible to establish a rest on tooth structure, and soft tissues must be used. Neither soft tissue rests nor distant hard tissue rests afford reliable control, and they reduce the force or power that can be used safely.

Occasionally, it is impossible to establish normal finger rests with the hand holding the instrument. Under these circumstances, instrument control may be gained using the forefinger of the opposite hand on the shank of the instrument or using an *indirect rest*, (i.e., the operating hand rests on the opposite hand, which rests on a stable oral structure).

Guards. Guards are hand instruments or other items, such as interproximal wedges, used to protect soft tissue from contact with sharp cutting or abrasive instruments (Fig. 8-10, *B*). (See the placement of wedges in Step 22 of Placement of the Rubber Dam in Chapter 11.)

Sharpening hand instruments

Selecting the proper hand cutting instrument and using the proper instrument grasp mean little if the instrument is not sharp. Instruments with dull cutting edges cause more pain, prolong operating time, are less controllable, and reduce quality and precision in cavity preparation. It is essential, therefore, that all cutting instruments be sharp. Resharpening requires little time and is very rewarding. The dentist or the assistant should habitually test for sharpness and sharpen when indicated the hand instruments before they are placed in the tray setup, thus preventing delays in starting or completing an operation (see Sharpness Test).

There are many types of sharpening equipment. These include stationary sharpening stones, mechanical sharpeners, and stones that are used in the handpiece. One type or design will usually not accommodate the full variety of dental instruments with their various shapes of cutting edges. For efficient and effective sharpening, the dentist must seek out the most suitable equipment.

Stationary sharpening stones. The most frequently used sharpening equipment consists of a block or stick of abrasive material called a "stone." The stone is supported on a firm surface and the instrument is oriented and held by hand while being stroked against the stone surface. Stationary stones are often called *oilstones* because of the common practice of applying a coating of oil to them as an aid to the sharpening process. Sharpening stones are available in a variety of grits, shapes, and materials.

Stationary *oilstones* are available in coarse, medium, or fine grit. Only a fine grit stone is suitable for the final sharpening of dental instruments to be used for cavity preparation. Coarse and medium grits may be used for initial reshaping of a badly damaged instrument or for sharpening other dental equipment such as bench knives. Coarser stones cut more rapidly but produce a rougher surface. If the use of two or more grits is required, the coarser is used as little as needed for reshaping and then the final sharpening is done with a fine stone.

Stationary stones can be obtained in a variety of shapes including flat, grooved, cylindrical, and tapered. The flat stones are preferred for sharpening all instruments which have straight cutting edges, the other shapes are most useful for sharpening instruments with curved cutting edges. Cylindrical stones are used for sharpening instruments with concave edges and the tapered stones permit using a portion of the stone with a curvature matching that of the instrument.

Sharpening stones are made from any of several natural or synthetic materials. The normal manufacturing process for the synthetic materials involves pressing carefully sized particles of an abrasive into the desired shape and heating to form a solid. In order to retain sharp edges on the particles, the process must result in a porous material. The properties of the stone depend on the volume and size of the pores as well as on the composition and size of the abrasive. Four types of materials are in common use for sharpening stones, Arkansas stone, silicon carbide, aluminum oxide, and diamond.

Arkansas stone is a naturally occurring form of microcrystalline quartz and has traditionally been the preferred material for fine sharpening stones. It is semitranslucent, white or gray in color, and is hard enough to sharpen steel but not carbide instruments. Arkansas stones are available in hard and soft varieties. The hard stone, although it may cut slower, is preferred because the soft stone scratches and grooves easily, rendering it useless. These stones should be lubricated with light machine oil before being used. This assists in the fineness of sharpening, prevents clogging of the stone pores, and avoids the creation of heat which alters the temper of the steel blade. In fact, an Arkansas stone should be covered with a thin film of oil when stored. During the sharpening of an instrument, the fine steel cuttings remain on the stone and tend to fill up the pores of the stone; therefore when the stone appears dirty, it should be wiped with a clean woolen cloth soaked in oil. If the stone is extremely dirty or difficult to clean, it may be wiped with a cloth soaked in alcohol.

Silicon carbide is widely used as an industrial abrasive. It is the most commonly used material for grinding wheels and "sandpapers" as well as for sharpening stones. It is hard enough to cut steel effectively but not hard enough to sharpen carbide instruments. Silicon carbide stones are available in many shapes in coarse and medium grits but not in fine grits. As a result they are not as suitable as other materials for final sharpening of dental instruments. Silicon carbide stones are normally of a dark color, often black or greenish black. These stones are moderately porous and require lubrication with a light oil to prevent clogging.

Aluminum oxide is increasingly used to manufacture sharpening stones. Stones commonly are produced in a variety of textures from different particle sizes of abrasive. Coarse and medium grit stones generally appear as speckled tan or brownish in color. Fine grit stones are usually white, have superior properties, and are less porous so that they require less lubrication during use. Either water or a light oil is adequate as a lubricant.

Diamond is the hardest available abrasive and is most effective for cutting and shaping hard materials. It is the only material routinely capable of sharpening carbide as well as steel instruments. *Diamond hones* are small blocks of metal with fine diamond particles impregnated in the surface. The diamonds are held in place by an electroplated layer of corrosion resistant metal. Most hones include grooved and rounded surfaces as well as a straight surface and are adaptable for sharpening instruments with curved blades. These hones are non-porous but the use of a lubricant will extend the life of the hones. They may be cleaned with a mild detergent and a medium-bristle brush.

Mechanical sharpeners. As high-speed rotary cutting instruments have been improved and their use has increased, the use of hand cutting instruments and the need for resharpening has decreased. As a result some dental office personnel do not do enough hand sharpening to remain confident of their proficiency. Under such circumstances the use of a *mechanical sharpener* (powered) is of great benefit.

One type of mechanical sharpener is represented by the Rx Honing Machine (Fig. 8-14, *A* to *F*). Basically this instrument moves a hone in a reciprocating motion at a slow speed while the instrument is held at the appropriate angulation and supported by a rest. This is much easier than having to hold the instrument at the proper angulation while moving it relative to the hone. Interchangeable aluminum oxide hones of different shapes and coarseness are available to accommodate the various instrument sizes, shapes, and degrees of dullness. Restoration of the cutting edge is accomplished more easily and in less time than by other sharpening methods. This type of sharpener is also very versatile and, with available accessories, can fill almost all instrument sharpening needs.

Handpiece sharpening stones. Mounted silicon carbide and aluminum oxide stones for use with both straight and angle handpieces are available in a variety of sizes and shapes (see Other Abrasive Instruments). Those intended for use in straight handpieces, particularly the cylindrical instruments with straight-sided silhouettes, are more useful for sharpening hand instruments than are the smaller points intended for intraoral use in the angle handpieces. Because of their curved periphery it is difficult to produce a flat surface using any of these instruments. These stones may also produce

somewhat inconsistent results because of the speed variables and the usual lack of a rest or guide for the instrument. However, satisfactory results can be obtained with minimal practice, especially on instruments with curved blades.

Principles of sharpening. The majority of operative hand cutting instruments can be sharpened successfully on either a stationary stone or the mechanical sharpener. The secret to easy and successful sharpening is to sharpen the instrument at the first sign of dullness and not wait until the edge is completely lost. If this procedure is followed, a fine cutting edge is restored with a few strokes on a stationary stone or a light touch to the mechanical sharpener. At the same time operating efficiency is not reduced by attempting to use an instrument that is getting progressively duller.

The choice of equipment used for sharpening is up to the dentist. In the use of any equipment there are several *basic principles of sharpening* that should be followed:

1. Sharpen instruments only after they have been cleaned and sterilized.
2. Establish the proper bevel angle (usually 45 degrees) and the desired angle of the cutting edge to the blade before placing the instrument against the stone and maintain these angles while sharpening.
3. Use a light stroke or pressure against the stone to minimize frictional heat.
4. Use a rest or guide whenever possible.
5. Remove as little metal from the blade as possible.
6. Lightly hone the unbeveled side of the blade after sharpening to remove the fine bur that may be created.
7. After sharpening, resterilize the instrument along with other items on the instrument tray setup.
8. Keep the sharpening stones clean and free of metal cuttings.

Mechanical techniques. When chisels, hatchets, hoes, angle formers, or gingival margin trimmers are sharpened on a reciprocating honing sharpener, the blade is placed against the steady rest, and the proper angle of the cutting edge of the blade is established before starting the motor. Light pressure of the instrument against the reciprocating hone is maintained with a firm grasp on the instrument. A trace of metal debris on the face of a flat hone along the length of the cutting edge is an indication that the entire cutting edge is contacting the hone (Fig. 8-14, *B*).

The mechanical sharpener is easily mastered with a little practice and is a quick method of sharpening hand instruments. Regardless of the type of mechanical sharpener used, the associated instructions for use should be thoroughly understood before an attempt is made to sharpen any type of instrument.

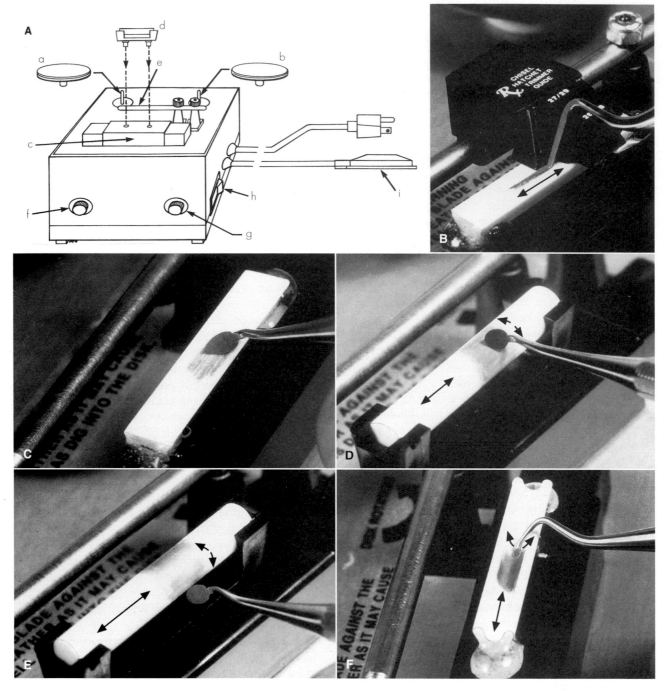

Fig. 8-14. Type of mechanical sharpener. **A,** R_x Honing Machine System II has: two spindle drives, one clockwise and other counter-clockwise, to which can be mounted diamond abrasive disk *(a),* RSC (rubberized silicon carbide) disk *(b),* or leather polishing disk; hone (reciprocating) carriage *(c)* to which can be mounted vitreous alumina (coarse) or ceramic alumina (fine) abrasive hone *(d);* angle guide (see **B**) slides onto bar *(e);* knob for selecting disk or hone drive *(f);* speed control knob *(g);* on/off switch *(h);* and foot activating switch *(i).* **B,** Sharpening enamel hatchet. Note instrument guide on bar, and track of sharpening debris on reciprocating *(two-headed arrow),* ceramic hone. Track width should equal length of cutting edge. **C,** Sharpening cleoid carver on same hone. **D** and **E,** Sharpening discoid carver on snap-in round, reciprocating *(two-headed arrow),* ceramic hone. Note track of sharpening debris as instrument is moved in arc by operator around hone *(arrows)* to sharpen desired length of blade edge. **F,** Sharpening small discoid excavator on grooved, reciprocating *(two-headed arrow),* ceramic hone. Again note operator arcing movement of blade *(arrows)* in hone to sharpen desired length of cutting edge.

Handpiece stones are used chiefly for instruments with curved blades, especially for the inside curve of such blades. The handpiece should be run at a low speed. The instrument is held lightly against the stone with a modified pen grasp, and, whenever possible, the ring and little fingers of each hand should be touching each other to act as a rest or steadying force. When this method of sharpening is used, care must be exercised not to overheat the instrument being sharpened. The use of some form of lubricant or coolant is desirable. If oil is used, care should be exercised not to throw oil from the stone during sharpening and the stone should be reserved for future use for sharpening only.

An instrument such as an amalgam or gold knife has a wide blade with a very narrow edge bevel, unlike the wide bevel of a chisel or hatchet. It is difficult to maintain the narrow edge bevel by using a mechanical sharpener or a handpiece stone; this instrument should be sharpened on a stationary stone.

Stationary stone techniques. The stationary sharpening stone should be at least 2 inches wide and 5 inches long, since a smaller stone is impractical. It should also be of medium grit for hand cutting instruments. Before the stone is used, a thin film of light oil should be placed on the working surface. In addition to establishing the proper 45-degree angle of the bevel and the cutting edge to the stone, there are several *fundamental rules* that apply to using the stationary stone:

1. Lay the stone on a flat surface and do not tilt the stone while sharpening.
2. Grasp the instrument firmly, usually with a modified pen grasp, so that it will not rotate or change angles while being sharpened.
3. To ensure stability during the sharpening strokes, use the ring and little fingers as a rest and guide along a flat surface or along the stone. This pre-

vents rolling or dipping of the instrument, which results in a distorted and uneven bevel.
4. Use a light stroke to prevent the creation of heat and the scratching of the stone.
5. Use different areas of the stone's surface while sharpening because this helps to prevent the formation of grooves on the stone that impair efficiency and accuracy of the sharpening procedure.

When sharpening *chisels, hatchets,* or *hoes* on the stationary stone, grasp the instrument with a modified pen grasp, place the blade perpendicular to the stone, and then tilt the instrument to establish the correct bevel (Fig. 8-15). Establishing and maintaining this correct bevel is the most difficult part of sharpening on a stationary stone. One method that assists in establishing the proper bevel angle is to observe the oil on the stone while the instrument is tilted in an effort to establish contact between the entire bevel and the stone. When oil is expressed evenly on all sides, then the entire bevel is touching the stone and the proper angle has been established to proceed with the sharpening strokes. If this alignment is altered during sharpening, discrepancies of the cutting edge and bevel will result. Using the finger rests and guides as illustrated in Fig. 8-15, the operator can slide the instrument back and forth along the stone. The motivating force should be from the shoulder so that the relationship of the hand to the plane of the stone is not changed during the stroke. Another technique is to move the stone back and forth while maintaining a constant position of the instrument.

The procedure for sharpening *angle formers* is essentially the same as that used for chisels, hatchets, or hoes, except that allowance must be made for the angle of the cutting edge to the blade.

The *gingival margin trimmers* require a little more orientation of the cutting edge to the stone before sharp-

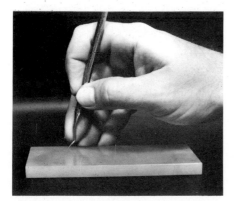

Fig. 8-15. Sharpening an instrument. Maintaining proper angle of bevel and angle of cutting edge to stone is aided by resting fingertips on stone.

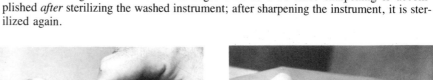

NOTE. Gloving is not illustrated in Figs. 8-15 to 8-17 since sharpening is accomplished *after* sterilizing the washed instrument; after sharpening the instrument, it is sterilized again.

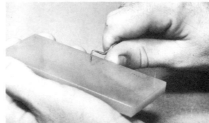

Fig. 8-16. Sharpening gingival margin trimmer. Palm-and-thumb grasp may be used while holding stone in opposite hand to establish proper cutting edge angle.

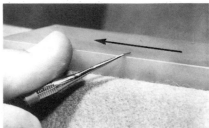

Fig. 8-17. Sharpening amalgam or gold knife. Place stone at edge of table so that blade may be tilted to form an acute angle with stone. Direction of sharpening movement of instrument along stone is indicated by arrow.

ening than a regular hatchet does. However, the same principle of establishing the proper bevel angle and cutting edge angle is the criterion for instrument position before sharpening. It may be expedient to use a palm-and-thumb grasp when sharpening a trimmer with a 95- or 100-centigrade cutting edge angle (Fig. 8-16).

When single-bevel instruments are sharpened, a thin, rough ridge of distorted metal, called a **burr** or *burr-edge,* collects on the unbeveled side of the blade. This burr is eliminated by a light stroke of the unbeveled side of the blade over the stone. This side of the blade is placed flat on the stone, and one short forward stroke is made. Burring can be kept to a minimum, however, if the direction of the sharpening stroke is only against the cutting edge of the blade and the cutting edge does not contact the stone during the return stroke. Thus the blade is touching the stone only on the forward sharpening stroke.

The *amalgam* or *gold knife* has a very thin blade tapering to the sharpened edge. There is a narrow edge bevel on both sides of the blade. In sharpening this instrument, only the edge bevels should be honed. If the entire side of the blade is worked each time, the thin blade will soon disappear or become so thin that it will

fracture under the slightest pressure. To sharpen the amalgam or gold knife, the blade is placed on the stone with the junction of the blade and shank immediately over the edge of the stone. The blade is then tilted to form a small acute angle with the surface of the stone, and the stroke is straight along the stone and toward the edge of the blade only (Fig. 8-17). The sharpening is accomplished on both sides of the blade with the stroke always toward the blade edge. This method will produce the finest edge and eliminate any burrs on the cutting edge.

The most difficult instruments to sharpen on a flat stone are the *spoon excavators* and *discoids*. Only the rounded outside surface of the spoon can be honed satisfactorily on a flat stone, and this involves a rotary movement accompanied by a pull stroke to maintain the curvature of the edge. The spoon is placed on the far end of the stone and held so that the handle is pointing toward the operator. As the instrument is pulled along the stone toward the operator, the handle is rotated gradually away from the operator until it is pointing away from the operator at the end of the stroke. The instrument is picked up and placed at the far end of the stone, and the motion is repeated until the edge is honed. The stone may either be placed on a flat surface or held in the hand for this procedure (Fig. 8-18). To hone the flat inside surface of the blade, a small cylindrical stone is passed back and forth over the surface (Fig. 8-19).

Other means of sharpening spoon excavators are by the use of the grooved stone, mounted discs, or stones for use with a straight handpiece. However, there is a

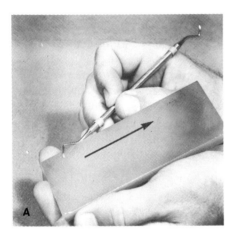

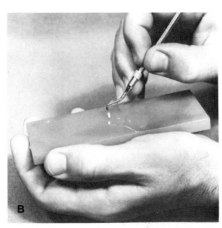

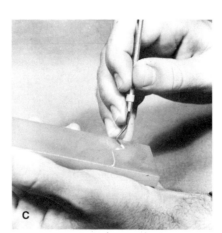

Fig. 8-18. Sharpening a spoon excavator. **A,** Beginning of stroke. **B,** Continuation of pull stroke while rotating handle in a direction opposite the stroke. **C,** Completion of stroke and handle rotation. Note that finger guides are used during entire stroke, which is in direction indicated by arrow.

NOTE. Gloving is not illustrated in Figs. 8-18 and 8-19, as explained in note for Figs. 8-15 to 8-17.

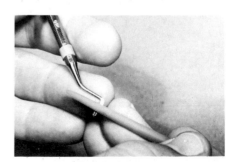

Fig. 8-19. Use of a small cylinder stone to hone inside surface of spoon excavators and discoid-cleoid instruments.

tendency to remove too much metal when handpiece stones are used.

Sharpness test. Sharpness of an instrument can be tested by lightly resting the cutting edge on a hard plastic surface. If the cutting edge digs in during an attempt to slide the instrument forward over the surface, the instrument is sharp. If it slides, the instrument is dull. Only very light pressure is exerted in testing for sharpness.

The principles and techniques discussed provide sufficient background for the operator to use proper methods in sharpening other instruments that are not discussed. *It cannot be stressed too often that sharp instruments are necessary for optimal operating procedures.* It has also been found prudent to have multiple tray setups so that a substitute instrument is available if necessary; or substitute sterile instruments should be available so that other sterile tray setups are not disrupted by borrowing of instruments.

Sterilization and storage of hand cutting instruments

The fact that hepatitis A and B viruses have been found in the saliva of infected persons and evidence of many hepatitis B infections among dental personnel emphasize the importance of proper equipment and procedures for instrument sterilization. Sterilization in dental offices can be accomplished by autoclaving, dry-heat procedures, ethylene oxide equipment, and chemical vapor sterilizers. Boiling and chemical solutions (cold disinfection) will not sterilize instruments and should be considered as disinfection procedures only. The thought that only instruments that puncture or cut soft tissue or are exposed to blood should be sterilized and others disinfected is no longer valid as a precaution against cross-infections. Aseptic techniques are presented in other subject areas and will not be detailed here. Sterilization procedures for operative dentistry are presented in Chapter 4. Storage of any hand cutting instrument should be in a sterile wrapped tray setup, or in an individual sterile wrapping.

POWERED CUTTING EQUIPMENT
Development of rotary equipment

The availability of some method of cutting and shaping of tooth structure is an essential for the restoration of teeth. Although there is archeological evidence of dental treatment as early as 5000 BC, little is known about the equipment and methods used then.[10] Early drills powered by hand are illustrated in Figs. 8-20 and 8-21. Much of the subsequent history leading to present *powered cutting equipment* can be seen as a search for improved sources of energy and means for holding and controlling the cutting instrument. This has culminated in the use of replaceable bladed or abrasive instruments

held in a rotary handpiece usually powered by compressed air.

A *handpiece* is a device for holding rotating instruments, transmitting power to them, and for positioning them intraorally. Handpieces and associated cutting and polishing instruments developed as two basic types, *straight* and *angle* (Fig. 8-22). Most of the development of methods for preparing teeth has occurred within the last 100 years;[26] and effective equipment for removal (or preparation) of enamel has been available only since 1947 when speeds of 10,000 rpm were first used along with newly marketed carbide burs and diamond instruments. Since 1953 continued improvements in the design and materials of construction for both handpieces and instruments have resulted in equipment that is efficient as well as sterilizeable, much to the credit of manufacturers and the profession alike. Table 8-1 summarizes some of the more significant developments of rotary dental equipment.

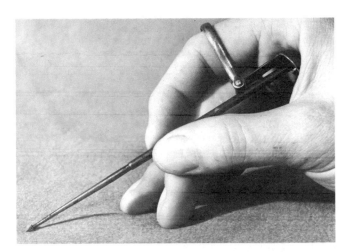

Fig. 8-20. Early straight hand drill for direct access cavities (circa 1800). Back end of bur shank fits into a finger ring while the front end is rotated with thumb and forefinger.

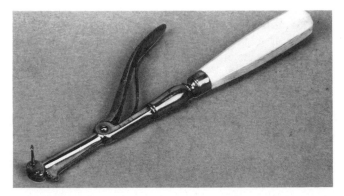

Fig. 8-21. Early angle hand drill for indirect access cavities (circa 1850). The bur is activated by squeezing spring-loaded handle.

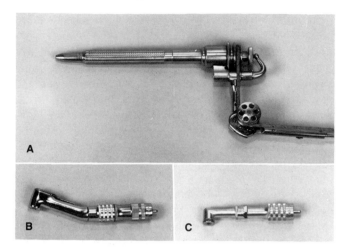

Fig. 8-22. Conventional designs of handpieces. **A,** Belt-driven straight handpiece. **B,** Gear-driven angle handpiece that attaches to front end of the straight handpiece. **C,** Gear-driven angle handpiece designed for cleaning and polishing procedures.

Table 8-1. Evolution of rotary equipment[26]

Date	Instrument	Speed (rpm)
1728	Hand-rotated instruments	300
1871	Foot engine	700
1874	Electric engine	1000
1914	Dental unit	5000
1942	Diamond cutting instruments	5000
1946	Old units converted to increase speed	10,000
1947	Tungsten carbide burs	12,000
1953	Ball bearings handpieces	25,000
1955	Water turbine angle handpiece	50,000
1955	Belt-driven angle handpiece (Page-Chayes)	150,000
1957	Air turbine angle handpiece	250,000
1961	Air turbine straight handpiece	25,000
1962	Experimental air bearing handpiece	(800,000)
1994	Contemporary air turbine handpiece	300,000

One of the most significant advancements was the introduction of the *electric motor* as a power source in 1874. It was incorporated into a *dental unit* in 1914.[27] The initial handpiece equipment and operating speeds (maximum of 5000 rpm) remained virtually unchanged until 1946 (Fig. 8-23). Steel burs that were used at the time could not cut enamel effectively even when applied with great force. With steel burs, increased speed and power resulted only in increased heat and instrument wear. Further progress was delayed until the development of instruments that could cut enamel. Diamond cutting instruments were developed in Germany around 1935, but were scarce in the United States until after World War II. In a 10-year period, starting in late

1946, cutting techniques were revolutionized. *Diamond instruments* and *tungsten carbide burs* capable of cutting enamel were produced commercially. Both instruments performed best at the highest speeds available and that prompted the development of higher speed handpieces. Obtaining speeds of 10,000 to 15,000 rpm was a relatively simple matter of modifying existing equipment by enlarging the drive pulleys on the dental engine. By 1950, speeds of 60,000 rpm and above had been attained by newly designed equipment employing speed-multiplying internal belt drives (Fig. 8-24).[26] They were found to be more effective for cutting tooth structure and for reducing perceived vibration.

The major breakthrough in the development of high-speed rotary equipment came with the introduction of *contra-angled handpieces with internal turbine drives* in the contra-angle head.[22] Early units were water-driven but subsequent units were air-driven (Figs. 8-25, 8-26, A). Although most current *air-turbine handpieces* (Fig. 8-27) have free-running speeds of approximately

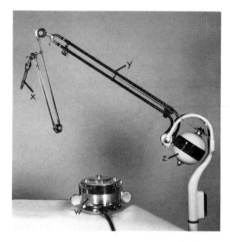

Fig. 8-23. Typical equipment when an electric motor is used as source of power: foot control with rheostat *(w)*, belt-driven straight handpiece *(x)*, three-piece adjustable extension arm *(y)*, and electric motor *(z)*.

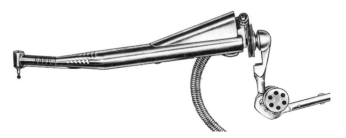

Fig. 8-24. Page-Chayes handpiece (circa 1955). The first belt-driven angle handpiece to operate successfully at speeds over 100,000 rpm.

300,000 rpm, the small size of the turbine in the head limits their power output. The speed can drop to 200,000 rpm or less with small lateral workloads during cutting, and the handpiece may stall at moderate loads.[28] This tendency to stall under high loads is an excellent safety feature for tooth preparation, since excessive pressure cannot be applied. Air-driven handpieces continue to be the most popular type of handpiece equipment because of the overall simplicity of design, ease of control, versatility, and patient acceptance. The external appearance of current handpieces is very similar to the earliest models.

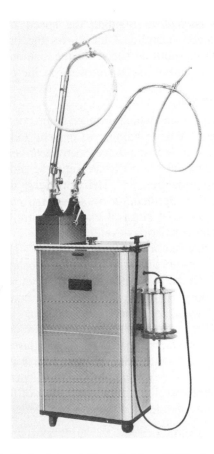

Fig. 8-25. Turbo-Jet portable unit (circa 1955). A small turbine in the head of the angle handpiece is driven by water circulated by a pump housed in the mobile base.

The low torque and power output of the contra-angle turbines made them unsuitable for some finishing and polishing techniques where large heavy instruments are needed. The application of the turbine principle to the *straight handpiece* eliminated the necessity of having an electric engine as part of a standard dental unit. The design of the straight handpiece turbine provided the desirable high torque for low-speed operation (Fig. 8-26, *B*).

Increasing concern about patient-to-patient transfer of infectious agents has put emphasis on other aspects of handpiece performance. Recent advancements in both straight and angle handpieces allow repeated sterilization by several methods (see Sterilization of Handpieces and Related Rotary Equipment, Chapter 4). However sterilization produces some damage to many parts of the handpiece thus requiring more frequent service and repair. Other improvements of the angle handpiece include smaller head sizes, more torque, lower noise levels, and better chucking mechanisms. Since 1955 angle handpieces have had an air-water spray feature to provide cooling, cleansing, and improved visibility[24](Fig. 8-27, *B*). Most modern angled handpieces also include fiberoptic lighting of the cutting site (Fig. 8-27, *B*).

Rotary speed ranges

The rotational speed of an instrument is measured in revolutions per minute (rpm). *Three speed ranges* are generally recognized: *low* or slow speeds (below 12,000 rpm), *medium* or intermediate speeds (12,000 to 200,000 rpm), and *high* or ultra-high speeds (above 200,000 rpm). The terms low, medium, and high are used preferentially in this textbook. Most useful instruments are rotated at either low or high speed.

The crucial factor for some purposes is the *surface speed* of the instrument, the velocity at which the edges of the cutting instrument pass across the surface being cut. This is proportional to both the rotational speed and the diameter of the instrument, with large instruments having higher surface speeds at any given rate of rotation.

Although intact tooth structure can be removed by an instrument rotating at low speeds, it is a traumatic expe-

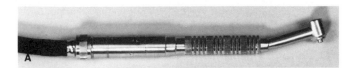

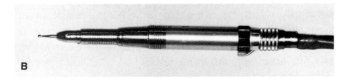

Fig. 8-26. Air turbine handpieces. **A,** Borden Airotor handpiece (circa 1957) was first clinically successful air turbine handpiece. Current airdriven handpieces are very similar in basic design. **B,** Air turbine straight handpiece (circa 1980).

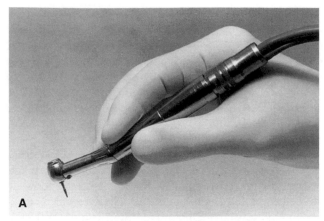

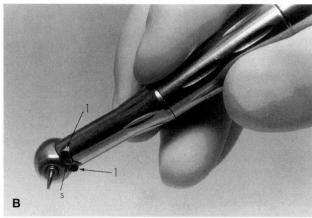

Fig. 8-27. Contemporary air turbine hand-piece (circa 1994). Most handpieces are being redesigned to withstand the rigors of routine sterilization. **A,** Contrangle air turbine handpiece connected to air-water supply line. **B,** Ventral view of handpiece (Star 430SWL) showing port for air-water spray (s) onto bur at cutting site, and epoxied end of fiber-optic bundle (1) to shine light at cutting site.

rience for both the patient and the dentist. Low-speed cutting is ineffective, time consuming, and requires a relatively heavy force application. This results in heat production at the operating site and produces vibrations of low frequency and high amplitude. Heat and vibration are the main sources of patient discomfort.[25] At low speeds burs have a tendency to roll out of the cavity preparation and mar the proximal margin or tooth surface. In addition, carbide burs do not last long because their brittle blades are easily broken at low speeds. Many of these disadvantages of low speed operation do not apply when the objective is some procedure other than cutting tooth structure. *The low speed range is used for cleaning teeth, occasional caries excavation, and finishing and polishing procedures.* At low speeds, tactile sensation is better and there is generally less chance for overheating cut surfaces. The availability of a low speed option is a valuable adjunct for many dental procedures.

At high speed, the surface speed needed for efficient cutting can be attained with smaller and more versatile cutting instruments. This speed is used for tooth preparation and removing old restorations. Other advantages are: (1) diamond and carbide cutting instruments remove tooth structure faster with less pressure, vibration, and heat generation; (2) the number of rotary cutting instruments needed is reduced because smaller sizes are more universal in application; (3) the operator has better control and greater ease of operation; (4) instruments last longer; (5) patients are generally less apprehensive because annoying vibrations and operating time are decreased; and (6) several teeth in the same arch can and should be treated at the same appointment.

Variable control to regulate the speed makes the handpiece more versatile. This allows the operator to easily obtain the optimal speed for the size and type of rotating instrument at any stage of a specific operation.

Laser equipment

Lasers are devices which produce beams of very high intensity light. A large number of current and potential uses of lasers in dentistry have been identified that involve the treatment of soft tissues and the modification of hard tooth structures.[21,31] The word *laser* is an acronym for *"light amplification by stimulated emission of radiation."* A crystal or gas is excited to emit light photons of a characteristic wavelength that are amplified and filtered to make a coherent light beam. The effects of the laser depend on the power of the beam and the extent to which the beam is absorbed. There are several types available (see Table 8-2) based on wavelengths. The lasers range from long wavelengths (infrared), through visible wavelengths, to short wavelengths (ultraviolet). *Excimers* are special ultraviolet lasers. At the present time, CO_2 and Nd:YAG lasers have shown the most promise. For any application it is important to select the correct wavelength for absorption of the energy and prevention of side-effects from heat generation.

Table 8-2. Laser types by source and wavelength

Type	Source	Wavelength	Mode	Output
Infrared	CO_2	10.60 μm	Continuous	1000 W
	CO_2	10.60 μm	Pulsed	1000 mJ/p
	Ho:YAG	2.06 μm	Pulsed	800 mJ/p
	Nd:YAG	1.06 μm	Pulsed	1000 mJ/p
	Nd:YAG	1.06 μm	Continuous	100 W
Visible	HeNe	633 nm	Continuous	25 W
	Argon	514, 488 nm	Continuous	20W
Ultraviolet (Excimer)	XeF	351 nm	Pulsed	50 mJ/p
	XeCl	308 nm	Pulsed	300 mJ/p
	KrF	248 nm	Pulsed	1000 mJ/p
	ArF	193 nm	Pulsed	800 mJ/p

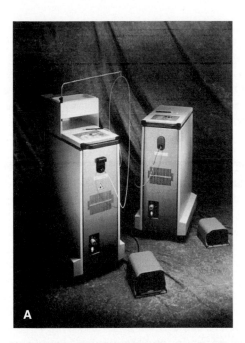

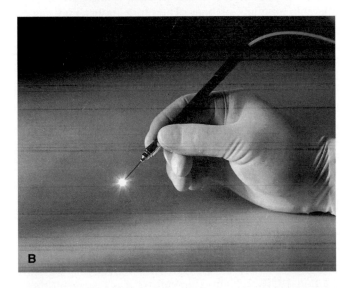

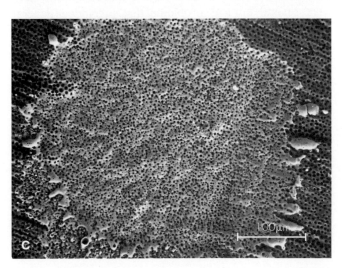

Scientific and commercial lasers produce highly collimated beams, but such a beam is potentially dangerous in clinical situations. The collimated beam is directed via a flexible fiber-optic light pipe or mirror train to the point of application where it is normally focused by a lens to a focal area near the tip.

Once the beam is focused, the total energy it delivers is a function of the intensity of the beam, the time of exposure, and the area affected. These are used to calculate the *exposure dose* (ED, Joules/cm^2). ED = (W)(t)/(A) where W is the power (watts) emitted from the light guide, t is the time (seconds) of the total exposure, and A is the area (cm^2) of the beam spot on the substrate.[19] The effect of this energy depends on whether or not the wavelength of the energy is absorbed by the surface. The absorption wavelengths for various hard and soft tissues are different. The best results are obtained when the laser wavelength is matched to an absorption band of the substrate. In some cases the substrate must be coated with an absorbing dye to facilitate beam interaction.

Interactions with the substrate can occur in photothermal, photo-chemical, or other ways. Generally dental lasers produce photo-thermal effects with soft or hard tissue being ablated by the action. At low temperatures, below 100° C, thermal effects denature proteins, produce hemolysis, cause coagulation, and cause shrinkage. Above 100° C, water in soft or hard tissues boils, producing explosive expansion. Above about 400° C, carbonization of organic materials is completed with the onset of some inorganic changes. As the temperature increases from 400° to 1400° C, inorganic constituents change in chemistry, may melt and/or recrystallize, and may vaporize. The actual temperatures depend on the initial composition of the tissue involved. When the laser and tissue are well matched, like the infrared lasers and enamel, energy can be absorbed very rapidly. Even low energy densities for short times can

Fig. 8-28. Example of laser use. **A,** Nd:YAG laser units, each with a power supply, control panel, foot controller, fiber optic wave guide, and probe. **B,** Laser probe and beam eminating from probe tip. **C,** Lased area on dentin (from Nd:YAG operated at 1.06 μm wavelength, 167 mJ/pulse, and 207 J/cm^2 power) showing physical modification produced by a single pulse. The hydroxyapatite crystals on the surface were melted and recrystallized with partial closure of the tubules. Surface roughness from tooth preparation was eliminated by the lasing. The area immediately adjacent to the lased site seemed to be unaffected. (**A** and **B,** compliments of Dr. Art Vassiliadis, Sunrise Technologies, Fremont, CA 94538; **C,** courtesy of Dr. Joel White, Department of Restorative Dentistry, UCSF School of Dentistry, San Francisco, California. See reference 30.)

cause enamel to melt and recrystallize. High energy densities and/or longer times produce vaporization with drilling or cutting of the surface. For dentin, the same effects occur at lower energy densities. An example of lased dentin is shown in Fig. 8-28. Such surfaces can be produced to seal the dentin and improve bonding of restorative materials.

While infrared lasers produce their effects by heating at the focal point, ultra-violet laser beams involve photon energies coincident with bond energies of cellular constituents and are capable of directly disrupting the bonds that hold the molecules together.[8] For this reason, it is necessary to avoid those wavelengths that are absorbed by proteins such as DNA and RNA.

For dental applications, excessive heat must be avoided to protect the dental pulp.[16] High surface temperatures for short periods of time are acceptable as long as there is sufficient time or path for heat dispersion. Lasers may be operated as continuous wave (cw) or pulsed (p) lasers. To control the beam energy it is common to pulse the beam. Normally the pulse rate (20 to 1000 Hertz or cycles per second) and pulse duration (1 to 50 microseconds) can be selected by the operator. Pulsing occurs rapidly and is not the same as the operator turning the beam on or off. Local temperatures during lasing can reach many hundreds of degrees C, but as long as the heat is dissipated effectively, then pulpal temperatures will not be affected. Clinical studies indicate that lasers can be used without causing pulpal damage.[30] Generally, pulpal temperature increases of more than 4.5° to 5.5° C are considered damaging.

There are a number of lasers which are of practical importance to medicine and dentistry (see Table 8-3). The ones of most current interest to dentistry are

Nd:YAG (Neodymium: yttrium-aluminum-garnet, wavelength = 1.064 μm; Fig. 8-28, A), Er:YAG (Erbium: yttrium-aluminum-garnet, wavelength = 2.94 μm), or CO_2 (carbon dioxide, maximum wavelength-10.6 μm). Argon, helium-neon, Ho:YAG, and excimer lasers are being evaluated as well. More than one wavelength of photon energy may be produced by a laser. In the case of CO_2 lasers, the 9.6 μm peak is much more readily absorbed by hydroxyapatite than the standard 10.6 μm peak. This wavelength may be selected by filtration to eliminate longer wavelengths.

It is no longer appropriate to question "whether lasers will be used by dentistry" but "when they will become commonplace." Current units are relatively expensive and must be used frequently in a dental practice to justify the expense. At the moment, lasers are used primarily for either soft tissue applications (see Table 8-3) or hard tissue surface modification (Fig 6-28, C). They are not used for cavity preparations because they are inefficient and awkward for removing large amounts of enamel or dentin, and that process would generate intolerable amounts of heat. Therefore, lasers may never replace a high-speed dental handpiece.

Lasers are regulated by the Food and Drug Administration (FDA) for safety and efficacy. They have been approved for soft tissue surgery but not for tooth preparation. Other safety precautions are prescribed. A door is required to close off the room involving lasers and appropriate signs are needed to indicate the presence of laser equipment. Eye protection is required for the operator, assistant, and patient to protect against any inadvertently reflected laser light. The FDA will most likely expand the number of sanctioned applications during the next few years.

Other equipment

There are alternative methods of cutting enamel and/or dentin that have been periodically assessed. In the mid-1950s, air-abrasive cutting was tested but there were several clinical problems that precluded general acceptance. Most importantly, there was no tactile sense associated with air-abrasive cutting of tooth structure. This made it difficult for the operator to determine the cutting progress within the cavity preparation. Additionally, the abrasive dust interfered with visibility of the cutting site and tended to mechanically etch the surface of the dental mirror. There was also the difficulty of preventing abrasive dust inhalation by the patient or office personnel. At the present time, air-abrasive equipment (e.g., KCP 2000) is being promoted for stain removal, debriding pit and fissures prior to sealing, and micro-mechanical roughening of surfaces to be bonded (enamel, cast metal alloys, or porcelain). These techniques do not involve conventional cavity preparation.

Table 8-3. Suggested dental applications for laser types

	CO_2	Ho:YAG	Nd:YAG	HeNe	Argon	Excimers
Cutting and coagulation	X	X	X		X	
Stimulation of healing				X		
Analgesia (low power)			X	X		
Fissure sealing	X	X	X			X
Caries treatment	X	X	X			X
Composite curing					X	
Surface modification	X	X	X			X
Root canal	X	X	X			X
Apicoectomy	X	X	X			
Root sealing	X	X				X
Gingivectomy	X	X				

ROTARY CUTTING INSTRUMENTS

The individual instruments intended for use with dental handpieces are manufactured in hundreds of sizes, shapes, and types. This variation is in part a result of the need for specialized designs for particular clinical applications or to fit particular handpieces, but much of the variation also results from individual preferences on the part of dentists. Since the introduction of high-speed techniques in clinical practice, there has been a rapid evolution of technique and an accompanying proliferation of new instrument designs. Nevertheless, the number of instruments essential for use with any one type of handpiece is comparatively small, especially in the case of the high-speed turbine handpieces.

Common design characteristics

In spite of the great variation that exists among rotary cutting instruments, they have certain design features in common. Each instrument consists of three parts: (1) shank, (2) neck, and (3) head (Fig. 8-29). Each has its own function, influencing its design and the materials used for its construction. *Note that there is a difference in the meaning of the term "shank" as applied to rotary instruments and to hand instruments.*

Shank design. The *shank* is the part that fits into the handpiece, accepts the rotary motion from the handpiece, and provides a bearing surface to control the alignment and concentricity of the instrument. The shank design and dimensions vary with the handpiece for which it is intended. The American Dental Association Specification No. 23 for dental excavating burs[1] includes five classes of instrument shanks. Three of these

(Fig. 8-30), the *straight handpiece shank,* the *latch-type angle handpiece shank,* and the *friction-grip angle handpiece shank,* are commonly encountered. The shank portion of the straight handpiece instrument is a simple cylinder. It is held in the handpiece by a metal chuck that accepts a range of shank diameters. Thus, precise control of the shank diameter is not as critical as for other shank designs. Straight handpiece instruments are now rarely used for preparing teeth, except for certain anterior restorations. However, they are commonly used for finishing and polishing completed restorations.

The more complicated shape of the latch-type shank reflects the different mechanisms by which these instruments are held in the handpiece. Their shorter overall length permits substantially improved access to posterior regions of the mouth in comparison with straight handpiece instruments. Handpieces that use latch-type burs normally have a metal bur tube within which the instruments fit as closely as possible while still permitting easy interchange. The posterior portion of the shank is flattened on one side so that the end of the instrument fits into a D-shaped socket at the bottom of the bur tube, and it is thus that the instrument is rotated. Latch-type instruments are not retained in the handpiece by a chuck but rather by a retaining latch that slides into the groove found at the shank end of the instrument. This type of instrument is used predominantly at low and medium speed ranges for finishing procedures. At these speeds the small amount of potential wobble inherent in the clearance between the instrument and the handpiece bur tube is controlled by the lateral pressure exerted during cutting procedures. At higher speeds the latch-type shank design is inadequate to provide a true-

Fig. 8-29. Normal designation of three parts of rotary cutting instruments.

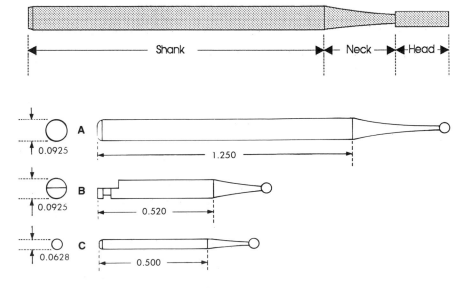

Fig. 8-30. Characteristics and typical dimensions (in inches) of three common instrument shank designs for: **A,** Straight handpiece; **B,** latch-type angle handpiece; and **C,** friction-grip angle handpiece.

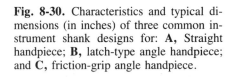

running instrument head, and as a result an improved shank design is required for these speeds.

The friction-grip shank design was developed for use with high-speed handpieces. This design is smaller in overall length than the latch-type instruments, thus providing a further improvement in access to the posterior regions of the mouth. The shank is a simple cylinder manufactured to very close dimensional tolerances. As the name implies, friction-grip instruments were originally designed to be held in the handpiece by friction between the shank and a plastic or metal chuck. Newer handpiece designs have metal chucks that close to make a positive contact with the bur shank. Careful dimensional control on the shanks of these instruments is important because for high-speed use even minor variations in shank diameter can cause substantial variation in instrument performance and problems with insertion, retention, and removal.

Neck design. As shown in Fig. 8-29, the **neck** is the intermediate portion of an instrument that connects the head to the shank. It corresponds to the part of a hand instrument called the shank. Except in the case of the larger, more massive instruments, the neck normally tapers from the shank diameter to a smaller size immediately adjacent to the head. The main function of the neck is to transmit rotational and translational forces to the head. At the same time it is desirable for the operator to have the greatest possible visibility of the cutting head and the greatest manipulative freedom. For this reason the neck dimensions represent a compromise between the need for a large cross section to provide strength and a small cross section to improve access and visibility.

Head design. The **head** is the working part of the instrument, the cutting edges or points of which perform the desired shaping of tooth structure. The shape of the head and the material used to construct it are closely related to its intended application and technique of use. The heads of instruments show greater variation in design and construction than either of the other main portions. For this reason the characteristics of the head form the basis on which rotary instruments are usually classified.

There are many characteristics of the heads of rotary instruments that could be used for classification. Most important among these is the division into bladed instruments and abrasive instruments. Material of construction, head size, and head shape are additional characteristics that are useful for further subdivision. Bladed and abrasive instruments exhibit substantially different clinical performances even when operated under nearly identical conditions. This appears to result from differences in the mechanism of cutting that are inherent in their design.

Dental burs

The term **bur** is applied to all rotary cutting instruments that have bladed cutting heads. This includes instruments intended for such purposes as finishing metal restorations and surgical removal of bone, as well as those primarily intended for tooth preparation.

Historical development of dental burs. The earliest burs, like that shown in Fig. 8-20, were handmade. Thus, they were both expensive and variable in dimension and performance. The shapes, dimensions, and nomenclature of modern burs are directly related to those of the first machine-made burs introduced in 1891.[27] Early burs were made of steel. **Steel burs** perform well cutting human dentin at low speeds, but dull rapidly at higher speeds or when cutting enamel. Once dulled, the reduced cutting effectiveness creates increased heat and vibration.

Carbide burs, which were introduced in 1947, have largely replaced steel burs for cavity preparation. Steel burs now are used mainly for finishing procedures. Carbide burs perform better than steel burs at all speeds and their superiority is greatest at high speeds.

All carbide burs have heads of cemented carbide in which microscopic carbide particles, usually of tungsten carbide, are held together in a matrix of cobalt or nickel. Carbide is much harder than steel, and thus less subject to dulling during cutting.

In most burs the carbide head is attached to a steel shank and neck by welding or brazing. This substitution of steel for carbide in those portions of the bur where greater wear resistance is not required has several advantages. It permits the manufacturer more freedom of design in attaining the characteristics desired in the instrument and at the same time allows economy in the cost of materials of construction.

Although most carbide burs have the joint located in the posterior part of the head, others are sold that have the joint located within the shank and thus have carbide necks as well as heads. Carbide is stiffer and stronger than steel, but it is also more brittle. A carbide neck subjected to a sudden blow or shock will fracture, whereas a steel neck will bend. A bur that is even slightly bent produces much increased vibration and over-cutting as a result of increased run-out. Thus, although steel necks reduce the risk of fracture during use, if bent they may cause severe problems. Either type can be satisfactory, and other design factors are varied to take maximal advantage of the properties of the material used.

Bur classification systems. In order to facilitate the description, selection, and manufacture of burs it is highly desirable to have some agreed-upon shorthand designation which represents all of the variables of a particular head design by some simple code. In the

United States dental burs traditionally have been described in terms of an arbitrary **numerical code** for head size and shape (e.g., 2 = 1.0 mm diameter round bur; 57 = 1.0 mm diameter straight fissure bur; 34 = 0.8 mm diameter inverted cone bur).[2] Despite the complexity of the system, it is still in common use. Other countries developed and used similarly arbitrary systems. Newer classification systems such as that developed by the International Dental Federation (FDI [Federation Dentaire Internationale]) and International Standards Organization (ISO) tend to use separate designations for shape, usually a shape name, and size usually a number giving the head diameter in tenths of a mm (e.g., round 010; straight fissure plain 010; inverted cone 008).[15,20]

Shapes. The term **bur shape** refers to the contour or silhouette of the head. The basic head shapes are: round, inverted cone, pear, straight fissure, and tapered fissure (Fig. 8-31).

A *round bur* is spherical. This shape customarily has been used for such purposes as initial entry into the tooth, extension of the preparation, preparation of retention potholes, and caries removal.

An *inverted cone bur* is a portion of a rather rapidly tapered cone with the apex of the cone directed toward the bur shank. Head length is about the same as the diameter. This shape is particularly suitable for providing undercuts in cavity preparations.

A *pear-shaped bur* is a portion of a slightly tapered cone with the small end of the cone directed toward the bur shank. The end of the head either is continuously curved, or is flat with rounded corners, where the sides and flat end intersect. A normal-length pear bur (length slightly greater than the width) is advocated for use in class I cavity preparations for gold foil. A long-length pear bur (length three times the width) is advocated for cavity preparations for amalgam.

A *straight fissure bur* is an elongated cylinder. This shape is advocated by some for amalgam cavity preparation. Modified burs of this design with slightly curved tip angles are available.

A *tapered fissure bur* is a portion of a slightly tapered cone with the small end of the cone directed away from the bur shank. This shape is used for inlay and crown preparations where freedom from undercuts is essential for successful withdrawal of patterns and final seating of cast restorations. Tapered fissure burs can have a flat end with the tip corners slightly rounded.

Among these basic shapes, variations are possible. Fissure and inverted cone burs may have half-round or domed ends. Taper and cone angles may be varied. The ratio of head length to diameter may be varied. In addition to shape, other features may be varied such as the number of blades, spiral versus axial patterns for blades, and continuous versus crosscut blade edges.

Sizes. In the United States, the number designating **bur size** also has traditionally served as a code for head design. This numbering system for burs was originated by the S. S. White Dental Manufacturing Company in 1891 for their first machine-made burs. It was both extensive and logical, so that other domestic manufacturers found it convenient to adopt it for their burs, as well. As a result, for over 60 years there was a general uniformity for bur numbers in the United States. Table 8-4 shows the correlation of bur head sizes with dimensions and shapes. It includes not only many bur sizes still in common use, but others that have since become obsolete.

The original numbering system grouped burs by 9 shapes and 11 sizes. The ½ and ¼ designations were added later when smaller instruments were included in the system. All original bur designs had continuous blade edges. Later, when crosscut burs were found to be more effective for cutting dentin at low speeds, crosscut versions of many bur sizes were introduced. This modification was indicated by adding 500 to the number of the equivalent non-crosscut size. Thus a No.

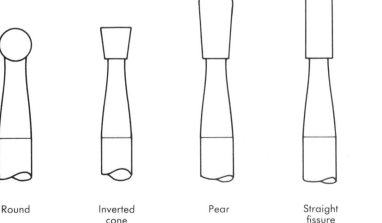

Fig. 8-31. Basic bur head shapes.

Round   Inverted cone   Pear   Straight fissure   Tapered fissure

Table 8-4. Original bur head sizes (1891 to 1954)

Head shapes	Head diameters in inches (mm*)												
	0.020 (0.5)	0.025 (0.6)	0.032 (0.8)	0.039 (1.0)	0.047 (1.2)	0.055 (1.4)	0.063 (1.6)	0.072 (1.8)	0.081 (2.1)	0.090 (2.3)	0.099 (2.5)	0.109 (2.8)	0.119 (3.0)
Round	¼	½	1	2	3	4	5	6	7	8	9	10	11
Wheel		11½	12	13	14	15	16	17	18	19	20	21	22
Cone		22½	23	24	25	26	27	28	29	30	31	32	33
Inverted cone		33½	34	35	36	37	38	39	40	41	42	43	44
Bud		44½	45	46	47	48	49	50	51				
Straight fissure (flat end)	55¼	55½	56	57	58	59	60	61	62				
Straight fissure (pointed end)		66½	67	68	69	70	71	72	73				
Pear		77½	78	79	80	81	82	83	84	85	86	87	88
Oval		88½	89	90	91	92	93	94	95				

Courtesy H.M. Moylan—S.S. White Dental Manufacturing Company.
*Millimeter values rounded to the nearest 0.1 mm.

Table 8-5. Standard bur head sizes—carbide and steel (1955 to present)

Head shapes	Head diameters in inches (mm*)													
	0.020 (0.5)	0.025 (0.6)	0.032 (0.8)	0.040 (1.0)	0.048 (1.2)	0.056 (1.4)	0.064 (1.6)	0.073 (1.9)	0.082 (2.1)	0.091 (2.3)	0.100 (2.5)	0.110 (2.8)	0.120 (3.0)	0.130 (3.3)
Round	¼	½	1	2	3	4	5	6	7	8	9	10	11	
Wheel		11½	12		14		16							
Inverted cone		33½	34	35	36	37	38	39	40					
Plain fissure		55½	56	57	58	59	60	61	62					
Round crosscut				502	503	504	505	506						
Straight fissure crosscut			556	557	558	559	560	561	562	563				
Tapered fissure crosscut				700	701		702		703					
End cutting fissure				957	958	959								
Round finishing				A	B	C	D		200		201		202	203
Oval finishing									218		219		220	221
Pear finishing									230		231		232	
Flame finishing				242	243	244	245	246						

Non-standard excavating and finishing burs are not shown in this table.
*Millimeter values rounded to the nearest 0.1 mm.

57 with crosscut was designated No. 557. Similarly, a 900 prefix was used to indicate a head design intended for end cutting only. Except for differences in blade design a No. 957, No. 557, and No. 57 bur all had the same head dimensions. These changes occurred gradually over time without disrupting the system. The sizes in common use in 1955 are shown in Table 8-5. The system changed rapidly thereafter but *where the numbers are still used the designs and dimensions remain the same*.

Modifications in bur design. As available handpiece speeds increased after 1950, particularly after the high-speed turbine handpieces were introduced, a new cycle of modification of bur sizes and shapes has occurred. In recent years, numerous other categories have arisen as new variations in blade number or design have been created. Some of the numbers assigned to those burs were arbitrarily selected. With the introduction of new bur sizes and elimination of older sizes, much of the logic in the system has no longer been maintained, and many dentists and manufacturers no longer recognize the original significance of the numbers used for burs. There has been a reduction in the number of standard sizes that have continued in use. This has been most obvious in the decreased popularity of large-diameter burs. The cutting effectiveness of carbide burs is greatly increased at high speeds.[6] This is particularly true of the small-diameter sizes, which did not have sufficient peripheral speed for efficient cutting when used at lower rates of rotation. As the *effectiveness of small burs has increased*, they have replaced larger burs in many procedures. *Three other major trends in bur design* are discernible: reduced use of crosscuts, extended heads on fissure burs, and rounding of sharp tip angles.

Crosscuts are needed on fissure burs to obtain adequate cutting effectiveness at low speeds, but at high speeds they are not needed. Because crosscut burs used at high speeds tend to produce unduly rough surfaces, many of the crosscut sizes originally developed for low-speed use have been replaced by non-crosscut instruments of the same dimension for high-speed use.[5] In many instances the non-crosscut equivalents were available, thus a No. 57 bur might be used at high speed, whereas a No. 557 bur was preferred for low-speed use. Non-crosscut versions of the 700 series burs have become popular, but their introduction precipitated a crisis in the bur numbering system, since no number had traditionally been assigned to burs of this type.

Carbide fissure burs have been introduced that have *extended head lengths* two to three times those of the normal tapered fissure burs of similar diameter. Such a design would never have been practical using a brittle material such as carbide if the bur were to be used at low speed. The applied force required to make a bur cut at speeds of 5000 to 6000 rpm would normally be sufficient to fracture such an attenuated head. The extremely light applied pressures that are needed for cutting at high speed, however, permit many modifications of burs that would have been impractical at low speed.

The third major trend in bur design has been toward *rounding of the sharp tip corners.* Early contributions to this trend were made by Markley and Sockwell.[26] Because teeth are relatively brittle, the sharp angles produced by conventional burs can result in high stress concentrations and increase the tendency of the tooth to fracture. Bur heads with rounded corners result in lower stresses in restored teeth, enhance the strength of the tooth by preserving vital dentin, and facilitate the adaptation of restorative materials. Both carbide burs and diamond instruments of these designs last longer because there are no sharp corners to chip and wear. Such burs facilitate the preparation of cavities with desired features of a flat cavity floor and rounded internal line angles.

Many of these new and modified bur designs simplify the techniques and reduce the effort needed for optimal results. Although the development of new bur sizes and shapes has greatly increased the number of different types in current use, the number actually required for clinical effectiveness has been reduced. Most instruments recommended in this text for the preparation of teeth are illustrated in Fig. 8-32. The selection

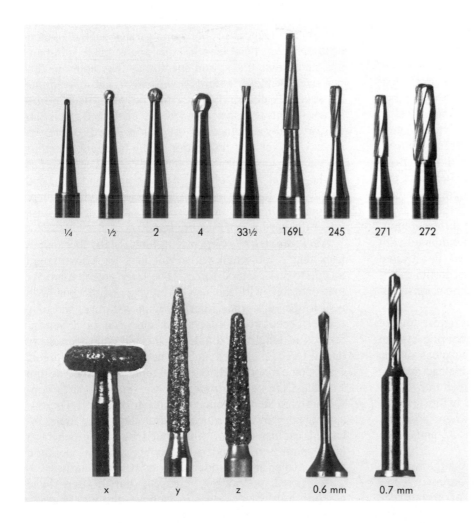

Fig. 8-32. Burs used in recommended procedures. Bur sizes ¼, ½, 2, 4, 33½, and 169L are standard carbide burs available from a variety of sources. The 245, 271, and 272 burs are non-standard carbide burs that do not conform to the current ADA standard numbering system. They are designed to combine rounded corners with flat ends and are available from several manufacturers. The diamond instruments shown are wheel (Star No. 110) (*x*), flame (Star No. 265-8F) (*y*), and tapered cylinder (R & R No. 770 x 7) (*z*). Two sizes of twist drill are illustrated. Particular drills are often provided as specified by manufacturers of pin-retention systems.

Table 8-6. Names and key dimensions of recommended burs

Manufacturer's size number	ADA size number	ISO size number	Head diameter (mm)	Head length (mm)	Taper angle (degrees)	Shape
¼	¼	005	0.50	0.40	—	Round
½	½	006	0.60	0.48	—	Round
2	2	010	1.00	0.80	—	Round
4	4	014	1.40	1.10	—	Round
33S*	—	006	0.60	0.45	12	Inverted cone
33½	33½	006	0.60	0.45	12	Inverted cone
169	169	009	0.90	4.3	6	Tapered fissure
169L†	169L	009	0.90	5.6	4	Elongated tapered fissure
329	329	007	0.70	0.85	8	Pear, normal length
330	330	008	0.80	1.00	8	Pear, normal length
245‡§	330L	008	0.80	3.0	4	Pear, long length
271‡	171	012	1.20	4.0	6	Tapered fissure
272‡	172	016	1.60	5.0	6	Tapered fissure

*Similar to the No. 33½ bur except that it is safe-sided end cutting only.
†Similar to the No. 169 bur except for greater head length.
‡These burs differ from the equivalent ADA size by being flat ended with rounded corners. The manufacturer's number has been changed to indicate this difference.
§Similar to the No. 330 bur except for greater head length.

includes standard head designs and modified designs of the types just discussed. Table 8-6 lists the significant head dimensions of these standard and modified burs.

There has been a long-standing international problem related to the dimensions and designations of rotary dental instruments that arose because each country developed its own system of classification. American dentists were not often aware of the problem because they predominantly used domestic products, and all U.S. manufacturers used the same system. The rapid rate at which new bur designs were introduced during the transition to high-speed techniques threatened to cause a *complete breakdown in the numbering system.* As different manufacturers developed and marketed new burs of similar design almost simultaneously, there was an increased risk of similar burs being given different numbers or different burs the same number. Combined with an increased use of foreign products in the United States, this has led to an increased interest in the establishment of international standards for dimensions, nomenclature, and other characteristics.

In recent years there has been slow progress toward the development of an international numbering system for basic shapes and sizes, under the auspices of the ISO. For other design features the trend instead appears to be toward the use of individual manufacturer's code numbers. Therefore, throughout the following text the traditional U.S. numbers will be used where possible. The few exceptions are shown in Fig. 8-32 and Table 8-6.

Additional features in head design. A large number of factors other than head size and shape are involved in determining the clinical effectiveness of a bur de-

sign.[13,14] Fig. 8-33 shows a lateral view and a cross-sectional view of a No. 701 crosscut tapered fissure bur in which a number of these factors are illustrated. The lateral view (Fig. 8-33, *A*) demonstrates neck diameter, head diameter, head length, taper angle, blade spiral angle, and crosscut size and spacing as they apply to this bur size. Of these features *head length* and *taper angle* are primarily descriptive and may be varied within limits consistent with the intended use of the bur. This bur was originally designed for use at low speeds in preparing cavities for cast restorations. The taper angle is thus intended to approximate the desired occlusal divergence of the lateral walls of the preparations, and the head length must be long enough to reach the full depth of the normal preparation. These factors do not otherwise affect the performance of the bur.

Neck diameter is important functionally because a neck that is too small will result in a weak instrument unable to resist lateral forces. Too large a neck diameter may interfere with the use of the part of the bur head next to the neck, may interfere with visibility, and may restrict access for coolants. As the head of a bur increases in length or diameter, the moment exerted by lateral forces increases and the neck needs to be larger.

In comparison with these factors, two other design variables, the *spiral angle* and *crosscutting,* have considerably greater influence on bur performance. There is a tendency toward reduced spiral angles on burs intended exclusively for high-speed operation where a large spiral is not needed to produce smooth operation and a smaller angle produces more efficient cutting.

As noted previously, crosscut bur designs have notches in the blade edges to increase cutting effective-

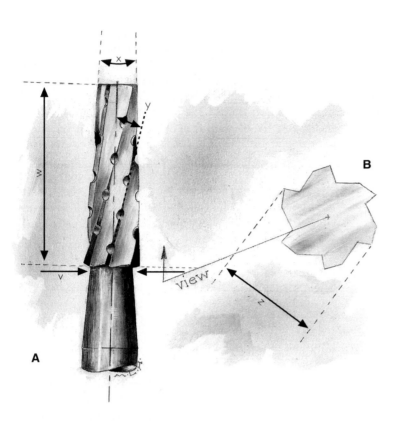

Fig. 8-33. Design features of bur heads (illustrated using No. 701 bur): **A,** Lateral view: neck diameter *(v)*, head length *(w)*, taper angle *(x)*, and spiral angle *(y)*. **B,** End view: head diameter *(z)*.

ness at low and medium speeds. A certain amount of perpendicular force is required to make a blade *dig in* and start cutting as it passes across a surface. The harder the surface, the duller the blade, and the greater its length, the more force is required to initiate cutting. By reducing the total length of bur blade that is actively cutting at any one time, the crosscuts effectively increase both the cutting pressure resulting from rotation of the bur and the perpendicular pressure holding the blade edge against the tooth.

As each crosscut blade cuts, it leaves small ridges of tooth structure standing behind the notches. Because the notches in two succeeding blades do not line up with each other, the ridges left by one blade are removed by the following one at low or medium speeds. However, at the high speed attained with air turbine handpieces the contact of the bur with the tooth is not continuous, and usually only one blade cuts effectively.[12] Under these circumstances, although the high cutting rate of crosscut burs is maintained, the ridges are not removed and a much rougher cut surface results.[5]

A cross-sectional view of the same No. 701 bur is shown in Fig. 8-33, *B*. This cross-section is made at the point of largest head diameter and is drawn as seen from the shank end. The bur has six blades uniformly spaced with depressed areas between them. These depressed areas are properly known as the ***flutes.*** The number of blades on a bur is always even because even numbers are easier to produce in the manufacturing pro-

cess, and instruments with odd numbers of blades cut no better than those with even numbers. The number of blades on an excavating bur may vary from 6 to 8 to 10. Burs intended mainly for finishing procedures usually have 12 to 40 blades. The greater the number of blades, the smoother will be the cutting action at low speeds; most burs are made with at least six blades because of the possibility that they may have to be used in this speed range. At the other extreme in the *high-speed range, it appears that no more than one blade cuts effectively at any one time,* and the remainder are in effect spares. The tendency for the bur to cut on a single blade is often a result of factors arising outside the bur itself; nevertheless it is important that the bur head be as symmetrical as possible. Two terms are in common use to measure this characteristic of bur heads: *concentricity* and *runout*.

Concentricity is a direct measurement of the symmetry of the bur head itself. It measures how closely a single circle can be passed through the tips of all of the blades. Thus concentricity is an indication of whether one blade is longer or shorter than the others. It is a static measurement not directly related to function. ***Runout,*** on the other hand, is a dynamic test measuring the accuracy with which all blade tips pass through a single point when the instrument is rotated. It measures not only the concentricity of the head but also the accuracy with which the center of rotation passes through the center of the head. Even a perfectly concentric head will exhibit substantial runout if the head is off center on the axis of the bur, if the bur neck is bent, if the bur is not held straight in the handpiece chuck, or if the chuck is eccentric relative to the handpiece bearings. The runout can never be less than the concentricity, and it is usually substantially greater. The runout is the more significant term clinically because it is the primary cause of vibration during cutting and is the factor that determines the minimum diameter of the hole that can be drilled by a given bur. It is because of runout errors that burs normally cut holes measurably larger than the head diameter.

Bur blade design. The actual cutting action of a bur (or a diamond) takes place in a very small region at the edge of the blade (or at the point of a diamond chip). In the high speed range this effective portion of the individual blade is limited to no more than a few thousandths of an inch adjacent to the blade edge. Fig. 8-34 is an enlarged schematic view of this portion of a bur blade. A number of terms used in the discussion of blade design are illustrated.

Each blade has two sides, the *rake face* (toward the direction of cutting) and *clearance face,* and three important angles, the *rake angle,* the *edge angle,* and the *clearance angle.* The optimal angles are dependent on such factors as the mechanical properties of the blade material, the mechanical properties of the material being cut, the rotational speed and diameter of the bur, and the lateral force applied by the operator to the handpiece and thus to the bur.

The rake angle is the most important design characteristic of a bur blade. For cutting hard, brittle materials, a negative rake angle minimizes fractures of the cutting edge, thereby increasing the tool life. A rake angle is said to be negative when the rake face is ahead of the radius (from cutting edge to axis of bur) as is illus-

trated in Fig. 8-34. Increasing the edge angle reinforces the cutting edge and reduces the likelihood for the edge of the blade to fracture. Carbide bur blades have higher hardness and are more wear resistant, but they are more brittle than steel blades and require greater edge angles to minimize fractures. The three angles cannot be varied independently of each other. An increase in the clearance angle, for example, causes a decrease in the edge angle. The clearance angle eliminates rubbing friction of the clearance face, provides a stop to prevent the bur edge from digging into the tooth structure excessively, and reduces the radius of the blade back of the cutting edge to provide adequate flute space or clearance space for the chips formed ahead of the following blade.

Carbide burs normally have blades with slight negative rake angles and edge angles of about 90 degrees. Their clearance faces either are curved or have two surfaces to provide a low clearance angle near the edge and a greater clearance space ahead of the following blade.

Diamond abrasive instruments

The second major category of rotary dental cutting instruments involves abrasive rather than blade cutting. *Abrasive instruments* are based on small, angular particles of a hard substance held in a matrix of softer material. Cutting occurs at a large number of points where individual hard particles protrude from the matrix, rather than along a continuous blade edge. This difference in design causes definite differences in the mechanisms by which the two types of instruments cut and in the applications for which they are best suited.

Abrasive instruments are generally grouped as diamond or other instruments. Diamond instruments have had great clinical impact because of their long life and great effectiveness in cutting enamel and dentin. Diamond instruments for dental use were introduced in the

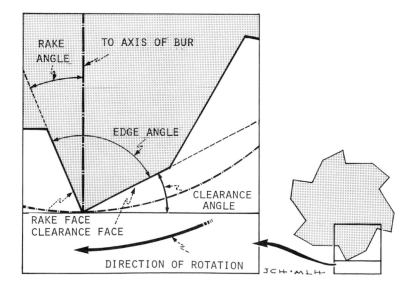

Fig. 8-34. Bur blade design. Schematic cross section viewed from shank end of head to show rake angle, edge angle, and clearance angle.

United States in 1942 at a time before carbide burs were available and at a time when interest in increased rotational speeds was beginning to emphasize the limitations of steel burs. The earliest diamond instruments were substitutes for previously used abrasive points of other types used for grinding and finishing. Their vastly superior performance in these applications led to their immediate acceptance. The shortage of burs as a result of wartime demands emphasized the relative durability of diamond points against enamel and promoted the development of operative techniques employing them.

Terminology. Diamond instruments consist of three parts: a metal blank, the powdered diamond abrasive, and a metallic bonding material that holds the diamond powder onto the blank (Fig. 8-35).[23] The *blank* in many ways resembles a bur without blades. It has the same essential parts: head, neck, and shank.

The shank dimensions, like those for bur shanks, depend on the intended handpiece. The neck is normally a tapered section of reduced diameter that connects the shank to the head, but for large disc or wheel-shaped instruments it may not be reduced below the shank diameter. The head of the blank is undersized in comparison with the desired final dimensions of the instrument, but its size and shape determine the size and shape of the finished instrument. Dimensions of the head make allowance for a fairly uniform thickness of diamonds and bonding material on all sides. Some abrasive instruments are designed as a mandrel and a detachable head. This is much more practical for abrasive disks that have very short lifetimes.

The diamonds employed are industrial diamonds, either natural or synthetic, that have been crushed to powder and then carefully graded for size and quality. The shape of the individual particle is important because of its effect on the cutting efficiency and durability of the instrument, but the careful control of particle size is probably of greater importance. The diamonds are attached to the blank by electroplating a layer of metal on the blank while holding the diamonds in place against it.

Classification. Diamond instruments are currently marketed in a profusion of head shapes and sizes and in all of the standard shank designs. This situation arose in part as a result of the relative simplicity of the manufacturing process. Because it is possible to make diamond instruments in almost any shape for which a blank can be manufactured, they are produced in many highly specialized shapes on which it would be impractical to cut blades. This has been a major factor in establishing applications for these points, which are not in direct competition with burs.

Head shapes and sizes. Diamond instruments are available in a wide variety of shapes and in sizes which correspond to all except the smallest diameter burs. The greatest difference lies in the diversity of other sizes and shapes in which diamond instruments are produced. For example, the standard list includes more than 70 subdivisions under discs, including groups such as flat, concave, perforated, non-perforated, safe-inside, and safe-outside in a wide variety of combinations. Even with this many subdivisions the size range within each group is very large in comparison with that found among the burs. Similar variations are found among the other shapes as well.

Because of their design with an abrasive layer over an underlying blank, the smallest diamond instruments cannot be as small in diameter as the smallest burs, but a wide range of sizes is available for each shape. No one manufacturer produces all sizes, but each will usually offer an assortment of instruments, including the popular sizes and shapes. Due to the lack of uniform nomenclature for diamond instruments, it is often necessary to select them by inspection to obtain the desired size and shape. It is *essential for the same reason to indicate the manufacturer when attempting to describe diamond instruments by catalogue number*.

Diamond particles factors. The clinical performance of diamond abrasive instruments depends on the *size, spacing, uniformity, exposure,* and **bonding** of the diamond particles. Increased pressure causes the particles to dig into the surface more deeply, leaving deeper scratches and removing more tooth structure.

Diamond *particle size* is commonly categorized as coarse (125 to 150 μm), medium (88 to 125 μm), fine (60 to 74 μm), and very fine (38 to 44 μm) for diamond excavating instruments.[23] These ranges correspond to standard sieve sizes for separating particle sizes. When

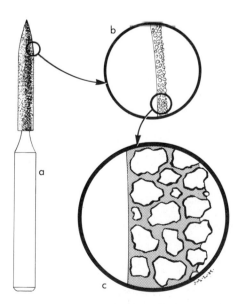

Fig. 8-35. Diamond instrument construction: overall view *(a)*, detail of abrasive layer *(b)*, and detail of particle bonding *(c)*.

using large particle sizes, the number of abrasive particles that can be placed on a given area of the head is decreased. Thus, for any given force that the operator applies, the pressure on each particle tip is greater. The resulting pressure also is increased if diamond particles are more widely *spaced* so that there are fewer in contact with the surface at any one time. The final clinical performance of diamond instruments is strongly affected by the technique used to take advantage of the design factors for each instrument.

Proper diamond instrument speed and pressure are the major factors determining service life.[7] Properly used diamond instruments will last almost indefinitely. Almost the only cause of failure of diamond instruments is loss of the diamonds from critical areas. This results from the use of excess pressure in an attempt to increase the cutting rate at inadequate speeds.[11]

Other abrasive instruments

Many types of abrasive instruments are used in dentistry in addition to diamond instruments. They were at one time extensively used for tooth preparation, but their use is now primarily restricted to shaping, finishing, and polishing restorations, both in the clinic and in the laboratory.

Classification. In these instruments, as in the diamond instruments, the cutting surfaces of the head are composed of abrasive particles held in a continuous matrix of softer material. Other than this and their use of standard shank designs, there is little similarity to diamond instruments in their construction. They may be divided into two distinct groups, molded instruments and coated instruments. Each uses a variety of abrasives and matrix materials.

Molded abrasive instruments have heads that are manufactured by molding or pressing a uniform mixture of abrasive and matrix around the roughened end of the shank, or cementing a pre-molded head to the shank. In contrast to diamond instruments, molded instruments have a much softer matrix and are expected to wear during use. The abrasive is distributed throughout the matrix so new particles are exposed by the wear. These instruments are made in a full range of shapes and sizes. The mounted heads are often termed *points* as well as *stones*. Hard and rigid molded instrument heads use rigid polymer or ceramic materials for their matrix. These are commonly used for grinding and shaping procedures. Other molded instrument heads use flexible matrix materials, such as rubber, to hold the abrasive particles. These are used predominantly for finishing and polishing procedures. Molded *unmounted discs* or *wheelstones* are made that attach by a screw to a mandrel of suitable size for a given handpiece which has a threaded hole in the end. This design permits the instruments to be changed easily and discarded economically.

The *coated abrasive instruments* are mostly discs that have a thin layer of abrasive cemented to a flexible backing. This construction allows the instrument to conform to the surface contour of a tooth or restoration. Most flexible discs are designed for reversible attachment to a mandrel. Coated abrasive instruments are used in the finishing/smoothing procedures of certain enamel walls (and margins) of cavity preparations for indirect restorations as well as in finishing procedures for restorations.

The abrasives are softer and less wear-resistant than diamond powder and as a result tend to lose their sharp edges and thus their cutting efficiency with use. When this happens to coated instruments, they are discarded. Molded instruments, in contrast, are intended to be partially regenerating by gradual loss of their worn outer layers but may require that the operator reshape them to improve their concentricity. This is accomplished by applying a truing or shaping stone against the rotating instrument.

Materials. The *matrix materials* usually are phenolic resins or rubber. Some molded points may be sintered but most are resin bonded. A *rubber matrix* is used primarily to obtain a flexible head on instruments to be used for polishing. A harder, *non-flexible rubber matrix* is often used for molded silicon carbide discs. The matrix bond of coated instruments is customarily one of the phenolic resins.

Synthetic or natural abrasives may be used, including silicon carbide, aluminum oxide, garnet, quartz, pumice, and cuttlebone. The hardness of the abrasive has a major effect on the cutting efficiency. Mohs hardnesses for important dental abrasives are shown in Table 8-7.

Silicon carbide (Carborundum^{TM}) is usually used in molded rounds, tree or bud shapes, wheels, and cylin-

Table 8-7. Hardness values of resorative materials, tooth structure, and abrasives

	Knoop hardness (KHN)	Brinell hardness (BHN)	Mohs hardness (value)
Dentin	68	48	3-4
Enamel	343	300	5
Dental composite	41-80	60-80	5-7
Dental amalgam	110	—	4-5
Gold alloy (Type III)	—	110	—
MGC Dicor	330	—	—
Feldspathic porcelain	460	—	6-7
Pumice	—	—	6
Cuttlebone	—	—	7
Garnet	—	—	6.5-7
Quartz	800	600	7
Aluminum oxide	1500	1200	9
Silicon carbide	2500	—	9.5
Diamond	7000+	5000+	10

ders of various sizes. These points are normally gray-green, are available in various textures, are usually fast cutting (except on enamel), and produce a moderately smooth surface. Molded unmounted discs are black or a dark color, have a soft matrix, wear more rapidly than stones, and produce a moderately rough surface texture. These discs are termed **Carborundum discs** or separating discs.

Aluminum oxide is used for the same instrument designs as silicon carbide. Points are usually white, rigid, fine textured, less porous, and produce a smoother surface.

Garnet (reddish) and **quartz** (white) are used for coated discs that are available in a series of particle sizes that ranges from coarse to medium-fine for use in initial finishing. These abrasives are hard enough to cut tooth structure and all restorative materials, with the exception of some porcelains.

Pumice is a powdered abrasive produced by crushing foamed volcanic glass into thin glass flakes. The flakes cut effectively, but break down rapidly. Pumice is used in rubber discs and wheels usually for initial polishing procedures.

Cuttlebone is derived from the cuttlefish, a relative of squid and octopus. It is becoming scarce and is gradually being replaced by synthetic substitutes. It is a soft white abrasive, used only in coated discs for final finishing and polishing. It is soft enough that it reduces the risk of unintentional damage to tooth structure during the final stages of finishing.

CUTTING MECHANISMS

For cutting it is necessary to apply sufficient pressure to make the cutting edge of a blade or abrasive particle dig into the surface. Local fracture occurs more easily if the strain rate is high (high rotary instrument surface speed) because the surface being cut responds in a brittle fashion.

The process by which rotary instruments cut tooth structure is complex and not fully understood. The following discussion of cutting will address cutting evaluations, cutting instrument design, proposed cutting mechanisms, and clinical recommendations for cutting.

Evaluation of cutting

Cutting can be measured in terms of both effectiveness and efficiency. Certain factors may influence one and not the other.[17] **Cutting effectiveness** is the rate of tooth structure removal (mm/min or mg/sec). Effectiveness does not consider potential side effects such as heat or noise. **Cutting efficiency** is the percentage of energy actually producing cutting. Cutting efficiency is reduced when energy is wasted as heat or noise. It is possible to increase effectiveness while decreasing efficiency. A

dull bur, for example, may be made to cut faster than a sharp bur by applying a greater pressure, but experience indicates that this results in a great increase in heat production, and thus reduced efficiency.[29]

There is general agreement that increased rotational speed results in increased effectiveness and efficiency. Adverse effects associated with increased speeds are heat, vibration, and noise. **Heat** has been identified as a primary cause of pulpal injury. Air-water sprays do not prevent the production of heat but do serve to remove it before it causes a damaging rise in temperature within the tooth.

Bladed cutting

The following discussion will focus on rotary bladed instruments but is applicable to bladed hand instruments as well. Tooth structure, like other materials, undergoes both brittle and ductile fracture. **Brittle fracture** is associated with crack production, usually by tensile loading. **Ductile fracture** involves plastic deformation of material, usually proceeding by shear. Extensive plastic deformation may also produce local work hardening and encourage brittle fracture as well. Low-speed cutting tends to proceed by plastic deformation prior to tooth structure fracture. High-speed cutting, especially of enamel, proceeds by brittle fracture.

The rate of stress application (or strain rate) affects the resultant properties of materials. In general, the faster the rate of loading, the greater will be the strength, hardness, modulus of elasticity, and brittleness of a material. A cutting instrument with a large diameter and high rotational speed will produce a high surface speed, and thus a high stress (or strain) rate.

Many factors interact to determine which cutting mechanism is active in a particular situation. The mechanical properties of tooth structure, the design of the cutting edge or point, the linear speed of the instrument's surface, the contact force applied, and the power output characteristics of the handpiece influence the cutting process in various ways.[6,18]

In order for the blade to initiate the cutting action, it must be sharp, must have a higher hardness and modulus of elasticity than the material being cut, and must be pressed against the surface with sufficient force. The high hardness and modulus of elasticity are essential to concentrate the applied force on a small enough area to exceed the shear strength of the material being cut.

As shown in Fig. 8-36, sheared segments accumulate in a distorted layer that slides up along the rake face of the blade until it breaks or until the blade disengages from the surface as it rotates. These chips will accumulate in the clearance space between blades until washed out or thrown out by centrifugal force.

Mechanical distortion of tooth structure ahead of the blade produces heat. Frictional heat is produced by the rubbing action of the cut chips against the rake face of the blade and that of the blade tip against the cut surface of the tooth immediately behind the edge.

This can produce extreme temperature increases in both the tooth and the bur in the absence of adequate cooling. The transfer of heat is not instantaneous, however, and the reduced temperature rise observed in teeth cut at very high speeds may in part be caused by removal of the heated surface layer of tooth structure by a following blade before the heat can be conducted into the tooth.

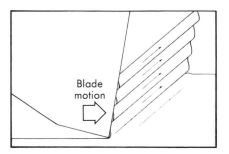

Fig. 8-36. Schematic representation of bur blade (end view) cutting a ductile material by shearing mechanism. Energy is required to deform the material removed and produce new surface.

Abrasive cutting

The following discussion is pertinent to all abrasive cutting situations, but diamond instruments will be used as the primary example.[9] The cutting action of diamond abrasive instruments is similar in many ways to that of bladed instruments but key differences result from the properties, size, and distribution of the abrasive. The very high hardness of diamonds provides superior resistance to wear. A diamond instrument that is not used abusively, has little or no tendency to dull with use. Individual diamond particles have very sharp edges, are randomly oriented on the surface, and tend to have large negative rake angles.

When diamond instruments are used to cut ductile materials, some material will be removed as chips, but much material will flow laterally around the cutting point and be left as a ridge of deformed material on the surface (Fig. 8-37). Repeated deformation work hardens the distorted material until irregular portions become brittle, break off, and are removed. This type of cutting is less efficient than that of a blade, and *burs are generally preferred for cutting ductile materials such as dentin.*

Diamonds cut brittle materials by a different mechanism. Most cutting results from tensile fractures that produce a series of subsurface cracks (Fig. 8-38). *Diamonds are most efficient when used to cut brittle materials and are superior to burs for the removal of dental enamel.*

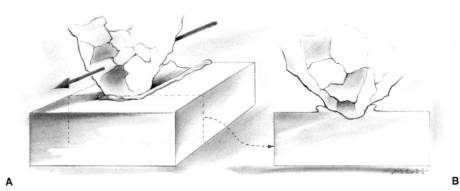

Fig. 8-37. Schematic representation of an abrasive particle cutting ductile material. **A,** Lateral view. **B,** Cross-sectional view. Material is displaced laterally by passage of an abrasive particle, work hardened, and subsequently removed by other particles.

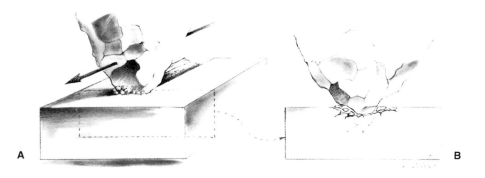

Fig. 8-38. Schematic representation of abrasive particle cutting brittle material. **A,** Lateral view. **B,** Cross-sectional view. Subsurface cracks caused by the passage of abrasive particles intersect, undermining small pieces of material, which are then easily removed by following abrasive particles.

Diamond abrasives are commonly used for milling disks or instruments for CAD/CAM or copy-milling applications (see Machined Restorations, in Chapter 6).

Cutting recommendations

Overall, the requirements for effective and efficient cutting include using a contra-angle handpiece, air-water spray for cooling, high operating speed (above 200,000 rpm), light pressure, and a carbide bur or diamond instrument. *Carbide burs* are better for end-cutting, produce lower heat, and have more blade edges per diameter for cutting. They are better for punch cuts to enter tooth structure, intra-coronal cavity preparation, amalgam removal, small preparations, and secondary retention features. Diamond instruments have higher hardness and coarse diamonds have very high cutting effectiveness. *Diamonds* are better for extra-coronal cavity preparation, beveling enamel margins on cavity preparations, and enameloplasty.

HAZARDS WITH CUTTING INSTRUMENTS

Almost everything done in a dental office involves some risk to the patient, dentist, and/or auxiliaries. For the patient, there are *pulpal dangers* from the cavity preparation and restoration procedures. There are also *soft tissue dangers.* Everyone is potentially susceptible to *eye, ear,* and *inhalation dangers.* However, careful adherence to normal *precautions* can eliminate or minimize most risks associated with cutting instrument use.

Pulpal precautions

The use of cutting instruments can harm the pulp by exposure to mechanical vibration, heat generation, desiccation and loss of dentinal tubule fluid and /or transection of odontoblastic processes. As the thickness of remaining dentin decreases, the pulpal insult (and response) from heat or desiccation increases. Slight to moderate injury produces a localized, protective pulpal response in the region of the cut tubules. In severe injury, destruction extends beyond the cut tubules, often resulting in pulpal abscess and death of the pulp. These pulpal sequellae (recovery or necrosis) take from 2 weeks to 6 months or longer, depending on the extent and degree of the trauma. Although a young pulp is more prone to injury, it also recovers more effectively when compared with an older pulp, in which the recuperative powers are slower and less effective.

Enamel and dentin are good thermal insulators and will protect the pulp if the *quantity of heat* is not too great and the *remaining thickness* of tissue is adequate. The longer the time of cutting and the higher the local temperature produced, the greater is the threat of thermal trauma. The remaining tissue is effective in protecting the pulp in proportion to the square of its thickness.

Steel burs produce more heat than carbide burs because of inefficient cutting. Burs and diamond instruments that are dull or plugged with debris do not cut efficiently, resulting in heat production. When used without coolants, diamond instruments generate more damaging heat than carbide burs.

The most common *instrument coolants* are *air, or air-water spray.* Air alone as a coolant is not effective in preventing pulpal damage since it needlessly desiccates the dentin and damages the odontoblasts (see Chapter 2, section on Dentin). An air coolant alone should be used only when visibility is a problem, such as during the finishing procedures of cavity preparations. At such times air coolant combined with both lower speed and light intermittent application should be used to enhance vision and minimize trauma. Air-water spray is universally used to cool, moisten, and clear the operating site during normal cutting procedures. In addition, the spray lubricates, cleans, and cools the cutting instrument, thereby increasing its efficiency and service life. A well-designed and properly directed air-water spray also helps to keep the gingival crevice open for better vision when gingival extension to this region is necessary. The use of a water spray and its removal by an effective high-volume evacuator are especially important when old amalgam restorations are removed in order to decrease mercury vapor release and to increase visibility.

During normal cutting procedures a layer of debris, described as a *smear layer,* is created that covers the cut surfaces of the enamel and dentin (see Chapters 2 and 6). The smear layer on dentin is moderately protective because it occludes dentinal tubules and inhibits the outward flow of tubular fluid and the inward penetration of microleakage contaminants. However the smear layer is still porous. When air alone is applied to dentin, local desiccation may produce fluid flow and affect the physiologic status of the odontoblastic processes in the underlying dentin (review Chapter 2 for hydrodynamic sequelae). *Air is applied only to the extent of removing excess moisture, leaving a glistening surface.*

Soft tissue precautions

The lips, tongue, and cheeks of the patient are the most frequent areas of soft tissue injury. The handpiece should never be operated unless there is good access and vision to the cutting site. A rubber dam is very helpful in isolating the operating site. When the dam is not used, the dental assistant can retract the soft tissue on one side with a mouth mirror, cotton roll, and/or evacuator tip. The dentist can usually manage the other side with a mirror and/or cotton roll. If the dentist must work alone, the patient can help by holding a retraction-type saliva ejector evacuator tip after it is positioned in the mouth.

With air turbine handpieces the rotating instrument does not stop immediately when the foot control is released. The operator must either wait for the instrument to stop or be extremely careful when removing the handpiece from the mouth so as not to lacerate soft tissues. The large disc is one of the most dangerous instruments used in the mouth. Fortunately such discs are seldom required. They should be used with light, intermittent application and with extreme caution.

The dentist and the assistant must always be alert to the patient during the cutting procedures. A sudden reflex movement by the patient such as gagging, swallowing, or coughing could result in serious injury. If an accident does occur in which soft tissue is damaged, the operator should remain calm and control any hemorrhage with a pressure pack. The patient should be told what has happened, and medical assistance should be obtained if needed.

The chance of mechanical pulpal involvement is greater if a hand excavator is used to remove the last portions of soft caries in a deep cavity. When the remaining dentinal wall is thin, the pressure exerted on the excavator may be sufficient to break into the pulp chamber. Therefore, a round bur may be used at a low speed with light, intermittent application for caries removal. Air turbine handpieces should be operated just above stalling speed to improve tactile sense for caries removal. Proceed with caution and inspect the area frequently.

Exercise care that the *biological width* of at least 2 mm is established or preserved for the junctional epithelium and connective tissue attachment located between the base of the gingival sulcus and the alveolar crest (see Chapter 5). In addition to this physiological dimension, the restoration margin should be as far away as possible from the gingival sulcus in order to maintain gingival health.

Eye precautions

The operator, assistant, and patient should wear glasses with side shields to prevent eye damage from flying particles during some operative procedures. When cut at high speeds, particles of old restorations, tooth structure, bacteria, and other debris are discharged at high speeds from the patient's mouth. Sufficiently strong high-volume evacuation applied by the dental assistant near the operating site helps to alleviate this problem. However, *protective glasses are always indicated*. The dentist is more likely to receive injury than is the assistant or the patient because of being in a more direct path of flying particles. If an eye is injured, it should be covered by a clean gauze pad until medical attention can be obtained.

In addition to routine air-borne debris, occasionally *there may be particles produced by matrix failure of molded abrasive cutting instruments*. Hard matrix wheels may crack or shatter into relatively large pieces. Soft abrasive wheels or points may increase in temperature during use, causing the rubber matrix to explosively debond from the abrasive into fine particles.

Furthermore, precautions must be taken for prevention of eye injury from unusual light sources, such as visible light-curing units and laser equipment. Dental personnel and patients should be protected from high intensity visible light using either colored plastic shields (attached to the fiber optic tip) or colored eyewear capable of blocking harmful wavelengths (see Chapter 18). Laser light can be inadvertently reflected from many surfaces in the dental operatory and, therefore, the operatory should be closed off and everyone should wear protective goggles (see Laser Equipment).

Ear precautions

Various sounds are known to affect people in different ways. Soft music or random sounds like rainfall usually have a relaxing or sedative effect. Loud noises are generally annoying and may contribute to mental and physical distress. A noisy environment decreases the ability to concentrate, increases accident proneness, and reduces overall efficiency. Extremely loud noises such as explosions, or continuous exposure to high noise levels can cause permanent damage to the hearing mechanism.

An objectionable high-pitched whine is produced by some air turbine handpieces at high speeds. Aside from the annoying aspect of this noise, there is some possibility that hearing loss can result from continued exposure.

Potential damage to hearing from noise depends on: (1) the intensity or loudness (decibels, db), (2) frequency (cps), and (3) duration (time) of the noise, as well as (4) the susceptibility of the individual. Increased age, existing ear damage, disease, and medications are other factors that can accelerate hearing loss.

Normal ears require that the intensity of sound reach a certain minimum level before the ear can detect it. This is known as the **auditory threshold.** It can vary with frequency and exposure to other sounds. When subjected to a loud noise of short duration, a protective mechanism of the ear causes it to lose some sensitivity temporarily. This is described as a *temporary threshold shift.* If sufficient time is allowed between exposures, recovery will be complete. Extended or continuous exposure is much more likely to result in a *permanent threshold shift* with persistent hearing loss. The loss may occur for all frequencies but often affects high frequency sounds more severely.

A certain amount of unnoticed noise (ambient noise

level) is present even in a quiet room (20 to 40 db). An ordinary conversation averages 50 to 70 db in a frequency range of 500 to 2500 cps.

Turbine handpieces with ball bearings, free running at 30 pounds air pressure, may have noise levels as high as 70 to 94 db at high frequencies. Noise levels in excess of 75 db in frequency ranges of 1000 to 8000 cps may cause hearing damage. There is considerable variation in noise levels among handpieces by the same manufacturer. Handpiece wear and eccentric rotating instruments can cause increased noise. Protective measures are recommended when the noise level reaches 85 db with frequency ranges from 300 to 4800 cps. Protection is mandatory in areas where the level transiently reaches 95 db. The effect of excessive noise levels depends on exposure times. Normal use of a dental handpiece is one of intermittent application that generally is less than 30 minutes per day. Earplugs can be used to reduce the level of exposure but have several drawbacks. Room soundproofing helps and can be accomplished with absorbing materials used on walls and floors.

Inhalation precautions

Aerosols and vapors are created by cutting tooth structure and restorative materials. Both aerosols and vapors are a health hazard to all present. The aerosols are fine dispersions in air of water, tooth debris, microorganisms, and/or filling materials. Both sub-micron particles and vapor are produced by cutting amalgams or composites. The particles that may be inadvertently inhaled have the potential to produce alveolar irritation and tissue reactions. Vapor from cutting amalgams is predominantly mercury and should be eliminated, as much as possible, by careful evacuation near the tooth being operated on. The vapors generated during cutting or polishing by thermal decomposition of polymeric restorative materials (sealants, acrylic resin, composites) are predominantly monomers. They may be efficiently eliminated by careful intraoral evacuation during the cutting or polishing procedures.

A rubber dam protects the patient against oral inhalation of aerosols or vapors, but nasal inhalation of vapor and finer aerosol may still occur. Disposable masks worn by dental office personnel filter out bacteria and all but the finest particulate matter. However, they do not filter out either mercury or monomer vapors. The biological effects of mercury hazards, as well as appropriate office hygiene measures, are discussed in Chapter 6.

REFERENCES

1. American Dental Association: Council on Dental Research adopts standards for shapes and dimensions of excavating burs and diamond instruments, *J Am Dent Assoc* 67:943, 1963.
2. American National Standards Institute: American Dental Association specification No. 23 for dental excavating burs, *J Am Dent Assoc* 104:887, 1982.
3. Black GV: *Operative dentistry,* ed 8, Woodstock, Ill, 1947, Medico-Dental Publishing.
4. Black GV: *The technical procedures in filling teeth,* 1899, Henry O. Shepard.
5. Cantwell KR, Aplin AW, Mahler DB: Surface characteristics of tooth structure after cutting with rotary instruments, *Dent Progr* 1(1):42-46, 1960.
6. Eames WB, Nale JL: A comparison of cutting efficiency of air-driven fissure burs, *J Am Dent Assoc* 86:412-415, 1973.
7. Eames WB, Reder BS, Smith GA: Cutting efficiency of diamond stones: effect of technique variables, *Oper Dent* 2(4):156-164, 1977.
8. Frentzen M, Koort HJ, Thiensiri I: Excimer lasers in dentistry: future possibilities with advanced technology, *Quint Int* 23:117-133, 1992.
9. Grajower R, Zeitchick A, Rajstein J: The grinding efficiency of diamond burs, *J Prosthet Dent* 42:422-428, 1979.
10. Guerini V: *A history of dentistry,* Philadelphia and New York, 1909, Lea & Febiger.
11. Hartley JL, Hudson DC: Modern rotating instruments: burs and diamond points, *Dent Clin North Am,* p 737, Nov 1958.
12. Hartley JL et al: Cutting characteristics of dental burs as shown by high speed photomicrography, *Armed Forces Med J* 8(2):209, 1957.
13. Henry EE: Influences of design factors on performance of the inverted cone bur, *J Dent Res* 35:704-713, 1956.
14. Henry EE, Peyton FA: The relationship between design and cutting efficiency of dental burs, *J Dent Res* 33:281-292, 1954.
15. International Standards Organization: Standard ISO 2157: head and neck dimensions of designated shapes of burs, Geneva, 1972, International Standards Organization.
16. Jeffrey IWM et al: CO_2 laser application to the mineralized dental tissues—the possibility of iatrogenic sequelae, *J Dent* 18:24-30, 1990.
17. Koblitz FF et al: *An overview of cutting and wear related phenomena in dentistry.* In Pearlman S, editor: *The cutting edge,* DHEW Publication No. (NIH) 76-670, Washington, DC, 1976, US Government Printing Office.
18. Lindhe J: Orthogonal cutting of dentine, *Odontol Revy* (Malma) 15(suppl 8):11-100, 1964.
19. Merritt R: Low-energy lasers in dentistry, *Brit Dent J* 172:90, 1992.
20. Morrant GA: Burs and rotary instruments: introduction of a new standard numbering system, *Brit Dent J* 147(4):97-98, 1979.
21. Myers TD: Lasers in dentistry, *J Am Dent Assoc* 122:46-50, 1991.
22. Nelson RJ, Pelander CE, Kumpula JW: Hydraulic turbine contra-angle handpiece, *J Am Dent Assoc* 47:324-329, 1953.

23. Nuckles DB: Status report on rotary diamond instruments, Council on deutal materials and devices, *J Am Dent Assoc* 97(2):233-235, 1978.
24. Peyton FA: Effectiveness of water coolants with rotary cutting instruments, *J Am Dent Assoc* 56:664-675, 1958.
25. Peyton FA: Temperature rise in teeth developed by rotating instruments, *J Am Dent Assoc* 50:629-630, 1955.
26. Sockwell CL: Dental handpieces and rotary cutting instruments, *Dent Clin North Am* 15(1):219-244, 1971.
27. SS White Dental Manufacturing Company: *A century of service to dentistry*. Philadelphia, 1944, SS White Dental Manufacturing.
28. Taylor DF, Perkins RR, Kumpula JW: Characteristics of some air turbine handpieces, *J Am Dent Assoc* 64:794-805, 1962.
29. Westland IN: The energy requirement of the dental cutting process, *J Oral Rehab* 7(1):51, 1980.
30. White JM et al: Effects of pulsed Nd:YAG laser energy on human teeth: a three-year follow-up study, *J Am Dent Assoc* 124:45-51, 1993.
31. Zakariasen KL, MacDonald R, Boran T: Spotlight on lasers—a look at potential benefits, *J Am Dent Assoc* 122:58-62, 1991.

Preliminary considerations for operative dentistry

Kenneth N. May, Jr.

Aldridge D. Wilder, Jr.

Roger E. Barton*

INFECTION CONTROL MEASURES

Before, during, and after any patient visit, appropriate *infection control measures must be instituted.* For this information the reader is referred to Chapter 4, Infection Control.

PATIENT AND OPERATOR POSITIONS

An appreciation of efficient patient and operator positions is essential for the welfare of both persons. The patient who is in a comfortable position is more relaxed, has less muscular tension, and is more capable of cooperating with the dentist. By using optimal operating positions and good posture, the operator experiences less physical strain and fatigue, and reduces the possibility of developing musculoskeletal disorders.

The practice of dentistry is demanding and stressful. Several physical problems are fostered through constant neglect of appropriate operating positions. Almost all restorative dental procedures can be accomplished while seated. *Positions that create unnecessary curvature of the spinal column or slumping of the shoulders should be avoided.* When the back and chest are held in an upright position with the shoulders squared, proper breathing and circulation are promoted. At times, circumstances prevent maintaining this position while operat-

ing, but it should remain the basic body position. Proper balance and weight distribution on both feet is essential when operating from a standing position. Generally, any uncomfortable or unnatural position that places undue strain on the body should be used only rarely. The health and fitness of the dentist are significant factors contributing to physical endurance and productivity.

Chair and patient positions

Modern dental chairs are designed to provide total body support in any chair position. An available chair accessory is an adjustable headrest or neckrest cushion, or an articulating headrest that is attached to the chair back. The contoured or lounge-type chair provides complete patient support and comfort. Chair design and adjustment permit maximal operator access to the work area. The adjustment control switches should be conveniently located. Some chairs are equipped with programmable operating positions. To improve infection control, chairs with a foot switch for patient positioning are recommended.

The patient should have direct access to the chair. The chair height should be low, the backrest upright, and the armrest adjusted to allow the patient to slide into the chair as though seated in a lounge chair. After the patient is seated, the armrest is returned to its normal position, and the headrest or neckrest cushion is positioned to support the head and to elevate the chin slightly away from the chest. In this position neck muscle strain is minimal and swallowing is facilitated. The chair is then adjusted to place the patient in a reclining position.

The most common patient positions for operative dentistry are almost supine or reclined 45 degrees (Fig. 9-1). The choice varies with the operator, the type of procedure, and the area of the mouth involved in the operation. In the almost supine position, the patient's head, knees, and feet are approximately the same level. The patient's head should not be lower than the feet. The head should be positioned lower than the feet only in an emergency, as when the patient is in syncope.

*This author is inactive this edition; see Preface.

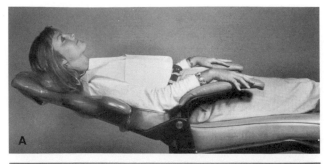

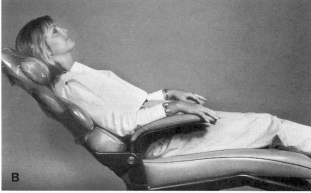

Fig. 9-1. Common patient positions. **A,** Supine and **B,** reclined 45 degrees. Both are recommended for sit-down dentistry. Use depends on arch being operated.

When the operation is completed, the chair should be placed in the upright position so that the patient can leave the chair easily and gracefully, preventing undue strain or loss of balance.

Operating positions

Operating positions may be described by the location of the operator or by the location of the operator's arms in relation to patient position. *For the right-handed operator, there are essentially three positions: right front, right, and right rear.* These are sometimes referred to as the 7, 9, and 11 o'clock positions (Fig. 9-2, *A*), respectively. *For the left-handed operator, the three positions are: left front, left, and left rear,* or the 5, 3, and 1 o'clock positions, respectively. A fourth position, *direct rear,* or 12 o'clock position, has application for certain areas of the mouth. All of the positions discussed may be used from the standing or seated operating position. To relieve stress on the operator's legs and to support the operator's back, most dental treatment is delivered from a seated position. The operating positions described below are for the right-handed operator. The left-handed operator should substitute *left* instead of *right*.

Right front position. This position facilitates examination and work on mandibular anterior teeth (Fig. 9-2, *B*), mandibular posterior teeth, especially the right side,

and maxillary anterior teeth. It is often advantageous to have the patient's head rotated slightly toward the operator.

Right position. Here the operator is directly to the right of the patient (Fig. 9-2, *C*). This position is convenient for operating on the facial surfaces of the maxillary and mandibular right posterior teeth and the occlusal surfaces of the mandibular right posterior teeth.

Right rear position. This is the position of choice for most operations. Most areas of the mouth are accessible and can be viewed directly or through the mouth mirror. The operator is behind and slightly to the right of the patient. The left arm is positioned around the patient's head (Fig. 9-2, *D*). When one is operating from this position, the lingual and incisal (occlusal) surfaces of the maxillary teeth are viewed in the mouth mirror. Direct vision may be used on mandibular teeth, particularly on the left side, but the use of a mouth mirror is advocated for light reflection, retraction, and viewing.

Direct rear position. This position has somewhat limited application and is primarily used for operating on the lingual surfaces of mandibular anterior teeth. The operator is located directly behind the patient and looks down over the patient's head (Fig. 9-2, *E*).

General considerations

The operator should not hesitate to rotate the patient's head backward or forward or from side-to-side to accommodate the demands of access and visibility of the operating field. Minor rotation of the patient's head is not uncomfortable to the patient and it allows the operator to maintain his or her basic body position. *As a rule, when operating in the maxillary arch, the maxillary occlusal surfaces should be oriented approximately perpendicular to the floor. When operating in the mandibular arch, the mandibular occlusal surfaces should be oriented approximately 45 degrees to the floor.* Patients are usually very cooperative in allowing the operator to position the head where it is most advantageous. Sacrificing good operating posture in most instances is unnecessary (Fig. 9-3).

The face of the operator should not come in close proximity to that of the patient. The ideal distance, such as that for reading a book, should be maintained. However, small, detailed, or inaccessible cavity preparations may require closer proximation for adequate viewing. Maintaining an appropriate working distance from the patient is important for the operator to master in the early stages of learning. Another important aspect of proper operating position is to minimize body contact with the patient. A good operator does not rest forearms on the patient's shoulders or hands on the patient's face or forehead. Unnecessary contact is unpleasant to many patients and should not be practiced.

From most positions the left hand should be free to

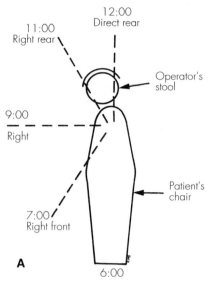

Fig. 9-2. Operating positions indicated by arm approach to the patient. A, Diagrammatic operator positions. B, Right front; C, right; D, right rear; and E, direct rear.

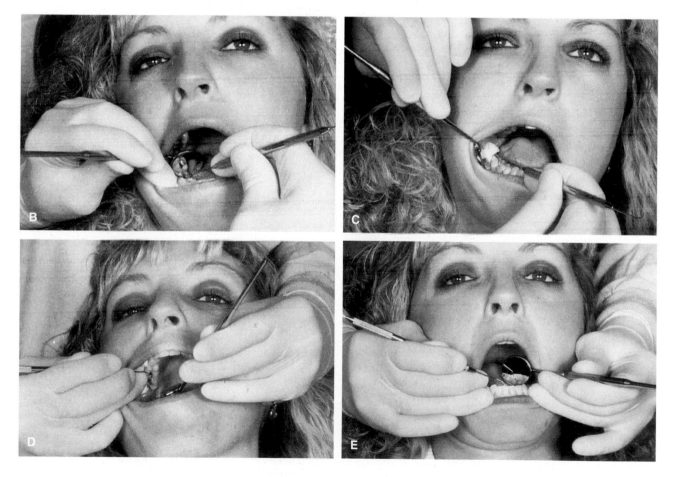

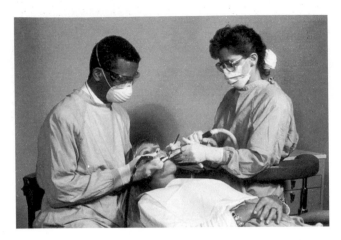

Fig. 9-3. Recommended seating positions for operator and chair-side assistant with height of the operating field slightly above elbow of operator.

hold the mouth mirror to reflect light onto the operating field to view the cavity indirectly, or to retract the cheek or tongue. In certain instances it is more appropriate to retract the cheek with one or two fingers of the left hand than to use a mouth mirror. However, it is often possible to reflect light and retract the cheek with the mouth mirror at the same time.

When operating for an extended period, the operator will find a certain amount of rest and muscle relaxation occur from changing operating positions.[1] Operating from a single position for an entire day, especially while standing, produces unnecessary fatigue. *Changing positions, if only for a short time, reduces muscle strain and lessens fatigue.* Although the sitting position is more relaxing and requires less expenditure of energy, an occasional shift to a standing position may be beneficial. Proper distribution of balance on both feet is essential when operating from a standing position.

Operating stools

There are a variety of operating stools for the dentist and the dental assistant. The design of the stool is important. The stool should be on casters for mobility. It should be sturdy and well balanced to prevent tipping or gliding away from the dental chair. The seat should be well padded with smooth cushion edges and should be adjustable up and down. The backrest should be adjustable forward and back as well as up and down. The assistant's stool should have a foot ring to permit proper leg position. Operator stools do not have a foot rest. Comfortable, well designed stools will help to reduce tension and fatigue.

Some of the advantage of sitting to work is lost if the operator uses the stool improperly. The operator should not be balanced on the stool using it as a third leg of a tripod. The operator should sit back on the cushion using the entire seat and not just the front edge. The upper body should be positioned so that the spinal column is straight or bent slightly forward. Some operator and assistant stools have backrests with curved extensions that offer additional body support. The thighs should be parallel to the floor, and the lower legs should be perpendicular to the floor. Feet should be flat on the floor. Of course, this ideal position cannot be maintained at all times, but it should be assumed as often as possible.

The seated work position for the assistant is essentially the same as for the operator except that the stool is 4 to 6 inches higher for maximal visual access. It is important, therefore, that the stool for the assistant have an adequate footrest so that a parallel thigh position can be maintained with good foot support.

When properly seated, both the operator and assistant are capable of continuous dental service throughout the day without an unnecessary decline in efficiency and productivity because of muscle tension and fatigue.

INSTRUMENT EXCHANGE

All instrument exchange between the operator and assistant should occur in the **exchange zone** below the patient's chin and several inches above the patient's chest. During the procedure the operator should anticipate and inform the assistant of the next instrument required. This will allow it to be brought into the exchange zone in readiness for a timely exchange. An experienced assistant will anticipate the operator's instrument needs before they are verbalized.

During proper instrument exchange it should not be necessary for the operator to remove his or her eyes from the operating field. The operator should rotate the instrument handle forward to cue the assistant to exchange instruments. Exchange any sharp instrument with appropriate *deliberation*. The assistant should take the instrument from the operator, rather than the latter dropping it into the former's hand, and vice versa. The exchange need not be forceful, nor should it be conducted as if the instrument were a feather. Each person should feel assurance that the other has a firm grasp on the instrument before it is released. To maximize operating efficiency whether treating one tooth or several, each instrument should be used completely before proceeding to the next instrument. This will minimize the number of instrument exchanges necessary for each appointment.

MAGNIFICATION

The success of clinical operative dentistry is dependent upon visual acuity. The operator must be able to see clearly in order to attend to the details of each pro-

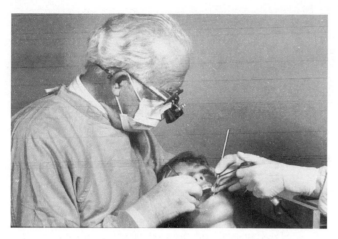

Fig. 9-4. Use of magnification by surgical telescopes.

cedure. Normal accommodation of the operator's eyes is necessary to maintain a proper working distance. The aging process causes a loss of accommodation. After age 40 operators may require magnifying lenses to compensate for this loss. Several types of magnification devices are available such as bifocal eyeglasses, loupes, and surgical telescopes (Fig. 9-4). The use of eyeglasses also provides some protection from eye injury.

REFERENCE

1. Shugars D et al: Musculoskeletal pain among general dentists, *Gen Dent* 35(4):272, 1987.

CHAPTER 10

Pain control

Clifford M. Sturdevant

Historically the public has associated *pain* with dental treatment. No longer should this be true, because materials, equipment, and techniques for the *elimination of pain* have been available for a number of years. Pain elimination, including atraumatic needle injection, is essential to a successful dental practice. Anesthesia must be at least as profound, and usually more so, in operative dentistry (or any phase of fixed restorative dentistry) as is required in any other health discipline. The following information, if understood and practiced, should eliminate pain associated with dental procedures. For additional information the reader is referred to a textbook on local anesthesia. The author of this chapter is grateful for a review and suggestions from Dr. Ronald D. Baker, Chairman, Department of Oral and Maxillofacial Surgery, University of North Carolina School of Dentistry.

LOCAL ANESTHESIA BY NEEDLE INJECTION OF ANESTHETIC AND EPINEPHRINE

Needle injection is the common modality for local anesthesia in fixed restorative dentistry. To eliminate pain and other unpleasantness (such as salivation) associated with tooth preparation and restoration, there should be few exceptions to the administration of local anesthesia of *all* tissues in the operating site for *all* patients.

A competent dentist must have a thorough knowledge of the patient's physical and emotional status as well as an understanding of the effects of these drugs (anesthetics and vasoconstrictors).

A *therapeutic dose* of a drug is the least amount that is effective when properly administered, and which does not cause adverse reactions. An *overdose* of a drug is an excessive, administered amount that results in overly elevated blood levels of the drug, and which causes adverse reactions.

The following *classification of patients* according to *physical status* is used by the American Society of Anesthesiology (ASA) and is appropriate for use by all health care personnel*:

I. Normal healthy individual
II. Patient with mild to moderate systemic disease
III. Patient with severe systemic disease that limits activity but is not incapacitating
IV. Patient with severe systemic disease that limits activity and is a constant threat to life
V. Moribund patient not expected to survive 24 hours with or without an operation

The normal healthy patient can safely receive as many as five to eight of the 1.8 ml cartridges containing anesthetic (2% lidocaine) and epinephrine 1/100,000 (number of cartridges increasing as body weight increases) per appointment. (There is merit to defining acceptable quantities in milligrams per pound of lean body weight.) Routine dental therapy for ASA II patients is permissible but with no more than two to four cartridges per appointment. ASA III or IV patients with significant health problems, such as congestive heart disease, but who are *ambulatory*, should not be administered more than two cartridges per appointment. ASA IV patients who are *not* ambulatory are neither candidates for local anesthesia (with or without vasoconstrictor) nor elective dental care. *All these doses presume proper administration, which includes extravascular, slow-deposition of the solution.*

Any special condition of the patient (such as pregnancy), or less than healthy status should be of *record*, particularly regarding the cardiovascular system, the central nervous system, the respiratory system, liver, kidneys, thyroid gland, age, and allergy. Thus a *medical history form* must be completed and signed by the patient (see Chapter 5).

Patient physical factors; relationship to anesthetic and epinephrine

The cardiovascular system (CVS). Before administering any drug the condition of the cardiovascular system (heart and blood vessels) must be assessed. A minimum physical examination of blood pressure, heart rate, and rhythm is recommended for all patients. A patient with *a pressure >200 systolic and/or >115 diastolic* (ASA IV) ought not to receive *invasive, elective clinical dental treatment* until the pressure is controlled (reduced).[3,p.122] Malamed also has suggested that any

resting patient with a heart rate below 60 or above 110 be further evaluated. Additionally, he emphasizes that five or more "missed beats" (premature ventricular contractions) per minute with no obvious cause is an indication for medical consultation.

Patients with *heart disease* (e.g., valvular defects) usually should be on an *antibiotic regimen* during dental treatment.

Overdose of the anesthetic drug (highly unlikely for properly administered 2% lidocaine) produces a *depression* of the myocardium and a lowering of blood pressure, sometimes resulting in unconsciousness from reduced oxygenation of the brain.

Overdose of epinephrine (very rare with 1/100,000 concentration, properly administered) causes a rise in blood pressure, elevated heart rate, and possible dysrhythmias. This latter effect happens not infrequently if retraction cord that is treated with epinephrine is applied to abraded gingivae. This results in a rapid, high uptake into the circulatory system. Careful operative dentistry should not result in abraded gingivae, even in subgingival (into the gingival sulcus) cavity preparations. (See Chapter 19, section on beveling and flaring.)

The central nervous system (CNS). The central nervous system (CNS) is more easily affected by *overdose of injected anesthetic drugs* than the cardiovascular system.[2,7] As with the cardiovascular system, anesthetics *depress* the CNS, but when administered properly for local anesthesia they cause very little to no clinical evidence of depression. However, at *minimum to moderate overdose levels*, the depression is manifested in *excitation* (such as talkativeness, apprehension, sweating, elevated blood pressure and heart rate, and elevated respiratory rate) or *drowsiness*. At *moderate to high overdose levels* there is *tonic-clonic seizure* activity, followed by *generalized CNS depression*, depressed blood pressure, reduced heart rate (less than 60/sec), and depressed respiratory rate, and then respiratory arrest.[3,pp.32,268]

With lidocaine and procaine, the usual progression of excitatory signs and symptoms described previously may *not* be seen, and the first clinical evidence of overdose may be *mild sedation* or *drowsiness* (more common with lidocaine).[3,pp.31,268]

The respiratory system. The respiratory system is not affected by therapeutic doses of anesthetic drug properly administered. The system, however, is depressed and may be arrested by central nervous system depression due to overdose.

Hepatic dysfunction. Hepatic dysfunction can lead to adverse effects from high anesthetic level in the blood, because the diseased liver has reduced capacity to biotransform the amide-type drugs (such as lidocaine). For these patients minimal effective volumes of anesthetic should be used. If the patient is ambulatory, how-

---

*Based on the classification used in McCarthy FM, Malamed SF: *J Am Dent Assoc* 99:181-184, 1979. Used with permission of the American Dental Association.[5]

ever, overdose is unlikely[3,p.263] if the anesthetic is properly administered. Significant heart disease may compromise the liver's opportunity to function properly due to reduced perfusion.

Renal dysfunction. Regarding renal dysfunction, Malamed states, "In actual clinical situations use of local anesthetics does not pose an increased risk for these patients" (with kidney trouble).[3,p.120] The patient being ambulatory would be a positive factor.

Thyroid disease. Patients with **uncontrolled hyperthyroidism** may show an exaggerated response to vasoconstrictors included in the anesthetic solution. This can be prevented or minimized by use of minimal concentrations of the vasoconstrictor as well as proper administration of the solution. *Controlled thyroidism* is not a contraindication for administration of an anesthetic drug with vasoconstrictor.

Age. For the extremes of age, the very young and very old patients, amounts and concentrations of anesthetic drugs and epinephrine should be *reduced* to the smallest doses that are effective. Body weight being small for the young, and reduced functional capacity of the organs in the very old, are reasons for this precaution.

Allergy. Malamed states, "One absolute contradiction exists for administration of local anesthetic: documented, reproducible allergy."[3,p.74] When any patient attests to a history of "sensitivity" or "reaction" from injected dental anesthetic, *the dentist must believe the patient* until further investigation (be it verbal questions and answers, or allergic testing in a sophisticated life support environment) disproves the patient's belief of an allergy. *Anaphylactic shock following an allergic reaction can be immediate and life-threatening.*

Overdose due to too much anesthetic injected too fast, or, more likely, an intravascular injection are reasons for many alleged allergic reactions.

Idiosyncrasy. Idiosyncrasy is a bizarre (nonpharmacological) clinical manifestation to an administered drug. Explanation is unknown, and treatment is basic life support.

Pregnancy. During the first trimester of pregnancy, elective dental treatment is not recommended. Communication with the physician (obstetrician) is recommended. Although it is safe to properly use anesthetics and vasoconstrictors, it is prudent to be conservative in the administration of drugs.

Patient psychological factors; relationship to anesthetic and epinephrine

The patient's psychological attitude affects responses to various stimuli. The *apprehensive* or *anxious patient* overreacts, and usually requires more anesthetic because the *pain threshold* is lowered. Such patient *stress* causes endogenous catecholamines (adrenalin) to enter the vascular system, and this coupled with the injection (deposition) of exogenous catecholamines (epinephrine) can result in overdose. This is particularly serious for the cardiovascularly impaired patient. Also, this *fearful patient* has a lowered threshold for convulsant seizure, which coupled with larger doses of adrenalin can precipitate serious overdose reactions. Bennett[2] reminds us that *the greater the medical risk of a patient the more important effective control of pain and anxiety becomes.*

Patients on prescribed **tricyclic antidepressants** should receive a *minimal dose of epinephrine* while, as always, the operator must avoid intravascular injection as well as deposit solution slowly.

These "problem" patients (about 1/500) especially require a dentist's empathetic patience, calmness, understanding, and an atraumatic injection technique, along with supine patient position and carefully chosen words of assurance that there will be no discomfort (notice: *no* reference to the word "pain") during the entire procedure. Elimination of pain in dental treatment for this patient is a challenge. Past unpleasant dental experiences and frightening remarks from relatives or "friends" regarding painful treatment are some reasons that explain why these patients are "conditioned" to expect pain.

Benefits of local anesthesia

Cooperative patient. When local anesthetic with epinephrine is properly administered (atraumatically, extravascularly, deposited *slowly,* etc.), patient anxiety and tenseness should be minimal. This maximizes rapport between dentist and patient throughout ensuing treatment. The appreciation and trust of the patient for the dentist (and dental assistant) is expressed in an almost relaxed and certainly **cooperative attitude.** Physically and emotionally, both patient and dentist benefit from this relatively calm environment.

Salivation control. It has been observed for years that complete anesthesia of all tissues (teeth *and* soft tissues) in the operating site results in a near cessation of salivation.[8] Conversely, whenever the patient as much as "feels" the touch of operator fingers or instruments there is flow of saliva. Salivation cessation is reason alone for profound anesthesia of *all* tissues involved, for *all* patients, with very few exceptions. When patients exclaim, "I don't need my teeth numbed because my teeth are not sensitive," or "I will be very still," or "I don't want the injection because I don't like the numb feeling," the dentist should explain, "I cannot properly prepare *your* tooth and cannot correctly restore it unless we stop all sensations to *you* for a short time;" and add further, "most patients have not been told by a dentist that such sensations cause great amounts of saliva to flow, and that this creates problems in making for *you* a good restoration." Notice the emphasis on "you" or "your," and putting the blame on dentists for not informing patients. Truly, sometimes a tooth is not sensitive and doesn't require anesthesia (e.g., when sclerotic dentin is under a restoration being replaced), but if *all* other sensations from the operating site are not eliminated, then salivation still will result.

Hemostasis. The term *hemostasis* as used in operative dentistry is the temporary reduction in blood flow and volume in the tissue *(ischemia)* where a *vasoconstrictor* is deposited or placed. The vasoconstrictor, usually epinephrine, causes constriction of the small blood vessels, and thus the affected tissue bleeds less if cut or abraded. (This condition is sought in the application of epinephrine-treated retraction cord, but as was mentioned in a previous section [The Cardiovascular System] regarding overdose of epinephrine, good operative dentistry does not produce abraded or cut gingiva.)

The *principle function of a vasoconstrictor in operative dentistry is the prolongation of anesthesia* due to reduced flow of blood *to* and *away from* the site of deposited anesthetic solution containing epinephrine, 1/100,000. Without epinephrine, anesthesia from 1 ml of deposited 2% lidocaine will last only 5 to 10 minutes, whereas with epinephrine the anesthesia will last 40 to 60 minutes. It is to be recognized further that this reduced blood flow helps in keeping the patient's blood level of both anesthetic and vasoconstrictor at a lower level by lowering the rate of absorption into the circulatory system.

Operator efficiency. Local anesthesia greatly benefits both dentist and patient, and is virtually indispensable for successful cavity preparation and restoration of the tooth. Usually the patient is calm, or nearly so (certainly after several previous appointments without a hint of pain), and is most cooperative. This reinforces the dentist's attitude of confidence and calmness, which fosters a "smooth," efficient manner. The lack of either distractions or management problems (such as heavy salivation) from the patient means that the dentist's thoughts and actions can be directed methodically and purposefully upon the treatment, which thereby should be completed successfully within a reasonable time frame.

Psychology in administering local anesthesia

Patients have varying degrees of concern about receiving an oral injection. Thus a concentrated effort is required of the dentist (and assistant) to make the procedure acceptable. Some psychology is desirable with all patients during this phase of dental treatment. Probably the greatest positive effect is achieved by a *caring manner,* rather than in what is said. Remember that words such as "pain," and "sting a little," and "hurt a little," are *not* to be used, because no matter what else is said, the patient will *only* remember these inappropriate

words (which may be evidence that an atraumatic, proper administration technique is not being used). The dentist who administers local anesthesia atraumatically (painlessly) will not have need for such hurtful and fear-provoking words. The operator must use a kind, considerate, and understanding approach. Every assurance should be made that comfort of the patient is paramount and that the teeth and soft tissues will be treated with care. Such assurances, confidently and "softly" spoken, are welcomed *during* the administration of local anesthesia. One example is, "I may be taking longer than you expected, but we are giving the solution *slowly to be kind to your tissues."* Conversely, *don't say,* "You may be *wondering* why I'm taking so long to *inject* the anesthetic; I am doing so to keep from *tearing* the tissue." Note the hurtful connotation of the words "wondering," "inject," and "tearing," versus in the former explanation the caring words, "kind to your tissues." Patients who *feel secure* (safe from pain and in caring hands) will gratefully accept local anesthesia.

The art of tactfully keeping the syringe and needle from view of the patient should be practiced. Here the chairside assistant can be a tremendous help.

Sequential steps and principles in technique

Profound, painless anesthesia of both the teeth and contiguous soft tissues is so important in operative dentistry that salient features of a recommended technique in infiltration anesthesia for a maxillary canine are presented. Also, **work practice controls and engineering controls** for infection control (particularly avoiding accidental needle stick) will be described. The following principles in needle injection of local anesthetic and epinephrine are applicable both for **infiltration anesthesia** (supraperiosteal or field block) where deposition is near the nerve ends in the operating site and for **conduction anesthesia** (nerve block) where deposition is near a nerve trunk at a distance from the operating site.

In this example of infiltration anesthesia, the needle *entry spot* and *direction* are different from that presented in some local anesthesia textbooks. Also, *aspiration* as well as *slow deposition* of solution will be emphasized.

For other local anesthesia injections, (e.g., inferior alveolar, Gow-Gates mandibular, posterior superior alveolar, infraorbital, mental, and periodontal ligament) the reader is referred to a textbook in local anesthesia.

Supine or semi-supine position of patient (see exceptions to supine). The routine supine position of the patient (the usual for operative dentistry) is an aid for preventing vasodepressor syncope, since it favors blood supply and pressure to the brain. A *precaution:* the upper torso should never be more than 10 degrees below the horizontal plane, as this may cause *respiratory distress* due to the force of viscera against the diaphragm.

On rare occasions patients may complain of difficulty in breathing except when sitting upright or standing (orthopnea), and a compromise in patient position is necessary. Another *exception* to the supine position is where symptoms suggest an epinephrine overdose, and then a semi-erect or sitting position is best since it minimizes any further elevation in cerebral blood pressure.[3,p.272] Some of these symptoms are fear, perspiration, weakness, pallor, palpitations, anxiety, and restlessness.

Aspirating syringe. A syringe must have an aspirating feature. In importance, probably aspiration is second only to slow deposition of solution in needle administration of anesthetic. For this purpose, the rod (piston) has on its cartridge end a *harpoon* and on the other end a *thumb ring* (Fig. 10-1, *H*). The harpoon engages the cartridge plunger, resulting in its reverse movement to create negative pressure when the operator's thumb (in ring) pulls gently in a backward direction.

Avoidance of infected tissue. Injection into infected tissue should be avoided because of risk of spreading the infection. Also, the anesthetic is less effective because the tissue is acidic rather than basic. Alternative approaches, such as nerve block, are to be used.

Sheathed and capped, new, sufficiently long, proper gauge, disposable needle. The *sheath* covers the injection needle and the cap covers the reverse-end (or cartridge-end) of the needle (note *s* and *c* in Fig. 10-1, *B*). For *each* patient (appointment) the dental assistant, if knowing the scheduled treatment, selects a sheathed, capped, new, disposable needle of desired length and gauge. The sheathed needle comes sterile from the manufacturer. The *needle remains sheathed, except for setting the harpoon and syringe preparedness testing* (see later principles) *until the moment of entry at the injection site*. This helps to prevent **accidental needle stick,** which among other things indicates needle replacement. Using for each patient appointment a new, sterile needle that is contaminated *only* by that patient's oral tissues eliminates cross-infection (from one person to another) via the needle, except for accidental needle stick of dental personnel during multiple injections. The sheath in place also means that the needle is "manufacturer sharp." A needle should not be inserted more than three times during the appointment, lest its point becomes dull. Also, when the needle touches, even if gently, the firmer periosteal tissue or bone (see later principle), a minute *barb* can be formed which will cause pain on withdrawal or during a subsequent entry and insertion.

The needle must be *sufficiently long* that its full length is never out-of-sight (never completely within tissue). This means that in the unlikely event a needle breaks at the hub junction (invariably the location of breakage) there will be some of the needle exposed for grasping and withdrawal.

Needles of 27-*gauge* are recommended, although some operators prefer the 30-gauge, short needle for infiltration anesthesia of the maxillary teeth. The 30-gauge needle may not allow aspiration, and it is believed by some authorities that it does not pierce or move in tissue easier than the 27-gauge needle. The 30-gauge, long needle may deviate during injection for conduction anesthesia (for the inferior alveolar nerve).

Insertion of sheathed end into prop/guard card. The *dental assistant* inserts the sheathed needle end into the prop/guard (STIK-SHIELD*) card (Fig. 10-1, *A* to *D*).

Removal of cap. The *dental assistant* removes the cap on the reverse-end of the needle (Fig. 10-1, *E*).

Attachment of sheathed needle to syringe. The *dental assistant* inserts the reverse end of the needle into the hole at the threaded end of the syringe and screws the sheathed needle to a full seating position against the nose of the syringe (Fig. 10-1, *F* and *G*). Guard card protects both hands (card will hit nose of syringe before needle could stick the hand holding the syringe).

Propped, assembled syringe. The *dental assistant* lays the propped (by card) syringe on a tray or countertop (Fig. 10-1, *H*) behind the patient for the *operator* to insert the cartridge, remove the sheath, set the harpoon *(h),* and test for preparedness (subsequent step-principles).

Fig. 10-1. A, Prop/guard (STIK-SHIELD) card. Note: Periphery of hole *(h)* is indexed *(i)* (four pairs of short cuts) to accept four external ridges *(r)* of sheath *(s)* shown in **B. B,** *Sheath (s)* covers injection portion of needle, and *cap (c)* covers reverse end (cartridge needle). Sheath and cap are joined by spot plastic weld *(w)*. Note external ridge *(r)*. **C,** With fingers of one hand holding prop/guard card printed-side-up as well as supporting it, the *dental assistant (DA)* uses ends of thumb, index, and middle fingers of other hand to press the end one third of sheath through hole while lining up external ridges to coincide with card indices. (Do *not* at this time jar cap (on reverse end) loose with hand.) **D,** *Dental assistant (DA)* applies thumb pressure *(arrow)* on end of cap to fully insert sheath to its collar. (Do *not* at this time loosen cap by any twisting motion.) **E,** *Dental assistant's (DA)* left hand holds sheath (card on sheath) and presses down on countertop in a "hard-stationary" position *(left arrow)* while fingers of right hand "twist-break" plastic weld at cap/sheath union and then deliberately move cap off reverse-end needle. Note horizontal right arrow depicting movement of hand (away from needle) which discards cap. **F,** *Dental assistant's (DA)* left hand still holding carded sheathed needle now inserts reverse-end needle into hole in threaded end of syringe held by other hand kept at last 3 inches away from card, and, **G,** then screws sheathed needle clockwise ("righty-tighty") onto syringe threads to a *full-seating position* against syringe nose. Note protection of both hands by guard card during such press-threading. Harpoon *(h)* is utilized later. **H,** *Dental assistant* lays prepared syringe (minus anesthetic cartridge) on countertop or tray behind patient, propped due to guard card and *ready for operator*. Note harpoon *(h)* on piston end.

*STIK-SHIELD®, Tacoma, Washington.

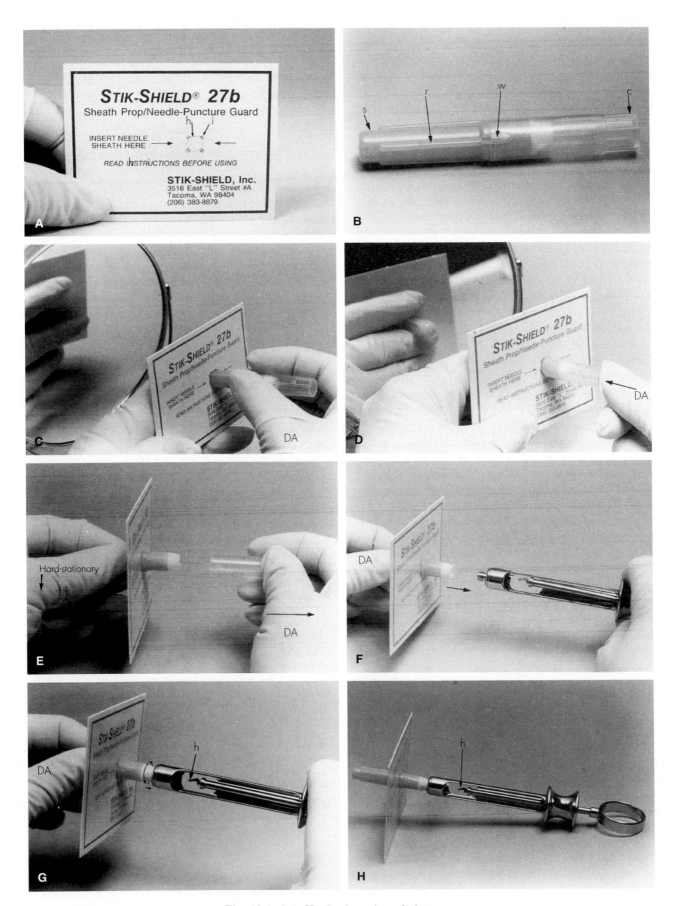

Fig. 10-1, A to **H.** For legend see facing page.

Fresh and new cartridge. A new cartridge for each patient is axiomatic; and it should be reasonably fresh by not being over 18 months old from the date of manufacture, since some ingredients do not have an extended shelf-life. Some manufacturers place an expiration date on the cartridge, and the expiration date is always on the packing container. The diaphragm end of the cartridge should not be contaminated by contact with suspect (infected) surfaces. The cartridge should *not* be immersed in a sterilizing solution (e.g., cold sterilizing solution, or alcohol) since this can diffuse through the diaphragm and cause tissue damage.[3,p.97] Cartridges should not be exposed to sunlight and should be stored at room temperature.

Weakest solution, yet effective anesthesia. Use the weakest solution of anesthetic that is still effective. Two percent lidocaine with 1/100,000 epinephrine (see next principle) is commonly used in operative dentistry and recommended. One milliliter (half a cartridge) will provide anesthesia for 40 to 60 minutes.

Vasoconstrictor (epinephrine). The addition of a vasoconstrictor (epinephrine 1/100,000 recommended) to the anesthetic solution is necessary to *prolong anesthesia* by decreasing the rate of absorption of the anesthetic into the blood. Moreover, by its action the potential of anesthetic toxicity is reduced. As described in a previous section (Hemostasis), epinephrine in the anesthetic solution administered infiltratively is useful in reducing occasional hemorrhage by producing slight, transient *ischemia* of cut (or abraded) soft tissue.

Diaphragm-centered needle. The *operator* picks up the syringe, and while holding the piston *fully* retracted inserts the cartridge (Fig. 10-1, *I* and *J*) and sees that the cartridge *needle is diaphragm-centered;* if not, the operator "finger-guides" the axial alignment of the cartridge by virtue of the syringe slots so that the needle does pierce the center of the diaphragm as the spring-loaded, retracted piston is slowly released. When this piercing occasionally occurs near the aluminum cap (periphery of diaphragm), gross leaking can happen as deposition is attempted, with most of the distasteful solution dripping freely into the patient's mouth. Injection then must be aborted for another cartridge to be placed properly in the syringe.

Removal of sheath. Sheath removal is by the operator (the person giving the injection), behind the patient, with fingers holding the sheath *moving it away from the needle* and syringe-holding hand, which is held stationary on the tray or countertop (Fig. 10-1, *K* and *L*). The prop/guard card protects the hand during sheath removal (Fig. 10-1, *I*), and then the card props the sheath from possibility of extraneous contamination (Fig. 10-1, *M*).

Set harpoon. Set the harpoon into the plunger by a sharp, but not too strong, thump from the palm of the hand onto the thumb ring (Fig. 10-1, *N*). (Too strong a rap may crack or break the cartridge!)

Test of syringe preparedness. Test the syringe preparedness by pressing (activating) the plunger forward 1 to 2 mm to verify that it slides easily, while also observing the emission of solution from the needle tip without leakage elsewhere (Fig. 10-1, *O*).

If preparation of the injection site has previously been accomplished by the gauze wiping of the entry site and the 2-minute placement of topical anesthetic (next principles), the injection procedure follows (see Needle Sheath Removal if in Place; Needle Entry Spot and Direction).

Gauze wipe. Prior to needle entry (see later section on needle entry spot) the mucosa of the injection site should be wiped free of debris and saliva by a sterile gauze wipe.

Topical anesthetic. After gauze wiping, apply a lidocaine topical anesthetic ointment for a minimum of 1 minute (ideal is 2 minutes) to the proposed entry spot (see later section on needle entry spot) using a cotton-tipped swab, *limiting the area to just that of the swab dimension.* (This procedure in a time sequence in experienced hands often is started immediately after positioning the patient in the chair and following the gauze wiping. The chairside assistant may be instructed to accomplish the gauze wipe and application of topical anesthetic.)

Needle sheath removal if in place; needle entry spot and direction. Remove the needle sheath if in place in a one-person procedure with the hand protected by the shield (review the section titled Removal of Sheath and Fig. 10-1, *K* and *L*). With the left hand (right-handed operator) gently raise the lip outward and upward to

---

Fig. 10-1—cont'd. I and **J,** *Operator* (behind patient), while *fully* retracting spring-loaded, moveable, rear cartridge seat of syringe by hand retraction of piston, inserts cartridge, rearward end first (**I**), and then "drops" the forward end (diaphragm end) of cartridge to position (**J**) without dragging across or bending reverse-end needle; then operator slowly releases piston retraction, moving rear cartridge seat and cartridge forward, allowing reverse-end needle to pierce diaphragm. (Leakage of cartridge during later attempted deposition is usually caused by bent, reverse-end needle poorly centered on diaphragm.) **K** and **L,** With syringe propped by card on countertop (or tray) behind patient, *operator* holds sheath by fingers of one hand (card protected) and syringe by other hand which is kept "hard-stationary" (**K**) as sheath is loosened and removed *away from needle* (**L**). **M,** Guard card now props sheath. **N,** *Operator* sets harpoon by gentle palm-thump of thumb ring, and then, **O,** tests syringe for preparedness by thumb pressure moving plunger forward 1 to 2 mm while verifying emission of solution *(s)* from needle without leakage at forward end of syringe body.

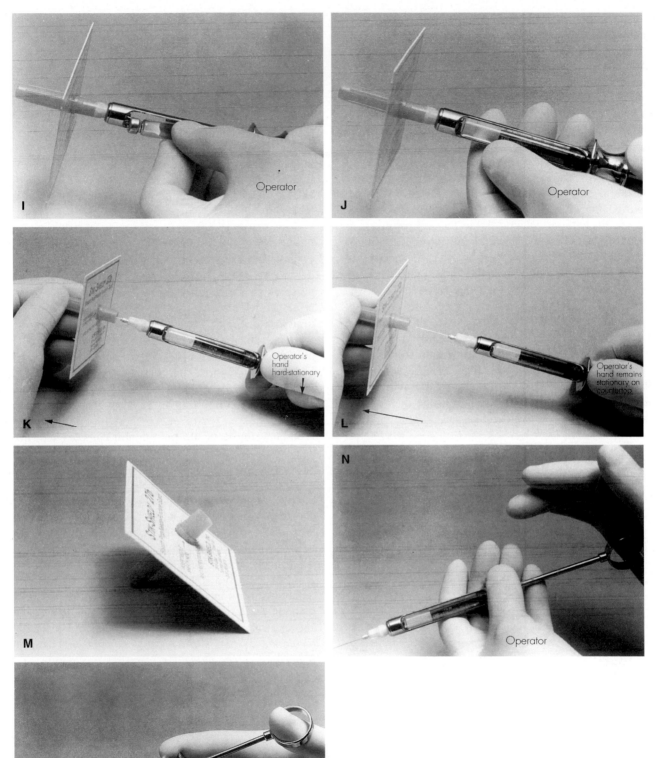

Fig. 10-1, I to O. For legend see facing page.

identify the vestibular fornix, or junction of the alveolar mucosa (fixed) with vestibular mucosa (loose) (Fig. 10-2). Continuing to gently hold the lip high enough, "visualize" the location of the root end, and mentally note on the vestibular loose mucosa the entry spot for the needle when it is held (1) at an angle (perpendicular, or nearly so) to the long axis of the tooth and (2) in the direction (lined-up) for insertion to a *periosteum target area* which is *slightly mesial to and at the level of the root end or slightly above it* (exception: slightly distal for maxillary central incisor) (Fig. 10-2). This entry spot should be 5 to 8 mm lateral of the fornix, thereby allowing some freedom for small movements of the entered needle without causing tissue tension (refer again to Fig. 10-2). These are important principles in an atraumatic and painless injection! If the needle is lined-up parallel to the tooth long axis, rather than at an angle as recommended, the tendency (especially for inexperienced operators) is to enter too close to the attached mucosa, and then to insert (slide) the needle too close to the very sensitive periosteal lining of the alveolar bone, thereby inviting pain from premature touching or tearing the periosteum. This can be prevented 100% of the time! The needle tip must not even be close to the periosteum until the final stage of insertion (see later principle, Periosteum Target, Aspiration, and Slow Deposition).

Entry and initial, slow, small deposition. Now, knowing the entry spot and with the needle directed properly, do two things simultaneously: (1) apply a *small, gentle tug* to the lip (outward and upward) to have the entry spot tissue slightly taut; and (2) *enter* the

needle into the mucosa about 3 mm (all the bevel under the epithelium). The small, gentle tug and tensing the tissue, coupled with topical anesthesia, masks for the patient any sensation from the needle entry (100% success!). After this, the lip tautness should be relaxed somewhat, just so long as operator visibility of the needle is maintained. Now *deposit slowly a small amount of solution* by only a 1- to 2-mm movement of the plunger over 10 seconds, while observing the patient and offering comforting words. Then wait 10 seconds more for further diffusion of the solution and anesthetization of tissue, while continuing patient observation and softly spoken assurances.

Periosteum target, aspiration, and SLOW deposition. Now, still maintaining proper needle direction, gently continue inserting the needle toward the periosteum target, being careful to sense the slight increase in resistance when the needle tip *first touches this lining of the bone,* at which time the needle is immediately withdrawn 1 to 2 mm. (The needle tip in fact often touches the bone, but should do so only *very gently.*) Occasionally, lip fascia may give slight resistance to insertion, before the periosteal target is reached; experience will teach the difference in resistance, the former being less resistant. It is important to be through such fascia and then *close to the periosteum,* otherwise complete or profound anesthesia of the pulp-dentin complex will not be achieved.

Now aspirate by a small (1 mm) reversing of the harpooned plunger by *gentle* backward movement of the thumb ring to verify (through negative pressure) that the needle end is not within a blood vessel. If blood appears into the cartridge (positive aspiration), immediately withdraw the needle 1 to 2 mm, and aspirate again to determine that it is negative.

After negative aspiration, *SLOWLY* deposit 1 mL (slightly more than half the cartridge) over the next 30 seconds (minimal time), while continually observing and assuring the patient. (One minute for 1 ml is the *ideal* rate of deposition.) *Slow deposition is the most important safety procedure* for the prevention of adverse reactions due to high blood levels of anesthetic or epinephrine.[3,p.267] Aspiration rates second in importance. Quoting Dr. RD Baker, "Often deposition is too rapid."[1] Dr. SF Malamed defines too rapid deposition as ≤30 seconds for 1.8 ml[3,p.265] (one cartridge). This rate separates tissue (too rapid to allow diffusion along normal tissue planes), and if intravascular can lead to serious adverse reactions, and is painful (or at least uncomfortable). Conversely, Dr. Malamed states that 1 minute for 1.8 ml of anesthetic (30 seconds for 1 ml or half a cartridge) will not cause tissue damage and will not lead to serious overdose reactions, even if accidentally intravascular.[3,p.140]

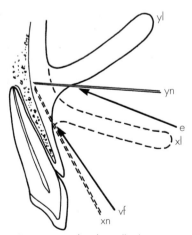

Lip position *yl* and needle direction *yn* recommended

Fig. 10-2. Recommended *entry spot e, direction of needle yn,* and lip position *yl* for infiltration anesthesia of maxillary canine. Direction of needle *xn* and lip position *xl* are not recommended. Vestibular fornix *vf* is junction of loose and fixed mucosa.

Smallest volume, yet effective anesthesia. An important principle is to deposit the smallest volume that will still provide effective anesthesia. One of the more common errors is to deposit so much anesthetic (with epinephrine) that overdose reactions occur.

Resheathed needle. After deposition, gently withdraw the needle and *resheath it in a one-handed procedure* by inserting partially into the propped sheath (left after the unsheathing procedure) and then uprighting the syringe (and sheath) upon the tray or countertop and pressing the needle fully into the sheath (Fig. 10-3, *A* and *B*). The sheathed syringe is left propped for possible reuse (discouraged; see Multiple Injections) or for later removal of the sheathed needle for its disposal (Fig. 10-3, *C*). Resheathing is *extremely important in the prevention of cross-infection to operator or other office personnel by needle stick.* The federal Occupational Safety and Health Administration (OSHA) stipulates that needle resheathing be a one-handed procedure.[6] It

is recommended that *needle resheathing also be by the same person who gave the injection. This eliminates the hazard of passing exposed needles.*

Multiple injections. Multiple injections using the same needle for a patient is permitted as regards infection control; however, *such multiple use is discouraged because the used needle and its lumen contents are infectious to dental personnel if accidental needle stick occurs.*

Continual observation of patient during and after administration. It is important that the patient be continually observed during and after the administration of local anesthesia. *Never* leave the anesthetized patient unattended and *unobserved.* Adverse reactions, if they occur, demand immediate attention by the *dentist.*

Removal and disposal of sheathed, used needle. Removal and disposal of the sheathed, used needle is *by the dental assistant* whose shield-protected hand carefully unscrews the *sheathed* needle from the syringe

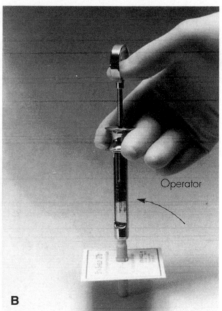

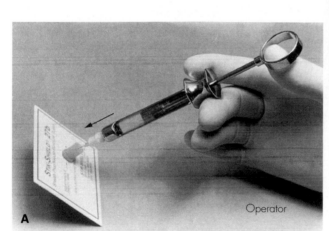

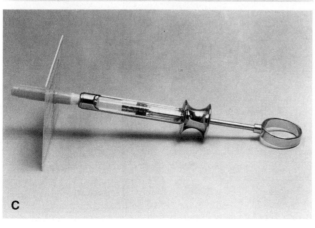

Fig. 10-3. A, Behind the patient, *operator* (person who gave injection) using *only* the syringe-holding hand inserts needle partially into sheath propped by prop/guard card, and then, **B,** uprights syringe and sheath upon the tray or countertop and presses needle fully into sheath. **C,** Operator lays resheathed syringe propped by card on countertop. Reuse of contaminated needle and remaining solution later in appointment is not recommended; rather, use new needle and cartridge.

Continued.

(Fig. 10-3, *D*), and then the hand still holding the sheathed needle *immediately moves it away* from the syringe (Fig. 10-3, *E*). *WARNING: Avoid any tissue contact with the uncapped "reverse-end" of a needle* (the short, "cartridge" needle). If the needle hub is too tight to remove with controlled finger pressure alone, use a suture-needle holder (or similar tool) to loosen the needle hub. *NEVER manually recap the "reverse-end" of the used needle.* The assistant's hands, of course, are gloved, either with treatment gloves (during patient ap-

pointment) or with utility gloves (after patient appointment).

Disposal of the sheathed, used needle immediately follows its removal from the syringe. With the hand still holding the unscrewed, sheathed needle (protective guard card still in place), convey it (reverse-end needle down) to a nearby (within a few feet) sharps disposal container, laying the attached card on the orifice rim (Fig. 10-3, *F); then with thumb only, push the shielded needle out of the card into the container (Fig. 10-3, *G*).

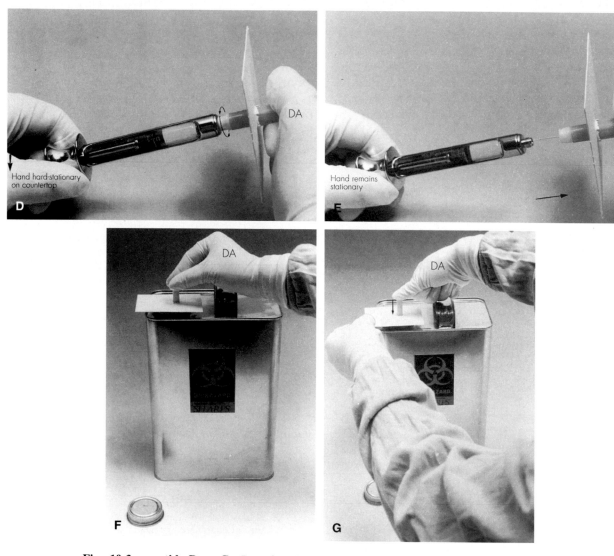

Fig. 10-3—cont'd. D to **G,** *Dental assistant,* after patient dismissal, holds syringe "hard-stationary" with fingers of one hand at least 2 inches away from guard card as fingers of stronger hand firstly unscrew counterclockwise ("lefty-loosey") the sheathed, used needle free from syringe **(D)** and secondly **(E)** *immediately move it (with reverse-end needle exposed) away from syringe* (distance from card to end of reverse-end needle is only 1 inch, and card will stop needle from sticking syringe-holding fingers, which are 2 inches or more away); thirdly, **(F)** dental assistant continues to hold the sheathed needle and conveys it to nearby (within a few feet) leakproof, hard-walled, OSHA biohazard-labeled container with suitable size orifice, gently laying on rim the guard card with the reverse-end needle down; and lastly, **(G)** steadies the card with fingers of one hand and presses with thumb of other hand the sheathed needle out of card to free-fall into container. Keep container upright, tightly closed between disposals of sharps, and out of reach of children.

CAUTION: This procedure should only be performed manually if the sheath is of a needle-impermeable material (i.e., hard plastic). The *sharps container* must be leakproof, hard-walled, and have the OSHA biohazard label.[6]

Emergency procedures

Adverse reactions occurring during or following administration of local anesthesia can lead to serious complications that call for emergency procedures. Cardinal among these are: (1) place the patient in a *supine* position (note exception), (2) apply *basic life support* (free airway, and cardiopulmonary resuscitation if needed), (3) monitor *vital signs,* and (4) summon *medical assistance.* The supine position, with legs (only) slightly elevated will increase the volume of circulating blood and aid in raising blood pressure; this procedure for the patient in syncope (or nearly so) should relieve hypoxia of the brain and return (or maintain) consciousness. However, the supine position should *not* be used when symptoms (such as fear, perspiration, weakness, pallor, palpitations) suggest an epinephrine overdose, and then a semi-erect or sitting position is best, since it minimizes any further elevation in cerebral blood pressure.[3,p.272]

ANALGESIA (INHALATION SEDATION)

The most appropriate method of preventing pain is by blocking the nerve pathways capable of conducting nerve impulses. However, for those patients who have a low threshold of pain and are apprehensive (hyperresponders), raising the threshold by inhalation sedation (nitrous oxide) is an aid to be coupled with anesthesia by needle injection.

Most textbooks on local anesthesia cover inhalation sedation in detail, and reference should be made to them. The operator must understand that this method of pain control has definite limitations when painful procedures are performed. Analgesia should not be thought of as general anesthesia in any stage or depth. It is simply a condition in which the pain threshold is elevated, and the patient is not in any way unmindful of the surroundings and activities.

HYPNOSIS

The fear of pain associated with dental procedures can sometimes be controlled by hypnosis. The favorable mental attitude must be established through suggestions of relaxation. Through hypnosis, the dentist, as well as the patient, derives certain benefits. The dentist has the opportunity to work on a more relaxed and cooperative patient and has control over patient habits such as talking, rinsing, and oral tissue tension. The patient who is relaxed is much less fatigued at the end of the appointment and has no marked recollection of having experienced discomfort.

This particular means of making the patient more receptive to dental operations has merit under certain circumstances and has produced satisfactory results for some practitioners when properly applied. However, before hypnosis is attempted the operator must know how to recognize and cope with conditions associated with psychological, emotional, and mental factors and must be thoroughly familiar with all of the principles involved in hypnosis.

Hypnosis is not to be regarded as a means of eliminating all other accepted means of minimizing dental pain or discomfort, but it may well be a valuable adjunct in improving accepted procedures.[4] Also, posthypnotic suggestion has been found to be successful in alleviating certain noxious dental habits.

REFERENCES

1. Baker RD: Personal communication, 1992.
2. Bennett CR: *Monheim's local anesthesia and pain control in dental practice,* ed 7, St Louis, 1984, Mosby.
3. Malamed SF: *Handbook of local anesthesia,* ed 3, St Louis, 1990, Mosby.
4. Marcus HW: The role of hypnosis and suggestions in dentistry, *J Am Dent Assoc* 59:1149, 1959.
5. McCarthy FM, Malamed SF: Physical evaluation system to determine medical risk and indicated dental therapy modifications, *J Am Dent Assoc* 99(2):181-184, 1979.
6. Occupational Safety and Health Administration: Bloodborne pathogens. Section 1910, 1030 (26 U.S.C. 635), Federal Register 56(235):64175-64181, 1991.
7. Scott DB: Toxicity caused by local anesthetic drugs, *Br J Anaesth* 53:553-554, 1981.
8. Sturdevant CM et al: *The art and science of operative dentistry,* ed 1, New York, 1968, McGraw-Hill; and ed 2, St Louis, 1985, Mosby.

CHAPTER 11

Isolation of the operating field

Aldridge D. Wilder, Jr.

Kenneth N. May, Jr.

William D. Strickland*

*This author is inactive this edition; see Preface.

CONCEPTUAL ELEMENTS OF OPERATING FIELD ISOLATION

For best results operative procedures require adequate isolation of the operating field. The *advantages of isolation* are (1) a dry, clean operating field, (2) access and visibility, (3) improved properties of dental materials, (4) protection of the patient and operator, and (5) operating efficiency. These advantages are discussed in later sections of this chapter. Isolation of the *operating field* involves several *conceptual elements:* moisture control, retraction, and harm prevention.

Moisture control

Operative dentistry cannot be executed properly unless the moisture in the mouth is controlled. *Moisture control refers to excluding sulcular fluid, saliva, and gingival bleeding from the operating field*. It also refers to preventing the handpiece spray and restorative debris from being swallowed or aspirated by the patient. The rubber dam, suction devices, and absorbents are varyingly effective in moisture control. These techniques and others are discussed in detail later.

Retraction and access

The details of the restorative procedure cannot be managed without proper retraction and access. This provides maximal exposure of the operating site. It usually involves maintaining mouth opening, and depressing or retracting the gingival tissue, tongue, lips, and cheek. The rubber dam, high-volume evacuator, absorbents, retraction cord, and mouth prop are used for retraction and access. Each of these are presented later in the chapter.

Harm prevention

An axiom taught to every member of the health profession is "Do no harm." *An important consideration of isolating the operating field is preventing the patient from being harmed during the operation.*[11,13] Excessive saliva and handpiece spray can alarm the patient. Small instruments and restorative debris can be aspirated or swallowed. Soft tissue can be damaged accidently. As with moisture control and retraction, the rubber dam, suction devices, absorbents, and occasional use of a mouth prop contribute not only to harm prevention but also to patient comfort and operator efficiency. Harm prevention is provided as much by the manner in which these devices are used as by the devices themselves.

LOCAL ANESTHETICS

Local anesthetics play a role in eliminating the discomfort of dental treatment and in controlling moisture. Use of these agents reduces salivation. This is apparently because the patient is more comfortable, less anxious, and less sensitive to oral stimuli, thus producing a lower salivary rate. Local anesthetics incorporating a vasoconstrictor also reduce blood flow, thus helping to control hemorrhage at the operating site (see Chapter 10 for details).

THE RUBBER DAM

In 1864 S.C. Barnum, a New York City dentist, introduced the rubber dam into dentistry. Use of the rubber dam ensures appropriate dryness of the teeth and improves the quality of clinical restorative dentistry.[5,19,23,24]

Purpose

The rubber dam is used to define the operating field by isolating one or more teeth from the oral environment. The dam eliminates saliva from the operating site and retracts the soft tissue. Most procedures in operative dentistry are performed better and with fewer interruptions when the rubber dam is used because dryness is ensured during cavity preparation and restoration. *When excavating a deep carious lesion risking pulpal exposure, use of the rubber dam is mandatory to prevent or minimize pulpal contamination from oral fluids.*

Advantages

The rubber dam is the most successful method of isolating the operating field. The advantages of the rubber dam are significant and become obvious as the operator gains proficiency with it.[26]

Dry, clean, operating field. *Rubber dam isolation is the preferred method of obtaining appropriate dryness.* The operator can best perform such procedures as caries removal, proper cavity preparation, and insertion of restorative materials in a dry field. Teeth prepared and restored using rubber dam isolation are less prone to postoperative problems related to contamination from oral fluids. The time saved by operating in a clean field with good visibility more than compensates for the time spent in applying the rubber dam.[9]

Access and visibility. The rubber dam provides maximal access and visibility. It controls moisture and retracts the soft tissue. Gingival tissue is retracted mildly to provide better access and visibility to gingival aspects of the cavity preparation. The dam also retracts the lips, cheeks, and tongue. Black rubber dam provides a dark, nonreflective background in contrast to the operating site. Because the dam remains in place throughout the operative procedure, access and visibility are maintained without interruption.

Improved properties of dental materials. The rubber dam prevents moisture contamination of restorative materials during insertion. Restorative materials will not achieve their maximal physical properties if used in a wet field.[2,3,27,29] The dentist is professionally obligated to provide the highest quality restoration possible, which can only be accomplished in a moisture-free environment. Because saliva interferes with fluoride uptake, reducing its effectiveness, topical fluoride may be applied prior to rubber dam removal.

Protection of the patient and operator. The rubber dam protects the patient from aspirating or swallowing small instruments or debris associated with operative procedures.[21] Immediate recovery of these items is facilitated by the rubber dam. A properly applied rubber dam protects the soft tissue from irritating or distasteful medicaments such as etching agents. The dam also offers some soft tissue protection from rotating burs and stones. In addition, the operator is afforded significant protection from infections present in the patient's mouth.[7,10,25,30]

Operating efficiency. Use of the rubber dam allows for operating efficiency and increased productivity. The time involved in letting the patient rinse and expectorate is eliminated. Excessive patient conversation is discouraged. The rubber dam retainer (see later section) helps to provide a moderate extent of mouth opening during the procedure. (For additional mouth-opening aids see later section, Mouth Prop.) Quadrant restorative procedures are facilitated. Many state dental practice acts permit the assistant to place the rubber dam, thereby saving the dentist additional time. Each of the rubber dam's advantages permits a more efficient operative procedure. The rubber dam can make the task easier and more comfortable for the patient, and create conditions that facilitate dental service of the highest possible quality.

Disadvantages

Time consumption and patient objection are the most frequently quoted disadvantages of the rubber dam. However, these claims are eliminated with the use of a simplified routine.[15,26] In most situations the rubber dam may be placed in 3 to 5 minutes. This is the approximate time necessary for onset of anesthesia. After the dam is applied, most patients are more relaxed knowing that water spray and debris from the procedure are isolated from them.

Certain conditions may preclude the use of the rubber dam: (1) teeth that have not erupted sufficiently to receive a retainer, (2) some third molars, and (3) extremely malpositioned teeth. In addition, patients suffering from asthma may not tolerate the rubber dam if breathing through the nose is difficult. Also, there are rare instances when the patient cannot tolerate a rubber dam because of psychological reasons. Reports of patients disliking the rubber dam are usually the result of awkwardness or ineptness of the dental team with its application.[12]

Materials and instruments

The materials and instruments necessary for the use of the rubber dam are available from most dental supply companies.

Rubber dam material. *Rubber dam material*, as with all rubber products, deteriorates over time, resulting in low tear strength. Therefore, material that is reasonably new from date of manufacture should be used. Dam material is available in 5 × 5 inch (12.5 × 12.5 cm) or 6 × 6 inch (15 × 15 cm) sheets. Sterile dam material is also available, packaged as individual sheets. The thicknesses or weights available are thin (0.006 inch [0.15 mm]), medium (0.008 inch [0.2 mm]), heavy (0.010 inch [0.25 mm]), extra heavy (0.012 inch [0.30 mm]), and special heavy (0.014 inch [0.35 mm]). Both light and dark dam material are available, but the dark color is preferred for contrast. Green and blue colors are also marketed. Fig. 11-1 illustrates rubber dam material. Rubber dam material has a shiny and a dull side. Because the dull side is less light reflective, it is generally placed facing the occlusal aspect. The thicker dam is more effective in retracting tissue, more resistant to tearing, and especially recommended for isolating Class V cavities in conjunction with a cervical retainer. The thinner material has the advantage of passing through the contacts easier, which is particularly helpful when they are tight. However, the thicker types generally are recommended.

Rubber dam holder. The *rubber dam holder* positions and holds the borders of the rubber dam. The Young holder is a U-shaped metal frame (Fig. 11-2), with small metal projections for securing the borders of the rubber dam. It is easily applied and comfortable for the patient. An optional adjustable neck strap (Fig. 11-3) positioned behind the patient's neck is attached to the two hooks, one in the middle of each side of the frame. The neck strap is lightly tightened to snug the dam and frame to the face to maximize retraction and provide access to the operating site.

Rubber dam retainer. The *rubber dam retainer (clamp)* consists of four prongs and two jaws connected by a bow (Fig. 11-4). The retainer is used to anchor the dam to the most posterior tooth to be isolated. Retainers are also used to retract gingival tissue. Many different sizes and shapes are available, with specific retainers designed for certain teeth (Fig. 11-5). Refer to Table 11-1 for suggested retainer applications. Experience will reduce the number of retainers necessary. *When po-*

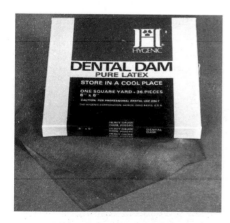

Fig. 11-1. Rubber dam material as supplied in sheets.

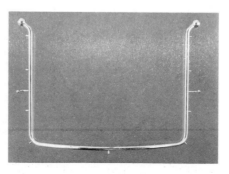

Fig. 11-2. The Young rubber dam frame *(holder)*.

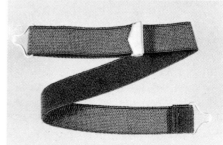

Fig. 11-3. Adjustable neck strap for use with the Young rubber dam frame.

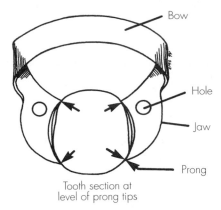

Fig. 11-4. Rubber dam retainer. Note four-point prong contact *(arrows)* with tooth.

Table 11-1. Suggested retainers for various anchor tooth applications

W56—	Retainer appropriate for most molar anchor teeth
W7—	Retainer appropriate for mandibular molar anchor teeth
W8—	Retainer appropriate for maxillary molar anchor teeth
W4—	Retainer appropriate for most premolar anchor teeth
W2—	Retainer appropriate for small premolar anchor teeth
W27—	Retainer appropriate for terminal mandibular molar anchor teeth requiring preparations involving the distal surface

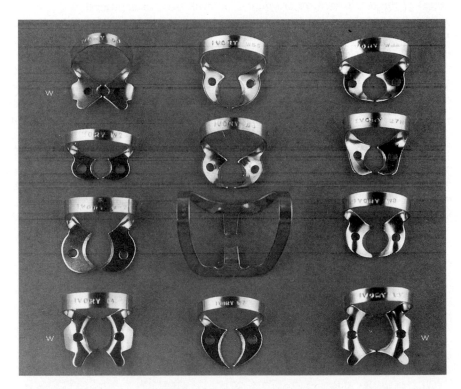

Fig. 11-5. Typical selection of rubber dam retainers. Note retainers with wings *(w)*.

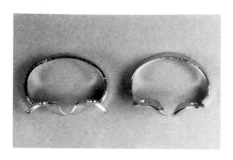

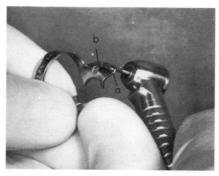

Fig. 11-6. Retainers with prongs directed gingivally are helpful when anchor tooth is only partially erupted.

Fig. 11-7. Removing anterior wings *(a)* on molar retainer. Lateral wings *(b)* are for holding lip of stretched rubber dam hole.

Fig. 11-6   **Fig. 11-7**

sitioned on a tooth, the properly selected retainer should contact the tooth in four areas, two on the facial surface and two on the lingual surface (Fig. 11-4). This four-point contact prevents rocking or tilting of the retainer. Movement of the retainer on the anchor tooth can injure the gingiva and tooth, resulting in postoperative soreness or sensitivity. The prongs of some retainers are gingivally directed (inverted) and are helpful when the anchor tooth is only partially erupted or when additional soft tissue retraction is indicated (Fig. 11-6). *Jaws of the retainer should not extend beyond the mesial and distal line angles of the tooth because (1) they may interfere with wedge placement, (2) a complete seal around the anchor tooth is more difficult to achieve, and (3) gingival trauma is more likely to occur.*

Wingless and **winged retainers** are available (Fig. 11-5). The winged retainer has both anterior and lateral wings (Fig. 11-7). The wings are designed to provide extra retraction of the rubber dam from the operating field and to allow attaching the dam to the retainer before conveying the retainer (with dam) to the anchor tooth (see Fig. 11-22), after which the dam is removed from the lateral wings. A disadvantage of the winged retainer is that wings often interfere with the placement of matrix bands, band retainers, and wedges. Most operators prefer the wingless retainer. As seen in Fig. 11-7, the anterior wings can be cut away if they are not wanted.

The retainer (except the No. 212, which is applied after the rubber dam is in place) should be *tied with dental floss* (Fig. 11-8) at least 12 inches (30.5 cm) in length before carrying into the mouth. The tie should be threaded through both holes in the jaws because the bow of the retainer could break. The floss allows retrieval of the retainer or its broken parts if accidentally swallowed or aspirated.

It is sometimes necessary to *recontour the jaws* of the retainer to the shape of the tooth by grinding with a mounted stone (Fig. 11-9).

A retainer usually is not required when the dam is applied for treatment of the anterior teeth except for the cervical retainer for Class V restorations.

Rubber dam punch. The *punch* is a precision instrument having a rotating metal table (disk) with six holes of varying sizes and a tapered, sharp-pointed plunger (Fig. 11-10). Care should be exercised when changing from one hole to another. The plunger should be centered in the cutting hole and the tip of the plunger should not be allowed to drag over the edges of the

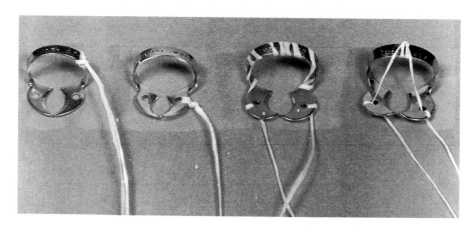

Fig. 11-8. Methods of tying retainers with dental floss.

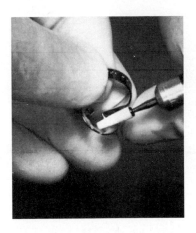

Fig. 11-9. Recontouring jaws of retainer with mounted stone.

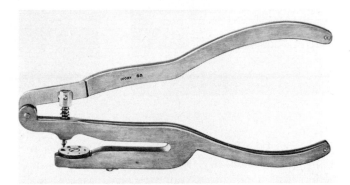

Fig. 11-10. Rubber dam punch.

holes. Otherwise, the cutting quality of the punch will be ruined as evidenced by incompletely cut holes. These holes will tear open easily when spread during application over the retainer or tooth.

Rubber dam retainer forceps. The *forceps* is used both for placement of the retainer and its removal from the tooth (Fig. 11-11).

Rubber dam napkin. The *napkin* that is placed between the rubber dam and the patient's skin has the following advantages: (1) prevents skin contact with rubber to reduce the possibility of allergic reactions in sensitive patients, (2) absorbs saliva at the corners of the mouth, (3) acts as a cushion, and (4) provides a convenient method of wiping the patient's lips on removal of the dam. The rubber dam napkin adds to the comfort of the patient, particularly when the dam must be used for long appointments. Most operators use commercially available napkins that are soft, absorbent, and disposable (Fig. 11-12).

Lubricant. A water-soluble *lubricant* applied in the area of the punched holes facilitates the passing of the dam through the proximal contacts. A satisfactory rubber dam lubricant is commercially available, but other lubricants, such as shaving cream or a soap slurry, are also satisfactory. Applying the lubricant to both sides of the dam in the area of the punched holes will aid in passing the dam through the contacts. Cocoa butter or petroleum jelly is often used at the corners of the patient's mouth to prevent irritation. These two materials, however, are not satisfactory rubber dam lubricants.

Modeling compound. Low-fusing *modeling compound* is sometimes used to secure the retainer to the tooth to prevent retainer movement during the operative procedure.

Anchors other than retainers. The proximal contact may be sufficient to anchor the dam on the tooth farthest from the posterior retainer (in the isolated field), thereby eliminating the need for a second retainer (see

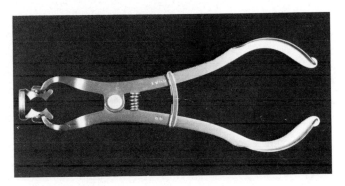

Fig. 11-11. Rubber dam retainer forceps engaging retainer.

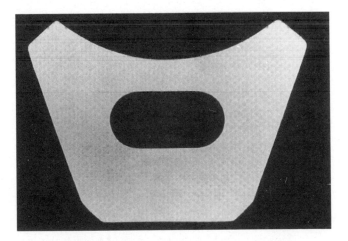

Fig. 11-12. Disposable rubber dam napkin.

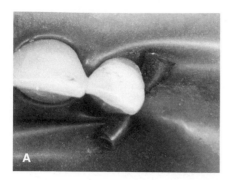 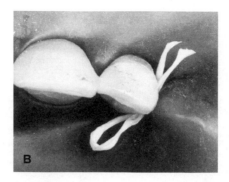

Fig. 11-13. A, Anchor formed from rubber dam material. B, Anchor formed from dental tape.

Placement of the Rubber Dam [Step 13]). To further secure the dam anteriorly or to *anchor the dam* on any tooth where a retainer is not indicated, pass a small piece of rubber dam material (cut from a sheet of dam) or dental tape through the proximal contact. The piece of dam material is first stretched, passed through the contact, and then released (Fig. 11-13, *A*). When dental tape is used, it should be passed through the contact, looped, and passed through a second time (Fig. 11-13, *B*). Once the anchor is in place, excess lengths of dam material or tape should be cut away to prevent interference with the operating site.

Hole size and position

Successful isolation of the teeth and maintenance of a dry, clean operating field largely depend on the *size and position of the holes* in the rubber dam.[14] Punch the holes following the arch form making adjustments for malpositioned or missing teeth. Most rubber dam punches have either five or six holes in the cutting table. Use the smaller holes for the incisors, canines, and premolars, and the larger holes for the molars. The largest hole is generally reserved for the posterior anchor tooth (Fig. 11-14). The following guidelines and suggestions are helpful when positioning the holes:

1. *(Optional)* Punch an *identification hole* in the upper left (patient's left) corner of the rubber dam for ease of location of that corner when applying the dam to the holder (see Fig. 11-16).
2. When operating on the *incisors and mesial surfaces of canines*, isolate from first premolar to first premolar. Metal retainers usually are not required for this isolation (Fig. 11-15, *A*). If additional access is necessary after isolating the teeth as described, a retainer can be positioned over the dam to engage the adjacent unisolated tooth, but care must be exercised not to pinch the gingiva beneath the dam (Fig. 11-15, *B* and *C*). When operating on a canine, it is preferred to isolate from the first molar to the opposite lateral incisor. To treat a Class V lesion on a canine, isolate posteriorly to include the first molar to

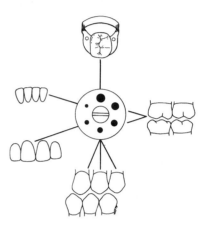

Fig. 11-14. Cutting table on rubber dam punch illustrating use of hole size.

provide access for the cervical retainer to the canine.

3. When operating on *posterior teeth*, it is beneficial to isolate anteriorly to include the lateral incisor on the opposite side of the arch from the operating site. In this case the hole for the lateral incisor will be the most remote from the hole for the posterior anchor tooth. Anterior teeth may be included in the isolation to provide (1) finger rests on dry teeth, and (2) better access and visibility for the operator and assistant.
4. When operating on the *premolars*, punch holes to include two teeth distally, and extend anteriorly to include the opposite lateral incisor.
5. When operating on the *molars*, punch holes as far distally as possible, and extend anteriorly to include the opposite lateral incisor.
6. Always isolate a *minimum of three teeth* except when root canal therapy is indicated, then only the tooth to be treated is isolated.
7. The *distance between holes* is equal to the distance from the center of one tooth to the center of the adjacent tooth, measured at the level of the gingival tissue. Generally, this is approxi-

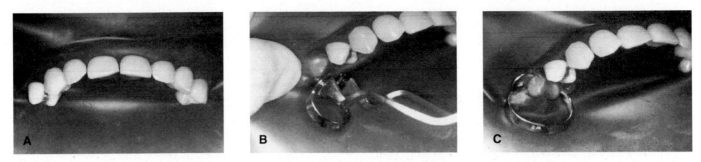

Fig. 11-15. A, Isolation for operating on incisors and mesial surface of canines. **B** and **C,** Increasing access by application of metal retainer over dam and adjacent nonisolated tooth.

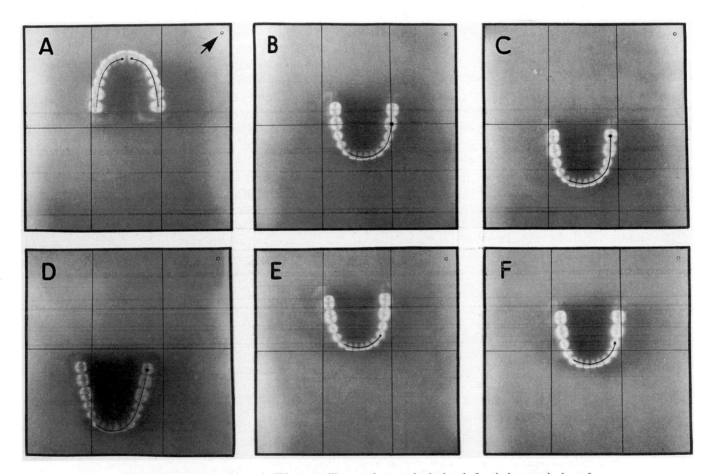

Fig. 11-16. Hole position. **A,** When maxillary teeth are to be isolated, first holes punched are for central incisors, approximately 1 inch (2.5 cm) from superior border. **B,** Hole position when anchor tooth is mandibular first molar. **C,** Hole position when anchor tooth is mandibular second molar. **D,** Hole position when anchor tooth is mandibular third molar. **E,** Hole position when anchor tooth is mandibular first premolar. **F,** Hole position when anchor tooth is mandibular second premolar. Note hole punched in each of these six representative rubber dam sheets for identification of the upper left corner *(arrow* in **A).**

mately ¼ inch (6.3 mm). *When the distance between holes is excessive, the dam wrinkles between the teeth. Conversely, too little distance between holes causes the dam to stretch open around the teeth, resulting in leakage.* When the distance is correct, the dam will intimately adapt to the teeth, and cover and slightly retract the interdental tissue.

8. When the rubber dam is applied to the *maxillary teeth,* the first holes punched (after the identification hole) are for the central incisors. These holes are positioned approximately 1 inch (25 mm) from the superior border of the dam (Fig. 11-16, *A*), providing sufficient material to cover the patient's upper lip. For a patient with a large upper lip or mustache, position the holes more than an inch from the edge. Conversely, for a child or an adult with a small upper lip, the holes should be positioned less than an inch from the edge. Once the holes for the incisors are located, the remaining holes are punched.

9. When the rubber dam is applied to the *mandibular teeth,* the first hole punched (after the identification hole) is for the posterior anchor tooth that is to receive the retainer. Mentally divide the rubber dam into three vertical sections: left, middle, and right. If the anchor tooth is the mandibular first molar, punch the hole for this tooth (the first hole to be punched) at a point halfway from the superior edge to the inferior edge and on the line that divides the right (left) and middle thirds (Fig. 11-16, *B*). If the anchor tooth is the second or third molar, the position

for the hole moves toward the inferior border and slightly toward the center of the rubber dam, compared with the hole for the first molar (Fig. 11-16, *C* and *D*). If the anchor tooth is the first premolar, the hole is placed toward the superior border, compared with the hole for the first molar, and also toward the center of the dam (Fig. 11-16, *E*). The farther posteriorly the mandibular anchor tooth, the more dam material is required to come from behind the retainer over the upper lip. Fig. 11-17 illustrates the difference in the amount of dam required comparing the first premolar and the second molar as anchor teeth. The distances may also be compared by noting the length of dam between the superior edge of the dam and the position of the hole for the posterior anchor tooth (see Fig. 11-16, *C* and *E*).

10. When a *cervical retainer* is to be applied to isolate a Class V lesion, the heavier rubber dam is usually recommended for better tissue retraction, and the hole for the tooth should be punched facially to the arch form to compensate for the extension of the rubber. The farther gingivally the lesion extends, the farther the hole must be positioned from the arch form. In addition, the hole should be slightly larger, and the distance between it and the holes for the adjacent teeth should be slightly increased (Fig. 11-18).

11. When the *thinner rubber dam* is used, smaller holes must be punched to achieve an adequate seal around the teeth because the thin dam has greater elasticity.

12. Until the above guidelines and suggestions related to hole position are mastered, the inexperienced operator may choose to use commercial products to aid in locating hole position (Fig. 11-19). A *rubber stamp* is available that im-

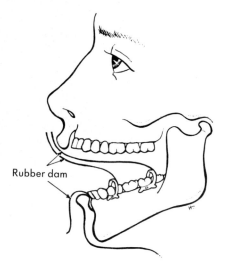

Fig. 11-17. The farther posteriorly the mandibular anchor tooth, the more dam material is required to come from behind retainer over upper lip.

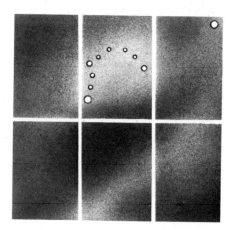

Fig. 11-18. Hole position for tooth (maxillary right canine) to receive cervical retainer is positioned facially to arch form.

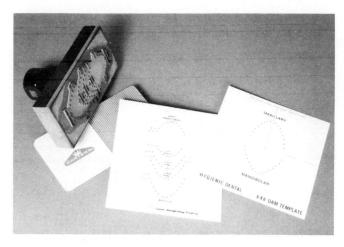

Fig. 11-19. Commercial products to aid in locating hole position.

prints both permanent and primary arch forms on the rubber dam, and several sheets of dam material can be stamped in advance. A *plastic template* can also be used to mark hole position. Experience will eliminate the need for these aids. Accurate hole location is best achieved by noting the patient's arch form and tooth position. Understanding the principles of hole punching is helpful in using a stamp or template.

Placement of the rubber dam

Before *placing the rubber dam*, the dental chair should be adjusted for optimal patient comfort and access for the operator and assistant. The patient's head and chest should not be lower than the feet. It may be necessary to remove debris and calculus from the teeth to be isolated.

Anesthesia precedes application of the rubber dam (see Chapter 10). This allows for the onset of profound anesthesia and more comfortable retainer placement on the anchor tooth. Occasionally, the posterior anchor tooth in the maxillary arch needs to be anesthetized if it is remote from the anesthetized operating site.

The technique for application of the rubber dam is presented by numerous authors.[5,6,8,18,26] The step-by-step application and removal of the rubber dam using the maxillary left first molar for the posterior retainer and including the maxillary right lateral incisor as the anterior anchor is described and illustrated below. The procedure is described as if the operator and assistant are working together. However, application and removal of the rubber dam is often the responsibility of a single person, and then the individual will perform the duties described for the operator and the assistant. Following the administration of the local anesthetic, many operators delegate rubber dam application to a second chairside assistant permitting the operator to treat another patient.

When compared to the alternative procedures discussed in a later section, the illustrated procedure allows the retainer and dam to be placed sequentially. This provides for maximal visibility when placing the retainer, which reduces the risk of impinging gingival tissue. For most operators this is a simpler procedure than placing the retainer and dam simultaneously. Isolating a greater number of teeth as illustrated in this procedure is indicated for quadrant operative procedures. For limited operative procedures it is often acceptable to isolate fewer teeth. The general rule for limited isolation is to include one tooth posterior and two teeth anterior to the tooth (teeth) being operated on (Fig. 11-20).

The application procedure is described for right-handed operators. Left-handed users should substitute left where right is described.

Step 1. The operator receives *dental floss* from the assistant to test the interproximal contacts and to remove debris from the teeth to be isolated. Passing (or attempts to pass) floss through the contacts identifies any sharp edges of restorations or enamel that must be smoothed or removed to prevent tearing the dam. The proximal portion of the tooth to be restored may be partially prepared to eliminate a sharp or difficult contact before the dam is placed. Tight contacts that are difficult to floss, but do not cut or fray the floss, may be wedged apart slightly to permit placement of the rubber dam. A blunt hand instrument may be used for wedging.

Step 2. It is recommended that the assistant *punch the holes* after careful study of the arch form and tooth alignment. However, some operators prefer to have the assistant prepunch the holes marked by a template or a rubber dam stamp.

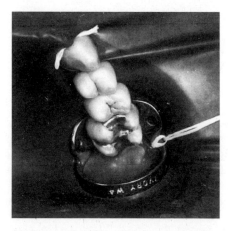

Fig. 11-20. Limited isolation for operating maxillary left second premolar.

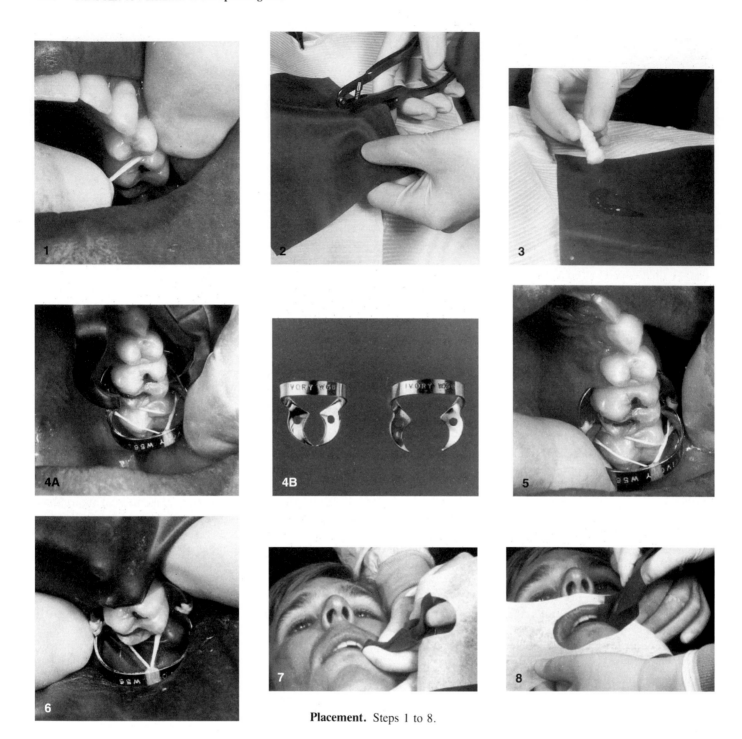

Placement. Steps 1 to 8.

Step 3. The assistant *lubricates* both sides of the rubber dam in the area of the punched holes using a cotton roll or fingertip to apply the lubricant. This facilitates passing the rubber dam through the contacts. The lips and especially the corners of the mouth may be lubricated with petroleum jelly or cocoa butter to prevent irritation.

Step 4. (A) The operator receives from the assistant the rubber dam retainer forceps with the selected re-

tainer and floss tie in position. The free end of the tie should exit from the cheek side of the retainer. *Try the retainer on the tooth* to verify retainer stability. If the retainer fits poorly, it is removed either for adjustment or selection of a different size.[22] Retainer adjustment, if needed to provide stability, is presented in a prior section, Rubber Dam Retainers. Whenever the forceps is holding the retainer, care should be taken not to open the retainer more than necessary to secure it in the forceps. Stretching the retainer open for extended periods will cause it to lose its spring. **(B)** Retainers that are "sprung" should be discarded. Note sprung retainer on right.

Step 5. If during trial placement the retainer seems acceptable, then remove the forceps. *Test the retainer's stability and retention* by lifting gently in an occlusal direction with a fingertip under the bow of the retainer. An improperly fitting retainer will rock or be easily dislodged.

Step 6. Before applying the dam, the floss tie may be threaded through the anchor hole, or it may be left on the underside of the dam. With the forefingers, *stretch the hole of the dam over the retainer* (bow first) and then under the jaws. The lip of the hole must pass completely under the jaws. The forefingers then may thin out to a single thickness the septal dam for the mesial contact of the retainer tooth and attempt to pass it through the contact, lip of the hole first. The septal dam must always pass through its respective contact in single thickness. If it does not pass through readily, it should be left to be passed through with dental tape later in the procedure.

Step 7. The operator now gathers the rubber dam in the left hand while the assistant inserts the fingers and thumb of the right (left) hand through the napkin's opening and grasps the bunched dam held by the operator.

Step 8. The assistant then *pulls the bunched dam through the napkin and positions it* on the patient's face. The operator helps by positioning the napkin on the patient's right side. The napkin helps to reduce skin contact with the dam.

Step 9. The operator *unfolds the dam*. (If an identification hole was punched, it is used to identify the upper left corner.) The assistant aids in unfolding the dam and, while holding the frame in place, attaches the dam to the metal projections on the left side of the frame. Simultaneously, the operator stretches and attaches the dam on the right side. The frame is positioned outside

the dam. The dam lies between the frame and napkin. Either the operator or assistant attaches the dam along the inferior border of the frame. *Attaching the dam to the frame* at this time controls the dam to provide access and visibility. Secure the free ends of the floss tie to the frame.

Step 10 (optional). The assistant attaches the *neck strap* to the left side of the frame and passes it behind the patient's neck. The operator then attaches it to the right side of the frame. Neck strap tension is adjusted to stabilize the frame and to hold the frame (and periphery of the dam) gently against the face and away from the operating field. If desired, contact of the patient's neck against the strap may be prevented by using soft tissue paper between the neck and strap.

Step 11. If there is a tooth distal to the retainer, the distal edge of the posterior anchor hole should be passed through the contact (single thickness, no folds) to ensure a seal around the anchor tooth. If necessary, use waxed dental tape to assist in this procedure (see Step 15 for use of tape). If the retainer comes off unintentionally as this is done or during subsequent procedures, passage of the dam through the distal contact anchors the dam sufficiently to allow easier reapplication of the retainer or placement of an adjusted or different retainer.

Step 12 (optional). If the stability of the retainer is questionable, low-fusing modeling compound may be used. The assistant heats the end of a stick of compound in an open flame and tempers it by holding it in water for a few seconds. While the assistant holds the unheated end, the operator pinches off a sufficient amount to form a cone about ½ inch (12.7 mm) long.

The assistant should ensure dryness by directing a few short bursts from the air syringe on the occlusal surface of the tooth before compound placement. The operator positions the compound cone on the ball of the forefinger, briefly resoftens the tip of the cone in the flame, and carries the compound to place, covering the bow of the retainer and part of the occlusal surface of

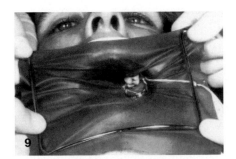
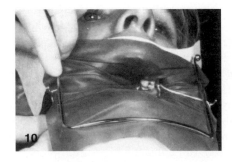
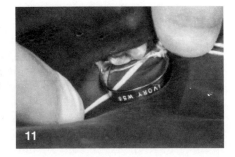

Placement. Steps 9 to 11.

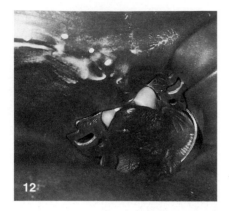

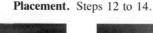

Placement. Steps 12 to 14.

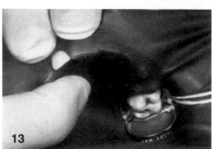

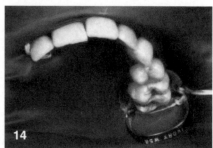

the tooth. The compound should not cover the holes in the jaws of the retainer. The compound will adhere to the tooth if the tooth is dry.

Step 13. The operator passes the *dam over the anterior anchor tooth,* anchoring the anterior portion of the rubber dam. Usually, the dam will pass easily through the mesial and distal contacts of the anchor tooth if it is passed in single thickness starting with the lip of the hole. Stretching the lip of the hole and sliding it back and forth will aid in positioning the septum. When the contact farthest from the retainer is minimal, an anchor may be required in the form of a double thickness of dental tape, or a narrow strip of dam material that is stretched, inserted, and released (see Fig. 11-13, *A* and *B*). If the contact is open, a rolled piece of dam material may be used as shown in Fig. 11-29.

Step 14. The operator passes the *septa through as many contacts as possible without the use of dental tape* by stretching the septal dam faciogingivally and linguogingivally with the forefingers. Each septum must not be allowed to bunch or fold. Rather, its passage through the contact should be started with a single edge and continued with a single thickness. Passing the dam through as many contacts as possible without using dental tape is urged because the use of tape always increases the risk of tearing holes in the septa. Slight wedging of the teeth is sometimes an aid when the contacts are extremely tight. Pressure from a blunt hand instrument (e.g., beaver-tail burnisher) applied in the facial embrasure gingival to the contact usually is sufficient to obtain enough separation to permit the septum to pass through the contact.

Step 15. *Use waxed dental tape to pass the dam through the remaining contacts.* Tape is preferred over floss because its wider dimension more effectively carries the rubber septa through the contacts. Also, tape is not as likely to cut the septa. The waxed variety makes passage easier and decreases the chances for cutting holes in the septa or tearing the edges of the holes. The leading edge of the septum should be over the contact ready to be drawn into and through the contact with the

tape. As before, the septal rubber should be kept in single thickness with no folds. The tape should be placed at the contact on a slight angle. With a good finger rest on the tooth, the tape should be controlled so that it slides (not snaps) through the proximal contact, thus preventing damage to the interdental tissues. Once the leading edge of the septum has passed the contact, the remaining interseptal dam can be carried through more easily.

Step 16 (optional). Often, several passes with dental tape are required to carry a reluctant septum through a tight contact. When this happens, previously passed tape should be left in the gingival embrasure until the entire septum has been successfully placed with subsequent passage of tape. This prevents a partially passed septum from being removed or torn.

Step 17. *Start inverting the dam* into the gingival sulcus to complete the seal around the tooth. Often, the dam inverts itself as the septa are passed through the contacts as a result of the dam being stretched gingivally. The operator should verify that the dam is inverted interproximally. Inversion in this region is best accomplished with dental tape.

Step 18. With the edges of the dam inverted interproximally, *complete the **inversion*** facially and lingually using an explorer or a beaver-tail burnisher while the assistant directs a stream of air onto the tooth. This is done by moving the explorer around the neck of the tooth facially and lingually with the tip perpendicular to the tooth surface or directed slightly gingivally. A dry surface will prevent the dam from sliding out of the crevice. Alternatively, the dam can be inverted facially and lingually by drying the tooth while stretching the dam gingivally and then releasing it slowly.

Step 19 (optional). The use of a saliva ejector is not routine because most patients are able, and usually prefer, to swallow excess saliva. Furthermore, salivation is greatly reduced when profound anesthesia is obtained. If salivation is a problem, the operator or assistant uses cotton pliers to pick up the dam lingual to the mandibular incisors and cuts a small hole through which the sa-

Placement. Steps 15 to 22.

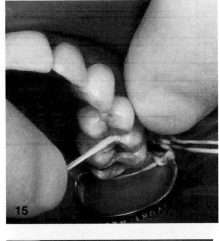

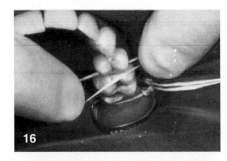

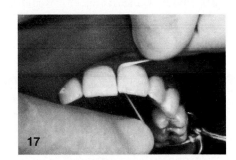

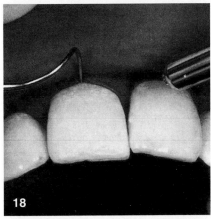

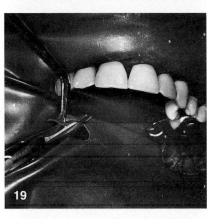

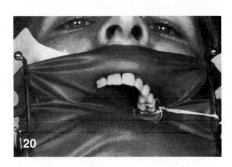

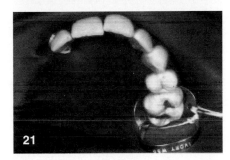

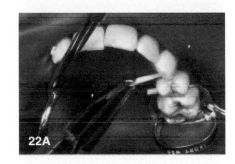

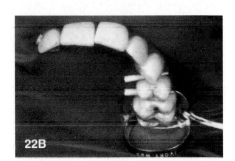

liva ejector is inserted. The hole should be positioned so that the rubber dam helps support the weight of the ejector, preventing pressure on the delicate tissues in the floor of the mouth.

Step 20. The properly applied rubber dam will be securely positioned and comfortable to the patient. The patient should be assured that the rubber dam does not prevent swallowing or closing the mouth (about halfway) when there is a pause in the procedure.

Step 21. Check to see that the completed rubber dam provides maximal access and visibility for the operative procedure.

Step 22. For Class II preparations, many operators *consider the insertion of interproximal **wedges** as the fi-nal step in rubber dam application*. Wedges are used in gingival embrasures adjacent to mesial and distal surfaces that are to be restored (see Chapter 12). Wedges are generally round toothpick ends about ½ inch (12.7 mm) in length that are snugly inserted into the gingival embrasures from the facial or lingual embrasure, whichever is greater, using No. 110 pliers.

(A) To facilitate wedge insertion, first stretch the dam slightly by fingertip pressure in the direction opposite wedge insertion, and then insert the wedge *while* slowly releasing the dam. This results in a passive dam under the wedge (dam will not rebound the wedge) as well as prevents bunching or tearing of the septal dam during wedge insertion. **(B)** Wedges inserted.

Removal of the rubber dam

Before removal of the rubber dam, rinse and suction away any debris that may have collected to prevent its falling into the floor of the mouth during the removal procedure. If a saliva ejector was used, remove it at this time.

Step 1. *Stretch the dam facially* pulling the septal rubber away from the gingival tissues and the tooth. Protect the underlying soft tissue by placing a fingertip beneath the septum. *Clip each septum* with blunt-tipped scissors, freeing the dam from the interproximal spaces, but leave the dam over the anterior and posterior anchor teeth.

Step 2. Engage the retainer with the retainer forceps. It is unnecessary to remove any compound, if used, since it will break free as the retainer is spread and lifted from the tooth. While the operator *removes the retainer,* the assistant *releases the neck strap,* if used, from the left side of the frame.

Step 3. Once the retainer is removed, *release the dam from the anterior anchor tooth, and remove the dam and frame simultaneously.* While doing this, caution the patient not to bite on newly inserted amalgam restorations until the occlusion can be evaluated.

Step 4. *Wipe the patient's lips* with the napkin immediately after the dam and frame are removed. This helps to prevent saliva from getting on the patient's face and it is comforting to the patient.

Step 5. *Rinse* the teeth and mouth using air-water spray and the high-volume evacuator. To enhance circulation, particularly around the anchor teeth, massage the tissue around the teeth that were isolated.

Step 6. Lay the sheet of rubber dam over a light-colored flat surface or hold it up to the operating light *to determine that no portion of the rubber dam has remained* between or around the teeth. Such a remnant will cause gingival inflammation.

Alternative methods for placing the rubber dam and retainer

The above procedure describes the method of sequentially placing the retainer and rubber dam on the anchor tooth. Some operators prefer alternative methods. In the hands of inexperienced operators, these methods may reduce visibility of the gingival tissues.

Method 1. The retainer and dam may be placed simultaneously to reduce the risk of the retainer being swallowed or aspirated before the dam is placed. Also, this solves the occasional difficulty of trying to pass the dam over a previously placed retainer, the bow of which is pressing against oral soft tissues.

In this method, first apply the posterior retainer to

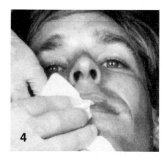
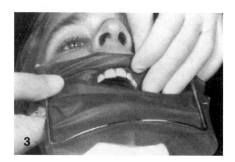
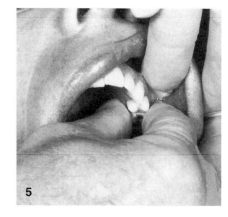
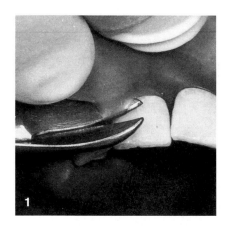
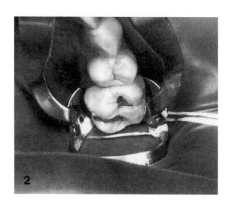
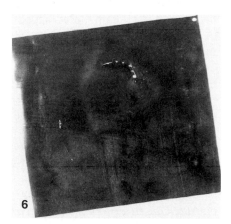

Removal. Steps 1 to 6.

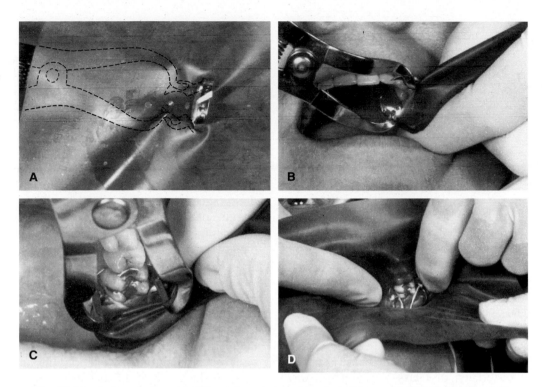

Fig. 11-21. A, Bow being passed through posterior anchor hole from underside of dam. **B,** Gathering dam to facilitate placement of retainer. **C,** Positioning retainer on anchor tooth. **D,** Stretching anchor hole borders over and under jaws of retainer.

verify a stable fit. Then remove the retainer, and with forceps still holding the retainer pass the bow through the proper hole from the underside of the dam (the lubricated rubber dam is held by the assistant). The free end of the floss tie may remain on the underside of the dam, or it may be threaded through the anchor hole before the retainer bow is inserted (Fig. 11-21, *A*). When using a retainer with lateral wings, place the retainer in the hole punched for the anchor tooth by stretching the dam to engage these wings (Fig. 11-22). Winged retainers are rarely used because the wings may interfere with subsequent procedures.

The operator grasps the handle of the forceps in the right hand and gathers the dam with the left hand, in order to visualize clearly the jaws of the retainer and facilitate its placement (Fig. 11-21, *B*).

The operator conveys the retainer (with dam) into the mouth and positions it on the anchor tooth. Care is necessary when applying the retainer to prevent the jaws from sliding gingivally and impinging on the soft tissue. The retainer should be opened slightly and moved occlusally when gingival tissue is trapped (Fig. 11-21, *C*).

The assistant gently pulls the inferior border of the dam toward the chin while the operator positions the superior border over the upper lip. As the assistant holds the borders of the dam, the operator uses the second or

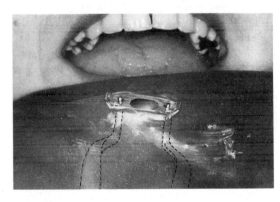

Fig. 11-22. Lip of hole for anchor tooth is stretched to engage lateral wings of retainer.

middle finger of both hands, one finger facial and the other finger lingual to the bow, to pass the anchor hole borders over and under the jaws of the retainer (Fig. 11-21, *D*). At this point, the application procedure continues as above beginning with Step 7.

Method 2. The dam may be stretched over the anchor tooth before the retainer is placed. The advantage of this method is not having to manipulate the dam over the retainer. The operator places the retainer, while the dental assistant stretches and holds the dam over the an-

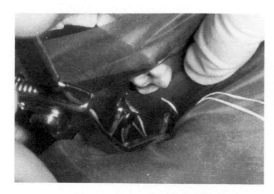

Fig. 11-23. Retainer applied after dam is stretched over posterior anchor tooth.

chor tooth (Fig. 11-23). The disadvantage is the reduction in visibility of underlying gingival tissue that may become impinged upon by the retainer.

Cervical retainer placement

Markley[16] recommends the use of the No. 212 cervical retainer for restoration of Class V cavity preparations. When punching the holes in the rubber dam, recall that the hole for the tooth to receive this retainer and a facial cervical restoration should be positioned facially (a few millimeters) to the arch form (Fig. 11-24, A). Also, the distance to the adjacent holes should be increased approximately 1 mm on each side. If the cervical retainer is to be placed on an incisor, recall that isolation should be extended to include the first premolars, and that metal retainers usually are not needed to anchor the dam (Fig. 11-24, B). If the cervical retainer is to be placed on a canine or a posterior tooth, remember to position the posterior retainer sufficiently posterior so as not to interfere with placement of the cervical retainer. If this is not possible, the posterior retainer should be removed before positioning the cervical retainer.

Before positioning the cervical retainer, have available a stick of low-fusing compound and a flame burner. Engage the jaws of the cervical retainer with the forceps, spread the retainer sufficiently, and position the lingual jaw against the tooth at the height of contour (Fig. 11-24, C). Then gently move the jaw gingivally, depressing the dam and soft tissue, until the jaw of the retainer is positioned slightly apical of the height of contour (Fig. 11-24, D). Exercise care not to allow the lingual jaw to pinch the lingual gingiva or to injure the gingival attachment. While positioning the lingual jaw, the index finger of the left hand (right-handed operator) should help in supporting and guiding the retainer jaw gingivally to the proper location.

While stabilizing the lingual jaw with the index finger, use the thumb of the left hand to pull the dam apically to expose the lesion and the gingival crest (Fig.

11-24, E). Then, position the facial jaw gingival to the lesion, and release the dam held by the thumb. Next, move the thumb onto the facial jaw to secure it (Fig. 11-24, F). Exercise care while positioning the facial jaw not to scar the enamel or cementum. The tip of each jaw should not be sharp and should conform to the contour of the engaged tooth surface. Do not position the jaw too close to the lesion because of the danger of collapsing carious or weak tooth structure. Such proximity would also limit access and visibility to the operating site. As a rule, the facial jaw should be 0.5 to 1 mm gingival to the anticipated location of the gingival margin of the completed cavity preparation. While maintaining the retainer's position with the fingers of the left hand, remove the forceps.

While the operator positions the retainer, the assistant heats and tempers the end of a stick of compound. Maintaining the retainer's position with the fingers of the left hand, the operator presses the softened compound under and over one bow. With a moistened thumb and forefinger, press the compound onto the incisal (occlusal) surface(s) and into the interproximal area(s), locking the compound in the embrasure(s) (Fig. 11-24, G). The cervical area should be examined for adequate isolation and access before the compound hardens. If additional retraction is necessary, engage the retainer and move the facial jaw gingivally while the compound is soft. Cool the compound with air. Only after the compound has been cooled and hardened should the fingers of the left hand be removed from the retainer. Apply compound in a similar manner to the other bow of the retainer (Fig. 11-24, H).

If the facial lip of the dam is not already inverted into the gingival sulcus, dry the tooth and tease the dam to proper position using a suitable, blunt instrument. Continuous inversion provides complete coverage of soft tissue, slight retraction as well as some protection of marginal gingiva, and isolation from oral fluids.

If it is necessary to move the facial jaw gingivally during the operation subsequent to the initial placement of the retainer, the retainer is easily removed with the retainer forceps and reapplied. Using compound to stabilize a cervical retainer is recommended because the retainer may be inadvertently bumped out of place during the operative procedure. Also, it is a convenient resting place for the operator's finger(s).

To remove the cervical retainer, engage it with the forceps, spread the jaws to free the compound support, and lift it incisally (occlusally) being careful to spread the retainer sufficiently to prevent the jaws from scraping the tooth or damaging the newly inserted restoration (Fig. 11-24, I). Free the embrasures of any remaining compound before removing the rubber dam.

A *modified No. 212 retainer** is recommended, es-

*S.S. White No. 212 cervical retainer (UNC modified).

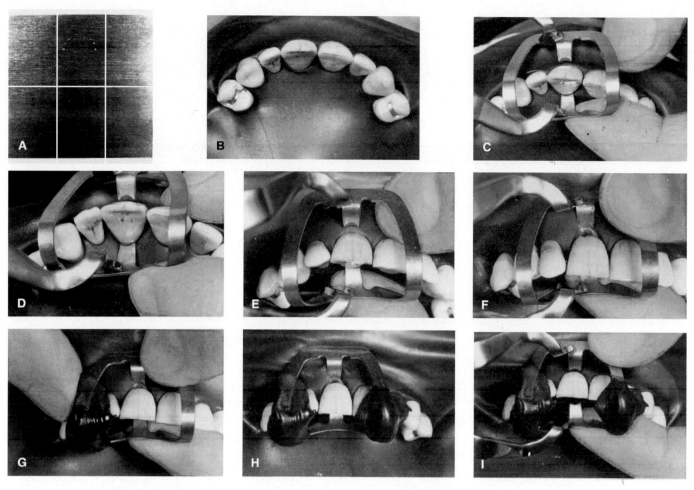

Fig. 11-24. Applying cervical retainer. **A,** Hole for maxillary right central incisor is punched facial to arch form. **B,** Isolation is extended to include first premolars; metal posterior retainers are unnecessary. **C,** First, position lingual jaw touching height of contour while keeping facial jaw from touching tooth; steady retainer with fingers of left hand using index finger under lingual bow and thumb under facial bow. **D,** Final position of lingual jaw after gently moving it apical of height of contour, with fingers continually supporting and guiding retainer and with facial jaw away from tooth. **E,** Facial rubber stretched apically by thumb to expose lesion and soft tissue, with forefinger maintaining position of lingual jaw and with the facial jaw not touching. **F,** Facial jaw having apically retracted tissue and dam, and in position against tooth 0.5 to 1 mm apical of lesion. Note that thumb has now moved from under facial bow to apply holding pressure, while index finger continues to maintain the lingual jaw position. **G,** Application of compound over and under bow and into the gingival embrasures, while fingers of left hand hold retainer's position. **H,** Application of retainer is completed by addition of compound to other bow and into gingival embrasures. **I,** Removal of retainer by ample spreading of retainer jaws before lifting from site of operation.

pecially for treatment of cervical lesions with greatly extended gingival margins. The modified version of the No. 212 retainer can be ordered, if specified, or the retainer can be modified by the operator. The modification technique involves heating each jaw of the retainer in an open flame, and then bending it with No. 110 pliers from its oblique orientation to a more horizontal one. Allowing the modified retainer to bench-cool will return it to its original hardened state. The principle in-

volved in the modification is illustrated in Fig. 20-20 (see Chapter 20).

Fixed bridge isolation

It is sometimes necessary to isolate one or more abutment teeth of a fixed bridge. Indications for fixed bridge isolation include restoration of an adjacent proximal surface and cervical restoration of an abutment tooth.

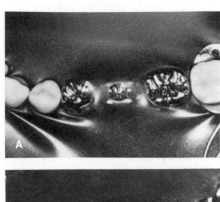
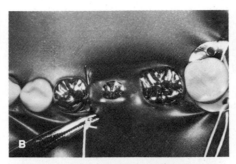
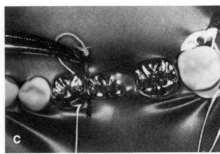
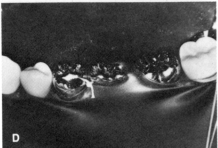
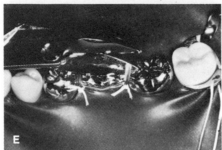

Fig. 11-25. Procedure for isolating a fixed bridge. **A,** Dam is applied except in area of fixed bridge. **B,** Threading blunted suture needle from facial to lingual aspect through anterior abutment hole, and then under anterior connector and back through same hole on lingual surface. **C,** Passing needle facially through hole for second bridge unit, and then under same connector and through hole for second unit. **D,** First septum has been tied off. **E,** Cutting posterior septum to initiate removal of dam.

The technique suggested for this procedure follows.[4] The rubber dam is punched as usual except for providing one large hole for each unit in the bridge. Fixed bridge isolation is accomplished after the remainder of the dam is applied (Fig. 11-25, *A*). A blunted, curved suture needle with dental floss attached is threaded from the facial aspect through the hole for the anterior abutment and then under the anterior connector and back through the same hole on the lingual side (Fig. 11-25, *B*). The needle's direction is then reversed as it is passed from the lingual side through the hole for the second bridge unit, then under the same anterior connector, and through the hole of the second bridge unit on the facial side (Fig. 11-25, *C*). A square knot is then tied with the two ends of the floss, thereby pulling the dam material snugly around the connector and into the gingival embrasure. The free ends of the floss should be cut closely so they neither interfere with access and visibility nor become entangled in a rotating instrument. Each terminal abutment of the bridge is isolated by this method (Fig. 11-25, *D*). If the floss knot on the facial aspect interferes with cervical restoration of an abutment tooth, the operator can tie the septum from the lingual. Removal of the rubber dam isolating a fixed bridge is accomplished by cutting the interseptal rubber over the connectors with scissors and removing the floss ties (Fig. 11-25, *E*). As always, after dam removal the operator needs to verify that no dam segments are missing and should massage the adjacent gingival tissue.

Substitution of a retainer with a matrix

When a matrix band must be applied to the posterior anchor tooth, the jaws of the retainer often prevent proper positioning and wedging of the matrix (Fig. 11-26, *A*). Successful application of the matrix can be accomplished by substituting the retainer with the matrix. Fig. 11-26, *B* to *D,* illustrates making this exchange on a mandibular right molar as the index finger of the operator depresses gingivally and distally the rubber dam adjacent to the facial jaw while the assistant similarly depresses the dam on the lingual side. After the band is placed, the tension is released on the dam allowing it to invert around the band. The matrix, unlike the retainer, has neither jaws nor bow, so there is a tendency for the dam to slip occlusally and over the matrix unless dryness is maintained.

The operator obtains access and visibility for insertion of the alloy by reflecting the dam distally and occlusally with the mirror. However, care must be exercised not to stretch the dam so much that it is pulled away from the matrix, permitting leakage around the tooth or slippage over the matrix.

Following condensation, the occlusal portion is carved before removing the matrix. To complete the procedure the operator has the choice of (1) removing the matrix, replacing the retainer, and completing the carving, or (2) removing the matrix and rubber dam, and completing the carving. To maintain isolation throughout the procedure, it is preferred to replace the retainer before completing the carving.

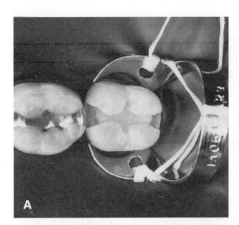
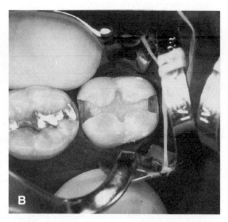
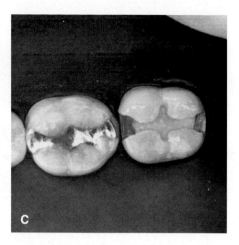

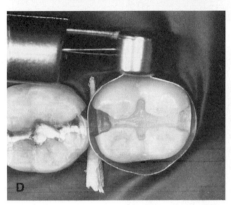

Fig. 11-26. Substituting retainer with matrix on terminal tooth. **A,** Completed cavity preparation of terminal tooth with retainer in place. **B,** Dentist and assistant stretch dam distally and gingivally as retainer is being removed. **C,** Retainer removed prior to placement of matrix. **D,** Completed matrix in place. To maximize access and visibility during condensation, the mouth mirror is used to reflect dam distally and occlusally.

Variations with age levels

The age of the patient often dictates changes in the procedures of rubber dam application. A few variations are described below:

1. Because young patients have smaller dental arches than adult patients, holes should be punched in the dam accordingly. For primary teeth, isolation is usually from the most posterior tooth to the canine on the same side. The sheet of rubber dam may be smaller (5 × 5 inch [12.5 × 12.5 cm]) for the young patient so that the rubber material does not cover the nose.

2. Some operators prefer to alter the procedure of application on the young patient. The unpunched rubber dam is attached to the frame, the holes are then punched, the dam with the frame is applied over the anchor tooth, and the retainer is applied (Fig. 11-27). Since the dam is generally in place for shorter intervals than for the adult patient, the napkin often is not used.

3. The jaws of the retainers used on primary and young permanent teeth need to be directed more gingivally because of short clinical crowns or because the anchor tooth's height of contour is below the crest of the gingival tissue. The *S.S. White No. 27 retainer* is recommended for pri-

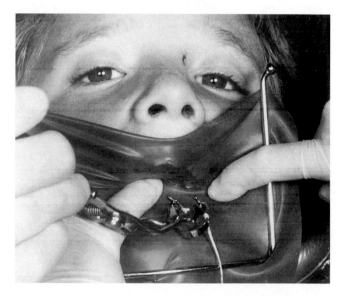

Fig. 11-27. On a child, rubber dam is often attached to frame before holes are punched. Dam is then positioned over anchor tooth before retainer is applied as in Fig. 11-23.

mary teeth. The *Ivory No. W14 retainer* is recommended for young permanent teeth.

4. Isolated teeth with short clinical crowns other than the anchor tooth may require ***ligation*** to hold the dam in position. Ligation is permissible, but should be used only when necessary because of the possible damage to gingival tissues. Ligatures should be removed first during the procedure of

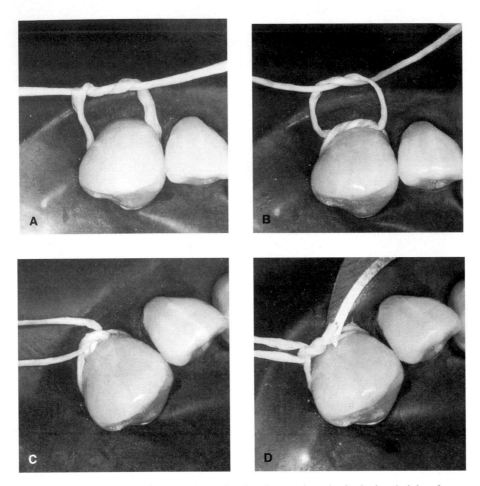

Fig. 11-28. Surgeon's knot. **A,** Dental tape is placed around tooth gingival to height of contour, and knot is tied by first making two loops with free ends, followed by single loop, **B. C,** Free ends are not cut but tied to frame to serve as reminder that ligature is in place. **D,** To remove ligature, simply cut tape with scalpel blade, amalgam knife, or scissors.

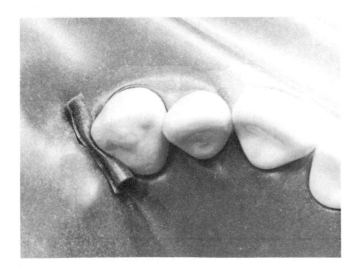

Fig. 11-29. A piece of rubber dam material may be rolled, stretched, and placed in diastema to serve as anterior anchor.

rubber dam removal. Generally, ligation is unnecessary if a sufficient number of teeth are isolated by the rubber dam. However, when ligatures are indicated, a surgeon's knot is used to secure the ligature (Fig. 11-28). Ligatures may be removed by teasing them occlusally with an explorer or by cutting them with a hand instrument or scissors.

5. A small piece of rubber dam material may be rolled, stretched, and placed into a diastema to serve as an *anterior anchor* (Fig. 11-29).

Errors in application and removal

Certain *errors in application and removal* can prevent adequate moisture control, reduce access and visibility, or cause injury to the patient.

Off-center arch form. A rubber dam punched off center may not adequately shield the patient's oral cavity, allowing foreign matter to escape down the patient's throat. An off-center dam can result in an excess of dam material superiorly that may occlude the patient's nasal airway (Fig. 11-30, *A*). If this happens, the superior border of the dam can be folded under, or can be cut from around the patient's nose (Fig. 11-30, *B* and *C*). Proper hole placement, however, will correctly position the dam. It is important to verify that the rubber dam frame has been applied so that its ends are not dangerously close to the patient's eyes.

Inappropriate distance between the holes. Too small a distance between holes precludes adequate isolation because the hole margins in the rubber dam will not fit snugly around the necks of the teeth. Conversely, too great a distance results in excess septal width causing the dam to (1) wrinkle between the teeth, (2) interfere with proximal access, and (3) not provide adequate tissue retraction.

Incorrect arch form of holes. If the punched arch form is too small, the holes will be stretched open around the teeth permitting leakage. If the punched arch form is too large, the dam will wrinkle around the teeth and thus may interfere with access.

Inappropriate retainer. A retainer may be inappropriate by (1) being too small resulting in occasional breakage when the jays are overspread, (2) being unstable on the anchor tooth, (3) impinging on soft tissue, or (4) impeding wedge placement. An appropriate retainer should maintain a stable four-point contact with the anchor tooth and not interfere with wedge placement.

Retainer-pinched tissue. The jaws and prongs of the rubber dam retainer usually slightly depress the tissue, but should not pinch or impinge on it.

Shredded or torn dam. Care should be exercised to prevent shredding or tearing the dam, especially during hole punching or passing the septa through the contacts. Moisture control is possible only if the dam is intact.

Incorrect location of hole for Class V lesion. If the hole for a Class V lesion is not punched facial to the arch form, circulation in the interproximal tissue will be diminished because of the added pressure on it once the dam and cervical retainer are in place.

Sharp tips on No. 212 retainer. Sharp tips on a No. 212 retainer should be sufficiently dulled to prevent damaging the cementum.

Incorrect technique for cutting septa. During removal of the rubber dam, not stretching the septa away from the gingiva or not protecting the lip and cheek with an index finger increases the risk of cutting soft tissue with the scissors as the septa are cut.

HIGH-VOLUME EVACUATORS; SALIVA EJECTORS
High-volume evacuators

When a high-speed handpiece is used, air-water spray is supplied through the head of the handpiece to wash the operating site and to act as a coolant for the bur and the tooth. High-volume evacuators are preferred for suctioning water and debris from the mouth (Fig. 11-31) because saliva ejectors remove water slowly and have little capacity for picking up solids. McWherter[17] showed that one type of evacuator would remove one pint (0.5 L) of water in 2 seconds, had a 75% to 95%

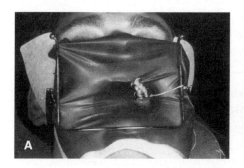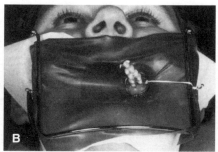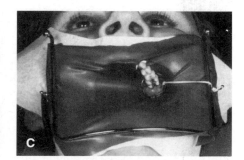

Fig. 11-30. **A,** Inappropriately punched dam may occlude patient's nasal airway. **B,** Excess dam material along superior border folded under to proper position. **C,** Excess dam material cut from around patient's nose.

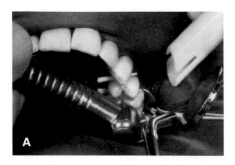
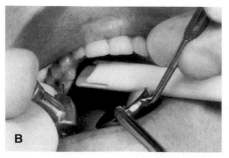

Fig. 11-31. Position of evacuator tip for maximal removal of water and debris in operating area. With rubber dam applied (**A**). With cotton roll isolation (**B**).

pickup of water in air, and would remove 100% of solids during cutting procedures. A practical test for adequacy of a high-volume evacuator is to submerge the evacuator tip in a 5-ounce cup (150 ml) of water. The water should disappear in approximately 1 second.

The combined use of water spray, or air-water spray, and a high-volume evacuator during cutting procedures has the following advantages:

1. Cuttings both of tooth and restorative material, as well as other debris, are removed from the operating site.
2. A washed operating field[28] improves access and visibility.
3. There is no dehydration of the oral tissues.[17]
4. Without an anesthetic the patient experiences less pain.
5. Pauses that are sometimes annoying and time-consuming are eliminated.[17]
6. Precious metals are more readily salvaged.
7. Quadrant dentistry is facilitated.

The assistant's responsibility is to place the evacuator tip as near to the tooth being prepared as possible. However, it should not obstruct the operator's access or vision. Also, the evacuator tip should not be so close to the handpiece head that the air-water spray is diverted from the rotary instrument. The assistant should place the evacuator tip in the mouth before the operator positions the handpiece and mirror. The assistant will usually place the tip of the evacuator just distal to the tooth to be prepared. The assistant's right hand holds the evacuator tip, and the left hand manipulates the air/water syringe. Hand positions are reversed if the operator is left-handed. When the operator needs to examine the progress of tooth preparation, the assistant will rinse and dry the tooth (teeth) using air from the air/water syringe in conjunction with the evacuator.

Saliva ejectors

Most patients do not require saliva ejectors for removal of saliva because salivary flow is greatly reduced when the operating site is profoundly anesthetized. The dentist or assistant will position the saliva ejector, if needed.

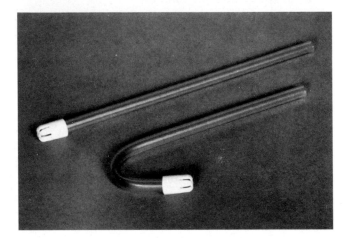

Fig. 11-32. Saliva ejectors.

The saliva ejector removes saliva that collects on the floor of the mouth. It is used in conjunction with sponges, cotton rolls, and the rubber dam. It should be placed in an area least likely to interfere with the operator's movements.

The tip of the ejector must be smooth and made from a nonirritating material. Disposable, inexpensive plastic ejectors that may be shaped by bending with the fingers are available (Fig. 11-32). The ejector should be placed to prevent occluding its tip with tissue from the floor of the mouth. Some ejectors are designed to prevent suctioning of tissue. It also may be necessary to adjust the suction for each patient to prevent this occurrence. A Svedopter is a helpful device which serves both as saliva ejector and as tongue retractor.

ABSORBENTS AND THROAT SHIELDS
Cotton roll isolation and cellulose wafers

Absorbents, such as cotton rolls and cellulose wafers (Fig. 11-33), are helpful for short periods of isolation (e.g., examination, polishing, sealant placement),[27,29] and topical fluoride applications. Absorbents are isolation alternatives when rubber dam application is impractical or impossible. Especially in conjunction with profound anesthesia, absorbents provide acceptable dryness for procedures such as impression-taking and cementation. Using a saliva ejector in conjunction with absorbents will further abate salivary flow. The assistant has the responsibility of keeping dry cotton rolls in the mouth. The assistant should change the cotton rolls when they become saturated. It is sometimes permissible to suction the free moisture from a saturated cotton roll in place in the mouth. This is done by placing the evacuator tip next to the end of the cotton roll while the cotton roll is secured by the operator.

Several commercial devices for holding cotton rolls in position are available (Fig. 11-34). It is generally necessary to remove the holding appliance from the mouth to change the cotton rolls. This is inconvenient and time-consuming. An advantage of *cotton roll holders* is that the cheeks and tongue are slightly retracted from the teeth, which enhances access and visibility. When dryness is required for an extended period, the rubber dam is indicated.

The maxillary teeth are isolated by placing a medium-sized cotton roll in the adjacent vestibule (Fig. 11-

35). The mandibular teeth are isolated by placing one medium-sized cotton roll in the vestibule and a larger one between the teeth and the tongue (Fig. 11-36). The teeth are then dried with short blasts from the air syringe. Cellulose wafers may be used to retract the cheek and provide absorbency. After the cotton rolls or cellulose wafers are in place, the saliva ejector may be positioned. When removing cotton rolls or cellulose wafers, it may be necessary to moisten them using the air/water

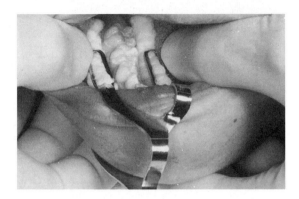

Fig. 11-34. A cotton roll holder in position.

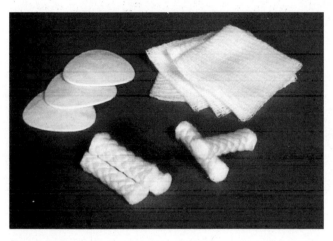

Fig. 11-33. Absorbents such as cotton rolls, cellulose wafers, and gauze sponges provide satisfactory dryness for short periods of time.

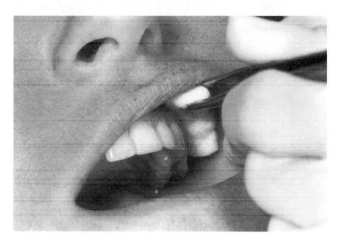

Fig. 11-35. Isolate maxillary posterior teeth by placing cotton roll in vestibule adjacent to teeth.

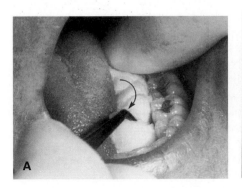

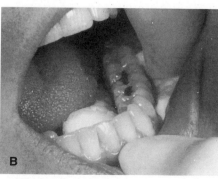

Fig. 11-36. A, Position large cotton roll between tongue and teeth by "rolling" it to place in direction of arrow. B, Properly positioned facial and lingual cotton rolls improve access and visibility.

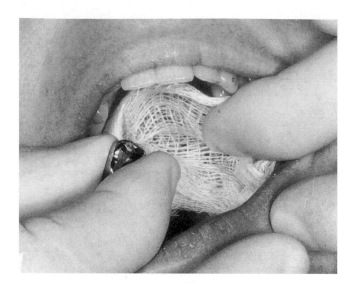

Fig. 11-37. A throat screen is used during try-in and removal of indirect restorations.

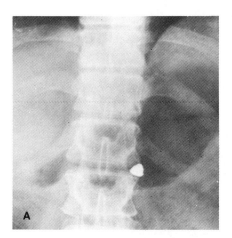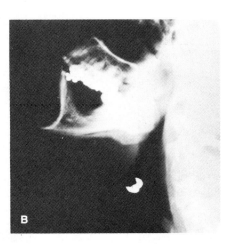

Fig. 11-38. A, Radiograph of swallowed casting in patient's stomach. **B,** Radiograph of casting lodged in patient's throat.

syringe to prevent inadvertent removal of the epithelium from the cheeks, floor of the mouth, or lips.

Throat shields

Throat shields are indicated when small instruments are being used without the rubber dam, or when indirect restorations are being inserted. This is particularly important when treating teeth in the maxillary arch. A gauze sponge (2 × 2 inch [5 × 5 cm]), unfolded and spread over the tongue and the posterior part of the mouth, is helpful in recovering a restoration should it be dropped (Fig. 11-37). Without a throat shield, it is possible for a restoration to be aspirated or swallowed (Fig. 11-38).[20]

ALTERNATIVE OR ADDITIONAL ISOLATION AIDS
Retraction cord

Retraction cord, properly applied, often can be used for isolation and retraction in the direct procedures of treatment of cervical lesions (exception: treatment using gold foil) and in facial veneering, as well as in indirect procedures involving gingival margins. When use of the rubber dam is impractical or inappropriate, retraction cord moistened with a noncaustic styptic (e.g., Hemodent*) may be placed in the gingival sulcus to control sulcular seepage and/or hemorrhage. Most brands of re-

*Hemodent, Premier Dental Products Company, Norristown, Pa.

traction cord are available with and without the vasoconstrictor, epinephrine, which acts also to control sulcular fluids. To achieve adequate moisture control, retraction cord isolation should be used in conjunction with **salivation control** by virtue of **profound anesthesia** of all tissues of the operating site. A properly applied retraction cord will improve access and visibility and help prevent abrasion of gingival tissue during cavity preparation. Retraction cord can restrict excess restorative material from the gingival sulcus.

Principles of using retraction cord are:

1. Insert the cord after attaining profound anesthesia and *before cavity preparation when treating cervical lesions and before removal of infected dentin when treating proximal lesions.* When the proper cord is correctly applied, its mild physical and chemical (noncaustic styptic) effects achieve *isolation* from fluids (along with cotton roll use), *access,* and *visibility,* and *does not cause harm.*

2. Choose the *diameter of cord* that can be gently inserted into the gingival sulcus and will produce lateral displacement (a few tenths of a millimeter) of the free gingiva ("opening" the sulcus) without blanching it (ischemia due to pressure). The *length of cord* should be sufficient to extend approximately 1 mm beyond the gingival width of the cavity preparation. Use a thin, blunt-edged instrument blade, or side of an explorer, to progressively insert the cord. To prevent displacement of previously inserted cord, the placement instrument should be moved slightly backward at each step as it is stepped along the cord (Fig. 11-39). Cord placement should not abuse the gingival tissue or damage the epithelial attachment. If ischemia of the gingival tissue is observed, an oversized cord has been placed and should be immediately replaced with a smaller cord. *The objective* is to obtain minimal yet sufficient lateral displacement of the free gingiva, and *not* to force it apically. Cord insertion will result in adequate *apical retraction* of the gingival crest in a short time.

3. Due to the delicate, thin dimension of the free gingiva *on the facial aspect of anterior and premolar teeth, the smallest diameter cord is often used.* If braided cord is used, it may be helpful at times to separate the strands of the smallest cord to custom-make a still smaller cord. A second, usually larger, cord may be placed over (not beside) the first if additional retraction is necessary.

4. When a *proximal crevice* is involved, it may be helpful to insert a second, usually larger, cord over the initially inserted cord. This may be indicated when isolating for an impression recording adjacent gingival margins and the gingival papilla is difficult to retract.

5. *In procedures for the indirect restoration* (e.g., onlay), insert the cord before the removal of infected dentin and placement of a liner and base. This provides isolation and opens the sulcus in readiness for any beveling of the gingival margins. Before beveling, the cord is removed temporarily. After beveling, the same cord may be reinserted and remain a few minutes to help assure an open sulcus when the cord is again removed just prior to the impression.

6. It is emphasized to insert cord before (or early) in cavity preparation *to prevent abrasion of the gingival tissue;* thereby there is no exposure of capillaries and minimal absorption of any medicament from the cord into the circulatory system.

7. The cord may be *moistened with a noncaustic styptic* prior to insertion if hemorrhage of fragile tissue is anticipated.

Specific uses of retraction cord are detailed and illustrated in Chapters 16, 18, and 19.

Mirror and evacuator tip retraction

A secondary function of the mirror and evacuator tip is to retract the cheek, lip, and tongue (Fig. 11-40).

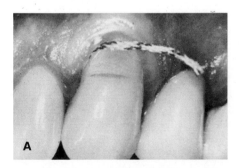 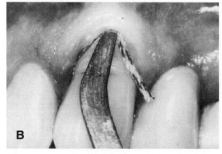 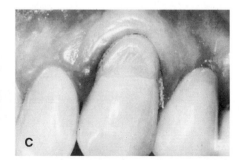

Fig. 11-39. Retraction cord placed in gingival crevice. **A,** Cord placement initiated. **B,** A thin, flat-bladed instrument is used for cord placement. **C,** Cord placed.

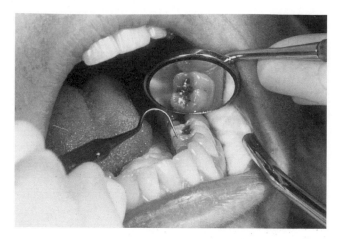

Fig. 11-40. Chairside assistant uses air syringe to dry teeth and to keep mirror free of debris.

This is particularly important when the rubber dam is not used.

Mouth prop

A decided aid to cavity preparation on posterior teeth during an extended procedure is a mouth prop (Fig. 11-41, *A*). A prop should establish and maintain suitable mouth opening, thereby relieving the muscles of this task which often produces fatigue and sometimes pain. Moreover, with the use of a prop, the patient is relieved of the responsibility of maintaining sufficient mouth opening, thereby permitting added relaxation.

The ideal characteristics of a mouth prop are as follows: (1) it should be adaptable to all mouths; (2) it should be capable of being easily positioned with no patient discomfort; (3) it should be easily adjusted, if necessary, to provide the proper mouth opening or to improve its position in the mouth; (4) it should be stable once it is applied; (5) it should be easily and readily removable by the operator or the patient in case of emergency; and (6) it should be either sterilizable or disposable.

Mouth props of different designs and different materials are available. They are generally available either as block type or ratchet type (Fig. 11-41, *B* and *C*). Although the ratchet type is adjustable, its size and cost are disadvantages. The convenience and cost of the block type commend it for use in operative procedures.

The use of a mouth prop is a decided benefit to both the operator and patient. The most outstanding benefits to the patient are relief of responsibility of maintaining adequate mouth opening and relief of muscle fatigue and muscle pain. For the dentist the prop ensures constant and adequate mouth opening and permits extended or multiple operations if desired.

Drugs

The use of drugs in restorative dentistry to control salivation is rarely indicated and is generally limited to **atropine.** As with any drug, the operator should be familiar with its indications, contraindications, and side effects. It is important to remember that atropine is contraindicated for nursing mothers and for patients with glaucoma.[1]

REFERENCES

1. *Accepted dental therapeutics,* ed 40, Chicago, 1984, American Dental Association.
2. ADA Council on Dental Materials, Instruments, and Equipment, Posterior composite resins, *J Am Dent Assoc* 112:707, May 1986.
3. Barghi N, Knight GT, Berry TG: Comparing two methods of moisture control in bonding to enamel: a clinical study, *Oper Dent* 16:130, 1991.
4. Baum L, Phillips RW, Lund MR: *Textbook of operative dentistry,* Philadelphia, 1981, WB Saunders.
5. Black GL: *Operative dentistry,* ed 8, vol 2, Woodstock, Ill, 1947, Medico-Dental.
6. Brinker HA: Access—the key to success, *J Prosthet Dent* 28:391, 1972.
7. Cochran MA, Miller CH, Sheldrake MA: The efficacy of the rubber dam as a barrier to the spread of microorganisms during dental treatment, *J Am Dent Assoc* 119:141, July 1989.

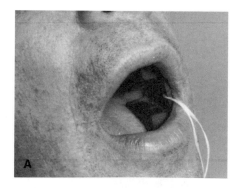
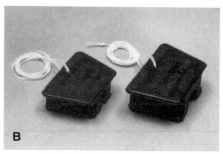
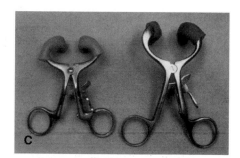

Fig. 11-41. Mouth props. **A,** Block-type prop maintaining mouth opening. **B,** Block-type prop. **C,** Ratchet-type prop.

8. Cunningham PR, Ferguson GW: The instruction of rubber dam technique, *J Am Acad Gold Foil Oper* 13:5, April 1970.

9. Dinin A: Rubber dam: a simple procedure, *Dent Items Interest* 73:113, 1951.

10. Forrest WR, Perez RS: The rubber dam as a surgical drape: protection against AIDS and hepatitis, *Gen Dent* 37(3):236, 1989.

11. Heling I, Sommer M, Kot I: Rubber dam—an essential safeguard, *Quintessence Int* 19(5):377, 1988.

12. Howard WW, Moller RC: *Atlas of operative dentistry,* ed 3, St Louis, 1981, Mosby.

13. Huggins DR: The rubber dam—an insurance policy against litigation, *J Indiana Dent Assoc* 65(3):23, 1986.

14. Ingraham R, Koser JR: *An atlas of gold foil and rubber dam procedures,* Buena Park, Calif, 1961, Uni-Tro College Press.

15. Jones CM, Reid JS: Patient and operator attitudes toward rubber dam, *ASDC J Dent Child* 55(6):452, 1988.

16. Markley MR: Amalgam restorations for Class V cavities, *J Am Dent Assoc* 50:301, 1955.

17. McWherter E: Modern method improvements and works simplification approach to clinical procedures of the washed field technic in dentistry, *Ark Dent J* 28:10, March 1957.

18. Medina JE: The rubber dam—an incentive for excellence, *Dent Clin North Am* p 255, March 1967.

19. Mosteller JH: Restoration of teeth with silver amalgam, *J Prosthet Dent* 11:288, 1961.

20. Nelson JF: Ingesting an onlay: a case report, *J Am Dent Assoc* 123:73, July 1992.

21. Nimmo A et al: Particulate inhalation during the removal of amalgam restorations, *J Prosthet Dent* 63:228, Feb 1990.

22. Peterson JE, Nation WA, Matsson L: Effect of a rubber dam clamp (retainer) on cementum and junctional epithelium, *Oper Dent* 11:42, 1986.

23. Phillips RW: *Skinner's science of dental materials,* ed 8, Philadelphia, 1982, WB Saunders.

24. Prime JM: Inconsistencies in operative dentistry, *J Am Dent Assoc* 24:82, 1937.

25. Samaranayake LP, Reid J, Evans D: The efficacy of rubber dam isolation in reducing atmospheric bacterial contamination, *ASDC J Dent Child* 56(6):442, 1989.

26. Stibbs GD: Rubber dam, *J Can Dent Assoc* 17:311, 1951.

27. Straffon LH, Dennison JB, More FG: Three-year evaluation of sealant: effect of isolation on efficacy, *J Am Dent Assoc* 110:714, May 1985.

28. Thompson ED: Clinical application of the washed field technic in dentistry, *J Am Dent Assoc* 51:703, 1955.

29. van Dijken JWV, Hörstedt P: Effect of the use of rubber dam versus cotton rolls on marginal adaptation of composite resin fillings to acid-etched enamel, *ACTA Odontol Scand* 45:303, 1987.

30. Wong RCK: The rubber dam as a means of infection control in an era of AIDS and hepatitis, *J Indiana Dent Assoc* 67(1):41, January/February 1988.

CHAPTER 12

Amalgam restorations for Class I cavity preparations

Aldridge D. Wilder, Jr.

Kenneth N. May, Jr.

William D. Strickland*

*This author is inactive this edition; see Preface.

Properly handled, *dental amalgam* produces a restoration that will provide many years of service. More posterior teeth are restored with amalgam than any other material. Understanding the physical properties of amalgam and the principles of cavity preparation is necessary to produce amalgam restorations that provide optimal service.

The success of amalgam restorations depends on many factors. This chapter deals with the techniques and procedures that affect the quality and longevity of amalgam restorations in Class I cavity preparations. Unfortunately, many amalgam failures occur though improved techniques and materials are available. Much time is spent replacing restorations that are failing as a result of recurrent caries, marginal deterioration (ditching), fractures, or poor contours.[20,21] However, attention to detail throughout the procedure can significantly decrease the incidence of failures and extend the life of the restoration.

INDICATIONS AND CONTRAINDICATIONS

The following items must be considered when selecting the restorative material for the Class I cavity preparation:

1. Extent of pit and fissure caries
2. Incidence of proximal surface caries
3. Age of the patient
4. Esthetics
5. Economics
6. Preventive procedures

Extent of pit and fissure caries

Dental amalgam is appropriate for conservative cavity preparations, for example, when pit and fissure caries is not extensive. When caries is extensive, or a large, failing restoration is treated, amalgam may not be the material of choice. If one or more cusps have been undermined, these should be included in the outline form. Cusp-capping preparations may be restored with amalgam, cast gold, laboratory-processed composite, or porcelain, and these restorations are discussed in Chapters 13, 15, 17, and 19. If the remaining tooth crown is subject to fracture because of extensive loss of tooth structure, restorations are indicated which provide adequate resistance form against postrestorative fracture of the tooth; these include crowns, gold onlays skirting the line angles, and tooth-bonded restorations of laboratory-processed composite or porcelain.

Incidence of proximal surface caries

When examination of the other teeth reveals numerous carious proximal surfaces or failing restorations and there are indications that the tooth in question may develop proximal caries within a few years, then a less expensive treatment procedure, such as an amalgam restoration, is indicated.

Age of the patient

Amalgam restorations for Class I cavity preparations are particularly indicated for those young patients who are thought to be at risk for carious proximal surfaces. Some clinicians choose amalgam for large cavity preparations when the life expectancy of the tooth is questionable, and also when "repair" dentistry is appropriate (e.g., for the medically compromised patient). Often, amalgam is the material of choice regardless of the age of the patient.

Esthetics

Some patients object to the metallic appearance of amalgam restorations. However, in the posterior teeth well-polished amalgam restorations should not be a deterrent to the esthetics-conscious patient, particularly when the facial surfaces are not involved. Obviously, in areas of esthetic concern the dentist should consider the use of a tooth-colored restorative material rather than amalgam. For patients in the public eye, the consideration of esthetics may supersede other considerations.

Economics

Cost to the patient for Class I amalgam restorations is less than for gold or tooth-colored restorations since less time is required. However, the dentist must consider the long-term cost to the patient and not use amalgam when another procedure is indicated. It is poor judgment to place a large amalgam restoration in a tooth that may subsequently fracture. Placing a large amalgam restoration that may have to be replaced with an onlay or crown in a few years is not cost-effective and may jeopardize the integrity of the tooth.

Preventive procedures

Caries occurs frequently in the pits and fissures of the posterior teeth. As a preventive or prophylactic procedure, the pits and fissures may be minimally prepared and restored with amalgam before visible attack by caries. Hyatt[15] referred to this procedure as *prophylactic odontotomy*. The dentist must consider the patient's caries rate, oral hygiene, and anatomy of the pits and fissures to determine when cavity preparation and restoration is indicated. Pits and fissures that "catch" an explorer tine and are in mouths with a high caries rate and a significant amount of plaque are usually indicated for this procedure.

Pits and fissures that are judged not to have dentinal caries but are at risk for caries may be treated by *fluoride, sealants, conservative resin restorations,*[37,42] or *enameloplasty.* (For fluoride, sealants, and conservative resin restorations, see Chapters 3 and 17. For enameloplasty see later section in this chapter.)

OCCLUSION

When the occlusal surfaces are involved in the cavity preparation, use articulating paper to register preoperatively the centric holding stops and excursive contacts so that these marked areas can be either excluded from the outline form or properly restored. *"Plunging cusps"* should be reduced (1) to improve the plane of occlusion, (2) to lessen the likelihood of fracture of the new restoration as a result of occlusal forces, (3) to reduce the steepness of involved occlusal inclines, and (4) to decrease the potential for interferences in eccentric tooth positions.

Occlusion of the dentition should be evaluated *before* establishing a treatment plan and instituting cavity preparation(s). (Refer to Chapter 2 for details on occlusion and to Examination of Occlusion in Chapter 5.)

LOCAL ANESTHESIA

Profound anesthesia of the operating site is usually a prerequisite for good dentistry. In addition to eliminating pain, local anesthesia usually greatly reduces salivation because the patient is less sensitive to stimulation of the oral tissues. This reduction of salivation is a critical factor contributing to excellence in operative dentistry. The operator is more efficient when the patient is comfortable.

CONSERVATIVE CAVITY PREPARATIONS

Conservative cavity preparation is recommended to protect the pulp,[11] preserve the strength of the tooth,[34,44] and reduce deterioration of the amalgam restoration.[26] This section describes conservative Class I cavity preparations for amalgam restoration of occlusal pits and fissures where caries is minimal to moderate. *Caries is moderate if the remaining dentin thickness after excavation is judged to be 1 mm or more.* The maxillary first premolar is used for illustration. Management of extensive occlusal caries is described in a later section, Cavity Preparation for Extensive Caries. Other Class I cavities are detailed in later sections of this chapter.

Isolation of the operating site

Generally, isolation with the rubber dam is recommended.[11] The few minutes it takes to apply the rubber dam allows time for onset of profound anesthesia before initiating the cavity preparation. For a single maxillary

tooth, where caries is not extensive, adequate moisture control may be achieved with cotton rolls and profound anesthesia. Removing deep caries that is judged to be less than a millimeter from the pulp should always be accomplished with rubber dam isolation. Moisture control is also necessary during amalgam condensation,[32] particularly when amalgam alloys containing zinc are used.[33,46] (For details on moisture control refer to Chapter 11 and to a later section in this chapter, Cavity Preparation for Extensive Caries.)

Initial cavity preparation

Recall from Chapter 7 that *initial cavity preparation is defined as establishing the outline form by extension of the external walls to sound tooth structure, maintaining a specified, limited depth, and providing resistance and retention forms.*

Outline, resistance, and retention forms. The outline form for the Class I occlusal cavity preparation should include all of the occlusal pits and fissures in such a manner that sharp angles in the marginal outline are avoided. Frequently, the marginal outline for maxillary premolars is butterfly-shaped because of extension to include the developmental fissures facially and lingually. The ideal outline form (Fig. 12-1, *A*) involves the following resistance form principles that are basic to all cavity preparations of occlusal surfaces (positioning margins in areas that are sound and subject to minimal forces, and conserving tooth structure to maintain the strength and health of the tooth): (1) going around the cusps to conserve tooth structure and prevent the internal line angles from approaching the pulp horns too

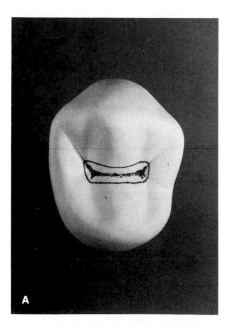
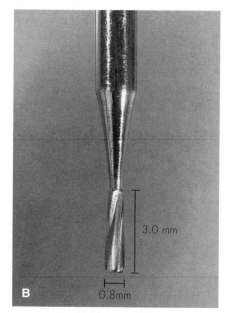
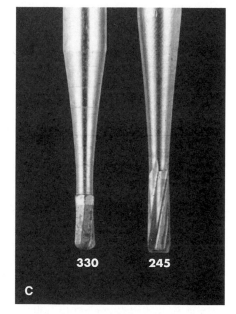

Fig. 12-1. For legend see facing page.

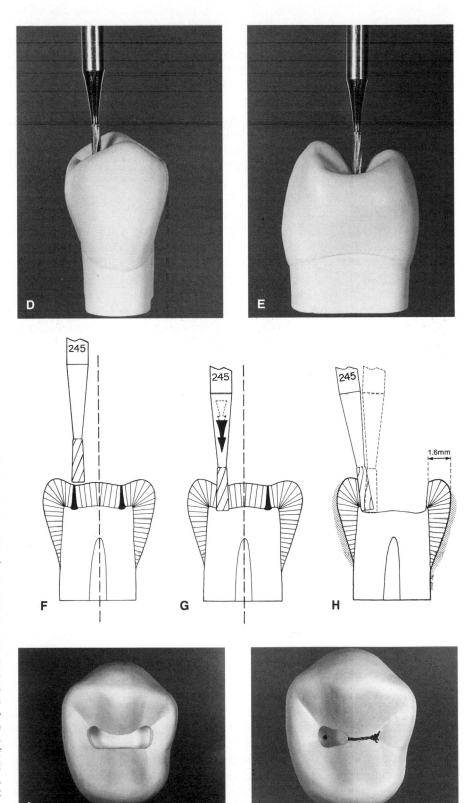

Fig. 12-1. Outline and entry. **A,** Ideal outline includes all occlusal pits and fissures. **B,** Dimensions of head of No. 245 bur. **C,** Nos. 330 and 245 burs compared. **D,** No. 245 bur oriented parallel to long axis of tooth crown for entry as viewed from lingual aspect. **E,** Bur positioned for entry as viewed from distal aspect. **F,** Bur positioned over more carious pit (distal) for entry. Distal aspect of bur is positioned over distal pit. **G,** Enter pit with punch cut to a depth of 1.5 to 2 mm or one-half to two-thirds the head length of bur. (The 1.5 mm depth is measured at central fissure; the measurement of same entry cut but of prepared external wall is up to 2.0 mm. See Fig. 12-2.) **H,** Incline bur distally to establish proper occlusal divergence to distal wall to prevent removal of dentin supporting marginal ridge enamel when pulpal floor is in dentin and distal extension is necessary to include a fissure or caries. For such an extension on premolars the distance from margin to proximal surface (imaginary projection) must not be less than 1.6 mm (two diameters of end of bur). **I,** Occlusal view of initial cavity preparation that has mesial and distal walls that diverge occlusally. **J,** Distofacial and distolingual fissures that radiate from pit are included before extending along central fissure.

closely, (2) not extending the facial and lingual margins more than halfway between the central groove and the cusp tips,[44] (3) extending the outline to include fissures, thereby placing the margins on relatively smooth, sound tooth structure,[10] (4) minimally extending into the marginal ridges (only enough to include the defect) without removing dentinal support, (5) eliminating a weak wall of enamel by joining two outlines that come close together (less than 0.5 mm apart), (6) extending the outline form to include enamel undermined by caries, (7) using enameloplasty on the terminal ends of shallow fissures to conserve tooth structure, and (8) establishing the optimal, conservative depth of the pulpal wall.

A *No. 245 bur* with a head length of 3 mm and a diameter of 0.8 mm is used to prepare the Class I cavity preparation (Fig. 12-1, *B*). A silhouette of this Sockwell-designed bur shows sides slightly divergent endwise, which produce an occlusal convergence to the facial and lingual walls, providing adequate retention form to the cavity preparation. The slightly rounded corners of the end of this bur produce slightly rounded internal line angles that render the tooth more resistant to fracture from occlusal force.[38] The *No. 330 bur* is a smaller and pear-shaped version of the No. 245 bur. It is indicated for the very conservative amalgam preparation (Fig. 12-1, *C*).

Begin the Class I occlusal cavity preparation by entering the deepest or most carious pit with a punch cut using the No. 245 carbide bur at high speed with airwater spray.[11,39] A ***punch cut*** is performed by orienting the bur so that its long axis parallels the long axis of the tooth crown (Fig. 12-1, *D* and *E*), and then inserting the bur directly into the faulty pit. When the pits are equally faulty, enter the distal pit as illustrated. The bur should be positioned so that its distal aspect is directly over the distal pit, thereby minimizing extension into the marginal ridge (Fig. 12-1, *F*). The bur should be rotating when it is applied to the tooth and should not stop rotating until it is removed from the tooth. *As the bur enters the pit, the proper depth of 1.5 to 2 mm (one-half to two-thirds the length of the cutting portion of the bur) should be established (Fig. 12-1, G). The 1.5 mm depth is measured at the central fissure. The 2 mm measurement is usually the depth of the prepared external walls* (refer to Fig. 12-2). *The desired pulpal depth is usually 0.1 to 0.2 mm into dentin.* The length of the blades of an unfamiliar entry bur should be measured before it is used as a depth gauge.

Distal extension into the distal marginal ridge to include a fissure or caries *sometimes indicates a slight tilting of the bur* distally (no more than 10 degrees) to create a slight occlusal divergence to the distal wall to prevent undermining the marginal ridge of its dentin support (Fig. 12-1, *H* and *I*). For premolars the distance from the margin of such an extension to the proximal

surface must not be less than 1.6 mm or two diameters of the end of the No. 245 bur measured from a tangent to the proximal surface.[41] For molars this minimal distance is 2 mm. A minimal distal (or mesial) extension often does not require changing the orientation of the bur's axis from being parallel to the long axis of the tooth crown, and thus the mesial and distal walls will be parallel to the long axis of the tooth crown, or slightly convergent occlusally.

While maintaining the bur's orientation and depth, extend the preparation distofacially or distolingually to include any fissures that radiate from the pit (Fig. 12-1, *J*). Care should be taken not to undermine the marginal ridge. When these fissures require extensions of more than a few tenths of a millimeter, consideration should be given to changing to a smaller diameter bur, such as a *No. 169L*, or to using enameloplasty (see next section). Both of these approaches conserve tooth structure and the strength of the tooth.

Continuing to maintain the bur's orientation and depth, and with intermittent pressure, extend along the central fissure toward the mesial pit. This will generally create a flat pulpal floor. However, in larger teeth with steep cuspal inclines the pulpal floor may follow the rise and fall of the occlusal surface in order to maintain a more uniform pulpal floor depth (Fig. 12-2). When the central fissure has minimal caries, one pass along the fissure at the prescribed depth provides the desired minimal width to the isthmus. Ideally, the width of the isthmus need be no more than the diameter of the bur.[10] Vale[44] concluded that an isthmus width of one fourth the distance between the cusp tips does not reduce the strength of the tooth. As previously described for the distal margin, the orientation of the bur should not change as it approaches the mesial pit if the mesial extension is minimal. If the fissure extends farther onto the marginal ridge, the long axis of the bur should be changed to establish a slight occlusal divergence to the mesial wall if the marginal ridge would be otherwise undermined of its dentinal support. Fig. 12-3, *A* to *C*, illustrates the correct and incorrect preparation of the mesial and distal walls. *It should be emphasized that minimal faciolingual width of the outline and minimal occlusal convergence of the facial and lingual walls is desired. This is ideally achieved when the bur makes only one pass along the central fissure.*

The remainder of the occlusal enamel defects are included in the outline,[10] and the facial and lingual walls are extended, if necessary, to remove enamel undermined by caries. *A strong, **ideal enamel margin** should remain: one that is made up of full-length enamel rods resting on sound dentin, supported on the cavity side by shorter rods also resting on sound dentin (Fig. 12-4).*

The conservative Class I cavity preparation should have an outline form with gently flowing curves and dis-

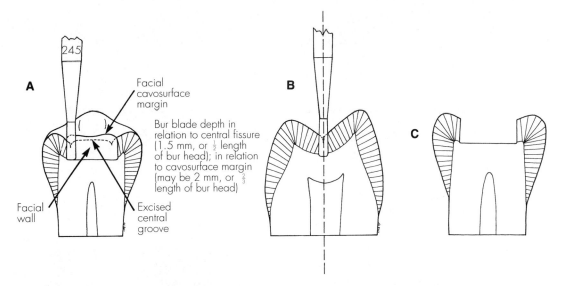

Fig. 12-2. A, Mesiodistal longitudinal seciton. Relationship of head of No. 245 bur to excised central fissure and cavosurface margin at ideal pulpal floor depth. **B,** Faciolingual longitudinal section. Dotted line indicates long axis of tooth and direction of bur. **C,** Mesiodistal longitudinal section. Pulpal floors are generally flat but may follow the rise and fall of occlusal surface.

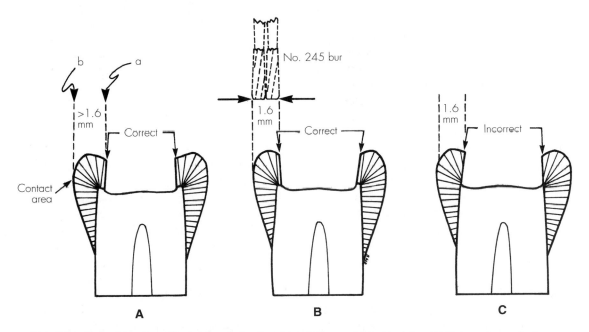

Fig. 12-3. Direction of mesial and distal walls is influenced by remaining thickness of marginal ridge as measured from mesial or distal margin (*a*) to proximal surface (imaginary projection of proximal surface, *b*). **A,** Mesial and distal walls should converge occlusally when distance form *a* to *b* is **greater than 1.6 mm. (B)** However, when operator judges that extension will leave only 1.6 mm thickness (two diameters of No. 245 bur) of marginal ridge (premolars) as illustrated both here and in Fig. 12-1, *H* and *I*, the mesial and distal walls must diverge occlusally to conserve ridge supporting dentin. **C,** Extending mesial or distal wall to two-diameter limit without diverging wall occlusally will undermine marginal ridge enamel.

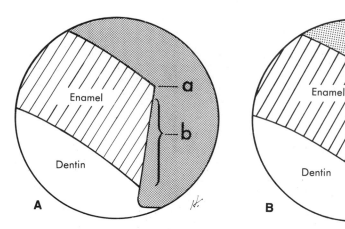

Fig. 12-4. Ideal enamel margin is formed by full-length enamel rods *(a)* resting on sound dentin supported on cavity side by shorter rods also resting on sound dentin *(b)*. This is true whether pulpal floor is in dentin **(A)** or enamel **(B)**.

tinct cavosurface margins. *A faciolingual width of no more than 1 to 1.5 mm and a depth of 1.5 to 2 mm are considered ideal.* The pulpal floor, depending on the enamel thickness, is usually in dentin (Fig. 12-1, *I*). Such conservation saves tooth structure, minimizing pulpal irritation and leaving the remaining tooth crown as strong as possible.[12,17] Although conservation of tooth structure is essential, *convenience form* requires that the extent of the preparation allows adequate access and visibility.

This completes the *initial cavity preparation. For the Class I amalgam cavity preparation, initial cavity preparation is defined as extension of the facial, lingual, mesial, and distal walls to sound tooth structure (enamel and dentin) at an ideal pulpal floor depth of 1.5 to 2 mm while providing adequate resistance and retention forms. Extension should ensure that all caries is removed from the peripheral dentinoenamel junction. For initial cavity preparation the pulpal floor should remain at ideal depth even if restorative material or caries remains* (i.e., the bur never enters deeper than described, even if its end may be in previously inserted restorative material, or infected dentin, or "AIR") (Fig. 12-5).

Resistance form is provided by (1) sufficient area(s) of relatively flat pulpal floor in sound tooth structure to resist forces directed in the long axis of the tooth, providing a strong stable seat for the restoration (refer to later section, Removal of Any Remaining Enamel Pit/Fissure and Infected Dentin); (2) minimal extension of external walls, and thus not weakening the tooth; (3) strong, ideal enamel margins (defined and illustrated previously); and (4) sufficient depth (1.5 mm) to result in adequate thickness of the restoration for its resistance to fracture and wear.

Retention form is provided by the parallelism or slight occlusal convergence of two (or more) opposing, external walls.

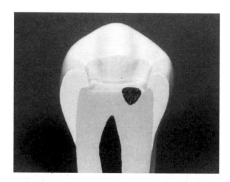

Fig. 12-5. Mesiodistal longitudinal section showing example when pulpal floor is in dentin and caries is exposed after initial cavity preparation. Note also that carious lesion is surrounded by sound dentin on the pulpal floor for resistance form.

Enameloplasty. Usually, the No. 245 bur is used for extensions into the mesiofacial and distofacial fissures. During such extensions the remaining length of the fissure can be viewed in cross section by looking at the wall being extended. When the remaining fissure is no deeper than one-quarter to one-third the thickness of the enamel, enameloplasty is indicated rather than further extension of the outline with the No. 245 bur. *Enameloplasty refers to eliminating the developmental fault by opening it using the side of a flame-shaped diamond stone leaving a smooth surface* (Fig. 12-6, *A* to *C*). This procedure frequently reduces the need for further extension into the fissures with the No. 245 bur, thereby conserving tooth structure. The extent to which enameloplasty should be used cannot be determined exactly until the process of extending into the fissured area occurs, at which time the depth of the fissure into the enamel can be observed. The surface left by enameloplasty should meet the cavity preparation wall with a cavosurface angle no greater than 100 degrees. This

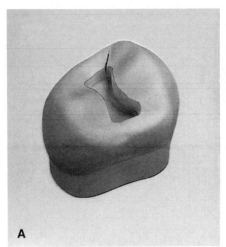
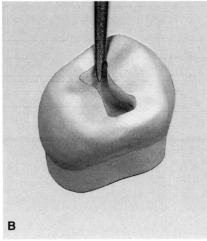
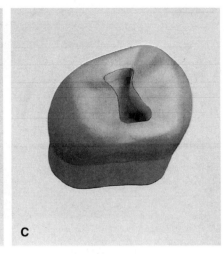

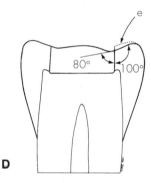

Fig. 12-6. Enameloplasty. **A,** Developmental fault at terminal end of fissure. **B,** Fine-grit diamond stone in position to remove fault. **C,** Smooth surface following enameloplasty. **D,** Cavosurface angle should not exceed 100 degrees, and marginal amalgam angle should not be less than 80 degrees. Enamel external surface *(e)* before enameloplasty.

would produce a distinct margin for amalgam of no less than 80 degrees (Fig. 12-6, *D*). During carving, amalgam should be removed from areas of enameloplasty.

If enameloplasty is unsuccessful in eliminating a mesial (or distal) fissure that extends to the crest of a marginal ridge or beyond, judgment will determine one of the following alternatives: (1) make no further change in the outline form, (2) extend through the marginal ridge when margins will be lingual to the contact (Fig. 12-7), or (3) include the fissure in a conservative Class II cavity preparation. The first alternative usually should be chosen, except for patients at high risk for caries. Enameloplasty is not indicated if a centric contact is involved. In which case, the choices are either to consider the preparation complete (an option for patients at low risk for caries) or to extend the preparation to include the fissure as previously described. (Refer to Enameloplasty, in Chapter 7.)

Final cavity preparation

Final cavity preparation includes removal from the pulpal wall any remaining defective enamel and infected dentin; pulp protection; procedures for finishing external walls; and final procedures of cleaning, inspecting, and varnishing.

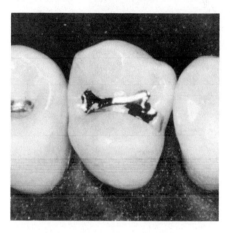

Fig. 12-7. Mesial fissure that cannot be eliminated by enameloplasty may be included in preparation if margins can be lingual of contact.

Removal of any remaining enamel pit/fissure and infected dentin. Any remaining enamel pit/fissure in the pulpal floor should be removed. If several enamel pit/fissure remnants remain in the floor, or if a central fissure remnant extends over most of the floor, deepen the floor with the No. 245 bur to eliminate the fault(s) or to uncover the caries to a maximal preparation depth of 2 mm (Fig. 12-8). However, if the pit and fissure remnants are few and small, remove them with a suitably sized, round carbide bur (Fig. 12-9). Removal of the remaining infected dentin (caries that extends pulpally from the established pulpal floor) is best accomplished using a discoid-type ***spoon excavator*** or a slowly re-

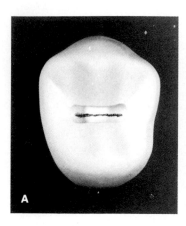
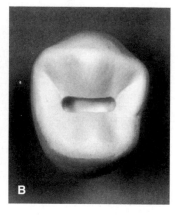

Fig. 12-8. Removal of enamel fissure extending over most of pulpal floor. **A,** Full-length occlusal fissure remnant remaining on pulpal floor after initial cavity preparation. **B** and **C,** Pulpal floor is deepened to maximal depth of 2 mm to eliminate the fissure or uncover dentinal caries.

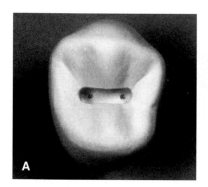
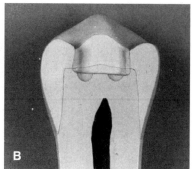

Fig. 12-9. Removal of enamel pit/fissure and infected dentin that is limited to a few small pit and fissure remnants. **A,** Two pit remnants remain on pulpal floor after initial cavity preparation. **B,** Defective enamel and infected dentin have been removed.

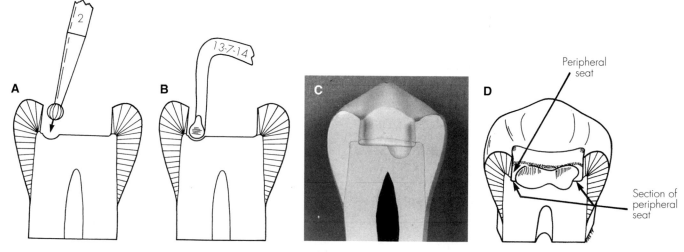

Fig. 12-10. Removal of dentinal caries is accomplished with round burs **(A)** or spoon excavators **(B). (C),** and **D,** Resistance form requires flat floor peripheral to excavated area(s).

volving, round carbide bur of appropriate size (Fig. 12-10, *A* and *B*). Using the largest instrument that fits the carious area is safest because it is least likely to penetrate the tooth uncontrollably. *When removing infected dentin, stop the excavation when a hard or firm feel to tooth structure is achieved (i.e., the same feel as sound dentin). This often occurs before all stained or discolored dentin is removed.[9] Ensure that caries is removed from the peripheral dentinoenamel junction where it is less visible than on the pulpal floor. A sharp explorer or hand instrument is more reliable than a rotating bur in judging the adequacy of removal of infected dentin.*

The removal of carious dentin should not affect resistance form if the restoration has a seat on a flat floor peripheral to the excavated area(s). It is emphasized that the flat floor should be at the ideal, previously described pulpal floor depth of 1.5 to 2 mm and in sound enamel or dentin (Fig. 12-10, *C*). If the flat seat cannot be established around the entire circumference of the excavation(s), then an attempt should be made to establish at least three flat seats with the No. 245 bur equally spaced around the periphery of the excavation to maintain satisfactory resistance form (Fig. 12-10, *D*).

Pulp protection. If the cavity preparation is of ideal depth, no *liner* or *base* is indicated. *In moderately deep carious excavations (where the remaining dentin thickness is judged to be 1 mm or more) place a thin layer (0.5 to 0.75 mm) of a quick-setting zinc oxide–eugenol cement.* The cement is picked up on the end of a blunt-tipped periodontal probe or cement-placing instrument and inserted in small increments. The cement should flow when it is touched to the dentin. It can be teased to place over the desired area (Fig. 12-11). The zinc oxide–eugenol cement liner provides insulation for the pulp from rapid thermal changes[14] and also acts as an obtundent.[39] Never cover an entire pulpal floor with zinc oxide–eugenol cement because the cement is not strong enough to support an amalgam restoration subjected to heavy occlusal forces. Recall that the amalgam

under occlusal loading should be supported by seats in sound tooth structure peripheral to the cement. No other base material is required.[3,27,36,47]

Procedures for finishing external walls. The external walls have already been finished during earlier steps in this conservative cavity preparation for amalgam. An occlusal cavosurface bevel is contraindicated in the cavity preparation for an amalgam restoration.[19] It is important to provide a 90- to 100-degree **cavosurface angle,**[10] which should result in 80- to 90-degree amalgam at the margins. Clinical experience has established that this butt joint margin of enamel and amalgam is the strongest. Amalgam is a brittle material with low edge strength and tends to chip under occlusal stress if its angle at the margins is less than 80 degrees.

Final procedures: cleaning; inspecting; varnishing. A final inspection of the preparation is advocated. The cavity preparation should be free of debris and visible moisture. It has been demonstrated that air-water spray is effective in removing bacteria from the cavity preparation. A cavity disinfectant is unnecessary.[45]

Apply two layers of **cavity varnish** *before inserting the amalgam.* Form a cotton pellet small enough to fit into the preparation. Holding the pellet with sterile (to prevent contamination of varnish in the bottle) cotton pliers, touch the surface of the varnish for absorption (do not "load" the beaks), blot the excess varnish from the pellet, and place the pellet into the preparation. Quickly, use an explorer tip to move the pellet over the cavity walls (enamel and dentinal) to apply an even coating (Fig. 12-12). After drying this coating with the air syringe, the procedure is repeated. It has been demonstrated that two applications of cavity varnish provide a more complete seal of the dentinal tubules.[32] Varnish that has become viscous should be thinned before use by adding acetone or solvent provided by the manufacturer.* The application of varnish reduces microleakage

*Copalite, Harry J. Bosworth Company, Skokie, Ill.

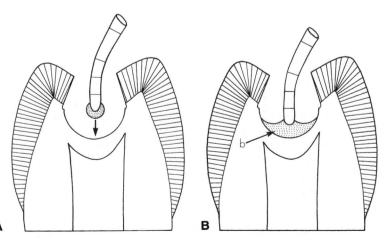

A   **B**

Fig. 12-11. Bases/liners. **A,** Inserting zinc oxide–eugenol cement with Williams periodontal probe. **B,** In moderately deep excavations a base *(b)* thickness of 0.5 to 0.75 mm is indicated.

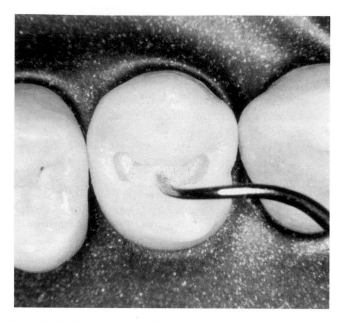

Fig. 12-12. Insert any required base/liner followed by two coats of cavity varnish. Use explorer tip to manipulate small cotton pellet, wet with varnish, throughout cavity preparation.

between the restoration and the cavity walls immediately after condensation.[2,8,32,47] Pashley has written that cavity varnish reduces microleakage whether or not the smear layer is removed.[30] Postoperative microleakage can result in tooth sensitivity and pulpal inflammation.

In lieu of cavity varnish, recent studies have indicated that it is possible to bond amalgam to the enamel and dentin preparation walls by new dentin adhesive systems[43] and other resin/metal adhesives containing 4-META. Bonding the amalgam can increase the fracture resistance of the restored tooth[7] and reduce microleakage.[2] Ben-Amar states that longevity of this bond in the oral environment should be evaluated; and further advises that most well-manipulated and well-placed amalgams (using cavity varnish) do not exhibit microleakage after a time.[2] More regarding resin bonding of amalgam is presented in Chapter 13. It is recognized that different from the application of cavity varnish, the *application of the resin-based bonding agent follows etching the preparation walls, rinsing, and removing excess water, whereupon immediately the freshly mixed amalgam is inserted and condensed, resulting in* the autopolymerizing bonding agent mechanically interlocking with the amalgam as well as the etched preparation surfaces.

CAVITY PREPARATION FOR EXTENSIVE CARIES

Caries is extensive if the distance between infected dentin and the pulp is judged to be less than 1 mm. The following treatment is indicated as soon as possible, as-

suming the pulp is vital and *not* severely diseased (not exhibiting irreversible pulpitis). (Refer to Chapters 2, 3, 5, and 7 for diagnosis of pulpitis.)

Isolation of the operating site

The rubber dam should be used for isolation of the operating site where caries is extensive.[11] If caries excavation exposes the pulp, capping the exposure will be more often successful in maintaining a vital pulp if the site is isolated with a properly applied rubber dam. Also, the dam will prevent moisture contamination of the amalgam mix during insertion.[32]

Initial cavity preparation

With extensive caries, concern during initial cavity preparation regarding outline, resistance, and retention forms is sometimes deferred until after the excavation of infected dentin and the insertion of a base. The reason is to protect the pulp as early as possible from the insult of cavity preparation.

Outline, primary resistance, and primary retention forms. Using a No. 245 bur at high speed with air-water spray and oriented with its long axis parallel to the long axis of the tooth crown, prepare the outline, primary resistance, and primary retention forms, *maintaining a depth of 1.5 to 2 mm* (measured 1.5 mm at any pit or fissure and up to 2 mm on the prepared external walls). The cutting is extended laterally to remove all enamel undermined by caries by alternately cutting and examining the lateral extension of the caries. It may be necessary to alter the bur's long axis to prepare a 90- to 100-degree cavosurface angle (Fig. 12-13, *A*).

Enameloplasty. If indicated, use enameloplasty. (Refer to Enameloplasty in previous section, Conservative Cavity Preparations.)

Final cavity preparation

Removal of remaining infected dentin. Remove the remaining infected dentin in the same manner as described previously for the conservative preparation with the following exception: cease removing caries in a pulpal direction if a pulpal exposure is expected. This may be determined with the aid of a radiograph and the appearance of a pinkish hue to the dentin. A pulpal exposure is undesirable because it often introduces foreign matter into the pulp and desiccates the pulp, thereby jeopardizing its health. If an exposure occurs, the operator must decide whether to apply a ***direct pulp cap*** of ***calcium hydroxide*** to the exposure or to treat the tooth by root canal therapy. (For factors influencing this decision, see Caries Control Restoration, Chapter 3.)

Pulp protection. *Use a nonpressure flow technique to insert a 0.5 to 0.75 mm minimal thickness of a quick-setting calcium hydroxide material as a base to cover all areas of near exposure or exposure (Fig. 12-13,*

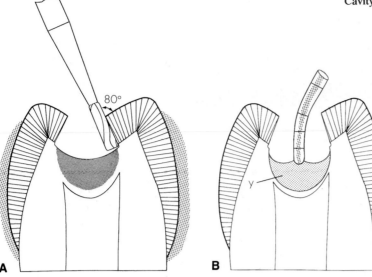

Fig. 12-13. A, Initial cavity preparation with extensive caries. When extending laterally to remove enamel undermined by caries, alter bur's long axis to prepare 90- to 100-degree cavosurface angle. A 100-degree cavosurface angle on cuspal incline will result in 80-degree marginal amalgam angle. **B,** In excavations having a potential or actual pulpal exposure, insert a quick-setting calcium hydroxide base *(y)* of 0.5 to 0.75 mm minimal thickness.

B).[25] Evidence indicates that Dycal* has the strength[3] and the thermal insulating capacity at that thickness[14,31] to serve as the sole base.[32] Furthermore, at a thickness of 1 mm over an exposure as wide as 2 mm, it will resist intrusion of the filling material into the pulp during amalgam condensation.[25] Insertion of a *spherical* type of *amalgam* is recommended in a tooth having a direct pulp cap because less condensation pressure is required.

Secondary resistance and retention forms. Recall that primary resistance form was obtained by extending the outline of the cavity preparation to include only undermined and defective tooth structure, while preparing strong enamel walls and allowing strong cuspal areas to remain. If the excavation of infected dentin has removed most or all of the flat pulpal floor that was initially prepared, establish at least three flat seats in dentin (0.2 mm from the dentinoenamel junction) somewhat equally spaced around the periphery of the excavation to provide *secondary resistance form* in sound tooth structure at the pulpal wall level.[41]

Primary *retention* was obtained by the occlusal convergence of the enamel walls. Secondary retention is undercut areas that are sometimes left in dentin following removal of infected dentin and that are not covered by the base.

Procedures for finishing external walls. Refer to earlier section, Procedures for Finishing External Walls, under Conservative Cavity Preparations.

Final procedures: cleaning; inspecting; varnishing. Attention to cleaning and inspecting the preparation is indicated, followed by application of two coats of varnish to the cavity preparation as described previously for the conservative cavity preparation.

The reader is referred to this same step in cavity preparation in the previous section, Conservative Cavity Preparations, for a discussion regarding the use of a resin-based bonding agent rather than varnish.

*Dycal, The L.D. Caulk Company, Milford, Del.

MERCURY HYGIENE

Because of concern about **mercury exposure** in the dental office, precautions should be taken to protect the patient and the dental staff.[5] When removing an amalgam restoration, a rubber dam should be in place and air-water spray and high-volume evacuation should be used. Air-water spray and high-volume evacuation should also be used when finishing an amalgam restoration. Glasses and disposable face masks should be worn to reduce hazards associated with flying particles and the inhalation of amalgam dust. Amalgam capsules that allow mercury leakage during trituration should not be used. Amalgamators that completely enclose the arms and amalgam capsule during trituration should be used. Free mercury and amalgam scraps should be stored in an unbreakable, tightly closed container away from any source of heat. Since mercury vaporizes at room temperature, operatories should be well ventilated to minimize the mercury level in the air. An annual mercury assessment for personnel regularly employed in the dental office is encouraged (see also Chapter 6, Mercury Management, in the Dental Amalgam section).

PREPARATION OF AMALGAM

Because of its superior clinical performance, **high-copper amalgam** is recommended. Amalgam should be triturated according to the manufacturer's directions. It is often necessary to make additional mixes (as needed) to complete the restoration, particularly for large preparations. Empty the triturated amalgam into a dappen dish or an amalgam well. It is not necessary to squeeze excess mercury from the mix when using controlled mercury systems (Fig. 12-14, *A*). Correctly mixed amalgam should not be dry and crumbly. It will have a minimal, yet sufficient, "wetness" to aid in achieving a homogeneous and well-adapted restoration.[32] Excess mercury in the mix is contraindicated. Nadal[26] has

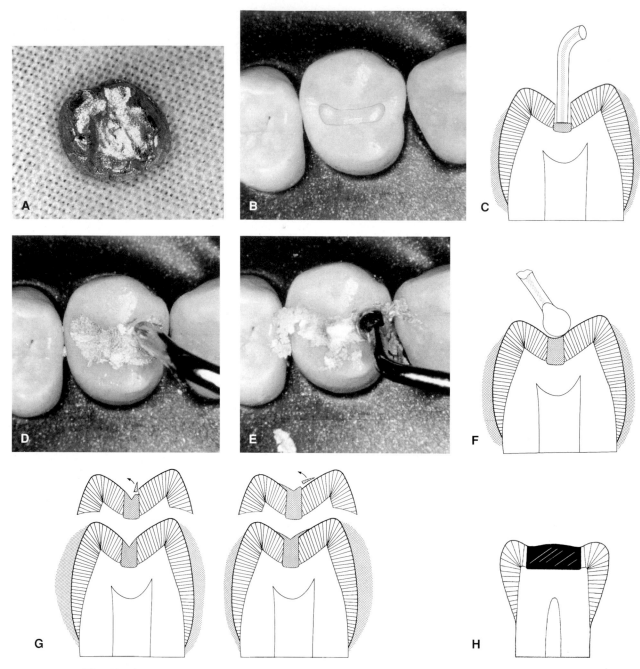

Fig. 12-14. Restoration of occlusal cavity preparation. **A,** Properly triturated amalgam is a homogeneous mass with slightly reflective surface. It flattens slightly if dropped on a table top. **B,** Operator should have a mental image of outline form of preparation before condensing amalgam to aid in locating cavosurface margins during carving procedure. **C,** Amalgam should be inserted incrementally and condensed with overlapping strokes. **D,** Cavity preparation should be overpacked to ensure well-condensed marginal amalgam that is not mercury rich. **E,** Precarve burnishing with large burnisher is a form of condensation. **F,** Carver should rest partially on external tooth surface adjacent to margins to prevent overcarving. **G,** Deep occlusal grooves invite chipping of amalgam at margins. Thin portions of amalgam left on external surfaces soon break away, giving the appearance that amalgam has grown out of cavity. **H,** Carve fossae slightly deeper than proximal marginal ridges.

shown that more marginal deterioration and surface roughness occur among restorations with a high mercury content.

INSERTION OF AMALGAM

Before inserting the amalgam, review the outline of the cavity preparation to form a mental image that will aid later in carving the amalgam to the cavosurface margin (Fig. 12-14, *B*). Use an *amalgam carrier* to transfer amalgam to the cavity preparation. *Increments extruded from the carrier should be smaller (often only half or less of a full carrier tip) for a small preparation, particularly during the initial insertion.* Use a flat-faced, circular, or elliptical **condenser** to condense the amalgam over the pulpal floor of the preparation. Be careful to condense the amalgam into the pulpal line angles (Fig. 12-14, *C*). *The initial condenser should be small enough to condense into the line angles, but large enough not to "poke holes" in the amalgam mass.* Usually a smaller condenser is used while filling the preparation and a larger one for overpacking. Thoroughly condense each portion extruded from the carrier before placing the next increment. Each condensed increment should fill only one-third to one-half the cavity depth. *Each condensing stroke should overlap the previous condensing stroke to ensure that the entire mass is well condensed.* The condensation pressure required will depend on the amalgam used and the diameter of the **condenser nib.** *Condensers with larger diameter nibs require greater condensation pressure.* The preparation should be overpacked 1 mm or more using heavy pressure (Fig. 12-14, *D*). This will ensure that the cavosurface margins are completely covered with well-condensed amalgam. Final condensation over cavosurface margins should be done perpendicular to the external enamel surface adjacent to the margins.

Condensation of a mix should be completed within the time specified by the manufacturer, which is usually 2½ to 3½ minutes. Otherwise, crystallization of the unused portion will be too advanced to react properly (chemically bond) with the condensed portion. Discard the mix if it becomes dry, and quickly make another mix to continue the insertion.

PRECARVE BURNISHING PROCEDURE

Precarve burnishing is a form of condensation. As stated previously, cavity preparations should be overfilled with amalgam. To ensure that the marginal amalgam is well condensed before carving, the overpacked amalgam should be burnished immediately with a large burnisher using heavy strokes mesiodistally and faciolingually. To maximize its effectiveness, the burnisher head should be large enough that in the final strokes it will contact the cusp slopes but not the margins (Fig. 12-14, *E*). Precarve burnishing produces denser amalgam at the margins of occlusal preparations restored with high-copper amalgam alloys.[1,18]

CARVING PROCEDURE

With care, carving may begin immediately following condensation. Sharp discoid-cleoid instruments of suitable radii are recommended carvers. Use the larger discoid-cleoid instrument (No. 3-6) first, followed by the smaller instrument (No. 4-5) in regions not accessible to the larger instrument. *All carving should be done with the edge of the blade perpendicular to the margins as the instrument is moved parallel to the margins. Part of the edge of the carving blade should rest on the unprepared tooth surface adjacent to the cavity margin* (Fig. 12-14, *F*). Using this surface as a guide helps to prevent overcarving the amalgam at the margins and to produce a continuity of surface contour across the margins.

Deep occlusal grooves should not be carved into the restoration, since these weaken the restoration and invite chipping of the thinned-out amalgam at the occlusal margins (Fig. 12-14, *G*). Undercarving leaves thin portions of amalgam on the unprepared tooth surface that will break away giving the appearance that the amalgam has expanded beyond the preparation. The mesial and distal fossae should be carved slightly deeper than the proximal marginal ridges (Fig. 12-14, *H*).

After carving, the outline of the amalgam margin should reflect the contour and location of the prepared cavosurface margin, revealing a regular (unragged) outline with gentle curves. It is important to recall the mental image of the preparation outline form. An amalgam outline that is larger or irregular is undercarved and requires further carving or finishing (Fig. 12-15). An amalgam restoration that is more than minimally overcarved (a submarginal defect greater than 0.2 mm) should be replaced.[35]

If total carving time is short enough, the smoothness of the carved surface may be improved by wiping with a small damp ball of cotton held in the operating pliers. All shavings from the carving procedure should be removed from the mouth with the aid of the oral evacuator.

POSTCARVE BURNISHING PROCEDURE

Postcarve burnishing is the light rubbing of the carved surface with a burnisher of suitable size and shape to improve smoothness and produce a satin (not shiny) appearance. Postcarve burnishing produces denser amalgam at the margins of occlusal preparations restored with conventional (low-copper) amalgam alloys.[16] Postcarve burnishing in conjunction with pre-

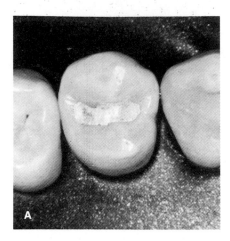
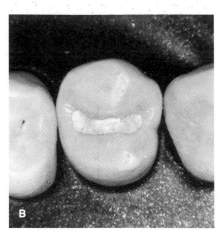

Fig. 12-15. **A,** Undercarved amalgam with flash beyond margins. Note that restoration outline is irregular and larger than cavity outline in Fig. 12-14, *B*. **B,** Correctly carved amalgam restoration.

carve burnishing of conventional alloys may serve as a viable substitute for conventional polishing.[22] With high-copper amalgams, postcarve burnishing is unnecessary because burnishing techniques have been shown to have no significant effect on the clinical performance of high-copper amalgams at 2 years.[23]

OCCLUSION OF RESTORATION

After completion of the carving and during the removal of rubber dam or cotton rolls, the patient is advised not to bite because of the danger of fracturing the restoration, which is weak at this stage. Even if the carving has been carefully accomplished, the restoration occasionally will be "high," indicating a premature occlusal contact. Whenever possible, visually inspect the contact potential of the restored tooth and assess the extent of closure. To ensure that the occlusion is correct, place a piece of articulating paper over the restoration, and instruct the patient to *close very lightly.* If anesthesia is still present, it may be difficult for the patient to tell when the teeth are in contact. High spots will be marked, which are then removed by additional carving. The process of light closure with articulating paper is repeated, and additional carving is accomplished until the patient can close the teeth to prerestoration occlusion. While carving, attempt to establish stable, centric-holding contacts where indicated. These contacts should be perpendicular to the direction of occlusal load where possible. If the contact area is on an incline (not perpendicular to occlusal load), try, when carving away excess amalgam, either to remove the undesirable portion of the contact area (that on an incline) or to carve a plateau perpendicular to the direction of load. Guard against carving centric contacts out of occlusion (Fig. 12-16). Finally, caution the patient to protect the restoration from any heavy biting pressure for several hours.

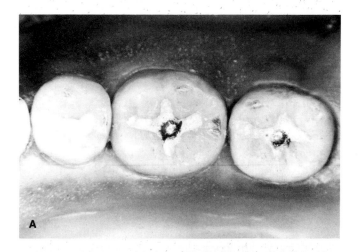
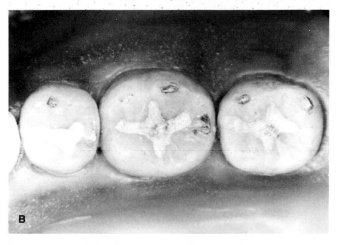

Fig. 12-16. Occluding the restoration. **A,** Heavy occlusal contacts on new amalgam should be avoided. Articulating paper will mark heavy contacts as dark areas and very heavy contacts as dark areas having shiny centers. **B,** Amalgam should not be carved out of occlusion. Rather, it should have light occlusal contact(s) as indicated by faint markings.

FINISHING AND POLISHING PROCEDURES

Not all amalgam restorations require finishing and polishing. However, these procedures are occasionally necessary (1) to complete the carving, (2) refine the anatomy, contours, and marginal integrity, and (3) enhance the surface texture of the restoration. Finishing and polishing procedures for amalgam restorations are not attempted within 24 hours of insertion, since crystallization is not complete.[32] Often, these procedures are delayed until all of the patient's restorations have been placed, rather than finishing and polishing periodically during the course of treatment. An amalgam restoration is less prone to tarnish and corrosion if a smooth, homogeneous surface is achieved.[10,32,46] Polishing of high-copper amalgams is less important[4,6,13,24,40] than with conventional amalgams, because high-copper amalgams are less susceptible to tarnish and marginal breakdown.[28,29]

During carving, the margins are located and the desired contours and occlusion are developed. Finishing and polishing significantly reduces the roughness of a carved restoration. These procedures must not leave the restoration undercontoured, and must not alter the centric holding contacts. The final anatomy of the polished restoration should be patterned after normal occlusal contours. After polishing is completed, the tip of an explorer should pass from the tooth surface to the restoration surface, and vice versa, without jumping or catching. There should be a perfect continuity of contour across the margin, which is a requirement of all restorations.

Begin the finishing procedure by marking the occlusion with articulating paper and evaluating the margins with an explorer. If the occlusion can be improved or there is not a perfect continuity of surface contour across the margins, a pointed, white, fused *alumina stone* or a green *carborundum stone* is used to correct the discrepancy (Fig. 12-17, *A*). The green stone is more abrasive than the white stone. *During surfacing of the amalgam, the stone's long axis is held at a right angle to the margins. Guard against reducing any centric holding area.* After the stone is used, the margins should be reevaluated with an explorer tine. If no discrepancy is detected, the area should be further surfaced using a light touch with a suitably shaped *finishing bur* (Fig. 12-17, *B*). If the groove and fossa features are not sufficiently defined, accentuate them by lightly using a small round finishing bur without reducing the centric holding areas. A flame-shaped finishing bur may be used on accessible margins. The bur should be held perpendicular to the margin to allow the unprepared tooth structure to guide the bur and prevent unnecessary removal of amalgam (Fig. 12-17, *C*). A smooth surface

should be achieved before the polishing procedure is initiated.

Initiate the polishing procedure by using a coarse, *rubber abrasive point* at low speed to produce an amalgam surface with a smooth, satiny appearance (Fig. 12-17, *D* and *E*). If the amalgam surface does not exhibit this appearance after only a few seconds of polishing, the surface was too rough at the start. In this instance, resurfacing with a finishing bur is necessary, followed with the coarse, rubber abrasive point to develop the satiny appearance. *It is important that the rubber points be used at low speed or "stall out" speed for two reasons: (1) the danger of the point disintegrating at high speeds, and (2) the danger of elevating the temperature of the restoration and the tooth.* An excessive temperature rise (above 140° F [60° C]) can cause irreparable damage to the pulp and/or restoration. When overheated, the surface of the amalgam will appear cloudy even though it may have a high polish. This cloudy appearance indicates that mercury has been brought to the surface, which results in corrosion of the amalgam and loss of strength.[32]

After polishing with the coarse, abrasive rubber point, there should be no deep scratches on the amalgam surface, only the moderately polished surface left by the rubber point. Also, there should be the perfect continuity of contour from tooth to restoration as tested by the explorer tip.

After the area is washed free of abrasive particles, a high polish may be imparted to the restoration with a series of medium- and fine-grit abrasive points (Fig. 12-17, *F*). As with the more abrasive points, the finer abrasive points must be used at low speed. *If a high luster does not appear within a few seconds, the restoration requires additional polishing with the more abrasive points.* The system that is illustrated includes coarse-, medium-, and fine-grit rubber abrasive points. Using these points in sequence from coarse to fine will produce an amalgam surface with a brilliant luster (Fig. 12-17, *G*). Instead of rubber abrasive points, final polishing may be accomplished using a rubber cup with *flour of pumice* followed by a high-luster agent, such as *precipitated chalk*.

Finishing may be indicated to improve the contour, margins, surface, or anatomy of older, existing restorations (Fig. 12-18, *A* and *B*). Occlusal contours of amalgam restorations that have expanded beyond the cavosurface margins, or that were originally undercarved may be corrected with abrasive stones and finishing burs. Margins exhibiting minimal ditching may be refined and rough surfaces smoothed. Round finishing burs are recommended to correct poorly defined anatomy. Polishing of older, existing restorations is infrequently indicated.

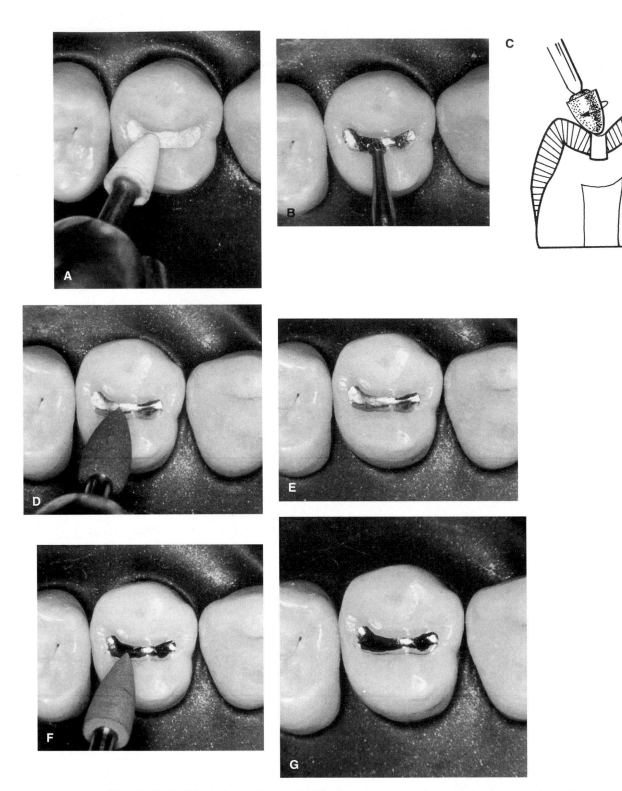

Fig. 12-17. Polishing the amalgam. **A,** When necessary, use fine-grit alumina or carborundum stone to develop continuity of surface from tooth to restoration. **B,** Surface the restoration with round finishing bur. **C,** The stone's or bur's long axis is held at a right angle to the margin. **D,** Initiate polishing with coarse, rubber abrasive point at low speed. **E,** Point should produce smooth, satiny appearance. **F,** Obtain high polish with medium- and fine-grit abrasive points. **G,** Polished restoration.

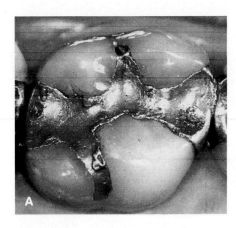 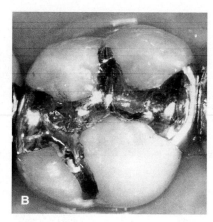

Fig. 12-18. A, Existing amalgam restoration exhibiting marginal deterioration and surface roughness. B, Same restoration after finishing and polishing.

OCCLUSOLINGUAL CAVITY PREPARATION AND RESTORATION
Isolation of the operating site

The advantages of using the rubber dam have been discussed in Chapter 10. Following evaluation of the occlusal contacts and local anesthesia, apply the rubber dam isolating enough teeth to provide access and visibility. Usually, when operating on the maxillary first molar, the operator isolates four teeth (second molar to first premolar). Some operators prefer to include the teeth from second molar around to the opposite lateral incisor in the isolation.

Initial cavity preparation

Outline, primary resistance, and primary retention forms. *The occlusolingual (OL) cavity preparation on maxillary molars* is indicated when the distal pit and distal oblique and lingual fissures are connected and carious or at caries-risk (Fig. 12-19). Accepted principles of *outline form* previously stated are to be observed

with special attention to the following: (1) the cavity preparation should be no wider than necessary (ideally the mesiodistal width should not exceed 1 mm, except for extension necessary to remove carious or undermined enamel or to include unusual fissuring), (2) when indicated, the cavity preparation should be cut more at the expense of the oblique ridge rather than centering over the fissure, (3) especially on smaller teeth, the occlusal portion may have a slight distal tilt (Fig. 12-20), and (4) the margins should extend as little as possible onto the oblique ridge, distolingual cusp, and distal marginal ridge. Such objectives help to conserve the dentinal support and strength of the tooth, aid in establishing an enamel cavosurface angle as close as possible to 90 degrees (not to exceed 100 degrees) (Fig. 12-21), and help to minimize marginal deterioration of the restoration by locating the margins away from enamel eminences where occlusal forces may be concentrated.

Using the mirror for indirect vision and the high-speed handpiece with air-water spray, enter the distal pit with the end of the No. 245 bur (Fig. 12-22, *A*). The

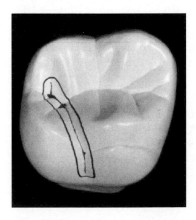

Fig. 12-19. Outline of margins for occlusolingual cavity preparation.

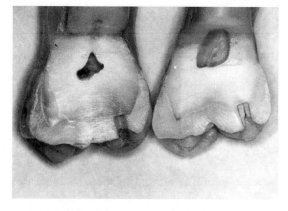

Fig. 12-20. Small distal inclination of bur on smaller teeth may be indicated to conserve dentinal support and strength of marginal ridge.

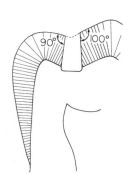

Fig. 12-21. Enamel cavosurface angles of 90 degrees are ideal and should not exceed 100 degrees.

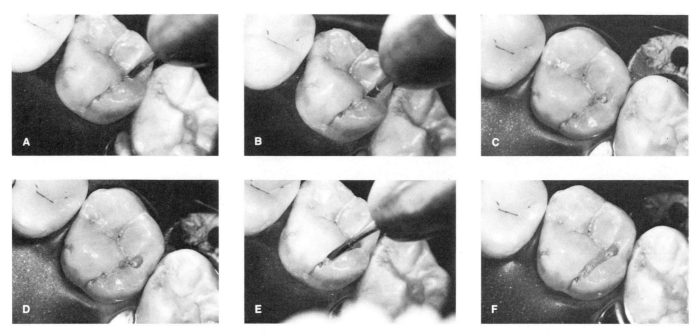

Fig. 12-22. Occlusolingual cavity preparation. **A,** No. 245 bur positioned for entry. **B,** Penetrate to minimal depth of 1.5 to 2 mm. **C,** Entry cut. **D,** Remaining fissures facial to point of entry are removed with same bur. **E** and **F,** Cut lingually along fissure until bur has extended the preparation onto lingual surface.

long axis of the bur usually should be parallel to the long axis of the tooth crown. *Remember to conserve the dentinal support and strength of the distal marginal ridge. Recall that this may indicate directing the bur so that it is cutting more of the tooth structure mesial to the pit rather than distal (e.g., 70/30 rather than 50/50).* For the same reason, on smaller teeth a small distal tilt to the bur is sometimes indicated. Penetrate to a depth of 1.5 to 2 mm as measured by the bur on the cut walls (1.5 mm at the fissure and 2 mm on the external walls) (Fig. 12-22, *B*). At this depth the pulpal floor may or may not be in dentin. Once the entry cut is made (Fig. 12-22, *C*), move the bur (always maintaining the established depth) to include any remaining fissures facial to the point of entry (Fig. 12-22, *D*). However, remember to utilize *enameloplasty* if indicated. Next, at the same depth, move the bur along the fissure toward the lingual surface (Fig. 12-22, *E*). Remember that a slight distal inclination of the bur will sometimes be indicated (smaller teeth) to conserve the dentinal support and strength of the marginal ridge as well as the distolingual cusp. To ensure adequate strength to the marginal ridge the distopulpal line angle must not approach the distal surface closer than 2 mm. On large molars the bur should remain parallel to the long axis of the tooth, particularly if the bur is offset slightly mesial to the center of the fissure. Remember, the objective is to conserve dentinal support of the oblique ridge and the

distal wall. Keeping the bur parallel to the long axis of the tooth creates a distal wall with a slight occlusal convergence providing favorable enamel and amalgam angles. Continue to move the bur lingually along the fissure, maintaining a uniform depth, until the bur has extended the preparation onto the lingual surface (Fig. 12-22, *F*). The pulpal floor should follow the contour of the occlusal surface and, depending on enamel thickness, usually will be in dentin.

The mesial and distal walls of this occlusal portion of the preparation should converge occlusally toward each other corresponding to the shape of the bur. This convergence provides sufficient retention form to the occlusal portion of the preparation. If the slight distal bur tilt was required, the mesial and distal walls should still converge relative to each other, although the distal wall may be divergent occlusally relative to the tooth's long axis.

Next, prepare the lingual portion with the bur's long axis parallel with the lingual surface (Fig. 12-23, *A* and *B*). The tip of the bur should be located at the gingival extent of the lingual fissure. Be careful to control the bur and not allow it to "roll out" onto the lingual surface, since this could "round over" or damage the cavosurface margin. Using the bur at high speed to prepare the lingual portion usually prevents this occurrence. The facial inclination of the bur must be altered as the cutting progresses to establish the axial wall of the lingual

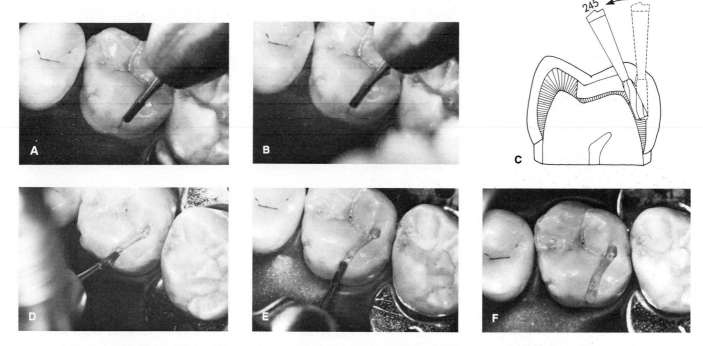

Fig. 12-23. Occlusolingual cavity preparation. **A,** Position of bur to cut lingual portion. **B,** Initial entry of bur for cutting lingual portion. **C,** Alter inclination of bur to establish correct axial wall depth. **D** and **E,** Direct bur perpendicular to axial wall to accentuate mesioaxial and distoaxial line angles. **F,** Axial wall depth should be maintained at 1.5 mm.

portion at a uniform depth of 1.5 mm (Fig. 12-23, *C*). The axial wall should follow the contour of the lingual surface of the tooth.

Use the No. 245 bur with its long axis perpendicular to the axial wall to accentuate (refine) the mesioaxial and distoaxial line angles and to make the mesial and distal walls slightly undercut (depthwise) due to the shape of the bur (Fig. 12-23, *D* and *E*). During this step the axial wall depth of 1.5 mm is not altered (Fig. 12-23, *F*).

Keeping the bur perpendicular to the tooth surface, round the axiopulpal line angle (Fig. 12-24). Leaving a sharp line angle increases the possibility of fracture of the restorative material because of inadequate preparation depth and because of stress concentration. Initial cavity preparation of the occlusolingual preparation is now complete.

Enameloplasty. If indicated, and as mentioned in the previous section, utilize enameloplasty to conserve tooth structure and limit extension.

Final cavity preparation

Removal of any remaining enamel pit/fissure and infected dentin. Remove any remaining enamel pit/fissure and infected dentin on the pulpal and axial walls (Fig. 12-25, *A* and *B*) by using a suitably-sized round bur or discoid-type spoon excavator, or both.

Pulp protection. Placing a base/liner in the occlusolingual cavity preparation is similar to the procedure previously described for the occlusal cavity preparation. Necessary base/liners for the axial and pulpal walls are placed by the flow technique.

Secondary resistance and retention forms. Removal of remaining caries in the dentin should not affect resis-

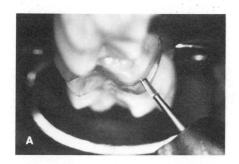
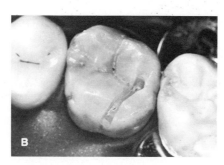

Fig. 12-24. A, Bur position for rounding axiopulpal line angle. **B,** Axiopulpal line angle rounded.

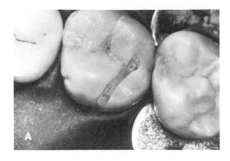

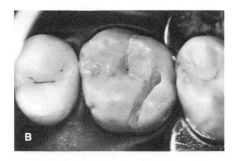

Fig. 12-25. A, Remove any remaining enamel pit/fissure and infected dentin on established pulpal and axial walls. B, Completed cavity preparation.

tance form if flat pulpal wall seats are present or prepared in sound tooth structure peripheral to the excavated areas.

If additional retention is required, the No. ¼ bur can be used to prepare locks into the mesioaxial and distoaxial line angles (Fig. 12-26, A). If these angles are in enamel the axial wall must be deepened to 0.2 mm pulpally of the dentinoenamel junction because the locks must be cut in dentin, and they must not undermine enamel. The depth of the locks at the gingival floor is the offset (minimum) to one-half the diameter of the No. ¼ bur. The cutting direction for each lock is the bisector of the respective line angle. The lock is slightly deeper pulpally than the correctly positioned axial wall and is 0.2 mm pulpal to the dentinoenamel junction. The locks should diminish in depth toward the occlusal surface terminating midway along the axial wall (Fig. 12-26, B). Test the adequacy of the lock by inserting the tine of an explorer into the lock and moving it lingually. The mesial or distal depth of the lock should prevent the explorer from being withdrawn directly to the lingual.

If unusual extension of a facial occlusal fissure dictated a slight divergence occlusally to the facial wall (to conserve support of the facial ridge), the side of a No. 33½ bur may be used to enhance retention form in the occlusal portion by preparing a small cove in the faciopulpal line angle (Fig. 12-26, C and D). The tip of the No. 245 bur held parallel to the long axis of the tooth crown may also be used to prepare this cove. Be careful not to undermine the occlusal enamel. This retentive cove is recommended if occlusal convergence of the mesial and distal walls of the occlusal portion is absent or inadequate.

Procedures for finishing external walls. Refer to earlier section, Procedures for Finishing External Walls, under Conservative Cavity Preparations.

Final procedures: cleaning; inspecting; varnishing. Careful inspection of the preparation may reveal areas that need cleaning or additional finishing. For example, any irregularities at the margins usually indicate weak enamel that should be smoothed by the side of the No. 245 bur rotating at slow speed. Fig. 12-25, B, illustrates the completed preparation that has received two applications of

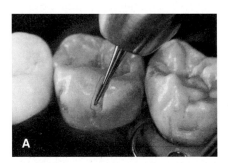

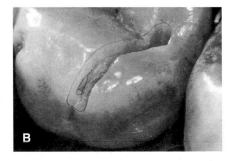

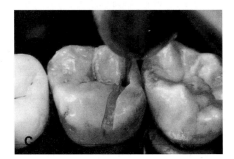

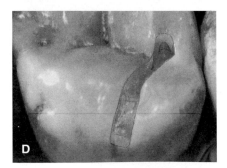

Fig. 12-26. Secondary retention form. A, Bur position for cutting lock in mesioaxial line angle. B, Completed lock. C, Bur position for retentive cove in faciopulpal line angle. D, Completed cove.

cavity varnish as previously described for the conservative occlusal cavity preparation.

Insertion and carving procedures

Using a rigid *matrix* to support the lingual portion of the restoration during condensation is desirable. A matrix is helpful to prevent "landsliding" during condensation and to ensure marginal adaptation and strength of the restoration. *A matrix should possess certain qualities. It should (1) be easy to apply and remove, (2) be rigid to resist condensation pressures, and (3) provide proper contour.* The *Tofflemire matrix retainer* is used to secure a matrix band to the tooth, as described in Chapter 13. Since this type of matrix band does not intimately adapt to the lingual groove area of the tooth (Fig. 12-27, *A*), an additional step may be necessary to provide a matrix that is rigid on the lingual portion of the cavity preparation. Cut a piece of stainless steel matrix material (0.002 inch [0.05 mm] thick, ⁵⁄₁₆ inch [8 mm] wide) that will fit between the lingual surface of the tooth and the band already in place (Fig. 12-27, *B*). Place the gingival edge of this segment of matrix material slightly gingival to the gingival edge of the band to help secure the band segment. Break off approximately ½ inch (12.7 mm) of a round toothpick, holding it in the beaks of the No. 110 pliers. Heat the end of a stick of green compound and cover the end of the toothpick wedge (Fig. 12-27, *C*). Immediately insert the compound-coated wedge between the Tofflemire band and the cut piece of matrix material (Fig. 12-27, *D*). While the compound is still soft, use a suitable burnisher to press the compound gingivally, thereby securing the matrix tightly against the gingival cavosurface margin and the lingual surface of the tooth to provide a rigid, lingual matrix (Fig. 12-27, *E* and *F*). A unique property of the lingual matrix is its ability to respond to needed change in contour by pressing a warmed, plastic instrument against the band from the cavity side. The heat is transferred through the matrix material to the compound, which may be reshaped to provide the proper contour. The use of this type of matrix for the occlusolingual amalgam restoration was first suggested by Barton.

Insertion of the filling material is accomplished as previously described for the Class I occlusal cavity preparation. Begin at the gingival wall. When the cavity is sufficiently overfilled, carving of the occlusal surface may begin immediately with suitable, sharp discoidcleoids. All carving should be done with the edge of the blade perpendicular to the margin and with the blade moving parallel to the margin. To prevent overcarving, the blade edge should be guided by the unprepared tooth surface adjacent to the margin. Use an explorer to remove excess amalgam adjacent to the lingual matrix

before matrix removal (Fig. 12-27, *G*). After the occlusal carving is complete, loosen the Tofflemire retainer from the band, and remove the retainer with No. 110 pliers. Push the free ends of the band one at a time lingually and occlusally through the contacts. As the band is freed from the tooth, the compound, wedge, and the cut segment of steel matrix material may be lifted away from the tooth. Complete the carving on the lingual surface. Only a slight excess should remain to carve away. With carving completed (Fig. 12-27, *H*), remove the rubber dam, and adjust the restoration for proper occlusion.

Finishing and polishing procedures

Finishing and polishing the amalgam restoration are not attempted within 24 hours following insertion. The procedures are accomplished as previously described for the Class I occlusal restoration. Fig. 12-27, *I*, illustrates the polished occlusolingual restoration.

ADDITIONAL CLASS I CAVITY PREPARATIONS

These cavity preparations are for restoring with amalgam the described pit or fissure that is *judged carious or at risk for caries.*

Facial pit of mandibular molar

Often, the facial surface of a mandibular molar has a developmental pit but no facial fissure (Fig. 12-28, *A*). Cavity preparation is accomplished with the No. 245 bur (high-speed and air-water spray) positioned perpendicular to the tooth surface (Fig. 12-28, *B*). When the defect is small, a No. 330 or 169L bur may be used. Enter the pit using a punch cut in one smooth insertion to a depth of 1.5 mm and immediately withdraw the bur, which should still be rotating. Penetration to a depth of 1.5 mm usually positions the axial wall just into dentin. Dry the cavity preparation and examine it for any remaining defect or caries which must be removed. It may be necessary to extend (widen) the outline of the cavity preparation to gain access for caries removal. If indicated, insert a base/liner. Maintaining the No. 245 bur perpendicular to the facial surface results in cavity walls that are parallel or slightly undercut and should eliminate the need for additional retention. However, if needed, a No. ¼ bur is used to make small undercuts in dentin that do not undermine the enamel. Such undercuts are indicated for the cavity preparation prepared with the No. 169L bur.

Lingual pit of maxillary incisor

A carious or caries-risk pit/fissure on the lingual surface of a maxillary anterior tooth may be restored with amalgam, since the fault generally is small and esthetics

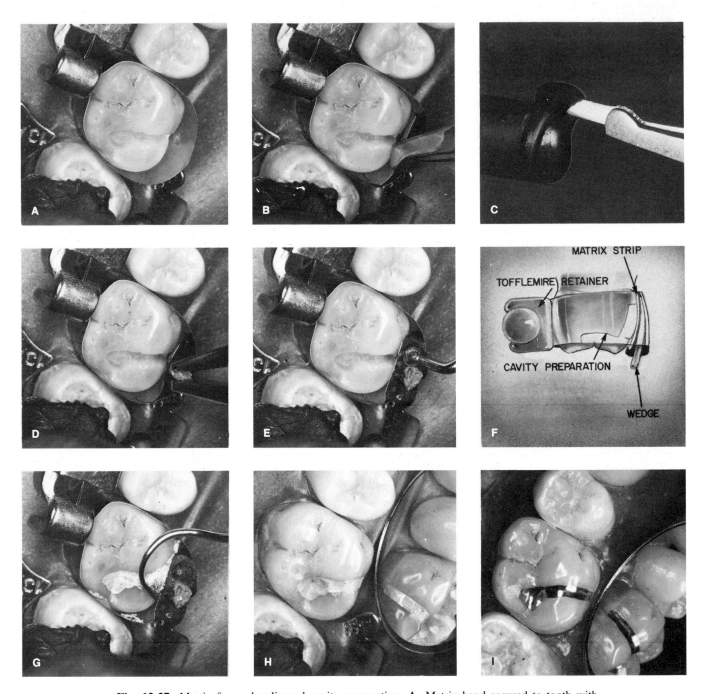

Fig. 12-27. Matrix for occlusolingual cavity preparation. **A,** Matrix band secured to tooth with Tofflemire retainer. **B,** Positioning small strip of stainless steel matrix material between tooth and band already in place. **C,** Covering wedge with softened compound. **D,** Inserting wedge and compound. **E,** Compressing compound gingivally, which in turn adapts steel strip to lingual surface. **F,** Cross section of cavity preparation and matrix construction. **G,** Using explorer to remove excess amalgam adjacent to lingual matrix. **H,** Carving completed. **I,** Polished restoration.

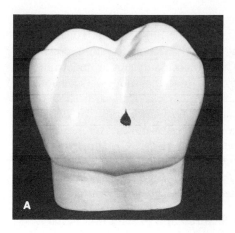
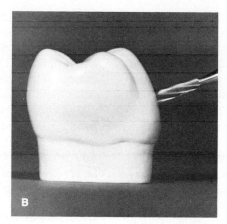
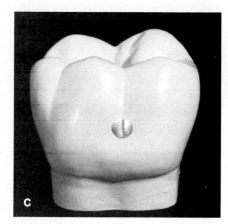

Fig. 12-28. Mandibular molar. A, Carious (or at caries-risk) facial pit. B, Position bur perpendicular to tooth surface for entry. C, Outline of restoration.

is not a factor (Fig. 12-29). Using the No. 245 bur, the direction of cutting follows the orientation of the pit which is often in an apical direction. The cavity outline should be extended, if necessary, to ensure 90-degree cavosurface margins. The preparation outline is governed by the extent of the caries, but is generally conservative. When the fault is small, some operators prefer to use the No. 330 or 169L bur. Since the lingual enamel is thinner, the depth of the initial penetration is 1 to 1.2 mm, which is shallower than for other pit and fissure cavity preparations. This depth will help avoid a pulpal exposure of the lingual pulp horn which may be present. Remove any enamel pit/fissure or infected dentin remaining on the pulpal wall using an appropriately sized round bur, and apply a base/liner if indicated. If needed, retention is placed using a No. ¼ bur as de-

scribed in the previous section for the facial pit preparation.

A maxillary lateral incisor sometimes has a developmental variation in the lingual pit referred to as *"dens in dente."* It appears as a deep invagination of the lingual pit (fissure) and usually can be seen radiographically (Fig. 12-30, *A*). Cavity preparation and restoration (Fig. 12-30, *B*) can be very difficult because the defect and/or caries often is very deep and extensive, and much care is necessary during the cavity preparation to avoid exposure of the pulp or perforation of the root surface. Establishing sound cavity walls, excavation of caries, and application of a base/liner is determined by the defect and the extent of the caries. Early prophylactic restoration of dens in dente may prevent loss of the tooth from caries.

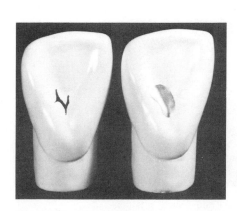

Fig. 12-29. Carious (or at caries-risk) lingual pit/fissure and restoration on maxillary lateral incisor.

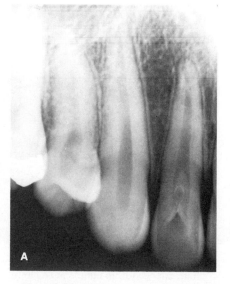
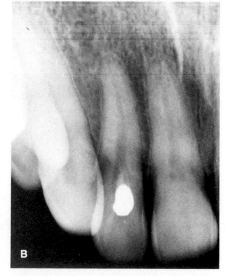

Fig. 12-30. Maxillary lateral incisor. A, Preoperative radiograph of dens in dente. B, Radiograph of restoration after 13 years. (Courtesy Dr. Ludwig Scott.)

Occlusal pits of mandibular first premolar

Many mandibular first premolars have no central occlusal fissure because of the very large facial cusp and its heavy transverse ridge of enamel. However, occlusal pits (mesial, distal, or both) may exist. Generally, these are easily restored by placing small "pit amalgam" restorations (Fig. 12-31, *A*). With a No. 245 bur properly tilted, enter the pit with the end of the bur, penetrating by a punch cut to the proper depth of 1.5 to 2 mm. Fig. 12-31, *B,* illustrates how to determine the extent of lingual tilt of the bur for entry into the tooth. This bur direction is maintained during cavity preparation. The resultant orientation of the pulpal wall (declines toward the lingual aspect) and lingual wall conserves the dentin over the prominent facial pulp horn, as well as the dentin supporting the small lingual cusp. In addition, the direction of the prepared facial wall will result in amalgam that approaches 90 degrees at the cavosurface margin.

This preparation is usually done more at the expense of the facial cusp than of the lingual cusp. Extend laterally to include any defective enamel or to uncover caries, if indicated. Care is necessary not to undermine the enamel at the proximal marginal ridges. Occasionally, when there is an existing central occlusal fissure, or the two occlusal pits are in close proximity, or both, preparing a conventional occlusal outline for the preparation may be indicated (Fig. 12-31, *C*). *If caries excavation is required, again be careful not to expose the large, prominent facial pulp horn, or unnecessarily undermine the enamel of the small lingual cusp.*

Occlusal pits and fissures of maxillary first molar

The cavity preparation for the distal pit and distal oblique and lingual fissure of a maxillary first molar has been previously described in this chapter. A cavity preparation that includes the mesial and central pits and a connecting fissure is illustrated in Fig. 12-32, *A.* The

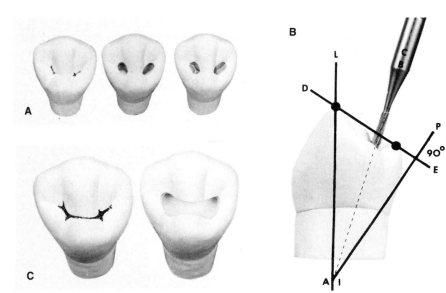

Fig. 12-31. A, Cavity design and restoration of carious or caries-risk occlusal pits on mandibular first premolar. **B,** Bur tilt for entry. Cutting instrument is held so that its long axis *(broken line, CI)* is parallel with bisector *(B)* of angle formed by long axis of tooth *(LA)* and line *(P)* that is perpendicular to plane *(DE)* drawn through facial and lingual cusp points. This dotted line *(CI)* is bur position for entry. **C,** Conventional outline including occlusal pits and central fissure.

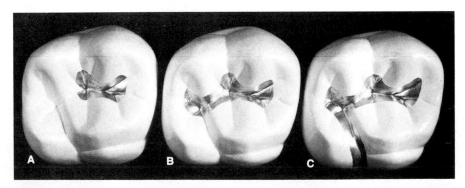

Fig. 12-32. Maxillary first molar. **A,** Outline necessary to include mesial and central pits connected by fissure. **B,** Cavity outline extended from outline in **(A)** to include distal pit and connecting deep fissure in oblique ridge. **C,** Cavity outline extended from outline in **(B)** to include distal oblique and lingual fissures.

heavy oblique ridge of enamel should not be crossed in cavity preparation unless the ridge is undermined by caries or intersected by a deep fissure. Leaving the oblique ridge intact will preserve the strength of the tooth crown. However, if it is necessary to extend through the oblique ridge, include the distal pit area in the outline form (Fig. 12-32, *B*), and also the distal oblique and lingual fissures if at caries-risk (Fig. 12-32, *C*).

Occlusal pits and fissures of mandibular second premolars and molars

Generally, the occlusal pit and fissure anatomy of the mandibular second premolar requires no special consideration for preparation outline form (Fig. 12-33, *A*). However, when two lingual cusps are present, the lingual developmental groove may be fissured and extend onto the lingual surface. During the cavity preparation of this tooth, extension along this fissure is permissible so long as the lingual ridge enamel is not undermined. To preserve the lingual ridge enamel, the linguopulpal line angle should be extended no closer than 2 mm to the lingual surface of the tooth crown. Recall that enameloplasty may sometimes eliminate the terminal portion of the fissure, thereby providing a smooth enamel surface on a previously fissured ridge. However, when the ridge enamel is weakened or the fissure extends through the ridge enamel, the preparation should include the fissure and extend onto the lingual surface (Fig. 12-33, *B*). The pulpal floor of the extension is 1.5 to 2 mm deep (1.5 mm at the fissure and 2 mm on external walls).

Like the mandibular first premolar, some second premolars do not have an occlusal fissure connecting the mesial and distal pits. If so, faulty or carious pits can be restored separately as with the first premolar.

Often on mandibular molars a facial occlusal fissure is continuous with a facial surface fissure (Fig. 12-34, *A*). When this occurs, the occlusal cavity preparation should be extended onto the facial surface to include the facial fissure.

To do this, extend through the facial ridge onto the facial surface with the No. 245 bur, maintaining a uniform depth of 1.5 to 2 mm (1.5 mm at the fissure and 2 mm on external walls) (Fig. 12-34, *B* and *C*). The gingival floor of the extension will be continuous with the pulpal floor of the occlusal portion of the cavity preparation (Fig. 12-34, *C*). As with the occlusolingual (OL) preparation of a maxillary molar, the pulpal floor of the facial extension will follow the contour of the enamel surface.

The facial surface portion of the preparation is prepared with the bur's long axis parallel to the facial surface (Fig. 12-34, *D*). As with the OL preparation, the orientation of the bur must be altered during preparation to ensure a uniform axial depth of 1.5 mm. Next, the mesioaxial and distoaxial line angles should be accentuated by the end of the bur with its long axis directed perpendicular to the facial surface (Fig. 12-34, *E*). The No. 169L bur may be directed as illustrated in Fig. 12-34, *F*, to define the line angles when access from a facial direction is limited.

A flat gingival seat to the extension is desirable for resistance form. If the mesial and distal walls of the facial extension are slightly undercut (as they should be after using the No. 245 bur held perpendicular to the axial wall), additional retention form is not required. Retention may be ensured by preparing locks as described previously for the occlusolingual cavity preparation on the maxillary first molar (Fig. 12-34, *G*). Fig. 12-34, *H*, illustrates the completed preparation.

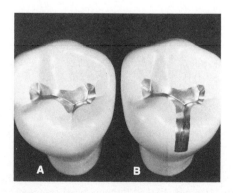

Fig. 12-33. Mandibular second premolar. **A,** Typical occlusal outline. **B,** Extension through lingual ridge enamel is necessary when enameloplasty does not eliminate lingual fissure.

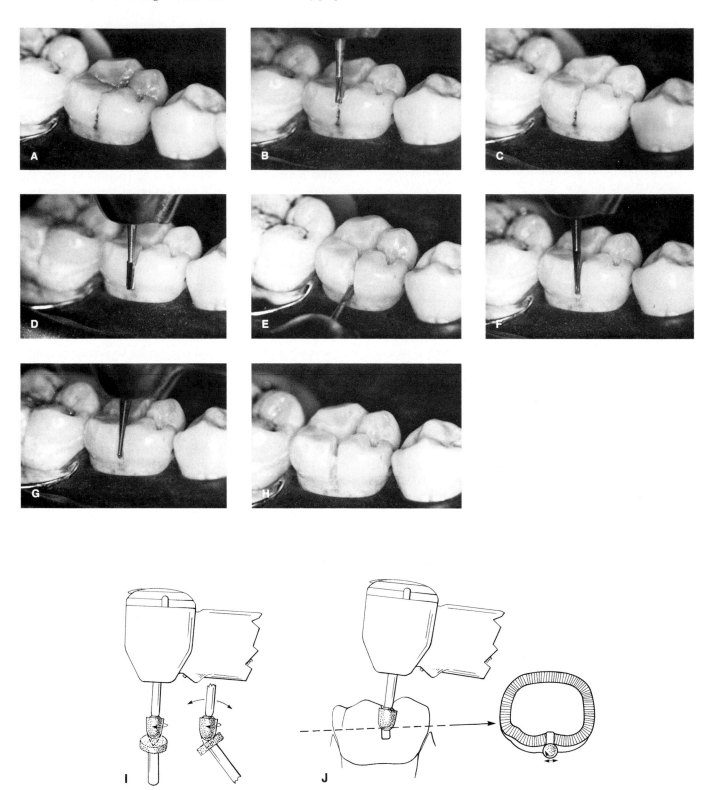

Fig. 12-34. Fissure extension. **A,** Facial occlusal fissure continuous with fissure on facial surface (fissures carious or at caries-risk). **B,** Extend through facial ridge onto facial surface. **C,** Appearance of cavity preparation following extension through ridge. **D,** Facial surface portion of extension is cut with side of bur. **E,** Sharpen line angles by directing bur from facial aspect. **F,** Sharpening line angles from occlusal direction with No. 169L bur. **G,** Ensuring retention form by cutting retention locks with No. ¼ round bur. **H,** Completed cavity preparation. **I,** Rubber polishing point may be trued and blunted on a coarse diamond wheel. **J,** Proper orientation of rubber point when polishing facial surface groove area.

REFERENCES

1. Bauer JG: A study of procedures for burnishing amalgam restorations, *J Prosthet Dent* 57(6):669, 1987.
2. Ben-Amar A: Reduction of microleakage around new amalgam restorations, *J Am Dent Assoc* 119:725, Dec 1989.
3. Chong WF, Swartz ML, Phillips RW: Displacement of cement bases by amalgam condensation, *J Am Dent Assoc* 74:97, Jan 1967.
4. Collins CJ, Bryant RW: Finishing of amalgam restorations: a three-year clinical study, *J Dent* 20:202, 1992.
5. Council on Dental Materials, Instruments and Equipment: Dental mercury hygiene: summary of recommendations in 1990, *J Am Dent Assoc* 122:112, 1991.
6. Drummond JL et al: Surface roughness of polished amalgams, *Oper Dent* 17:129, 1992.
7. Eakle WS, Staninec M, Lacy AM: Effect of bonded amalgam on the fracture resistance of teeth, *J Prosthet Dent* 68:257, 1992.
8. Fanian F, Hadavi F, Asgar K: Marginal leakage of dental amalgams: effect of cavity varnish and burnishing, *J Can Dent Assoc* 6:484, 1984.
9. Fusayama T: Two layers of carious dentin: diagnosis and treatment, *Oper Dent* 4(2):63, 1979.
10. Gilmore HW: Restorative materials and cavity preparation design, *Dent Clin North Am* 15(1):99, 1971.
11. Gilmore HW: Pulpal considerations for operative dentistry, *J Prosthet Dent* 14:752, 1964.
12. Goel VK et al: Effect of cavity depth on stresses in a restored tooth, *J Prosthet Dent* 67(2):174, 1992.
13. Hadavi F, Caffesse RG, Charbeneau GT: A study of the gingival response to polished and unpolished amalgam restorations, *J Can Dent Assoc* 3:211, 1986.
14. Harper RH et al: In vivo measurements of thermal diffusion through restorations of various materials, *J Prosthet Dent* 43(2):180, 1980.
15. Hyatt TP: Prophylactic odontotomy: the ideal procedure in dentistry for children, *Dent Cosmos* 78:353, 1936.
16. Karai S: Structure studies of amalgam II. Effect of burnishing on the margins of occlusal amalgam fillings, *ACTA Odontol Scan* 24:47, May 1966.
17. Lagouvardos P, Sourai P, Douvitsas G: Coronal fractures in posterior teeth, *Oper Dent* 14:28, 1989.
18. Lovadino JR, Ruhnke LA, Consani S: Influence of burnishing on amalgam adaptation to cavity walls, *J Prosthet Dent* 58(3):284, 1987.
19. Mahler DB, Terkla LG: Analysis of stress in dental structures, *Dent Clin North Am* p 789, Nov 1958.
20. Maryniuk GA: In search of treatment longevity—a 30-year perspective, *J Am Dent Assoc* 109:739, Nov 1984.
21. Maryniuk GA, Kaplan SH: Longevity of restorations: survey results of dentists' estimates and attitudes, *J Am Dent Assoc* 112:39, Jan 1986.
22. May KN, Wilder AD, Leinfelder KF: Burnished amalgam restorations: a two-year evaluation, *J Prosthet Dent* 49(2):193, 1983.
23. May KN, Wilder AD, Leinfelder KF: Clinical evaluation of various burnishing techniques on high-copper amalgam, *J Prosthet Dent* 61:213, 1982 (abstract).
24. Mayhew RB, Schmeltzer LD, Pierson WP: Effect of polishing on the marginal integrity of high-copper amalgams, *Oper Dent* 11:8, 1986.
25. Mitchum JC: The potential of amalgam condensation causing intrusion of capping materials into the pulp, *J Prosthet Dent* 26:506, 1971.
26. Nadal R, Phillips RW, Swartz ML: Clinical investigation on the relation of mercury to the amalgam restoration, *J Am Dent Assoc* 63:488, 1961.
27. Novickas D, Fiocca VL, Grajower R: Linings and caries in retrieved permanent teeth with amalgam restorations, *Oper Dent* 14:33, 1989.
28. Osborne JW, Norman RD: 13-year clinical assessment of 10 amalgam alloys, *Dent Mater* 6:189, July 1990.
29. Osborne JW et al: Two independent evaluations of ten amalgam alloys, *J Prosthet Dent* 43(6):622, 1980.
30. Pashley DH, Depew DD: Effects of the smear layer, Copalite, and oxalate on microleakage, *Oper Dent* 11:95, 1986.
31. Peters DA, Ausburger RA: In vitro cold transference of bases and restorations, *J Am Dent Assoc* 102:642, 1981.
32. Phillips RW, editor: *Skinner's science of dental materials,* ed 9, Philadelphia, 1991, WB Saunders.
33. Phillips RW, Swartz ML, Boozayaangool R: Effect of moisture contamination on the compressive strength of amalgam, *J Am Dent Assoc* 49:436, 1954.
34. Prime JM: A plea for conservatism in operative procedures, *J Am Dent Assoc* 15:1234, 1928.
35. Restoration of cavity preparations with amalgam and tooth-colored materials: Project ACCORDE student syllabus, Washington, DC, 1974, US Department of Health, Education, and Welfare.
36. Robbins JW: The placement of bases beneath amalgam restorations: review of literature and recommendations for use, *J Am Dent Assoc* 113:910, Dec 1986.
37. Simonsen RJ: The preventive resin restoration: a minimally invasive, nonmetallic restoration, *Compend Contin Educ Dent* VIII(6):428, 1987.
38. Sockwell CL: Dental handpieces and rotary cutting instruments, *Dent Clin North Am* 15:219, Jan 1971.
39. Stanley HR: Personal communication, 1983.
40. Straffon LH, Dennison JB, Asgar K: A clinical evaluation of polished and unpolished amalgams: 36-month results, *Pediatr Dent* 6(4), 1984.
41. Sturdevant CM et al: *The art and science of operative dentistry,* ed 2, St Louis, 1985, Mosby.
42. Swift EJ: Preventive resin restorations, *J Am Dent Assoc* 114:819, June 1987.
43. Triolo PT Jr, Swift EJ Jr: Shear bond strengths of ten dentin adhesive systems, *Dent Mater,* 8:370, Nov 1992.
44. Vale WA: Cavity preparation and further thoughts on high speed, *Br Dent J* 107:333, 1979.
45. Vlietstra JR, Sidaway DA, Plant CG: Cavity cleansers, *Br Dent J* 149:293, 1980.
46. Wing G: Modern concepts for the amalgam restoration, *Dent Clin North Am* 15:43, Jan 1971.
47. Yates JL, Murray GA, Hembree JH Jr: Cavity varnishes applied over insulating bases: effect on microleakage, *Oper Dent* 5(2):43, 1980.

CHAPTER 13

Amalgam restorations for Class II cavity preparations

Aldridge D. Wilder, Jr.

Kenneth N. May, Jr.

William D. Strickland*

Amalgam restorations that restore one or both of the proximal surfaces of the tooth provide years of service to the patient when the (1) cavity preparation is correct, (2) matrix is suitable, (3) rubber dam is used, and (4) filling material is manipulated properly. Inattention to one or more of these criteria produces inferior restorations prone to early failure. This chapter deals with the principles, techniques, and procedures necessary to produce quality **amalgam restorations in Class II cavity preparations**.

INDICATIONS AND CONTRAINDICATIONS

When caries occurs on the proximal surface(s), the following factors must be considered in the selection of the restorative material for the Class II cavity preparation:

1. Incidence and extent of proximal, facial, and lingual surface caries
2. Age of patient
3. Esthetics
4. Economics

*This author is inactive this edition; see Preface.

5. Galvanism
6. Abutment teeth for removable partial denture

Incidence and extent of proximal, facial, and lingual surface caries

When there are indications that the patient's caries rate is high, the amalgam restoration is chosen over the more expensive gold restoration until the caries rate is brought under control. However, when the proximal carious lesion is extensive, consideration should be given to the cast gold restoration because: (1) its superior physical properties along with proper cavity design better protect the remaining tooth structure from fracture; and, (2) it facilitates development of ideal tooth contours. The presence of facial or lingual caries is usually an indication for the amalgam restoration. However, extensive facial and lingual caries usually warrants consideration of a full crown restoration.

Amalgam is the material of choice for treatment of small proximal lesions because cavity preparation can and should be conservative, resulting in restorations that should have extended service life and that do not jeopardize the strength of the remaining tooth.

Age of patient

When amalgam is the material of choice, it is used regardless of the age of the patient. Amalgam is appropriate in both young and geriatric patients who are susceptible to caries (and recurrent caries) because of a caries-inducing diet and/or poor oral hygiene. Root caries is common in geriatric patients, and proximal root surface lesions on the posterior teeth of these patients are indications for the use of amalgam (see Slot Preparation).

Esthetics

Although amalgam is the most used and useful restorative material for posterior teeth, its use is sometimes contraindicated in esthetic areas of the mouth in patients who object to its metallic appearance. Patients in the public eye often fall into this category. Tooth-colored alternatives to amalgam (see Chapters 16 and 17) are typically more technique-sensitive. Amalgam is indicated for the routine conservative restoration of permanent posterior teeth.

Large cavity preparations and/or overextension of the mesiofacial wall of maxillary premolars and first molars result in restorations that are more publicly visible, compared with conservative preparations. Because esthetics is important to the patient, the dentist should be as conservative as possible when removing tooth structure. *However, principles of cavity preparation should not be routinely compromised to satisfy the esthetic factor.*

Economics

Cost to the patient for amalgam restorations is less than for gold restorations because less time is required and material cost is less. Patients should not feel that their dental treatment is inferior because the fee for an amalgam restoration is less than for other types of restorations. A skillfully accomplished amalgam restoration is the most appropriate restoration for the conservative Class II cavity preparation. Such a restoration requires operating time deserving an appropriate fee, especially since service life will often exceed that of other materials.

A resin-bonded amalgam (or composite) restoration is an option versus the usually more expensive indirect restoration for treating a weak tooth that is subject to fracture. The indirect restoration is preferred assuming that it circumferentially braces the remaining tooth structure.

Galvanism

Complete rehabilitation of the posterior teeth with amalgam is appropriate for many patients when conditions indicate the use of amalgam. When the restoration of some of the posterior teeth with gold is necessary, the continued use of the same material may be indicated to eliminate possible galvanic activity between dissimilar metals. Although galvanic action does sometimes occur and is uncomfortable to the patient, it is generally short-lived and should not influence the dentist's choice of an appropriate restorative material. Few patients experience difficulty from dissimilar metals in their teeth. An amalgam restoration in juxtaposition with a cast gold restoration often has a black, surface corrosion, but this is not clinically significant where esthetics is not a factor.

Abutment teeth for removable partial denture

When a tooth is planned to be an abutment for a removable denture, a full veneer crown is often considered the most desirable restoration, particularly if the facial (and lingual) surface(s) is(are) involved with caries, previous restoration, and/or undesirable contours. The crown best allows development of the rest seat(s), guide-plane(s) (for modification spaces), and retentive contours. If the condition of the tooth permits the option of restoring the proximal surface(s) with amalgam, modifications of the cavity preparation are indicated and these are presented later in the section, Modifications in Cavity Design.

OCCLUSION

Centric holding stops and excursive contacts should be marked preoperatively with articulating paper so that these areas can either be excluded from the outline form or, if included, be properly restored. The operator should also view the teeth as they are closed in centric contact, noting intercuspation and contacts of cusps on marginal ridges. The contact pattern can be used for reference to indicate full closure of the teeth after carving the amalgam. Also, an opposing "plunging cusp" should be recontoured both to lessen the likelihood of fracture of the new restoration as a result of occlusal forces and to reduce the potential for excursive interferences, especially nonfunctional interferences.

LOCAL ANESTHESIA

Local anesthesia of the tooth to be treated, as well as the adjacent soft tissues, is usually a prerequisite for good dentistry. In addition to eliminating pain, local anesthesia usually reduces salivation because the patient is less sensitive to stimulation of the oral tissues. The operator is more efficient when the patient is comfortable. (Refer to Local Anesthesia, in Chapter 10.)

ISOLATION OF THE OPERATING SITE

Before initiating the cavity preparation, it is desirable to place the rubber dam, which usually can be applied in the time necessary for onset of profound anesthesia. Occasionally, when replacing an existing restoration that has a very rough proximal contact surface that may damage the septal dam, removing the restoration prior to application of the dam is a suggested procedure. All phases of cavity preparation and restoration can be performed more safely, comfortably, and efficiently with the rubber dam in place. Infected carious dentin should be removed with the rubber dam in place, especially if a pulpal exposure is a possibility. Moreover, final procedures of the cavity preparation are best accomplished when there is no visible moisture on tooth surfaces (refer to Chapter 11 for rubber dam procedures). Insertion of *interproximal wedges* is the last step in rubber dam application when Class II cavity preparations are scheduled. A gingival wedge should be inserted into each involved interproximal space from the facial or lingual embrasure, whichever is larger. *The wedge depresses and protects the rubber dam and underlying soft tissues, separates the teeth slightly, and can serve as a guide to prevent gingival overextension of proximal boxes.*

If necessary to prevent friction between the septal dam and wedge during wedge insertion, stretch the dam slightly away from the teeth (wedge insertion side), and insert the wedge *while* slowly releasing the dam. This results in a passive dam under the wedge and tends to prevent bunching or tearing of the septal dam during wedge insertion. (Refer to Placement of the Rubber Dam, Step 22, in Chapter 11.)

TWO-SURFACE CAVITY PREPARATION FOR A PROXIMAL LESION

This portion of the chapter introduces most of *the principles and techniques of Class II cavity preparation for an amalgam restoration* of a carious, cavitated ("broken surface") lesion on the proximal surface. For descriptive purposes a mesioocclusal (MO) cavity preparation on a mandibular second premolar that also has precarious or carious occlusal pits and fissures is presented. Moderate advancement of caries (to dentinoenamel junction and slightly deeper) is assumed in this example.

Initial cavity preparation

Occlusal outline form (occlusal step). Outline form of the occlusal step of a Class II cavity preparation for amalgam is similar to the outline form for the Class I cavity preparation as described in Chapter 12. Appropriate differences are described in this section.

Using high speed with air-water spray, enter the pit nearest the involved proximal surface with a *punch cut* using a *No. 245 bur* oriented as illustrated in Fig. 13-1, *A* and *B*. The bur should be rotating when applied to the tooth and should not stop rotating until removed. *Viewed from the proximal and lingual (facial) aspects, the long axis of the bur and the long axis of the tooth crown should remain parallel during cutting procedures. Proper depth for the initial entry cut is 1.5 to 2 mm (one-half to two-thirds the length of the cutting portion of a No. 245 bur), 1.5 mm as measured at the central fissure, and 2 mm on the prepared external walls.* The operator should measure and be familiar with each bur's dimensions to prevent being misled by varying bur sizes. *This pulpal depth is usually 0.1 to 0.2 mm into the dentin.* While maintaining the same depth and bur orientation, move the bur to extend the outline to include the central fissure and the opposite pit (the distal pit in this example) (Fig. 13-1, *C* and *D*). *Unless otherwise indicated, the isthmus width should be as narrow as possible*[1] *and no wider than one-quarter the intercuspal distance.*[17,23] *Ideally, it should be the width of the No. 245 bur. The pulpal floor should be prepared to a uniform, previously described depth and is usually flat.* However, the pulpal floor of the preparation should follow the slight rise and fall of the central fissure region of the occlusal surface in teeth with prominent triangular ridges.

Maintaining the bur parallel to the long axis of the tooth crown creates facial, lingual, and distal walls with a slight occlusal convergence, which provides favorable amalgam angles at the margins. It is necessary to tilt the bur to diverge occlusally the distal wall only when extension of the distal margin would undermine the marginal ridge of its dentinal support (see Fig. 12-1, *H* and

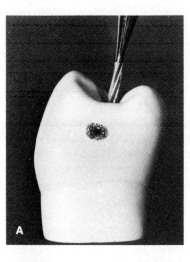

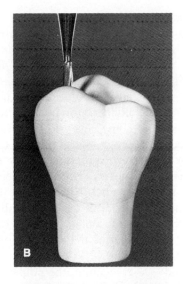

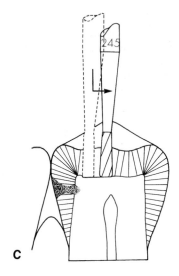

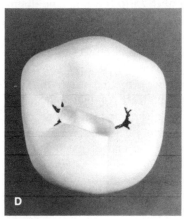

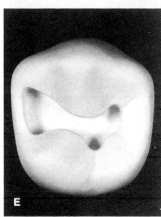

Fig 13-1. Entry and occlusal step. **A,** Bur position for entry, as viewed proximally. Note slight lingual tilt of bur. **B,** Bur position as viewed lingually. **C,** Enter tooth with punch cut, and extend distally along central fissure at uniform depth of 1.5 to 2 mm (1.5 mm at fissure; because of inclination of unprepared tooth surface, corresponding measurement on prepared wall is 2.0 mm). **D,** Occlusal view of **C. E,** Completed occlusal step.

1). During development of the distal pit area of the preparation, extension to include any distofacial and distolingual developmental fissures radiating from the pit provides ***dovetail retention form*** against mesial displacement of the completed restoration. This type of retention form is also provided by any extension of the central fissure preparation that is not in a straight direction from pit to pit (Fig. 13-1, *E*).

Enameloplasty should be utilized where indicated to conserve tooth structure. (Refer to Enameloplasty, in Chapter 11.)

Before extending into the involved proximal marginal ridge (the mesial ridge in this example), visualize the final location of the facial and lingual walls of the proximal box relative to the contact area. This will prevent overextension of the occlusal outline form to accommodate poor planning in joining the occlusal outline form (step) with the proximal outline form (box) (Fig. 13-2, *A* and *B*).

While maintaining the established pulpal depth and with the bur parallel to the long axis of the tooth crown, extend the preparation mesially, stopping 0.8 mm (the

diameter of the end of the bur) short of cutting through the marginal ridge into the contact area. The occlusal step in this region is made slightly wider faciolingually than in the Class I preparation because additional width is necessary for the proximal box. It should be emphasized, however, that the proper depth of the occlusal portion of the cavity is a more important factor contributing to the strength of the restoration than is the faciolingual width. Fig. 13-1, *E*, illustrates the completed *occlusal outline form.*

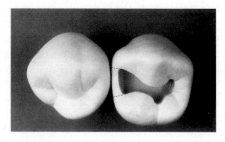

Fig. 13-2. Visualize final location of proximoocclusal margins *(dotted lines)* before preparing proximal box.

Proximal outline form (proximal box). Again visualize the desired final location of the facial and lingual walls of the proximal box or proximal outline form, relative to the contact area.

Proximal ditch cut. The initial procedure in preparing the outline form of the proximal box is the isolation of the proximal (mesial) enamel by the *proximal ditch cut.* This is a critically important procedure in conservative cavity preparation and is presented purposely in much detail. With the same orientation of the bur, position it over the pulpal floor next to the remaining mesial marginal ridge (Fig. 13-3, *A*). *Allow the end of the bur to cut a ditch gingivally along the exposed dentinoenamel junction, two thirds at the expense of dentin and one third at the expense of enamel. The 0.8 mm diameter bur end is cutting 0.5 to 0.6 mm into dentin and 0.2 to 0.3 mm into enamel.* Pressure is directed gingivally and lightly toward the mesial surface to keep the bur against the proximal enamel, while the bur is moved facially and lingually along the dentinoenamel junction. As a rule, extend the ditch gingivally just beyond the caries or the contact width, whichever is greater (Fig. 13-3, *B*). Because dentin is softer and cuts easier than enamel, the bur should be cutting away the dentin immediately supporting the enamel. The harder enamel acts to guide the bur, thus creating an axial wall that faciolingually follows the contour of the proximal surface and the dentinoenamel junction (Fig. 13-3, *D*).

As a further guide for the facial and lingual extension of the ditch, visualize the completed mesiofacial and mesiolingual margins as right-angle projections of the facial and lingual limits of the ditch (Fig. 13-3, E). *When preparing a tooth with a small lesion, these margins should clear the adjacent tooth by only 0.2 to 0.3 mm.*[23] *A guide for the gingival extension is the visualization that the finished gingival margin will be only slightly gingival to the gingival limit of the ditch. This margin should clear the adjacent tooth by only 0.5 mm in a small cavity preparation* (Fig. 13-3, *F*). Clearance of the proximal margins (mesiofacial, mesiolingual, and gingival) greater than 0.5 mm is excessive unless indicated to include caries, undermined enamel, or existing restorative material.[5] See Fig. 13-66 for conservative extension of proximal margins. Since the location of final proximal margins is often established with hand instruments (chisels, hatchets, or trimmers), the position of proximal walls (facial, lingual, and gingival) should not be overextended with the No. 245 bur, considering the additional extension provided by hand instruments (see Fig. 13-3, *E*). Extending gingival margins into the gingival sulcus should be avoided where possible because subgingival margins may be a contributing factor to periodontal disease.[14,15,31] (See Figs. 13-24 and 13-58 for conservative extension of proximal margins.)

The proximal ditch should be sufficiently deep into dentin (0.5 to 0.6 mm) that the retentive locks (see Secondary Resistance and Retention Forms) can be prepared into the axiolingual and axiofacial line angles without undermining the proximal enamel. When all of the proximal ditch cut is in dentin, the axial wall usually is too deep. Because the proximal enamel becomes thinner from occlusal to gingival, the end of the bur will come closer to the external tooth surface as the cutting progresses gingivally (see Fig. 13-3, *B*). Premolars may have proximal boxes that are shallower pulpally than molars because premolars typically have thinner enamel. However, in the tooth crown the ideal *dentinal* depth of the axial wall of proximal boxes of premolars and molars should be similar (two-thirds to three-fourths the diameter of the No. 245 bur, or 0.5 to 0.6 mm).[23] When extension places the gingival margin in cementum, the pulpal depth of the axiogingival line angle should be a minimum of 0.75 to 0.8 mm (the diameter of the tip end of the No. 245 bur is 0.8 mm), and never more. Note in Fig. 13-3, *C,* that the bur may shave the side of the wedge which is protecting the rubber dam and underlying gingiva.

The gingival depth of the proximal ditch may be measured by first noting the depth of the nonrotating bur in the ditch. Then remove the bur from the preparation and hold it in the facial embrasure at the same level to observe the relationship of the end of the bur to the contact.

The proximal ditch cut is diverged gingivally so that the faciolingual dimension at the gingival is greater than at the occlusal (Fig. 13-3, *G*). This gingival divergence contributes to retention form and provides for desirable extension of the facial and lingual proximal margins to include carious tooth structure at the gingival level while conserving the marginal ridge and providing for 90-degree amalgam at the margins on this ridge.[5,17]

To conserve tooth structure, do not overextend the ditch facially and lingually. Occasionally, it is permissible *not to extend* the outline facially and lingually beyond the proximal contact. An example of this modification is a narrow proximal lesion where there is broad proximal contact in a clean mouth.

Completion of proximal extensions. Next, make two cuts, one starting at the facial limit of the proximal ditch and the other starting at the lingual limit, extending toward and perpendicular to the proximal surface until the bur is nearly through the enamel at contact level (Fig. 13-3, *H*). The side of the bur may emerge slightly through the surface at the level of the gingival floor (Fig. 13-3, *I*). This weakens the remaining enamel by which the isolated portion is held. If this level is judged to be insufficiently gingival, additional gingival extension should be accomplished at this time, using the isolated proximal enamel that is still in place to guide the bur. This prevents the bur from marring the proxi-

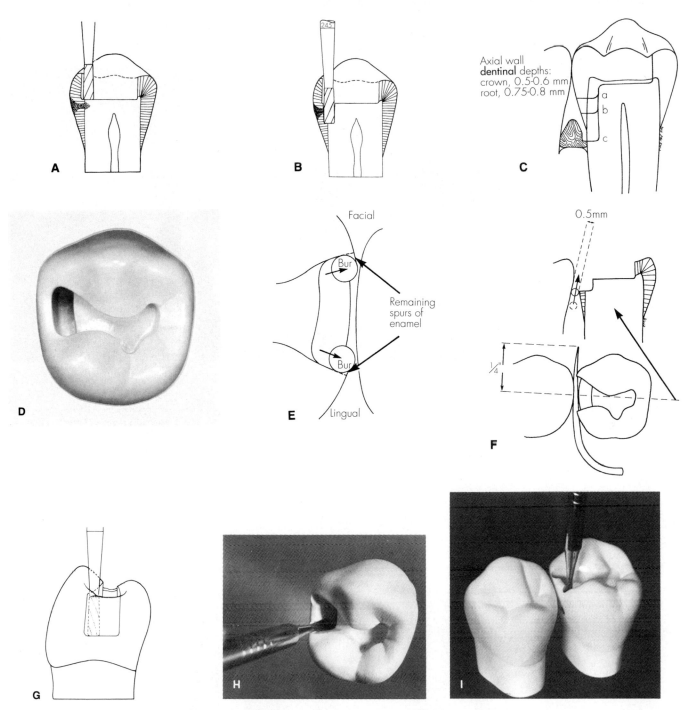

Fig. 13-3. Isolation of proximal enamel. **A,** Bur position to begin proximal ditch cut. **B,** Proximal ditch is extended gingivally to desired level of gingival wall (floor). **C,** Variance in pulpal depth of axiogingival line angle as extension of gingival wall varies: *a,* at minimal gingival extension; *b,* at moderate extension; *c,* at extension that places gingival margin in cementum whereupon pulpal depth is 0.75 to 0.8 mm and bur may shave side of wedge. **D,** Proximal ditch cut results in axial wall that follows outside contour of proximal surface. **E,** Position of proximal walls (facial, lingual, and gingival) should not be overextended with No. 245 bur considering additional extension provided by hand instruments once remaining spurs of enamel are removed. (From ACORDE [A Consortium on Restorative Dentistry Education].) **F,** When small lesion is prepared, gingival margin should clear adjacent tooth by only 0.5 mm. This clearance may be measured with side of explorer. Five-tenths millimeter is diameter of tine of No. 23 explorer ¼ inch (6.3 mm) from its tip. **G,** Faciolingual dimension of proximal ditch is greater at gingival than at occlusal level. **H,** To further isolate and weaken proximal enamel, bur is moved toward and perpendicular to proximal surface (parallel to direction of enamel rods). **I,** Side of bur may emerge slightly through proximal surface at level of gingival floor *(arrow).*

Fig. 13-4. Removing isolated enamel. **A,** Using spoon excavator to fracture out weakened proximal enamel. **B,** Occlusal view with proximal enamel removed. **C,** Proximal view with proximal enamel removed.

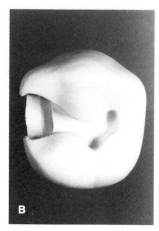
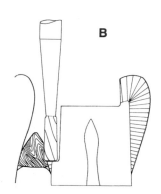
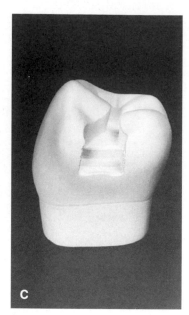

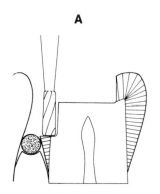
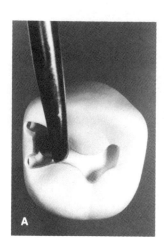

Fig. 13-5. Wedging. **A,** Round toothpick wedge placed in gingival embrasure protects gingiva and rubber dam during preparation of proximal box. **B,** Triangular wedge is indicated when deep gingival extension of proximal box is anticipated because wedge's greatest cross-sectional dimension is at its base. Consequently, it will more readily engage the remaining clinical tooth surface.

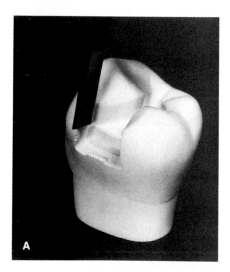
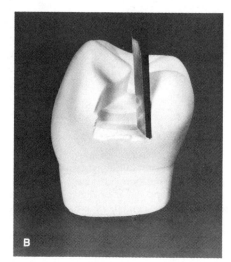
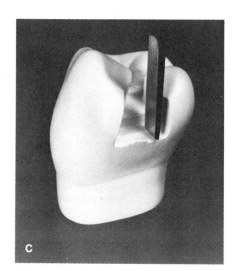

Fig. 13-6. Removing remaining undermined proximal enamel with enamel hatchet on facial proximal wall **(A),** lingual proximal wall **(B),** and gingival wall **(C).**

mal surface of the adjacent tooth. At this stage, however, the remaining wall of enamel often breaks away during cutting, especially when high speed is used. At such times, if additional use of the bur is indicated, a matrix band may be used around the adjacent tooth to prevent marring its proximal surface. The isolated enamel, if still in place, is fractured out with a spoon excavator (Fig. 13-4).

To protect the gingiva and the rubber dam when extending the gingival wall gingivally, a **wooden wedge** should already be in place in the gingival embrasure to depress the soft tissue and rubber dam.[17] A *round toothpick wedge* is preferred unless a deep gingival extension is anticipated (Fig. 13-5, *A*). A *triangular (anatomic) wedge* is more appropriate for deep gingival extensions because the greatest cross-sectional dimension of the wedge is at its base (Fig. 13-5, *B*). As the gingival wall is cut, the bur's end corner may at times slightly shave the wedge (Fig. 13-5, *B*). For wedge insertion refer to previous section, Isolation of the operating site.

*With the **enamel hatchet (10-7-14)** or the **binangle chisel (12-7-8)**, or both, cleave away the remaining undermined proximal enamel (Fig. 13-6, A and B), establishing the proper direction to the mesiolingual and mesiofacial walls. Proximal margins having cavosurface angles of 90 degrees are indicated.*[17] Exercise care not to thrust the cutting edge against the gingival wall, since this can cause a craze line (fracture) that extends gingivally in the enamel, often to the cervical line. Fig. 13-7 shows the importance of the correct direction of the mesiofacial and mesiolingual walls, dictated by enamel rod direction and physical properties of the amalgam. *Ideally, the mesiofacial and mesiolingual margins of the conservative preparation should clear the adjacent tooth by only 0.2 to 0.3 mm (see Fig. 13-66).*

Also, remove the weakened enamel along the gingival wall by using the enamel hatchet in a scraping motion (Fig. 13-6, *C*). *Ideally, the minimal clearance of the completed gingival margin with the adjacent tooth is 0.5 mm.* This may be measured by passing an explorer tine of this diameter between the margin and adjacent tooth (see Fig. 13-3, *F*).

Viewed from the occlusal, the direction of the mesiofacial enamel wall is parallel to the enamel rod direction, thus usually creating a **reverse curve** in the outline (Fig. 13-8).[23] Note that the curve is sufficient only to permit 90-degree amalgam at the mesiofacial margin. Lingually, a reverse curve usually is unnecessary, or is minimal.

When the isolation of the proximal enamel has been properly executed, the proximal box can be completed easily with hand cutting instruments. Otherwise, more cutting with rotary instruments may be indicated. High speed equipment has reduced the use of hand instruments. However, the value of sharp hand cutting instruments should not be underestimated.

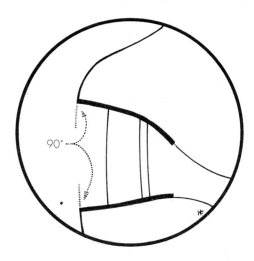

Fig. 13-8. Reverse curve in occlusal outline is usually created when mesiofacial enamel wall is parallel to enamel rod direction. Lingually, reverse curve is very slight, often unnecessary.

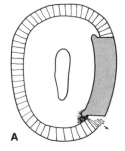 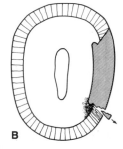 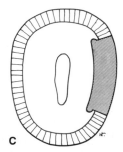

Fig. 13-7. Direction of mesiofacial and mesiolingual walls. **A,** Failure caused by weak enamel margin. **B,** Failure caused by weak amalgam margin. **C,** Proper direction to proximal walls results in full-length enamel rods and 90-degree amalgam at cavity margin. Note also that retention locks have been cut 0.2 mm inside dentinoenamel junction, and their direction of depth is parallel to dentinoenamel junction.

When a rotary instrument is used in a proximal box after the proximal enamel is removed, there is a danger of the instrument either marring the adjacent proximal surface or "crawling out" of the box into the gingiva or across the proximal margins. The latter misfortune produces a rounded cavosurface angle, which, if not corrected, will result in an amalgam margin of much less than 90 degrees. The danger of this occurring is markedly reduced when high speeds are used. When finishing enamel margins by rotary instrument, use intermittent application of the bur along with air coolant to improve vision.

Primary resistance and retention forms. Primary resistance form is provided by (1) the pulpal and gingival walls being relatively flat and perpendicular to forces directed with the long axis of the tooth, (2) restricting extension of the walls to allow strong cusps and ridge areas to remain with sufficient dentin support, (3) restricting the occlusal outline form where possible to areas receiving minimal occlusal contact,[21] (4) slightly coving the internal line angles to reduce stress concentration in tooth structure (automatically created by bur design), and (5) providing enough thickness of restorative material to prevent its fracture under mastication.

Primary retention form is provided by the occlusal convergence of facial and lingual walls, as well as by the dovetail design of the occlusal step.

This completes the *initial cavity preparation.* Recall from Chapter 7 that *initial cavity preparation for the Class II cavity preparation is defined as extension of external walls at a specified limited depth to reach sound tooth structure, to resist fracture of the tooth or restorative material from forces directed with the long axis of the tooth, and to retain restorative material in the tooth. Axial and pulpal walls should be prepared to this ideal depth whether cutting in existing restorative material or caries (or* AIR!*).*

After completing the initial cavity preparation, the adjacent proximal surface should be evaluated. An adjacent proximal restoration may require recontouring and smoothing to develop proper contact, contour, and embrasure form for the new restoration. Detection of caries would indicate restoration of the proximal surface or replacement of the existing restoration. Minimal damage to the adjacent proximal surface during initial cavity preparation can be corrected with abrasive strips and disks.

Final cavity preparation

Removal of any remaining defective enamel and infected carious dentin. Removing any remaining enamel pit/fissure and infected carious dentin on the pulpal wall in Class II preparations is accomplished in the same manner as in the Class I preparation. *The presence of infected carious dentin on a portion of either the pulpal wall (floor) or axial wall does not indicate deepening the entire wall.* Infected carious dentin is removed with a slowly revolving round bur of appropriate size or a discoid-type spoon excavator, or both. Stop excavating when a hard or firm feel with an explorer or small spoon excavator is achieved. This often occurs before all of the stained or discolored dentin is removed. *Removing any remaining enamel pit/fissure and infected carious dentin should not affect resistance form. To maintain good resistance form, the occlusal step should have at least two pulpal seats at normal level, perpendicular to the long axis of the tooth, in sound tooth structure, opposite one another and peripheral to the excavated area(s)* (Fig. 13-9).

Any old restorative material (including base/liner) remaining should not be removed if there is no evidence of recurrent caries (there being no border gaps or softness) and the tooth pulp is symptomless for disease. (With proper outline form the pulpal and axial line angles are always in sound dentin.) This concept is particularly important if removal of all remaining restorative material might increase the risk of pulpal exposure.

As seen in Fig. 13-10, caries in the axial wall does not dictate cutting the entire axial wall toward the pulp. Recall that in initial cavity preparation, the facial, lingual, and gingival walls of the proximal box are extended as necessary until each wall is located in sound dentin. In all such extensions the pulpal depth of the axiofacial, axiolingual, and axiogingival line angles should never be altered because of the presence of caries in the axial wall "central" of these line angles. Infected carious dentin in the axial wall is then removed with suitably sized round burs or spoon excavators, or both.

After completion of the minimal gingival extension (gingivoaxial line angle is in sound dentin), a remnant of the enamel portion of a carious lesion may remain on the gingival floor (wall), seen in the form of a white, chalky area bordering the margin (Fig. 13-11). This dictates extending a part or all the gingival floor gingivally to place it in sound tooth structure. Extension of the entire gingival wall to include a large carious lesion may place the gingival margin so deep that proper matrix application and, particularly, wedging are extremely difficult. Fig. 13-12, *A,* illustrates an outline form that extends gingivally in the central portion of the gingival wall to include caries that is deep gingivally, while leaving the facial and lingual gingival corners at a more occlusal position. This *partial extension of the gingival wall* will permit wedging of the band where otherwise it may be difficult and damaging to the soft tissue. In this instance, a small portion of the band may not be tightly supported by the gingival wedge. Special care must then be exercised by placing small amounts of amalgam in this area first and condensing lightly but thoroughly.

Fig. 13-9. Management of small to moderate size carious lesion on pulpal wall. **A,** Infected carious dentin extending beyond ideal pulpal wall position. **B,** Incorrect lowering of pulpal wall to include infected carious dentin. **C,** Correct extension facially and lingually beyond infected carious dentin. Note that excavation below ideal pulpal wall level has been lined with zinc oxide–eugenol base and that facial and lingual seats are at ideal pulpal wall level.

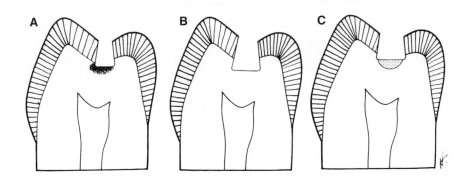

Fig. 13-10. Management of moderate to extensive size carious lesion. Infected carious dentin on axial wall does not call for cutting axial wall toward pulp as shown by dotted lines. Infected carious dentin extending pulpally of ideal axial wall position is removed with round bur. A zinc oxide–eugenol liner is placed in any excavation judged not to have a near or actual exposure, whereas a calcium-hydroxide base is placed when there is a near or actual pulpal exposure.

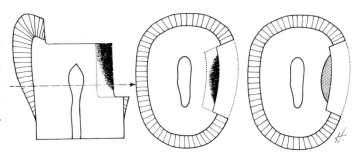

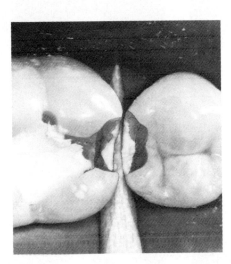

Fig. 13-11. Remnant of carious lesion bordering the enamel margin after insufficient gingival extension. Such a lesion indicates extending part or all of gingival floor gingivally to place it in sound tooth structure. (Courtesy Dr. C.L. Sockwell.)

In addition, care is exercised in carving the restoration in this area to remove any excess that may have extruded gingivally during condensation.

Fig. 13-12, *B,* illustrates a carious excavation facially and gingivally beyond the conventional marginal position. Such minor variations from ideal cavity form permit conservation of tooth structure. A ***partial extension of a facial or lingual wall*** is permissible if (1) the entire wall is not weakened, (2) the extension remains accessible and visible, (3) sufficient gingival seats remain to support the restoration, and (4) a butt joint fit at the amalgam/enamel margin (90-degree amalgam/90-degree cavosurface angle) is possible.

Pulp protection. Insertion of a calcium hydroxide or zinc oxide-eugenol ***base/liner*** in excavations on the axial wall is similar to the procedures followed for excavations on the pulpal wall. (Refer to Chapter 12 for the philosophy and procedure of placing a base/liner, in the sections Conservative Cavity Preparations and Cavity Preparation for Extensive Caries.)

The viscosity of the base material should be as high as possible but still permit flowing it to place. The viscosity of cavity liners is typically thinner. The ***Williams periodontal probe*** or a cement placing instrument is suitable to convey the material to the excavated area. If access is limited, other small instruments, such as the back side of a small spoon excavator or a broken explorer, may be used.

Secondary resistance and retention forms. Secondary resistance form in final cavity preparation involves both resistance of the remaining tooth structure against fracture from oblique forces and resistance of restorative material against fracture. The former is provided by restricting extensions of external walls. The latter is enhanced by using the *gingival margin trimmer* to bevel or round the axiopulpal line angle (Fig. 13-13).[16] Thereby the restorative material in this region is stronger by increasing its bulk and decreasing stress concentration. Proximal locks (discussed later) also increase the fracture resistance of the amalgam restoration.[18,19]

Secondary retention form for the occlusal and proximal portions of the preparation should be independent of each other.[1] The occlusal convergence of the facial

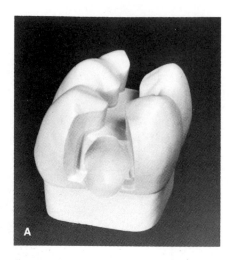
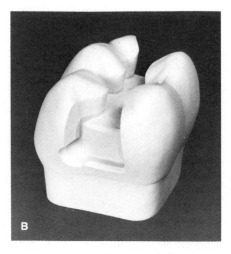
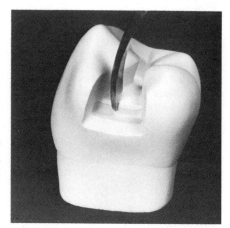

Fig. 13-12. A, Outline form that permits extension of center portion of gingival wall to facilitate proper matrix construction and wedging in situations where caries extends deep gingivally. **B,** Outline form that permits partial wall extension facially and gingivally to conserve tooth structure.

Fig. 13-13. Beveling axiopulpal line angle.

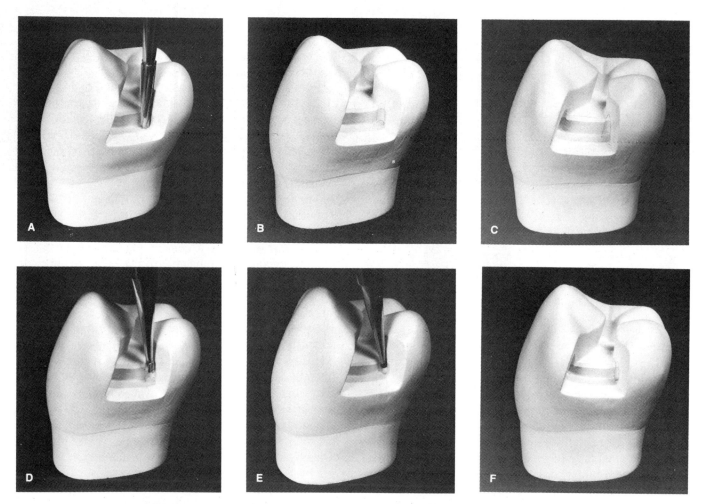

Fig. 13-14. Proximal retention locks. **A,** Position of No. 169L bur to prepare retentive lock as bur is moved lingually and pulpally. **B,** Lingual lock. Note dentin support of proximal enamel. **C,** Completed locks. **D,** Locks prepared with No. 33½ bur. **E,** Locks prepared with No. ¼ bur. **F,** Completed locks.

and lingual walls and the dovetail design provide sufficient retention form to the occlusal portion of the cavity preparation. The occlusal convergence of the mesiofacial and mesiolingual walls offers retention in the proximal portion of the preparation against displacement occlusally. To enhance retention form of the proximal portion, ***proximal locks*** are prepared to counter proximal displacement.[6,17] Using a No. 169L bur with air coolant (to improve vision) and reduced speed (to improve tactile "feel" and control), prepare a retentive lock in the axiolingual line angle as the bur is tilted slightly in a direction opposite to the direction of translation, and then moved (translated) lingually and pulpally (Fig. 13-14, *A*) (or parallel to the dentinoenamel junction as illustrated in Fig. 13-15). The bur is tilted to allow cutting to the depth of the diameter of the end of the bur at the point angle (0.5 mm) and permit the lock to diminish in depth occlusally, terminating at the axiolinguopulpal point angle. In a similar manner prepare the facial lock in the axiofacial line angle. When the axiofacial and axiolingual line angles are less than 2 mm in length, tilt the bur slightly less so that the proximal locks are extended occlusally to disappear midway between the dentinoenamel junction and the enamel margin (Fig. 13-14, *B* and *C*). *There are four characteristics of proximal locks: (1) position, (2) translation, (3) depth, and (4) occlusogingival orientation* (see Fig. 13-15). *Position* refers to the axiofacial and axiolingual line angles of initial cavity preparation (0.2 mm axial to dentinoenamel junction). *Translation* refers to the direction of movement of the axis of the bur. *Depth* refers to the extent of translation (0.5 mm at gingival floor level). *Occlusogingival orientation* refers to the tilt of the No. 169L bur, which dictates the occlusal height of the lock, given a constant depth.

Some operators prefer using the No. 33½ bur or No. ¼ bur to cut the proximal locks. The rotating bur is carried into the axiolinguogingival (axiofaciogingival) point angle, and then moved parallel to the dentinoenamel junction to the depth of the diameter of the bur. It is then drawn occlusally along the axiolingual (axiofacial) line angle, allowing the lock to become shallower and to terminate at the axiolinguopulpal (axiofaciopulpal) point angle, or more occlusally if the line angles are less than 2 mm in length (see Fig. 13-14, *D* to *F*).

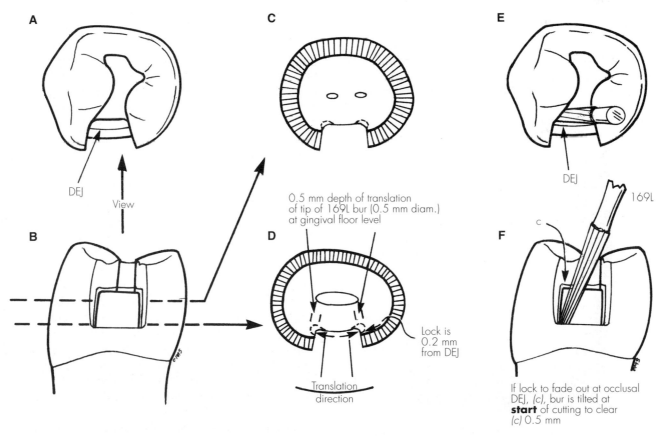

Fig. 13-15. Four characteristics of retentive locks. **A,** Occlusal view of mesioocclusal preparation before placement of retention locks. **B,** Proximal view of mesioocclusal preparation. **C** and **D,** Position, translation, and depth. **E** and **F,** Occlusogingival orientation.

The distance between the facial and lingual proximal walls affects the depth of the proximal locks, as well as the requirement for additional retention form. Narrow proximal boxes permit shallow proximal locks. Wide proximal boxes require deeper locks.

Slots in the gingival floor may be used to provide additional retention in an extensive proximal box that has facial and lingual walls extending to or beyond the proximal line angles of the tooth crown. Slot dimension will depend on the size of the proximal box. *Generally, slots are prepared with a No. ¼ or ½ bur 0.5 to 1 mm deep gingivally, 2 to 3 mm in length faciolingually, and 0.2 to 0.3 mm inside the dentinoenamel junction* (Fig. 13-16). *"Pot-holes"* in the gingival floor may also be used to provide additional retention. They are usually prepared with a No. 1/2 or 1 bur 0.5 to 1 mm deep gingivally and 0.2 to 0.3 mm inside the dentinoenamel junction.

Regardless of the method used in placing the locks, extreme care is necessary to prevent the removal of dentin that immediately supports the proximal enamel. Also, it is essential not to prepare the locks entirely in the axial wall (incorrect translation, i.e., moving the bur only in a pulpal direction), since no effective retention is obtained, and there is a risk of pulpal involvement.

An improperly positioned axiofacial or axiolingual line angle must not be used as a positional guide for the proximal lock. If the axial line angle is too shallow, the lock may undermine the enamel of dentinal support. If the line angle is too deep, preparation of the lock may result in exposure of the pulp.

Mondelli and others[18,19] have demonstrated that proximal retentive locks in the axiofacial and axiolin-

gual line angles significantly strengthen the isthmus of a Class II restoration. Also, these locks are significantly superior to axiogingival grooves in increasing the restoration's fracture strength. Galan, Phillips, and Swartz[11] and Terkla, Mahler, and Van Eysden[30] have shown that "mesioocclusodistal deformation" and the extent of proximal extrusion of a Class II amalgam restoration are related to the *creep value* of the amalgam alloys. The higher the material's creep value, the greater the proximal extrusion and mesioocclusodistal deformation or marginal breakdown. These studies indicate that proximal retentive locks should be used, as well as an amalgam with a low creep value, to maximize strength of the restoration and to minimize marginal breakdown. *It is recommended that the creep value of amalgam not exceed 1%.*[22] *The high copper amalgam available today satisfies this requirement.* Summitt and others have suggested that retention locks located occlusal to the axiopulpal line angle provide more resistance than conventional grooves.[28] Contrasting the studies cited above, Sturdevant and others have demonstrated that *with high-copper amalgams, proximal retentive locks are unnecessary in preparations that include dovetails.*[26] This contrasting view is further supported by Moore.[20]

Procedure for finishing external walls. The cavity walls and margins should not have unsupported enamel and marginal irregularities, which, if present, would indicate correction. Khera and Chan[12] demonstrated that less marginal leakage occurred if the margins were straight and smooth (not ragged [Editor's note]). No occlusal cavosurface bevel is indicated in the cavity preparation for amalgam. Ideally, there should be a 90-degree cavosurface angle (maximum of 100 degrees). This angle aids in obtaining a marginal amalgam angle of 90 degrees (no less than 80 degrees). *Clinical experience has established that this "butt joint" relationship of enamel and amalgam creates the strongest margin.*[17] *Amalgam is a brittle material and tends to chip away under occlusal stress if its angle at the margin is less than 90 degrees.*

Use the mesial gingival margin trimmer, 13-85-10-14, R and L, to establish a slight cavosurface bevel (6 centigrades [or 20 degrees] declination gingivally) at the gingival margin if it is in enamel. The bevel is no steeper than necessary to ensure full-length enamel rods forming the gingival margin and is no wider than the enamel (Fig. 13-17). *When the gingival margin is positioned gingival to the cementoenamel junction, the bevel is not indicated.*[17] (When beveling the gingival margin on the distal surface, use the distal gingival margin trimmer 13-95-10-14, R and L).

Final procedures: cleaning; inspecting; varnishing. The cavity preparation may need *cleaning* with the air/water spray, a wet cotton pellet, or a 3% solution of hydrogen peroxide.[2] Then, a few short pulses of air from the

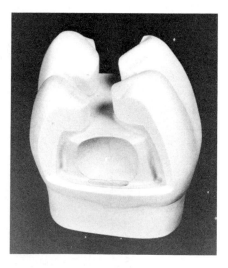

Fig. 13-16. Slot prepared 2 to 3 mm in length in gingival floor may be used to provide additional retention in extensive proximal box that has facial and lingual walls extending to or beyond proximal line angles of tooth crown.

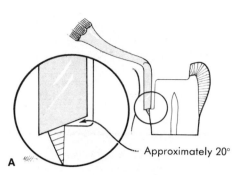

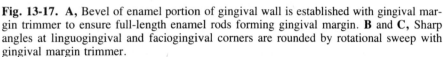

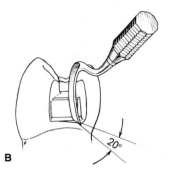

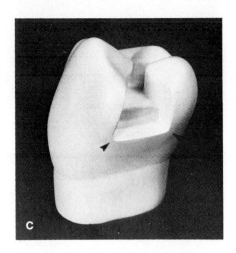

Fig. 13-17. A, Bevel of enamel portion of gingival wall is established with gingival margin trimmer to ensure full-length enamel rods forming gingival margin. **B** and **C,** Sharp angles at linguogingival and faciogingival corners are rounded by rotational sweep with gingival margin trimmer.

air syringe are applied to remove any visible moisture from the preparation walls, being careful not to desiccate the dentin. *Inspect* the cavity preparation for detection and removal of debris or of base/liner where unwanted; and examine for final approval or correction of all cavo-surface angles and margins.

Two applications of *cavity varnish* are applied to cavity preparations for amalgam restorations (see next paragraph for exception) as described in Conservative Cavity Preparations, in Chapter 12. *To prevent pooling of the varnish at the junction of the matrix band and proximal margins, application of cavity varnish prior to matrix application is preferable.*

Recently, in lieu of varnish, adhesive resin systems have been suggested for bonding amalgam to the preparation walls.[3] (Refer to Chapter 12, the section, Conservative Cavity Preparations, and also in this chapter to a later section, Insertion of Amalgam.)

VARIATIONS OF SINGLE PROXIMAL SURFACE CAVITY PREPARATIONS
Mandibular first premolar

In a Class II cavity preparation for amalgam for the mandibular first premolar the conventional approach and technique must be modified because the morphological structure of this tooth is different from the other posterior teeth, particularly due to the diminished size of the lingual cusp. In this tooth, as in all teeth, the principles of cavity preparation for amalgam must be correlated with the physical properties of the restorative material and the anatomical structure of the tooth. The relationship of the pulp chamber to the dentinoenamel junction and the relatively small size of the lingual cusp are illustrated in Fig. 13-18. It is easily understood that injudicious cutting in the central groove area could weaken the lingual cusp and that excessive cutting in a facial direction could approach or expose the facial pulp

horn. Therefore, while preparing the occlusal portion, tilt the bur slightly lingually to establish the correct pulpal wall direction (see Fig. 12-31, *B*). Fig. 13-18 also illustrates the correct position of the pulpal wall and how it differs in direction as compared to the second premolar.

The mandibular first premolar presents a variety of occlusal patterns, most of which exhibit a large transverse ridge of enamel. Often such a ridge has no connecting fissure between the mesial and distal pits, and in the preparation of a Class II cavity this indicates an outline form that does not extend to, or across, the ridge (Fig. 13-19, *A*). If the opposite pit is faulty, it is restored with a separate restoration.

For the *preparation that does not cross the transverse ridge,* prepare the proximal box before the occlusal portion to prevent cutting away the tooth structure that is to form the isthmus between the occlusal dovetail and the proximal box. Enter the pit adjacent to the involved proximal surface with the No. 245 bur. Immediately following the entry, direct the bur into the proximal marginal ridge and then pulpally if necessary until the proximal dentinoenamel junction is visible. Isolate the proximal enamel, and complete the proximal box as

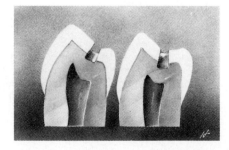

Fig. 13-18. When mandibular first and second premolars are compared, note differences in size of pulp chambers, lingual cusps, and direction of pulpal walls.

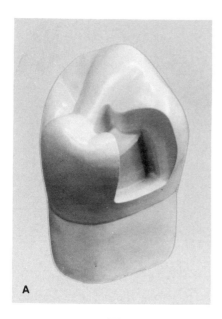

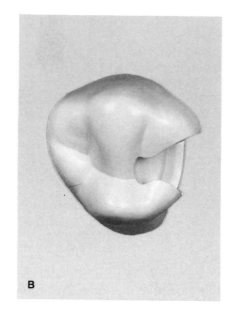

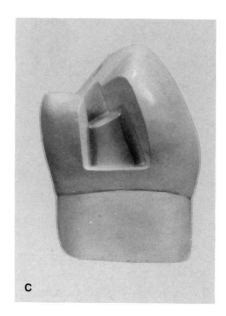

Fig. 13-19. Mandibular first premolar with sound transverse ridge. **A,** Two-surface cavity preparation that does not include opposite pit. **B,** Occlusal outline form. **C,** Proximal view of completed preparation.

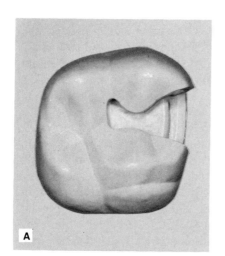

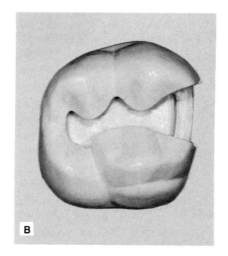

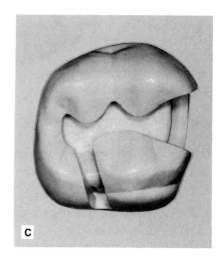

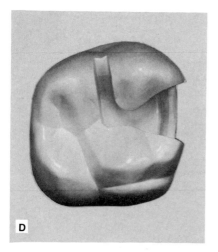

Fig. 13-20. Maxillary first molar. **A,** Conventional mesioocclusal preparation. **B,** Mesioocclusal preparation extended to include distal pit. **C,** Mesioocclusolingual preparation including distal pit, and distal oblique and lingual fissures. **D,** Mesioocclusal preparation with facial fissure extension.

previously described for the mandibular second premolar. Return the bur to the area of entry, and prepare the occlusal step with a dovetail. When preparing the occlusal portion, the bur is tilted slightly lingual to establish the correct pulpal wall direction, which maintains dentin support for the small lingual cusp and prevents encroachment on the facial pulp horn. *The primary difference in cavity preparation on this tooth when compared with the preparation on other posterior teeth is the facial inclination of the pulpal wall.* Broaden the isthmus to sufficient width, but do not make it so wide as to remove the dovetail retention form. Fig. 13-19, *B*, illustrates the correct occlusal outline form. Removing any remaining caries (if present) and inserting necessary bases/liners precede the placement of proximal locks and finishing of the enamel margins to complete the preparation (Fig. 13-19, *C*).

Maxillary first molar

When mesial and distal proximal surface restorations are indicated on the maxillary first molar that has an unaffected oblique ridge, separate two-surface cavity preparations are indicated rather than a mesioocclusodistal preparation, since the strength of the tooth crown is significantly greater when the oblique ridge is intact.[17]

The *mesioocclusal cavity preparation* is generally uncomplicated (Fig. 13-20, *A*). Extension into the enamel oblique ridge is avoided whenever possible to maintain the cross-splinting strength it provides to the tooth. Occasionally, extension through the ridge and into the distal pit is necessary because of the extent of caries. Also, examine the distal oblique and lingual grooves, and include them in the outline when they are fissured, carious, or at risk of caries. The outline of this occlusolingual pit and fissure portion is similar to that of the Class I occlusolingual preparation. Fig. 13-20, *B* and *C*, illustrates the *mesioocclusal preparation extended to include the distal pit, and the outline form that includes the distal oblique and lingual fissures.*

When the occlusal fissure extends into the facial cusp ridge and it cannot be removed by enameloplasty, the defect should be eliminated by extension of the cavity preparation. Sometimes this can be accomplished by tilting the bur to create an occlusal divergence of the facial wall in this region while maintaining the dentin support of the ridge. If this fault cannot be eliminated without extending the margin to the height of the cusp ridge or undermining the enamel margin, extend the preparation facially through the ridge (Fig. 13-20, *D*). The pulpal wall of this facial extension may have remaining enamel, but a depth of 1.5 to 2 mm is necessary to provide sufficient bulk of material for adequate strength. *For the best esthetic results minimal extension of the proximal mesiofacial margin is indicated.*

The distoocclusal cavity preparation may take one of several outlines depending on the occlusal anatomy. The occlusal outline is determined by the pit and fissure pattern, as well as by the amount and extension of caries. An extension onto the lingual surface to include a lingual fissure should be prepared only after the distolingual proximal margin is established. This permits the operator to maintain sufficient tooth structure between the distolingual wall and the lingual fissure extension for strength of the distolingual cusp by preparing the lingual fissure extension more at the expense of the mesiolingual cusp than the distolingual cusp when indicated. Nevertheless, the distolingual cusp on many maxillary molars (particularly maxillary second molars) may be weakened during such a distoocclusolingual cavity preparation because of the small cuspal portion remaining between the lingual fissure preparation and the distolingual proximal wall. In addition, caries excavation may weaken the cusp. Capping of the distolingual cusp is then necessary to provide proper resistance form. The procedure is described in a later section, Capping Cusps (see Fig. 13-33).

Maxillary first premolar

A Class II cavity preparation involving the mesial surface of a maxillary first premolar requires special attention because the mesiofacial embrasure is esthetically important. *The occlusal to gingival direction of the facial wall of the mesial box should be parallel to the long axis of the tooth since divergence of this wall gingivally may result in an unesthetic display of amalgam in the faciogingival corner of the restoration.* Facial extension of the mesiofacial wall with a No. 245 bur should be minimal so that the mesiofacial proximal margin of the preparation will minimally clear the contact as the margin is finished with an appropriate enamel hatchet or chisel (Fig. 13-21).

If the mesial proximal involvement (1) is limited to a caries-risk fissure in the marginal ridge, (2) is not treatable by enameloplasty, and (3) does not involve the proximal contact, the proximal portion of the cavity preparation is prepared by extending through the fault with the No. 245 bur so that the margins are lingual to the contact. Often this means that the proximal box will be the faciolingual width of the bur and the gingival floor may be at the same depth as the pulpal floor or somewhat occlusal to it. Retention form for this extension is provided by the slight occlusal convergence of the facial and lingual walls (see Fig. 12-7).

If proximal caries is limited to the mesiolingual embrasure, do not involve the mesial proximal contact in the cavity preparation. If only the lingual aspect of the mesial proximal contact is carious, it is permissible not to include the entire contact in the preparation for the sake of esthetics.

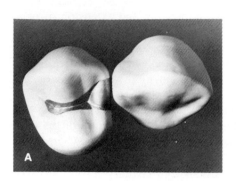

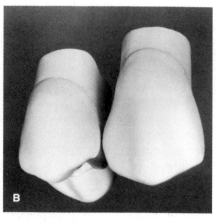

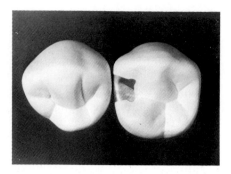

Fig. 13-21. To produce inconspicuous margin on maxillary first premolar, mesiofacial wall does **not** diverge gingivally, and facial extension with No. 245 bur should be minimal so that mesiofacial proximal margin of preparation will minimally clear the contact as margin is finished. **A,** Occlusal view. **B,** Facial view.

Fig. 13-22. Simple box restoration without occlusal step is permissible when restoring small proximal lesion in tooth without either occlusal fissures or previously inserted occlusal restoration and when involved marginal ridge does not support occlusal contact. Note that proximal locks extend to occlusal surface.

A Class II cavity preparation involving the distal surface of the maxillary first premolar is treated much like the mandibular second premolar described earlier.

Modifications in cavity design

Simple box preparation. When restoring a small, cavitated, proximal lesion in a tooth with neither occlusal fissures nor a previously inserted occlusal restoration, Almquist, Cowan, and Lambert[1] and Markley[17] recommend a ***proximal box preparation*** without an occlusal step. *To maximize retention, preparations with facial and lingual walls that almost oppose each other are advised.* Therefore this type of preparation should be limited to a proximal surface with a narrow interproximal contact allowing minimal facial and lingual extensions. As in the conventional preparation the facial and lingual proximal walls converge occlusally. *To compensate for the lack of an occlusal dovetail, the proximal retentive locks should have a 0.5 mm depth at the gingival point angle, tapering to a depth of 0.3 mm at the occlusal surface (Fig. 13-22).* In contrast, recall that for a conventional proximoocclusal preparation having an axial wall less than 2 mm occlusogingivally, the locks extended occlusally to disappear midway between the dentinoenamel junction and the occlusal margin.

Slot preparation for root caries. Older patients who have gingival recession exposing the cementum often experience caries on the proximal root surface that is appreciably gingival to the proximal contact (Fig. 13-23, *A*). *Assuming that the contact does not need restoring, the* **cavity preparation** *is usually approached from the facial and has the form of a slot (Fig. 13-23, B). A lingual approach is used when the caries is limited to the linguoproximal surface.*

After isolation of the operating field, prepare initial cavity outline form from a facial approach with a No. 2 or 4 bur using high speed and air-water spray. *Outline form* extension of the external walls to sound tooth structure is at a limited depth pulpally, 0.75 to 1 mm at the gingival aspect (if no enamel), increasing to 1 to 1.25 mm at the occlusal wall (if margin in enamel) (Fig. 13-23, *B*). During this extension, the bur should not remove from the pulpal wall any infected carious dentin deeper than the outline form limited depth. This remaining infected carious dentin will be removed in final cavity preparation (Fig. 13-23, *C*). External walls should form a 90-degree cavosurface angle. With a facial approach the lingual wall should face facially as much as possible. This will aid condensation of amalgam during its insertion. The facial wall must be extended to provide access and visibility, or *convenience form* (Fig. 13-23, *D*).

In final cavity preparation use the No. 2 or 4 bur to *remove any remaining infected carious dentin* on the axial wall. If indicated, apply a *base/liner* as described for the Class I or II cavity preparation.

Prepare *retention grooves* with a No. 1/4 bur depthwise into the occlusal and gingival walls at the axial line angles, 0.2 mm inside the dentinoenamel junction or 0.3 to 0.5 mm from the cemental margin. The depth of these grooves is one-half the diameter of the bur head (0.25 mm).

Varnish is applied as usual. The *matrix* for inserting amalgam is similar to that depicted in Fig. 13-23, *F*.

For those instances where root caries encircles the tooth, the proximals can be restored as described previously. Subsequently, Class V preparations are prepared and abutted with the proximal restorations. Alternatively, the Class V portions can be restored first. When

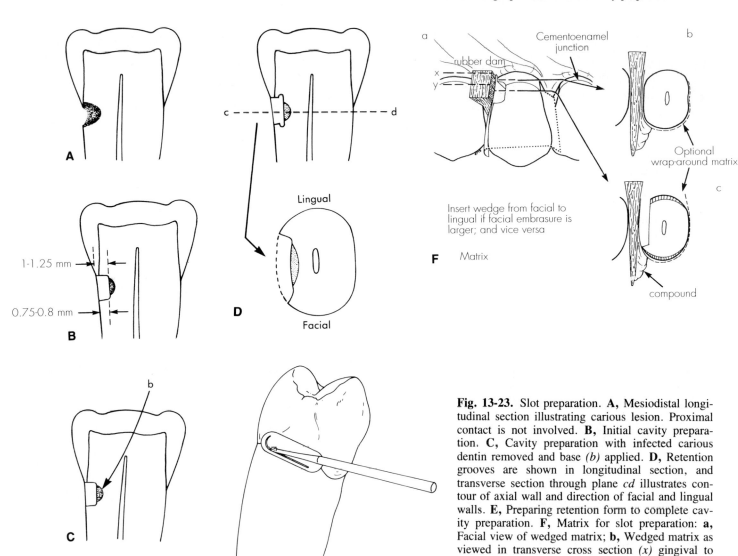

Fig. 13-23. Slot preparation. **A,** Mesiodistal longitudinal section illustrating carious lesion. Proximal contact is not involved. **B,** Initial cavity preparation. **C,** Cavity preparation with infected carious dentin removed and base *(b)* applied. **D,** Retention grooves are shown in longitudinal section, and transverse section through plane *cd* illustrates contour of axial wall and direction of facial and lingual walls. **E,** Preparing retention form to complete cavity preparation. **F,** Matrix for slot preparation: **a,** Facial view of wedged matrix; **b,** Wedged matrix as viewed in transverse cross section *(x)* gingival to gingival floor; **c,** Wedged matrix as viewed in transverse cross section *(y)* occlusal to gingival floor.

the proximals are restored first, the mesial and distal walls of the Class V preparations would be in amalgam. Doing the "encircled restoration" in segments allows proper condensation of amalgam. These patients should be counseled to improve oral hygiene and use fluoride rinses.

Rotated teeth. Cavity preparation for rotated teeth follows the same principles as cavity preparation for normally aligned teeth. The outline form for a mesioocclusal cavity preparation on the rotated mandibular second premolar illustrated in Fig. 13-24, *A,* differs from normal in that its proximal box is displaced facially because the proximal caries involves the mesiofacial line angle of the tooth crown.

When the tooth is rotated 90 degrees and the "proximal" lesion is on the facial (or lingual) surface, and/or orthodontic correction is declined or ruled out, the preparation may require an isthmus that includes the cuspal eminence (Fig. 13-24, *B*). If the lesion is small, consideration should be given to the slot preparation. In this instance, the occlusal margin may be in the contact area or slightly occlusal to it (Fig. 13-24, *C*).

Unusual outline forms. Outline forms should conform to the restoration requirements of the tooth and not necessarily to the classic example of a Class II cavity preparation. For example, a dovetail feature is not required in the occlusal step of a single proximal surface preparation unless it is indicated by a fissure emanating from an occlusal pit. Without a dovetail the step should not be in a straight direction to ensure retention form. Another example is an occlusal fissure that is segmented by coalesced enamel. This should be treated with isolated amalgam restorations if the preparations are separated by approximately 0.5 mm or more of sound tooth structure[1,27] (Fig. 13-25).

Adjoining restorations. *It is permissible to repair or*

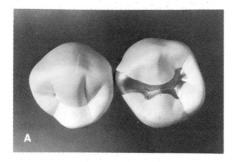

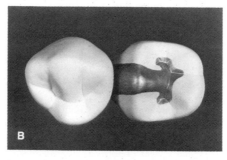

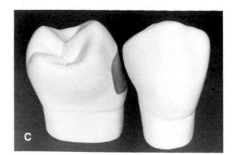

Fig. 13-24. Restoration outlines for rotated teeth. **A,** Mesioocclusal outline for mandibular premolar with 45-degree rotation. **B,** Mesioocclusal outline for mandibular premolar with 90-degree rotation. **C,** Slot preparation outline for restoration of a small mesial lesion involving proximal contact of mandibular premolar with 90-degree rotation.

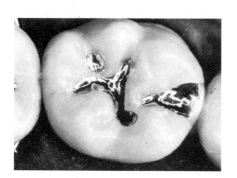

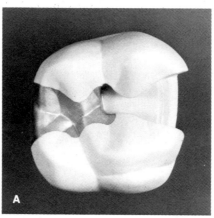

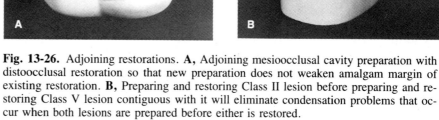

Fig. 13-25. Restoration of mesioocclusal cavity preparation with central fissure segmented by coalesced enamel.

Fig. 13-26. Adjoining restorations. **A,** Adjoining mesioocclusal cavity preparation with distoocclusal restoration so that new preparation does not weaken amalgam margin of existing restoration. **B,** Preparing and restoring Class II lesion before preparing and restoring Class V lesion contiguous with it will eliminate condensation problems that occur when both lesions are prepared before either is restored.

replace a defective portion of an existing amalgam restoration if the remaining portion of original restoration retains adequate resistance and retention form. Adjoining restorations on the occlusal surface occurs more often in molars because the dovetail of the new restoration can usually be prepared without eliminating the dovetail of the existing restoration. Where the two adjoin, care should be taken that the outline of the second restoration does not weaken the amalgam margin of the first (Fig. 13-26, *A*). The intersecting margins of the two restorations should be at right angles as much as possible. The decision to adjoin two restorations implies that the first restoration, or a part of it, does not need replacing and assumes that the procedure for the single proximal restoration when compared to a mesioocclusodistal restoration is less complicated, especially in matrix application.

Occasionally, preparing an amalgam restoration in two or more phases is indicated, such as for a Class II lesion that is contiguous with a Class V lesion. Preparing both lesions before placing restorative material introduces condensation problems that can be eliminated by preparing and restoring the Class II lesion before preparing and restoring the Class V lesion (Fig. 13-26, *B*). A butting wall of the first preparation that is carious, for example, is a better wall against which to condense amalgam than no wall at all.

Abutment teeth for removable partial denture. When the tooth is an abutment for a planned removable partial denture, the occlusoproximal outline form adjacent to the edentulous region may need additional extension if a rest seat is planned, such as for the tooth-borne partial denture. This additional extension must be sufficient facially, lingually, and pulpally to allow preparing the rest seat in the restoration without jeopardizing its strength. *The facial and lingual proximal walls and re-*

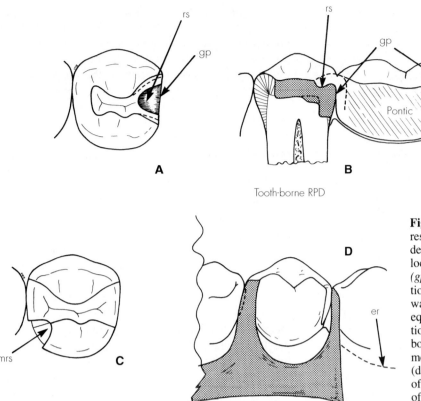

Tooth-borne RPD

Fig. 13-27. Abutment teeth with Class II restorations designed for removable partial denture (RPD). **A,** Occlusal view showing location of rest seat *(rs)* and guiding plane *(gp)* for a tooth-borne RPD. **B,** Cross-sectional view illustrating deepened pulpal wall in area of rest seat *(rs)* to provide adequate thickness of amalgam. Note relationship of guiding planes *(gp)* to tooth-borne RPD. **C,** Occlusal view showing mesial rest seat *(mrs)* for tissue-borne (distal extension) RPD. **D,** Lingual view of tissue-borne RPD showing relationship of RPD to Class II restoration and edentulous ridge *(er).*

spective occlusal margins must be extended so that the entire rest seat can be prepared in amalgam without encroaching the occlusal margins. There should be a minimum of 0.5 mm of amalgam between the rest seat and the margins (Fig. 13-27, *A*). *The portion of the pulpal wall apical to the planned rest seat is deepened 0.5 mm so that the total depth of the axiopulpal line angle measured on the facial and lingual wall is 2.5 mm* (Fig. 13-27, *B*). A rest seat on the mesiolingual of an abutment tooth, such as for a tissue-borne (distal extension) partial denture, usually involves both enamel and amalgam when the mesial is restored with amalgam. No modification of the outline form of the cavity preparation is indicated (Fig. 13-27, *C*). Fig. 13-27, *D*, illustrates the relationship of the tissue-borne removable partial denture with the abutment tooth shown in Fig. 13-27. *C.*

CAVITY PREPARATIONS INVOLVING BOTH PROXIMAL SURFACES

The uncomplicated ***mesioocclusodistal (MOD) cavity preparation for amalgam*** is similar to the two-surface cavity preparation for a single proximal surface except that both proximal surfaces are included. The cavity preparation follows the same sequence as the two-surface procedure. To preserve the strength of the tooth the operator should maintain ideal pulpal floor depth and

occlusal isthmus width whenever possible. Khera and others have demonstrated that excessive pulpal floor depth is more contributory to tooth fracture than isthmus width.[13] El-Sherif and others have concluded that the strength of the tooth decreases in proportion to the isthmus width.[10] The ***mesioocclusodistal cavity preparation in the mandibular second premolar*** is illustrated in Fig. 13-28. Compare this outline with the mesioocclusal (MO) preparation, and note the similarity.

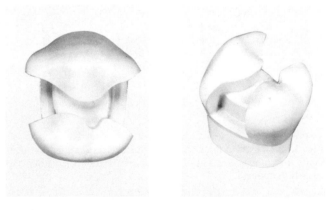

Fig. 13-28. Mesioocclusodistal preparation on mandibular second premolar.

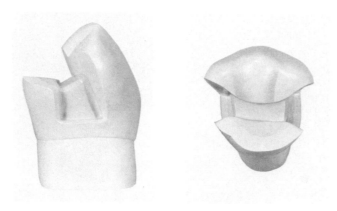

Fig. 13-29. Mandibular first premolar with lingual cusp reduced for capping.

Mandibular first premolar

When a *mesiooclusodistal cavity preparation* is necessary for the mandibular first premolar, the support of the small lingual cusp may be conserved by preparing the occlusal step more at the expense of tooth structure facial to the central groove than lingual. Also, recall that the bur is tilted slightly lingual to establish the correct pulpal wall direction. Despite these precautions, the lingual cusp may need to be reduced for capping if the lingual margin of the occlusal step extends more than two-thirds the distance from the central fissure to the cuspal eminence (Fig. 13-29). Special attention is given to such cusp reduction because retention is severely diminished when the reduction nearly eliminates the lingual wall of the occlusal portion of the cavity preparation. *Depth gauge cuts* of 1 mm will aid the operator in establishing the correct amount of cusp reduction and conserving a small portion of the lingual wall in the occlusal step. *Nonfunctional cusps such as the lingual cusp of the mandibular first premolar require only a minimal amalgam capping of 1.5 mm. Cusps in occlusion require a minimal reduction of 2 mm for amalgam.* It is acceptable when restoring diminutive nonfunctional cusps such as the lingual cusp of a mandibular first premolar to reduce the cusp only 0.5 to 1 mm, and then restore the cusp to achieve 1.5 mm amalgam thickness. This procedure conserves more of the lingual wall of the isthmus for added retention form. For the correct lingual tilt of the bur to establish the appropriate pulpal wall orientation, refer to Fig. 12-31.

Maxillary first molar

The mesioocclusodistal cavity preparation of the maxillary first molar requires extending through the oblique ridge to unite the proximal preparations with the occlusal step. *Cutting through the oblique ridge is indicated only if (1) the ridge is undermined with caries, (2) it is crossed by a deep fissure, or (3) occlusal portions of the separate mesioocclusal and distoocclusal outline forms leave less than 0.5 mm of tooth structure between them.* The remainder of the outline form is similar to the two-surface outline forms described previously in this chapter. Fig. 13-30 illustrates several typical three- and four-surface restorations (see Capping Cusps and Fig. 13-33 for the preparation of the distolingual cusp for capping).

Maxillary second molar with caries on distal portion of facial surface

Close examination of the distal portion of the facial surface of the maxillary second molar occasionally reveals a condition of decalcification and cavitation. When the enamel is only slightly cavitated (softened and rough), polishing with sandpaper discs may elimi-

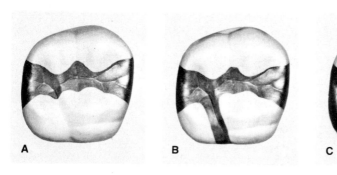

Fig. 13-30. Typical three- and four-surface restorations for maxillary first molar. See Fig. 13-33 for preparation of distolingual cusp for capping.

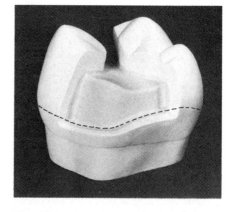

Fig. 13-31. Mesioocclusodistofacial preparation of maxillary second molar showing extension to include moderate to extensive caries in distal half of facial surface. Outline includes distofacial cusp and facial groove. Dotted line represents soft tissue level.

nate the fault, and careful brushing technique in addition to daily use of fluoride (toothpaste and/or rinses) and periodical applications of a topical fluoride preparation may prevent further breakdown. However, when such decalcification is as deep as the dentinoenamel junction and distal proximal caries is also present, the entire distofacial cusp may need to be included in a mesioocclusodistofacial cavity preparation. The facial lesion may be restored separately if it is judged that the distofacial cusp would not be significantly weakened if left unrestored (uncapped) by amalgam. The mesioocclusodistal cavity would then be prepared and restored first, followed by preparation and restoration of the facial lesion. When such sequential preparations are contraindicated, the cavity outline (Fig. 13-31) includes the distofacial cusp gingivally just beyond the caries and mesially to include the facial groove. The No. 245 bur should be used to create a gingival floor (shoulder) perpendicular to the occlusal force by extending the distal gingival floor to include the affected facial surface. Including the distofacial caries often indicates a gingival margin that follows the gingival tissue level as illustrated. The width of the shoulder should be approximately 1 mm. Resistance form is partially supplied by the shoulder. A retention lock should be placed in the axiofacial line angle of this distofacial extension, similar to the locks placed in the proximal boxes. For additional retention a slot in the gingival floor similar to that shown in Fig. 13-16 may also be indicated.

PROCEDURES FOR THE DISTAL CUSP OF THE MANDIBULAR FIRST MOLAR

The distal cusp on the mandibular first molar frequently presents a problem when positioning the disto-

facial wall and margin. Facial extension of the distofacial margin to clear the distal contact often places the occlusal outline in the center of the cusp. This dictates relocation of the margin to provide a sound enamel wall and 90-degree amalgam. When the distal cusp is small or weakened, or both, extension of the distal gingival floor and distofacial wall to include the distal cusp places the margin just mesial to the distofacial groove. Compare in Fig. 13-32 the ideal distofacial extension *(A)* with that necessary to include the distal cusp *(B)*.

Capping the distal cusp is an alternative to extending the entire distofacial wall when the occlusal margin crosses the cuspal eminence (Fig. 13-32, *C*). A minimal reduction of 2 mm should result in the minimal 2 mm thickness of amalgam for capping the cusp (Fig. 13-32, *D*). The cusp reduction should be such that a butt joint between the tooth structure and the amalgam results. Whenever possible, capping the distal cusp is more desirable than extending the distofacial margin because the remaining portion of the cusp helps in applying the matrix for the development of proper embrasure form. It also conserves more tooth structure.

REDUCTION OF CUSP(S) FOR CAPPING

When caries is extensive, reduction of one or more of the cusps for capping may be indicated. *When the facial (lingual) extension is two-thirds from a primary fissure toward the cusp tip, reduction of the cusp(s) for amalgam capping is mandatory for the development of adequate resistance form,* just as in preparations for cast gold restorations (see Capping Cusps, in Chapter 19). Reduction should be accomplished early in cavity preparation because it greatly improves access and visibility for subsequent steps. Make **depth gauge cuts** (2

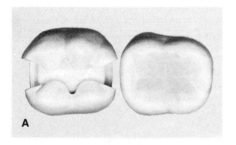
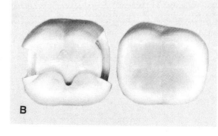
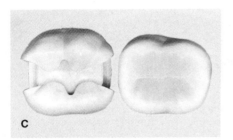
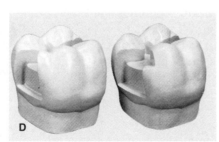

Fig. 13-32. Mandibular first molar. **A,** Ideal distofacial extension. **B,** Entire distal cusp included in cavity outline form. **C,** Capping of distal cusp is indicated when occlusal margin crosses cuspal eminence. **D,** *Left,* Distofacial view of distal cusp shown in C before reduction for capping; *right,* distal cusp after reduction. Reduction of 2 mm is necessary to provide for minimal 2 mm thickness of amalgam.

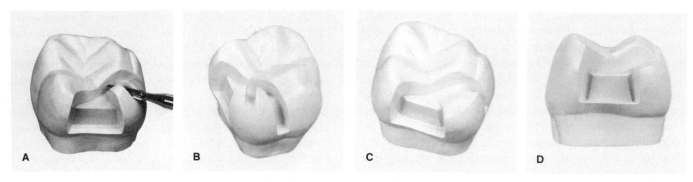

Fig. 13-33. Reduction of distolingual cusp of maxillary molar. **A,** Cutting depth gauge groove with side of bur. **B,** Completed depth gauge groove. **C** and **D,** Completed cusp reduction.

mm minimum for functional cusps and 1.5 mm minimum for nonfunctional cusps)[17] on each cusp to be capped using the side of a carbide fissure bur or a suitable diamond instrument (Fig. 13-33, *A* and *B*). Uniform reduction is ensured using the depth gauge cuts as a guide. Slightly round any sharp external corners at the junction of the cusp-reduced surface with contiguous prepared surfaces to decrease stress concentration in the capping amalgam and thus improve its resistance to occlusal forces. The procedure for reducing the distolingual cusp of a maxillary first molar for capping is illustrated in Fig. 13-33. (Extending the facial or lingual wall of a proximal box to include the entire cusp is indicated only when necessary to include weak or carious tooth structure or existing restorative material, and examples are illustrated in Figs. 13-31 and 13-32.)

Cusp reduction significantly decreases retention form caused by loss of height of the vertical walls. When additional retention is indicated, slots and potholes can be prepared along the gingival floor 0.2 mm pulpally from the dentinoenamel junction. Also, retention may be increased by inserting pins in carefully positioned pinholes. Chapter 15 describes the procedure for the use of metal pins for gaining retention in badly broken-down teeth.

MATRICES FOR TWO- AND THREE-SURFACE RESTORATIONS

Unfortunately, dentistry does not have a truly satisfactory manufactured *matrix for amalgam restorations.* In 1957, Brass[4] stated that no retainer in use provided in any material way to the support, form, and necessary separation essential for good amalgam condensation. Most matrices available to the profession have some good qualities but do not meet all the requisites. The primary function of the matrix is to restore anatomical contours and contact areas. Qualities of a good matrix include (1) rigidity, (2) establishment of proper anatom-

ical contour, (3) restoration of correct proximal contact relation, (4) prevention of gingival excesses, (5) convenient application, and (6) ease of removal.

Universal matrix

The Universal matrix system (Fig. 13-34), *designed by B.R. Tofflemire, is ideally indicated when three surfaces (mesial, occlusal, and distal) of a posterior tooth have been prepared. Also, it is commonly used for the two-surface Class II restoration.* A definite advantage of the **Tofflemire matrix retainer** is that it may be positioned on the facial or lingual aspect of the tooth. Lingual positioning (Fig. 13-35), however, requires the contra-angled design of the retainer (which can be used on the facial aspect as well). The retainer and band are generally stable when in place. The retainer is easily separated from the band to expedite removal of the band. Bands (see Fig. 13-34) with varying occlusogingival measurements are available; however, each must be properly contoured. The retainer is available in a small size, which may be used on the primary dentition.

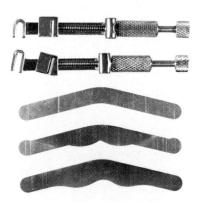

Fig. 13-34. Straight and contra-angled Universal (Tofflemire) retainers. Bands are available with varying occlusogingival measurements.

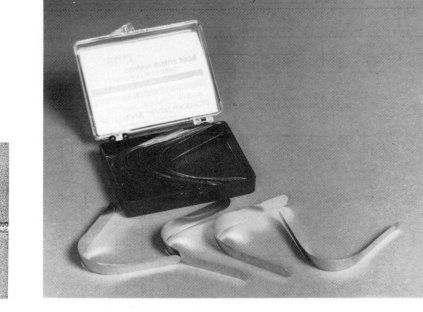

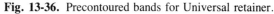

| Fig. 13-35. Lingual positioning requires contra-angled Universal retainer. | Fig. 13-36. Precontoured bands for Universal retainer. |

Even though the Universal retainer is a versatile instrument, it still does not meet all the requirements of the ideal retainer and band. *The conventional, flat (unburnished) Tofflemire band must be reshaped to achieve proper contour and contact.* Proximal surfaces restored using the Tofflemire band may require more carving than those restored with the compound-supported matrix (presented next). Precontoured bands for the Universal retainer are available commercially and need little or no adjustment before placing in the retainer (Fig. 13-36). Also, these bands are simpler to use because they usually require little or no adjustment or modification after positioning around the tooth. Although precontoured bands are more expensive, the difference in cost seems justified because they require less chairtime. The noncontoured bands are available in two thicknesses, 0.002 (0.05 mm) and 0.0015 (0.038 mm) inch. Burnishing the thinner band to contour is more difficult. It is also less likely to maintain its contour when tightened around the tooth.

Dryness during insertion of the amalgam is essential to the success of the restoration. Rubber dam procedures are discussed in Chapter 11. When cotton roll isolation is the only option, the Tofflemire retainer will help to hold the cotton roll in place (Fig. 13-37).

To prepare the retainer to receive the band, turn the larger of the knurled nuts until the locking vise (Fig. 13-38, *A*) is a short distance (¼ inch [6 mm]) from the end of the retainer. Next, while holding the large nut, move the small knurled nut counterclockwise until the pointed spindle is free of the slot in the locking vise

(Fig. 13-38, *B*). If a flat band is used, place it on a resilient paper pad, and burnish the proximal areas as illustrated (Fig. 13-38, *C* and *D*). The large **egg-shaped burnisher** is well suited for this task. When a precontoured band is available, burnishing is unnecessary. Fold the matrix band end to end, forming a loop (Fig. 13-38, *E*). *Notice that when the band is folded, the gingival edge has a smaller circumference than the occlusal edge. This design accommodates the difference in tooth circumferences at the contact and gingival levels. Position the band in the retainer so that the slotted side of the retainer is always directed gingivally to permit easy separation of the retainer from the band in an oc-*

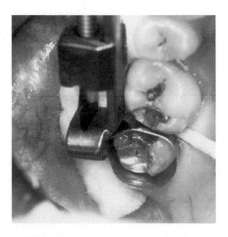

Fig. 13-37. Tofflemire retainer maintaining cotton roll in maxillary vestibule during condensation.

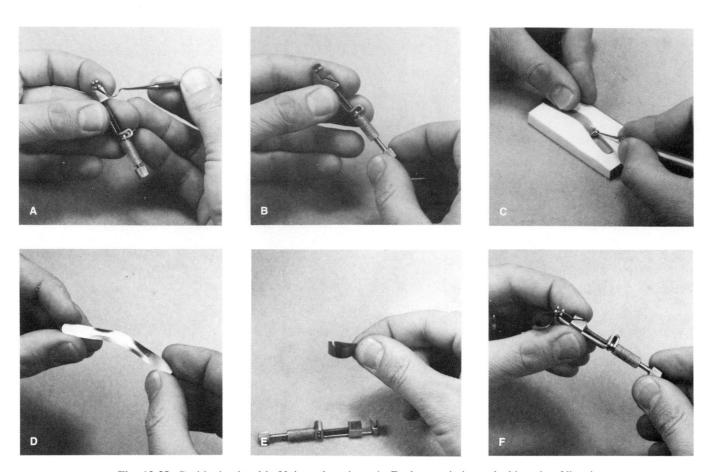

Fig. 13-38. Positioning band in Universal retainer. **A,** Explorer pointing to locking vise. View is showing gingival side of vise. **B,** Pointed spindle is released from locking vise by turning small knurled nut counterclockwise. **C,** Contour band with egg-shaped burnisher. **D,** Contoured band. **E,** Fold band to form loop, and position in retainer, occlusal edge of band first. **F,** Tighten spindle against band in locking vise.

clusal direction (later procedure). This is accomplished by placing the occlusal edge of the band in the correct guide channel (right, left, or parallel to the long axis of the retainer) depending on the location of the tooth. The two ends of the band are placed in the slot of the locking vise, and the smaller of the knurled nuts is turned clockwise to tighten the pointed spindle against the band (Fig. 13-38, *F*). Slip the matrix band over the tooth allowing the gingival edge of the band to be positioned beyond the gingival margin at least 1 mm, but do not damage the gingival attachment. The larger of the knurled nuts is turned counterclockwise to obtain a larger loop, if needed, to fit over the tooth. *Be careful not to trap rubber dam between the band and the gingival margin.* If the dam material is trapped between the band and the tooth, stretch the septum of the dam and depress it gingivally to reposition the dam material. *Next, turn the larger knurled nut clockwise to tighten the band slightly and use an explorer along the gingival margin to determine that the gingival edge of the band extends beyond the preparation.* Once the band is cor-

rectly positioned, tighten the band securely around the tooth.

When one of the proximal margins is deeper gingivally than the other, the Tofflemire mesioocclusodistal band may be modified to prevent damage to the gingival tissue or attachment on the shallow side. Fig. 13-39 illustrates how a band may be trimmed for the shallow gingival margin, permitting the matrix to extend farther gingivally for the deeper gingival margin on the other proximal surface.

Next, evaluate the band by viewing the proximal contour(s) of the band, and note the contact level. With the mirror facial/lingual to the tooth, position the reflecting surface to view through the interproximal space the contour of the strip (see Fig. 13-37, *P*). The occlusogingival contour should be convex, with the height of contour at proper contact level and contacting the adjacent tooth. Next, observe the matrix from an occlusal view, and evaluate the position of the contact area in a faciolingual direction. It may be necessary to remove the retainer and reburnish the band for additional con-

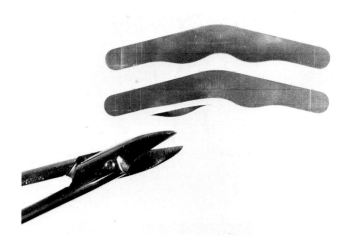

Fig. 13-39. Band may be trimmed for the shallower gingival margin, permitting matrix to extend farther gingivally for the deeper gingival margin on the other proximal surface.

touring. Minor alterations in contour and contact may be accomplished without removal from the tooth. The back side of the blade of the 15-8-14 spoon excavator is an excellent instrument for improving both contour and contact. If a smaller burnishing instrument is used, exercise care not to create a grooved or bumpy surface that will result in a restoration with an uneven proximal surface.

A minor modification of the matrix may be indicated for restoring the proximal surface that is planned for a guide-plane for a removable partial denture. Abutment teeth for a *tooth-supported removable partial denture* must provide amalgam contour to allow defining (carving, or later discing) a guide-plane extending from the marginal ridge 2.5 mm gingivally (see Fig. 13-27, *B*). However, *normal proximal contour,* rather than overcontour, is usually sufficient and best for development of a guide-plane. This favors a resultant gingival embrasure (denture-tooth) that is less open and less likely to trap food (see Fig. 13-27, *B*).

Abutment teeth adjacent to the residual ridge for a *tissue-supported (distal extension) removable partial denture* are carved to provide normal morphology. Suf-

ficient gingival embrasure should be provided to allow for the difference between the compression under load of the ridge soft tissues and that of the periodontal membrane even though a small area guide-plane may be provided (see Fig. 13-27, *D*). Compare this embrasure in *(D)* to that in *(B)*.

Wedge placement. Break off approximately ½ inch (1.2 cm) of a round toothpick. Have a small amount of rubber dam lubricant available. Grasp the broken end of the wedge with the No. 110 pliers, and lightly "wet" the gingival aspect of the wedge with the lubricant. *Insert the pointed tip from the facial or lingual embrasure, whichever is larger, slightly gingival to the gingival margin, wedging the band tightly against the tooth and margin* (Fig. 13-40, *A*). If the wedge is occlusal to the gingival margin, the band will be pressed into the preparation, creating an abnormal concavity in the proximal surface of the restoration (Fig. 13-40, *B*). The wedge should not be so far apical to the gingival margin that the band will not be held tightly against the gingival margin. This improper wedge placement will result in a gingival excess (*"overhang"*) caused by the band moving slightly away from the margin during condensation of the amalgam. Such an overhang often goes undetected and causes irritation of the gingiva. If the wedge is significantly apical of the gingival margin, a second, usually smaller, wedge may be "piggy-backed" on the first to wedge adequately the matrix against the margin (Fig. 13-41, *C* and *D*). *To be effective, a wedge should be positioned as near to the gingival margin as possible without being occlusal to it.* **"Piggy-back" wedging** is particularly useful in patients with recession of interproximal tissue level.

The gingival wedge should be tight enough to prevent any possibility of an overhang of amalgam in at least the middle two thirds of the gingival margin (Fig. 13-41, *A* and *B*). Occasionally, **double-wedging** is permitted, if access allows, to secure the matrix when the proximal box is wide faciolingually. Double-wedging refers to inserting two wedges—one from the lingual and a second from the facial embrasure (Fig. 13-41, *E* and *F*). Two wedges help to ensure that the gingival corners of a wide proximal box can be properly con-

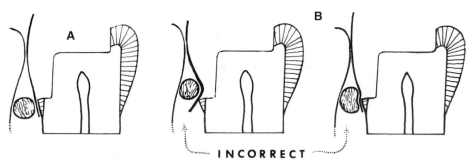

Fig. 13-40. A, Correct wedge position. **B,** Incorrect wedge position.

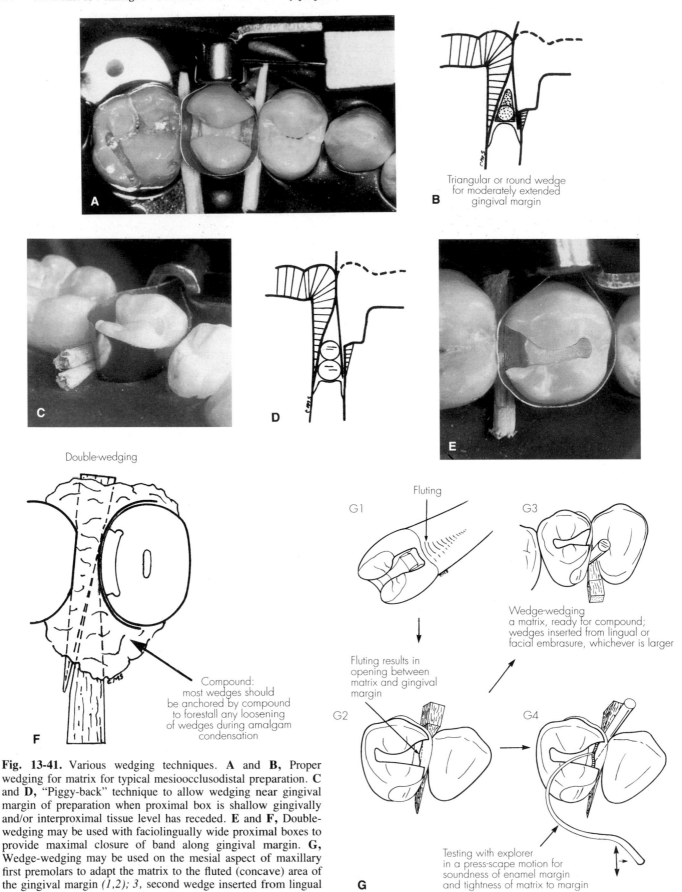

Fig. 13-41. Various wedging techniques. **A** and **B,** Proper wedging for matrix for typical mesioocclusodistal preparation. **C** and **D,** "Piggy-back" technique to allow wedging near gingival margin of preparation when proximal box is shallow gingivally and/or interproximal tissue level has receded. **E** and **F,** Double-wedging may be used with faciolingually wide proximal boxes to provide maximal closure of band along gingival margin. **G,** Wedge-wedging may be used on the mesial aspect of maxillary first premolars to adapt the matrix to the fluted (concave) area of the gingival margin (*1,2*); *3,* second wedge inserted from lingual embrasure; *4,* testing adaptation of band after insertion of wedges from facial.

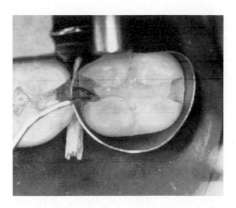

Fig. 13-42. With pressure, use explorer tip to ensure proper adaptation of the band to gingival margin. Also, press-drag the tip along gingival margin in both directions to ensure removal of any friable enamel.

densed as well as to minimize gingival excess. However, double-wedging should be used only if the middle two thirds of the proximal margins can be adequately wedged. *Because the facial and lingual corners are accessible to carving, proper wedging is important to prevent gingival excess of amalgam in the middle two thirds of the proximal box* (Fig. 13-41, *B*).

Occasionally, a concavity may be present on the proximal surface gingivally of the contact and extending as a fluting onto the root (e.g., the mesial of the maxil-

lary first premolar) (Fig. 13-41, *G1*). A gingival margin located in this area will be similarly concave (Fig. 13-41, *G2*). To wedge a matrix band tight against such a margin, a second pointed wedge can be inserted between the first wedge and the band by *wedge-wedging* (Fig. 13-41, *G3* and *G4*).

The wedging action between the teeth should provide enough separation to compensate for the thickness of the matrix band. This will ensure a positive contact relationship after the matrix is removed following the condensation and initial carving of the amalgam. ***Test for tightness of the wedge*** by pressing the tip of an explorer firmly at several points along the middle two-thirds of the gingival margin to verify that the matrix cannot be moved away from the gingival margin (Fig. 13-42). While directing a gentle stream of air, press-drag the tip of the explorer along the gingival margin in both directions to remove any friable enamel. As an additional test, attempt to pull out the wedge using the explorer with moderate pressure, first having set the explorer tip into the wood near the broken end. Moderate pulling should not cause dislodgement. Gingival overhangs of amalgam can inadvertently occur as a result of wedges becoming loose during amalgam condensation.

Often, the rubber dam has a tendency to loosen the wedge. This is caused by rebounding of the dam from having been stretched as the wedge was inserted. This problem can be prevented by stretching the interproxi-

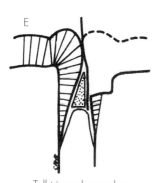

Tall triangular wedge
incorrect for minimally
extended gingival margin

A

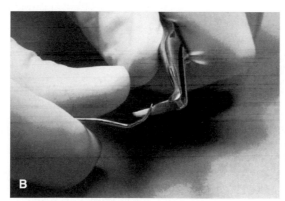

B

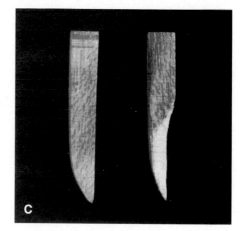

C

Corrective
trimming
of wedge

D

Fig. 13-43. Modified triangular (anatomical) wedge. **A,** Depending on proximal convexity, triangular wedge may distort matrix contour. **B,** A sharp-bladed instrument may be used to modify the triangular steepness of the wedge. **C,** Modified and unmodified wedges compared. **D,** Properly modified triangular wedge prevents distortion of matrix contour.

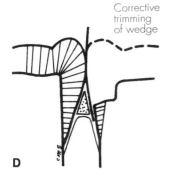

mal dam in the direction opposite the wedge insertion before and during the placement of the wedge, along with lubricating the wedge as described previously. The stretched dam is released after the wedge is inserted.

Some operators prefer a triangular shaped wedge because it can be modified (by knife or scalpel blade) to conform to the approximating tooth contours (Fig. 13-43). However, *the round toothpick wedge is preferred with conservative proximal boxes because its wedging action is more occlusal (nearer the gingival margin) than with the triangular wedge (Fig. 13-44, A and B).*

The triangular (anatomic) wedge is especially recommended for the deep gingival margin. It is usually indicated with the Tofflemire mesioocclusodistal band. The triangular wedge is positioned similarly to the round wedge, and the result is the same. When the gingival margin is deep, the base of the triangular wedge will more readily engage enough tooth gingival to the margin without causing excessive soft tissue displacement. *The anatomic wedge is preferred for deeply extended gingival margins because its greatest cross-sectional dimension is at its base (Fig. 13-44, C and D).*

To maintain gingival isolation attained by an anatomic wedge placed before the preparation of a deeply extended gingival margin, it may be appropriate to withdraw the wedge a small distance to allow passage of the band between the loosened wedge and the gingival margin. Tilting (canting) the matrix into place helps the gingival edge of the band slide between the loosened wedge and gingival margin. The band is then tightened

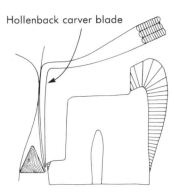

Fig. 13-45. Supporting matrix with blade of Hollenback carver during wedge insertion. (Demonstrated by Dr. Miles Markley at UNC School of Dentistry.)

and the same wedge is firmly reinserted.

Markley[16,17] demonstrated the effectiveness of supporting the matrix material by the **blade of a Hollenback carver** during the insertion of the wedge for the difficult deep gingival restoration. The tip of the blade is placed between the matrix and gingival margin, and then the "heel" of the blade is leaned against the matrix and adjacent tooth (Fig. 13-45). In this position the blade supports the matrix to help both in positioning the wedge sufficiently gingivally and preventing the wedge from pushing the matrix into the preparation. After the wedge is properly inserted, the blade is gently removed.

Assess all aspects of the band, and make any desired corrections, once the wedge is placed. Using a mirror,

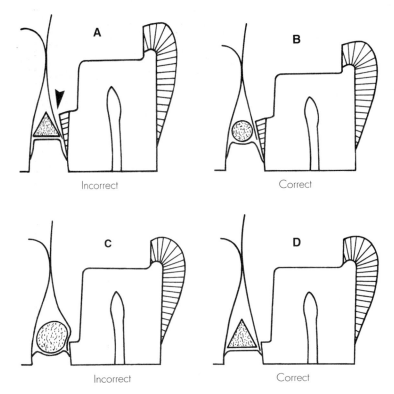

Fig. 13-44. Indications for round toothpick versus triangular (anatomic) wedges. **A,** As a rule, the triangular wedge will not firmly support the matrix band against the gingival margin in conservative Class II preparations *(arrow).* **B,** The round toothpick wedge is preferred with these preparations because its wedging action is nearer the gingival margin. **C,** In Class II preparations with deep gingival margins, the round toothpick wedge will crimp the matrix band contour if its diameter is above the gingival margin. **D,** the triangular wedge is preferred with these preparations because its greatest width is at its base.

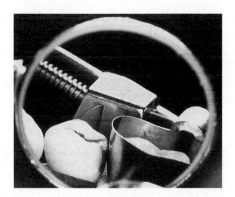

Fig. 13-46. Using mirror from facial or lingual position to evaluate proximal contour of matrix band.

again view facially and lingually the proximal aspects of the matrix band to verify that it touches the adjacent tooth and that proper contour has been achieved. Reflected light must not be seen in the contact area between the band and the adjacent tooth (Fig. 13-46). Carefully position the mirror to prevent a false impression of contact resulting from visual overlap of the band and the adjacent tooth. If the band does not reach the adjacent contact area(s) after contouring and wedging, release the tension of the band a small amount by turning the larger knurled nut counterclockwise. If loosening the loop of a Tofflemire band still does not allow contacting an adjacent tooth, a ***custom-made band*** with a smaller angle can be used. The smaller the angle (Fig. 13-47), the greater the difference in length of the gingival and occlusal edges (circumferences). After cutting a suitable length of matrix material, fold it as shown in Fig. 13-47. Then, burnish for appropriate occlusogingival contour (in the contact areas), and insert the band into the Tofflemire retainer. To maximize the advantage of either this custom band or the loosened Tofflemire band, compound should be applied as described in the next section, Compound-Supported Matrix.

A suitably trimmed ***tongue blade*** can wedge a matrix where the intraarch spacing between teeth is large (Fig.

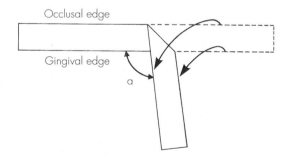

Fig. 13-47. Custom-made matrix strip is folded as indicated by arrows. The smaller angle *(a)* compared to angle of commercial strip increases difference between length of gingival and occlusal edges.

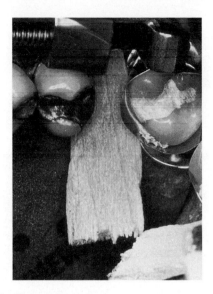

Fig. 13-48. Custom-made tongue-blade wedge may be used when excessive space exists between adjacent teeth.

13-48). Sometimes, however, it is impossible to use a wedge to secure the matrix band. The band must be sufficiently tight to minimize the gingival excess of amalgam. Because the band is not wedged, special care must be exercised by placing small amounts of amalgam in the gingival floor and condensing the first 1 mm of amalgam lightly but thoroughly in a gingival direction. Next, carefully continue condensation in a gingival direction using a larger condenser with firm pressure. Condensation against an unwedged matrix will cause the amalgam to extrude grossly beyond the gingival margin. (Obviously, without a wedge there will be some excess amalgam at the proximal margins and some overcontour, requiring correction by a suitable carver immediately after matrix removal.)

Matrix removal. Following insertion of the amalgam and carving the occlusal portion, especially the occlusal embrasure(s) (procedures described in a later section), ***remove the retainer*** from the band after turning the small knurled nut counterclockwise to retract the pointed spindle. The end of the index finger may be placed on the occlusal surface of the tooth to stabilize the band as the retainer is removed. Next, remove any compound that was applied to support the matrix. When the amalgam has hardened enough to avoid fracture of the marginal ridge during band removal, use the No. 110 pliers to tease the band free from one contact area at a time by pushing or pulling the band in a linguoocclusal (or facioocclusal) direction, and if possible in the direction of wedge insertion (Fig. 13-49). Leave the wedge(s) in place to provide separation of the teeth while the matrix band is removed. By maintaining slight interdental separation, the wedge reduces the possibility of the amalgam fracturing. Avoid a straight occlusal direction to prevent breaking the marginal ridges.

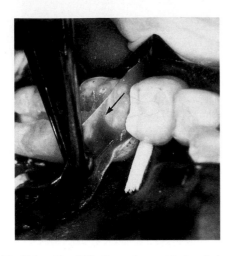

Fig. 13-49. Using No. 110 pliers, the matrix band should be removed in a linguoocclusal (as illustrated) or facioocclusal direction, *not* in a strickly occlusal direction.

Remove the wedge(s), and complete the carving procedures, as described in a later section.

Compound-supported matrix

An alternative to the Universal matrix is the compound-supported matrix. The wedged matrix supported by compound as described by Sweeney[29] provides most of the essential qualities of a good matrix, especially when used for two-surface proximal restorations. It is more rigid than commercial matrices, provides better contact and contour, is virtually trouble free during proper removal, and requires very little proximal carving after the matrix strip is removed.

Using $\frac{5}{16}$ inch (8 mm) wide, 0.002 inch (0.05 mm) thick stainless steel matrix material, cut a length sufficient to cover one third of the facial surface, and extending through the proximal to cover one third of the lingual surface. To prevent the matrix material from impinging on the facial and lingual gingiva, trim the gingival edge as shown in Fig. 13-50, *A*. Note that the re-

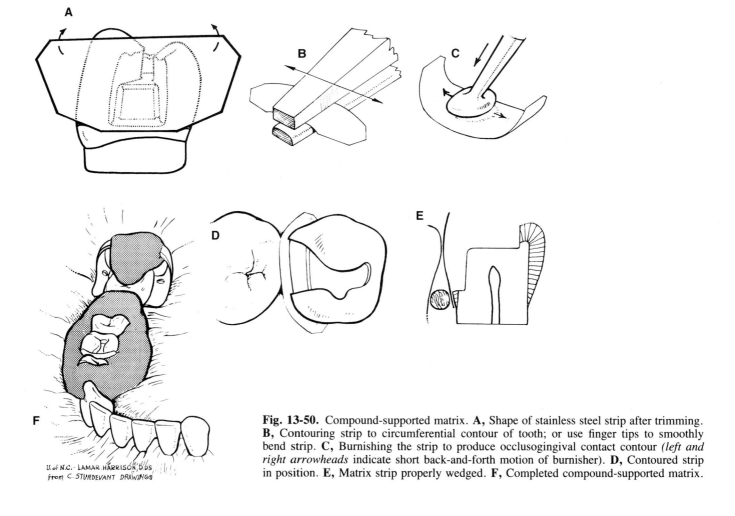

U. of N.C.- LAMAR HARRISON, DDS
from C. STURDEVANT DRAWINGS

Fig. 13-50. Compound-supported matrix. **A,** Shape of stainless steel strip after trimming. **B,** Contouring strip to circumferential contour of tooth; or use finger tips to smoothly bend strip. **C,** Burnishing the strip to produce occlusogingival contact contour *(left and right arrowheads* indicate short back-and-forth motion of burnisher). **D,** Contoured strip in position. **E,** Matrix strip properly wedged. **F,** Completed compound-supported matrix.

maining untrimmed gingival edge is longer than the length of the gingival margin of the cavity preparation. With contouring pliers, or fingers, contour the strip to conform to the circumferential contour of the tooth (Fig. 13-50, *B* and *D*). When contouring with pliers, exercise care to produce a smoothly curved surface. Contour the strip occlusogingivally with the egg-shaped burnisher using a short back-and-forth motion (see *arrows*) (Fig. 13-50, *C*). This is best accomplished with the strip laid on a resilient paper pad, which provides a yielding surface. Burnish with sufficient pressure to shape the steel strip to the desired contact contour. Contours vary both faciolingually and occlusogingivally because some teeth are more bulbous than others.

Commercially available metal strips (Palodent*) are precontoured and ready for application to the tooth (Fig. 13-51). *Palodent strips* have limited application because of their rounded contour. They usually are most suitable for mandibular first premolars and the distal surface of maxillary canines. The contact area of the adjacent tooth occasionally is too close to allow placement of the contoured Palodent strip without causing a dent in the strip's contact area, making it unusable.

The smoothness of the proximal surface of the restoration is determined by the smoothness of the steel matrix. Little finishing of the proximal surface is necessary when the matrix is smooth and properly contoured.

Position the steel strip (Fig. 13-50, *D* and *E*), carefully inserting the gingival edge into the gingival crevice about 1 mm beyond the gingival margin. The occlusal edge of the strip should extend no less than 1 mm and no more than 2 mm occlusally to the adjacent mar-

---

*Palodent, Palodent Company, Portola Valley, Calif.

ginal ridge. Visually inspect the occlusogingival contour of the strip. Sometimes the strip cannot be properly evaluated until after it is stabilized by placing the gingival wedge. Wedging is described in the next section.

It may be necessary to remove the strip for reburnishing when the contour is incorrect. After reburnishing, insert the strip, and, using a mirror, evaluate the matrix from the lingual (facial) and occlusal for correctness. Fig. 13-50, *E,* illustrates the correct occlusogingival contour. The strip should be shaped so that proper facial and lingual embrasure form will be established after compound application (Fig. 13-52). If these embrasures are too open, food impaction and injury to underlying tissues may occur; if too closed with a broad contact, proper scouring by food movement or by the toothbrush is hindered.

Wedge placement. Position the gingival wedge interproximally (see Fig. 13-50, *D*) to secure the band tightly at the gingival margin to prevent an excess of amalgam ("overhang"). The wedge also separates the teeth slightly to compensate for the thickness of the band material. Variations in wedge design and details on wedge placement, including tests for tightness, have been described previously in the section, Universal Matrix. The application of compound is indicated with this matrix system to develop proper proximal contacts, proximal contours, embrasure form, and stability (rigidity) (Figs. 13-50, *F,* and 13-53, *D*).

Compound application. The steps of applying low-fusing compound are: (1) soften a piece of low-fusing compound in a bunsen flame; (2) shape into a cone; (3) slightly glaze the base by a quick pass through the edge of the flame; (4) attach the base to the end of the appropriate forefinger; (5) glaze the tip of the cone by a pass through the side of the flame (Fig. 13-53, *A*); (6) immediately press the softened tip into the facial (lingual) embrasure (into whichever side the wedge was inserted) formed by the matrix and adjacent tooth, forcing the compound into the gingival embrasure; and (7) see that some of the compound is extended against the facial

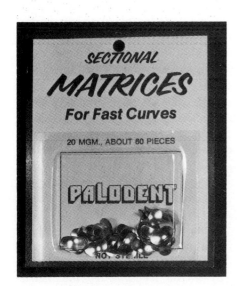

Fig. 13-51. Commercially manufactured, precontoured metal strips.

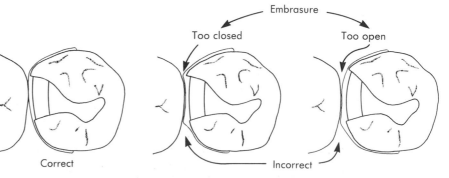

Fig. 13-52. Correct or incorrect facial and lingual embrasure form is determined by shape of matrix strip.

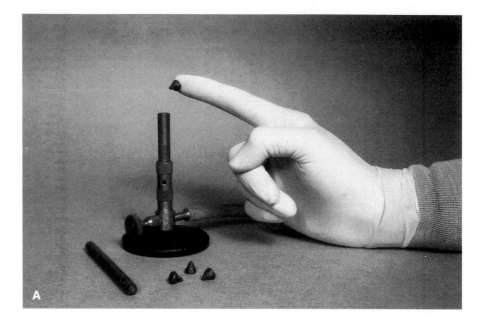

Fig. 13-53. Compound-supported matrix. **A,** Glazing tip of compound cone. **B,** Compound applied facially. **C,** Compound applied lingually. **D,** Stability of matrix ensured by uniting facial and lingual compound with additional compound over the occlusal surface of adjacent tooth.

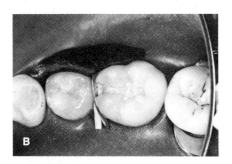

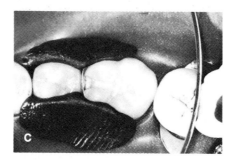

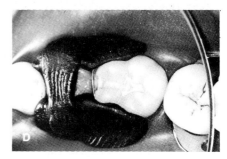

(lingual) surfaces of the operated tooth (past the edge of the matrix) and adjacent tooth (Fig. 13-53, *B*). These steps, except for the softening of the compound, should take only a few seconds. Now, repeat this application of compound for the opposite side (the side showing the tip of the wedge) (Fig. 13-53, *C*).

With experience, making and placing compound cones require very little time. When these compound cones are manipulated correctly, the consistency of the base portion (somewhat soft and moldable) forces the more fluid tip portion into the gingival embrasure and then out over half of the facial (lingual) surfaces of the teeth. Practice is required to achieve the correct consistency and placement of the compound. An experienced operator may apply both facial and lingual cones simultaneously—one cone attached to the thumb and the other to the index finger. Compound softened and applied as described will stick securely to clean, dry, tooth surfaces. However, stability is enhanced by the compound having been adapted properly to the facial and lingual tooth surfaces. Do not allow compound to encroach on the occlusal surface of the matrixed tooth or on the adjacent marginal ridge of the tooth that will be forming the proximal contact with the restoration. *A*

common error is to apply too much compound, which results in a bulky matrix that is sometimes loosened by movements of the tongue or cheek or by the flexing of the rubber dam. Stability of the matrix may be ensured (optional) by uniting the facial and lingual compound by addition of compound over the occlusal surfaces of adjacent teeth (not over the adjacent marginal ridge) (see Figs. 13-50, *F,* and 13-53, *D*). Harden the compound by cooling with a stream of air.

If proper contact and contour are not established initially, they can be corrected. A unique property of the compound-supported matrix is its ability to respond to needed change in contour by the application of a warm burnishing instrument (back side of a 15-8-14 spoon excavator) pressed against the band from the cavity side (Fig. 13-54). *This step should be routine to assure the operator that the compound has not moved the matrix away from the adjacent tooth.* As warmth of the instrument is transferred readily through the metal strip to soften the compound immediately adjacent to the strip, a burnishing movement of the instrument with moderate pressure *confirms (by tactile feel through the instrument) the contact of the strip against the adjacent tooth.* A small amount of compound often exudes occlusal to

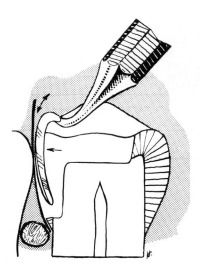

Fig. 13-54. Contour of compound-supported matrix may be altered by applying warm burnishing instrument against band from cavity side.

the contact to reveal that compound was (but is no longer) between the strip and adjacent tooth. Do not release the pressure against the strip until the instrument, strip, and compound have been cooled with an air syringe. The proximal contour is determined by the shape of the matrix band against which the amalgam will be condensed. *It is much easier, as well as more efficient and effective, to establish proper contours in the matrix prior to amalgam condensation rather than in the amalgam after matrix removal.*

Two features of proximal surface contour should be considered. One feature is the normal slight convexity between the occlusal and middle thirds of the proximal surface when viewed from the lingual (or facial) aspect. Correct and incorrect contours are illustrated in Fig. 13-55, *A* to *C*. Proximal surface restorations *often* display an occlusogingival proximal contour that is too straight, whereupon the contact relationship is located too far occlusally with little or no occlusal embrasure (Fig.

13-55, *C*). This condition allows food impaction between the teeth with resultant injury to the interproximal gingiva and supporting tissues and invites caries.

The second feature of proximal surface contour is alteration of the matrix, when indicated, to provide the correct form to the proximofacial line angle region (Fig. 13-56). With a warm burnishing instrument, provide this feature to the matrix. This contour feature may be present already if the first shaping of the matrix was correct before compound was placed. If this contour is not present, the facial embrasure of the restoration will be too open, inviting food impaction and injury to underlying supporting tissues.

The matrix should be tight against the facial and lingual margins on the proximal surface so that the amalgam can be well condensed at the cavity margins. Also, when the matrix is tight against the tooth, minimal carving is necessary on the proximal margins after the matrix is removed. However, *it must be emphasized that a matrix which is tight against the margins requires thorough condensation of the amalgam into the matrix-tooth corners to prevent amalgam voids at the proximal margins.*

As a last step before condensation, press-drag the tip of an explorer tine along the gingival margin in both directions to loosen and displace any weak portions of enamel. Use the air syringe to clear all debris from the preparation, and recheck the matrix for correctness.

Matrix removal. Removing the compound-supported matrix follows condensation of the amalgam and carving the occlusal surface, especially the occlusal embrasure (subjects described in a later section). First break away the compound from the facial and lingual surfaces with a stiff explorer tine. Carefully loosen and remove any compound remaining in the gingival embrasure (Fig. 13-57). Assuming the wedge was inserted from the lingual, grasp with No. 110 pliers the facial edge of the matrix and remove it facially until free of the contact (Fig. 13-58). To maintain the interdental separation, always remove the matrix in the same direction as

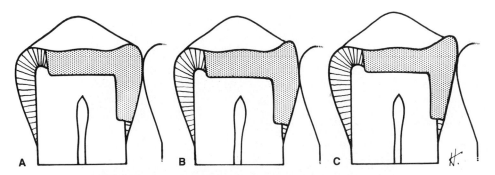

Fig. 13-55. Proximal contour. **A,** Correct proximal contour. **B,** Incorrect marginal ridge height and occlusal embrasure form. **C,** Occlusogingival proximal contour too straight, contact too high, and incorrect occlusal embrasure form.

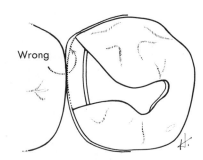

Fig. 13-56. Alteration of matrix contour to provide correct form to proximofacial line angle region.

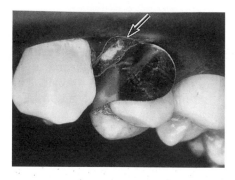

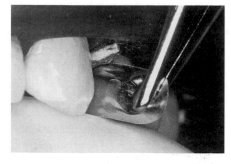

Fig. 13-57

Fig. 13-58

Fig. 13-57. Carefully remove any compound remaining in gingival embrasure *(arrow)* before matrix removal.

Fig. 13-58. Remove metal strip of compound-supported matrix by pulling it facially.

that in which the wedge was inserted. The matrix strip should never be moved occlusally, since breakage of the marginal ridge may occur. Being able to withdraw the strip without any occlusal vector is a noteworthy advantage. Because the matrix strip is thin and smooth, it will easily slip out past the wedge. Also, as long as the wedge remains in place, no bleeding will occur. This feature (control of possible hemorrhage) can be helpful when the operator judges that further carving is indicated to improve the form of embrasures before removal of the rubber dam. Using the No. 110 pliers, remove the wedge in the direction opposite that of insertion.

The proximal surface should be nearly complete, requiring minimal carving except to remove a possible small amount of excess amalgam at the facial and lingual margins and faciogingival and linguogingival marginal corners. The explorer is a suitable instrument for carving these areas if done before the amalgam is too hard. These margins may be refined with *"amalgam knives" (scalers, No. 34 and No. 35)* (Fig. 13-59). Amalgam knives are indicated if the amalgam is too hard to carve with an explorer. Carving strokes, as always, should be parallel to the margins, using the surface enamel to guide the carver. The back edges of the knife blade also are often helpful, using either a push stroke or a pull stroke.

Automatrix

The Automatrix* is a retainerless matrix system with four types of bands, designed to fit all teeth regardless of circumference (Fig. 13-60). The bands vary in height from $^3/_{16}$ to $^5/_{16}$ inch (4.7 to 7.9 mm) and are supplied in two thicknesses, 0.0015 inch (0.038 mm) and 0.002 inch (0.05 mm). The indicated use of this matrix is for extensive Class II preparations, especially those replacing two or more cusps. As with all matrix systems, it

*Automatrix, The L.D. Caulk Company, Milford, Del.

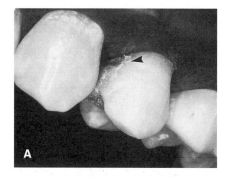

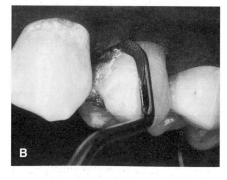

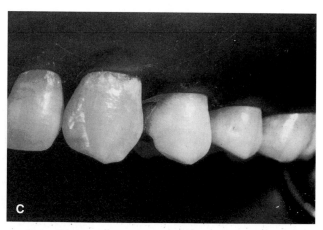

Fig. 13-59. Removal of gingival excess of amalgam. **A,** Excess of amalgam *(arrow)* at gingival corner of restoration. **B,** Use of amalgam knife for removal of gingival excess. **C,** Gingival corner of restoration with excess removed.

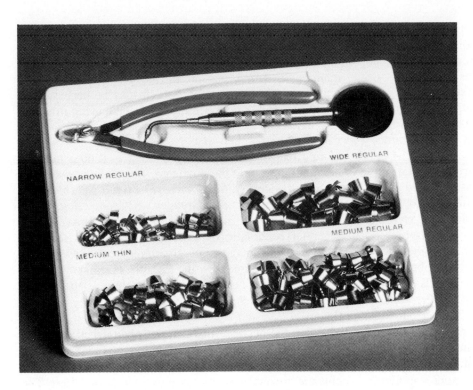

Fig. 13-60. Automatrix system.

has advantages and disadvantages. One advantage is that the auto-lock loop can be positioned either on the facial or lingual surface with equal ease. A disadvantage is that the bands are not precontoured, and development of physiological proximal contours is difficult. For a complete description of the Automatrix and its use, see Chapter 15.

PROCEDURES FOR INSERTING AND CARVING THE RESTORATION
Insertion of amalgam

The principle objectives during insertion of amalgam are: (1) condensation to adapt the amalgam to the cavity walls and matrix, and produce a restoration free of voids; and (2) to have as low as possible mercury content in the restoration to improve strength and decrease corrosion. Condensers should be selected that are best suited for use in each part of the cavity preparation and that can be used without binding. Condensation of amalgam that contains spherical particles requires larger condensers than are commonly used for admixed amalgam because smaller condensers penetrate the mass, resulting in little or no effective force to compact or adapt the amalgam within the preparation.

*If a **resin-based bonding system** is used in lieu of cavity varnish, carefuuly follow the manufacturer's instructions regarding tooth surface conditioning and bonding agent application.* Amalgam "bonding agents" are auto-cured resins which are mixed and applied to the cavity walls with a small brush or small sponge-like

applicator. Immediately the amalgam is mixed and condensed into the cavity preparation, mixing and mechanically interlocking with the auto-polymerizing resin. Some amalgam bonding agents will adhere to the stainless steel matrix band unless the band has been coated with a separating agent. After matrix removal and before carving the proximal amalgam, check the gingival sulcus for any excess bonding resin, which, if present, must be removed. Resin interlocks with the preparation walls as well as the amalgam. Ben-Amar reported that the amalgam restoration is bonded to the tooth structure and exhibits a significant reduction in microleakage, and states that *the longevity of this bond in the oral environment should be evaluated*.[3] Staninec found that amalgam which was bonded to the tooth resulted in a restoration that was more resistant to displacement than was conventionally placed amalgam retained with proximal grooves or dovetails;[24] Eakle adds, "If this finding holds true in clinical trials, then the bonding of amalgams to tooth structure will permit more conservative cavity preparations."[8] Eakle reported in a study that a bonded amalgam restoration of a Class II cavity preparation in a premolar significantly increased resistance of the restored tooth to fracture.[8] He adds, "It is not known whether microleakage, recurrent caries, or retention of the amalgam is a problem if the resin fatigues and breaks down. Long term clinical trials are needed to assess these factors. . ." He further states, "It is our opinion that bonded intracoronal restorations should not be substituted for circumferential reinforcement of teeth when the operator judges that the teeth are weak and susceptible to fracture."[8] Refer to Chapter 19 for circumferential reinforcement of the weak tooth by a gold alloy onlay restoration which skirts the coronal transitional line angles.[26]

However, since the indirect restoration usually is more expensive (more time consuming), the bonded amalgam restoration is an option for a patient when economics is a factor (editorial comment by C. Sturdevant).

Select an alloy certified by the American Dental Association and developed for the Eames-controlled mercury technique (low mercury/alloy ratio).[9] Alloys are commercially available in powder, tablet, and preproportioned forms. Most operators prefer the disposable capsules for (1) consistency of mix because the alloy and mercury are preweighed, and (2) the contribution to mercury hygiene. Some precapsulated brands require activation of the capsules before trituration. Preproportioned disposable capsules are available in sizes ranging from 400 to 800 mg. Triturate (according to the manufacturer's directions) a capsule containing enough alloy to fill a small or medium-sized preparation. Large cavity preparations often require two or more capsules. Convey the mix either to an amalgam cloth, a dappen dish, or an amalgam well. *Fill the amalgam carrier, and transfer into the proximal portion of the cavity preparation only the amount of amalgam that when condensed will fill the gingival 1 mm (approximately) of the proximal box.* **Condense the amalgam** along the gingival floor with the previously selected condenser. Move the condenser in a gingival direction with sufficient force to adapt the amalgam to the gingival floor. *Carefully condense the amalgam against the proximal margins of the preparation, as well as into the proximal locks.* This is accomplished by firm, laterally directed pressure of the condenser at the same time as exertion of gingivally-directed force (Fig. 13-61).

Continue the procedure of adding amalgam and con-

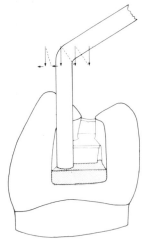

Fig. 13-61. Lateral and occlusogingival force is necessary to properly condense amalgam into proximal locks and into angles at junction of matrix band with margins of preparation.

densing until the filling material reaches the level of the pulpal wall. Change condensers (usually to a larger one), if indicated, and condense amalgam in the remaining proximal portion of the preparation concurrently with the occlusal portion. It may be necessary to return to a smaller condenser when condensing in a narrow extension of the preparation or near the proximal margins. Remember that a smaller condenser face is more effective at condensing as long as it does not significantly penetrate the amalgam. *Because the area of a circular condenser face increases by the square of the diameter, doubling the diameter will require four times more force for the same pressure on a unit area.*

Either pneumatic or hand condensation is satisfactory. A disadvantage of the **pneumatic condenser** is the possibility of damaging the enamel margins with the condenser points. A second disadvantage is the risk of inadequate condensation in conservative cavity preparations.[7]

When the occlusal margins are approached, exercise care not to injure the enamel margins. Exert maximal pressure with the hand condenser as the occlusal margins are covered and overpacked by at least 1 mm. The exertion of this maximal pressure may be accompanied by a slight rocking motion. Using a large condenser, make sure that the occlusal margins are well-condensed.

Condensation should be completed within the working time for the alloy being used. Condensation should be accomplished in 3 to 4 minutes (more or less time depending on the alloy). Otherwise, crystallization of the new amalgam matrix in the unused portion will be too advanced to permit (1) proper coherence and homogeneity with minimal voids in the restoration, (2) the development of the maximal strength and minimal flow (creep) in the completed restoration, and (3) the desired adaptation of the material to the walls of the preparation and matrix during condensation. Therefore, when inserting amalgam into large preparations and the mix is nearing 3 minutes old, a new mix should be made. While condensing, the operator should monitor the plasticity and slight wetness of the amalgam mass. To allow proper condensation, the mix should be neither wet (mercury rich) nor dry (mercury lean) and crumbly.

Procedure for carving the occlusal portion

Before carving procedures are initiated, some operators **precarve-burnish** the occlusal portion with a large egg-shaped or ball burnisher large enough to preclude undercontouring the restoration (Fig. 13-62). Use pressure about equal to the force used when condensing the amalgam. Move the burnisher mesiodistally and faciolingually until it contacts the enamel surfaces external to the margins. Burnishing should not continue after this since some amalgam should remain for carving procedures.

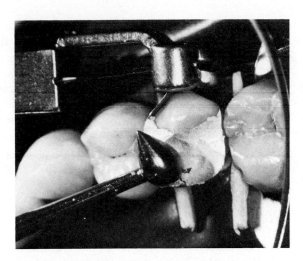

Fig. 13-62. Precarve burnish with large burnisher.

With the matrix band still in place, careful carving of the occlusal portion should begin immediately following condensation and burnishing. Sharp discoid instruments of suitable radii are recommended carvers. Use the larger discoid first, followed by the smaller in regions not accessible to the larger instrument (see Carving Procedure, Chapter 12).

While the matrix is in place, *give special attention to carving the marginal ridge* (Fig. 13-63). Use an explorer or small Hollenback carver to define carefully (open) the occlusal embrasure. This step will significantly lessen the danger of marginal ridge fracture during removal of the matrix.

Recall that occlusal contacts were evaluated before cavity preparation. Remembering the pattern of occlusal contacts, observing the height of the adjacent marginal ridge, and knowing where the preparation cavosurface margins are located will aid the operator in completing carving of the occlusal surface, including the marginal ridge and occlusal embrasure.

Removal of matrix band and completion of carving

As described in previous sections, depending on the type of matrix used, remove the compound or the matrix retainer, or both, and remove the matrix band (or strip) followed by the wedge(s). The *proximal surface* should be nearly completed, with proper contact evident and minimal *carving* required except to remove a possible small amount of excess amalgam at the proximal facial and lingual margins and at the faciogingival and linguogingival corners. The side of the explorer, the Hollenback carver No. 3, or the amalgam knives (scalers No. 34 and 35) are suitable instruments for carving these areas. Recall that the secondary (or "back") edges on the blades of these knives are sometimes helpful, using either a pull or push stroke. Carving, as always, should be parallel to the margins using the tooth surface external and contiguous to the margin to guide the carver. If, because of an incorrect matrix, appreciable excess is present at the gingival margin, or if the excess has hardened so much that the side of the explorer cannot carve effectively, remove it with the amalgam knives (Fig. 13-64). Again, the back edges of these knives are useful as previously mentioned.

On the proximal surface where a guide-plane is planned for a removable partial denture, do not overcarve the surface extending from the marginal ridge 2.5 mm gingivally. Development of normal tooth contour before defining the guide-plane is usually the best procedure.

When carving is completed, some operators *postcarve burnish* the amalgam surface using a small burnisher (Fig. 13-65). This is accomplished by lightly rubbing the surface until a satin finish appears. Do not

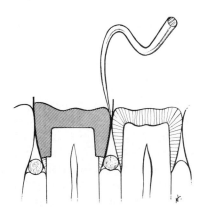

Fig. 13-63. Define marginal ridge and occlusal embrasure with explorer.

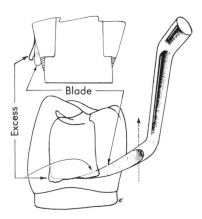

Fig. 13-64. Gingival excess may be removed with amalgam knives (see Fig. 13-59).

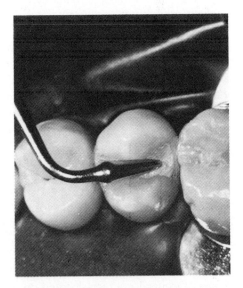

Fig. 13-65. When carving procedures are completed, postcarve burnish with small burnisher.

rub the surface hard enough to produce grooves in the amalgam. Cease burnishing if the amalgam has hardened to a point that burnishing creates a shiny or reflective surface (see Postcarve Burnishing, in Chapter 12.) If the amalgam is not too hard, the smoothness of the restoration can be improved by wiping with a small, damp ball of cotton held in the operating pliers.

While removing the rubber dam, advise the patient not to close because of the possibility of fracturing the newly condensed restoration if the restoration is "high". During the final procedure in rubber dam removal remind the patient again not to close until further instructions are given, since the first closure of the jaws must be observed. While these instructions are given, the operator's fingers should be in the patient's mouth, thereby preventing premature closure. Separating the patient's lips for visibility, instruct the patient to *CLOSE SLOWLY AND LIGHTLY and to stop closing when the teeth barely touch.*

During this first closure look for features of the occlusal relationship that offer clues suggesting the restoration is high: (1) cusp tips of the adjacent teeth are not in occlusal contact with certain mated areas when it is known from the preoperative occlusal survey that they should be touching, and (2) the cusp that occludes with a marginal ridge of the restoration is prematurely high. Occasionally, when the carving is done carefully no further occlusal adjustments will be necessary. If a marginal ridge of the restoration is high, reduce the high aspects of the carving. Observing the space (short of touching) between certain occlusally mated surfaces of nearby teeth indicates how much to reduce when carving. For example, if these opposing surfaces are 0.5 mm apart (estimating by eyesight), then reduce the high marginal ridge almost by this amount. This expedites occlusal adjustment, as compared with making an insufficient, shallower carving adjustment, and then having to repeat closure and carving again and again. If these preoperatively mated surfaces of nearby opposing teeth are not touching and, also, the cusp(s) opposing the carved marginal ridge(s) is not touching, then the prematurely high area(s) of the carving will be found in a more central fossa region or on an obscure cuspal region (of a cusp-capping restoration). To find these areas, look for a shiny spot, or ask the patient to lightly close on *articulating paper*. This should disclose the interfering area. After making the first occlusal adjustment, repeat the sequence of closure, observation, and carving until the appropriate surfaces of the opposing teeth are touching. When **carving for occlusion,** attempt to establish stable centric contacts of cusps to opposing surfaces that are perpendicular to occlusal forces. Occlusal contacts located on a cuspal incline or ridge slope are undesirable because they cause a deflective force on the tooth and should be adjusted until the resulting contact is stable (i.e, the force vector of centric occlusal contacts should be one that parallels the long axis of the tooth).

Notice that until now (1) the patient has only closed from a hinge-axis relationship (centric and no excursions), and (2) articulating paper usually has not been used. Articulating paper usually should not be used when adjusting marginal ridges because it (1) masks some of the sense of touch (teeth touching) of the patient, and (2) obscures the operator's vision of not only the offending high region(s) but also the occlusally mated surfaces of other teeth (this eliminates operator assessment of how much the carved surface should be reduced).

While holding the lips open and viewing the teeth, ask the patient to *"lightly* close the teeth and *lightly* slide them from side to side." *Observe* whether occlusal interferences occur during lateral excursions, and make appropriate adjustments.

Now, with the aid of articulating paper, evaluate the occlusion, and make any indicated adjustments. These should be small if the previous procedures have been satisfied. *Test objectively* for any highness using the articulating paper, even if the patient does not testify to a sense of highness. Any interference can be recognized on the restoration by the depth of color imparted by the paper, and especially if the colored area has a silvery center. Adjust (reduce) the deeper-colored or shiny-centered area(s) until all markings are uniformly of a light hue (and with no shiny centers). Guard against overcarving the restoration into infraocclusion, especially trying not to overcarve desired centric holding contacts. Before the patient is dismissed, thin dental floss may be passed through the proximal contacts one time to remove any amalgam shavings on the proximal surface of the restoration. Passing the floss through a contact more than once may weaken it. It is important that these shavings be removed to eliminate the possibility of a rough proximal surface. When carving is completed, rinse and evacuate all debris from the mouth.

Caution the patient not to use the new restoration for biting or chewing for a few hours.

FINISHING AND POLISHING PROCEDURES

Finishing of amalgam restorations may be necessary to correct a marginal discrepancy or improve the contour. However, evidence suggests that polishing of high-copper amalgams is unnecessary. They are less prone to corrosion and marginal deterioration than their low-copper predecessors. Nevertheless, many operators prefer to polish all amalgam restorations to maximize their clinical performance.

Polishing the amalgam restoration is not attempted within 24 hours following insertion since crystallization is not complete. Usually, finishing and polishing are delayed until all proposed restorations have been placed, rather than being done periodically during the course of treatment. (Refer to Finishing and Polishing Procedures, in Chapter 12.)

Finish and polish the occlusal portion similar to the procedures for the Class I restoration. Finishing and polishing of the proximal surface is indicated where the proximal amalgam is accessible. This includes the facial and lingual margins and the amalgam occlusal to the contact. The remainder of the proximal surface is inaccessible, and sufficient smoothness has been imparted to it by the matrix band.

If the amalgam along the facial and lingual proximal margins was slightly overcarved, the enamel margin can be felt as the explorer tip passes from amalgam across the margin onto the external enamel surface. When this occurs and/or where the proximal amalgam is accessible, use *sandpaper discs,* rotating at slow speed, to smooth the enamel-amalgam margin. Inappropriate use of sandpaper discs will "ledge" the restoration around the contact, resulting in poor contours. Sandpaper discs can also be used to smooth and contour the marginal ridge.

In very conservative preparations the facial and lingual proximal margins are generally inaccessible for finishing and polishing. However, fine cuttle discs or the tip of sharpened rubber polishing points should be used to polish any part of the proximal portion that is accessible. When proximal margins are inaccessible to finishing and polishing with discs or rubber polishing points and there is some excess amalgam (such as at the gingival corners and margins), use the amalgam knives to trim the amalgam back to the margin and to normal contour. Remember that the secondary (or "back")

edges of the blades of these instruments can be used with push or pull stroke, as well as the primary edge, to smooth the amalgam and make minor contour alterations. Such light surfacing can produce a smooth surface.

Some polishing techniques include using dental tape and a polishing agent on the proximal surface. With the polishing agent pressed into the facial and lingual embrasures, pass dental tape through the contact. Then press-slide the tape sideways in both directions several times against the proximal surface gingival to the contact. Exercise care not to traumatize the soft tissue. In addition, accessible facial and lingual proximal margins may be polished using the edge of a rubber cup and a polishing agent.

Final polishing of the occlusal surface and accessible areas of the proximal surface may be accomplished with a fine-grit rubber polishing point or by the rubber cup with flour of pumice followed by a high-luster agent, such as precipitated chalk. Figs. 13-66 and 13-67 illustrate examples of properly finished and polished amalgam restorations.

QUADRANT DENTISTRY

When several teeth are to be restored, experienced dentists usually treat them by quadrants rather than individually. Quadrant dentistry implies more efficient production for the dentist and less chairtime for the patient. The use of the rubber dam is particularly important when quadrant dentistry is planned. When a quadrant of amalgam cavity preparations is indicated, each rotary or hand instrument should be used on every tooth where it is needed before being exchanged.

When restoring a quadrant of Class II amalgam cav-

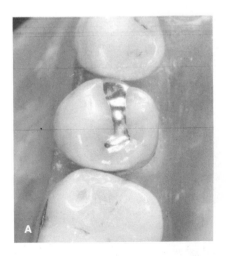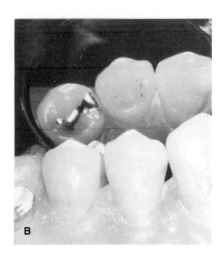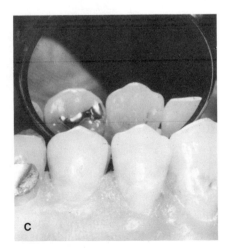

Fig. 13-66. Polished mesioocclusal amalgam restoration. Note conservative extension. **A,** Occlusal view. **B,** Mesiofacial and occlusal views of mesiofacial margin. **C,** Facial and occlusal views of proximal surface contour and location of proximal contact.

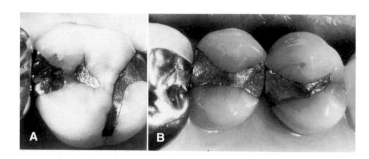

Fig. 13-67. Amalgam restorations. The amalgam restorations in **A** and **B** are 58 years old. They were inserted in 1934 by Dr. Miles Markley. (Photos courtesy of Drs. John Osborne and James Summitt.)

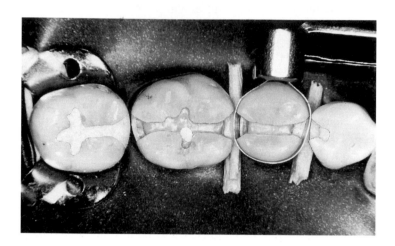

Fig. 13-68. Quadrant dentistry. Unless otherwise indicated, a quadrant of Class II preparations with similarly sized proximal boxes can be restored using two bands simultaneously if they are placed on every other prepared tooth. It is recommended to restore the most posterior tooth first.

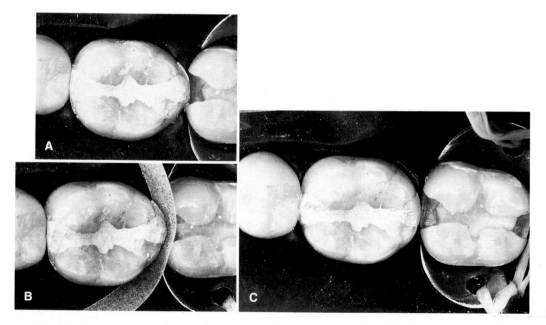

Fig. 13-69. When the first of two adjacent Class II preparations is restored, proper contour can be established using a finishing/contouring strip before restoring the second. **A,** Before using the strip. **B,** Applying the strip. **C,** Verification of proper contour can be achieved by viewing the restoration with a mirror from the occlusal and facial/lingual positions. Proximal contour can also be evaluated after matrix placement by noting the symmetry between the restored surface and the burnished matrix band.

ity preparations, it is permissible to apply matrix bands on alternate preparations in the quadrant, and restore the teeth two at a time. Banding adjacent preparations requires excessive wedging to compensate for the double thickness of band material and makes the control of proximal contours and interproximal contacts virtually impossible. Extensive cavity preparations may need to be restored one at a time. If proximal boxes differ in size, teeth with smaller boxes should be restored first because often their proximal margins are inaccessible to carving if the larger adjacent box is restored first. Also, smaller boxes can be more quickly and accurately restored, since more tooth structure remains to guide the carver. If the larger box is restored first, there is a risk of damaging the gingival contour of the restoration when the wedge is inserted to secure the matrix band for the second (smaller) restoration. If the adjacent proximal boxes are similar in size, start the banding of alternate preparations with a most posterior preparation, since this allows the patient to close slightly as subsequent restorations are being inserted (Fig. 13-68).

The operator should carefully establish the proximal contour of the first of two adjacent restorations (the first half of each interproximal contact) because its anatomy will serve as the guide to establish proper contact size and location of the second restoration as well as good embrasure form. A *finishing strip* often can be used to refine the contour of the proximal amalgam (Fig. 13-69). However, the finishing strip is indicated only where the proximal contact is open. Using a finishing strip between contacting amalgam restorations may lighten or eliminate the proximal contact.

REFERENCES

1. Almquist TC, Cowan RD, Lambert RL: Conservative amalgam restorations, *J Prosthet Dent* 29:524, 1973.
2. Baum L, Phillips RW, Lund MR: *Textbook of operative dentistry,* Philadelphia, 1981, WB Saunders.
3. Ben-Amar A: Reduction of microleakage around new amalgam restorations, *J Am Dent Assoc* 119:725, Dec 1989.
4. Brass GA: An amalgam technic, *Illinois Dent J* 26:539, 1957.
5. Bronner FJ: Mechanical, physiological and pathological aspects of operative procedures, *Dent Cosmos* 73:577, 1931.
6. Crockett WD et al: The influence of proximal retention grooves on the retention and resistance of class II preparations for amalgam, *J Am Dent Assoc* 91:1053, 1975.
7. Duncalf WV, Wilson NHF: Adaptation and condensation of amalgam restorations in Class II preparations of conventional and conservative design, *Quintessence Int* 23(7):499, 1992.
8. Eakle WS, Staninec M, Lacy AM: Effect of bonded amalgam on the fracture resistance of teeth, *J Prosthet Dent* 68:257-60, 1992.
9. Eames WB: Preparation and condensation of amalgam with a low mercury alloy ratio, *J Am Dent Assoc* 58:78, 1959.
10. El-Sherif MH et al: Fracture strength of premolars with Class 2 silver amalgam restorations, *Oper Dent* 13:50, 1988.
11. Galan J, Phillips RW, Swartz ML: Plastic deformation of the amalgam restoration as related to cavity design and alloy system, *J Am Dent Assoc* 87:1395, 1973.
12. Khera SC, Chan KC: Microleakage and enamel finish: *J Prosthet Dent* 39:414, 1978.
13. Khera SC et al: Parameters of MOD cavity preparations: a 3-D FEM study. II. *Oper Dent* 16:42, 1991.
14. Leon AR: The periodontium and restorative procedures, a critical review, *J Oral Rehab* 4(2):105, 1977.
15. Loe H: Reactions of marginal periodontal tissues to restorative procedures, *Int Dent J* 18:759, 1968.
16. Markley MR: Postgraduate course, Chapel Hill, NC, Oct 1982, University of North Carolina.
17. Markley MR: Restorations of silver amalgam, *J Am Dent Assoc* 43:133, 1951.
18. Mondelli J et al: Influence of proximal retention on the fracture strength of Class II amalgam restorations, *J Prosthet Dent* 46(4):420, 1981.
19. Mondelli J et al: Fracture strength of amalgam restorations in modern Class II preparations with proximal retentive grooves, *J Prosthet Dent* 32:564, 1974.
20. Moore, DL: Retentive grooves for the Class 2 amalgam restoration: necessity or hazard? *Oper Dent* 17:29, 1992.
21. Osborne JW, Gale EN: Failure at the margin of amalgams as affected by cavity width, tooth position, and alloy selection, *J Dent Res* 60:681, 1981.
22. Phillips RW: *Skinner's science of dental materials,* ed 9, Philadelphia, 1991, WB Saunders.
23. Rodda JC: Modern class II amalgam cavity preparations, *NZ Dent J* 68:132, April 1972.
24. Staninec M: Retention of amalgam restorations: undercuts versus bonding, *Quintessence Int* 20:347-351, 1989.
25. Sturdevant JR, Sturdevant CM: Gold inlay and onlay restorations for Class II cavity preparations. In Sturdevant CM, Barton RE, Sockwell CL, Strickland WD, editors: *The art and science of operative dentistry,* St Louis, 1985, Mosby.
26. Sturdevant JR et al: Conservative preparation designs for Class II amalgam restorations, *Dent Mater* 3:144, 1987.
27. Summitt JB, Osborne JW: Initial preparations for amalgam restorations: extending the longevity of the tooth-restoration unit, *J Am Dent Assoc* 123:67, 1992.
28. Summitt JB et al: Effect of grooves on resistance form of conservative Class 2 amalgams, *Oper Dent* 17:50, 1992.
29. Sweeney JT: Amalgam manipulation: manual vs. mechanical aids. II. Comparison of clinical applications, *J Am Dent Assoc* 27:1940, 1940.
30. Terkla LG, Mahler DB, Van Eysden J: Analysis of amalgam cavity design, *J Prosthet Dent* 29:204, Feb 1973.
31. Waerhaug J: Histologic considerations which govern where the margins of restorations should be located in relation to the gingivae, *Dent Clin North Am* 4:161, March 1960.

Note: The references in this chapter refer specifically to amalgam restorations for Class II cavity preparations. Refer to Chapters 12, 14, and 15 for other references on amalgam preparation and restoration.

CHAPTER 14

Amalgam restorations for Classes III, V, and VI cavity preparations

Kenneth N. May, Jr.

Aldridge D. Wilder, Jr.

William D. Strickland*

Amalgam restorations for Classes III and V cavity preparations can present the operator with special problems requiring good clinical judgment, patience, and ingenuity to solve. The Class V preparation and restoration can be especially difficult because of location, extent of caries, and limited access and visibility. The procedures for Class VI cavity preparation and restoration are generally uncomplicated. Indications and procedures for *amalgam restorations of Classes III, V, and VI* cavity preparations are presented in this chapter.

CLASS III CAVITY PREPARATION AND RESTORATION
Indications and contraindications

The selection of restorative material for the Class III cavity preparation involves the following considerations:
1. Tooth location
2. Service
3. Size and position of the carious lesion
4. Esthetics
5. Age of the patient
6. Economics

Tooth location. The most common area for an amalgam restoration in a Class III cavity preparation is the distal surface of maxillary and mandibular canines. When additional surfaces of the canine are extensively carious or contain large restorations, a full crown may be the indicated treatment to achieve maximal resistance form. For esthetic reasons amalgam is rarely indicated for the proximal surfaces of incisors and the mesial surface of canines.

Service. Amalgam restorations provide longer service to the patient than tooth-colored restorations,

*This author is inactive this edition; see Preface.

which tend to wear and stain. Therefore, composite resin is recommended for the distal surface of canines involving the proximal contact only when esthetics is an overriding factor. Glass ionomer cements are susceptible to dehydration and their long-term clinical performance is unknown.

Size and position of the carious lesion. Amalgam may be used when the carious lesion is small, has not involved the facial surface, and has not undermined the incisal corner. Access for the cavity preparation is generally from the lingual approach to conserve the enamel facial to the proximal contact. When the incisal corner is involved, a more complex cavity preparation is necessary, and a different restorative material is indicated for esthetics and retention, except for the distal surface of canines.

Esthetics. Well-polished amalgam restorations in areas that do not show in normal mouth movements should not be objectionable to the esthetics-conscious patient. The facial margin is usually not visible when the cavity preparation is approached from the lingual surface. Tooth-colored restorative materials provide immediate esthetic results, but in time may lose this quality because of staining and loss of contour. Tooth-colored veneers can be placed as inserts in areas where esthetics is important.

Age of the patient. Amalgam restorations rather than more expensive gold restorations are usually indicated for the adolescent because the caries rate in these patients is generally greater than in older patients. In the medically compromised patient, young or old, the use of amalgam may be more appropriate than restorative materials involving more complicated treatment procedures even though amalgam may not be the ideal material. When amalgam is indicated, it may be used regardless of the age of the patient.

Economics. Cost to the patient for amalgam restorations is less than for gold restorations because less time is required to restore the tooth, and the cost of the restorative material is less.

Local anesthesia

Local anesthesia of the tooth to be operated, as well as the adjacent soft tissues, is usually a requirement for better dentistry. In addition to pain control, anesthesia generally reduces salivation because the patient is less sensitive to stimulation of the oral tissues. Assurance of the patient's comfort is a major factor contributing to optimal performance of the operator. (Refer to Pain Control, Local Anesthesia, in Chapter 10.)

Isolation of the operating site

Before initiating the cavity preparation, it is desirable to apply the rubber dam. Its advantages and application are presented in Chapter 11. The last step in application

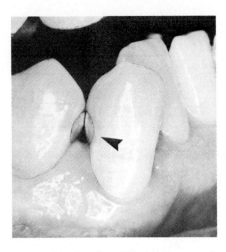

Fig. 14-1. Restoration for Class III cavity preparation using facial approach on mandibular canine. Restoration is 5 years old. (Courtesy Dr. C.L. Sockwell.)

of the rubber dam is placement of a wedge for the preparation of cavities having a proximal gingival margin. (Refer to Placement of the Rubber Dam, Step 21, in Chapter 11.) *Isolation with **cotton rolls** is occasionally permissible, but **rubber dam isolation,** which includes wedge placement, is ideal.*

Distal cavity preparation for the maxillary or mandibular canine

The distal cavity preparation of the maxillary canine is presented. The preparation for a distal amalgam restoration on the mandibular canine is identical except when the lesion is more facial than lingual. In that instance, a facial approach is indicated because the restoration usually is not visible even at conversational distance (Fig. 14-1).

Initial cavity preparation; outline form. The *outline form* of the Class III cavity preparation for amalgam on canines is similar to that for the conventional Class III cavity preparation for direct tooth-colored restorative material. Usually, the outline form includes only the proximal surface. A lingual dovetail is not indicated unless it existed previously or is necessary to enhance retention form for the cavity preparation with maximal incisal extension.

Enter the tooth with a No. 2 bur on the distolingual marginal ridge. A No. 1/2 or 1 bur should be used when the tooth is small for conservation of tooth structure. The bur is positioned so that the entry cut will penetrate into the carious lesion, which is usually gingival to and slightly into the contact area. The bur is held so that its long axis is perpendicular to the lingual surface of the tooth (Fig. 14-2, *A* and *B*). Penetration through the enamel should place the bur in such a position that additional cutting will both isolate the proximal enamel af-

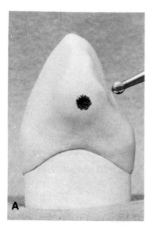
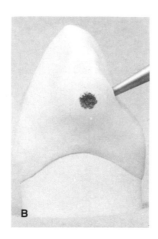
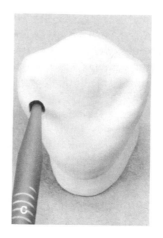
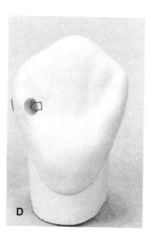

Fig. 14-2. Entry for Class III cavity preparation on maxillary canine. **A,** Bur position is perpendicular to enamel surface at point of entry. **B,** Initial penetration through enamel is directed toward cavitated, carious lesion. **C,** Initial entry should isolate proximal enamel. **D,** Initial cutting reveals dentoenamel junction *(arrow).*

fected by caries and remove some or all of the infected dentin, and *will be at a limited depth* 0.5 to 0.6 mm pulpally of the dentinoenamel junction (Fig. 14-2, *C* and *D)* or at a 0.75 to 0.8 mm depth pulpally where the gingival margin will be in cementum (on root surface) (see Fig. 14-8). This 0.75 mm pulpal depth allows 0.25 mm (the diameter of the No. $^{1/4}$ bur is 0.5 mm) distance between the retention groove and the gingival margin (see later section, Resistance and Retention Forms). Infected dentin that is deeper than this limited pulpal depth is removed later in final cavity preparation.

Ideally and for a small lesion, the facial margin is extended 0.2 to 0.3 mm into the facial embrasure, with a curved outline from the incisal to the gingival margin, resulting in an inconspicuous margin. The lingual out-

line blends with the incisal and gingival margins in a smooth curve, creating a preparation with little or no lingual proximal wall. The cavosurface angle should be 90 degrees at all margins. The facial, incisal, and gingival walls should meet the axial wall at a right angle. The lingual wall meets the axial wall at an obtuse angle or may be continuous with the axial wall (Figs. 14-3 and 14-4). The axial wall should be uniformly deep into dentin and follow the faciolingual contour of the external tooth surface (Fig. 14-4).

The axial wall of initial cavity preparation outline form with limited pulpal depth may be in sound dentin (shallow lesion), or with some infected dentin remaining (moderate-depth lesion), or in AIR except for axial line angles in sound dentin (deep lesion).

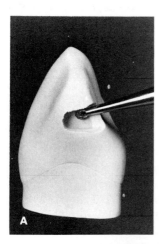
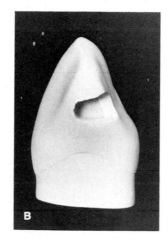

Fig. 14-3. Class III cavity preparation on maxillary canine. **A,** Round bur shaping incisal area. Note that incisal angle remains. **B,** Initial shape of preparation accomplished with round bur.

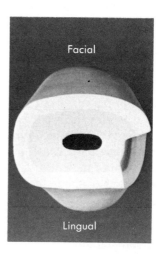

Fig. 14-4. Transverse section of mandibular lateral incisor illustrating that lingual wall of Class III cavity preparation may meet axial wall at an obtuse angle and that axial wall is a uniform depth into dentin and follows faciolingual contour of external tooth surface.

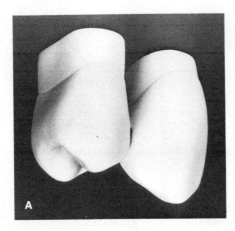 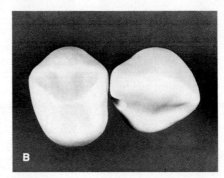

Fig. 14-5. Distofacial (**A**) and incisal (**B**) views of canine to show curved proximal outline necessary to preserve distoincisal corner of tooth. Incisal margin of this preparation example is located slightly incisally of proximal contact, but whenever possible the margin may be in contact area.

Incisal extension to remove carious tooth structure may eliminate the proximal contact (Fig. 14-5). It is important to conserve as much tooth structure as possible at the distoincisal corner *(canopy)*. Where removal of carious or undermined enamel permits, it is better to leave the incisal margin in the contact, just as with a conservative preparation for tooth-colored material (see Chapter 16). The importance of retaining as much of the distoincisal corner as possible for retention, longevity, and esthetics cannot be overemphasized.

When preparing a gingival wall that is near the level of the dam, or apical of it, it is especially important to have a wedge placed in the gingival embrasure to depress and protect the soft tissue and rubber dam. As the bur is cutting along the gingival wall, it occasionally may be lightly shaving the wedge. Remember that a triangular (anatomical) wedge rather than a round wedge is used for the deep gingival margin.

Complete the initial cavity preparation by using a No. ½ bur to accentuate the axial line angles (Fig. 14-6, *A* and *B*), particularly the axiogingival. The No. ½ bur may also be used to smooth the roughened, undermined enamel produced at the gingival and facial margins by the No. 2 bur (Fig. 14-6, *C*). The incisal margin of the minimally extended preparation is not accessible to the bur without marring the adjacent tooth (Fig. 14-6, *D*). (Finishing the incisal margin is presented later in Procedures for Finishing External Walls.) This completes the initial cavity preparation.

Final cavity preparation. Final cavity preparation involves the steps of removal of any remaining infected dentin, pulp protection, developing resistance and retention forms, finishing external walls (includes margins), and the final procedures of cleaning, inspecting, and varnishing.

Removal of any remaining infected dentin. Remove

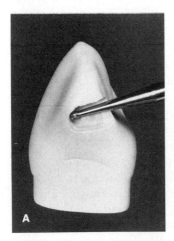 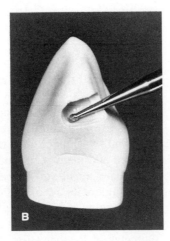 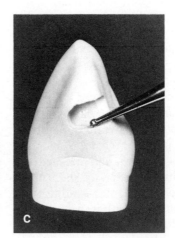 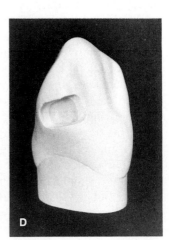

Fig. 14-6. Refining proximal portion. **A, B,** and **C,** Small round bur is used to shape cavity walls, define line angles, and initiate removal of undermined enamel along gingival and facial margins. **D,** Cavity preparation completed except for final finishing of enamel margins and providing retention form.

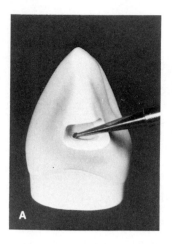
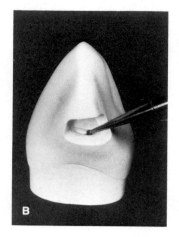
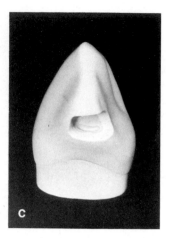

Fig. 14-7. Preparing gingival retention form. **A,** Position of No. ¼ bur in axiofaciogingival point angle. **B,** Advancing bur lingually to prepare groove along axiogingival line angle. (See Fig. 14-8 regarding location, depth direction, and direction depth of groove.) **C,** Completed gingival retention groove.

any remaining infected carious dentin (caries that extends pulpally from the established axial wall) using a slowly revolving round bur (No. 2 or 4) or discoid-type spoon excavators, or both.

Pulp protection. Refer to sections in Chapter 12 titled, Pulp Protection, for conservative cavity preparation, and Cavity Preparation for Extensive Caries, for procedures regarding bases/liners.

Resistance and retention forms. Resistance form of tooth structure against postrestorative fracture is provided by cavosurface angles of 90 degrees and enamel walls supported by sound dentin. *Resistance form of the restoration* against postrestorative fracture is provided by amalgam with (1) marginal angles of 90 degrees, (2) sufficient bulk (minimal 1 mm thickness), and (3) no sharp internal angle at the junction of the proximal and lingual portions, reducing stress concentration (see subsequent section, Lingual Dovetail).

Provide *retention form* by preparing a gingival groove and an incisal cove, and for some extensive proximal cavity preparations an additional retention feature, the lingual dovetail.

Prepare the *gingival retention groove,* by placing a No. ¼ bur rotating at low speed in the axiofaciogingival point angle and move it lingually along the axiogingival line angle with the depthwise direction of cutting mostly gingival and slightly pulpal (Figs. 14-7 and 14-8). The diameter of the bur is 0.5 mm, and the depth of the groove should be half this diameter, or 0.25 mm. Note in Fig. 14-8 the location and depthwise direction of the groove where the gingival wall is partially of enamel. If the axiogingival line angle is ideally located, directing the groove depthwise as described should not undermine the enamel. When cutting the groove where the gingival wall is entirely in dentin, the distance from

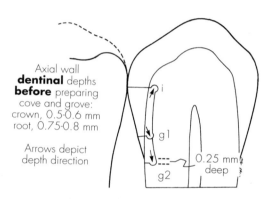

Fig. 14-8. Mesiodistal longitudinal section showing location, depth direction *(arrows),* and direction depth of retention form in Class III cavity preparations of different gingival depths. *i,* Incisal cove; *g1,* gingival groove, enamel margin; *g2,* gingival groove, root surface margin. Distance from outer aspect of *g2* groove to margin is 0.25 to 0.3 mm; bur head diameter is 0.5 mm; direction depth of groove is half this diameter, or 0.25 mm.

the margin to the groove will be 0.25 mm (Fig. 14-8). Extreme care is necessary to prevent the removal of dentin that immediately supports the gingival enamel. Care is exercised not to prepare the groove directly into the axial wall, since no effective retention form is developed and there is risk of pulpal involvement.

Prepare an *incisal retention cove* at the axioincisal point angle with a No. ¼ bur in dentin being careful not to undermine the enamel. It is directed facioincisopulpally into the incisal point angle and cut to one-half the diameter of the bur (Fig. 14-9). The facial and pulpal components of the direction of cutting help to prevent undermining the incisal enamel and corner of the tooth.

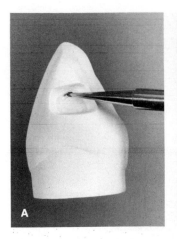
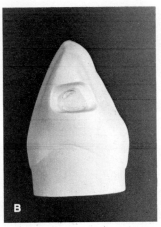

Fig. 14-9. Preparing incisal retention cove. **A,** Position of No. ¼ bur in axioincisal point angle. **B,** Completed incisal cove.

For the maxillary canine the ***palm-and-thumb grasp*** may be used to direct more easily the bur facioincisally (Fig. 14-10). This completes the distal surface preparation (Fig. 14-11).

Refer to the section titled, Class V Cavity Preparation and Restoration (under Retention Form) for a brief discussion of new dentin (and enamel) adhesive systems for bonding amalgam to the cavity preparation. Christensen reports that dentists using the new dentinal adhesive systems have observed elimination of the occasional sensitivity following an amalgam restoration; but he suggests that until these adhesives have been proven to provide sufficient retention in clinical longevity studies, it is wise to prepare mechanical retention even if using an adhesive system.[2]

Lingual dovetail. The lingual dovetail is not required in small or moderately sized Class III cavity preparations. It is reserved for large preparations, especially those with excessive incisal extension in which additional retention form is needed. Even in large preparations, the dovetail may not be necessary if incisal retention can be judiciously and effectively accomplished.

Prepare the lingual dovetail only after preparation of the proximal portion has been completed (Fig. 14-12). The dovetail should not be prepared earlier because the tooth structure needed for the isthmus between the proximal portion and the dovetail might be removed when the proximal outline form is prepared. The lingual dovetail should be conservative, generally not extending beyond the mesiodistal midpoint of the lingual surface. This will vary according to the extent of the proximal caries. The pulpal depth of the dovetail should approximate 1 mm, and the pulpal wall should be parallel to the lingual surface of the tooth. This wall may or may not be in dentin. Position the No. 245 bur in the proximal portion at the correct depth and angulation, and move the bur in a mesial direction (Fig. 14-13, *A* and *B*). The correct angulation is such that the long axis of the bur is perpendicular to the lingual surface. Move the bur to the point that corresponds to the most mesial extent of the dovetail (Fig. 14-13, *C* and *D*). Next, move the bur incisally and gingivally to create sufficient incisogingival dimension to the dovetail (approximately 2.5 mm) (Fig. 14-13, *E* and *F*). Then, prepare the incisal and gingival walls of the isthmus in smooth curves connecting the dovetail to the proximal outline form (Fig. 14-13, *G* and *H*).

The gingival margin trimmer is used to bevel (or round) the axiopulpal line angle. This increases the strength of the restoration at the junction of the proximal and lingual portions by providing bulk and reducing stress concentration.

The lingual convergence of the dovetail's external walls prepared with the No. 245 bur usually provides sufficient retention form. However, retention coves, one

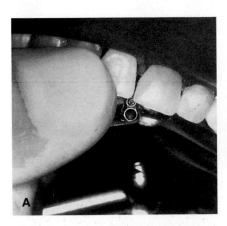
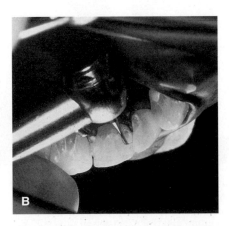

Fig. 14-10. Use of palm-and-thumb grasp to place incisal retention cove. **A,** Hand position showing thumb rest. **B,** Handpiece position for preparing incisal retention.

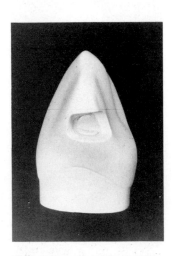

Fig. 14-11. Completed Class III cavity preparation for amalgam restoration.

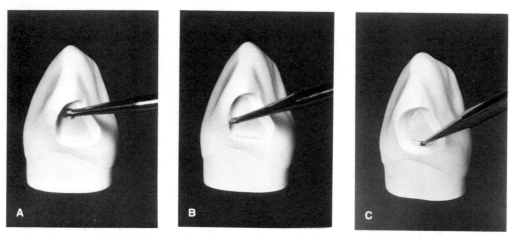

Fig. 14-12. Extensive Class III cavity preparation. **A,** Initial cavity preparation with No. 2 bur. **B,** Defining line angles and removing undermined enamel with No. ½ bur. **C,** Placing retention groove using No. ¼ bur. Note completed incisal cove.

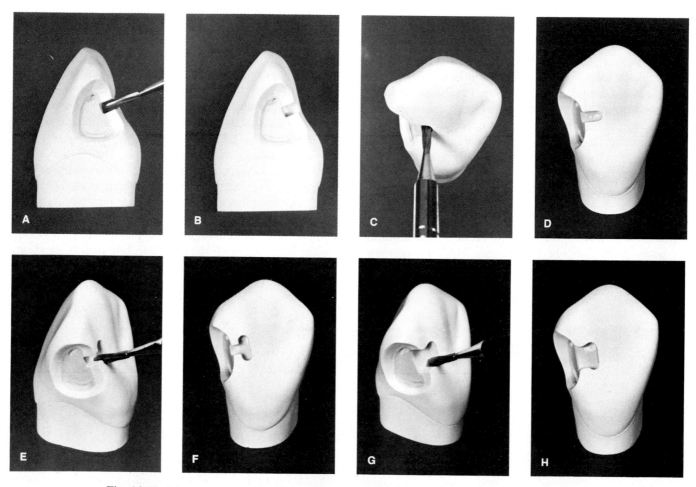

Fig. 14-13. Lingual dovetail providing additional retention for extensive amalgam restoration. **A,** Bur position at correct depth and angulation to begin cutting. **B,** Initial cut in beginning dovetail. **C,** Bur moved to most mesial extent of dovetail. **D,** If possible, cutting should not extend beyond midlingual position. **E,** Bur cutting gingival extension of dovetail. **F,** Incisal and gingival extensions of dovetail. **G,** Completing isthmus. Note that proximal and lingual portions are connected by incisal and gingival walls in smooth curves. **H,** Completed lingual dovetail.

in the incisal corner and one in the gingival corner (Fig. 14-14), may be placed in the dovetail to enhance retention. The coves are prepared with the No. 33½ bur and are entirely in dentin that does not immediately support the lingual enamel.

Procedures for finishing external walls. Remove any unsupported enamel, smooth enamel walls and margins, and refine the cavosurface angles where indicated. The *8-3-22 hoe* is recommended for finishing minimally extended margins (see Fig. 14-17, *B*). If the gingival margin is in enamel, a slight bevel is necessary to ensure full-length enamel rods forming the margin (see Fig. 14-8). As previously indicated, the walls of the preparation should meet the external tooth surface to form a right angle (butt joint) (Figs. 14-11 and 14-15). Various steps in a clinical procedure with the dovetail are shown in Fig. 14-16.

Final procedures: cleaning; inspecting; varnishing. Using air/water spray, clean the cavity preparation of debris if present. Using the air syringe, remove visible moisture (do not desiccate the tooth), carefully inspect the cavity preparation for detection and removal of debris or unwanted base/liner, and examine for final approval or correction of the cavosurface angles and margins. Two applications of cavity varnish should be applied. *Varnish is applied prior to matrix placement to prevent pooling at the enamel-matrix interface.*

For a brief discussion of new dentin (and enamel) adhesive systems for sealing amalgam against microleakage, refer to varnishing in later section, Class V Cavity Preparation and Restoration.

Cavity preparation for the mandibular incisor

The rare *Class III cavity preparation for an amalgam restoration for mandibular incisors* is similar to that for maxillary canines. Obviously, for esthetic reasons amalgam is best suited for the smaller carious lesion that can be placed from lingual access rather than for the cavity preparation that extends onto the facial surface.

Preliminary procedures for operating, such as anesthesia, isolation of the operating site, and wedging are presented in Chapter 11.

Initial cavity preparation. To prepare the *outline form,* enter the tooth from lingual approach (preferred) or facial approach using a small, appropriate-size round bur at high-speed with air-water spray, limiting the depth pulpally 0.5 to 0.6 mm from the dentinoenamel junction, or 0.75 to 0.8 mm where the gingival margin will be in cementum (or root surface) (Fig. 14-17, *A*). The choice of lingual or facial approach depends on the position of the tooth, the location of the carious lesion, and esthetics. The entry is generally made from the surface that requires the least removal of tooth structure except for conserving the facial tooth structure for esthetics. Once entry has been made to the carious lesion, use the bur to extend the cavity preparation farther to form the *facial wall,* maintaining the limited depth. Prepare the facial wall as near 90 degrees to the external surface as possible, extending the wall and margin only enough to be in sound tooth structure. *Incisally,* do not involve the proximal contact anymore than is necessary to extend to sound tooth structure. Usually, the incisal

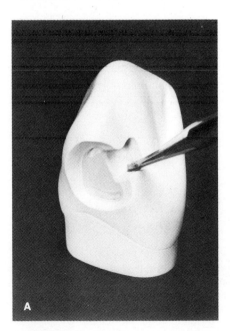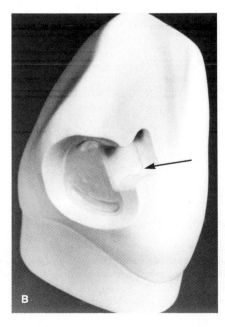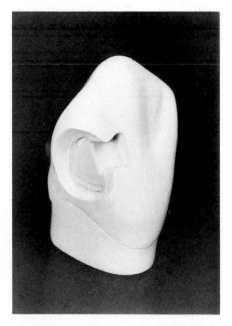

Fig. 14-14. Ensuring retention in lingual dovetail (often optional). **A,** Position of No. 33½ bur for cutting retention cove. **B,** Note that preparation of cove has not removed dentinal support of lingual enamel *(arrow).*

Fig. 14-15. Completed distolingual Class III cavity preparation for amalgam.

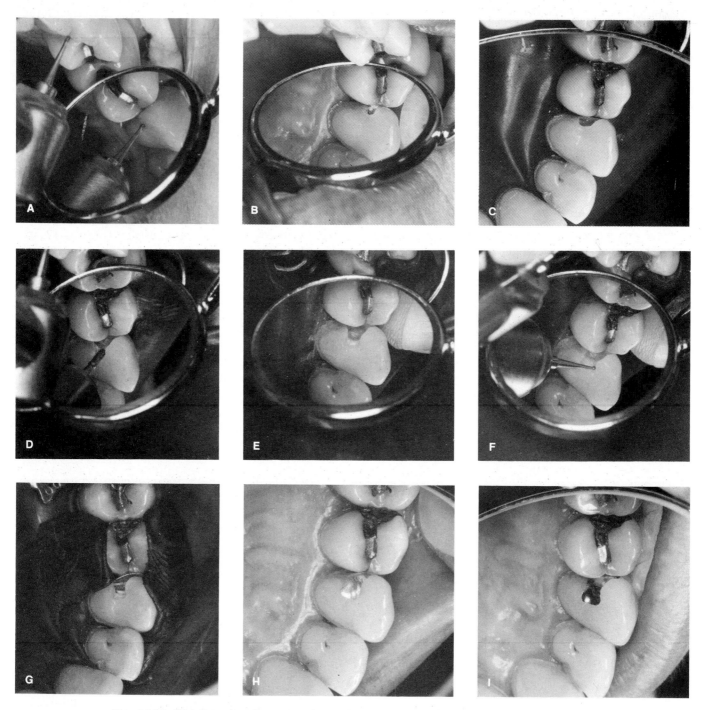

Fig. 14-16. Distolingual cavity preparation and restoration. **A,** Bur position for entry. **B,** Penetration made through lingual enamel to caries. **C,** Proximal portion completed except for retention form. **D,** Preparing dovetail. **E,** Completed preparation except for retention groove and coves. **F,** Bur position for incisal cove in dovetail. **G,** Compound matrix and cement base ready for insertion of amalgam. **H,** Carving completed and rubber dam removed. **I,** Polished restoration.

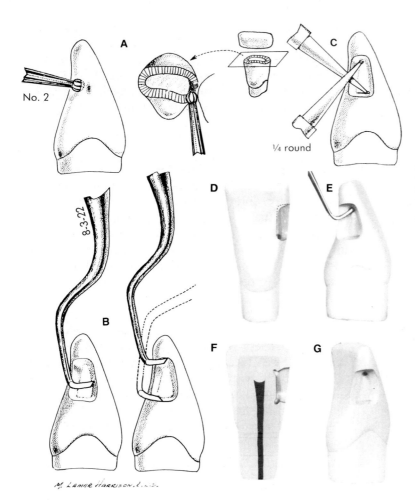

Fig. 14-17. Class III cavity preparation for amalgam restoration on mandibular incisor. **A,** Entering tooth from lingual approach. **B,** Finishing facial, incisal, and gingival enamel margins with a 8-3-22 triple-angle hoe. Note how the reverse bevel blade is used on the gingival enamel. **C,** Placing incisal and gingival retention forms with No. ¼ bur. **D,** Dotted line indicates outline of additional extension sometimes necessary for access in placing incisal retention cove. **E,** Position of bibeveled hatchet 3-2-28 to place incisal retention cove. **F,** Axial wall forms convex surface over pulp. **G,** Completed cavity preparation. Note gingival retention groove.

margin will be in the contact area for small and moderate size lesions. Extend the *gingival wall,* still maintaining the limited depth, only enough to be in sound tooth structure. All external walls, when completed in final cavity preparation (next section), will form 90-degree cavosurface angles.

When preparing the gingival wall that is near the level of the dam, or apical of it, it is especially important to have a wedge placed in the gingival embrasure to depress the soft tissue and the rubber dam. The wedge protects the rubber dam and gingival tissue as the bur is cutting along the gingival wall. The bur may slightly shave the wedge as the wall is prepared.

The *lingual outline* must be extended sufficiently to permit access and visibility for instrumentation during cavity preparation and insertion of the restorative material. The *axial wall* as previously described is positioned into dentin 0.5 mm from the dentinoenamel junction, or 0.75 mm deep where the gingival margin will be in cementum, and follows the general contour faciolingually of the external tooth surface. *Infected carious dentin that is deeper pulpally than this position is excavated later in final cavity preparation.*

Final cavity preparation. Now, with a slowly revolving round bur or with a hand excavator *remove any infected carious dentin* remaining on the axial wall, and apply a *base/liner,* if indicated.

The cavosurface angles should be 90 degrees to provide a butt joint of amalgam to the cavosurface margin. An 8-3-22 hoe is helpful on the incisal and facial (lingual) enamel walls to remove unsupported enamel at the margins (Fig. 14-17, *B*). Because the gingival embrasure is usually sufficiently large at the level of the gingival margin, this margin often can be completed with the round bur. However, use of the reverse beveled blade of the 8-3-22 hoe ensures removal of unsupported gingival enamel (Fig. 14-17, *B*). A slight cavosurface bevel of the enamel on the gingival floor may be indicated to produce a sound gingival margin.

Ensure the *retention form* by preparing an incisal cove and a gingival groove as described in the previous section on cavity preparation for the distal surface of canines (Fig. 14-17, *C* and *F*). Frequently it is difficult to direct the No. ¼ bur properly for preparing the cove at the axioincisal point angle. Often, this difficulty can be alleviated by additional extension of the incisal portion of the lingual wall (Fig. 14-17, *D*). The use of the **bibeveled hatchet, 3-2-28,** sometimes is useful for preparing the cove (Fig. 14-17, *E*). Place the blade of the hatchet in the axioincisal point angle, and by rotary motion enlarge and deepen the point angle in a facioincisopulpal direction until a retention cove is produced. Be careful not to undermine the facial or incisal enamel. Final cavity preparation is now complete (Fig. 14-17, *G*).

Clean the cavity preparation, if indicated, and *inspect* it for any corrections. Two applications of *cavity varnish* are placed at this time rather than after matrix placement to prevent pooling at the enamel-matrix interface.

Matrix for Class III preparations

The wedged, *compound-supported matrix* is best for the Class III amalgam cavity preparation. (Refer to Chapter 13 for a detailed procedure of placing this matrix.)

Insertion of the filling material in the Class III cavity preparation is from the lingual (or facial) direction. Thus, it is essential to trim the lingual (facial) portion of the strip matrix material correctly to avoid covering the preparation and blocking access for insertion of the filling material. Using $5/16$ inch (8 mm) wide, 0.002 inch (0.05 mm) thick, ribbon, stainless steel matrix material, cut a length to cover one third of the facial surface and to extend through the proximal to the lingual surface. Trim the lingual portion by cutting the strip on an angle to correspond approximately to the slope of the lingual surface of the tooth (Fig. 14-18). Next, use fingers to contour the strip to approximate the circumferential contour of the tooth. Then lay the strip on a resilient paper pad and burnish using an egg-shaped burnisher the desired contact contour of the strip. Place the strip in position, and insert the wedge from the facial or lingual embrasure, whichever is greater. Now, stabilize the facial portion of the strip with low-fusing compound. A smaller amount of compound may be used lingually to position and stabilize the matrix material against the linguogingival corner (Fig. 14-16, *G*). The experienced operator may coat the tip of the wedge with softened compound before the wedge is inserted, and position the wedge and compound simultaneously. Precontoured Palodent* matrices may be used instead of custom-made matrices if the contour of the Palodent matrix coincides with that of the proximal surface being restored.

Procedures for inserting, carving, and polishing the restoration

Insertion of the amalgam, initial carving, matrix removal, wedge removal, and final carving are similar to the same procedures on posterior teeth (see Chapter 13). If a dentin adhesive system is to be used (in lieu of cavity varnish), refer to the brief discussion regarding the use of this system in Chapter 13, under Insertion of Amalgam. Polishing the restoration should follow at least a 24 hour delay. Restorations on the distal surface of canines are inconspicuous in conservative cavity preparations when correctly placed and polished (Fig. 14-19). The mercury in precapsulated high-copper amalgams is less likely to stain ("blue") the restored tooth since less mercury is used than with conventional amalgams and the precapsulated form allows for a controlled mercury-alloy ratio. Proximal restorations on the mandibular incisors that are extended facially to be visible are not as esthetic as tooth-colored restorations but may provide a longer service (Fig. 14-20).

CLASS V CAVITY PREPARATION AND RESTORATION

Cervical caries usually develops because the affected tooth surface is unclean and the patient has a caries-inducing diet. Incipient, smooth-surface enamel caries appears as a "milky white" line just occlusal or incisal to the crest of the marginal gingiva, usually on the facial surface (Fig. 14-21). These areas are often overlooked in the oral examination unless the teeth are free of debris, isolated with cotton rolls, and dried with the air syringe. When this form of incipient caries has not decalcified the enamel sufficiently to allow the explorer to

*Palodent, Palodent Company, Portola Valley, Calif.

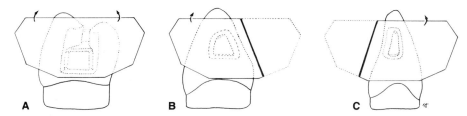

Fig. 14-18. Matrix strip design. **A,** Design required for compound-supported matrix for Class II cavity preparations. **B,** Alteration necessary for Class III preparation on maxillary canine. **C,** Alteration necessary for mandibular incisor. Note that strip material is cut to approximate slope of lingual surface.

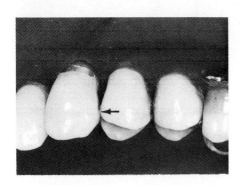

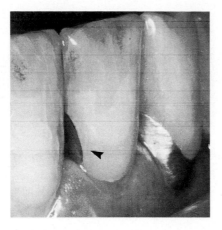

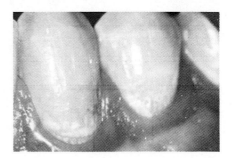

Fig. 14-19. Inconspicious facial margin of Class III amalgam restoration on maxillary canine.

Fig. 14-20. Class III amalgam restoration on mandibular incisor *(arrow)*.

Fig. 14-21. Incipient carious lesions of enamel appear as **white spots.** The affected surface may be smooth (noncavitated). Carious white spots are more visible when dried.

detect a break or roughness in the surface (noncavitated), the lesion may be reversed by *remineralization* resulting from altered diet, improved oral hygiene, and fluoride treatment (see Diagnosis and Prevention, in Chapter 3). An affected enamel surface that has a small break or roughness (cavitated) can be successfully treated occasionally by smoothing with sandpaper discs, polishing, and treating with a fluoride preparation, thereby preventing further caries that would require cavity preparation and restoration. Obviously, this prophylactic, preventive treatment cannot be instituted if caries has progressed to decalcify and soften the enamel to an appreciable depth. In this instance, a Class V cavity preparation and restoration is indicated, particularly if caries has penetrated to the dentinoenamel junction (Fig. 14-22, *A*). When a large number of cervical lesions are present (Fig. 14-22, *B*), particularly on the lingual surface, a relatively high caries index is obvious, and the patient should be instructed and encouraged to improve oral hygiene and diet.

Indications and contraindications

Because of limited access and visibility, many Class V restorations are difficult and present special problems during both the preparation and restorative procedures. The quality of a dentist's restorative treatment may be best judged by the quality of Class V restorations (C. Sturdevant, editor). The selection of amalgam as a restorative material for the Class V cavity preparation should involve the following considerations:

1. Caries
2. Erosion or abrasion, or both
3. Sensitive areas at, or apical to, the cementoenamel junction
4. Service
5. Economics
6. Abutment teeth for removable partial dentures
7. Esthetics

Caries. When there are indications that the caries rate is high, amalgam is chosen over more expensive types of materials. Periodic oral examinations should detect early caries, thereby permitting the best treatment in the form of prevention or the next best treatment in the form of conservative cavity preparation. Extensive, deep cervical preparations weaken the tooth. When Class V caries is of such magnitude, a full crown resto-

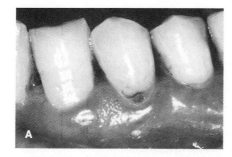

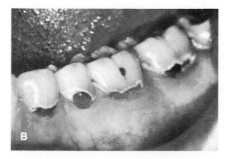

Fig. 14-22. Cervical caries. **A,** Cavitation involving both enamel and dentin. **B,** Relatively high caries index is obvious when large number of cervical lesions are present.

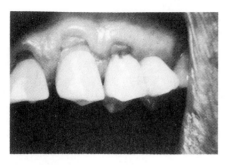

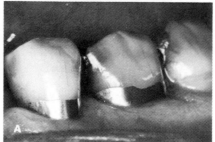

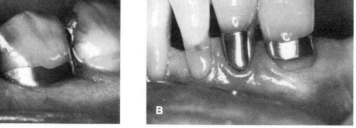

Fig. 14-23. Severe cervical abrasion/erosion lesions.

Fig. 14-24. A, Six-year-old cervical restorations. **B,** After 16 years some abrasion/erosion is evident at gingival margin of lateral incisor and canine restorations.

ration should be considered for protection of the tooth against possible fracture. If the Class V lesion is on a tooth that also is affected by extensive Class II caries or has a large, failing restoration, then a full crown often is the best treatment.

Erosion or abrasion, or both. It is sometimes necessary to restore "notched-out" areas caused by erosion or abrasion, or both, and possibly by occlusal forces flexing the tooth (Fig. 14-23). There usually is no caries in these lesions. The lesion should be restored when one (several or all) of the following conditions is(are) manifest: (1) uncontrollably sensitive; (2) deep enough to jeopardize the future health of the pulp; (3) deep enough that further erosion or abrasion may severely weaken the tooth; and (4) deep enough to prevent adequate homecare. As stated in the previous section, the treatment of choice often is a full crown if other surfaces of the tooth are extensively involved by caries and/or restoration(s).

Sensitive areas at, or apical to, the cementoenamel junction. Because of gingival recession or periodontal surgery, or both, the root surface may be extremely sensitive. When conservative methods of desensitizing the area fail, cavity preparation and restoration are necessary. Because of the difficulty of sealing a cemental margin with composite resin (see Chapter 16), amalgam is generally the filling material of choice in Class V preparations except when esthetics is of primary concern. (For details on dentinal hypersensitivity, see Indications for Operative Treatment, under Treatment Planning in Chapter 5; also see The Pulp-Dentin Complex, in Chapter 2.)

Service. One measure of clinical success of cervical amalgam restorations is the length of time the restoration serves without failing (Fig. 14-24; see also Fig. 5-19, *B*). Many Class V amalgams are seen clinically that are well contoured, with smooth margins, and obviously will continue to be clinically acceptable for many years. On the other hand, clinicians often observe cervical amalgam restorations that show evidence of failure even after a short period of time. *Inattention to*

cavity preparation principles, improper manipulation of the material, and moisture contamination all contribute to early failure. Extended service depends on the operator's care in following accepted treatment techniques, as well as proper homecare by the patient.

Economics. The patient's economic situation may influence the selection of amalgam over more expensive treatments using other restorative materials whose use is often more labor intensive. Advantages and disadvantages of these alternative treatments should be explained to the patient. However, the patient should not feel that restoration with amalgam compromises treatment or the health of a tooth, when in fact, the use of amalgam is often the treatment of choice even when the patient could afford any treatment choice.

Abutment teeth for removable partial dentures. Amalgam is usually preferred over composite resin materials when placed on partial denture abutment teeth because amalgam is more resistant to wear as clasps move over the restoration. Furthermore, contours prepared in the restoration to provide rests and retentive areas for the clasp tips may be obtained more easily and maintained longer when the restoration is amalgam, as compared with the composite materials.

Esthetics. Some patients object to metal restorations that are visible during conversation. However, a well-polished amalgam restoration is not objectionable to many patients (Fig. 14-25). Generally, Class V amalgams placed on the facial surface of mandibular canines, premolars, and molars are not visible. Those placed on maxillary premolars and first molars may be visible. The patient's view of esthetics should be considered when planning treatment in areas of esthetic concern. Improvements in tooth-colored materials and techniques are resulting in restorations showing an extended service life, and their use in Class V restorations, compared with amalgam, is increasing.

Local anesthesia

Profound anesthesia of the tooth and surrounding tissues is a requirement for restoring Class V cavities. In

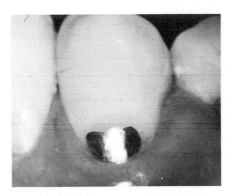

Fig. 14-25. Polished amalgam is esthetically acceptable to many patients.

addition to pain control, anesthesia significantly reduces salivation.

Isolation

Isolation prevents moisture contamination of the operating site, improves asepsis, and provides access and visibility. *Moisture in the form of saliva, gingival sulcular fluid, or gingival hemorrhage must be excluded during caries removal, base/liner and varnish application, and insertion and carving of amalgam.* Moisture impairs visual assessment, may contaminate the pulp during caries removal (especially with a pulpal exposure), and negatively affects the physical properties of restorative materials. The gingival margin of Class V cavity preparations is often apical to the gingival crest. This necessitates retraction of the free gingiva to protect it

and provide access while also eliminating seepage of sulcular fluid into the cavity preparation or restorative materials.

These isolation objectives are met by local anesthesia and isolation by (1) cotton roll(s) and retraction cord, or (2) the rubber dam and suitable cervical retainer.

Cotton roll(s) and retraction cord. *Isolation by cotton roll(s) and retraction cord is satisfactory when properly accomplished, practical, and probably the approach most often used.*

The *styptic (noncaustic) treated cord* should be placed in the sulcus *before* initial cavity preparation to reduce the possibility of cutting instruments contacting the free gingiva. (The technique of cord placement is presented in the following paragraphs.) The cord should produce a temporary, adequate, nontraumatic apical retraction and lateral deflection of the free gingiva. Cord usually is treated with epinephrine, and this drug on abraded gingiva can be rapidly absorbed into the circulatory system, causing a rise in blood pressure, elevated heart rate, and possible dysrhythmias. Gentle placement of cord and absence of trauma to the free gingiva should preclude such systemic sequelae. *Careful operative dentistry should not abrade the gingiva to open capillaries, even in cavity preparations extending subgingivally.* Cord untreated with epinephrine is available for patients at risk for cardiac problems.

Place the cotton roll(s) and dry the area with the air syringe. Cut retraction cord of suitable diameter to a length ¼ inch (6 mm) longer than the gingival margin. The diameter of the cord should be that which the gingival sulcus can easily accommodate. Some operators

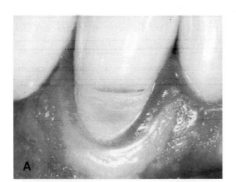
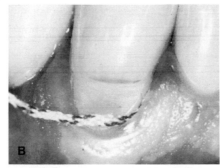
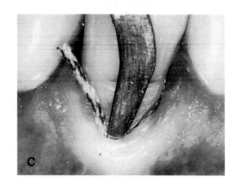
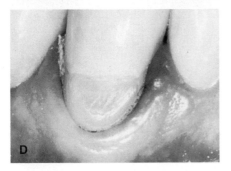

Fig. 14-26. Use of retraction cord for isolation of Class V lesion. **A,** Preoperative view. **B,** Cord placement initiated. **C,** Cord placement using a thin, flat-bladed instrument. **D,** Cord placement completed.

prefer to place the cord in a dappen dish, wet it with a drop of Hemodent*, and then blot it with a 2 × 2 inch (5 × 5 cm) gauze to remove excess liquid. Next, the cord is twisted tightly to further remove excess liquid while reducing the cord diameter. A larger cord can be later inserted over the first cord if indicated. Using a thin, blunt-edged instrument blade, or side of an explorer tine, gently insert the cord progressively to place. A slight backward direction of the instrument as it steps along the cord will help prevent dislodgement of previously inserted cord (Fig. 14-26). Also, using a second instrument stepping along behind the first instrument can help prevent dislodgement of cord. Additionally, using the air syringe or cotton pellets to reduce or absorb the sulcular fluid in the cord already placed is helpful during the cord placement. The effects of the cord will result in adequate retraction in a short time. *If significant blanching of the free gingiva is observed, excessive cord has been placed and should be immediately exchanged with a cord of smaller diameter.* The cord usually remains in place throughout cavity preparation and insertion and carving of amalgam.

Usually, insert the smallest diameter cord into the sulcus on the facial of anterior and premolar teeth because the free gingiva is thin, delicate, and tight. Sometimes in this instance, a single strand of unbraided cord can be separated and twisted into a still smaller cord.

The cord can be moistened before or after placement with a styptic solution (e.g., Hemodent™) if slight hemorrhage is anticipated or observed.

While carving amalgam at the gingival margin, the presence of the cord may cause difficulty in feeling the unprepared tooth surface to prevent undercarving of the margin which results in overcontour and marginal excess.

*Hemodent, Premier Dental Products Company, Norristown, Pa.

cess. In this instance, after carving gross excess, the cord can be teased from place before completing the carving.

Occasionally, the carious lesion extends gingivally enough that a soft tissue flap must be reflected for adequate access and visibility (Fig. 14-27). Proper surgical procedures must be followed including sterile technique, careful soft tissue management, and complete debridement of the operating site prior to wound closure.

Rubber dam and suitable cervical retainer. Rubber dam isolation using a suitable cervical retainer is sometimes preferred (Fig. 14-28). (Refer to Cervical Retainer Placement, in Chapter 11.)

Definition and principles of outline form

Outline form for Class V cavity preparations is extending the external walls (and margins) to sound tooth structure while maintaining a limited depth pulpally of 0.5 mm from the dentinoenamel junction and 0.75 mm from the cementum (or root surface). The outline form for the Class V cavity preparation is primarily determined by the location and size of the carious area. Historically, cervical restorations were accomplished with outlines that were grossly overextended. Presently, most operators have adopted a more conservative philosophy resulting in smaller restorations with outline forms that are dictated primarily by the size of the lesion. Clinical judgment determines final cavity outline, especially when the cavosurface margins approach or extend into areas of enamel decalcification. The operator must observe the prepared enamel wall to evaluate the depth of the decalcified enamel, as well as use the explorer to ascertain a break in the enamel surface (cavitation). When no cavitation has occurred and when the decalcification does not extend appreciably into the

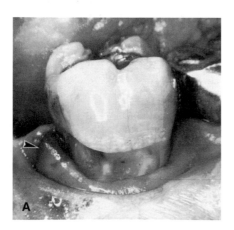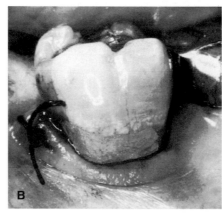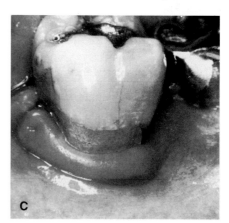

Fig. 14-27. Surgical access. **A,** Class V preparation requiring flap procedure with relaxing incision (*arrow*). **B,** Completed restoration with suture in place. **C,** One-week postoperative with suture removed.

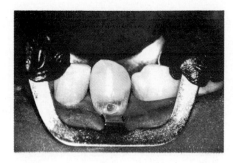

Fig. 14-28. The rubber dam and No. 212 retainer may be required to properly isolate carious area.

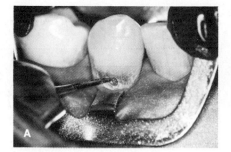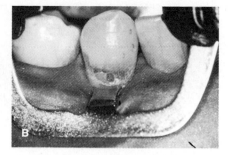

Fig. 14-29. Starting Class V cavity preparation. **A,** Bur positioned for entry into carious lesion. **B,** Entry cut is the beginning of outline form having a limited 1-mm pulpal depth. (The end of bur in center of lesion may be in carious tooth structure or air!)

enamel, extension of the outline form often should cease. Topical fluoride application and a rigid home care program may prevent further breakdown of the decalcified areas and result in remineralization.

Mandibular canine

Initial cavity preparation; outline form. Using a tapered fissure bur of suitable size, enter the carious lesion (or existing restoration) to a limited pulpal depth of 0.5 mm from the dentinoenamel junction (1 to 1.25 mm total crown depth) to 0.75 mm from cementum (root depth) (Fig. 14-29). When entering a carious lesion the entry should be off the center of the lesion enough that the bur's depth can be related to the original tooth contour (before cavitation). The end of the bur at the described *limited depth* is in dentin, or infected carious dentin, or old restorative material, or AIR, depending

on conditions! Using the edge of the end of the bur to penetrate the area is more efficient than using the flat end of the bur and reduces the possibility of the bur's "crawling." Once the entry is made, endeavor to maintain the bur so that all external walls are perpendicular to the external tooth surface and thereby parallel to the enamel rods (Fig. 14-30). *Extend the preparation incisally, gingivally, mesially, and distally until all external walls are positioned in sound tooth structure at pulpal depths ranging from 0.75 mm at the gingival wall to 1.25 mm at the incisal wall.* When extending mesially and distally, protect the rubber dam from the bur by placing a flat-bladed instrument over the dam (Fig. 14-31). The axial wall is in sound dentin except for any remaining infected caries or old restorative material, and because of uniform depth, it follows mesiodistally the contour of the facial surface of the tooth. The axial

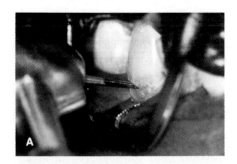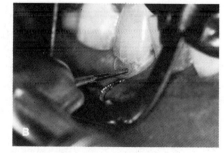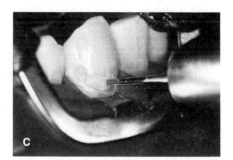

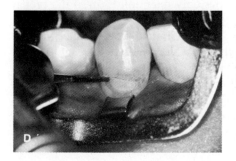

Fig. 14-30. When extending incisally **(A),** gingivally **(B),** mesially **(C),** and distally **(D),** position bur to prepare these walls perpendicular to external tooth surface.

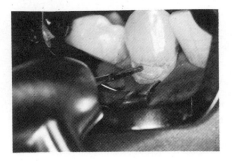

Fig. 14-31. Flat-bladed instrument protects rubber dam for bur.

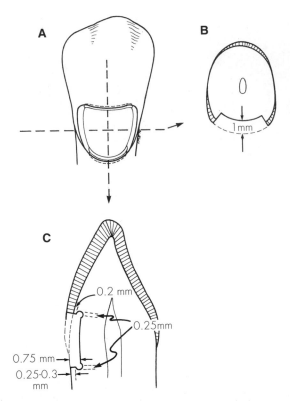

Fig. 14-32. A, Extended Class V cavity preparation with axial wall following dentoenamel junction (DEJ) contour mesiodistally **(B)** and incisogingivally **(C)**. Note axial wall pulpal depth of 1 mm in crown and 0.75 mm in root. Also note location and direction depth (0.25 mm) of retention grooves, as well as dimension of gingival wall (0.25 mm) from root surface to retention groove.

wall, therefore, usually will be convex mesiodistally. *It should be emphasized that the axial wall will be slightly shallower pulpally at the gingival wall with little or no enamel (approximately 0.75 to 1 mm in depth) than at the incisal wall with more enamel (1 to 1.25 mm in depth).* A 1.25 mm depth incisally may be necessary to place the incisoaxial line angle deep enough into the dentin to prevent undermining the enamel when placing the retention groove. This subtle difference in depth serves also to increase the thickness of the remaining dentin (between the axial wall and the pulp) in the gingival aspect of the preparation to aid in protecting the pulp. For the cavity preparation that is very extended incisogingivally, the axial wall should be slightly convex as it follows the contour of the dentinoenamel junction, and the depth of the incisal wall will be 1.5 mm or slightly more due to the additional thickness of the enamel and the requirement for a 0.5 mm dentinal wall for placement of the incisal retention groove (Fig. 14-32). If there is inadequate access for the tapered fissure bur, the initial cavity preparation can be accomplished with round burs as described later in the section, Extended Cervical Restoration that Includes Transitional Line Angle(s). This will complete the initial cavity preparation.

Final cavity preparation. Final cavity preparation involves removal of any remaining infected dentin, pulp protection, retention form, finishing external walls, and final procedures of cleaning, inspecting, and varnishing.

Removal of any remaining infected dentin. Remove any remaining infected dentin with a No. 2 or 4 bur. Any old restorative material (including base/liner) remaining should not be removed if there is no evidence of recurrent caries and the tooth is symptomless for disease. (With proper outline form the axial line angles are always in sound dentin.)

Pulp protection. Apply appropriate base/liner. (Refer to Pulp Protection sections in Chapters 12 and 13.)

Retention form. The mesial, distal, gingival, and incisal walls of the cavity preparation, being perpendicular to the external tooth surface, diverge outward. Thus,

retention form must be provided. Using a No. ¼ bur prepare two retention grooves, one directed depthwise mostly occlusally (slightly pulpally) and along the incisoaxial line angle, and the other directed depthwise mostly gingivally (slightly pulpally) and along the gingivoaxial line angle (Fig. 14-33). Alternatively, four retention coves may be prepared, one each in the four axial point angles of the preparation (Fig. 14-34). Using four coves instead of two full length grooves conserves dentin protecting the pulp, reducing the possibility of a pulp exposure. Depth of the grooves should approximate 0.25 mm, which is half the diameter of the bur. It is important that the retention grooves be adequate, since they provide the only retention form to the preparation. However, the grooves should not be so large or so positioned that dentin immediately supporting the enamel is removed or that the axial wall is significantly deepened. It is emphasized that depthwise the incisal groove is directed more incisally than pulpally, and that the gingival groove is directed more gingivally than pulpally, just as in conventional Class V cavity preparations for direct tooth-colored restorative materials (see Fig. 16-47).

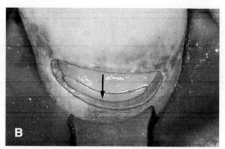

Fig. 14-33. Retention form. **A,** No. ¼ bur positioned to prepare gingival retention groove. **B,** Gingival retention groove *(arrow)* prepared along gingivoaxial line angle and directed depthwise mostly gingivally and slightly pulpally. An incisal retention groove is prepared along incisoaxial line angle and directed depthwise mostly incisally and slightly pulpally. (See Fig. 13-32, *C.*)

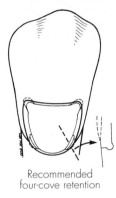

Recommended
four-cove retention

Fig. 14-34. Large Class V preparation with retention coves prepared in the four axial point angles.

Alternate methods of placing retention form include the use of the 7-85-2½-6 angle-former chisel or the No. 33½ bur. When properly placed, such retention grooves will be angular, positioned in the same location and approximately to the same depth as when the No. ¼ bur is used.

The rounded retention form placed with the No. ¼ bur is preferred because insertion of the amalgam into rounded areas may be more complete than into sharpened areas, resulting in better adaptation into the retention grooves.

In the very large cervical preparation, one that is wide incisogingivally (occlusogingivally) and mesiodistally, retention form may be enhanced by extending the retention groove around the internal line angles of the entire cavity preparation (circumferentially).

In vitro studies of *new dentin (and enamel) adhesive systems* report category III shear bond strengths of approximately 20 MPa that only fail cohesively.[3-6] These systems show promise for bonding amalgam to cavity preparations without mechanical retention form. Confirmation of these findings by longevity clinical studies can result in conservation of tooth structure. Refer to earlier subsection, Resistance and Retention Forms, in the section, Distal Cavity Preparation for Canines, for Christensen's[2] advice to use mechanical retention while using the adhesive for eliminating microleakage sensitivity.

Procedures for finishing external walls. Using suitable hand instruments (chisels or margin trimmers), lightly plane the enamel margins testing for soundness and reevaluating for 90-degree cavosurface angles.

Final procedures; cleaning; inspecting; varnishing. Rinse the preparation, if indicated, using air/water spray and evacuation. Using the air syringe to remove visible moisture (do not desiccate tooth structure), inspect the cavity preparation for detection and removal of debris or unwanted base/liner. Next, apply two coats of cavity varnish to the cavity preparation.

In lieu of cavity varnish, new dentin adhesive systems are applied immediately before insertion of the amalgam (see later section). Ben-Amar reported that the amalgam restoration is bonded to the tooth structure and exhibits a significant *reduction in microleakage,* and states that *the longevity of this bond in the oral environment should be evaluated.*[1]

Extended cervical restoration that includes transitional line angle(s)

Caries on the facial (lingual) surface will often extend beyond the transitional line angles of the tooth. The maxillary molars, particularly the second molars, are most commonly affected (Fig. 14-35, *A*). In this example, if the remainder of the distal surface is sound and the distal caries is accessible facially, the facial restoration should extend around the angle, thereby preventing the necessity of a proximal restoration to include the caries on the distal surface. Complete as much of the preparation as possible with a fissure bur. Then, using a round bur approximately the same diameter as the fissure bur, block out (roughly prepare) the distal portion of the preparation (Fig. 14-35, *B* and *C*). Use smaller round burs to further accentuate the internal line angles. Preparing the facial portion first provides access and visibility to the distal portion. Occasionally, hand cutting instruments may be useful for completing the distal half of the preparation when space for the handpiece is limited (Fig. 14-35, *D* to *F*).

Retention grooves along the entire length of the occlusoaxial and gingivoaxial line angles ensure retention of the restoration. Use the No. ¼ bur as previously described to prepare the retention grooves. A gingival margin trimmer or a 7-85-2½-6 angle-former chisel often can be used in the distal half of the preparation to

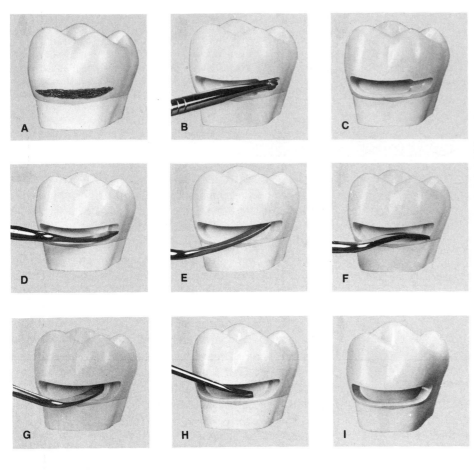

Fig. 14-35. Cavity preparation on maxillary molar. **A,** Caries extending around distofacial corner of tooth. **B** and **C,** Distal extension is accomplished with round bur. **D, E,** and **F,** Gingival margin trimmer may be useful in completing distal half of preparation when handpiece access is limited. **G,** Gingival margin trimmer may be used to provide retention grooves. **H,** Angle-former chisel may be used to prepare retention grooves in distal portion of preparation. **I,** Completed cavity preparation.

provide retention form when access for the handpiece is limited (Fig. 14-35, *G* and *H*).

Because of the proximity of the coronoid process, access to the facial surfaces of maxillary molars, particularly second molars, is often limited. Having the patient close midway and shift the mandible toward the tooth being operated will improve access and visibility (Fig. 14-36).

If the Class V outline form approaches an existing proximal restorations, it is best to extend slightly into the bulk of the proximal restoration rather than to leave a thin section of tooth structure between the two restorations (Fig. 14-37). In this illustration, the previously placed amalgam served as the distal (mesial) wall of the preparation.

When treatment requires that both a Class II and Class V preparation must be accomplished on the same tooth, the operator is advised to first complete the Class II preparation and restoration before initiating the Class V. If the Class V were restored first, it might be damaged by the matrix band and wedge needed for restoring the Class II preparation.

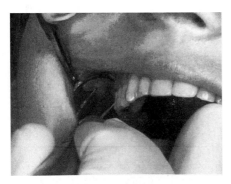

Fig. 14-36

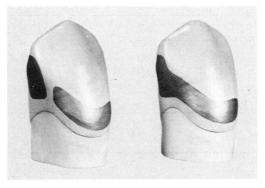

Fig. 14-37

Fig. 14-36. Mandible shifted laterally for improved access and visibility.

Fig. 14-37. When Class V outline form closely approaches an existing restoration, extend the preparation to remove remaining thin enamel wall, resulting in adjoining restorations.

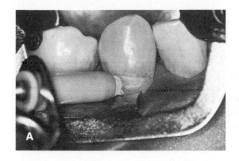

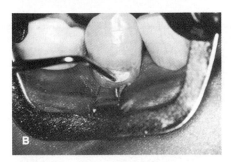

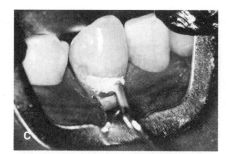

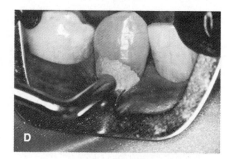

Fig. 14-38. Inserting amalgam. A, Place amalgam into preparation in small increments. B, Condense first into retention grooves with small condenser. C, Next condense against mesial and distal walls. D, Overfill and provide sufficient bulk to allow for carving.

Insertion of amalgam

If a dentin adhesive system is to be used (in lieu of cavity varnish), refer to Insertion of Amalgam, in Chapter 13, for a brief discussion regarding the use of this system.

Most Class V amalgam restorations are placed without the use of any type of matrix. Using the amalgam carrier, *insert the mixed amalgam* into the preparation in small increments (Fig. 14-38, *A*), and condense first into the retention areas with an appropriately sized condenser (Fig. 14-38, *B*). Next, condense against the mesial and distal walls of the preparation (Fig. 14-38, *C*). Finally, build the central portion to sufficient bulk to allow for carving (Fig. 14-38, *D*). As the surface of the restoration becomes more convex, condensation becomes increasingly difficult. The operator must guard against the amalgam's "landsliding" during overpacking. Often, a large condenser or plastic instrument held against the amalgam may help to offer resistance from pressure applied elsewhere on the restoration (Fig. 14-39).

The most difficult gingival cavity preparation to condense is the one with an axial wall that is very convex mesiodistally. Two alternative methods for insertion may be considered. The preferred method is the application of a matrix to confine the amalgam in the mesial and distal portions of the preparation (Fig. 14-40). Short lengths of stainless steel matrix material, one each for the mesial and distal surfaces, are passed through the proximal contacts, carefully guided into the gingival sulcus, and wedged. The strips must be wide enough to extend occlusally through the respective contacts and long enough to extend slightly past the facial (lingual) line angles. The strip usually requires compound for stability and rigidity. It is often helpful to apply a small amount of softened compound on the tip of the wedge before wedge insertion. The steel strips offer support

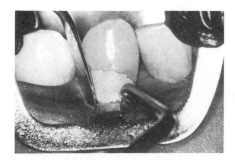

Fig. 14-39. Use large condenser or flat-bladed instrument to offer resistance to condensation pressure applied elsewhere on restoration.

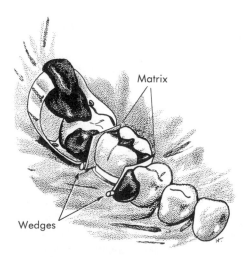

Fig. 14-40. Application of matrix to confine amalgam in mesial and distal extensions of preparation.

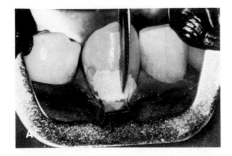

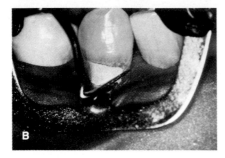

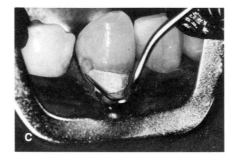

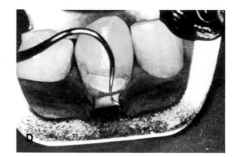

Fig. 14-41. Carving and contouring restoration. **A,** Begin carving procedure by removing excess and locating incisal margin. **B** and **C,** Explorer may be used to remove excess and locate mesial and distal margins. **D,** Finally, remove excess and locate gingival margin.

for condensing the mesial and distal portions, which in turn provide support for condensing the center of the restoration. The gingival edge of the steel strip often must be trimmed to conform to the circumferential contour (level) of the base of the gingival sulcus to prevent soft tissue damage. Rather than using two short pieces of steel strip, the operator may choose to use a sufficient length that may be passed through one contact, extended around the lingual (facial) surface, and passed through the other contact, forming a U-shaped matrix. Trimming the gingival edge to conform to the interproximal soft tissue anatomy usually is more difficult with one matrix strip than when two strips are used.

Alternatively, the cavity may be prepared and restored in sections. Each successive section of the preparation should be extended slightly into the previously condensed portion to ensure caries removal. This procedure is time consuming, but effective.

Procedures for carving and contouring the restoration

Carving may begin immediately following insertion of the amalgam (Fig. 14-41). All carving should be done parallel to the margins, using the side of the explorer tine or a Hollenback No. 3 carver. Also, the edge of the carving instrument should always rest on external tooth *surface* adjacent to the margin. This helps to prevent overcarving (uncovering portions of the cavity walls). Begin the carving procedure by removing excess amalgam and locating the incisal (occlusal) margin. Continue removing excess to locate the mesial and distal margins. Finally, carve away excess at the gingival margin. Carving should establish contours desired in the finished restoration. Improper use of the carving instru-

ments will result in a poorly contoured restoration. Note in Fig. 14-42 how carving instruments are positioned to preserve amalgam for developing desired gingival contours. It is important that no excess is left beyond margins, since feathered excess may break away, creating a fault or defect at the margin.

There are instances when it is appropriate to change facial contours because of altered soft tissue levels, as with cervical lesions in periodontally treated patients. Facial contours may be increased (or relocated) only enough to prevent food impaction into the gingival sulcus and to provide access for the patient to clean the area. Overcontouring must be avoided, as it will result in a lack of normal stimulation and cleansing of the gingiva during mastication.

When isolation is by rubber dam and cervical retainer, use air/water spray and evacuation followed by air to remove any amalgam particles, particularly in the sulcus. Remove the No. 212 retainer using care to open the jaws of the retainer wide enough to prevent marring

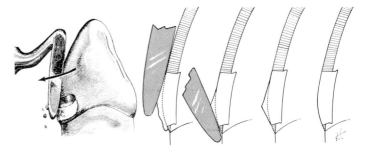

Fig. 14-42. Position of carving instrument to prevent overcarving amalgam and to develop desired gingival contours.

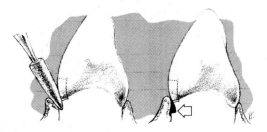

Fig. 14-43. Incorrect use of pointed stone at gingival margin results in removal of cementum or notching of tooth structure gingival to margin, or both.

the surface of the restoration. Remove the rubber dam and again ensure that no amalgam particles remain in the sulcus, using an explorer tine and air.

When retraction cord is used for isolation, it may interfere with the carving of excess amalgam at the gingival margin. In this instance, carve away gross excess, and carefully remove the cord before final carving along the margin.

Procedures for finishing and polishing the restoration

Finishing of amalgam restorations may be necessary to correct a marginal discrepancy or improve the contour. However, evidence suggests that polishing of high copper amalgams is unnecessary. They are less prone to corrosion and marginal deterioration than their low copper predecessors. Nevertheless, many operators prefer to polish all amalgam restorations to maximize their clinical performance.

Finishing and polishing procedures for amalgam restorations are generally not attempted within a 24-hour period following insertion. It is more efficient to delay these procedures until all proposed restorations have been placed, rather than proceed periodically during the course of treatment. Finishing and polishing should not

undercontour the restoration, and when completed, the tine of the explorer should pass from the tooth surface onto the restoration, and vice versa, in a smooth manner. There should be perfect continuity of surface contour—a requirement for all restorations.

First, perfect the contour if necessary, using small, fine-grit, pointed stones in the contra-angle handpiece. If carving procedures were performed correctly, little or no stone finishing will be required. Extreme care is necessary when using stones or any rotating cutting instrument on margins positioned below the cementoenamel junction because of the possibility of removing cementum or notching the tooth structure gingival to the margin, or both (Fig. 14-43). Begin the polishing procedure by using a tapered rubber polishing point of medium grit in the contra-angle handpiece at relatively low speed. When the high speed handpiece is used, the speed of the rotating instrument should be just above the stalling point. It is best to use light, intermittent strokes to prevent overheating the restoration and tooth. The surface of the restoration should appear smooth with a "satiny" finish. When the rubber point becomes worn, it may be reshaped by running it against the surface of a carborundum or diamond disc (Fig. 14-44). Rubber polishing points that are eccentric should be "trued" against the same disc before use. Sandpaper discs may be substituted for, or used in conjunction with, the rubber point when finishing the restoration. A high polish (shiny surface) is obtained using a fine grit polishing point as just described (Fig. 14-45). If a high luster does not appear in a few seconds, the restoration requires additional finishing.

An alternate method of finishing is to first use the prophylaxis handpiece, rubber cup, and pumice. Polishing is accomplished using a rubber cup and prepared chalk or tin oxide. Special care is necessary when using rubber cups to avoid overheating the amalgam and/or removing cementum gingival to the restoration.

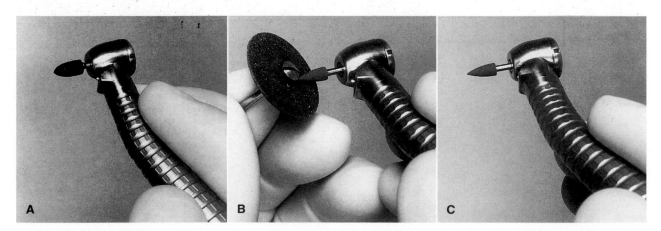

Fig. 14-44. Reshaping rubber abrasive point.

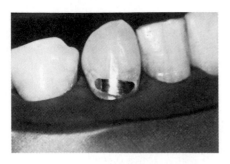

Fig. 14-45. Fine-grit polishing point produces highly polished surface.

CLASS VI CAVITY PREPARATION AND RESTORATION

The Class VI cavity preparation is used to restore the incisal edge of anterior teeth or the cusp tip regions of the posterior teeth. Such cavity preparations are frequently indicated where attritional wear (loss of tooth substance from the occluding of food, abrasives, and opposing teeth) has removed the enamel to expose the underlying dentin (Fig. 14-46, *A*). Such a wear pattern occurs more often in geriatric patients. Once the softer dentin is exposed, it wears faster than the surrounding enamel, resulting in "cupped-out" areas. As the dentin support is lost the enamel begins to fracture away, exposing more dentin and often causing sensitivity. Sensitivity to temperature change is a frequent complaint, and some patients are bothered by food impaction in the deeper depressions. Enamel edges become jagged and sharp to the tongue, lips, or cheek. Lip, tongue, or cheek biting is sometimes a complaint. Rounding and smoothing such inciso(occluso)axial edges is an excellent service to the patient. Early recognition and resto-ration of these lesions is recommended to limit the loss of dentin as well as subsequent loss of enamel supported by this dentin.

The Class VI cavity preparation also is indicated to restore the *hypoplastic pit* occasionally found on cusp tips (Fig. 14-47). Such developmental faults are vulnerable to caries, especially in high-risk patients, and should be restored as soon as they are detected. Rarely is caries found in the dentin where attritional wear has removed the overlying enamel (and dentin).

Cavity preparation in treatment of either of the previously described conditions is similar. Enter the area with a small tapered fissure bur, extending to a sufficient size to place the cavosurface margin on enamel that has sound dentin support (Fig. 14-46, *B*). A depth of 1.5 mm is sufficient to provide bulk of material for strength. Retention of the restoration is ensured by the creation of small undercuts along the internal line angles. Be careful not to remove dentin that is immediately supporting the enamel. Conservative cavity preparation is particularly important with Class VI preparations because it is easy to undermine enamel on incisal edges and cusp tips. Inserting, carving, and polishing are similar to procedures described for Class I cavity preparations for amalgam. Esthetic consideration may indicate the use of improved tooth-colored materials in small Class VI cavity preparations, particularly for the hypoplastic pit. (Refer to Class VI Cavity Preparation, in Chatper 17.)

Some geriatric patients have excessive occlusal wear of most of the teeth in the form of large concave areas with much exposed dentin. Generally, such dentitions require fixed prosthodontics beyond the scope of this textbook.

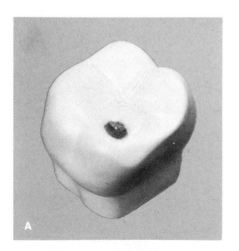

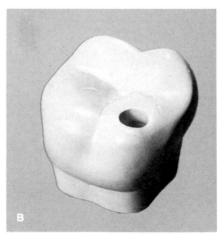

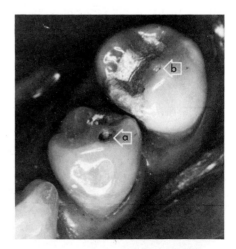

Fig. 14-46. Class VI preparation. **A,** Exposed dentin on mesiofacial cusp. **B,** Cavity preparation necessary to restore involved area.

Fig. 14-47. Class VI lesions. Carious cusp tip fault on first premolar *(a)*. Non-carious fault on second premolar *(b)*.

REFERENCES

1. Ben-Amar A: Reduction of microleakage around new amalgam restorations, *J Am Dent Assoc* 119:725, Dec 1989.
2. Christensen G: Personal communication to C. Sturdevant, editor, June 1993.
3. Eick JD et al: The dentinal surface: its influence on dentinal adhesion. II. *Quintessence Int* 23:43-51, 1992.
4. Eick JD et al: The dentinal surface: its influence on dentinal adhesion. I. *Quintessence Int* 22:967-977, 1991.
5. Nakabayashi N, Watanabe A, Gendusa NJ: Dentin adhesion of "modified" 4-META/MMA-TBB resin: function of HEMA, *Dent Mater* 8(4):259-264, Jul 1992.
6. Van Meerbeek B et al: Morphological aspects of the resin-dentin interdiffusion zone with different dentin adhesive systems, *J Dent Res* 71:1530-1540, 1992.

CHAPTER 15

Complex amalgam restorations

Kenneth N. May, Jr.

Aldridge D. Wilder, Jr.

INDICATIONS AND CONTRAINDICATIONS

Complex restorations, as defined in this chapter, involve the use of amalgam restorative material to replace missing tooth structure of teeth severely involved with caries or existing restorative material. When determining the appropriateness of a complex restoration, the following *factors* must be considered:
1. Resistance and retention forms
2. Status and prognosis of the tooth
3. Role of the tooth in the overall treatment plan
4. Occlusion, esthetics, and economics
5. Age and health of the patient

Resistance and retention forms

In a tooth severely involved with caries or existing restorative material, any undermined enamel or weak tooth structure subject to fracture must be removed and restored. Often, a weakened tooth is best restored with a properly designed cast restoration that will prevent tooth fracture caused by the forces of mastication (see Chapter 19). However, in selected cases, preparations may be designed for amalgam that improve the resistance form of a tooth (Fig. 15-1).

When conventional retention locks cannot be prepared because of insufficient tooth structure, *slots* and *pins* may be used to enhance retention form. The num-

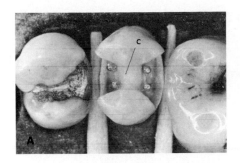 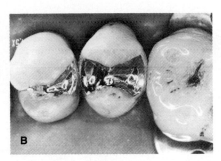

Fig. 15-1. Maxillary second premolar weakened both by extensive caries and by the small fracture line extending mesiodistally on the center of the excavated dentinal wall. **A,** Minikin pins placed in the gingival floor will improve resistance form after amalgam has been place. Note calcium hydroxide base *(c)*. **B,** Restorations polished.

ber of retention features used depends on the amount of tooth structure remaining and the tooth being restored. Pins also can provide desired resistance form.

Status and prognosis of the tooth

Complex restorations may be used as (1) control restorations in teeth which are symptomatic preoperatively, (2) control restorations in teeth with acute and severe caries, (3) final restorations, or (4) foundations. A control restoration is indicated when a tooth's prognosis is questionable. A tooth which is grossly decayed, which may require root canal therapy or crown-lengthening, or whose periodontal prognosis is uncertain is often treated initially with a control restoration. This helps to (1) isolate the pulp from oral fluids, (2) provide an anatomic contour against which the gingival tissue may heal, (3) facilitate control of caries and plaque, and (4) provide some resistance against tooth fracture or propagation of an existing fracture. A tooth which is asymptomatic and requires no root canal or periodontal therapy may be treated by a complex restoration as a definitive restoration or foundation. For the definition and description of foundations, refer to the section titled, Foundations.

The size, number, and placement of retention features will be determined by the status and prognosis of the tooth. Larger restorations generally require more retention. However, the size, number, and location of retention features demand greater care in smaller teeth, in teeth that have been significantly excavated, and in teeth that are symptomatic. Carelessness can risk pulpal irritation or exposure.

Role of the tooth in the overall treatment plan

The treatment of choice for a tooth will be influenced by its role in the overall treatment plan. Complex restorations are not only an occasional alternative to cast restorations but are often indicated. Abutment teeth for fixed prostheses may utilize a complex restoration as a foundation. Extensive caries or previous restorations on abutment teeth for removable prostheses generally indicate a cast restoration for resistance and retention forms as well as for development of external surface contours for retention of the prosthesis. A tooth may be treated

with a complex restoration if adequate resistance and retention forms can be provided. For periodontal and orthodontic patients the complex restoration may be the restoration of choice until the final phase of treatment when cast restorations may be preferred.

Occlusion, esthetics, and economics

Complex restorations are sometimes indicated as interim restorations for teeth that require elaborate occlusal alterations ranging from vertical dimension changes to correcting occlusal plane discrepancies.

When esthetics is a primary consideration, a complex restoration particularly with amalgam may not be the treatment of choice because of the display of metal. However, an esthetic result can be obtained by inserting a composite resin veneer (see Chapter 18).

When cost to the patient is a major factor, the complex restoration is appropriate providing that adequate resistance and retention forms are provided.

Age and health of the patient

For some geriatric and debilitated patients the complex restoration may be the treatment of choice over the more expensive and time-consuming cast restoration.

CAPPING CUSPS
Indications

When caries is extensive, reduction of one or more of the cusps for capping may be indicated. Robbins and others[47] and Smales[49] have documented the longevity of complex amalgam restorations involving one or more capped cusps. *When the facial (lingual) extension is two-thirds from a primary groove toward the cusp tip, reduction of the cusp(s) for amalgam capping is mandatory for the development of adequate resistance form* (Fig. 15-2, *A*), just as in preparations for cast gold restorations (see Fig. 19-22, *A*). Reduction should be accomplished early in cavity preparation because it greatly improves access and visibility for subsequent steps. *If the cusp(s) to be capped is (are) located at the correct occlusal height prior to preparation, make depth cuts (2 mm minimum for functional cusps and 1.5 mm minimum for nonfunctional cusps)[10] on the remaining occlusal*

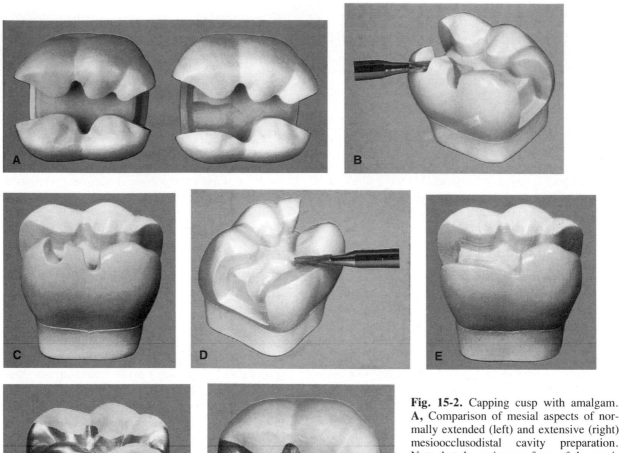

Fig. 15-2. Capping cusp with amalgam. **A,** Comparison of mesial aspects of normally extended (left) and extensive (right) mesioocclusodistal cavity preparation. Note that the resistance form of the mesiolingual cusp of extensive preparation is compromised and indicated for capping with amalgam. **B,** Preparing depth cuts. **C,** Depth cuts prepared. **D,** Reducing cusp. **E,** Cusp reduced. **F** and **G,** Final restoration.

surface of each cusp to be capped using the side of a carbide fissure bur or a suitable diamond instrument (Fig. 15-2, *B*). *If the cusp(s) is (are) located less than the correct occlusal height, the depth cuts may be less. If the cusp(s) is (are) located at more than the correct occlusal height, the depth cuts will be deeper.* Careful evaluation of the tooth preoperatively will help ensure that the final restoration has restored cusps with a minimal thickness of 2 mm of amalgam for functional cusps and 1.5 mm of amalgam for nonfunctional cusps (Fig. 15-2, *C*). The reduction is completed using the depth cuts as a guide to provide for a uniform reduction of tooth structure (Fig. 15-2, *D*). Slightly round any sharp external corners of the cavity preparation formed at the junction of prepared surfaces to reduce stress concentration in the amalgam and thus improve its resistance to fracture from occlusal forces (Fig. 15-2, *E*). Fig. 15-2, *F* and *G* illustrates the final restoration. The

procedure for capping the distolingual cusp of a maxillary first molar is illustrated in Fig. 13-33. Extending the facial or lingual wall of a proximal box to include the entire cusp is indicated only when necessary to include carious tooth structure or existing restorative material. The typical extension of the proximal box for restoring an entire cusp is illustrated in Figs. 13-31 and 13-32, *B*.

Retention form

In this textbook, the word *longitudinal* is used in lieu of the word *vertical* to describe cavity preparation walls and other preparation aspects that are approximately parallel to the long axis of the tooth; and the word *transverse* is used in lieu of the word *horizontal* to describe the walls and other aspects that are approximately perpendicular to the long axis of the tooth.

Cusp reduction significantly diminishes retention

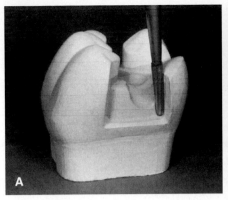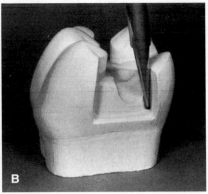

Fig. 15-3. Placement of retention locks. **A,** Position of No. 169 bur to prepare retention lock. **B,** Lock prepared with No. ¼ bur.

form by decreasing the height of the longitudinal walls. Whenever possible, use a No. 169L or ¼ bur to place conventional retention locks in dentin (Fig. 15-3, *A* and *B*). When additional retention is indicated, slots can be prepared along the gingival floor pulpal to the dentinoenamel junction. (Refer to the section, Slot and Lock Retention.) Also, retention may be increased by inserting pins in carefully positioned pinholes. (Refer to the section, Pin-retained Amalgam Restorations.)

SLOT AND LOCK RETENTION; "DENTIN CHAMBER" RETENTION

*For a complex restoration, a **slot** is a retention groove whose length is in a transverse plane and in dentin (Fig. 15-4). A **lock** is a retention groove whose length is in a longitudinal plane and in dentin (Fig. 15-5). Slot and lock retention may be used in conjunction with pin retention or as an alternative to it. Because of the varying cavity forms of teeth requiring complex restorations, the operator should be familiar with both slot and lock retention and pin retention. Slot and lock retention is used more in preparations with longitudinal walls which allow locks to oppose one another. Pin retention is used more in preparations with few or no longitudinal walls.*

Although pins are the primary source of retention for the illustrated preparation, the use of a No. ¼ bur to place slots in appropriate locations remote from the pulp can provide adequate retention (Fig. 15-6). Proximal locks, as described in Chapter 13, are placed in the proximal box and in other locations where sufficient longitudinal tooth preparation will permit (Fig. 15-7).

Gingival slots can serve as an alternative to pins or as auxiliary retention when pins are used. A No. 33½ or No. 169L bur is used to place a continuous slot in the gingival floor 0.5 mm pulpal of the dentinoenamel junction (see Fig. 15-4). The slot is at least 0.5 mm in depth and 1 or more mm in length depending on the distance between the vertical walls. McMaster has shown that shorter slots provide as much resistance to trans-

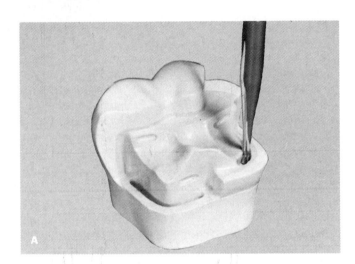

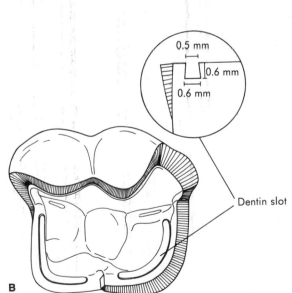

0.5 mm

0.6 mm

0.6 mm

Dentin slot

Fig. 15-4. Slots. **A** and **B,** With No. 33 ½ bur, prepare dentinal slots approximately 0.6 mm deep and 0.5 mm inside dentinoenamel junction.

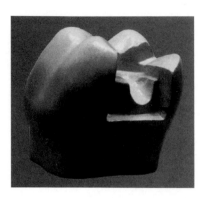

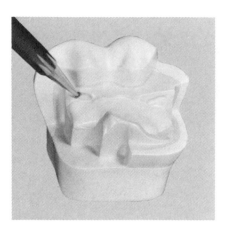

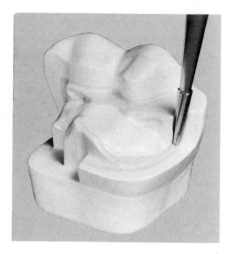

Fig. 15-5. Retention lock is a prepared groove whose length is in a longitudinal plane, and it is in dentin.

Fig. 15-6. Prepare transverse slots in dentin with No. ¼ bur where appropriate.

Fig. 15-7. Prepare longitudinal locks in dentin with No. 169L bur where appropriate.

verse force as do longer slots.[36] In this illustration no pins were used. *The success of all amalgam restorations depends on the stability of the matrix during condensation.* Assuming matrix stability, studies have shown that the retention provided by slots and locks and by self-threading pins is comparable.[2,44] A 2-year clinical study[20] has confirmed that there is no statistically significant difference in the retention of amalgams retained by self-threading pins and those retained by dentinal slots. Therefore, clinical experience will determine whether the slot-retained amalgam is more appropriate than the pin-retained amalgam. Compared with pin placement, more tooth structure is removed preparing slots. However, slots are less likely to perforate the tooth.

A second alternative to pin placement is the **amalgapin technique** described by Shavell.[48] Several *"dentin chambers"* are prepared with the No. 245 bur parallel to the external surface of the tooth to a depth of ap-

proximately 2 mm (Fig. 15-8, *A*). An appropriately sized round bur is used to "bevel" the junction of the pulpal floor and the walls of the chamber to provide additional bulk of amalgam (Fig. 15-8, *B*). Amalgam is carefully condensed into the chambers and the restoration completed. As with slots, the matrix must be rigid and stable to prevent premature shearing of the bulk of the amalgam from the amalgam in the dentin chambers prior to matrix removal. The potential for tooth perforation is greater with amalgapins than with slots. Amalgapins probably do not provide as much retention as do slots or pins.

PIN-RETAINED AMALGAM RESTORATIONS

A pin-retained restoration may be defined as any restoration requiring the placement of one or more pins in the dentin to provide adequate resistance and retention forms. Pins are used whenever adequate resistance and

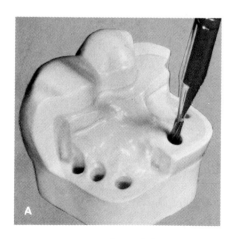

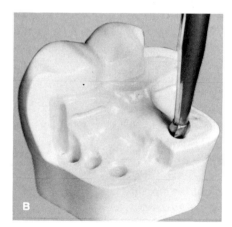

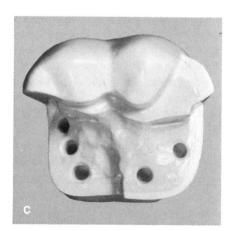

Fig. 15-8. Preparation of "dentin chambers" for modified amalgapin technique. **A,** Prepare chambers with No. 245 bur. **B,** Use appropriately sized round bur to "bevel" chambers. **C,** Completed preparation.

retention forms cannot be established with slots, locks, or undercuts. The pin-retained restorations described and illustrated in this section are amalgam restorations.

Because of the relatively small size of anterior teeth and the potential for enamel and dentin bonding, pins are rarely used in anterior teeth and with tooth-colored (composite) restorative materials.

Advantages

Conservation of tooth structure. The preparation of pinholes is more conservative than for slot and lock retention. Also, the pin-retained amalgam preparation is more conservative than the preparation for a cast restoration.

Appointment time. The pin-retained restoration can be completed in one appointment. The cast restoration requires at least two appointments.

Resistance and retention forms. Resistance and retention forms may be significantly increased by the use of pins (see Fig. 15-1).

Economics. Compared to a cast restoration, the amalgam restoration is a relatively inexpensive restorative procedure. When economics is a factor, the pin-amalgam restoration may provide the patient with the only alternative to extraction of the severely broken-down tooth.

Disadvantages

Dentinal microfractures. Drilling pinholes and placing pins may create craze lines or fractures, as well as internal stresses in the dentin.[5,52,57] Such craze lines and internal stress may have little or no clinical significance but are important when minimal dentin is present.

Microleakage. Microleakage around all types of pins has been demonstrated.[38] However, such microleakage is no greater than that occurring at the interface of the restorative material and the cavity walls. (Use of new dentin-adhesive systems may significantly reduce microleakage. [Comment by C. Sturdevant, editor.])

Decreased strength of amalgam. Pins do not reinforce amalgam and therefore do not increase its strength. The compressive strength of the amalgam material is not increased, and the tensile strength and transverse strength are significantly decreased.[23,58]

Resistance form. Resistance form is more difficult to develop than when preparing a tooth for an onlay (skirting axial corners of the tooth) or a full crown.

Perforations. Pin retention increases the risk of perforating into the pulp or the external tooth surface. Perforations should be recognized immediately and appropriate treatment instituted. Refer to the section titled, Penetration into the Pulp and Perforation of the External Tooth Surface.

Tooth anatomy. Proper contours and occlusal contacts are sometimes difficult to achieve.

Types of pins

The most frequently used pin type is the self-threading pin. Friction-locked and cemented pins are still available but are rarely used (Fig. 15-9).

Self-threading pins. The pin-retained amalgam restoration using self-threading pins was described by Going in 1966.[22] The diameter of the prepared pinhole is 0.0015 inch to 0.004 inch (0.038 to 0.1 mm) smaller than the diameter of the pin (Table 15-1). The pin is retained by the threads engaging the dentin as it is inserted. The elasticity (resiliency) of the dentin allows insertion of a threaded pin into a hole of smaller diameter.[45] Although the threads of self-threading pins do not engage the dentin for their entire width, the self-threading pin is the most retentive of the three types of pins (Fig. 15-10).[46] It is 3 to 6 times more retentive than the cemented pin.[37,56] Lateral and apical stresses can be generated in the dentin when a self-threading pin is inserted. Although some studies[14,52] have shown that insertion of self-threading pins produces more dentinal craze lines than insertion of either of the other two types, Pameijer and Stallard[45] have shown that self-threading pins do not create dentinal crazing and that the crazing demonstrated in other studies may be caused by the technique used for preparation of the specimen. Pulpal stress is maximal when the self-threading pin is inserted perpendicular to the pulp.[54] Use of cavity var-

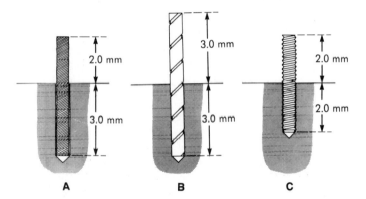

Fig. 15-9. Three types of pins. **A,** Cemented. **B,** Friction-locked. **C,** Self-threading.

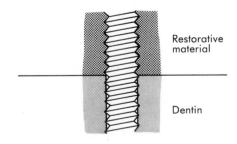

Fig. 15-10. Complete width of threads of self-threading pins does **not** engage dentin.

†able 15-1. TMS pins

Name	Illustration (not to scale)	Color code	Pin diameter (in/mm*)	Drill diameter (in/mm)	Total pin length (mm)	Pin length extending from dentin (mm)
Regular (standard)		Gold	0.031/0.78	0.027/0.68	7.1	5.1
Regular (self-shearing)		Gold	0.031/0.78	0.027/0.68	8.2	3.2
Regular (two-in-one)		Gold	0.031/0.78	0.027/0.68	9.5	2.8
Minim (standard)		Silver	0.024/0.61	0.021/0.53	6.7	4.7
Minim (two-in-one)		Silver	0.024/0.61	0.021/0.53	9.5	2.8
Minikin (self-shearing)		Red	0.019/0.48	0.017/0.43	7.1	1.5
Minuta (self-shearing)		Pink	0.015/0.38	0.0135/0.34	6.2	1.0

*1 mm = 0.03937 in.

ñish in the pinhole does not reduce the retentive ability of the self-threading pin. The depth of the pinhole varies from 1.3 to 2 mm depending on the diameter of the pin used.[13] Several styles of self-threading pins are available. Because of its (1) versatility, (2) wide range of pin sizes, (3) color-coding system, (4) greater retentiveness,[18,26] and (5) gold-plated pins, which may eliminate the possibility of corrosion, the Thread Mate System* (TMS) is the most widely used self-threading pin.

Cemented pins. In 1958 Markley[34] described a technique for restoring teeth with amalgam and cemented pins using threaded (or serrated) stainless steel pins cemented into pinholes prepared 0.001 to 0.002 inch (0.025 to 0.05 mm) larger than the diameter of the pin. The cementing medium may be either zinc phosphate or polycarboxylate cement.

Friction-locked pins. In 1966 Goldstein[24] described a technique for the friction-locked pin in which the diameter of the prepared pinhole is 0.001 inch (0.025 mm) smaller than the diameter of the pin. The pins are tapped to place, retained by the resiliency of the dentin, and are 2 to 3 times more retentive than cemented pins.[37]

Factors affecting the retention of the pin in dentin and amalgam[10]

Type. In the order of retentiveness, the self-threading pin is the most retentive,[37] the friction-locked pin is intermediate, and the cemented pin is the least retentive.

Surface characteristics. Retention of the pin in amalgam is influenced by the number and depth of the elevations on the pin. Therefore, the self-threading pin

*Thread Mate System, Whaledent, Inc., New York, NY.

has the greatest retention value. With the use of spherical or admixed amalgams, the adaptation of amalgam to the pins is greatly improved.[9,32]

Orientation, number, and diameter. Retention provided by pins is increased by placing them in a nonparallel manner. Excessive bending of pins to improve retention in amalgam is not desirable, since bends may interfere with adequate condensation of amalgam around the pin and thereby decrease the retention. Excessive bending also weakens the pin.

Within limits, increasing the number of pins increases the retention in dentin and amalgam. The benefits of increasing the number of pins must be weighed against the potential problems created as the number of pins increases. As the number of pins increases, (1) the crazing of the dentin and the potential for fracture increase, (2) the amount of available dentin between the pins decreases,[31] and (3) the strength of the amalgam restoration decreases.[59]

Within limits, as the diameter of the pin increases, the retention in dentin and amalgam increases. As the number, depth, and diameter of pins increase, the danger of perforating into the pulp or the external tooth surface increases. A large number of long pins can severely compromise condensation of the amalgam and the amalgam's adaptation to the pins. *A pin technique should be used that permits optimal retention with minimal danger to the remaining tooth structure.*[10]

Extension into dentin and amalgam. For self-threading pins there is no significant increase in retention when the length of embedment into dentin exceeds 2 mm. A laboratory study has demonstrated that the 0.024 inch (0.61 mm) self-threading pin fractures when removal from an embedment greater than 2 mm is attempted. Removal of the 0.031 inch (0.78 mm) self-threading pin results in fracture of the dentin.[37]

When the length of a 0.024 inch (.61 mm) self-threading pin extends into the amalgam more than 2 mm and removal is attempted, the pin fractures. Removal of the 0.031 inch (0.78 mm) self-threading pin extending more than 2 mm into the amalgam results in fracture of the amalgam.[37] *Pin extension into dentin and amalgam greater than 2 mm is unnecessary for pin retention, and contraindicated to preserve the strength of the dentin and the amalgam.*

Pin-retained Class II amalgam restorations

Mozer and Watson[40] point to the significance of pins in amalgam restorations. The pin-retained amalgam is an important adjunct in the restoration of badly decayed or broken teeth. Every general practitioner should be able to place large, pin-retained amalgam restorations.

Patient education. Treatment options should be discussed with the patient. Before the preparation for a pin-retained amalgam restoration begins, an explanation of the procedure should be given to the patient. The possible complications that might occur during the procedure and the limitations of the restoration itself should also be presented.

Initial cavity preparation. Evaluate occlusal factors, administer local anesthetic, apply the rubber dam, and perform initial cavity preparation (refer to Chapter 13).

Final cavity preparation. After initial cavity preparation of a severely involved tooth, there is need for excavation of any remaining infected carious dentin or removal of remaining old restorative material, pulp protection, additional retention or resistance form features, finishing of external walls, and final procedures including application of varnish. For a concept regarding the removal of any remaining old restorative material, refer to Cavity Preparation for Extensive Caries; Final Cavity Preparation in Chapter 12.

Removal of remaining infected carious dentin. Remove any remaining infected carious dentin (or remaining old restorative material). (Refer to Removal of Remaining Defective Enamel and Infected Carious Dentin; Final Cavity Preparation, in Chapter 13.)

Pulp protection. Apply base/liners, if needed. The base material should not be applied closer than 1.5 mm to the dentinoenamel junction or closer than 2 mm to the external surface of the tooth, especially in locations where pinholes are to be prepared.

Resistance and retention forms. Final cavity preparation resistance and retention forms are provided by preparing locks, slots, and pinholes for pins.

Locks. As described in Chapter 13, prepare retentive locks in the axial line angles in a longitudinal plane (Fig. 15-11, *A*). These locks should be prepared before preparing pinholes and inserting pins.

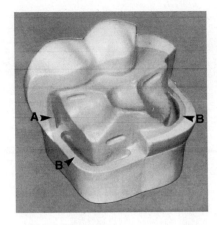

Fig. 15-11. Locks (**A**) and slots (**B**).

Slots. Prepare slots, if desired, when dentinal walls allow for them in addition to the planned pinholes (Fig. 15-11, *B*). Certain slots, depending on location, can enhance resistance form as well as retention form.

Pins. Properly placed self-threading pins ensure adequate retention form, and also provide resistance form. Factors and technique for proper placement are presented.

Pin size. Four sizes of pins are available (Fig. 15-12), each with a corresponding color-coded drill (see Table 15-1). Familiarity with drill sizes and their corresponding color is necessary to ensure the proper size of pinhole is prepared for the desired pin. It is difficult to specify a particular size of pin that is always appropriate for a particular tooth. Two determining factors for selecting the appropriate size pin are (1) the amount of dentin available to safely receive the pin and (2) the amount of retention desired. In the Thread Mate System the pins of choice for severely involved posterior teeth are the Minikin (0.019 inch [0.48 mm]) and the Minim (0.024 inch [0.61 mm]). Both sizes of pins can be used in the same tooth depending on the dentin available in the area where the pins are to be inserted. The Minuta (0.015 inch [0.38 mm]) pin is usually too small to provide adequate retention in posterior teeth. Again, the retention of a pin increases as the diameter of the pin increases. However, the Regular (0.031 inch [0.78 mm]) or largest diameter pin should not be used because a significant amount of stress and crazing in the enamel may be created during its insertion.[14,16]

Number of pins. Several factors must be considered when deciding how many pins are required: (1) the amount of missing tooth structure, (2) the amount of dentin available to receive pins safely, (3) the amount of retention required, and (4) the size of the pins. *As a rule, one pin per missing axial line angle should be used.* Certain factors may cause the operator to alter this rule. The fewest pins possible should be used to achieve

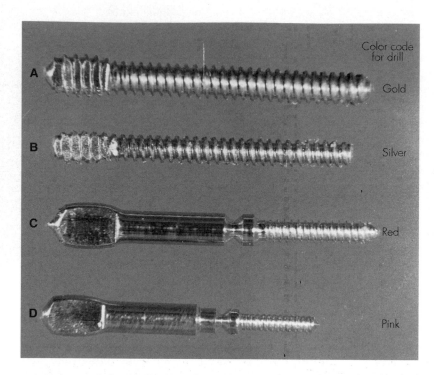

Fig. 15-12. Four sizes of TMS pins. **A,** Regular (0.031 inch [0.78 mm]). **B,** Minim (0.024 inch [0.61 mm]). **C,** Minikin (0.019 inch [0.48 mm]). **D,** Minuta (0.015 inch]0.38 mm]).

the desired retention for a given restoration. *When only 2 to 3 mm of the occlusogingival height of a cusp has been removed, no pin is required because enough tooth structure remains to prepare conventional retention* (see Fig. 15-2, *B* and Fig. 15-13).

As stated previously, the retention of the restoration increases as the number of pins increases. However, an excessive number of pins can fracture the tooth and significantly weaken the amalgam restoration.

Location. Several factors aid in locating pinholes: (1) knowledge of normal pulp anatomy and external tooth contours, (2) a current radiograph of the tooth, (3) a periodontal probe, and (4) the patient's age. Although the radiograph is only a two-dimensional picture of the tooth, it can give an indication of the position of the pulp chamber, and the contour of the mesial and distal surfaces of the tooth. Consideration must also be given to the placement of pins in areas where the greatest bulk of amalgam will occur to minimize the weakening effect of the pins.[39] Areas of occlusal contacts on the restoration must be anticipated, since a pin oriented longitudinally and positioned directly below an occlusal load weakens the amalgam significantly.[8]

Several attempts have been made to identify the ideal location of the pinhole. Caputo and Standlee[6] state that, ideally, pinholes should be located halfway between the pulp and the dentinoenamel junction or external surface of the tooth root. Standlee and others[52] have shown that there should be at least 1 mm of sound dentin around the circumference of the pinhole. Such location assures the proper stress distribution of occlusal forces. Felton and others have demonstrated that pin placement allow-

ing at least 1 mm of remaining dentin thickness elicits minimal pulpal inflammatory response.[19] Because it is difficult to fulfill these conditions, the following philosophy may be more practical. In the cervical one third of molars and premolars (where most pins are located), pinholes should be located near the line angles of the tooth, except as described later.[10,25] *The pinhole should be positioned no closer than 1 mm to the dentinoenamel junction and no closer than 1.5 mm to the external surface of the tooth* (Fig. 15-14). *Before the final decision is made about the location of the pinhole, the operator*

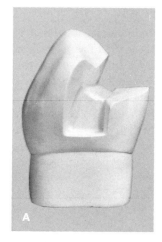
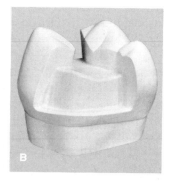

Fig. 15-13. Examples illustrating reduction of cusps **without** need for pin or pins. **A,** Mandibular first premolar with lingual cusp reduced for capping. **B,** Maxillary second molar prepared for restoration of mesial and distal surfaces and distofacial cusp.

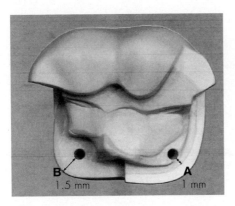

Fig. 15-14. Pinhole position. **A,** Position relative to dentinoenamel junction. **B,** Position relative to external tooth surface.

should carefully probe the gingival crevice to determine if any abnormal contours exist that would predispose the tooth to an external perforation.

The position of a pinhole must not result in the pin being so close to a longitudinal wall of tooth structure that condensation of amalgam against the pin or wall is jeopardized (Fig. 15-15, *A*). It may be necessary to prepare first a "cove" into the vertical wall with the No. 245 bur to permit pinhole preparation as well as to provide a minimum of 0.5 mm clearance around the circumference of the pin for adequate condensation of amalgam (Fig. 15-15, *B* and *C*).

Pinholes should be located on a flat surface that is perpendicular to the proposed direction of the pinhole. Otherwise, the drill may slip or "crawl," and a depth-limiting drill (to be discussed later) cannot prepare the hole as deeply as intended (Fig. 15-16).

Whenever three or more pinholes are placed, they should be located at different levels on the tooth if possible. This will prevent stresses resulting from pin placement in the same transverse plane of the tooth.

Spacing between pins, or the interpin distance, must be considered when two or more pinholes are prepared. The optimal *interpin distance* depends on the size of pin to be used. The minimal interpin distance is 3 mm for the Minikin (0.019 inch [0.48 mm]) pin and 5 mm for the Minim (0.024 inch [0.61 mm]) pin.[31] Maximal interpin distance results in lower levels of stress in dentin.[7]

Several posterior teeth have anatomical features that may preclude safe pinhole placement. *External perfo-*

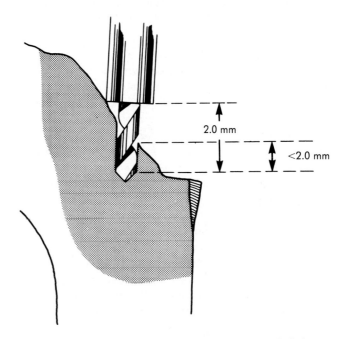

Fig. 15-16. Use of depth-limiting drill to prepare pinhole in surface that is not perpendicular to direction of pinhole will result in pinhole of inadequate depth.

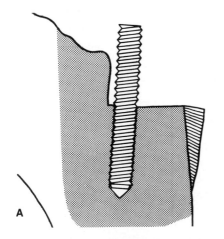
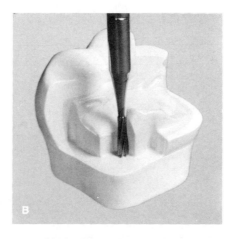
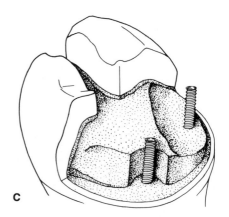

Fig. 15-15. A, Pin placed too close to longitudinal (vertical) wall such that adequate condensation of amalgam is jeopardized, **B** and **C,** Prepare cove in longitudinal wall of mandibular molar with No. 245 bur to provide adequate space for amalgam condensation around pin.

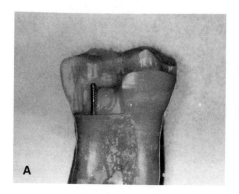

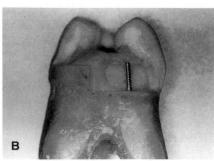

Fig. 15-17. Note distal root angulation of mandibular molar (**A**) and palatal root angulation of maxillary molar (**B**). Root angulation should be considered before pinhole placement.

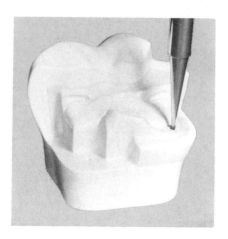

Fig. 15-18. Prepare pilot hole with No ¼ bur.

ration may result from pinhole placement (1) over the prominent mesial concavity of the maxillary first premolar, (2) at the midlingual and midfacial bifurcations of the mandibular first and second molars, and (3) at the midfacial, midmesial, and middistal furcations of the maxillary first and second molars. ***Pulpal penetration*** may result from pin placement at the mesiofacial corner of the maxillary first molar and the mandibular first molar.

Whenever possible, the location of pinholes on the distal surface of mandibular molars and lingual surface of maxillary molars should be avoided. Obtaining the proper direction for preparing a pinhole in these locations is difficult because of the abrupt angulation of the roots just apical to the cementoenamel junction (Fig. 15-17). If the pinhole is placed parallel to the external surface of the crown in these areas, penetration into the pulp is likely.[25] (Refer to the section, Penetration into

the Pulp and Perforation of the External Tooth Surface.)

When the pinhole locations have been determined, use a No. ¼ bur to prepare a ***pilot hole*** (dimple) approximately one-half the diameter of the bur at each location (Fig. 15-18). The purpose of this hole is to allow more accurate placement of the twist drill and to prevent the drill from "crawling" once it has begun to rotate.

Pinhole preparation. The ***Kodex drill*** (a twist drill) should be used for drilling pinholes (Fig. 15-19, *A*). The drill is made of a high-speed tool steel that is swaged into an aluminum shank. The aluminum shank, which acts as a heat absorber, is color coded so that it can be easily matched with the appropriate pin size (Tables 15-1 and 15-2). The drill shanks for the Minuta and

Table 15-2. TMS Link Series and Link Plus pins

Name	Illustration (not to scale)	Color code	Pin diameter (in/mm*)	Drill diameter (in/mm)	Pin length extending from sleeve (mm)	Pin length extending from dentin (mm)
Link series						
Regular (single shear)		Gold	0.031/0.78	0.027/0.68	5.5	3.2
Regular (double shear)		Gold	0.031/0.78	0.027/0.68	7.8	2.6
Minim (single shear)		Silver	0.024/0.61	0.021/0.53	5.4	3.2
Minim (double shear)		Silver	0.024/0.61	0.021/0.53	7.6	2.6
Minikin (single shear)		Red	0.019/0.48	0.017/0.43	6.9	1.5
Minuta (single shear)		Pink	0.015/0.38	0.0135/0.34	6.3	1.0
Link plus						
Minim (double shear)		Silver	0.024/0.61	0.021/0.53	10.8	2.7

*1 mm = 0.03937 in.

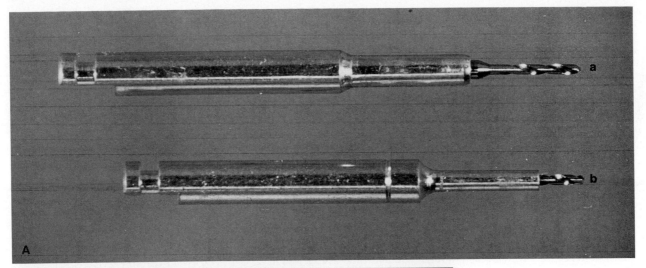

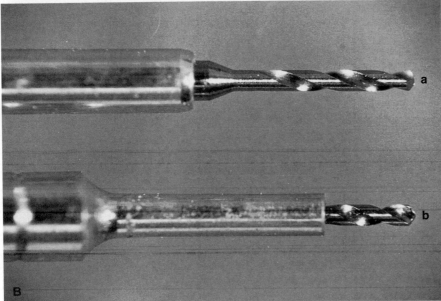

Fig. 15-19. A, Two types of Kodex twist drills: standard *(a)* and depth-limiting *(b).* **B,** Drills enlarged: standard *(a)* and depth-limiting *(b).*

Minikin pins are tapered to provide a built-in "wobble" when placed in a latch-type contra-angle handpiece. This wobble allows the drill to be "free floating" and thus align itself as the pinhole is prepared to minimize dentinal crazing or breakage of the small drills.

Because the optimal depth of the pinhole into the dentin is 2 mm (only 1.5 mm for the Minikin pin), the depth-limiting drill should be used to prepare the hole (Fig. 15-19). Only when this type of drill prepares a hole on a flat surface that is perpendicular to the drill will it prepare a hole 2 mm deep (see Fig. 15-16). When the location for starting a pinhole is neither flat nor perpendicular to the desired pinhole direction, either correct the location area or use the *standard twist drill* (Fig. 15-19, *A*), whose blades are 4 to 5 mm in length, to prepare a pinhole that has an effective depth of 2 mm. To minimize guessing when using the standard twist drill, the *Omni-Depth gauge* can be used to measure accurately the pinhole depth (Fig. 15-20).

With the drill in the latch-type contra-angle hand-

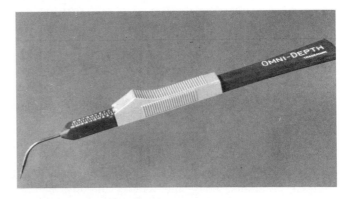

Fig. 15-20. Omni-Depth gauge is used to measure depth of pinhole(s).

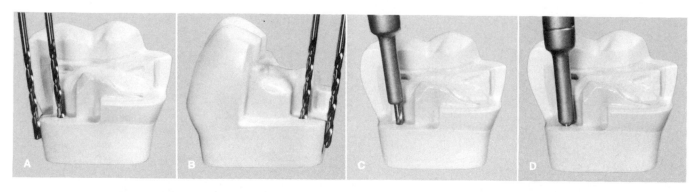

Fig. 15-21. Determining angulation for twist drill. **A,** Place drill in gingival crevice, and position it flat against tooth. Move it occlusally into position without changing angulation obtained. **B,** Repeat **A** while viewing drill from position 90° to that viewed in **A**. **C** and **D,** With twist drill at correct angulation, prepare pinhole in one or two thrusts until depth-limiting portion of drill is reached.

piece, place the drill in the gingival crevice opposite the location for the pinhole, position it until it lies flat against the external surface of the tooth, and then, without changing the angulation obtained from the crevice position, move the handpiece occlusally and place the drill in the previously prepared pilot hole (Fig. 15-21, *A*). Now, view the drill from a position 90 degrees to the previous viewing position to ascertain that the drill is also correctly angled in this plane (Fig. 15-21, *B*). Incorrect angulation of the drill may result in pulpal exposure or external perforation. (Refer to the section, Penetration into the Pulp and Perforation of the External Tooth Surface.) Should the proximity of an adjacent tooth interfere with placement of the drill into the gingival crevice, place a flat, thin-bladed hand instrument into the crevice and against the external surface of the tooth to indicate the proper angulation for the drill.[12] With the handpiece rotating at very low speed (300 to 500 rpm), apply pressure to the drill and prepare the pinhole in one or two movements until the depth-limiting portion of the drill is reached (Fig. 15-21, *C* and *D*). *Using more than one or two movements, tilting the handpiece during the drilling procedure, or allowing the drill to rotate more than very briefly at the bottom of the pinhole will result in a hole that is too large.* A steady stream of air should be applied to the drill to dissipate heat. *The drill should never stop rotating from insertion to removal from the pinhole to prevent the drill from breaking while in the hole.* (Refer to the section, Broken Drills and Broken Pins.)

Dull drills used to prepare pinholes can cause increased frictional heat and cracks in the dentin. Standlee, Collard, and Caputo[51] have demonstrated that a twist drill becomes too dull for use after cutting 20 pinholes or less, and the signal for discarding the drill is the need for increased pressure on the handpiece.

Unique situations require extra care in determining

pinhole angulation. The distal aspect of mandibular molars and the lingual aspect of maxillary molars have been mentioned previously as areas of potential problems because of the abrupt angulation of the roots just apical to the cementoenamel junction (see Fig. 15-17). The mandibular posterior teeth with their lingual crown tilt, teeth that are rotated in the arch, and teeth that are abnormally tilted in the arch deserve careful attention before and during pinhole placement. For mandibular second molars that are severely tilted mesially, care must be exercised to orient properly the drill to prevent external perforation on the mesial surface and pulpal penetration on the distal surface (Fig. 15-22). Because of limited interarch space, it is sometimes difficult to orient correctly the twist drill when placing pinholes at the distofacial or distolingual line angles of mandibular second and third molars (Fig. 15-23).

Pin design. For each of the four sizes of pins several designs are available: ***standard, self-shearing, two-in-one, Link Series,*** and ***Link Plus*** (Fig. 15-24). *The Link Series and Link Plus pins are recommended.* TMS pins are available in titanium or stainless steel plated with gold.

The Link Series pin is contained in a color-coded plastic sleeve that fits a latch-type contra-angle handpiece, or the specially designed ***plastic hand wrench*** (see Fig. 15-28, *D*). The pin is somewhat free floating in the plastic sleeve to allow it to align itself as it is threaded into the pinhole (Fig. 15-25). When the pin reaches the bottom of the hole, the top portion of the pin shears off, leaving a length of pin extending from the dentin. The plastic sleeve is then discarded. The Minuta, Minikin, Minim, and Regular pins are available in the Link Series. The Link Series pins are recommended because of their versatility, self-aligning ability, and retentiveness.[18]

The Link Plus pins are self-shearing and are avail-

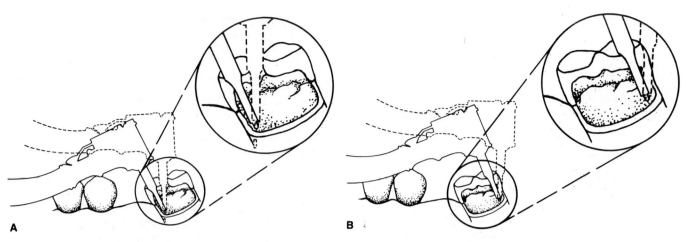

Fig. 15-22. Care must be exercised when preparing pinholes in mesially tilted molars to prevent external perforation on mesial surface (**A**) and pulpal penetration on the distal surface (**B**). Broken line is **incorrect** angulation of twist drill.

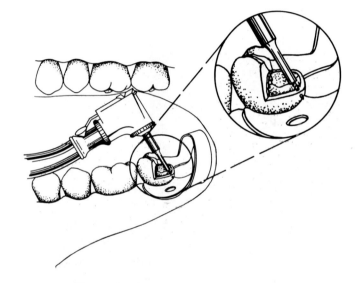

Fig. 15-23. When limited interarch space exists, care must be exercised when placing pinholes in molars to prevent external perforation on distal surface.

Fig. 15-24. Five designs of TMS pins. **A**, Standard. **B**, Self-shearing. **C**, Two-in-one. **D**, Link Series. **E**, Link Plus.

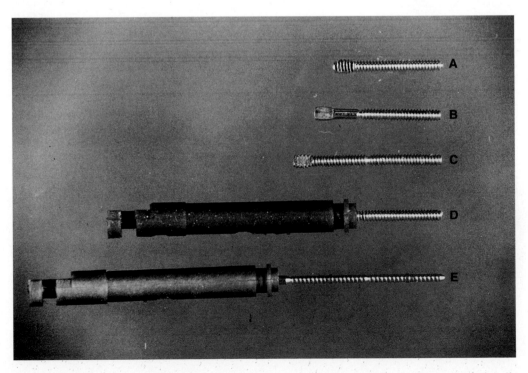

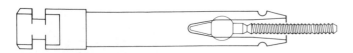

Fig. 15-25. Cross-sectional view of Link Series pin.

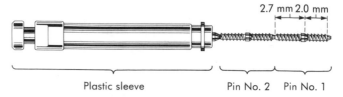

Fig. 15-26. Link Plus pin.

able as a single or two-in-one pin contained in a color-coded plastic sleeve (Fig. 15-26). This design has a sharper thread, a shoulder stop at 2 mm, and a tapered tip to more readily fit the bottom of the pinhole as prepared by the twist drill. It also provides a 2.7 mm length of pin to extend out of the dentin. Theoretically, and as suggested by Standlee, Caputo, and Collard,[50] these innovations should reduce the stress created in the surrounding dentin as the pin is inserted and reduce the apical stress at the bottom of the pinhole. Kelsey, Blankenau, and Cavel[30] have demonstrated that both the first and second pins seat completely into the pinhole before

shearing. The Link Plus pins are recommended because of their thread design, shoulder stop, tapered tip, and self-aligning ability.

The standard pin is approximately 7 mm long with a flattened head to engage the hand wrench or the appropriate handpiece chuck, and is threaded to place until it reaches the bottom of the pinhole as judged by tactile sense. One advantage of the standard design pin is that it can be reversed one-fourth to one-half turn following insertion to full depth to reduce stress created at the apical end of the hole[27] (Fig. 15-27).

The self-shearing pin has a total length that varies ac-

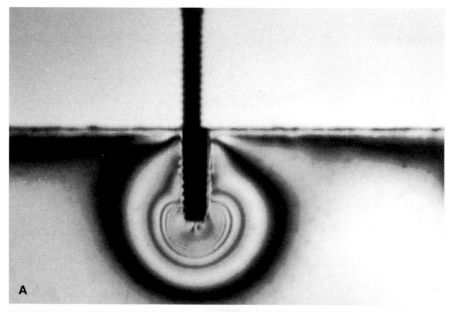

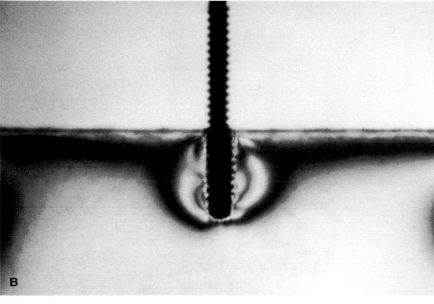

Fig. 15-27. Stress created by self-threading pin as illustrated in a photoelastic study. **A,** Pin fully seated in pinhole. **B,** Pin reversed one-quarter turn. (Photographs courtesy Dr. Alan W. Irvin.)

cording to the diameter of the pin (see Table 15-1). It also consists of a flattened head to engage the hand wrench or the appropriate handpiece chuck for threading into the pinhole. When the pin approaches the bottom of the hole, the head of the pin shears off, leaving a length of pin extending from the dentin.

The two-in-one pin is actually two pins-in-one, with each one being shorter than the standard pin. The two-in-one pin is approximately 9.5 mm in length and also has a flattened head to aid in its insertion. When the pin approaches the bottom of the pinhole, it shears approximately in half, leaving a length of pin extending from the dentin with the other half remaining in the hand wrench or the handpiece chuck. This second pin may be positioned in another pinhole and threaded to place in the same manner as the standard pin. The designs available with each size of pin are shown in Tables 15-1 and 15-2.

All of the pin designs can be inserted with an appropriate hand wrench (Fig. 15-28). A conventional latch-type contra-angle handpiece with the appropriate chuck (Fig. 15-29) can be used to insert any of the pins except the standard design.

Selection of a particular pin design (see Tables 15-1 and 15-2) is influenced by the size of the pin being used, the amount of interarch space available, and operator preference. The Minuta and Minikin are available only in the self-shearing and Link (also self-shearing) design. With minimal interarch space the two-in-one

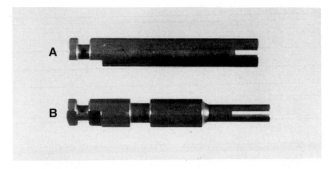

Fig. 15-29. Handpiece chucks for (**A**) TMS regular self-shearing and Minikin pins, and (**B**) TMS Minuta pins.

design is undesirable because of its length. Studies have shown that the two-in-one pin and the self-shearing pin may sometimes fail to reach the bottom of the pinhole.[3,4,20] A study by May and Heymann[35] found that 93% of Link Series and Link Plus two-in-one pins extended to the optimal depth of 2 mm. Eames and Solly[18] demonstrated no significant difference between the retention of the self-shearing pin and the standard design pin. However, Newitter and Schlissel[42] have shown that more force is required to dislodge the standard design pin than the self-shearing pin.

Pin insertion. Two instruments for insertion of threaded pins are available: conventional latch-type contra-angle handpiece (Fig. 15-30), and TMS hand wrenches (see Fig. 15-28). Studies conflict as to which method of pin insertion produces the best results.* The latch-type handpiece is recommended for the insertion of the Link Series and the Link Plus pins. The hand wrench is recommended for the insertion of standard pins.

When using the latch-type handpiece, insert a Link Series or a Link Plus pin into the handpiece and place the pin in the pinhole. Activate the handpiece until the plastic sleeve shears from the pin. Then, remove the sleeve and discard it.

A standard design pin is placed in the appropriate

*References 4,11,18,20,30,40.

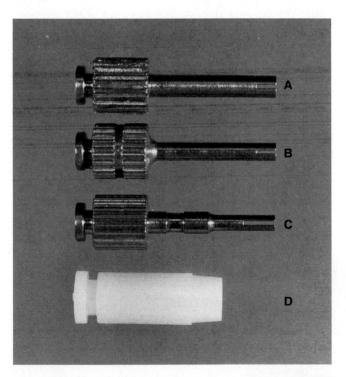

Fig. 15-28. Hand wrenches for TMS pins. **A,** Regular and Minikin. **B,** Minim. **C,** Minuta. **D,** Link Series and Link Plus.

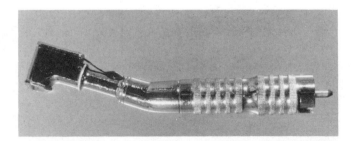

Fig. 15-30. Conventional latch-type contra-angle handpiece.

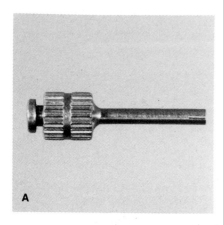
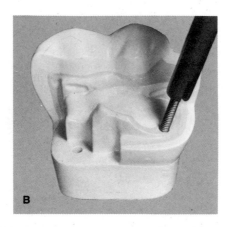
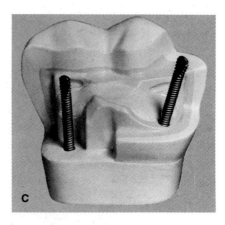

Fig. 15-31. **A,** Use of hand wrench to place pin. **B,** Thread pin to bottom of pinhole, and then reverse wrench one-quarter to one-half turn. **C,** Evaluate length of pin extending from dentin.

wrench (Fig. 15-31) and slowly threaded into the pinhole until a definite resistance is felt when the pin reaches the bottom of the hole (see Fig. 15-27). The pin should then be rotated one-fourth to one-half turn counterclockwise to reduce the dentinal stress created by the end of the pin pressing the dentin.[27] Carefully remove the hand wrench from the pin.

If the hand wrench is used without rubber dam isolation, a gauze *throat shield* must be in place, and a strand of dental tape approximately 12 to 15 inches (30 to 38 cm) in length should be securely tied to the end of the wrench (Fig. 15-32). These precautions will prevent the patient from swallowing or aspirating the hand wrench should it be dropped accidentally.

Once the pins are placed, evaluate their length (see Fig. 15-31, *C*). *Any length of pin greater than 2 mm should be removed. Recall that 2 mm of pin length into amalgam is appropriate.* Also, whenever possible, it is desirable to have at least 2 mm of amalgam over the end of the pin to prevent unnecessary weakening of the restoration. To cut off the excess length of pin, use at high speed a sharp No. ¼, ½, or 169L bur oriented perpendicularly to the pin (Fig. 15-33, *A*). If oriented otherwise, the rotation of the bur may loosen the pin by rotating it counterclockwise. During cut-off, the assistant should apply a steady stream of air to the pin and have the evacuator tip positioned to remove the pin seg-

ment. Also during cut-off, the pin may be stabilized with a small hemostat or cotton pliers. Test the pin for tightness. See if it can be wiggled or easily withdrawn. Refer to the section, Loose Pins.

Using a mirror, view the preparation from all directions (particularly from the occlusal) to determine if any pins need to be bent to position them within the contour of the final restoration and to provide adequate bulk of amalgam between the pin and the external surface of the final restoration (Fig. 15-33, *B* and *C*). *Pins are not to be bent to make them parallel or to increase their retentiveness.* Occasionally, bending a pin may be necessary to allow for condensation of amalgam occlusogingivally. When pins require bending, the *TMS bending tool* (Fig. 15-34, *A*) must be used. Place the bending tool on the pin where the pin is to be bent, and with firm controlled pressure rotate the bending tool until the desired amount of bend is achieved (Fig. 15-34, *B* to *D*). Use of the bending tool allows placement of the fulcrum at some point along the length of the exposed pin. *A hand instrument such as an amalgam condenser or Black spoon excavator should not be used to bend a pin because the location of the fulcrum will be at the mouth of the pinhole.* These hand instruments may cause crazing or fracture of the dentin, and the abrupt or "sharp" bend increases the chance of breaking the pin (Fig. 15-35). Also, when pressure is applied with a hand instru-

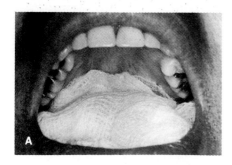
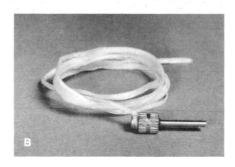

Fig. 15-32. Precautions must be taken if rubber dam is not used. **A,** Gauze throat shield. **B,** Hand wrench with 12 to 15 inches (30 to 38 cm) of dental tape attached.

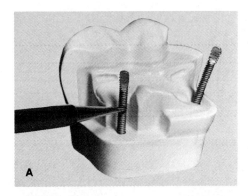

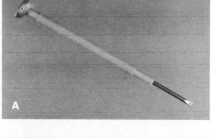

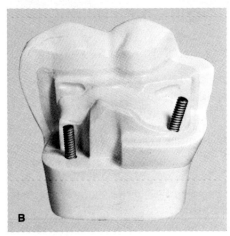

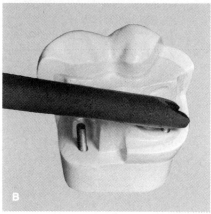

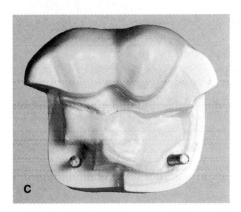

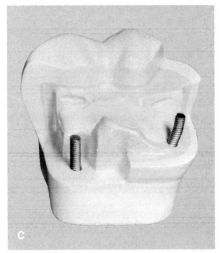

Fig. 15-33. A, Use sharp No. ¼ bur held perpendicular to pin to shorten pin. **B** and **C,** Evaluate preparation to determine need for bending pin(s).

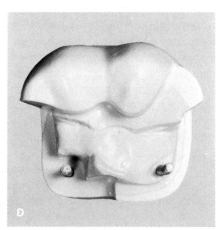

Fig. 15-34. A, TMS bending tool. **B,** Use bending tool to bend pin. **C** and **D,** Pin is bent to position that provides adequate bulk of amalgam between pin and external surface of final restoration.

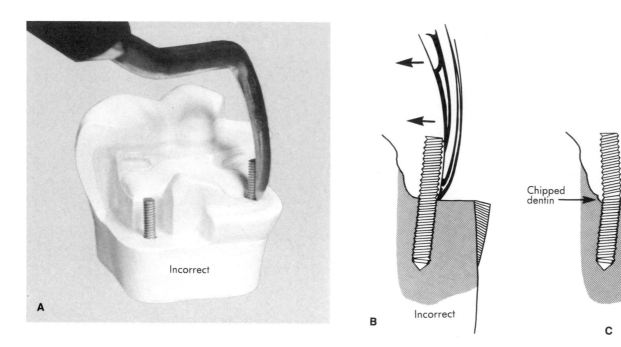

Fig. 15-35. A, Do **not** use Black spoon excavator or other hand instrument to bend pin. **B** and **C,**
Use of hand instruments may create sharp bend in pin and chip dentin.

ment there is less control, and the chance of slipping is increased. Refer to the section, Broken Drills and Broken Pins.

Cemented pins. Pinholes are prepared in dentin 3 to 4 mm deep using a twist drill with a diameter of 0.027 inch (0.68 mm) or 0.021 inch (0.53 mm) (Fig. 15-36, *A*). Threaded stainless steel wire with a diameter of 0.025 inch (0.64 mm) is used for the 0.027 inch pinhole and 0.020 inch (0.51 mm) wire for the 0.021 inch pinhole (Fig. 15-36, *B* to *F*). The pins are cemented into place with zinc phosphate or polycarboxylate cement using a Lentulo spiral instrument (Fig. 15-36, *G* and *H*).

Procedure for finishing external enamel walls. Evaluate the enamel margins for soundness and a correct cavosurface angle of 90 degrees. An enamel margin with a cavosurface angle less than 90 degrees usually is friable if tested by a rubbing-pressure applied from the side of an explorer tine. Correct where indicated.

Final procedures: cleaning; inspecting; varnishing. Rinse the preparation if indicated with air/water spray and dry to remove visible moisture without desiccating the tooth. Inspect for detection and removal of any debris or unwanted base/liner. To prevent pooling of the varnish at the margin-matrix interface, apply cavity varnish prior to matrix placement. Two applications of cavity varnish are recommended. As mentioned previously, the use of new dentin-adhesive systems (in lieu of varnish) may reduce microleakage. Longevity clinical studies are needed to demonstrate their efficacy.

Matrices. One of the most difficult steps in restoring

a severely involved posterior tooth is development of a satisfactory matrix.

Universal matrix. For the majority of posterior teeth the Tofflemire retainer and band described in Chapter 13 can be used successfully (Fig. 15-37, *O*). Use of the Tofflemire retainer requires that sufficient tooth structure is available to retain the band after it is applied.

When the open aspect of the Tofflemire matrix is located next to prepared tooth structure, a closed system can be developed as illustrated in Fig. 15-38. Cut a strip of matrix material that is long enough to extend from the mesial to the distal corners of the tooth. The strip must extend into these corners enough that the band, when tight, will hold the strip in position, but it must not extend into the proximal areas or a ledge will result in the restoration contour when the matrix is removed. Loosen the Tofflemire retainer one-half turn, and insert the strip of matrix material next to the opening and between the matrix band and the tooth. Tighten the retainer, and complete the matrix as described previously in Chapter 13. Sometimes it is helpful to condense a small amount of softened compound between the strip and open aspect of the band-retainer to stabilize and support the strip further (Fig. 15-38, *G* and *H*).

Regardless of the type of matrix system used, it must be stable. If the matrix for a pin amalgam restoration is not stable during condensation, a homogeneous restoration cannot be developed, and the restoration will be weak and may disintegrate when the matrix is removed.

When very little tooth structure remains and deep gingival margins are present, the Tofflemire matrix can-

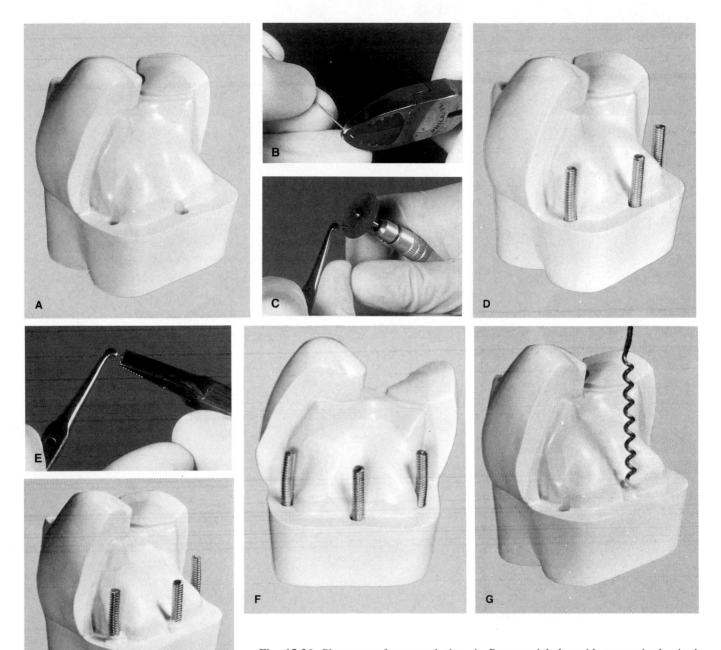

Fig. 15-36. Placement of cemented pins. **A,** Prepare pinholes with appropriately sized twist drill. **B,** Cut proper length of pin with wire-cutting pliers. **C,** Slightly round the end of the pin with rotating carborundum disc. **D,** Place pins in tooth, and evaluate need for bending. **E,** Hold pin with two pairs of pliers, and bend as necessary. **F,** Pins bent. **G,** Convey cement into pinholes with a Lentulo spiral instrument. **H,** Pins cemented.

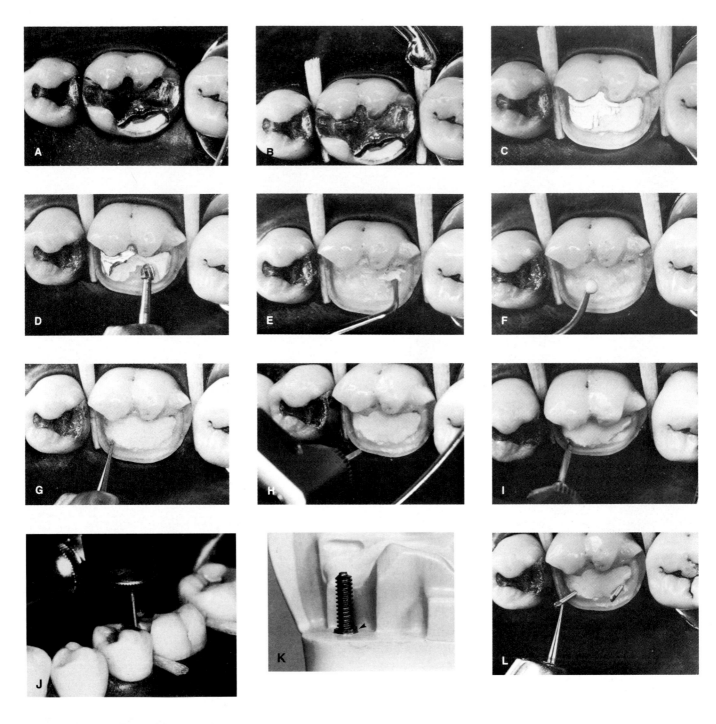

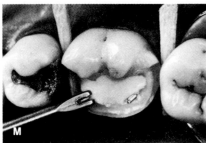

Fig. 15-37. A, Mandibular first molar with fractured distolingual cusp. B, Insert wedges. C, Initial cavity preparation. D and E, Excavate any infected dentin; if indicated, remove and/or any remaining old restorative materials. F, Apply base (if necessary). G, Prepare pilot holes. H, Align twist drill with external surface of tooth. I, Prepare pinholes. J, Insert Link pins with slow-speed handpiece. K, Note depth-limiting shoulder (arrow) of inserted Link Plus pin. L, Use No ¼ bur to shorten pins.

Continued.

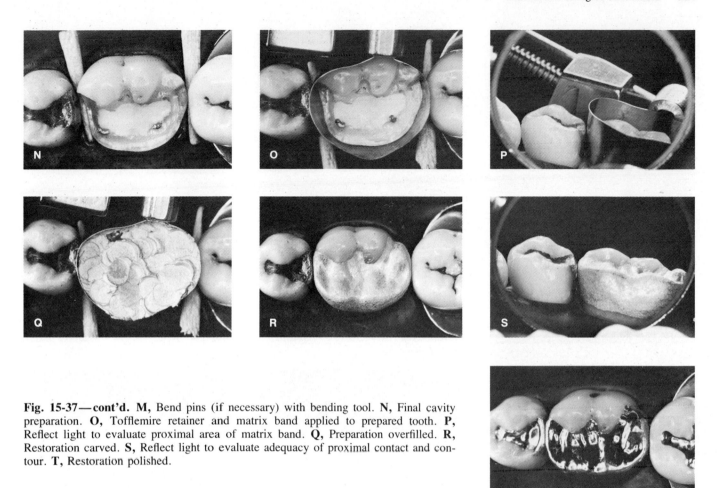

Fig. 15-37—cont'd. M, Bend pins (if necessary) with bending tool. **N,** Final cavity preparation. **O,** Tofflemire retainer and matrix band applied to prepared tooth. **P,** Reflect light to evaluate proximal area of matrix band. **Q,** Preparation overfilled. **R,** Restoration carved. **S,** Reflect light to evaluate adequacy of proximal contact and contour. **T,** Restoration polished.

not be used successfully. In the following sections the compound-supported copper band (Fig. 15-39) and the Automatrix* (Fig. 15-40) are presented for use when minimal tooth structure is available.

Compound-supported copper band matrix. The compound-supported copper band matrix may be used when the Tofflemire matrix cannot be used successfully. Fabrication of the copper band matrix can be time-consuming, but when done properly satisfies the requirements of a good matrix. Fig. 15-39 illustrates the fabrication of a compound-supported copper band matrix. A seamless, annealed copper band is used for the matrix. The band can be annealed by heating it red-hot and then immediately immersing it in water. Select the smallest copper band that will fit over the circumference of the tooth and still touch or nearly touch the proximal surfaces of the adjacent teeth. Before trying a band on the tooth, festoon the gingival end with *curved crown and bridge scissors* to correspond to the level of the gingival attachment, smooth any rough edges by a sandpaper disc or mounted rubber wheel, and contour the cut end

*The LD Caulk Co., Milford, Del.

with *No. 114 contouring pliers* (Fig. 15-39, *B* to *F*). Slightly withdraw the wedges placed during preparation of the tooth. This will allow teasing the band between the wedges and gingival margin. Continue to try the band, and adjust the gingival end until the band extends approximately 1 mm past the gingival margins. No. 114 contouring pliers can be used to develop some contour to the proximal, facial, and lingual aspects of the band and to improve its gingival adaptation. With the band in place on the tooth, use a sharp explorer to scribe a line around the outer surface of the band to indicate the correct occlusal height (Fig. 15-39, *G*). This line should be 1 to 2 mm above the marginal ridges of adjacent teeth and should provide adequate occlusal height on the facial and lingual surfaces to allow for restoration of reduced cusps. Remove the band, cut it with scissors along the scribed line, and smooth any rough edges by a sandpaper disc or mounted rubber wheel (Fig. 15-39, *H* and *I*). To help ensure adequate proximal contact with the adjacent teeth, reduce the thickness of the band (but do not penetrate) by relieving the outer surface in the area of each contact using a rotating sandpaper disc or suitable mounted stone (Fig. 15-39, *J*). Replace the

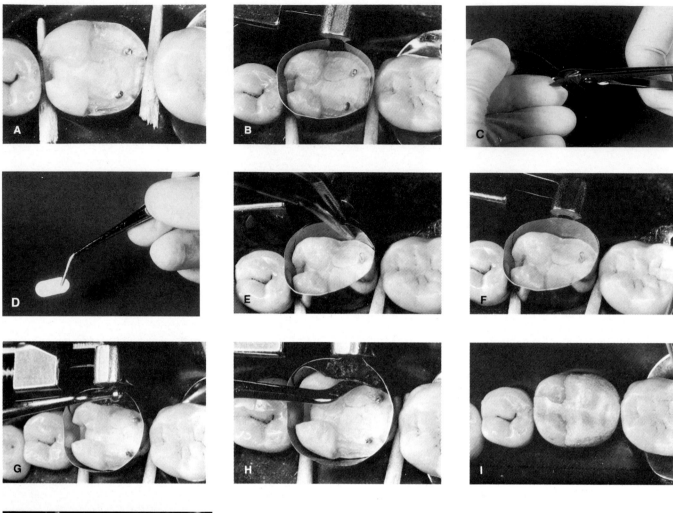

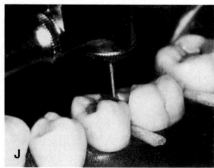

Fig. 15-38. Technique for closing open space of Tofflemire matrix system. **A,** Tooth preparation with wedges in place. **B,** Open aspect of matrix band next to prepared tooth structure. **C** and **D,** Cut appropriate length of matrix material. **E,** Insert strip of matrix material. **F,** Closed matrix system. **G** and **H,** Place compound between strip and matrix band, and contour if necessary. **I,** Restoration carved. **J,** Restoration polished.

band, and reinsert the wedges. To further adapt the band to the tooth, crimp the facial surface in the gingival one third using No. 110 pliers (Fig. 15-39, *L* and *M*). Evaluate proximal contacts and contour, making adjustments if indicated. Apply compound to stabilize the band and improve its adaptation to the tooth in the gingival aspect of the facial and lingual surfaces (Fig. 13-39, *N*). (Refer to Compound-supported Matrix, in Chapter 13.) Again, evaluate the matrix for adequate adaptation and contour, and make corrections where indicated. *Routinely burnish the cavity side of the matrix with a warmed, suitably shaped burnisher in the contact areas to ensure that no compound is between the band and the adjacent teeth (at the contacts) and to assess tactilely that the band is touching the adjacent teeth* (Fig. 15-39, *O*).

Condense the amalgam, and initiate carving (Fig. 15-39, *P*). (Refer to Procedures for Inserting and Carving the Restoration, in Chapter 13.) Following carving of the occlusal aspect of the restoration, break away the compound with an explorer or Black spoon excavator. To remove the band, carefully cut a groove occlusogingivally on the facial and lingual surfaces of the band with a No. 2 bur (Fig. 15-39, *Q*). Tear the band apart

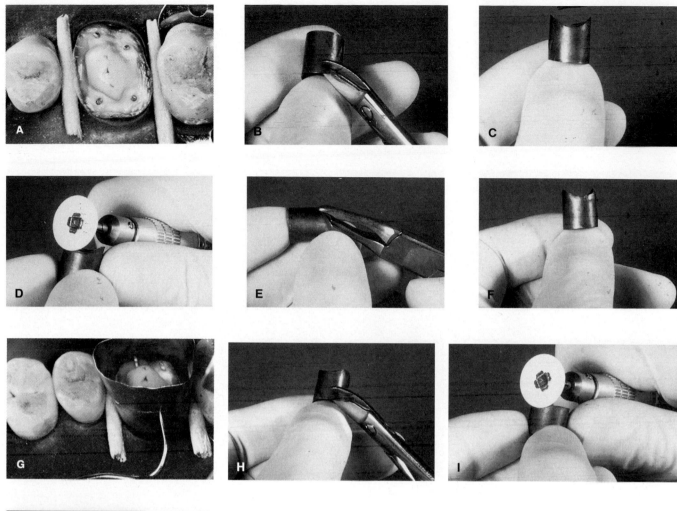

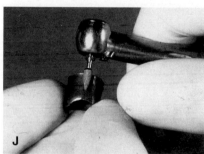

Fig. 15-39. Compound-supported copper band matrix for developing pin-retained "amalgam crown" on maxillary first molar. **A,** Tooth preparation with wedges in place. **B,** Festoon gingival end of band with curved crown and bridge scissors. **C,** Festooned band. **D,** Smooth any rough edges with rotating sandpaper disc. **E,** Contour gingival end of band with No. 114 contouring pliers. **F,** Contoured band. **G,** With band in place, use explorer to scribe a line around band at correct occlusal height. **H** and **I,** Remove band, trim at scribed line, and smooth any rough edges with rotating sandpaper disc. **J,** Thin the proximal contact areas with green stone.   *Continued.*

along these grooves with an explorer, and remove the two sections in an oblique direction occlusolingually or occlusofacially (Fig. 15-39, *R*). Complete the carving of the restoration (Fig. 15-39, *S*).

Automatrix. The Automatrix (Fig. 15-40) is a retainerless matrix system designed for any tooth regardless of its circumference. The Automatrix bands are supplied in three widths: ³⁄₁₆, ¼, and ⁵⁄₁₆ inch (4.8, 6.35, and 7.79 mm). The medium band is available in two thicknesses (0.0015 and 0.002 inch [0.038 and 0.05 mm]). The ³⁄₁₆ and ⁵⁄₁₆ inch band widths are available in the 0.002 inch thickness only. Advantages of this sys-

tem include (1) convenience, (2) improved visibility because of absence of a retainer, (3) ability to place the autolock loop on the facial or lingual surface of the tooth, and (4) decreased time for application as compared to the copper band matrix. The development of proper proximal contours and contacts can be difficult with the Automatrix bands. Refer to the manufacturer's directions for the use of this matrix system. Use of the Automatrix system is illustrated in Fig. 15-41.

Procedures for inserting and carving the restoration. A spherical or admixed high-copper alloy is strongly recommended for the pin amalgam restoration because

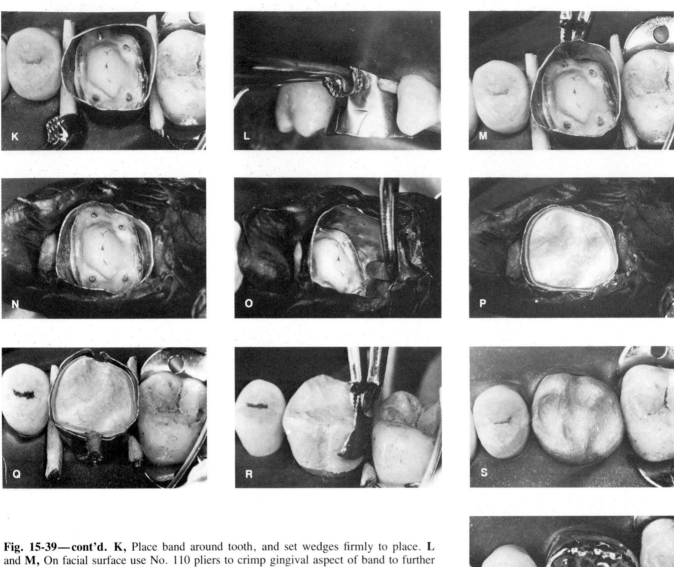

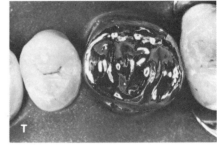

Fig. 15-39—cont'd. K, Place band around tooth, and set wedges firmly to place. **L** and **M,** On facial surface use No. 110 pliers to crimp gingival aspect of band to further adapt it to tooth. **N,** Apply green compound. **O,** Contour band with back of warm black spoon excavator. **P,** Overfill preparation, and carve occlusal aspect. **Q,** Break away compound, and section band occlusogingivally on facial and lingual surfaces. **R,** Remove sections in oblique direction (facially with some occlusal vector). **S,** Restoration carved. **T,** Restoration polished.

of excellent clinical performance,[33,43] higher early compressive strengths,[17] and better adaptation to the pin(s).[9,32] An alloy with an extended working time is also recommended to allow sufficient time for condensation, removal of the matrix band, and final carving.

Triturate a mix of amalgam according to the manufacturer's directions, and transfer some of the amalgam to the gingival portion of the preparation. Using appropriately sized condensers, condense each increment of amalgam. *Care must be taken to condense the amalgam adequately around the pins.* If a mix of amalgam be-

comes dry or crumbly, immediately triturate a new mix. Layering and therefore weakening of the restoration can be minimized by using multiple mixes of amalgam. Continue condensation until the preparation is overfilled (Fig. 15-37, *Q*). Define the occlusal embrasures and marginal ridges with the tine of an explorer. A marginal ridge must be at or near the same height as the adjacent marginal ridge to reduce the likelihood of fracturing when the matrix is removed. Remove the bulk of excess amalgam on the occlusal surface, and develop the anatomy with a discoid carver. With the wedges remaining in place to maintain passive pressure on the band from

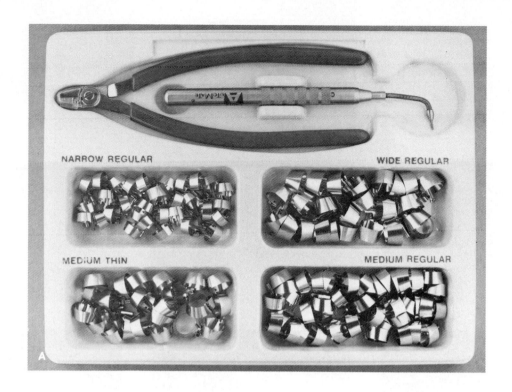

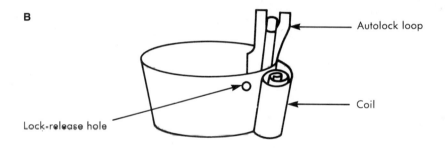

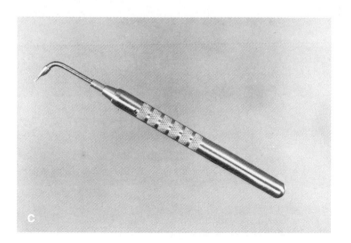

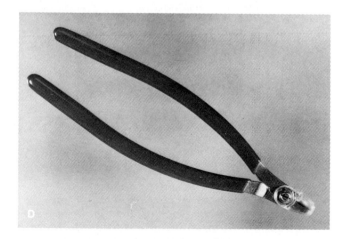

Fig. 15-40. A, Automatrix retainerless matrix system. **B,** Automatrix band. **C,** Automate II tightening device. **D,** Shielded nippers. (**A,** Courtesy The L.D. Caulk Company, Milford, DE)

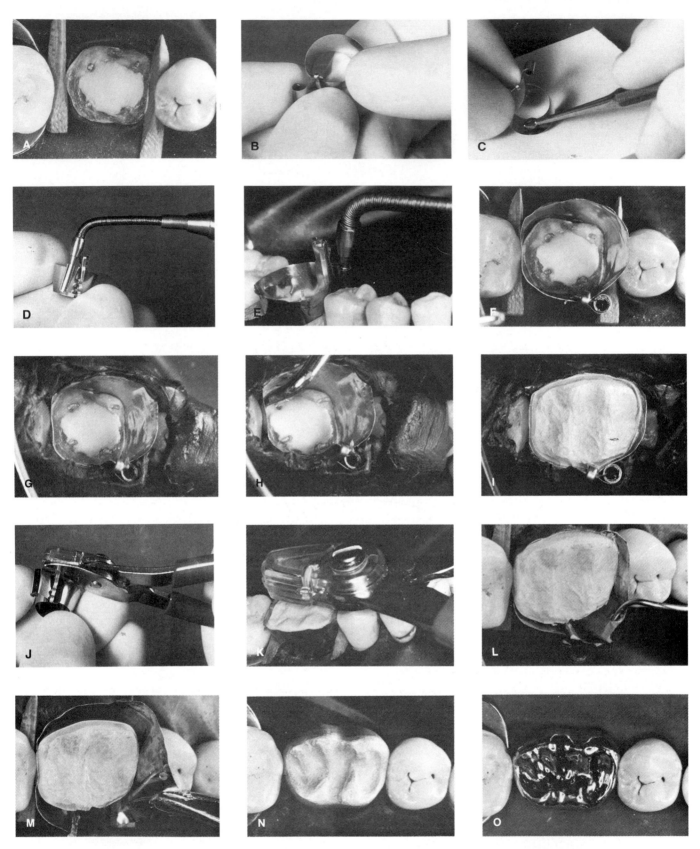

Fig. 15-41. Application of Automatrix for developing pin-retained "amalgam crown" on mandibular first molar. **A,** Tooth preparation with wedges in place. **B,** Enlarge circumference of band if necessary. **C,** Burnish band with egg-shaped burnisher. **D to F,** Place band around tooth, tighten with Automate II tightening device, and set wedges firmly to place. **G,** Apply green compound. **H,** Contour band with back of warm Black spoon excavator. **I,** Overfill preparation, and carve the occlusal aspect. **J** and **K,** Use shielded nippers to cut autolock loop. **L,** Separate band with explorer. **M,** Remove band in oblique direction (facially with some occlusal vector). **N,** Restoration carved. **O,** Restoration polished.

the adjacent tooth, remove the Tofflemire retainer from the band. Then remove each end of the band by sliding it in an oblique direction (i.e., move the band facially or lingually while simultaneously moving it in an occlusal direction). Moving the band obliquely toward the occlusal surface minimizes the possibility of fracturing the marginal ridge. Every effort should be made to remove the matrix band in the same direction as wedge placement to prevent dislodging the wedges. Next, remove the wedges and any interproximal gingival excess with an explorer or an amalgam knife. Develop facial and lingual contours with an explorer or Hollenback carver to complete the carving (Fig. 15-37, R). Sometimes it may be necessary to use rotary instruments to complete the occlusal carving if the amalgam has set to a hardness that the force needed to carve with hand instruments might fracture portions of the restoration. Appropriate round burs, flame-shaped burs, and tapered fissure burs can be used to develop occlusal anatomy.

Evaluate the margins with an explorer, and correct any discrepancy. Evaluate the adequacy of each proximal contact by using a mirror to assure that no light can be reflected between the restoration and the adjacent tooth at the level of the proximal contact (Fig. 15-37, S). When the proper contour and contact cannot be achieved in the initial restoration, it is often possible to correct this problem by preparing an "ideal" two-surface cavity preparation within the pin amalgam and then restoring the proper proximal surface. Any amalgam forming the walls of this "ideal" preparation must have sufficient bulk to prevent future fracture.

Remove the rubber dam and evaluate the occlusal contacts by observing the restoration and adjacent cusp-fossa relationships as the patient slowly closes. If no gross discrepancies can be seen, use articulating paper to mark the occlusal contacts. Adjust the restoration as needed to maintain harmony with the remaining teeth. For the procedure of obtaining desired occlusal contacts, refer to Removing the Matrix Band and Completing the Carving in Chapter 13. Before the patient is dismissed, dental floss may be passed through the proximal contacts one time to remove any amalgam shavings on the proximal surface of the restoration. Passing the floss through a contact more than once may weaken a

contact. It is important that these shavings be removed to eliminate the possibility of a rough proximal surface. Caution the patient not to use the restoration for several hours.

Finishing and polishing procedures. Finish and polish the amalgam restoration according to procedures described in Chapters 12 and 13 (Fig. 15-37, T).

Pin-retained Classes IV and V amalgam restorations

Class IV. The indication for pins in a Class IV restoration is rare. The use of pins may be considered for the large Class IV preparation on the distal surface of a canine that involves a significant amount of the distoincisal corner (Fig. 15-42). Pins placed in the gingival aspect may provide the needed retention for the restoration. However, use of a lingual dovetail as described in Chapter 14 is an alternative to pin retention if enough lingual tooth structure is available for preparation of the dovetail.

Class V. There is rarely a need to place pins for a Class V restoration. Adequate retention can usually be achieved by the placement of a transverse groove in the gingival and occlusal aspect of the preparation. Jorgensen, Matono and Shimokobe[28] have shown that teeth flex in the gingival area when an occlusal force is applied. The most severe flexure of a cusp occurs when a large Class V preparation and a mesioocclusodistal preparation are present in the same tooth. The placement of pins in a gingival and occlusal direction in the extensive Class V preparation has been suggested to reduce the amount of flexure.[21] However, the need for such placement of pins has not been demonstrated clinically.

PIN-RETAINED DIRECT TOOTH-COLORED RESTORATIONS

With the development of the acid etch technique, the need for pins in cavity preparations for direct tooth-colored restorations has virtually been eliminated. Proper use of the acid etch technique and selectively placed retention locks usually provide adequate retention for tooth-colored restorations. The use of pins may be considered for a tooth that has little or no enamel present

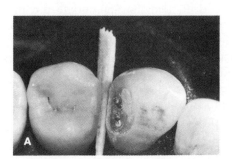
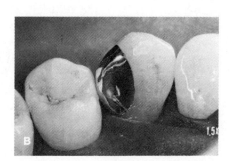

Fig. 15-42. A, Maxillary canine with extensive loss of tooth structure requiring placement of pins for adequate retention form. **B,** Restoration polished.

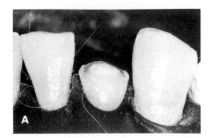
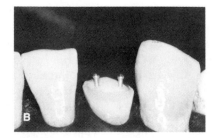
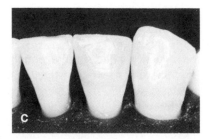

Fig. 15-43. Using light-activated composite to restore fractured mandibular lateral incisor. **A,** Cavosurface bevel prepared at 45 degrees to external enamel surface, and base of calcium hydroxide applied. **B,** Minikin pins placed and enamel etched. **C,** Restoration completed.

for acid etching and no appropriate place to prepare adequate retention locks (Fig. 15-43). Ideally, such a tooth should be restored with a tooth-colored crown. However, economics or time constraints may dictate the placement of a direct tooth-colored restoration. (Refer to Chapters 16 and 17 for description of cavity preparations for direct tooth-colored restorations.)

FAILURE OF PIN-RETAINED RESTORATIONS

The failure of pin-retained restorations might occur at any of five different locations (Fig. 15-44). Failure can occur (1) within the restoration (restoration fracture), (2) at the interface between the pin and the restorative material (pin-restoration separation), (3) within the pin (pin fracture), (4) at the interface between the pin

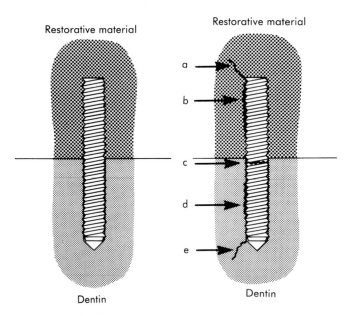

Fig. 15-44. Five possible locations of failure of pin-retained restorations. *a,* Fracture of restorative material; *b,* separation of pin from restorative material; *c,* fracture of pin; *d,* separation of pin from dentin; *e,* fracture of dentin.

and the dentin (pin-dentin separation), and (5) within the dentin (dentin fracture). Failure is more likely to occur at the pin-dentin interface than at the pin-restoration interface. The operator must keep these areas of potential failure in mind at all times and apply the necessary principles to minimize the possibility of an inadequate restoration.

BROKEN DRILLS AND BROKEN PINS

Occasionally, a twist drill will break if it is stressed laterally or allowed to stop rotating before being removed from the pinhole. Use of sharp twist drills will help to eliminate the possibility of drill breakage. The standard pin usually breaks if turned more than needed to reach the bottom of the pinhole. Pins may also break during bending if care is not exercised. The treatment for both broken drills and broken pins is to choose an alternate location at least 1.5 mm away from the broken item and prepare another pinhole. Removal of a broken pin or drill is difficult if not impossible and usually should not be attempted. The best solution for these two problems is prevention.

LOOSE PINS

Self-threading pins sometimes do not properly engage the dentin because the pinhole was inadvertently prepared too large or a self-shearing pin failed to shear resulting in stripped out dentin. The pin should be removed from the tooth and the pinhole reprepared with the next-largest size drill, and the appropriate pin inserted. Drilling another pinhole of the same size 1.5 mm from the original pinhole is also acceptable.

As described earlier, a properly placed pin can be loosened while being shortened with a bur if the bur is not held perpendicularly to the pin and stabilized. If loose, remove the pin from the pinhole by holding a rotating bur parallel to the pin and lightly contacting the surface of the pin. This will cause the pin to rotate counterclockwise out of the pinhole. Try to insert another pin of the same size. If the second pin fails to engage the dentin tightly, redrill a larger hole, and insert the appropriate pin. Drilling another pinhole of the same size 1.5 mm from the original pinhole is also acceptable.

PENETRATION INTO THE PULP AND PERFORATION OF THE EXTERNAL TOOTH SURFACE

Either penetration into the pulp or perforation of the external surface of the tooth is obvious if there is hemorrhage in the pinhole following removal of the drill. Usually, the operator can tell when a penetration or perforation has occurred by an abrupt loss of resistance of the cutting drill to hand pressure. Also, if a standard or Link Series pin continues to thread into the tooth beyond the 2 mm depth of the pinhole, this is an indication of a penetration or perforation. A pulpal penetration might be suspected if the patient is anesthetized and has had no sensitivity to tooth preparation until the pinhole is being completed or the pin is being placed. However, with profound anesthesia some patients may not feel pulpal penetration.

Radiographs can verify that a pulpal penetration has not occurred if the view shows dentin between the pulp and the pin. A radiograph projecting the pin in the same region as the pulp does not confirm a pulpal penetration because the pin and the pulp may be superimposed as a result of angulation. In contrast, a radiograph showing a pin projecting outside the tooth confirms external perforation. However, a radiograph showing the pin inside the projected outline of the tooth does not exclude the possibility of an external perforation.

In an asymptomatic tooth a pulpal penetration is treated as any other small mechanical exposure. If the exposure is discovered following preparation of the pinhole, control the hemorrhage, if any. Then, place calcium hydroxide over the opening of the pinhole, and prepare another hole 1.5 to 2 mm away. If the exposure is discovered as the pin is being placed, remove the pin and control any hemorrhage. Place calcium hydroxide over the pinhole, and prepare another hole 1.5 to 2 mm away. Although certain studies have shown that the pulp will tolerate pin penetration when placed in a relatively sterile environment,[1,15] it is not recommended that pins remain in place when a pulpal penetration has occurred. If the pin were left in the pulp, (1) the depth of the pin into pulpal tissue would be difficult to determine, (2) considerable postoperative sensitivity might ensue, and (3) the pin location might complicate subsequent root canal therapy. Regardless of the method of treatment rendered, the patient must be informed of the perforation or pulpal penetration at the completion of the appointment. The affected tooth should be periodi-

cally evaluated using appropriate radiographs. The patient should be instructed to inform the dentist if any discomfort develops.

Because most teeth receiving pins have had extensive restorations and/or caries, the health of the pulp is probably compromised to some extent. Therefore, the ideal treatment of a pulpal penetration for such a compromised tooth generally is root canal therapy. Root canal treatment should be strongly considered when such a tooth is to receive a cast restoration.

An external perforation might be suspected if an unanesthetized patient senses pain when a pinhole is being prepared or a pin is being placed in a tooth that has had root canal therapy. Observation of the angulation of the twist drill or the pin should indicate whether a pulpal penetration or external perforation has occurred.

Perforation of the external surface of the tooth can occur occlusal or apical to the gingival attachment. Location of a perforation must be accurately diagnosed by careful probing and radiographic examination. The method of treatment for a perforation often depends on the experience of the operator and the particular circumstances of the tooth being treated.

Three options are available for perforations located occlusal to the gingival attachment: (1) the pin can be cut off flush with the tooth surface and no further treatment rendered, (2) the pin can be cut off flush with the tooth surface and the preparation for a cast restoration extended gingivally beyond the perforation, or (3) the pin can be removed, if present, and the external aspect of the pinhole enlarged slightly and restored with amalgam. Surgical reflection of the gingival tissue may be necessary to render adequate treatment. The location of perforations occlusal to the attachment often determines the option to be pursued.

Two options are available for perforations located apical to the attachment: (1) reflect the tissue surgically, remove the necessary bone, enlarge the pinhole slightly, and restore with amalgam; or (2) perform a crown-lengthening procedure, and place the margin of a cast restoration gingival to the perforation (Fig. 15-45). As with those perforations located occlusal to the gingival attachment, the gingivoapical location of the perforation and the design of the present or planned restoration determine which option to pursue. As with pulpal penetration, the patient must be informed of the perforation and proposed treatment. The prognosis of external perforations is favorable when they are recognized early and treated properly.

The occurrence of pulpal penetrations and external perforations during the use of pins can be substantially reduced by having a thorough knowledge of pulpal and external anatomy of the teeth, by having an accurate representation of the tooth radiographically, and by following the techniques described in this chapter.

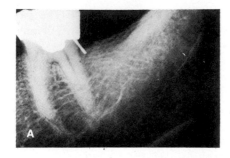
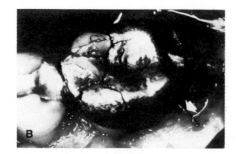
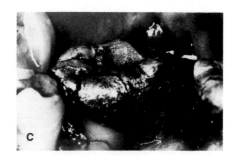
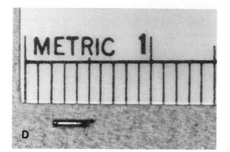

Fig. 15-45. External perforation of pin. **A,** Radiograph showing external perforation of pin. **B,** Surgical access to extruding pin *(arrow)*. **C,** Pin cut flush with tooth structure and crown-lengthening procedure performed. **D,** Length of pin removed.

BONDED AMALGAM RESTORATIONS

Amalgam adhesives are available which bond amalgam to tooth structure. Laboratory studies have shown that amalgam adhesives provide adequate retention and decrease microleakage of amalgam restorations.[53,55] Clinical research may demonstrate eventually a reduced need for conventional forms of retention when amalgam adhesives are used. The adhesive is used in lieu of cavity varnish.

FOUNDATIONS

A foundation is an initial restoration (usually amalgam) of a severely involved tooth in such a manner that the restorative material will serve in lieu of tooth structure in subsequent procedures for developing the final restoration.

A foundation may serve as a temporary or control restoration, but a temporary or control restoration cannot serve as a foundation if the retention and resistance forms are unknown by the operator or if known to be inadequate. A foundation may be indicated for teeth that are severely broken down and lack the resistance and retention forms for a cast restoration. When a foundation is indicated, it is placed prior to the preparation of a tooth for a cast restoration. It is designed to provide sufficient dimension to enhance the resistance and retention forms to the final preparation for the casting. *A foundation should be independently retentive, and ideally should also provide resistance form against forces that otherwise might fracture the remaining tooth structure. Unlike a conventional amalgam restoration, a foundation should not depend on remaining coronal tooth structure for support.*

A temporary or control restoration is used to restore a tooth temporarily and/or to control caries in a tooth (1) when definitive treatment is uncertain, or (2) when several teeth require immediate attention for control of caries. It may be used also when a tooth's prognosis is questionable. A temporary or control restoration often may not enhance the resistance or retention form. Instead, it depends on the remaining coronal tooth structure for support. When preparing a tooth for a foundation or temporary (control) restoration, remaining unsupported enamel may be left, except at the gingival, to aid in forming a matrix for amalgam condensation. There may be occasions when providing a temporary or control restoration that the operator will elect to provide sufficient retention and resistance forms to satisfy requirements of a foundation.

Restorative materials

The restorative materials used for foundations include amalgam, composite resin, glass ionomer-silver cermets, prefabricated posts, and cast post-and-cores. *Of the direct filling materials, amalgam is preferred because it is stronger and less prone to microleakage than composite resin or cermets in conventional amalgam cavity preparations.* The use of post-and-cores is limited to root canal–treated teeth and is used generally on anterior teeth or single-canal premolars with little or no remaining coronal tooth structure.

Vital vs root canal–treated teeth

Amalgam, composite resin, and glass ionomer-silver

cermets are used for foundations in vital or root canal–treated teeth. *The prefabricated post or cast post-and-core is used occasionally for a foundation in root canal–treated tooth. Amalgam foundations are the treatment of choice for posterior teeth when sufficient tooth structure remains. Slots, locks, and threaded pins can be used for retention in vital or root canal–treated teeth. Slots and locks are recommended if there are remaining longitudinal walls in which to prepare these retention forms. Pin retention is often used if few or no longitudinal walls remain.* A self-threading pin larger than the Minikin pin should not be used in root canal–treated teeth because they may be more subject to crazing.

Retention forms

Care must be exercised in placing both slot and lock retention and pin retention. Slot and lock retention removes more tooth structure than pin retention, but is less likely to create microfractures in the dentin and to perforate the pulp or the external tooth surface. Preparations utilizing slot and lock retention require absolute matrix stability to prevent fracture of the amalgam.

Slot and lock retention. Slots are placed in the gingival floor of a preparation with a No. 33½ or 169L bur and occasionally in a transverse plane on longitudinal dentinal walls (see Fig. 15-4). Locks are placed in remaining longitudinal walls with a No. 169L or ¼ bur as illustrated in Fig. 15-5. For foundations both slots and locks are placed slightly more pulpal than indicated for conventional amalgam preparations. This more pulpal positioning depends on the type of preparation for a casting that is planned. The preparation for the casting should not eliminate or cut into the retentive features. The indication for slots is determined by the number of remaining longitudinal walls. Slots are used to oppose lock retention in vertical walls or to provide retention where no vertical walls remain. Slots are generally 0.5 to 1 mm in depth and the width of the No. 33½ or 169L bur. Their length is usually 2 to 4 mm depending upon the distance between the remaining vertical walls.

Pin retention. Severely broken-down teeth with few or no longitudinal walls where a cast restoration is indicated usually require a pin-retained foundation. *The main difference between the use of pins for foundations and the use of pins in "permanent" restorations is the location of the pinholes from the external surface of the tooth. For foundations the pinholes must be located farther from the external surface of the tooth, and more bending of the pins may be necessary to allow for adequate axial reduction of the foundation without exposing the pins.* Any removal of the restorative material from the circumference of the pin will compromise its retentive effect. If the material is removed from more than one half the diameter of the pin, any retentive ef-

fect of the pin has probably been eliminated. *The location of the pinhole from the external surface of the tooth for foundations depends (1) on the occlusogingival location of the pin (external morphology of the tooth), (2) the type of restoration to be placed (a porcelain-fused-to-metal preparation requires more reduction than a full gold crown), and (3) the type of margin to be prepared.* As much retention as possible in the form of slots and locks should be used. The length of the pins must also be considered to allow for adequate occlusal reduction without exposing the pins.

If a fast-setting high-copper amalgam is used, the final preparation can be initiated within 30 to 45 minutes of insertion of the foundation. Composite resin or silver cermets might be the material of choice when an adequate matrix cannot be adapted to the tooth in the gingival aspect, such as a furcation area, assuming the area can be isolated from oral fluids. Oral fluids will interfere with the bonding of these materials to tooth structure, and with the setting of silver cermets. As with amalgam, mechanical retention in addition to bonding should be employed. If necessary, these materials can be positioned without a matrix, thus avoiding gingival overhangs that might result from condensation of amalgam. When these materials are used for a foundation, they should be a color or shade that is distinctly different from tooth structure. This will aid in determining when tooth structure is being prepared, especially in the area of margination, and thereby prevent the unintentional location of a margin on the foundation material.

TMS Minikin pins (0.019 inch [0.48 mm]) are generally recommended for all pin applications. Minim pins (0.024 inch [0.61 mm]) are occasionally used in molar teeth and in holes for Minikin pins that are no longer retentive. The smaller self-threading pins create less stress than the larger self-threading pins. Link Plus and Link Series pin designs are generally recommended. A self-threading pin larger than the Minikin pin should not be used in root canal–treated teeth because they may be more subject to crazing.

Alternative technique. An alternative technique has been described by Nayyar, Walton, and Leonard for developing foundations in multi-rooted root canal–treated teeth.[41] This technique is advocated only when (1) there is adequate dimension to the pulp chamber to provide retention and bulk of amalgam, and (2) there is adequate dentin thickness in the region of the pulp chamber to provide rigidity and strength to the tooth. Kane and others demonstrated that extension into the root canal space 2 to 4 mm is recommended when the pulp chamber height is 2 mm or less. When the pulp chamber height is 4 to 6 mm, no advantage is gained from extension into the root canal space.[29] *After matrix application, amalgam is then thoroughly condensed into the pulp canals, the pulp chamber, and the coronal portion* *of the tooth. Natural undercuts in the pulp chamber and the divergent canals provide necessary retention form.* Resistance form against forces that otherwise may cause tooth fracture is satisfied by gingival extension of the preparation for a full crown a minimum of 2 mm onto tooth structure, and this extension must not have a total taper of opposing walls of more than 10 degrees. Following tooth preparation, a cast restoration is fabricated and cemented. If these criteria cannot be met, the use of prefabricated posts or cast post-and-core, or pins, should be considered. Pins may be effective in foundations for root canal–treated teeth to provide resistance form against post-restorative fracture of the remaining tooth structure.

REFERENCES

1. Abraham G, Baum L: Intentional implantation of pins into the dental pulp, *J South Cal Dent Assoc* 40:914, 1972.
2. Bailey JH: Retention design for amalgam restorations: pins versus slots, *J Prosthet Dent* 65:71, 1991.
3. Barkmeier WW, Cooley RL: Self-shearing retentive pins: a laboratory evaluation of pin channel penetration before shearing, *J Am Dent Assoc* 99:476, 1979.
4. Barkmeier WW, Frost DE, Cooley RL: The two-in-one, self-threading, self-shearing pin: efficacy of insertion technique, *J Am Dent Assoc* 97(1):51, 1978.
5. Boyde A, Lester KS: Scanning electron microscopy of self-threading pins in dentin, *Oper Dent* 4(2):56, 1979.
6. Caputo AA, Standlee JP: Pins and posts—why, when, and how, *Dent Clin North Am* 20:299, 1976.
7. Caputo AA, Standlee JP, Collard EW: The mechanics of load transfer by retentive pins, *J Prosthet Dent* 29::442, 1973.
8. Cecconi BT, Asgar K: Pins in amalgam: a study of reinforcement, *J Prosthet Dent* 26(2):159, 1971.
9. Chan KC, Fuller JL, Khowassah MA: The adaptation of new amalgam and composite resin to pins, *J Prosthet Dent* 38:392, 1977.
10. Courtade GL, Timmermans JJ: *Pins in restorative dentistry*, St Louis, 1971, Mosby.
11. Currens WE, Korostoff E, von Fraunhofer JA: Penetration of shearing and nonshearing pins into dentin, *J Prosthet Dent* 44:430, 1980.
12. Dilts WE, Coury TL: A conservative approach to the placement of retentive pins, *Dent Clin North Am* 20:397, 1976.
13. Dilts WE, Welk DA, Stovall J: Retentive properties of pin materials in pin-retained silver amalgam restorations, *J Am Dent Assoc* 77:1085, 1968.
14. Dilts WE et al: Crazing of tooth structure associated with placement of pins for amalgam restorations, *J Am Dent Assoc* 81:387, 1970.
15. Dolph R: Intentional implanting of pins into the dental pulp, *Dent Clin North Am* 14:73, Jan 1970.
16. Durkowski JS et al: Effect of diameters of self-threading pins and channel locations on enamel crazing, *Oper Dent* 7(3):86, 1982.
17. Eames WB, MacNamara JF: Eight high copper amalgam alloys and six conventional alloys compared, *Oper Dent* 1(3):98, 1976.
18. Eames WB, Solly MJ: Five threaded pins compared for insertion and retention, *Oper Dent* 5(2):66, 1980.
19. Felton DA et al: Pulpal response to threaded pin and retentive slot techniques: a pilot investigation, *J Prosthet Dent* 66:597, 1991.
20. Garman TA et al: Self-threading pin penetration into dentin, *J Prosthet Dent* 43:298, 1980.
21. Gilmore HW et al: *Operative dentistry,* ed 4, St Louis, 1982, Mosby.
22. Going RE: Pin-retained amalgam, *J Am Dent Assoc* 73:691, 1966.
23. Going RE et al: The strength of dental amalgam as influenced by pins, *J Am Dent Assoc* 77:1331, 1968.
24. Goldstein PM: Retention pins are friction-locked without use of cement, *J Am Dent Assoc* 73:1103, 1966.
25. Gourley JW: Favorable locations for pins in molars, *Oper Dent* 5(1):2, 1980.
26. Hembree JH: Dentinal retention of pin-retained devices, *Gen Dent* 29:420, 1981.
27. Irvin AW, White JT, Holland GA: Analysis of stress induced by insertion of self-threading pins, *J Dent Res* 61:534, 1982 (abstract).
28. Jorgensen KD, Matono R, Shimokobe H: Deformation of cavities and resin fillings in loaded teeth, *Scand J Dent Res* 84(1):46, 1976.
29. Kane JJ, Burgess JO, Summitt JB: Fracture resistance of amalgam coronal-radicular restorations, *J Prosthet Dent* 63:607, 1990.
30. Kelsey WP III, Blankenau RJ, Cavel WT: Depth of seating of pins of the Link Series and Link Plus Series, *Oper Dent* 8(1):18, 1983.
31. Khera SC, Chan KC, Rittman BR: Dentinal crazing and interpin distance, *J Prosthet Dent* 40:538, 1978.
32. Khowassah MA, Denehy GE: A qualitative study of the interface between different dental amalgams and retentive pins, *J Prosthet Dent* 30:289, 1973.
33. Leinfelder KF: Clinical performance of amalgams with high content of copper, *Oper Dent* 5(3):125, 1980.
34. Markley MR: Pin reinforcement and retention of amalgam foundations and restorations, *J Am Dent Assoc* 56:675, 1958.
35. May KN, Heymann HO: Depth of penetration of Link Series and Link Plus pins, *Gen Dent* 34:359, 1986.
36. McMaster DR et al: The effect of slot preparation length on the transverse strength of slot-retained restorations, *J Prosthet Dent* 67:472, 1992.
37. Moffa JP, Razzano MR, Doyle MG: Pins—a comparison of their retentive properties, *J Am Dent Assoc* 78:529, 1969.
38. Moffa JP, Razzano MR, Folio J: Influence of cavity varnish on microleakage and retention of various pin-retaining devices, *J Prosthet Dent* 20:541, 1968.
39. Mondelli J, Vieira DF: The strength of Class II amalgam restorations with and without pins, *J Prosthet Dent* 28(2):179, 1972.
40. Mozer JE, Watson RW: The pin-retained amalgam, *Oper Dent* 4(4):149, 1979.
41. Nayyar A, Walton RE, Leonard LA: An amalgam coronal-radicular dowel and core technique for endodontically treated posterior teeth, *J Prosthet Dent* 43:511, 1980.

42. Newitter DA, Schlissel ER: Evaluation of four instruments for inserting self-threading pins, *Oper Dent* 5(4):142, 1980.

43. Osborne JW, Binon PP, Gale EN: Dental amalgam: clinical behavior up to eight years, *Oper Dent* 5(1):24, 1980.

44. Outhwaite WC, Garman TA, Pashley DH: Pin vs. slot retention in extensive amalgam restorations, *J Prosthet Dent* 41:396, 1979.

45. Pameijer CH, Stallard RE: Effect of self-threading pins, *J Am Dent Assoc* 85:895, 1972.

46. Perez RE, Schoeneck AG, Yanahara MH: The adaptation of noncemented pins, *J Prosthet Dent* 26:631, 1971.

47. Robbins JW, Summitt JB: Longevity of complex amalgam restorations, *Oper Dent* 13:54, 1988.

48. Shavell HM: The amalgapin technique for complex amalgam restorations, *J Cal Dent Assoc* 8(4):48, 1980.

49. Smales RJ: Longevity of cusp-covered amalgams: survivals after 15 years, *Oper Dent* 16:17, 1991.

50. Standlee JP, Caputo AA, Collard EW: Retentive pin installation stresses, *Dent Pract Dent Rec* 21:417, 1971.

51. Standlee JP, Collard EW, Caputo AA: Dentinal defects caused by some twist drills and retentive pins, *J Prosthet Dent* 24(2):185, 1970.

52. Standlee JP et al: Analysis of stress distribution by endodontic posts, *Oral Surg* 33:952, 1972.

53. Staninec M: Retention of amalgam restorations: undercuts versus bonding, *Quintessence Int* 20(5):347, 1989.

54. Trabert KC et al: Stress transfer to the dental pulp by retentive pins, *J Prosthet Dent* 30:808, 1973.

55. Varga J, Matsumura H, Masuhara E: Bonding of amalgam filling to tooth cavity with adhesive resin, *Dent Mater J* 5(2):158-64, 1986.

56. Vitsentzos SI: Study of the retention of pins, *J Prosthet Dent* 60:447, 1988.

57. Webb EL, Straka WF, Phillips CL: Tooth crazing associated with threaded pins: a three-dimensional model, *J Prosthet Dent* 61:624, 1989.

58. Welk DA, Dilts WE: Influence of pins on the compressive and transverse strength of dental amalgam and retention of pins in amalgam, *J Am Dent Assoc* 78:101, Jan 1969.

59. Wing G: Pin retention amalgam restorations, *Aust Dent J* 10:6, Feb 1965.

CHAPTER 16

Direct tooth-colored restorations for Classes III, IV, and V cavity preparations

Harald O. Heymann

Theodore M. Roberson

Clarence L. Sockwell*

INTRODUCTION TO ESTHETIC DENTISTRY

The search for an ideal esthetic material for conservative restorations has resulted in improvements in materials and techniques, particularly in recent years. Synthetic resins (and composites) and the acid etch technique represent major advances.[2,4,5,39] Adhesive materials that have a stronger bond to enamel and dentin further simplify restorative techniques.[1,36,37,44] The possibilities for innovative uses are exciting and almost unlimited. Many of these applications are presented in this chapter and in Chapters 17 and 18.

The choice of a material to restore carious lesions and other defects in teeth where esthetics is a factor

---

*This author is inactive this edition; see Preface.

continues to be a controversial subject. Tooth-colored materials such as silicate cement, fused porcelain, glass ionomer, acrylic resin, and composite have been used in all types and sizes of cavity preparations. These restorations may be accomplished with a minimal loss of tooth structure, little or no discomfort, relatively short operating time, and modest expense to the patient as compared to porcelain crowns. However, when a tooth is significantly weakened by extensive defects (especially in areas of heavy function) and esthetics is of primary concern, the best treatment usually is a porcelain crown.

An interpretation of esthetics primarily is determined by an individual's perception and is subject to wide variances. What is pleasing for one patient may be completely unacceptable to another. For example, some people have no objection to gold or other types of unharmonious restorations in their front teeth, while others find these restorations unesthetic.

It is the dentist's responsibility to present all logical restorative alternatives to the patient, but the patient should be given an opportunity to help make the final decision regarding which alternative will be selected. Explaining and showing the patient color photographs and models of teeth that have been restored by various methods is helpful. *Computer simulation* of possible treatment outcomes is also helpful using computer imaging technology. Many patients are not aware that some of the teeth or parts of the teeth are not visible in normal lip movements. For example, the patient in Fig. 16-1 does not show the gingival portion of the teeth even with a broad smile. Deeply abraded cervical areas were restored with gold inlays, which have been in service for over 20 years. Other examples of restoring anterior teeth with metal restorations are presented in the chapters on amalgam, gold inlays, and direct gold.

Most people want their teeth to look natural, including areas of the dentition that normally do not show. In 1959 Skinner[40] wrote, "The esthetic quality of a restoration may be as important to the mental health of the patient as the biological and technical qualities of the restoration are to his physical or dental health."

The lifespan of an esthetic restoration depends on many factors, including the nature of the initial problem, the treatment procedure, the restorative material utilized, operator skill, as well as patient factors such as oral hygiene, occlusion, and adverse habits. Failures can result from a number of causes, such as trauma, improper cavity preparation, inferior materials, and misuse of dental materials. The dentist is responsible for performing or accomplishing each operative procedure with meticulous care and attention to detail. Furthermore, patient cooperation is of utmost importance in maintaining the clinical appearance and influencing the longevity of any restoration. Long-range clinical suc-

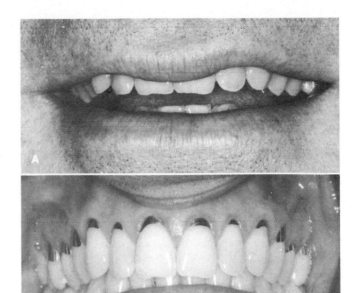

Fig. 16-1. A, Many patients do not normally show gingival third of anterior teeth. **B,** Patient in **A** with gold cervical restorations.

cess requires that the patient be knowledgeable of the causes of dental diseases and be motivated to practice preventive measures, including a proper diet, good oral hygiene, and maintenance recall visits to the dentist.

This chapter deals mainly with the properties and clinical uses of composite materials, since they have largely replaced other types of tooth-colored materials used for conservative esthetic restorations. The glass ionomer restorative material also is presented. However, it is appropriate that a brief discussion of other materials be included, not only to provide a historical perspective, but also because they are still available commercially and some dentists prefer their use. With widespread use in the past, such restorations will be encountered almost on a daily basis in the dental office. Many of these restorations are still clinically sound after years of service.

IMPORTANT ESTHETIC MATERIAL FACTORS
Important properties of esthetic materials

There are considerations regarding various properties of composites that must be understood if a successful composite restoration is to be done. These properties generally require that specific technique actions be incorporated into the restorative procedure, either in the cavity preparation or the application of the material. The following factors are presented, with additional information provided in the individual sections on technique as well as in Chapter 6.

Coefficient of thermal expansion. The coefficient of thermal expansion is the rate of dimensional change of a material per unit change in temperature. The closer the linear coefficient of thermal expansion (LCTE) of the material is to the LCTE of enamel, the less chance for creating voids or openings at the junction of the material and the tooth when temperature changes occur. The LCTE of improved composites is approximately 3 times that of tooth structure, and that for hybrid glass ionomer is 1½ to 2 times that of tooth structure. Bonding a composite to etched tooth structure reduces the potential negative effects of a difference between the LCTE of tooth structure and that of the material.

Water absorption. Water absorption is the amount of water that a material absorbs over a period of time per unit of surface area or volume. When a restorative material absorbs water its properties change and therefore its effectiveness as a restorative material may be diminished. All of the available tooth-colored materials exhibit some water absorption. Materials with higher filler contents exhibit lower water absorption values.

Polymerization shrinkage. Composite materials shrink while hardening. This is referred to as polymerization shrinkage. This cannot be avoided and there are important clinical procedural techniques which must be incorporated to offset the potential problems associated with a material pulling away from the cavity preparation walls as it hardens. Careful control of the amount and insertion point of the material, as well as acid etching the walls to improve bonding, will reduce these problems.

Wear resistance. Wear resistance refers to a material's ability to resist surface loss as a result of rubbing contact with tooth structure, restorative material, food boli, and such items as toothbrush bristles and toothpicks. The filler particle size, shape, and content affect the potential wear of the currently available tooth-colored restorative materials. Also affecting the potential wear of these materials are the restoration location in the dental arch and occlusal contact relationships.

Surface texture. Surface texture refers to the smoothness of the surface of the restorative material. Some restorations, especially those in close approximation to gingival tissues, require smoothness for maximum effectiveness. The size and amount of the filler particles will determine the potential smoothness of a restoration, as will the proper finishing and polishing procedures.

Method of polymerization. The method of polymerization of a composite material may affect the technique of insertion, the direction of polymerization shrinkage, the finishing procedure, color stability, and the amount of internal porosity in the material. There are two polymerization methods, namely, self-cured and light-cured using visible light. The *self-cured materials* require mixing two material components which then react to cause the material to polymerize. Since the components are mixed, there is greater chance for air inclusion in the mixture and therefore greater internal porosity. Also the working time to insert the material is restricted by the chemical reaction and may result in the necessity of increased finishing time. It also may be observed that the color stability of self-cured materials is less due to the eventual breakdown of the polymerization initiating chemical ingredients. Direction of polymerization shrinkage is toward the warmer cavity walls against which the material first polymerizes. This helps to maintain adaptation that prevents microleakage. *Light-cured materials* require the use of light sources that are expensive. The use of light sources may also cause retinal damage unless appropriate precautions are taken. However, the light-cured materials do provide increased working time during the insertion of the material and therefore less finishing time. They also have greater color stability and less potential internal porosity. A disadvantage is that polymerization shrinkage is toward the external surface of the light-exposed material since this surface is the first portion to polymerize. This creates stresses that tend to disrupt adaptation and result in microleakage. This can be partially compensated by an incremental insertion (and curing) technique. Also, there are some situations where application of sufficient light is difficult or compromised.

Radiopacity. Sufficient radiopaque components should be in restorative material so that caries around or under a restoration can be more easily interpreted in a radiograph.

Modulus of elasticity. Modulus of elasticity is the stiffness of a material. A material having a higher modulus is more *rigid;* conversely, a lower modulus is more *flexible.* A composite material with enough flexibility may serve better in certain Class V restorations (notch lesion restorations) than if it were more rigid.[18,20]

Solubility. Solubility is the loss in weight per unit surface area or volume due to dissolving or disintegrating in oral fluids of a material over a unit of time at a given temperature.

Esthetic materials

Silicate cement. Silicate cement, the first translucent filling material, was introduced in 1878 by Fletcher in England.[8] It was used extensively to restore cavities in the anterior teeth for over 60 years. Silicate cement powder is composed of acid-soluble glasses, and the liquid contains phosphoric acid, water, and buffering agents. Although silicate cement is rarely used as a restorative material today, the practitioner still may encounter silicate restorations, especially in older patients.

Silicate cement was recommended for small cavities in the anterior teeth of patients with a high caries activity.[46] By virtue of the high fluoride content, as well as

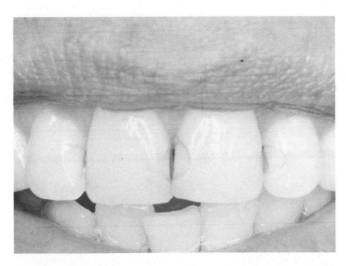

Fig. 16-2. Failed silicate cement restorations displaying discoloration and loss of contour.

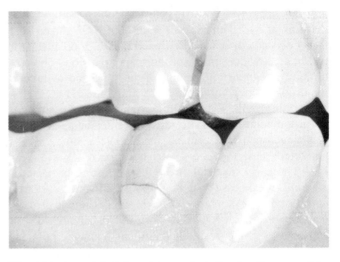

Fig. 16-3. Porcelain inlay with marginal discoloration caused by washed-out cement.

solubility of this restorative material, the adjacent enamel was rendered more resistant to recurrent caries. Cavity preparations for silicate cement were of the conventional type (boxlike form, see section titled, Cavity Preparation for Composite Restorations). A butt joint was required at the cavosurface margin because the material is brittle and has poor edge strength. Mechanical retention was necessary in the cavity preparation because the material does not adhere to the tooth structure. A liner or base was required under silicate cement to protect the pulp tissue from irritation due to the initial low pH of the material.

Tooth-matching ability, ease of manipulation, and an anticariogenic quality were favorable characteristics of silicate cement. It was also a good insulator, and its coefficient of thermal expansion approached that of enamel. The average life of a silicate cement restoration was approximately 4 years;[32] however, some of these restorations have been reported to last for 10 years and longer in some patients.[12]

Failures of silicate cement are easy to detect because of discolorations and loss of contour (Fig. 16-2). When examined with an explorer tip, silicate cement is rough and has the feel of ground glass. Old composite restorations may also exhibit a similar surface texture and discoloration (Fig. 16-6), but they are less subject to extensive ditching or loss of contour. Unlike silicate cement, conventional composite restorative materials exhibit a gray discoloration when scratched by the tip of an explorer or metal instrument.

Fused porcelain. The fused (baked) porcelain inlay dates from 1908 when John Byram described several designs of cavity preparations for its use.[6,8] Since the development of adhesive resin cements with acid etching of enamel walls there is renewed interest in using fused por-

celain for inlays and onlays in posterior teeth as well as for laminate veneers in anterior teeth.[7,15,35,45] Many of these restorations are fabricated in a dental laboratory with materials and equipment similar to that used for other types of fused porcelain. However, sophisticated CAD/CAM systems are available that fabricate porcelain restorations at chairside, eliminating the need for impressions, temporary restorations, laboratory procedures and costs, and additional appointments[23,28,29] (see Chapters 6 and 17).

Cavity preparation for the porcelain inlay is similar to that of the gold inlay with the following exceptions: (1) no cavosurface bevel is placed because a butt joint is required for strength of the material, and (2) the pulpal wall must be slightly deeper to obtain sufficient retention form and to enhance the strength and color-matching properties of the restoration.

Following completion of the cavity preparation for an *indirectly fabricated porcelain restoration*, an impression is made, a temporary filling placed, and the restoration is made in the laboratory. A second appointment is made for try-in and cementing the restoration. In the past, silicophosphate cement, a highly irritating material, was used as the luting agent. Unfortunately this type of cement washed out with time, and discoloration often occurred at the margins of the inlay (Fig. 16-3). Resin cements are now available that are less irritating to the pulp, less soluble in oral fluids, and adhesive with proper conditioning of the cavity preparation walls.

When seen clinically, the porcelain restoration has a highly glazed surface that is extremely hard and smooth like enamel. In some instances there is a visible cement line and a perceptible catch at the margins. When properly done, fused porcelain restorations are very esthetic, and the response of soft tissue adjacent to subgingival margins is excellent (see Chapter 17). The glazed surface does not discolor; the material is a good insulator and has a low coefficient of thermal expansion. The restoration is expensive because of the time and technique required for its completion.

Acrylic resin. Self-curing (chemically activated at room temperature) acrylic resin for anterior restorations was developed in Germany in the 1930s but was not marketed until the late 1940s because of World War II.[31] The early materials were disappointing because of inherent weaknesses such as poor activator systems, high polymerization shrinkage, high coefficient of thermal expansion, and lack of abrasion resistance. These weaknesses could result in marginal leakage, pulp injury, recurrent caries, color changes, and excessive wear.[31,38] Improvements in materials and procedures reduced the severity or occurrence of most of these problems. Acrylic resin restorations are rarely used today, but, as with silicate cement restorations, may be seen in older patients.

The cavity preparation for acrylic resin usually was either the conventional or beveled conventional type described later for composites. As a restoration, acrylic resin was most successful in protected areas where temperature change, abrasion, and stress were minimal.[41] Also it was used as an esthetic veneer on the facial surface of Class II and Class IV metal restorations and for facings in crowns and bridges. Today one of the most frequent uses of acrylic resin is for making temporary restorations in operative and fixed prosthodontic procedures requiring two or more appointments. Satisfactory temporary restorations that are esthetic, comfortable, and adequately wear resistant can be made quickly with acrylic resin.

Instructions for mixing acrylic resin must be followed carefully. When the powder and liquid are mixed, polymerization occurs at a rapid rate, resulting in some shrinkage and a slight rise in temperature as the material hardens.

Several unfavorable physical properties prevent acrylic resin from being an ideal restorative material. Because of poor wear resistance, it will not maintain its contour in areas subject to abrasion or attrition. It is not indicated for high-stress areas, since the material has low strength and will flow under load. Its high polymerization shrinkage and coefficient of thermal expansion may cause microleakage and eventual discoloration at the margins as a result of percolation (Fig. 16-4).[31] This problem can be largely overcome by providing adequate internal retention in the cavity preparation, acid etching the enamel, and inserting the material with a non-pressure technique.

The clinical appearance of an acrylic resin restoration is usually smooth and polished. When tested with an explorer tip, the material is relatively soft as compared

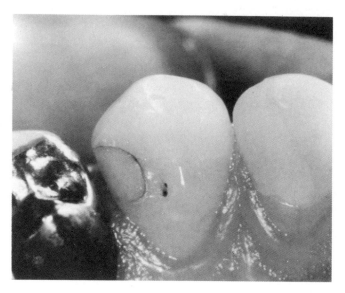

Fig. 16-4. Acrylic resin restoration displaying marginal discoloration after several years of service.

to enamel. After a few years a thin brown line may develop around the restoration, indicating microleakage (Fig. 16-4). However, such discoloration of properly inserted restorations does not indicate recurrent caries, and the objectionable brown line on the surface of an esthetic-sensitive area can be eliminated easily by a small-repair veneer restoration.

Composite. In an effort to improve the physical characteristics of unfilled acrylic resins, Bowen of the National Bureau of Standards (now called the National Institute of Standards Technology) developed a polymeric dental restorative material reinforced with silica particles.[3,10] The introduction of this filled resin material in 1962 became the basis for restorations that are generically termed *composites*.

Composites are presently the most popular tooth-colored materials, having largely replaced silicate cement and acrylic resin. Basically, composite restorative materials consist of the continuous polymeric or resin matrix in which an inorganic filler is dispersed (see Chapter 6, Dental Composites). This inorganic phase significantly enhances the physical properties of the composite compared to previous tooth-colored materials by increasing the strength of the restorative material and reducing the coefficient of thermal expansion.[2] Composites possess coefficients of thermal expansion that are one-half to one-third the value typically found for unfilled acrylic resins and therefore are nearer to that of tooth structure. (See Chapter 6 for details on components and properties.)

For a composite to have good mechanical properties a strong bond must exist between the organic resin matrix and inorganic filler. This bond is achieved by coating the filler particles with a ***silane coupling agent.***[9]

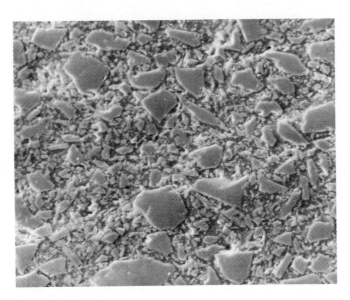

Fig. 16-5. Scanning electron micrograph of polished surface of a conventional composite (×300).

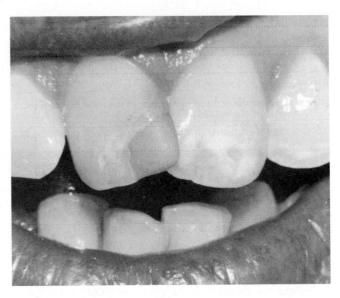

Fig. 16-6. Typical appearance of an extrinsically stained composite restoration.

This not only increases the strength of the composite, but also reduces its solubility and water absorption.[2]

Composites are divided into three types based primarily on the size, amount, and composition of the inorganic filler: (1) conventional composites, (2) microfill composites, and (3) hybrid composites.

Conventional composites. Conventional composites generally contain approximately 75% to 80% inorganic filler by weight. The average particle size of conventional composites in the 1980s was approximately 8 μm.[14] The particle size of contemporary conventional composites usually ranges from 1 to 10 μm with the average being approximately 3 μm. However, variations in particle size are also related to the composition of the filler. Because of the relatively large size and extreme hardness of the filler particles, conventional composites typically exhibit a rough surface texture. This characteristic can be clearly seen in the scanning electron micrograph in Fig. 16-5 (see also Fig. 6-50). The resin matrix wears at a faster rate than the filler particles, resulting further in a roughened surface. Unfortunately this type of surface texture causes the restoration to be more susceptible to discoloration from extrinsic staining (Fig. 16-6). *Conventional composites have a higher amount of initial wear at occlusal contact areas than do the microfill or hybrid types.*

The composition of the inorganic filler in conventional composites also affects the degree of surface roughness. A "soft" or "friable" glass such as strontium or barium glass yields a smoother surface than those with a filler of quartz. Also, it should be noted that when strontium or barium glasses are incorporated in sufficient amounts, the composite is made *radiopaque*. As stated in a preceding section, this is an important

Fig. 16-7. Scanning electron micrograph of polished surface of a microfill composite (×300).

characteristic in that caries around or under a composite restoration can be more easily interpreted in a radiograph.

Microfill composites. In the late 1970s the microfill composites or "polishable composites" were introduced. These materials were designed to replace the rough surface characteristic of conventional composites with a smooth, lustrous surface similar to tooth enamel. Instead of containing large filler particles typical of the conventional composites, the microfill composites have colloidal silica particles whose average diameter ranges from 0.02 to 0.04 μm. As illustrated in the scanning electron micrograph in Fig. 16-7, this small particle size results in a smooth, polished surface in the finished restoration that is less receptive to plaque or extrinsic staining. However, because of the greater surface area per unit volume of these microfine particles, the microfill composites cannot be as heavily filled (see Chapter 6, Classification).[9] Typically, microfill composites have an inorganic filler content of approximately 35% to 60% by weight. Because these materials contain considerably less filler than do conventional composite resins, their physical and mechanical characteristics are somewhat inferior. (See Table 6-14 for more details on properties.) Nonetheless, microfill composites are very wear resistant clinically. Also, their low modulus of elasticity allows microfill composite restorations to flex during tooth flexure. This quality makes microfill composites a good choice for restoring Class V cervical lesions or defects, where cervical flexure can be significant.[18]

Hybrid composites. In an effort to combine the good physical and mechanical properties characteristic of conventional composites with the smooth surface typical of the microfill composites, the hybrid types of composite were developed. These materials generally have an inorganic filler content of approximately 70% to 80% by weight. The filler is a mixture of conventional and microfill particles that has a smaller average particle size than that of conventional composites. Because of the relatively high content of inorganic fillers, the physical and mechanical characteristics are similar to those of conventional composites. Also, the presence of submicron-sized particles interspersed among the larger particles allows a smooth surface texture to be attained in the finished restoration.

Glass ionomer restorative materials. Glass ionomers were first developed by Wilson and Kent in 1972.[48] Like their predecessors, silicate cements, the original glass ionomer restorative materials were powder/liquid systems. Glass ionomers enjoy the same favorable characteristics of silicate cements, namely, they release fluoride into the surrounding tooth structure yielding an anticariogenic effect and possess a favorable coefficient of thermal expansion.[30,43] Unlike the silicate cements that have a phosphoric acid liquid, glass ionomers use polyacrylic acid which renders the final restorative material less soluble.

Although glass ionomers are relatively technique sensitive regarding mixing and insertion procedures, they are excellent materials for the restoration of root surface caries because of their inherent anticariogenic quality and adhesion to dentin. Similarly, glass ionomers are often indicated for other anterior restorations in patients exhibiting high caries activity. Because of their low resistance to wear and relatively low strength when compared to composite or amalgam, glass ionomers are not presently recommended for the restoration of occlusal aspects of posterior teeth. Glass ionomer cements also have been widely advocated for permanent cementation of crowns.

Like other cements, glass ionomer systems traditionally have required hand mixing of a powder and liquid with a spatula. However, some glass ionomers are available in encapsulated forms that are mixed by trituration. The capsule containing the mixed material is subsequently placed in an injection syringe for easy insertion into the cavity preparation. Additionally, light-cured glass ionomer materials have been developed which incorporate a resin component. These light-cured versions offer improved physical properties (greater compressive strength, resistance to dehydration, etc.), better esthetic qualities (less opaque), and are more easily placed than traditionally mixed and inserted glass ionomers.

GENERAL CONSIDERATIONS FOR DIRECT COMPOSITE RESTORATIONS

Concerns regarding esthetics and protection of the environment are increasing and valid. Fortunately, the use of composite restorative materials is established due to continuing improvements in the materials and restorative techniques.

Cavity preparations for composite materials should be as conservative as possible. The extent of the preparation is usually determined by the size, shape, and location of the defect and whatever extensions are necessary to provide access for vision and instrumentation. Acid etch techniques, effective bonding systems, and improved composites have significantly affected cavity preparation and expanded the scope of restorations of teeth.

The design of the cavity preparation to receive a composite restoration may vary depending on several factors. Therefore three types of cavity design (conventional, beveled conventional, and modified) will also be discussed in this section and later described in detail under individual classes of cavity preparation.

Indications for direct composite restorations

The need for an esthetically pleasing restoration is still the predominant indication for using composite materials. However, the strong bond developed between the etched enamel and bonding agent (and composite) also promotes additional indications for these restorations. As will be discussed in this chapter, as well as Chapters 17 and 18, the small tooth defect or carious lesion can be restored more conservatively with composite than with amalgam. Furthermore, the strong bond established between composite and enamel has the capacity to strengthen remaining, unprepared tooth structure in larger, more extensive restorations.[27] However,

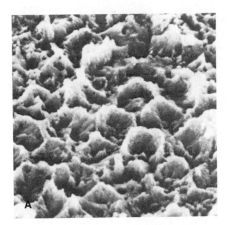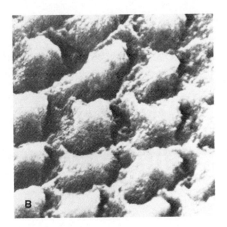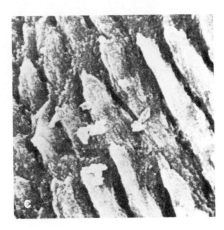

Fig. 16-8. Etching patterns of tooth enamel. **A,** Etching pattern characterized by removal of prism core. **B,** Etching pattern showing loss of prism periphery. **C,** Both etching patterns are evident. (**B** and **C,** Courtesy Dr. Leon Silverstone.)

when use of composite is considered for use in a posterior tooth, a careful judgement of potential wear must be made from an assessment of the patient's occlusion.

With increasing concerns about the use of amalgam as a dental restorative material (primarily regarding the environmental effects of disposal), the use of composite may continue to increase. However, as this chapter and Chapters 17 and 18 discuss, *the successful placement of a composite restoration requires meticulous attention to detail regarding cavity preparation, restorative material manipulation, and moisture control.*

Acid etch phenomenon

An innovative method of removing the enamel smear layer and obtaining micro-mechanical retention for resin restorations by acid etching the enamel was developed by Buonocore and reported in 1955.[4] Basically the technique consists of applying a solution or gel of 30% to 50% phosphoric acid to the enamel for 30 to 60 seconds, followed by thorough rinsing and drying of the area. The acid solution affects the prismatic structure of the enamel by preferential removal of either the prism core or periphery. This process results in an enamel surface characterized by numerous microscopic undercuts and irregular peaks in the enamel (Fig. 16-8). When a resin of low viscosity is applied to this acid-conditioned surface, it flows into the minute undercuts and polymerizes to form a *resin-enamel micro-mechanical bond* (Fig. 16-9). These penetrations of resin into the enamel have been described as "resin tags." (See Chapter 6, Bonding Systems, for specific details.) A detailed description of the clinical procedure is provided later in this chapter in the section titled, Procedures for Microretention from Acid Etching Enamel and Conditioning Dentin.

The use of composites retained by acid-etched enamel has provided a major advancement in operative dentistry. With modified cavity designs, more tooth structure is conserved with minimal pulpal irritation. The micro-mechanical bond produced between the resin and the enamel enhances marginal integrity and *reduces microleakage.*[34] Also, esthetics is improved when the butt joint marginal configuration is eliminated.

Enamel/dentin bonding systems

Low viscosity resins used for the adhesion to enamel and/or dentin are generally referred to as ***bonding agents.*** As noted earlier, acid etching of enamel results in numerous microscopic undercuts and irregular surface features into which a fluid resin can be applied and cured to produce a micro-mechanical bond. *Acid etching and the use of a fluid resin bonding agent is the basis for the retention, as well as marginal seal against microleakage, of virtually every composite restoration placed in cavity preparations involving enamel margins.*

Dentin, as well, can be pre-treated or *conditioned* much like enamel to produce a surface that is more retentive.[11,33] In most dentin bonding systems, a low viscosity hydrophilic resin, often referred to as the "primer" (an adhesion promoting agent), is used following application of a specific surface conditioning material, referred to as the ***conditioner.*** This ***primer*** is usually hydrophilic in nature to ensure optimal wetting and bonding to the hydrated dentinal surface. Once the dentin is conditioned and primed, a low viscosity resin adhesive ***bonding agent*** is applied to the dentin. These components are collectively referred to as a ***dentin bonding system.*** Although the term *dentin bonding agent* connotes a material used exclusively for bonding to dentin, the same low-viscosity resin used for bonding to dentin (following some type of conditioning and priming of the dentinal surface) is used for bonding to etched enamel. This bonding resin is sometimes termed

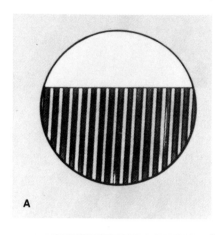

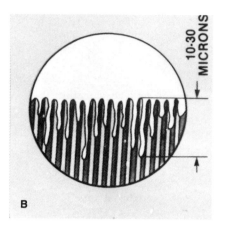

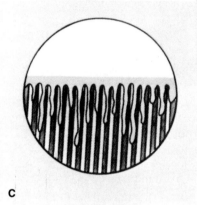

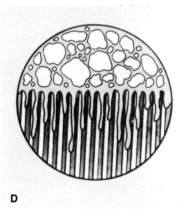

Fig. 16-9. Acid etching phenomenon. **A,** Enamel rods unetched. **B,** Enamel rods etched, creating numerous microundercuts. **C,** Fluid bonding agent engaging microundercuts, creating "resin tags" for mechanical bond to tooth. **D,** Composite material chemically bonded to bonding agent.

an *adhesive*. The clinical application of this system is presented later in the section, Procedures for Micro-retention from Acid Etching Enamel and Conditioning Dentin.

As previously stated, the dentin bonding system generally consists of a conditioning agent, a low viscosity hydrophilic resin primer, and a resin adhesive. The conditioning agent is used first to remove or solubilize the *smear layer,* a thin layer of dentinal debris produced by rotary instrumentation.[21] (The smear layer is considered an impediment in the bonding of resin to dentin and therefore must be removed or penetrated.) Following conditioning, the low viscosity resin primer is applied to the dentin surface and is usually followed by the application of the adhesive resin with most systems. Most bonding resins are light-cured; however, self-cured versions are still available.

It should be pointed out that although general similarities exist in the make-up of dentin bonding agent systems, *significant differences* are evident in the composition of the conditioning agents, primers, and adhesive resins employed by the various manufacturers. *Manufacturer's directions for their specific product must be followed closely to ensure optimal results. Ingredients from one manufacturer should not be used with ingredients from another manufacturer.*

Pulp protection

Protection of the dental pulp during cavity preparation and from irritating materials is a primary objective in maintaining tooth vitality. For this reason, many steps in the clinical procedure are incorporated to optimize pulpal health. These include: (1) proper isolation of the operating site to minimize bacterial infiltration, (2) removal of infected dentin, and (3) placement of a protective liner or base on deeply excavated areas.

Placing liners and/or bases under composite restorations usually is not necessary for: (1) shallow or normal depth preparations; (2) preparations in older patients whose teeth manifest receded, smaller pulps, and more peritubular dentin (smaller or occluded tubules); or (3) shallow preparations in teeth having had a previous restoration that is removed with little or no cutting of the underlying dentin. The protection provided by a liner or base becomes increasingly important as the dentin thickness between the cavity and the pulp decreases, especially in young patients in whose teeth the dentinal tubules are more open. Recall from Chapter 2 that the tubules also are more in number (per unit area) near the pulp. Also, for patients with preoperatively hypersensitive dentin, such as in cervical areas, a protective liner may help reduce postoperative sensitivity.

Liners. A liner is a material used in a thin protective

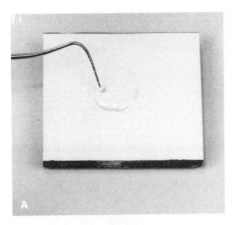
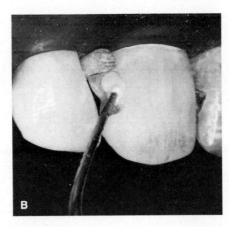
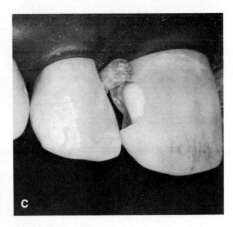

Fig. 16-10. Applying liner. **A** and **B,** Tip of Williams periodontal probe conveys small amount of liner to cavity preparation, using pressureless technique. **C,** A uniform liner of sufficient thickness has been added to axial wall.

film and in most cases is applied to dentin to produce a specific pulpal response. Liners used with composite restorations include, but are not limited to, glass ionomer cements, calcium hydroxide preparations, and certain resin materials. They are available in light-cured and self-cured types. Copal varnish, indicated under some materials such as silicate cements and amalgams, should not be placed under composites because it prevents retention to the underlying etched enamel and conditioned dentin. Likewise, a zinc oxide eugenol liner (or base) should not be used with a composite restoration because such a liner has potential to inhibit polymerization of the composite material. Although liners may be placed for specific purposes (i.e. protection against inadvertent acid etching, anticariogenic qualities, etc.) they are generally not indicated for routine use in shallow, easily accessible preparations whose margins are in enamel. The application of an enamel-dentin bonding system is usually sufficient to seal dentinal tubules in these cases.

A Williams periodontal probe, with the terminal 1 or 2 mm of the tip bent slightly, is an ideal instrument for applying the liner (or base). Other specially designed insertion instruments are available, but often are not small enough for small cavity preparations. With experience, the proper amount of material can be picked up on the very tip of the probe (Fig. 16-10) and artfully placed on the axial wall without accidental placement on shallower dentin, retentive areas, or enamel walls. If any liner (or base) is placed inadvertently on undesired locations, allow it to harden to simplify removal.

Bases. A base generally is defined as a material that is used in a thicker layer (than a liner) over dentin to provide necessary bulk for *thermal or mechanical protection to the pulp* (see Chapter 6, Liners and Bases). These materials are indicated when the thickness of dentin has been reduced (from caries excavation) to a point where it is judged there is less than ½ to 1 mm of

remaining dentin thickness between the restorative material and the pulp. Bases thicker than 1 mm are strong enough to resist pressure from occlusion (Class IV) or matrix closure during insertion of composite. Base materials used with composite restorations primarily include calcium hydroxide materials and glass ionomer cements. Both materials are available in light-cured and self-cured types. Calcium hydroxide bases are primarily indicated for deep caries excavations (within ½ mm of the pulp) or when a pulpal exposure exists. Glass ionomer cements are preferred as bases when greater strength or anticariogenicity is advisable, but never should be placed in direct contact with the pulp. Materials containing eugenol should not be used as bases under any type of composite restoration because of interference with the polymerization reaction.

Cavity preparation designs

Three designs of cavity preparations for composite restorations may be used, sometimes in combination. These include (1) *conventional,* (2) *beveled conventional,* and (3) *modified* preparation designs. All three designs are described in detail later under individual classes of cavity preparation. However, a discussion of general characteristics follows.

Conventional cavity preparation. Conventional cavity preparations usually are prepared entirely with carbide burs and hand instruments. Outline form is necessary extension of external walls at an initial, limited, uniform, dentinal depth, and the external cavity walls follow the direction of the enamel rods where present. If the margins are on root surface, the external walls should meet the root surface at a right angle. In all conventional cavity preparations the **butt joint marginal configuration** and **retention grooves** and **coves** in dentin are distinguishing features. These preparation designs were used extensively in the past and may be encountered when restoration replacement is indicated. It

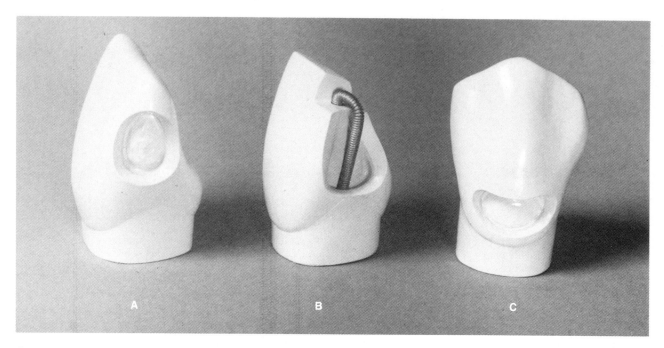

Fig. 16-11. Old conventional cavity designs for Class III (**A**), Class IV (**B**), and Class V (**C**) preparations. Butt joint marginal configuration and retention grooves in dentin characterized this cavity design. Currently this preparation design is used only on root surfaces.

should be noted that the previous use of the conventional preparation for composites was not restricted to the root surface only. Fig. 16-11 illustrates models of conventional cavity designs for Classes III, IV, and V preparations.

The conventional cavity design is necessary for brittle materials with limited edge strength such as silicate cement, amalgam, and porcelain. Although it may be used for composite, it is not the preferred cavity design. Acid etching the enamel in a conventional preparation improves the marginal seal and reduces marginal discoloration with resin materials. However, because retention and marginal seal are improved by beveling enamel margins (beveling increases favorable end-on etching of prisms), few conventional preparations will be indicated for composite restorations. *The primary indication for the conventional cavity preparation in composite restorations is when margins are located on root surfaces* (non-enamel areas). In these areas, the butt joint design provides a better cavity configuration into which the groove and cove retention form can be placed. This design facilitates a better seal between the composite and the dentin or cementum surfaces as well as ensures retention of the composite material in the tooth. Relying only on dentin bonding agents for retention of the restoration in non-enamel areas may not be successful, especially in Class V preparations.

Beveled conventional cavity preparation. Beveled conventional cavity preparations are similar to conventional preparations in that the outline form has external, "box-like" walls, but with *beveled enamel* margins. The principles of conventional outline form with the limited initial depth of the axial line angles are followed. This preparation design typically is indicated when a composite restoration is being used to replace an existing restoration exhibiting a conventional cavity preparation design with enamel margins. The old material is removed; or may be only partially removed if the remaining material is judged an acceptable base (radiographically negative for caries and the tooth pulp is symptomless). To facilitate better marginal sealing and bonding, all enamel margins are beveled and acid etched. Diamond instruments are used to prepare the bevel. Fig. 16-12 illustrates drawings of beveled conventional cavity designs for Classes III, IV, and V preparations.

The advantage of the enamel bevel is that the ends of the enamel rods (exposed by beveling) are more effectively etched than otherwise occurs when only the sides of the enamel rods are exposed to the acid etchant (Fig. 16-13).[10,24] Also, the increase in etched surface area results in a stronger enamel-to-resin bond, which increases the retention of the restoration and reduces marginal leakage and marginal discoloration.[47] For these reasons this type of preparation is especially suited for resin restorative materials that possess high coefficients of thermal expansion, such as acrylic resin and microfill composites, to help counter their poorer physical properties. Furthermore, the incorporation of a cavosurface

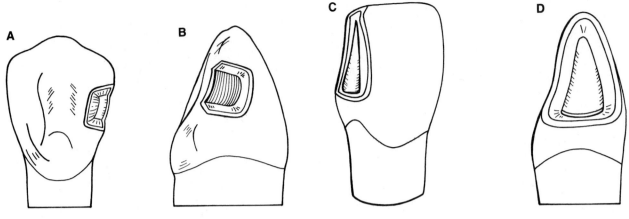

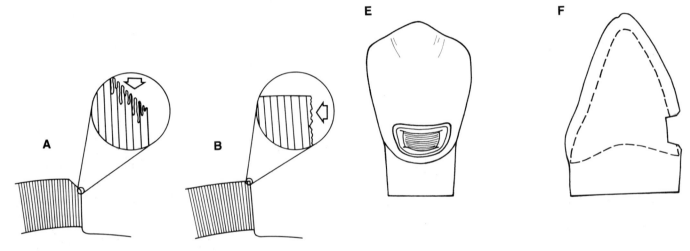

Fig. 16-12. Beveled conventional cavity designs for Class III **(A, B)**, Class IV **(C, D)**, and Class V **(E, F)** preparations.

Fig. 16-13. Ends of enamel rods **(A)** are more effectively etched, producing deeper microundercuts than when only sides of enamel rods are etched **(B)**.

bevel enables the restoration to blend more esthetically with the coloration of the surrounding tooth structure. A white line or "halo" is often seen clinically at the tooth-restoration interface when a butt joint marginal configuration characteristic of conventional cavity preparations is prepared (Fig. 16-14). This white line often is caused by microfracture of the marginal enamel during finishing of the restoration.

Modified cavity preparation. Modified cavity preparations for composite restorations have neither specified cavity wall configurations nor specified pulpal depth, and have enamel margins. The objective is to remove the fault as conservatively as possible and rely on the etched enamel to retain the restoration in the tooth. Modified cavity preparations conserve more tooth structure since retention is obtained by acid etching the sur-

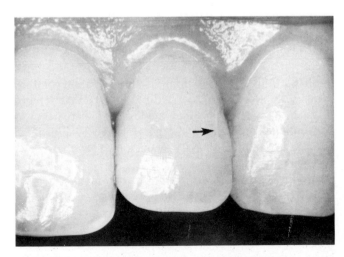

Fig. 16-14. White line or halo is seen around restoration on distal surface of lateral incisor. Butt joint marginal configuration typical of conventional cavity design was used in preparation.

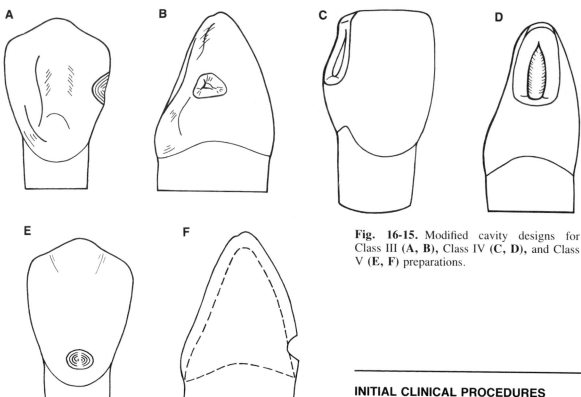

Fig. 16-15. Modified cavity designs for Class III **(A, B)**, Class IV **(C, D)**, and Class V **(E, F)** preparations.

rounding enamel rather than by preparation of groove (or cove) retention form in dentin. Unlike conventional preparations, modified preparations are not prepared to a uniform dentinal depth. Both the extension of the margins and the depth of a modified cavity preparation are dictated solely by the extent (laterally) and the depth of the carious lesion or other defects. Round burs or diamond stones are used to prepare this type of preparation, resulting in a marginal design similar to a beveled preparation yet less tooth structure is removed in the internal portions of the preparation. Often, the preparation appears to have been "scooped out" rather than having distinct internal cavity line angles characteristic of a conventional preparation design. Fig. 16-15 illustrates drawings of modified cavity designs for Classes III, IV, and V preparations.

Modified preparations primarily are indicated for the initial restoration of small, new, cavitated, carious lesions surrounded by enamel and for correcting enamel defects. However, they can be successful for larger restorations as well. For the restoration of large carious lesions, retention grooves, coves, or locks may be indicated in addition to the retention afforded by the etched enamel.

INITIAL CLINICAL PROCEDURES

It is necessary that a complete examination, diagnosis, and treatment plan be finalized before the patient is scheduled for operative appointments (emergencies excepted). A brief review of the chart, treatment plan, and radiographs should precede each restorative procedure. At the beginning of each appointment also carefully examine the operating site and *assess the occlusion,* particularly of the tooth (teeth) scheduled for treatment.

Local anesthesia

Local anesthesia is advocated *almost routinely* for operative procedures as cited in Chapter 10. It is especially indicated for Class V cavities because of sensitivity and the need for isolation from the gingival tissue and fluids, since isolation may otherwise at times be slightly uncomfortable. Profound anesthesia contributes to a pleasant and uninterrupted operation and usually results in a *marked reduction in salivation.* These effects of local anesthesia contribute to better operative dentistry.

Preparation of the operating site

Clean the operating site to remove calculus, plaque, pellicle, and superficial stains while waiting for the onset of anesthesia. Prophy pastes containing flavoring agents, glycerine, or fluorides act as *contaminants* and should be avoided to prevent a possible conflict with the acid etch technique. A slurry of pumice is recommended for this procedure (Fig. 16-16).

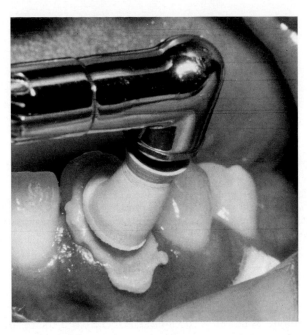

Fig. 16-16. Cleaning operating site with slurry of flour of pumice.

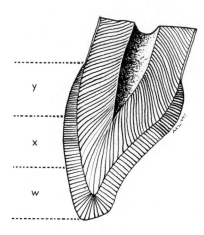

Fig. 16-17. Cross section of anterior tooth showing three color zones. Incisal third *(w)* is a lighter shade and more translucent than gingival third *(y)*, whereas middle third *(x)* represents blending of incisal and gingival thirds.

Shade selection

Special attention should be given to matching the color of the natural tooth since this is the main reason for using a tooth-colored material. *Determine the shade of the tooth before the teeth are subjected to any prolonged drying, because dehydrated teeth become lighter in shade as a result of a decrease in translucency.*

Normally, teeth are predominantly white with varying degrees of grey, yellow, or orange tints. The color also will vary with the translucency, thickness, and distribution of enamel and dentin, as well as the age of the patient. Other factors such as fluorosis, tetracycline staining, and endodontic treatment also affect tooth color. With so many variables it is necessary to match the individual surface of the tooth to be restored. A cross-section of an anterior tooth (Fig. 16-17) illustrates why there are color zones. The incisal third *(w)* is lighter and more translucent (mostly enamel) than the cervical third *(y)* (mostly dentin), whereas the middle third *(x)* is a blend of the incisal and cervical colors. Additional information on color can be found in Chapter 18.

Most manufacturers provide shade guides for their specific materials, which usually are not interchangeable with materials from other manufacturers. There are variations among the different manufacturers in the number of shades available. It should be noted, however, that recently more and more manufacturers are also cross-referencing their shades with those of the

VITA Shade Guide,* a universally adopted shade guide. Also, most composite materials are available in enamel and dentin shades as well as translucent and opaque shades. The translucency of the composite material selected depends on the translucency of the tooth structure in the area of the tooth to be restored. Enamel shades are more translucent and typically are indicated for restoration of translucent areas such as incisal edges.

Good lighting, either natural or artificial, is necessary when the color selection is made. Natural light is preferred for selection of shades. However, if no windows are present affording natural daylight, color-corrected operating lights or ceiling lights are available to facilitate accurate shade selection. If the dental operating light is used, it should be moved away to decrease the intensity, thus allowing the effect of shadows to be seen.

In choosing the appropriate shade, hold the entire shade guide near the teeth to determine general color. Then select and hold a specific shade tab alongside the area of the tooth to be restored (Fig. 16-18). The shade tab should be partially covered with the patient's lip or operator's thumb to create the natural effect of shadows. The cervical area is usually darker than the incisal area. Make the selection as rapidly as possible, since physiologic limitations of the color receptors in the eye make it increasingly difficult to distinguish between similar colors after approximately 30 seconds. If more time is needed, the eyes should be rested by looking at a blue or violet object for a few seconds.[17,42] These are the complimentary colors of orange and yellow, which are the predominant colors in teeth. By looking at the complimentary color, the color receptors in the eye are

*VITA Shade Guide, VitaZahnfabrik, Germany.

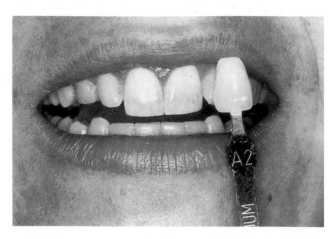

Fig. 16-18. Shade slection. Shade tab is held near the area to be restored.

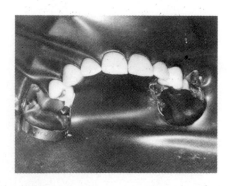

Fig. 16-19. Isolating anterior teeth with rubber dam. More access is provided for lingual instrumentation if premolars are included. Still more access may be provided by placing retainers over rubber dam and premolars.

revitalized and are re-sensitized to perceiving minor variations in yellow and orange. Some dentists request that their assistants select or assist in shade selection. This practice saves time for the dentist, and the assistant, when adequately trained to select shades, feels a greater sense of responsibility and involvement. Final shade selection also can be verified by the patient with the use of a hand mirror.

Most teeth can be matched from manufacturers' basic shades. If additional shades are needed, they may be obtained by mixing two or more of the available shades together or by adding color modifiers that are often available from the manufacturers. Record the shade on the patient's chart; however, teeth darken with age, and a different shade or material may be required if a replacement becomes necessary. It is better to err on the barely perceptible darker side to allow for this age-darkening; however, if bleaching to whiten the teeth is contemplated, it should be done before any restorations (see Bleaching in Chapter 18).

To be certain of the proper shade selection, place a small amount of material of the selected shade directly on the tooth, in close proximity to the area to be restored, and cure. This is a more accurate assessment of the selected shade. If the shade is correct, an explorer is used to remove the cured material from the tooth surface.

A more comprehensive review of factors affecting the esthetic considerations of tooth restoration is presented in Chapter 18.

Isolation of the operating site

Complete instructions for the control of moisture are given in Chapter 11. Isolation for tooth-colored restorations can be accomplished with (1) a rubber dam or (2) cotton rolls and retraction cord. Regardless of the

method, isolation of the area is imperative if the desired bond is to be obtained. Contamination of etched enamel (or conditioned dentin) by saliva results in a significantly decreased bond; likewise, contamination of the composite material during insertion results in degradation of physical properties.

Some operators prefer to "rough out" the cavity outline, using a carbide bur and air-water spray, before isolating the area in order to observe the level of the gingival tissue relative to the lesion. Subsequent steps in the procedure are optimal only if performed in an isolated area. If a pulp exposure occurs, the chances for successful treatment are better when the exposure and its treatment occur in an uncontaminated field.

Rubber dam. A heavy rubber dam is an excellent means of acquiring superb access, vision, and moisture control. For proximal surface cavities of the anterior teeth, the dam should isolate at least two teeth mesial and two teeth distal to the operating site. If a lingual approach is indicated, it is better to isolate all of the anterior teeth and include the first premolars to provide more access to the lingual area (Fig. 16-19). For Class V cavities and other facial or lingual defects, apply a **No. 212 retainer** (clamp) and stabilize with impression compound (Fig. 16-20). Stabilization with compound is important to prevent movement of the retainer and subsequent injury to the tooth and soft tissue.

If a proximal cavity involves all of the contact area and/or extends subgingivally, insert a **wedge** in the gingival embrasure. The wedge (1) depresses the interproximal soft tissue, (2) shields the dam and soft tissue from injury during the operative procedure, and (3) produces slight separation of the teeth to compensate for matrix thickness. Before placing the wedge from the facial approach (facial or lingual wedge placement depends on the operator's judgment, but usually the wedge is in-

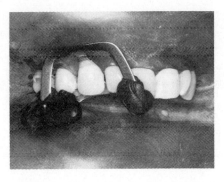

Fig. 16-20. Isolation of Class V cavity with rubber dam and No. 212 clamp. Impression compound stabilizes the retainer.

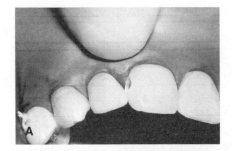

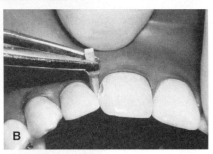

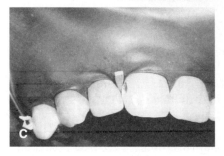

Fig. 16-21. Using triangular-shaped wood wedge to expose gingival margin of large proximal cavity. **A,** Dam is stretched facially and gingivally with fingertip. **B,** Insertion of wedge (dam is released during wedge insertion). **C,** Wedge in place.

serted into the larger embrasure), stretch the portion of the rubber dam that covers the interproximal papilla facially and gingivally (stretch lingually and gingivally if inserting the wedge from the lingual). Accomplish this by using a fingertip, first pressing firmly on the dam and underlying soft tissue near the teeth and then pulling the dam as the finger is slightly moved away from the teeth. While holding the dam in this stretched condition (Fig. 16-21, *A*), begin the insertion of the wedge (Fig. 16-21, *B*); then during the insertion, allow the stretched dam to slowly slide under the finger back to the normal position (Fig. 16-21, *C*). This procedure helps to prevent catching the rubber dam (or even piercing it) with the tip of the wedge and decreases the tension of the stretched dam under the wedge (which may dislodge the wedge). For additional details on isolation by rubber dam, see Chapter 11.

Cotton rolls and retraction cord. An alternate method of obtaining a dry operating field is the use of a cotton roll or rolls and a retraction cord. When the gingival margin of a cavity preparation is to be positioned subgingivally, or near the gingiva, a chemically treated cord can be used to both temporarily retract the tissue and reduce seepage of tissue fluids into the operating site. Gingival retraction cords are most commonly treated with epinephrine. A few patients are highly sensitive to epinephrine or may have cardiovascular contraindications to its use. For such patients untreated cord or cord treated with other agents is available.

After the initial cavity preparation and placement of cotton roll(s), *dry the area* with an air syringe. Tissue retraction in Class V areas using a treated cord is not difficult if properly done. A piece of cord approximately 0.5 to 1 mm in diameter (cords are usually available in various dimensions) and 8 to 10 mm long is usually sufficient depending on the dimension of the involved gingival crevice. For a synergistic effect in controlling hemorrhage, the cord may be moistened with a

small amount of *astringent*, such as Hemodent.* A simple way to accomplish this is to dip the closed beaks of sterilized cotton pliers (not the cord itself) into the bottle to pick up a small amount of liquid. Then touch the cord with the tip of the beaks to transfer the liquid to the cord. Some operators prefer to place the cord in a dappen dish, wet it with a drop of Hemodent, and then blot it with a 2 × 2 inch (5 × 5 cm) gauze to remove excess liquid. Next, the cord may need to be twisted in order to distribute the liquid and to make the cord more compact. However, many available cords are braided and do not require twisting. Now tuck the cord into the gingival crevice with the side of a No. 2 explorer or the end of an FP3 plastic instrument starting interproxi-

*Hemodent, Premier Dental Products Co., Norristown, Pa.

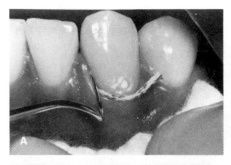
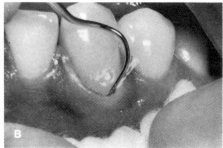
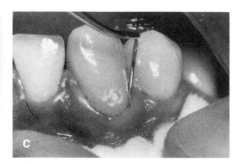

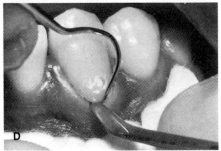

Fig. 16-22. Isolating Class V cavity with cotton roll and treated cord. **A,** One end of cord is tucked into gingival crevice with side of No. 2 explorer. **B,** Procedure is continued. **C,** Cord in place. **D,** Two instruments may be used to place cord in difficult cases. No. 2 explorer used to tuck, while small, blunt instrument used to hold cord in place.

mally at one end (Fig. 16-22, *A*). Continue cord placement along the gingival margin (Fig. 16-22, *B*) and slightly beyond the opposite extent of the cavity outline (Fig. 16-22, *C*). If difficulty is encountered during placement, a "holding" instrument such as a periodontal probe or a blade of a suitable plastic instrument may be used to keep the submerged portion of the cord in the crevice during placement of the free end (Fig. 16-22, *D*). As the tucking or packing procedure is continued, it may be necessary to follow with the holding instrument in a step-like manner. A slight "backward" vector to the insertion direction also helps to keep the previously inserted cord in place. When additional tissue displacement is needed, place a second cord on top of the first in the same manner. Remember that the cord is always inserted into the crevice, not on top of the gingiva! Any retraction cord placement must be done judiciously to avoid blunt dissection of the gingival tissue or periodontal attachment. Also, *do not over-pack to cause ischemia* of the gingiva (seen as a blanching), resulting in tissue damage and recession. Gently insert the cord (with astringent) which in a few minutes will cause the marginal gingiva to move laterally and apically approximately 0.5 mm away from the cavity preparation. Do not leave any loose strands of the cord, which may result in a cutting instrument catching and dislodging the cord. (A cord can become tightly tangled on a bur in a split second!) Occasionally observe the displaced and retracted tissue during subsequent procedures to ascertain that tissue strangulation is not occurring.

CAVITY PREPARATION FOR DIRECT COMPOSITE RESTORATIONS

The following sections describe Classes III, IV, and V cavity preparations for direct composite restorations. While each Class of cavity preparation is different because of its location in the tooth, the same principles of cavity preparation apply to each. The usual format of this section for each Class and design will be first a presentation or overview of concepts and features, followed by detailed cavity preparation stages and steps.

Class III cavity preparations for composite

Class III cavity preparations, by definition, are located on the proximal surfaces of anterior teeth. Such locations have been the predominant sites for the use of composite restorations because of the typical need for esthetically pleasing restorations in the front of the mouth.

When a proximal surface of an anterior tooth is to be restored and there is a choice between facial or lingual entry into the tooth, the lingual approach is preferable. The small carious lesion should always be treated from the lingual approach unless such an approach would necessitate excessive cutting of tooth structure because of irregular alignment of the teeth or facial positioning of the lesion.

Advantages of restoring the proximal cavity from the *lingual approach* include:
  1. The facial enamel is conserved for enhanced esthetics.

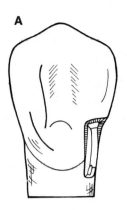 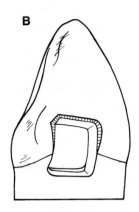

Fig. 16-23. (A, B), Combination cavity design for a Class III preparation that extends onto root surface. The root surface portion is a conventional cavity design preparation utilizing butt joint marginal configuration and retention groove in dentin. The coronal portion is a beveled conventional cavity design preparation.

2. Some unsupported, but not friable, enamel may be left on the facial wall of a Class III or Class IV preparation.
3. Color matching of the composite is not as critical.
4. The lingual area is less subject to thermal changes (important with materials possessing a high coefficient of thermal expansion).
5. Discoloration or deterioration of the restoration is less visible.

Indications for a *facial approach* include:
1. The carious lesion is positioned facially such that facial access would significantly conserve tooth structure.
2. There is an irregular alignment of teeth, making lingual access undesirable.
3. There is extensive caries extending onto the facial surface.
4. A faulty restoration which was originally placed from facial approach needs to be replaced.

When both the facial and lingual surfaces are involved, use the approach that provides the best access for instrumentation.

Prepare and restore approximating carious lesions or faulty restorations on adjacent teeth at the same appointment. Usually one of the cavities will be larger (more extended outline form) than the other. When the larger outline form is developed first, the second preparation usually can be more conservative because of the improved access provided by the larger preparation. The reverse order would be followed when the restorative material is inserted.

Conventional Class III cavity preparation. As stated earlier, the *primary indication* for this type of preparation is for the *restoration of root surfaces*. Thus, it

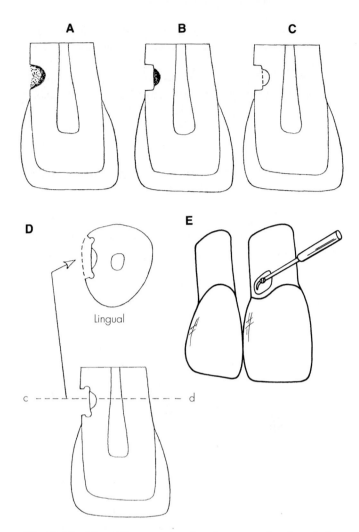

Fig. 16-24. Class III conventional cavity preparation for a lesion entirely on root surface. **A,** Mesiodistal longitudinal section illustrating carious lesion. **B,** Initial cavity preparation. **C,** Cavity preparation with infected carious dentin removed. **D,** Retention grooves and liner are shown in longitudinal section, and transverse section through plane *cd* illustrates contour of axial wall and direction of facial and lingual walls. **E,** Preparing retention form to complete cavity preparation.

would be unusual to have an entire preparation of the conventional type. More likely, only a portion of a cavity preparation would be prepared in this manner: that portion that is on the root surface and has no enamel margin (Fig. 16-23). The design of the preparation then would be a *combination of a modified or a beveled conventional preparation with conventionally prepared root surface area.* The exception would be when all of a lesion, fault, or defective restoration is located on the root surface of a tooth which would result in the entire preparation being the conventional type and exhibiting butt joint margins (Fig. 16-24). The preparation would be identical to the slot preparation for amalgam illustrated and described in Chapter 13, Slot Preparation for Root Caries.

When preparing the *conventional portion of a preparation* (on root surface), the form of the cavity walls is the same as that of an amalgam preparation. The cavosurface margins exhibit a 90-degree cavosurface angle and provide *butt joints* between the tooth and the composite material. Thus the external walls are prepared perpendicular to the root surface. In this conventionally prepared area of the tooth, which is apical of the cervical line, the external walls will be entirely of dentin. These walls must be prepared to a sufficient depth pulpally to provide for (1) adequate thickness for strength of the restorative material, and (2) the placement of retention grooves. This wall depth (depth to axial line angles) ideally will be 0.75 mm into dentin assuming no additional caries excavation is required. *Groove retention form* is necessary in non-enamel, root surface preparations to both increase the retention of the material in the tooth and to optimize the seal of the material at the junctional interface.

The *crown areas of the preparation* (where enamel margins are present) are prepared having a *beveled marginal configuration* (from either a beveled conventional or modified cavity preparation) and a pulpal depth dictated by either the extent of the existing restoration being replaced or the extent of the infected portion of the carious lesion. Typically the retention of the material in the crown portion of the preparation would be provided primarily by the bond afforded by *acid etching the enamel surfaces of the preparation, and by conditioning, priming, and bonding to dentinal surfaces.*

The specific cavity design for the **conventional Class III cavity preparation** can be reviewed in Chapter 14 in the section on Class III cavity preparation for amalgam, and is presented for composite in the following sections, which present the *stages and steps* of this root surface cavity preparation.

Initial cavity preparation stage. The steps of this stage follow:

Outline form. Using a No. ½, 1, or 2 round bur, prepare the outline form, extending the external walls to sound tooth structure while preparing to a limited depth (pulpally) of 0.75 mm. (This depth allows in a subsequent step the preparation of the retention grooves by the No. ¼ round bur [diameter of 0.5 mm] in the inner portion of the external walls without weakening the remaining outer portion.) Recall that the bur at this limited depth is touching dentin, or previous restorative material, or carious tooth structure, or air. Prepare the external walls perpendicular to the root surface, thus forming a 90-degree cavosurface angle. These walls may require further definition with appropriate hand instruments, such as the 8-3-22 hoe or the 7-85-2½-6 and

12-85-5-8 angle-forming chisels. *It is emphasized that during this step in cavity preparation the bur's cutting edges are moved to this limited pulpal depth and no deeper.*

Primary retention form. The "box-like" design is considered a part of retention form; however, at this stage in cavity preparation the external walls may be retentive due to opposing wall parallelism or slight undercuts, or nonretentive due to slight divergence outwardly.

Convenience form. If approach is facial, the facial wall may be extended facially to provide access and visibility; if approach is lingual, the lingual wall may be extended for the same reason.

Final cavity preparation stage. The steps of this stage follow:

Removal of remaining infected dentin or old restorative material. Remove all infected dentin using round burs or small spoon excavators, or both. Remaining old restorative material on the axial wall should be removed if any of the following conditions are present: (1) the old material is amalgam and its color would negatively affect the color of the new restoration, (2) there is radiographic evidence of caries under the old material, (3) the tooth pulp was symptomatic preoperatively, or (4) the periphery of the remaining restorative material is not intact (i.e., there is some breach in the junction of the material with the adjacent tooth structure which may indicate caries under the material). *If none of these conditions is present, the operator may elect to leave the remaining restorative material to serve as a base, rather than risk unnecessary (1) excavation nearer to the pulp or (2) irritation or exposure of the pulp.*

Pulp protection. Apply a calcium hydroxide **liner** or **base,** if indicated, following the removal of infected dentin or old restorative material. For details refer to a previous section, General Considerations for Direct Composite Restorations; Pulp Protection.

Secondary retention form. As stated previously, groove retention must be used in root surface preparations to ensure that the material is retained in the tooth. The **retention groove** created also will help in minimizing the potential negative effects of polymerization shrinkage (the composite pulling away from the margin) when inserting the composite incrementally. Additionally, this groove will enhance the marginal seal by resisting flexural forces (from tooth flexure) placed on the cervical portion of the restoration.

Prepare a continuous retention groove in the internal portion of the external walls using a No. ¼ round bur. The groove is located 0.25 mm (half the diameter of the No. ¼ round bur) from the root surface and is prepared to a depth of 0.25 mm (half the diameter of the No. ¼ round bur). This groove depthwise is directed mostly in the direction of the external walls (gingivally on gingival wall, incisally on incisal walls, etc.) and slightly

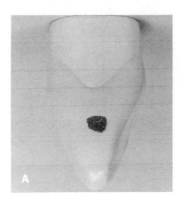
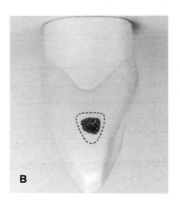
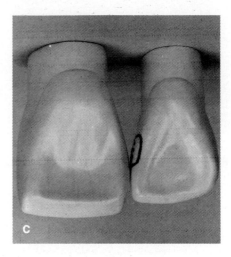

Fig. 16-25. A, Small proximal carious lesion on mesial surface of maxillary lateral incisor. **B,** Dotted line indicates normal outline form dictated by shape of carious lesion. **C,** Extension (convenience form) required for preparing and restoring cavity from lingual approach when teeth are in normal alignment.

pulpally (see Fig. 16-24, *D* and *E*). For its entire length the groove should extend parallel to the root surface. Use the side of the No. ¼ round bur for cutting retention form whenever possible to control retention depth.

Final procedures; cleaning; inspecting. Clean the preparation of any visible debris and inspect for final approval.

Beveled conventional Class III cavity preparation. The beveled conventional cavity preparation for composite restorations is indicated primarily for replacing an existing defective restoration in the crown portion of the tooth. However, it may also be used when restoring a large carious lesion where the need for increased retention form is anticipated. The cavity preparation takes the shape of the existing restoration along with any extensions necessary to include recurrent caries, friable tooth structure, or defects. Any extensions that are required may be prepared with a modified cavity preparation, as discussed in the next section. The beveled conventional preparation is characterized by external walls that are perpendicular to the enamel surface, and the margin is beveled. The axial line angles may or may not be of uniform pulpal depth, varying as the thickness of the enamel portion of the external walls varies. If part of the tooth to be restored is located on the root surface, a conventional cavosurface configuration should be used in this area as described in the preceding section resulting in a combination of two cavity preparation designs, a conventional type in the root portion and a beveled conventional type in the crown portion.

The cavity preparation for the replacement restoration will have the same general form of the previous

(old) cavity preparation and often the existing restoration will have utilized a conventional cavity preparation. Usually retention is obtained only by acid etching the enamel wall along with its cavosurface bevel around the entire cavity preparation, and no groove retention is necessary. However, when replacing a large restoration or restoring a large Class III lesion, the operator may decide that retention should be enhanced by placing groove (at gingival) and cove (at incisal) retention features in addition to the etched enamel periphery. Etching will be the first step in the application of restorative materials in a later section.

Lingual access, initial cavity preparation stage. Since indirect vision is usually required, a clean, unscratched front surface mirror is recommended to provide a clear, undistorted view. Sometimes direct vision may be used to advantage by tilting the patient's head.

After the procedures of local anesthesia, cleaning the area, shade selection, and isolation, use a round carbide bur (No. ½, 1, or 2), the size depending on the extent of the caries or defective restoration, to prepare the *outline form* (Fig. 16-25). Before contacting the tooth, the bur is positioned for entry and rotated at high speed using air-water spray. The assistant directs air on the mirror surface and positions the evacuator tip near the operating site. The point of bur entry is within the incisogingival dimension of the carious lesion or defective restoration and as close to the adjacent tooth as possible without contacting it (Fig. 16-26, *A*). Direct the bur perpendicular to the enamel surface, but at an entry angle that places the neck aspect of the bur as far into the embrasure (next to the adjacent tooth) as possible; use light pressure and intermittent cutting (brush stroke) to

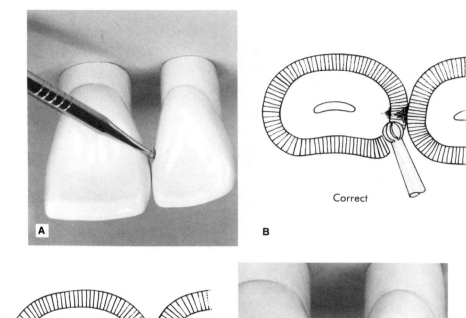

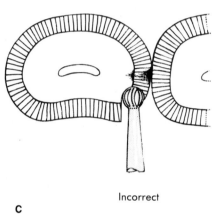

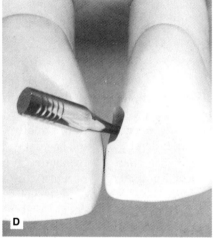

Fig. 16-26. Beginning Class III conventional cavity preparation, lingual approach. **A,** Bur is held perpendicular to enamel surface, and initial opening is made close to adjacent tooth at incisogingival level of caries. **B,** Correct angle of entry is parallel to enamel rods on mesiolingual angle of tooth. **C,** Incorrect entry overextends lingual outline. **D,** Same bur is used to enlarge opening for caries removal and convenience form while establishing initial axial wall depth.

gain access into the cavity. Incorrect entry overextends the lingual outline into potential stress areas and unnecessarily weakens the tooth (Fig. 16-26, *B* and *C*). The same bur may be used to enlarge the opening sufficiently to allow for the later described caries removal, completion of the preparation, and insertion of the restorative material (Fig. 16-26, *D*).

Extend the external walls during preparation of the outline form, which always is to a limited prescribed depth, to sound tooth structure. This extending should be as minimal as possible, dictated by the extent of caries and/or of old restorative material on these walls. Unless absolutely necessary, do not include the proximal contact area, or extend onto the facial surface or subgingivally. *The axial wall depth at this initial stage of cavity preparation is limited* to approximately 0.75 to 1.25 mm (the larger being incisally where enamel is thicker) with the axial wall outwardly convex, following normal external tooth contour and the dentinoenamel junction both incisogingivally and faciolingually (Fig. 16-27, *A* and *B*). Usually the axial line angles should be positioned at an initial depth of 0.2 mm into dentin. How-

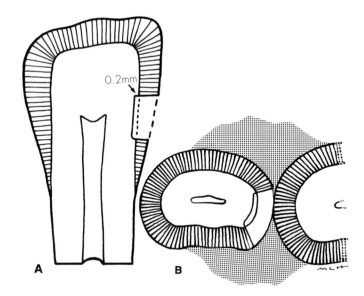

Fig. 16-27. Ideal initial axial wall preparation depth. **A,** Incisogingival section showing axial wall 0.2 mm into dentin. **B,** Faciolingual section showing facial extension and axial wall following contour of tooth.

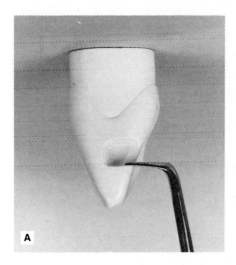
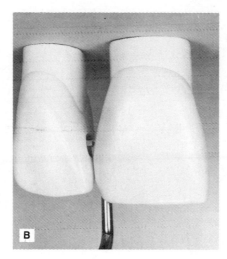
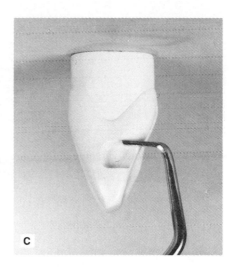

Fig. 16-28. Finishing enamel walls. **A,** Incisal wall is planed from lingual surface to facial wall with 8-3-22 hand instrument. **B,** Facial wall is finished with same instrument. **C,** If gingival margin is in close proximity to adjacent tooth, opposite end of 8-3-22 hoe with reverse bevel is used.

ever, if a retention groove is to be placed, the axial wall must be 0.5 mm into dentin at retention locations to prevent undermining enamel where the retention form is prepared. As noted previously when the cavity outline extends gingivally onto the root surface, the depth of the axial wall at the gingivoaxial line angle should be 0.75 mm, thus providing adequate dimension for composite strength, placement of a retention groove, and maintenance of strength of the gingival wall and margin. This depth must not be exceeded at this initial stage of cavity preparation even if the bur is cutting in air, caries, or old, restorative material. Any remaining infected dentin or old, defective restorative material on the axial wall will be removed during the final cavity preparation stage.

Prepare the enamel walls perpendicular to the external tooth surface. Use an instrument such as an 8-3-22 hoe with the distal bevel to plane the incisal wall, moving from the lingual surface to the facial wall (Fig. 16-28, *A*). Use the same instrument on the facial wall (Fig. 16-28, *B*). The gingival floor and lingual wall are usually finished with the same round bur that was used to prepare the outline form. If there is not an ample gingival embrasure space to avoid marring the adjacent tooth with the bur, use the opposite end of the 8-3-22 hoe with the reverse (mesial) bevel to finish the gingival floor (Fig. 16-28, *C*).

Once the outline form and initial axial wall depth have been established, the initial cavity preparation stage is completed and the final stage of cavity preparation begins.

Lingual access, final cavity preparation stage

Removal of remaining infected dentin or old restorative material. Remove all infected dentin using round burs or small spoon excavators, or both. Some undermined enamel can be left in nonstress areas, but very friable enamel at the margins should be removed. Remaining old restorative material on the axial wall should be removed if any of the following conditions are present: (1) there is radiographic evidence of caries under the old material, (2) the tooth pulp was symptomatic preoperatively, or (3) the periphery of the remaining restorative material is not intact (i.e., there is some breach in the junction of the material with the adjacent tooth structure which may indicate caries under the material). If none of these conditions is present, the operator may elect to leave the remaining restorative material to serve as a base, rather than risk unnecessary (1) excavation nearer to the pulp, or (2) irritation or exposure of the pulp.

Pulp protection. Apply a calcium hydroxide liner or base, if indicated.

Secondary retention form. If retention features are indicated, prepare them incisally and along the gingivoaxial line angle with a No. ¼ bur. The No. ½ bur is too large for this purpose (Fig. 16-29, *A*). Occasionally retention may be provided by undercuts left from caries removal. No purposeful attempt is made to provide retentive undercuts along the linguoaxial and facioaxial line angles, inasmuch as these areas are not needed to retain composites and might unnecessarily weaken the lingual and facial enamel walls and margins. Particular

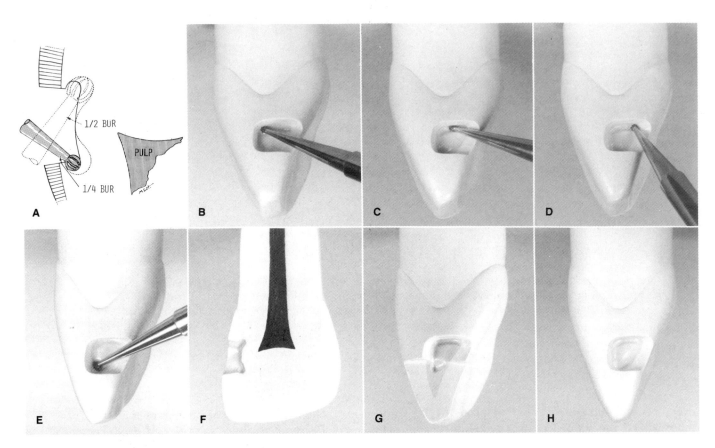

Fig. 16-29. Preparation of gingival retention groove and incisal retention cove. **A,** A No. ¼ bur should be used to cut retention. No. ½ bur is usually too large. **B,** Gingival groove is started at faciogingivoaxial point angle and extended incisally slightly along facioaxial line angle. **C,** Groove is extended lingually along gingivoaxial line angle. **D,** Groove is continued into linguo-gingivoaxial point angle. **E,** Position of No. ¼ bur for cutting incisal retention cove. **F and G,** Sections showing facioincisopulpal direction and depth of completed incisal cove. **H,** Completed gingival groove and incisal cove.

care must be exercised not to weaken the walls or incisal angles that are subject to masticatory forces.

Prepare a ***retention groove*** along the gingivoaxial line angle. Care should be exercised to prepare this groove approximately 0.2 mm inside the dentinoenamel junction to a depth of 0.25 mm (half the diameter of the No. ¼ bur) so as not to undermine the enamel portion of the gingival wall. The *depthwise direction of the groove* is directed primarily gingivally and slightly pulpally. Low handpiece speed with air coolant for this step provides better tactile sensation and vision. Start the gingival groove at the faciogingivoaxial point angle (Fig. 16-29, *B*) and extend along the gingivoaxial line angle to the linguogingivoaxial point angle (Fig. 16-29, *C* and *D*). The *lengthwise direction of the groove* parallels the dentinoenamel junction without undermining the enamel of its dentinal support.

Prepare the ***incisal retention cove*** with the No. ¼ bur at the axioincisal point angle with the bur oriented

in a facioincisopulpal direction, 0.2 mm inside the dentinoenamel junction and 0.25 mm deep (Fig. 16-29, *E*). Then extend it slightly into the facioaxial line angle where it fades out (Fig. 16-29, *F* and *G*). Care should be exercised not to take away dentinal support from the enamel. It is emphasized that the incisal retention is directed facioincisopulpally, where possible, rather than incisopulpally. Sometimes this feature is critical in preserving the strength of a weak incisal corner of a tooth. The completed gingival retention groove and incisal retention cove for a Class III beveled conventional cavity preparation are illustrated in Fig. 16-29, *H*.

The placement of incisal retention is not always as easy in the mouth as illustrated because of handpiece size and angulation problems caused by the anatomy of the maxilla and tooth positions. When teeth are rotated or abnormally aligned, additional extension of the incisal portion of the lingual wall may be necessary to provide the ***convenience form*** necessary to prepare the

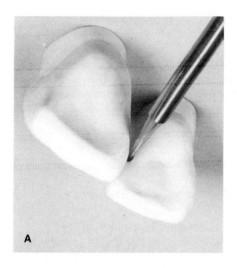

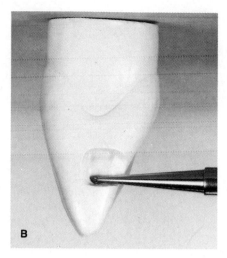

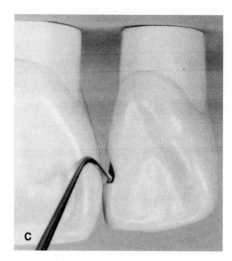

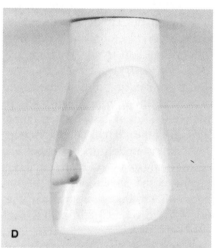

Fig. 16-30. Increasing lingual incisal access. **A,** Cutting incisal retention through lingual wall extension. **B,** Position of No. ¼ bur in **A. C,** Alternative method of cutting incisal retention cove with 3-2-28 bibeveled hatchet. **D,** Completed preparation.

incisal retention with the No. ¼ bur (Fig. 16-30, *A* and *B*). Also, extension of the bur out of the handpiece often enhances visibility and access in these circumstances. Another method is to use a bibeveled hatchet (3-2-28) with delicate shaving strokes in a facioincisopulpal direction, removing small amounts of dentin until the area is retentive (Fig. 16-30, *C*). This is an excellent instrument for testing to see that the incisal retention is positive, regardless of the method used to obtain the retention. Fig. 16-30, *D,* illustrates the completed gingival retention groove and retention cove in a Class III beveled conventional cavity preparation with added convenience form at the lingual incisal region.

Procedures for finishing external walls. Class III beveled conventional cavity preparations are prepared as conventional preparations with the incorporation of a **cavosurface bevel** of the enamel rather than a butt joint margin (Fig. 16-31). The cross-sectional view in Fig. 16-32 illustrates the cavosurface bevel that provides more surface area for end-on etching of the enamel rods. The cavosurface bevel is best prepared with a

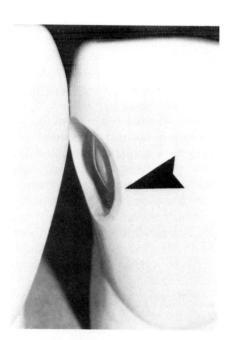

Fig. 16-31. Class III beveled conventional cavity preparation. Note cavosurface bevel *(arrow).*

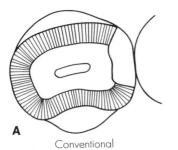

A Conventional

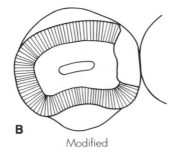

B Modified

Fig. 16-32. A, Cross section of facial approach Class III conventional cavity preparation with 90-degree cavosurface angle. **B,** Beveled conventional cavity preparation showing 45-degree cavosurface bevel on facial margin.

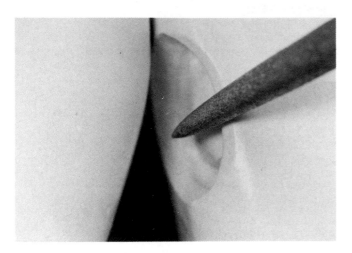

Fig. 16-33. Beveling. Cavosurface bevel is prepared with coarse, flame-shaped diamond oriented 45 degrees to external tooth surface contiguous with margin.

coarse, flame-shaped diamond instrument, oriented approximately 45 degrees to the external tooth surface (Fig. 16-33). A bevel width of 0.25 to 0.5 mm is considered sufficient unless the operator elects to increase the retention form by preparing a wider bevel which will increase the surface area to be etched and therefore the retention form. All accessible enamel margins usually are beveled, with the exception of the gingival margin. This margin is not usually beveled if little or no enamel is present or access is difficult for finishing procedures. If the preparation extends gingivally onto root structure, no bevel is placed on cementum and the area is prepared as a conventional cavity preparation. In addition, bevels may not be recommended on lingual surface margins that are in areas of centric contact or subjected to heavy masticatory forces, because composite does not have the wear resistance of enamel for withstanding heavy attritional forces.

Final procedures: cleaning; inspecting. Clean the preparation of any visible debris and inspect for final approval.

Facial access, initial cavity preparation stage. With a few exceptions, the same stages and steps of cavity preparation are followed as with lingual access. The procedure is simplified because direct vision is used and the lesion or faulty restoration is usually larger.

A large Class III lesion on the distal surface of a maxillary right central incisor is illustrated (Fig. 16-34, *A*). The rubber dam is placed after the anesthetic has been administered and the shade has been selected. A wedge is inserted in the gingival embrasure to depress the rubber dam and underlying soft tissue, thus improving gingival access (Fig. 16-34, *B*).

Using a No. 2 carbide bur rotating at high speed and with air-water spray, prepare the *outline form* with appropriate extension, as well as the initial, limited pulpal depth previously described in the lingual approach preparation (Fig. 16-34, *C*). Some undermined enamel can be left if it is not in a high-stress area. Enamel margins not immediately adjacent to the next tooth can be finished with a round bur. Other walls are completed with angle formers such as 7-85-2½-6 or 12-85-5-8 (Fig. 16-34, *G* and *H*).

When a proximal carious lesion or faulty restoration extends onto both the facial and lingual surfaces, instrumentation may be accomplished from either a facial or lingual approach. An example of an extensive Class III initial cavity preparation that allows such choice is illustrated in Fig. 16-35. Recall that if the preparation extends gingivally onto root structure, no bevel is placed on cementum and the area is prepared as a conventional cavity preparation.

Facial access, final cavity preparation stage. Remove any remaining infected dentin with a round bur rotating at low speed or a small spoon excavator, or both (Fig. 16-34, *D*). The point of a No. 2 explorer is excellent for detecting and removing traces of caries at the dentinoenamel junction (Fig. 16-34, *E*). If *old restorative material remains on the axial wall* after preparing the outline form, follow the procedure previously described in the lingual access preparation. Apply a calcium hydroxide *liner or base* if indicated for pulp protection (Fig. 16-34, *F*). Prepare *groove or cove retention,* if indicated, using a No. ¼ bur, or undercuts remaining from caries removal may suffice (Fig. 16-34, *I* and *J*). The preparation ready for beveling is shown in Fig. 16-34, *K. Bevel* accessible enamel margins with a

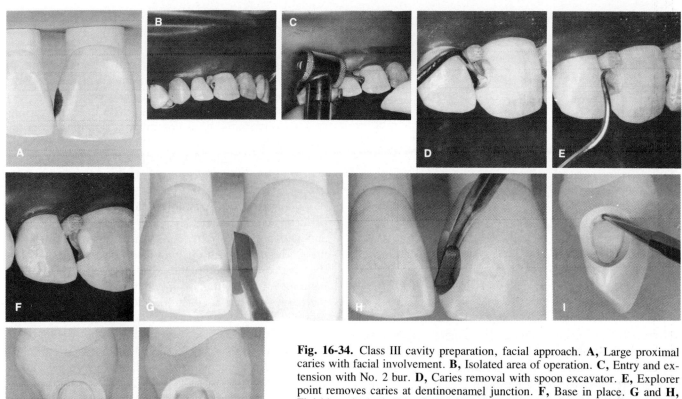

Fig. 16-34. Class III cavity preparation, facial approach. **A,** Large proximal caries with facial involvement. **B,** Isolated area of operation. **C,** Entry and extension with No. 2 bur. **D,** Caries removal with spoon excavator. **E,** Explorer point removes caries at dentinoenamel junction. **F,** Base in place. **G** and **H,** Finishing gingival, lingual, and incisal enamel walls with 12-85-5-8 hand instrument. **I,** Gingival retention being cut with No. ¼ bur. **J,** Cutting incisal retention. **K,** Completed conventional Class III preparation with facial approach. This is a beveled conventional preparation if accessible margins are beveled (see Fig. 16-36).

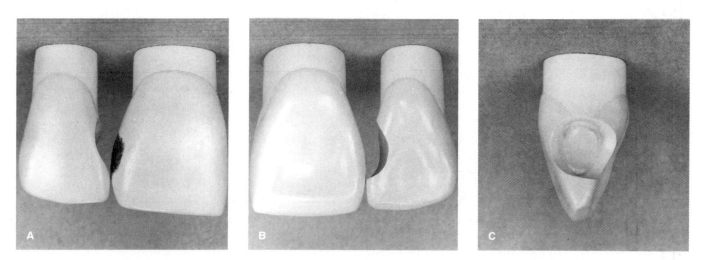

Fig. 16-35. Large Class III cavity preparation extending onto root surface. **A,** Facial view. **B,** Lingual view. **C,** Mesial view showing gingival and incisal retention. Cavity preparation is now ready for beveling the enamel walls.

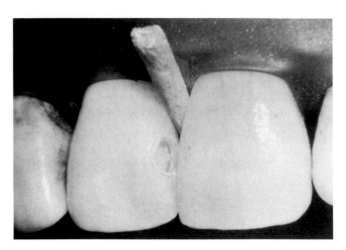

Fig. 16-36. Completed Class III beveled conventional cavity preparation, facial approach.

coarse, flame-shaped diamond instrument oriented approximately 45 degrees to the external tooth surface. A bevel of 0.25 to 0.5 mm is considered sufficient. The completed Class III facial approach preparation is illustrated in Fig. 16-36. Final preparation procedures are *cleaning* and *inspecting*.

Modified Class III cavity preparation. A modified Class III cavity preparation is indicated for a small-to-moderate size lesion or fault and is designed to be as conservative as possible. The cavity design is dictated by the extent of the fault or defect and is prepared from lingual approach wherever possible with an appropriate size round bur or diamond instrument. No effort is made to produce cavity walls that have specific shapes or forms. The extension pulpally also is dictated by the fault or lesion and usually will not be uniform in depth. Weakened, friable enamel is removed while preparing the cavosurface margins in a beveled configuration. Usually no groove (or cove) retention form is indicated since the retention of the material in the tooth will be obtained by the bond created between the composite material and the etched peripheral enamel. Thus, the cavity design appears to be scooped.

Modified cavity preparations can be made more conservative because retention is enhanced by "end-on" acid etching of the enamel. Unlike conventional cavity preparations, Class III modified preparations do not routinely extend into dentin. When the lesion or defect does not extend pulpally into dentin, the entire cavity preparation may be in enamel. In such cases no attempt is made to prepare internal cavity preparation line angles and no retention grooves or coves are prepared. Retention is obtained solely by acid etching all of the prepared enamel. Etching is the first step in applying the restorative materials in a later section.

Most initial composite restorations will utilize the modified cavity preparation. Because a carious lesion that requires a restoration will usually extend into dentin, many modified preparations will be prepared to an initial axial wall depth of 0.2 mm into dentin. However, no attempt is made to prepare distinct cavity walls, but rather, the objective is to include the infected carious area as conservatively as possible by "scooping" out the defective tooth structure. Additional caries excavation (deeper than the initial stage of 0.2 mm pulpal of the dentinoenamel junction) or marginal refinement may be necessary.

Initial cavity preparation stage. After the procedures of local anesthesia, cleaning the area, shade selection, and isolation, begin the preparation from lingual approach by making an opening using a round carbide bur (No. ½, 1, or 2) or diamond instrument, the size depending on the extent of the lesion. Before contacting the tooth, the bur is positioned for entry and rotated at high speed using air-water spray. The assistant directs air on the mirror surface and positions the evacuator tip near the operating site. The point of entry is within the incisogingival dimension of the lesion or defect and as close to the adjacent tooth as possible without contacting it (see Fig. 16-26, *A*). Direct the bur perpendicular to the enamel surface, but at an entry angle that places the neck aspect of the bur or diamond instrument as far into the embrasure (next to the adjacent tooth) as possible; use light pressure and intermittent cutting (brush stroke) to gain access into the cavity. Incorrect entry overextends the lingual outline into potential stress areas and unnecessarily weakens the tooth (Fig. 16-26, *B* and *C*). The same bur may be used to enlarge the opening sufficiently to allow in subsequent steps caries removal, completion of the preparation, and insertion of the restorative material (Fig. 16-26, *D*).

No effort is made to prepare cavity walls that are perpendicular to the enamel surface; in fact, for small preparations the cavity walls may diverge externally from the internal aspect in a scoop shape resulting in both: (1) a beveled marginal design, and (2) conservation of internal tooth structure (Fig. 16-37, *A*). For larger modified cavity preparations, the initial cavity preparation will still be prepared as conservatively as possible, but the cavity walls may not be as divergent from the axial wall. The term *axial wall* is now advisably used since in more extensive preparations at this initial preparation stage there should be an axial wall of limited depth 0.2 mm internal of the dentinoenamel junction (it may be in dentin, caries, or air). Subsequent beveling of accessible enamel areas may be required. However, the objective of initial cavity preparation is the same for both situations: to *prepare the tooth as conservatively as possible* by extending the outline form only the amount necessary to include the peripheral ex-

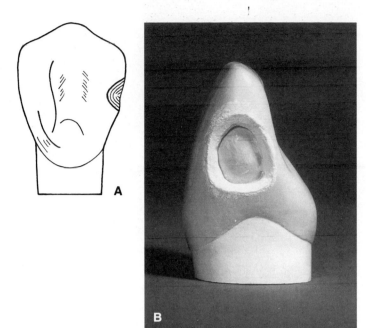

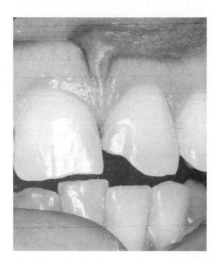

Fig. 16-38. Mesioincisal angle fractured on central incisor.

Fig. 16-37. Class III modified cavity preparations. **A,** Drawing of a small, scoop-shaped Class III modified cavity preparation. **B,** Model showing a large Class III modified cavity preparation.

tent of the lesion. Note that sometimes the incorporation of an enamel bevel also may be used to extend the final outline form to include the carious lesion (Fig. 16-49).

Extensions should be minimal, only that which is required by the extent of caries or defect. Some undermined enamel can be left in nonstress areas, but very friable enamel at the margins should be removed. If possible, the outline form should not: (1) include the entire contact area, (2) extend onto the facial surface, or (3) be extended subgingivally.

Usually the axial wall will not be uniform in depth but must allow (in subsequently described steps) the removal of infected dentin and the application of conditioner, bonding agent, and composite. If the cavity outline extends gingivally onto the root surface, the gingival wall should form a cavosurface angle of 90 degrees and the depth of the gingivoaxial line angle should be 0.75 mm for reasons discussed previously. This depth should not be exceeded in this initial stage of cavity preparation.

Final cavity preparation stage. When completed, the initial stage for the modified cavity preparation extends the outline form to include all of the fault unless it is anticipated that the incorporation of an enamel bevel will complete that objective. Small preparations already may have a beveled marginal configuration from the initial cavity preparation. Therefore, there may be little to do in the final cavity preparation stage for these preparations. If infected dentin remains (deeper than the ini-

tial axial wall depth), remove it, by suitably sized round burs and/or small spoon excavators. If indicated, place a calcium hydroxide ***liner or base*** over only the deepest portion of the excavated area, so that a maximum of dentinal surface is still exposed for bonding the restorative material. (See section on Liners and section on Bases.)

Larger preparations that are extended into dentin may require beveling of the accessible enamel walls. Bevel these enamel margins with a coarse, flame-shaped diamond instrument. Prepare the bevel by orienting the diamond instrument at a 45-degree angle to the external surface and to a width of 0.25 to 0.5 mm. Recall that if the gingival floor has been extended gingivally to a position where the remaining enamel thickness is minimal or non-existent, the bevel is omitted from this area to preserve the remaining enamel margin. Likewise, a bevel on the lingual enamel margin of a maxillary incisor may be precluded by the presence of occlusal contact, for reasons previously noted. A large completed modified cavity preparation is seen in Fig. 16-37, *B.*

Thus, final cavity preparation steps for a modified cavity preparation are, when indicated: (1) ***removal of infected dentin,*** (2) ***pulp protection,*** (3) ***bevel placement*** on accessible enamel margins, and (4) ***final procedures*** of ***cleaning,*** and ***inspecting.***

Class IV cavity preparations for composite

The Class IV composite restoration has provided the profession with a conservative treatment to restore fractured (Fig. 16-38), defective, or cariously involved anterior teeth when, previously, a porcelain crown may have been the treatment of choice. A brief description of the three types of cavity preparations will be presented. However, the conventional cavity preparation design has no clinical application except in those areas of a Class IV restoration that have margins located on root surfaces. The beveled conventional cavity preparation is usually indicated for large Class IV areas, while the modified cavity preparation is indicated for smaller Class IV needs. If a large amount of tooth structure is missing, groove retention form may be indicated even when the preparation periphery is entirely in enamel. Also, to provide additional retention in these high stress areas, the enamel bevels may be increased in width to provide greater surface area for etching, resulting in a stronger bond between the composite and the tooth. Last, in order to provide appropriate resistance form, the cavity walls may need to be prepared in such a way as to resist occlusal forces. This often requires proximal facial and lingual cavity walls that form 90-degree cavosurface angles, which are subsequently beveled, and a gingival floor prepared perpendicular to the long axis of the tooth. This box-like form may provide greater resistance to fracture of the restoration and tooth from masticatory forces.

Conventional Class IV cavity preparation. As noted above, there are no indications for this cavity preparation form except for any portion(s) of the restoration extending onto the root. The typical conventional preparation design with 90-degree cavosurface margins will be included in the following section on beveled conventional cavity preparations. Remember, however, any portion of any Class IV restoration that extends onto the root requires a 90-degree cavosurface margin and groove retention form regardless of whether either a beveled conventional or modified preparation design is used for the portion of the preparation in the crown of the tooth.

Beveled conventional Class IV cavity preparation. The beveled conventional Class IV cavity preparation is indicated for restoring large proximal areas which also involve the incisal surface of an anterior tooth. In addition to the etched enamel margin (described in a later section on applying restorative materials), retention of the composite restorative material in beveled conventional Class IV cavity preparations may be obtained by groove or other shaped undercuts, dovetail extensions, threaded pins, or a combination of these. All of these features would be part of the final stage of cavity preparation. Gingival and incisal retentive undercuts are indicated in large Class IV cavity preparations and are similar to those used in the Class III cavity preparation in which rounded undercuts are placed in the dentin along line angles and into point angles wherever possible without undermining the enamel. A dovetail extension onto the lingual surface of the tooth may enhance both the restoration's strength and retention, but is less conservative. Incisal and gin-

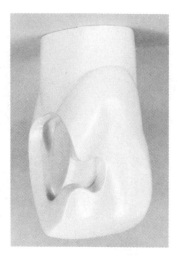

Fig. 16-39. Incisal and gingival retention grooves and dovetail extension in a large Class IV beveled conventional cavity preparation prior to beveling.

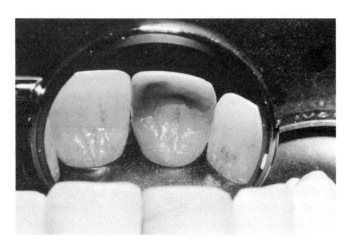

Fig. 16-40. Tooth and restoration discoloration caused by microleakage and subsequent corrosion of pin.

gival retention and dovetail extension are illustrated in Fig. 16-39.

Although pin retention is sometimes necessary, the use of pins in composite restorations is discouraged for several reasons: (1) the placement of pins in anterior teeth involves the risk of perforation either into the pulp or through the external surface; (2) pins do not enhance the strength of the restorative material;[13] and (3) some pins may corrode because of microleakage of the restoration, resulting in significant discoloration of the tooth and restoration (Fig. 16-40). Despite these disadvantages, when a large amount of tooth structure is missing, pin retention may be necessary to retain the composite restoration.

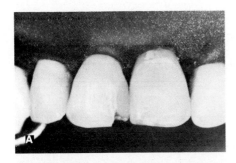
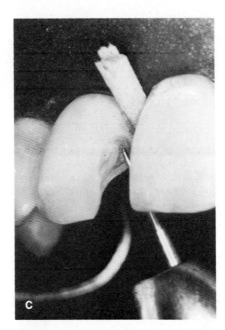
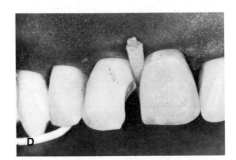
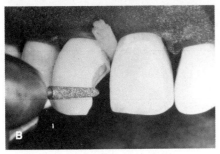

Fig. 16-41. Class IV beveled conventional cavity preparation. **A,** Large defective Class III restoration with resulting fractured incisal angle. **B,** Beveling cavosurface. **C,** Gingival retention groove. **D,** Completed Class IV beveled conventional cavity preparation.

Initial cavity preparation stage. A maxillary right central incisor is illustrated with a large defective Class III restoration and a fractured mesioincisal corner which upon removal necessitates a Class IV restoration (Fig. 16-41, *A*). Class IV beveled conventional cavity preparations are characterized by an outline form resulting when the cavity walls are prepared as much as possible perpendicular or parallel to the long axis of the tooth, resulting in a design which provides greater resistance to those biting forces that could cause fracture of the tooth or restorative material. Using an appropriate size round carbide bur at high speed with air-water coolant, prepare the ***outline form.*** Remove all weakened enamel and establish the initial axial wall depth at 0.5 mm into dentin (because groove retention form will be utilized). Prepare the cavity walls as much as possible parallel and perpendicular to the long axis of the tooth.

Final cavity preparation stage. Excavate any ***remaining infected dentin*** as the first step of final cavity preparation. If necessary, apply a calcium hydroxide liner or base. Bevel the cavosurface margin of all accessible enamel margins of the preparation. The bevel is prepared at a 45-degree angle to the external tooth surface with a coarse, flame-shaped diamond instrument (Fig. 16-41, *B*). The width of the bevel should be 0.25 to 2 mm, depending on the amount of tooth structure missing and the retention perceived to be necessary. Retention form is provided by both retentive undercuts and acid etching of the prepared enamel (which is the first procedure in the restoration phase). Prepare a gingival retention groove using a No. ¼ round bur 0.2 mm inside the dentinoenamel junction at a depth of 0.25 mm

(half the diameter of the No. ¼ bur). This groove should extend the length of the gingival floor and slightly up the facioaxial and linguoaxial line angles (Fig. 16-41, *C*). No retentive undercut is needed at the incisal area where mostly enamel exists. Fig. 16-41, *D* illustrates the completed Class IV beveled conventional cavity preparation.

Modified Class IV cavity preparation. The modified Class IV preparation for composite is indicated for small- or moderate-sized Class IV lesions or traumatic defects. The objective of the cavity preparation is to remove as little tooth structure as possible while providing for appropriate retention and resistance forms. Remove any existing lesion or defective restoration with a suitable size round bur or diamond instrument and prepare the ***outline form*** to include weakened, friable enamel. Usually little or no initial cavity preparation is indicated for fractured incisal corners. The cavosurface margins are prepared with a beveled configuration similar to that previously described. The pulpal depth is dependent on the extent of the lesion, previous restoration, or fracture. Usually no groove or cove retention form is indicated. Instead, the retention is obtained primarily from the etched enamel and, perhaps, from conditioned dentin. Etching enamel and conditioning dentin is covered later as the first step in applying restorative materials.

The treatment of teeth with minor traumatic fractures requires less preparation than the beveled conventional example. If the fracture is confined to enamel, adequate retention can usually be attained by simply beveling sharp cavosurface margins in the fractured area with a

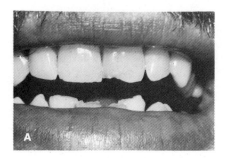
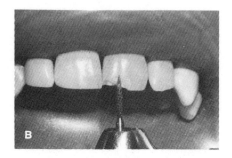
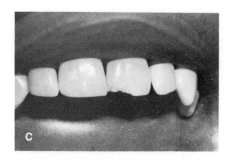

Fig. 16-42. Class IV modified cavity preparation. **A,** Minor traumatic fracture. **B,** Fractured enamel is roughened with coarse, flame-shaped diamond instrument. **C,** Completed Class IV modified cavity preparation.

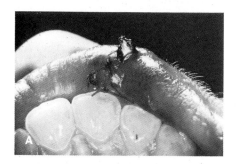
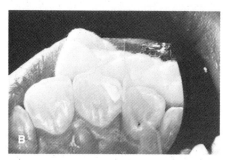

Fig. 16-43. Class IV modified cavity preparation. **A,** Extensive traumatic fracture exposing dentin. **B,** Completed Class IV modified cavity preparation.

coarse, flame-shaped diamond instrument followed by acid etching (Fig. 16-42).

Figure 16-43, *A,* illustrates a maxillary central incisor with a more extensive traumatic fracture exposing dentin. The enamel margins may be beveled as previously described for the beveled conventional Class IV preparation. Additional retention may be provided by a gingival retention groove, as noted earlier. Fig. 16-43, *B,* illustrates the final cavity preparation after acid etching (acid etching is later described as the first step in applying materials for the restoration).

Class V cavity preparations for composite

Class V cavity preparations, by definition, are located in the gingival one-third of the facial and lingual tooth surfaces. Because of esthetic considerations, composite materials most frequently are used for the restoration of Class V lesions in anterior teeth. However, composite may not always be the material of choice. Except when esthetics is the primary concern, a more durable, more easily placed amalgam restoration or a glass ionomer with inherent anti-cariogenic properties may be indicated. Numerous factors must be taken into consideration in material selection including esthetics, caries activity, access to the lesion, moisture control, and patient age. In fact, *increased patient age* is particularly important when considering the treatment of Class V root surface lesions (see Chapter 6, Effects of Aging, discussed in Biomechanics for Restorative Dentistry).

As stated in Chapter 1, the elderly component of the U.S. population will continue to increase. Furthermore, the elderly will retain more of their teeth as they age and consequently will experience more gingival recession. With more elderly having more root surfaces exposed, the *prevalence of root caries and/or cervical erosion or abrasion defects will increase.* Therefore the number of indicated Class V restorations also will increase. Because most of these restorative needs will involve root surfaces, careful consideration should be given to the restorative material to be used. As noted earlier, amalgam or glass ionomer may be preferred. The consideration for use of materials other than composite is intensified when it is realized that the elderly patient may present other factors that further complicate the use of composite on the root surfaces. These factors would include decreased salivary function, decreased motivation and ability for homecare, increased difficulty in adequately isolating the operating area, and increased difficulty in performing the operative procedure due to physical or medical problems of the patient. In spite of these concerns, the use of composite as a restorative material for Class V lesions will still predominate in areas of esthetic concern. Subsequently the various cavity preparation options are presented.

Before the cavity preparation is initiated, select the shade of the composite material as previously discussed and then isolate the operating area. During shade selection remember that the tooth is darker in the cervical

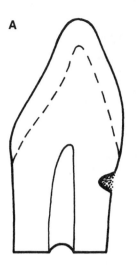
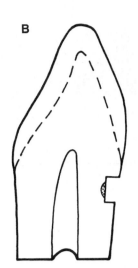
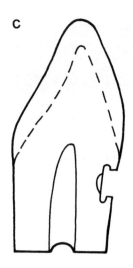

Fig. 16-44. Conventional Class V cavity preparation. **A,** Lesion entirely on root surface. **B,** Initial cavity preparation with 90-degree cavosurface margins and axial wall depth of 0.75 mm. **C,** Remaining infected dentin excavated, liner placed, and incisal and gingival retention form prepared.

third. Isolation may be achieved by a rubber dam and No. 212 retainer or with a cotton roll(s) and retraction cord as previously described. Usually microfill composites are selected for restoring Class V defects because their composition results in (1) increased restoration smoothness, and (2) restoration flexibility when the tooth undergoes cervical flexure. It is thought the restoration can flex rather than debond when the tooth flexes under occlusal forces.[18]

Conventional Class V cavity preparation. The conventional Class V cavity preparation for composite is indicated for that portion of a carious lesion or defect entirely or partially on the facial or lingual root surface of a tooth. The preparation form would be similar to that described in Chapter 14 (Class V Amalgam). The features of the cavity preparation include a *90-degree cavosurface angle, uniform depth of the axial line angles, and groove retention form.*

Since many Class V carious lesions or defects will have some enamel at the incisal (occlusal) and possibly the mesial and/or distal margins, the conventional composite cavity preparation design is indicated only for the portion of the lesion/defect extending onto the root surface. The enamel marginal areas are prepared using either a beveled conventional or modified cavity preparation design as described in the following sections of this chapter. However, occasionally a Class V lesion/defect is located entirely on the root of the tooth requiring the use of a conventional cavity preparation design exclusively. The following description of a conventional cavity preparation pertains to such a restoration that is located *entirely on the root surface of a tooth* (Fig. 16-44, *A*).

Initial cavity preparation stage. A tapered fissure carbide bur (No. 700, 701, or 271) is used at high speed with air-water spray. If access interproximally or gingivally is limited, a No. 1 or 2 round bur may be used to

prepare the cavity. When a tapered fissure bur is used, make entry at a 45-degree angle to the tooth surface by tilting the handpiece distally; but as the cutting progresses distally, maneuver the handpiece to thereafter maintain the bur's long axis perpendicular to the external surface of the tooth during preparation of the *outline form* which should result in *90-degree cavosurface margins.* At this initial cavity preparation stage, the pulpal depth should only be 0.75 mm (Fig. 16-44, *B*). The tip of the bur may be rotating in air, caries, or old restorative material while establishing this initial depth. Any infected dentin remaining on this initial axial wall will be removed during the final stage of cavity preparation. Any old restorative material remaining may or may not be removed according to the concepts stated previously in the section titled, Removal of Remaining Infected Dentin or Old Restorative Material. The 0.75 mm axial wall depth will provide adequate external wall width for: (1) strength of the cavity wall, (2) strength of the composite, and (3) placement of a retention groove. When the desired distal extension is obtained, move the bur mesially, incisally (occlusally), and gingivally for indicated extensions, while maintaining the proper initial depth and keeping the bur's long axis perpendicular to the root surface. The axial wall should follow the original contour of the facial surface, which is convex outward mesiodistally. The outline form extension of the mesial, distal, occlusal (incisal), and gingival walls is dictated by the extent of the caries, defect, or old restorative material indicated for replacement (sometimes the new material will abut a still satisfactory old restoration!).

If necessary, an angle former, 7-85-2½-6 or 12-85-5-8, may be used to better define the walls. A pushing and scraping motion will define the margin, develop a smooth outline, and maintain a 90-degree cavosurface angle. All of the external cavity walls of a Class V con-

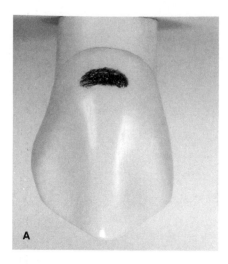
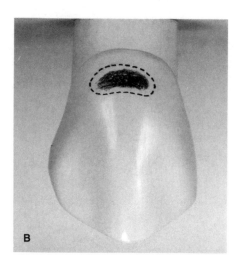

Fig. 16-45. A, Class V caries. **B,** Typical outline form.

ventional cavity preparation will be visible when viewed from a facial position (outwardly divergent walls).

Final cavity preparation stage. Final cavity preparation for the conventional preparation consists of the following steps: (1) *removing remaining infected dentin or old restorative material* (if indicated) on the initial axial wall, (2) applying a calcium hydroxide *liner or base* for pulp protection, if necessary, and (3) preparing *groove retention form.*

Prepare retention grooves with a No. ¼ bur along the full length of the gingivoaxial and incisoaxial (occlusoaxial) line angles. These grooves are prepared 0.25 mm in depth (half the bur head deep) into the external walls and next to the axial wall. This should leave between the groove and the margin sufficient remaining wall dimension (0.25 mm) to prevent fracture (Fig. 16-44, *C*). It is helpful while preparing the grooves to observe that this remaining wall dimension is equal to half the diameter of the bur head (0.5 mm). The incisal (occlusal) groove is directed depthwise mostly incisally (occlusally) and slightly pulpally. The gingival groove is directed depthwise mostly gingivally and slightly pulpally. *Clean* the preparation, if indicated, and *inspect* for final approval.

Beveled conventional Class V cavity preparation. The beveled conventional Class V cavity preparation has *beveled enamel margins* and is indicated either for (1) the replacement of an existing, defective Class V restoration which initially utilized a conventional cavity preparation or (2) for a large, new carious lesion for which the operator preoperatively believes a gingival retention groove will be necessary. The beveled conventional Class V cavity preparation *initially* will exhibit 90-degree cavosurface margins (that subsequently will be beveled) and axial line angles that are uniform in depth into the dentin only 0.2 mm when groove reten-

tion is judged unnecessary, or 0.5 to 0.6 mm where a retention groove is planned and the margin is enamel. Groove retention usually is not indicated when the periphery of the cavity preparation is located in enamel. Many of these preparations will be a combination of beveled enamel margins and 90-degree root surface (non-enamel) margins, with the root surface areas having groove retention (combined beveled conventional and conventional preparations). As stated previously, for the preparation portion on root surface the depth of the axial line angles should be 0.75 mm.

The advantages of the beveled conventional cavity preparation as compared to the conventional cavity preparation are: (1) increased retention due to the greater surface area of etched enamel afforded by the bevel, (2) decreased microleakage due to the enhanced bond between the material and the tooth, and (3) decreased need for groove retention form (and consequently less removal of tooth structure).

Initial cavity preparation stage. The typical outline form for a Class V lesion in enamel is seen in Fig. 16-45. Prepare the *outline form* as described in the preceding section except that the initial depth is only 0.2 mm into dentin when groove retention is unnecessary (Fig. 16-46).

Final cavity preparation stage. Complete the following steps of final cavity preparation: (1) *remove any remaining infected dentin,* and, *if indicated remove any old restorative material,* (2) apply a calcium hydroxide *liner* or *base,* if necessary, (3) prepare a gingival retention groove if either the gingival margin is located on the root surface or the preparation is large enough to warrant groove retention form (Fig. 16-47), and (4) bevel the enamel margins. The bevel on the enamel margin is accomplished with a coarse flame-shaped diamond instrument, angled at approximately 45 degrees to the external tooth surface and prepared to a width of

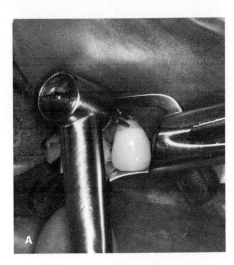
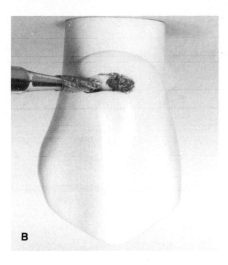
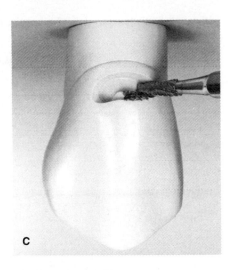

Fig. 16-46. Initiating a beveled conventional Class V cavity preparation. **A,** Operating position and equipment. Entry with No. 701 bur held at 45-degree angle to tooth surface. **B,** As cutting proceeds distally (0.2 mm into dentin), bur shank is held perpendicular to enamel surface. **C,** Mesial extension, keeping bur shank perpendicular to surface and maintaining initial depth.

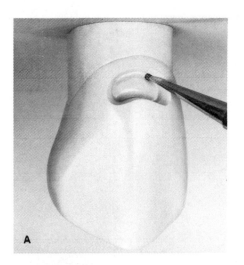
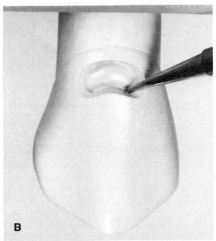

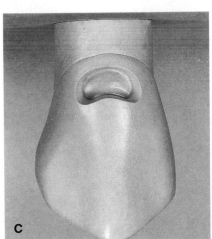
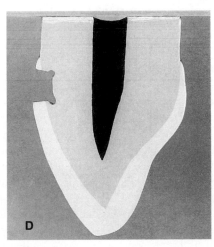
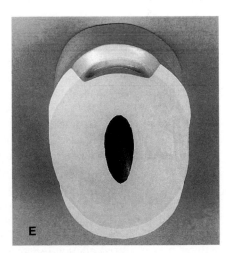

Fig. 16-47. Placement of retention grooves. **A** and **B,** Groove is placed with No. ¼ bur along gingivoaxial and incisoaxial line angles 0.2 mm inside the dentinoenamel junction and 0.25 mm deep. Note slight pulpal inclination of shank of No. ¼ bur. **C,** Facial view. **D,** Incisogingival section. Note that grooves depthwise are directed mostly incisally (gingivally) and slightly pulpally. **E,** Mesiodistal section.

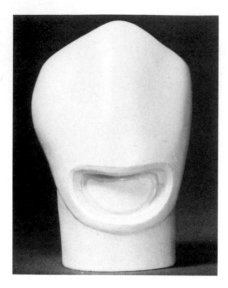

Fig. 16-48. Completed beveled conventional Class V preparation.

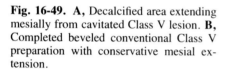

Fig. 16-49. A, Decalcified area extending mesially from cavitated Class V lesion. **B,** Completed beveled conventional Class V preparation with conservative mesial extension.

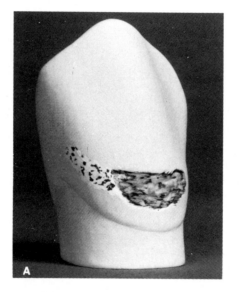
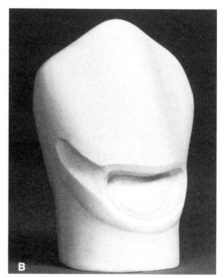

0.25 to 0.5 mm. A completed beveled conventional Class V cavity preparation is shown in Fig. 16-48.

An even more conservative approach may be used when extending the outline form of beveled conventional Class V preparations. Fig. 16-49, *A,* illustrates a path of a decalcified enamel lesion (in enamel only) having a broken, rough surface that often extends mesially and/or distally from the cavitated lesion (or failing existing restoration). After preparation of the cavitated lesion (or failing restoration), extend the margins of the preparation to include these areas of decalcification by using a coarse, round diamond instrument to prepare the cavosurface margin in the form of a chamfer extended only in the enamel. A completed beveled conventional cavity preparation of this type is illustrated in Fig. 16-49, *B.*

When a large Class V carious lesion or faulty restoration extends onto the *root surface,* the gingival wall is prepared in the same manner as a conventional Class V cavity preparation (i.e., butt joint with a dentinal retention groove). The depth of the *initial* preparation on the root surface should be only 0.75 mm. Only the enamel cavosurface margins are beveled. A completed combination of a Class V beveled conventional with a conventional cavity preparation extending onto the root surface is illustrated in Fig. 16-50.

Modified Class V cavity preparation. The modified Class V cavity preparation is indicated for the restoration of new Class V lesions or defects that are small to moderate in size. The objective is to restore the lesion or defect as conservatively as possible. Therefore, there is no effort to prepare the cavity walls as butt joints and

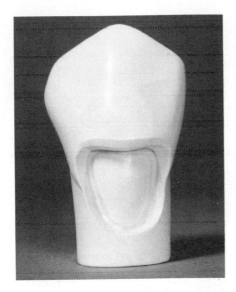

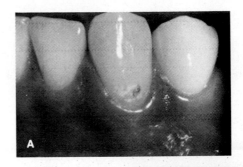

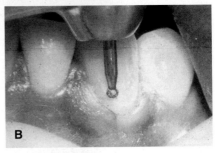

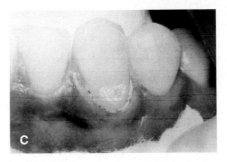

Fig. 16-50. Completed beveled conventional Class V cavity preparation extending onto the root.

Fig. 16-51. Modified Class V cavity preparation. **A,** Small cavitated Class V lesion. **B,** Surrounding enamel defect is prepared with round diamond instrument. **C,** Completed modified cavity preparation after acid etching.

usually no groove retention is incorporated. The lesion or defect is "scooped" out, resulting in a cavity form that may have a divergent cavity wall configuration and an axial surface that usually is not uniform in depth. Class V modified preparations are ideal for small enamel defects or small but cavitated (with broken surface) lesions that are largely or entirely in enamel (Fig. 16-51, *A*). These include decalcified and hypoplastic areas located in the cervical one-third of the teeth.

Initial cavity preparation stage. After the usual preliminary procedures, prepare initial cavity preparation with a round or elliptical diamond instrument (Fig. 16-51, *B*), eliminating all of the enamel lesion or defect. The preparation is only extended into dentin when the defect warrants such extension, which at this initial stage is prepared no deeper than 0.2 mm into dentin (since no groove retention form will be used). No effort is made to prepare 90-degree cavosurface margins.

Final cavity preparation stage. If *infected dentin* remains, it is removed with a round bur or spoon excavator. Apply a calcium hydroxide liner or base, but only if indicated. The completed preparation with etched enamel can be seen in Fig. 16-51, *C* (etching will be described later as the first step in applying restorative materials).

Class V cavity preparation for abrasion/erosion lesions. Class V modified cavity preparations are also used *to restore abraded or eroded cervical areas. Abrasion,* in the form of a notch, often V-shaped, is a loss or wearing away of tooth structure due to *mechanical forces,* such as strenuous toothbrushing with a hard bristle toothbrush or abrasive toothpaste.[25] *Erosion,* of-

ten a saucer-shaped notch, occurs primarily as a result of *chemical dissolution* (e.g., sustained exposure to citric acid [juices] or vomitus).[19] *Idiopathic erosion* may occur due to flexure of the cervical area under heavy occlusal stress, beginning with microfracture of the thin enamel tooth structure occlusal of the cementoenamel junction, which combined with abrasive toothbrushing could explain a "notched" defect (see Chapter 6, Strain within Tooth Structure, discussed in Biomechanics for Restorative Dentistry).[22] These notches are progressive, enlarging with time if the causative factor is not eliminated. When notching occurs (see Fig. 16-52, *A)* the operator first must decide, with input from the patient, whether or not the area needs to be restored. The decision to restore is based on the following considerations:

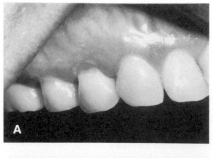
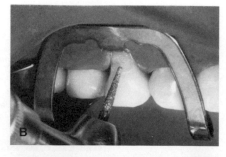
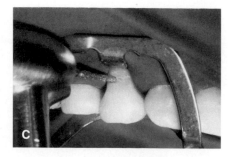

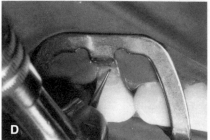
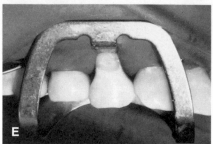

Fig. 16-52. Class V cavity preparation for abrasion/erosion lesions. **A,** Preoperative notched lesion. **B, C, D,** Beveling the enamel margin, roughening the internal walls, and placing retention groove. **E,** Completed preparation with etched enamel.

Caries. If caries is present, the defect should be restored unless the lesion is incipient and very superficial. For the incipient root caries lesion, treatment may consist only of minor recontouring of the area (cementoplasty) and application of a topical fluoride. (Most erosion and abrasion notches are not carious.)

Gingival health. If the notched defect is determined to be causing gingival inflammation (i.e., plaque retention) and/or further gingival recession is anticipated, the notched defect should be restored. (Usually, gingival health is excellent, with the notching having occurred after gingival recession.)

Esthetics. If the notched area is in an esthetically critical position, the patient may elect to have the area restored with a tooth-colored restoration.

Sensitivity. If the notched area is very sensitive, application of a dentin bonding agent may, at least temporarily, reduce or eliminate the sensitivity. Continuing sensitivity may require restoration of the area.

Pulp protection. If the notched area is very large and deep pulpally, the restoration of the defect may be indicated to avoid further defect development that may cause a pulpal exposure.

Tooth strength. If the notched area is very large or deep, the strength of the tooth at the cervical area may be compromised. Placement of a bonded restoration will eliminate further progression of the defect and may restore some of the lost strength.

The cavity preparation for a Class V abrasion or erosion area usually requires only roughening of the internal cavity walls, beveling all enamel margins, and plac-

ing a retention groove in non-enamel areas (Fig. 16-52, *B, C,* and *D*). If necessary, prepare the root surface cavosurface margins to approximately 90 degrees. Often the inherent form of an abraded/eroded lesion will result in no need for further preparation of root surface cavosurface margins. Although some success may be obtained without placement of the groove retention form, greater restoration retention is provided when the retentive groove is utilized. Moreover, greater resistance to marginal leakage results from groove placement, because this retentive feature assists in resisting the effects of polymerization shrinkage and tooth flexure.[26] The completed preparation with etched enamel is seen in Fig. 16-52, *E* (etching will be described later as the first step in applying restorative materials).

Cavity preparation for aberrant smooth surface pit fault. Occasionally a tooth surface that normally is smooth will have a pit in the enamel (Fig. 16-53, *A*). Most aberrant pit faults in enamel are restored best with use of a modified cavity preparation. For such a preparation for an aberrant pit fault, the *outline form* (includes extensions and depth) is dictated by the extent of the fault and/or caries lesion. Faults existing entirely in enamel are prepared with an appropriately sized round diamond instrument by merely eliminating the defect (Fig. 16-53, *B*). Adequate retention is obtained by acid etching (the first step in applying restorative materials). When the defect includes carious dentin, the *infected portion* is removed with a round bur; *liner* or *base* is placed, if needed; and the enamel margin is *beveled* with a diamond instrument.

Fig. 16-53. A, Faulty pit on facial surface of maxillary incisor. **B,** Modified cavity preparation for enamel pit defect.

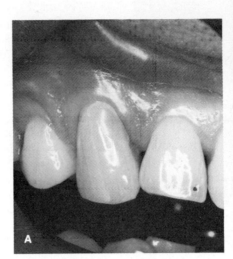
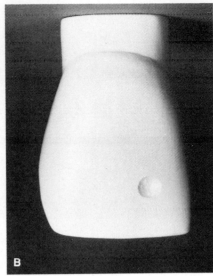

PROCEDURES FOR MICRO-RETENTION FROM ACID ETCHING ENAMEL AND CONDITIONING DENTIN

This section describes the procedures for developing micro-retention by acid etching enamel and conditioning dentin. These procedures usually precede application of the matrix, if necessary (subsequent section), which then may be followed by insertion of the bonding agent and composite. The exact sequence for applying the enamel/dentin conditioner, primer, adhesive bonding agent, and the matrix is dependent on the operator. Some operators prefer matrix application first, followed by enamel/dentin conditioner, primer, adhesive bonding agent, and finally insertion of the composite. This sequence may provide the best isolation of the cavity preparation for maximum enamel/dentin conditioning and adhesion. It also allows an assessment of any enamel fracture (upon insertion of the proximal wedge) prior to conditioning that area. If the matrix is applied first, care must be taken to avoid pooling of the conditioning and especially the adhesive materials. *Placing the matrix first in the sequence is especially beneficial when the cavity preparation is extensive gingivally.*

Other operators prefer to complete all enamel/dentin conditioning and adhesive application prior to matrix placement. The primary reasons for this sequence are to minimize pooling potential and maximize conditioning and adhesive placement at the cavosurface margins. Either sequence may be used as long as meticulous technique is followed. This chapter and Chapter 17 present several options for this sequence.

Procedure for acid etching enamel

Review the section titled, Acid Etch Phenomenon. The acid etch technique for enamel requires that a very exacting sequence be followed if optimal results are to be obtained, including isolation from fluids (saliva and sulcular weepage) by using either the rubber dam or cotton roll(s) and retraction cord (see Isolation of the Operating Site). Both liquid and gel etchants are available in concentrations of 37% or 50% phosphoric acid. Generally, liquid etchants are used when large surface areas are to be etched, such as placing full veneers (see Chapter 18). Thixotropic gels are preferred by most practitioners for the controlled application of etchant to enamel walls, including bevels and margins. The etchant gels may be placed carefully with hand instruments, brushes, or with endodontic paper points held in cotton pliers, but usually a syringe applicator is used to inject the gel etchant directly onto the enamel. Do not allow etched surfaces to be contaminated by mouth fluids (saliva or sulcular weepage), because such contamination dictates a repeat of the etching procedure.

Liquid etchants. Liquid etchants are used primarily to etch large surface areas of enamel, such as for veneers or sealants. (see Chapters 17 and 18). Common types of applicators include small cotton pellets, foam sponges, and brushes.

Gently apply the acid to the appropriate enamel surfaces to be restored, keeping the excess to a maximum of 0.5 mm past the anticipated extent of the restoration. For preparations involving the proximal area, place a polyester matrix strip before applying the acid to prevent inadvertent etching of the adjacent tooth. Repeat the application of acid every 10 to 15 seconds to keep the area moist for 30 seconds. Exercise care not to flood the area with acid or to rub the enamel. Then rinse the area with water for 10 to 15 seconds, starting on the ad-

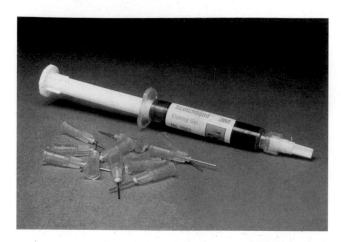

Fig. 16-54. Syringe used to dispense gel etchant.

jacent tooth to prevent possible splashing of acid-rich water onto the patient, dentist, or assistant. If cotton rolls were used for isolation, replace them at this time, ensuring that the cavity preparation does not become contaminated with saliva. Now dry the area for 20 seconds with clean, dry air. Enamel that has been properly acid-conditioned is described as having a ground glass or lightly frosted appearance. If this appearance is not apparent, re-etch for an additional 30 seconds. Note the statement at the close of the next section (Gel Etchants) warning against contamination of etched surfaces.

Gel etchants. For application of a gel etchant, use a brush, paper point, instrument, or syringe to place the etchant onto the prepared enamel wall and only 0.5 mm of the unprepared enamel beyond the cavosurface margin, and leave untouched for 30 seconds. Rinse for 20 to 30 seconds (a longer rinse time because the gel is more difficult to remove). Gel etchants are more easily applied with a small syringe. Various etchant syringes are available and provide advantages of easier and more precise control of the etchant. A typical etchant syringe is seen in Fig. 16-54.

If the patient has high caries activity, the enamel will usually etch very easily. Enamel that is resistant to acid etching may require doubling or tripling the usual 30-second etching time. Care should be exercised not to etch adjacent teeth or remote areas. Even though etched areas of enamel appear normal after several days, scanning electron microscopy has shown that etched enamel is not completely remineralized even after 90 days.[16]

Once the area is etched, washed, and dried (with clean, dry air), keep it immaculately clean and dry until the bonding agent resin is applied. This precaution is critical to the success of the operation. *If saliva or sulcular weepage accidently contacts the cavity preparation, reapply the acid etchant for 10 seconds to clean the area followed by thorough rinsing and drying.*

Procedure for conditioning dentin

As noted previously, most dentin bonding systems rely on some type of dentin conditioning and priming to maximize adhesion (see Enamel/Dentin Bonding Systems). Dentin conditioners typically remove or solubilize the smear layer in order to achieve optimal adhesion to the underlying dentin. However, there is no one established regimen for the application of dentin conditioners because they may be very different from one product to another. Dentin conditioners and primers should be *applied strictly in accordance with manufacturer's instructions.* The same applicators (paper points, foam sponges, cotton pellets, brushes, etc.) may be used for application of these materials. *If only enamel is to be etched and bonded, the dentin conditioning and priming steps are omitted.*

MATRIX APPLICATION

A *matrix* may be applied and stabilized by a *wedge* (and compound if used) before application of the enamel/dentin conditioner, primer, and bonding adhesive (the bonding system). Placing the matrix first provides an opportunity to assess that the gingival cavosurface tooth structure is sound and not fractured due to wedge insertion. However, care must be taken to avoid pooling of these materials.

Not only will a matrix aid in placing, confining, and contouring the composite restorative material but it may also aid in isolating the cavity preparation, thereby enhancing the potential effectiveness of the enamel/dentin bonding system (if done after matrix application). A proper matrix also reduces the amount of excess material, thereby minimizing the finishing time. A properly contoured and wedged matrix is a prerequisite for a restoration involving entirely a proximal contact area.

No matrix is needed for restoring preparations where the contour can be controlled as the composite restorative material is being inserted, such as in the Class V restoration. This is especially true when using light-cured materials whose extended working time allows the operator to initiate contouring of the restoration in the unpolymerized state.

A matrix for the proximal surface of an anterior tooth should be made of a thin inert material, such as polyester or metal, that can be contoured. There are two types of matrices: (1) a polyester strip matrix and (2) a compound-supported metal matrix.

Polyester strip matrix for proximal restorations

A properly contoured polyester strip matrix is used for most Class III and Class IV cavity preparations. Since the proximal surface of a tooth is usually convex incisogingivally and the strip is flat, it is necessary to shape the strip to conform with the desired tooth con-

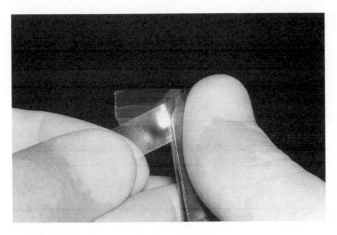

Fig. 16-55. Contouring polyester strip matrix by drawing it over rounded back end of operating pliers.

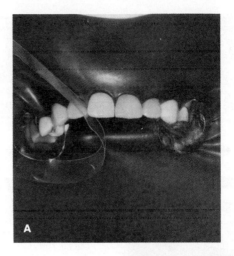

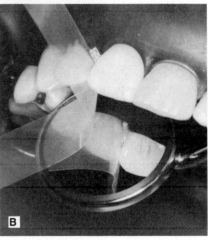

Fig. 16-56. Inserting and wedging polyester strip matrix. **A,** Strip with concave area next to cavity is positioned between teeth. **B,** Strip in position and wedge inserted.

tour by drawing it across a hard, round object such as the rounded, back end of operating pliers (Fig. 16-55). The amount of convexity placed in the strip depends on the size and contour of the anticipated restoration. Several pulls of the strip with heavy pressure across the rounded end of the operating pliers may be required to obtain enough convexity.

Position the contoured strip between the teeth so that the convex area conforms to the desired tooth contour (Fig. 16-56, *A*). Extend the matrix strip at least 1 mm beyond the prepared gingival and incisal margins. Sometimes the strip will not slide through or is distorted by a tight contact or cavity margin. In such instances a wedge is lightly positioned in the gingival embrasure before the strip is inserted. Once the strip is past the binding area it may be necessary to loosen the wedge in order to place the strip past the gingival margin (between the wedge and margin). Then reinsert the wedge tightly.

Usually *a wedge is needed at the gingival margin* to (1) help hold the strip in position, (2) to provide slight separation of the teeth, and (3) to prevent a gingival overhang of the composite resin material. A wedge is required when all of the proximal contact is involved because the wedge must separate the teeth sufficiently to compensate for the thickness of the matrix if the completed restoration is to properly contact the adjacent tooth.

Several types of commercial wedges are available in assorted sizes. A *triangular-shaped wedge* (in cross section) is ideal and indicated for preparations with margins that are deep in the gingival sulcus. An end of a *round wood toothpick* approximately ⅜ inch (9 mm) long usually is an excellent wedge. The wedge is kept as short as possible to avoid conflict with access during

insertion of the restorative material and holding procedures.

Place the wedge using No. 110 pliers from the facial approach for lingual access cavities (and vice versa for facial access) just gingival to the gingival margin. When isolation is accomplished with the rubber dam, wedge placement is aided by a small amount of water-soluble lubricant on the tip of the wedge. The rubber dam is first stretched gingivally (on the side from which the wedge is inserted) and then released gradually during wedge insertion (Fig. 16-56, *B*). Subsequently a trial opening and closing of the matrix strip is helpful. It must open enough for access to insert the enamel/dentin bonding agent (if necessary) and composite material, and close sufficiently to ensure proper contour. It may be necessary to shorten the wedge or insert it from the opposite embrasure to optimize access. Wedge placement may result in fracture of the proximal cavosurface

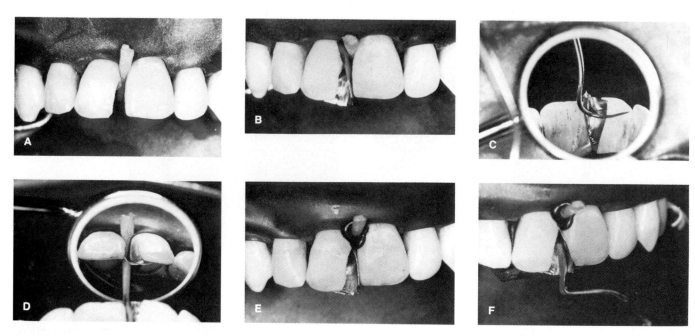

Fig. 16-57. Compound-supported metal matrix. **A,** Class IV cavity preparation to be restored. **B,** Dead soft metal matrix strip is positioned interproximally. **C,** Metal matrix strip is adapted to lingual margin of cavity preparation. Note that strip extends over lingual margin but does not cover all of lingual surface of tooth. **D,** Proximal contour of matrix is inspected incisally. **E,** Toothpick carrying a small amount of softened impression compound is positioned interproximally. **F,** Compound is applied from lingual approach to matrix and tooth, and then back side of warmed spoon excavator can be used from facial approach to make any necessary corrections to lingual and proximal contours of matrix strip. **G,** Finished compound-supported matrix with facial access.

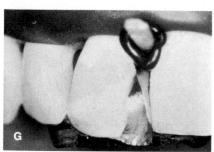

tooth structure. If this occurs, reconditioning of that area must occur.

The polyester strip matrix can also be used for most Class IV preparations, although the strip's flexibility makes control of the matrix somewhat difficult. This may result in an overcontoured or undercontoured restoration and/or open contact. Also, composite material will extrude incisally, but this excess can be easily removed when finishing.

Commercially available preformed plastic or celluloid crown forms are usually too thick and therefore are not recommended. Gingival overhangs and open contacts are common with techniques that do not employ gingival wedging.

Compound-supported metal matrix for Class IV restorations

If the operator does not have sufficient experience in using the more flexible polyester strip matrix, the compound-supported matrix may be the most appropriate for large Class IV preparations. To ensure correct proximal contour, a nonyielding compound-supported metal matrix that provides an access area for insertion of the restorative material may be utilized. A Class IV cavity preparation, facial approach, serves as an example for the application of this type of matrix (Fig. 16-57, *A*). Cut a ribbon of dead-soft metal matrix material* (.0015 inch [0.04 mm] thick and ⅜ inch [8 mm] wide) to a length of ⅝ inch (16 mm). Then orient, trim, and adjust this strip so that the facial edge protrudes just flush with the facial surface of the tooth (vice versa for lingual access) and the gingival and incisal edges extend beyond the cavity margins at least 1 mm (Fig. 16-57, *B*). For facial access the lingual portion of the strip is adapted to the lingual surface of the tooth and a wedge is placed from the facial or lingual embrasure, whichever is greater (Fig. 16-57, *C* and *D*). Burnish proximal contour into the strip with the side of a No. 2 explorer or the back side of a Black spoon excavator. An optional wedge is a toothpick that is positioned while carrying a small amount of softened impression compound (Fig. 16-57, *E*).

Soften more impression compound over a Bunsen burner and form a small cone. Lightly flame the base

*Dead Soft Metal Matrix, DenMat Corp., Santa Maria, Calif.

and attach to the index finger. Without delay, soften the cone tip over the flame and then press over the lingual area and into the gingival embrasure. It is helpful to hold the strip against the adjacent contact area with a burnisher while the compound is applied. Observe the adaptation of the matrix to the lingual cavity margin through the open facial access and, if needed, correct the proximal contour using the back side of a spoon excavator while the compound is still moldable (Fig. 16-57, *F*). If the compound has hardened, it may be necessary to soften the compound by using a warmed burnishing instrument on the cavity side of the strip. Also, if a small amount of compound is pressed between the matrix strip and the adjacent tooth, the compound is easily expressed by the application of a warm burnisher on the cavity side of the matrix in the contact area. It is best to always do this to assure that the strip is touching the adjacent tooth at contact area. This precaution, coupled with the separation by the wedge, assures proper contour and proximal contact of the restoration after removal of the matrix. Any compound that may contact the composite during insertion should be removed, since it may cause discoloration.

Ample opening is left in the completed matrix to insert the enamel/dentin bonding agent and composite from facial approach as illustrated in Fig. 16-57, *G*. If a Class IV cavity preparation is to be filled from lingual approach, the position of the matrix is reversed.

INFORMATION PRELIMINARY TO APPLICATION OF BONDING AGENT AND INSERTION OF COMPOSITE
Enamel/dentin bonding agent; relationship to composite placement

The composite restoration usually will be placed in two stages: first, a bonding agent (adhesive) will be applied (if not already placed during enamel and dentin conditioning procedures) and then the composite restorative material inserted. The free flowing bonding agent engages the numerous microundercuts produced in the etched enamel as well as bonds to the conditioned and primed dentin to provide micro-retention. When the composite restorative material is added, a chemical union occurs with the adhesive bonding agent, thus forming a strong attachment between the tooth and the composite. *If used in conjunction with enamel etching and dentin conditioning/priming, along with a bonding agent, most composite restorations produce an effective seal.*[39] Recall that two types of composites exist: self-cured and light-cured.

Polymerization types; relationship to dispensing and preparation of restorative materials

Self-cured composites. Typically, both the bonding agent and composite are supplied in individual containers of a *catalyst* and a *base*. Whereas additional shades of the composite base material are available, the catalyst remains the same. Items needed for mixing include a disposable plastic spatula, foam sponge, mixing pads, and operating pliers. For small cavity preparations the foam sponge applicator for applying the bonding agent should be sectioned into small pieces.

Because the mixing and application of the adhesive bonding agent and then the mixing and insertion of composite should follow a rapid sequence, the materials are dispensed in advance. Equal amounts of the composite catalyst and base (pastes) are placed on the pad first, since they do not have a tendency to run together. The setting time can be controlled by varying the proportion of catalyst and base. Variations as great as 2:1 of either catalyst or base to the other can be tolerated without an appreciable effect on the physical properties. However, it is always best to follow the manufacturer's instructions because of variations from one brand to another. The total amount of material dispensed depends on the size of the cavity preparation and method of insertion. This material is expensive, and needless waste often occurs. A new disposable plastic spatula is used to remove the pastes from the jars. To prevent cross contamination of the contents in the jars, it is important to use one end of a new spatula for dispensing the catalyst paste and the other end for base paste. This same spatula is placed adjacent to the pad so that it will be handy for mixing.

The bonding agent (adhesive) is dispensed last and mixed first. It is a liquid with low surface tension and has a tendency to run together. Usually one drop of each component (catalyst and base) is dispensed onto a second mixing pad, leaving a space of ¼ inch (6 mm) between the drops. The sponge is picked up with the operating pliers and used to stir the components of the bonding agent together for 5 seconds. The saturated sponge should be quickly blotted against a paper towel to remove excess and the bonding agent immediately applied to the etched enamel and conditioned dentin.

The composite material is mixed next with the same disposable plastic spatula that was used to dispense the materials. An assistant should mix the composite while the operator is mixing and applying the bonding agent. To initiate mixing, one paste is picked up with the spatula and placed on top of the other. With a wiping and folding motion, the catalyst and base are blended together for 30 seconds to obtain a homogeneous mixture. A stirring motion should be avoided because of the tendency to incorporate air into the mixture. Approximately 1 minute of working time remains for insertion of the material into the cavity preparation.

Light-cured composites. Many types of visible light units and brands of light-cured composites are commercially available. Light-cured materials usually include

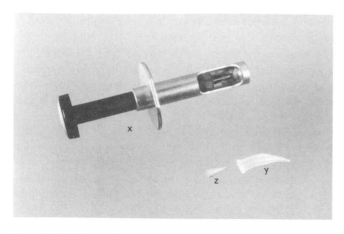

Fig. 16-58. Composite injection syringe *(x)* with disposable tip *(y)* and stopper *(z)*.

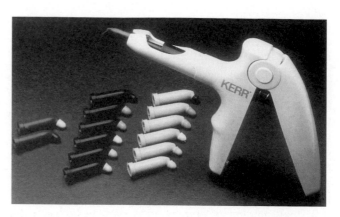

Fig. 16-59. Examples of pistol grip syringe and pre-loaded composite compule.

an enamel/dentin bonding agent and numerous syringes or self-contained syringe tips of various shades of composite.

No mixing of the visible light-cured materials is necessary unless a shade modification is desired (see Shade Selection). The operator should not dispense either the bonding agent or the composite until they are ready to be used. Both of these materials will begin to harden when exposed to daylight or other lights in the operatory.

Insertion instrumentation

A hand instrument or syringe can be used for inserting self-cured or light-cured composite. Both methods and materials will be presented in detail under insertion instructions for individual cavity preparations (in Application of Bonding Agent and Insertion of Composite).

Hand instrument. The use of a hand instrument is a popular method for placing composites because it is easy and fast. In addition to the simplicity of hand instrument insertion, a smaller amount of composite material is required, as compared to the amount needed for the syringe method. A disadvantage of hand instrument insertion is that air can be trapped in the cavity preparation and/or incorporated into the material during the insertion procedure. Experience and care in insertion, which is described later, will minimize this problem.

Syringe. An example of a syringe used for injecting composites is shown in Fig. 16-58 with its disposable tip and stopper. Black tips that are impervious to light penetration are also available for storing and injecting light-cured composite. The syringe technique is popular because it provides a convenient means for transporting the composite to the cavity preparation and reduces the possibility of trapping air. Many manufacturers produce pre-loaded syringe tips with a light-cured composite

(Fig. 16-59). Most are color coded for easy shade identification.

The syringe technique can present a problem in small cavity preparations with limited access because the syringe tip may be too large. When the cavity opening is questionable, an empty syringe tip should first be tried into the cavity preparation. When a syringe is used for self-cured composites, more material must be mixed than is required when inserting with a hand instrument.

The injectability of composites varies because of differences in viscosity and inorganic filler. Some microfill composites cannot be injected. Therefore this property of the material should be evaluated before clinical use.

APPLICATION OF BONDING AGENT AND INSERTION OF COMPOSITE
Class III, lingual access, polyester strip matrix, self-cured composites

The matrix is in place as previously described. Whenever possible, tilt the patient's head for direct vision, but most of the time indirect vision is required. With the mirror, hold the lingual portion of the strip away from the cavity opening to reflect light and to provide a clear view for inserting the composite (Fig. 16-60). Leave the facial end of the strip free.

With self-cured composites the time interval between mixing and polymerization is very short. Therefore mixing and application of materials must be carefully coordinated for optimal results. Everything must be in a "ready-to-go" position before mixing is initiated. Materials are inserted in two steps: bonding agent first and composite material second.

Hand instrument insertion. The mesial surface of a maxillary left lateral incisor serves as an example for this procedure (Fig. 16-61, *A*).

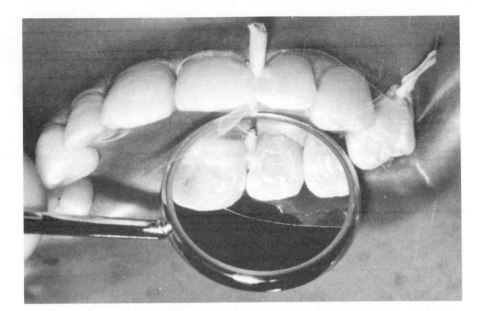

Fig. 16-60. Mirror is used to hold lingual portion of strip away from preparation, reflect light, and provide clear view for insertion of composite.

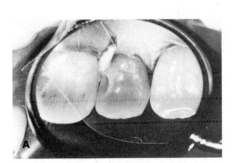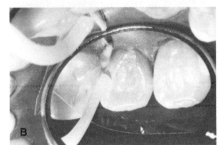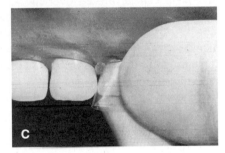

Fig. 16-61. Hand instrument insertion of composite. **A,** Class III lingual approach cavity preparation is to be restored. **B,** Composite is wiped into cavity preparation with blade end of hand instrument. **C,** Matrix strip is closed and held until composite is polymerized.

Mix the previously dispensed bonding agent with a foam sponge held in the beaks of operating pliers and blot against a paper towel to remove excess that would flood the cavity preparation. During application, cover the entire preparation (etched enamel and conditioned/primed dentin) with the adhesive bonding agent. Use a gentle stream of air to distribute the bonding agent in an even, thin layer. It is not necessary to wait for the bonding agent to set before placing the composite, since the outer surface of the bonding agent does not harden in the presence of air. If placement of the composite is delayed, this sticky film need not be removed because it will polymerize when air is excluded by the composite that is subsequently placed over it.

Mix the composite material as previously described. Most self-cured composite restorations require approximately 4 ½ minutes for the complete procedure: 30 seconds for mixing, 1 minute for insertion, and 3 minutes undisturbed time for final setting. Insert the mixed resin in two stages. First, pick up a small amount (approximately one-half the cavity size) on the blade end of the hand instrument and wipe into the cavity preparation (Fig. 16-61, *B*). Then use the plugger end to press the material into the retentive areas. If the composite has a tendency to stick to the instrument, a sparing amount of bonding agent can be used as a lubricant. This is easily obtained by touching the tip of the instrument to the bonding material left on the mixing pad or in the foam sponge applicator. Apply a second increment of composite to completely fill the cavity and provide a slight excess so that positive pressure can be applied with the matrix strip. Remove quickly any gross excess with the blade of the insertion instrument or an explorer tine before closing the matrix.

Set the mirror aside, and close the lingual end of the strip over the composite and hold with the index finger. Next, close the facial end of the strip over the tooth with the thumb and index finger of the other hand,

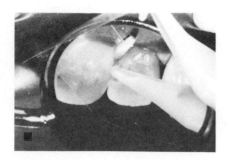

Fig. 16-62. Syringe injection of composite. Air entrapment is minimized by injecting composite starting in remote corner of preparation, as well as by slowly withdrawing tip while it is kept in restorative material during injection.

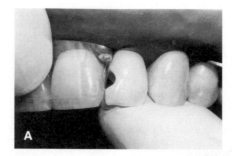

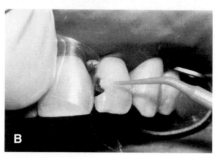

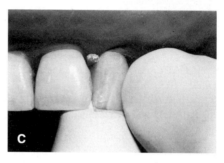

tightening the gingival aspect of the strip ahead of the incisal portion. The matrix can be held in this manner until polymerization is complete, or the thumb of the first hand can be placed over the facial of the strip to hold it without movement during final polymerization (Fig. 16-61, *C*). This latter maneuver frees the other hand for testing the hardening of the unused composite remaining on the mixing pad. After the composite hardens, remove the wedge and matrix strip before finishing the restoration (described in section on Finishing Technique for Composite).

Syringe injection. Mix the bonding agent and apply with a foam applicator in the usual manner. Following mixing of the composite, fill the syringe tip by pressing the large open end of the tip repeatedly into the composite mixture ("cookie-cutting") and then insert the stopper to force the material forward. Quickly place the filled syringe tip into the barrel of the injection syringe, and engage the plunger and press to extrude some of the composite out of the tip.

Starting in the most remote area of the cavity preparation, steadily inject the composite, being sure that the tip remains in the filling material while slowly withdrawing the syringe (Fig. 16-62). Fill the preparation to slight excess so that positive pressure can be applied by the matrix strip. Before the matrix strip is closed, remove any gross excess with a hand instrument. Close and secure the matrix strip as described previously.

Class III, facial access, polyester strip matrix, self-cured composites

Hold the polyester strip on the lingual aspect of the tooth to be restored with the index finger while the thumb reflects the facial end out of the way. If the wedge protrudes enough to interfere with access, shorten it and/or reposition.

Mix and apply the bonding agent as previously described. Follow the same insertion technique with a

Fig. 16-63. Insertion of light-cured composite. **A,** Lingual aspect of strip is secured with index finger while facial portion is reflected away for access. Bonding agent is applied **(B),** thinned with gentle stream of clean, dry air, and cured. **C,** Following insertion of composite, matrix strip is closed and material is cured through strip.

hand instrument or syringe for the facial approach as with the lingual approach. The procedure is simplified in that direct vision can be used.

Class III, facial access, polyester strip matrix, light-cured composites

The mesial surface of a maxillary left lateral incisor is used to demonstrate facial insertion of a light-cured composite. The matrix strip is contoured, placed interproximally, and wedged at the gingival margin. Secure the lingual aspect of the strip with the index finger while the thumb reflects the facial portion out of the way (Fig. 16-63, *A*). Light-cured materials do not have to be mixed and are not dispensed until ready for use.

Apply the adhesive bonding agent to the etched

enamel and conditioned/primed dentin with a small foam sponge or brush (Fig. 16-63, *B*). Distribute this material evenly and blow off any excess using a gentle stream of air. Cure the bonding agent with the visible light source for 10 to 20 seconds, with the tip near the preparation but not touching the tooth. Now insert the composite by hand instrument or syringe, close the strip and hold without movement while curing the composite with the light through the strip for 20 seconds (Fig. 16-63, *C*). Do not touch the strip with the tip of the light initially, since it could distort the contour of the restoration. Then remove the index finger and light-cure on the lingual surface an additional 20 seconds. Longer exposure to the light is required for the polymerization of dark and opaque shades. If the restoration is undercontoured, more composite can be added over the first and cured. No etching or bonding agent is required between layers if the surface is still the oxygen-inhibited layer. *With large restorations it is better to add and cure the composite in several increments to reduce the effects of polymerization shrinkage and to ensure more complete curing in remote regions.*

Class IV, polyester strip matrix, self-cured or light-cured composites

For most Class IV preparations a polyester strip matrix may be used as previously described. Following application of the resin bonding agent, insert the composite either with a hand instrument or syringe as described earlier for Class III restorations. Care must be taken when closing the strip not to pull with excessive force, since the soft material will be extruded incisally and result in an undercontoured restoration. If this happens, add composite to restore proper contour and contact.

Class IV, compound-supported matrix, self-cured or light-cured composites

A compound-supported matrix as previously described is much more appropriate for large Class IV cavity preparations. Apply (and cure for light-cured) the resin bonding agent first. When restoring with a *self-cured composite,* insertion is best accomplished by injecting the material with a syringe. Care must be taken to provide a slight excess of material at the exposed margins to ensure proper contour of the restoration after finishing.

Light-cured composites also can be used with compound-supported matrices for Class IV restorations. After the adhesive bonding agent has been applied and cured, insert the composite and cure in increments to ensure complete polymerization and to reduce the effects of polymerization shrinkage. Insertion is best accomplished with a hand instrument, although a syringe can be used. Because light-cured composites possess the advantage of an extended working time, the material

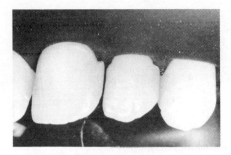

Fig. 16-64. Adjacent restorations restored simultaneously displaying faulty contours and gingival overhangs.

can be manipulated and shaped to a considerable degree before curing. Following polymerization, remove the supporting compound and strip. Finishing is described in a later section.

Adjacent proximal cavity preparations, self-cured or light-cured composites

Adjacent proximal cavity preparations should be restored one at a time. Techniques have been suggested for inserting two approximating restorations simultaneously, but these procedures generally result in matrix movement, poor adaptation, open contact, overhangs, and faulty contours (Fig. 16-64).

Restore the cavity preparation with the least access first. The matrix strip has been placed and wedged. Now apply the adhesive bonding agent (and cure for light-cured). Again, depending on the individual circumstance and operator, insert the composite (self-cured or light-cured) with either a hand instrument or syringe. If there is too much convexity present on the first restoration, the excess must be removed before the second restoration is inserted. If too little contour is present, more material is added to correct the contour. The first restoration should be contoured completely before the second one is started.

Since there will be some contamination of the second cavity preparation, it will need to be cleaned and etched before the composite is inserted. During these procedures, a strip should be in place to protect the first restoration and tooth.

Class V cavity preparations, self-cured or light-cured composites

No matrix is used when restoring Class V preparations because the contour of the restoration can be controlled during insertion. A self-cured or light-cured composite can be inserted with a hand instrument or syringe. Recall that microfill composites are recommended for most Class V restorations.

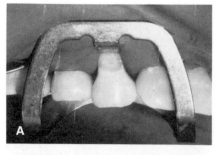
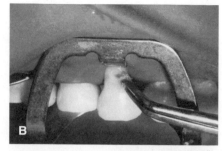
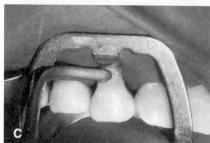
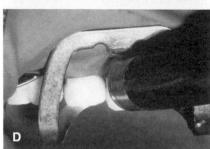

Fig. 16-65. Restoration of abrasion/erosion lesion. **A,** Cavity preparation. **B,** Bonding agent applied. **C,** Material is inserted incrementally. **D,** Restoration cured with visible light source.

Self-cured composites, hand instrument insertion. Since no matrix is used, care must be exercised to avoid having excess bonding agent, because it tends to act as a lubricant in the preparation. Wipe a small portion of mixed composite into the preparation with the blade of the hand instrument and jiggle to place with the plugger end. The tip can be lubricated with a sparing amount of bonding agent. Usually a second increment is needed and sufficient to slightly overfill the cavity. Remove the excess first at the gingival cavosurface margin with the tine of a No. 2 explorer. If the composite begins to harden before contouring is complete, further contouring should not be attempted at this stage.

Self-cured composites, syringe injection. Until experience is gained with hand insertion, injecting the composite with a syringe may be much easier for insertion into Class V cavity preparations. Follow the same procedures described in a previous section for applying the bonding agent, mixing the composite, and inserting it by syringe into Class III preparations.

Light-cured composites, hand instrument or syringe. A light-cured material is recommended for Class V preparations because of the extended working time and control of contour before polymerization. Less finishing is usually required. This feature is particularly valuable when dealing with large preparations or preparations with margins located on cementum, because rotary instrumentation can easily damage contiguous tooth structure.

The restoration of an abrasion/erosion lesion (Fig. 16-65, *A*) will illustrate proper insertion techniques. Following etching and conditioning/priming steps for enamel and dentin (per manufacturer's instructions), place a thin layer of adhesive bonding agent and cure (Fig. 16-65, *B*). Then insert the composite incrementally with a hand instrument or syringe (Fig. 16-65, *C*). Fill deep cavity preparations having retentive undercuts in at least two increments. First, insert a small amount of material in the retentive undercuts. Second, fill the outer portion of the preparation and shape the material as close to the final contour as possible. An explorer is useful in removing excess material from the cervical margin and obtaining the final contour. Then apply the light source for polymerization (Fig. 16-65, *D*). The restoration should require very little finishing.

FINISHING TECHNIQUE FOR COMPOSITE

Good technique and experience in inserting composites significantly reduce the amount of finishing required. Usually a slight excess of material is present that must be removed to provide the final contour and smooth finish. Coarse diamond instruments are not generally recommended for finishing composites because of the high risk of inadvertently damaging contiguous tooth structure. They also leave a rough surface on the restoration and tooth, as compared to finishing burs and discs. However, special diamond finishing instruments are available commercially and can be used to obtain excellent results if the manufacturer's instructions are followed. Care must be exercised with all rotary instruments to prevent damage to the tooth structure, especially at the gingival marginal areas.

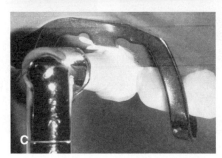
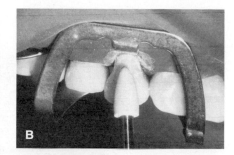
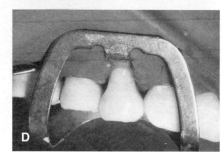

Fig. 16-66. Finishing and polishing. **A,** Flame-shaped finishing bur removing excess and contouring. Rubber polishing point **(B)** and aluminum oxide polishing paste **(C)** used for final polishing. **D,** Completed restoration.

Facial areas

A flame-shaped carbide finishing bur is recommended for removing excess composite on facial surfaces (Fig. 16-66, *A*). Use medium speed with light intermittent brush strokes and an air coolant for contouring. Final finishing and polishing are achieved with a rubber polishing point (Fig. 16-66, *B)* and an aluminum oxide polishing paste (Fig. 16-66, *C* and *D*).

For some locations a sandpaper disc (degree of abrasiveness depends on the amount of excess to be removed) mounted on a Moore mandrel* in an angle handpiece at low speed can be substituted for or used after the finishing bur (Fig. 16-67, *A*). No lubricant is placed on the bur or disc, since it is easier to see the composite and evaluate contours without it. The disc is rotated at low speed. The external enamel surface should act as a guide for proper contour. A constant shifting motion will aid in contouring and preventing the development of a flat surface. Do final polishing with a fine grit disc.

Another type of disc system known as Sof-Lex† is available for contouring and polishing. These discs are flexible and are produced in several diameters and abrasive textures. Also, Pop-On‡ discs and mandrels are available. This unique design provides a much smaller metal center and allows the disc to be placed on and removed from the mandrel without the need for proper orientation. Thin discs with small diameters, such as Super Snap* discs, will fit into embrasure areas more easily and are especially useful in contouring and polishing gingival areas.

Use rotary instruments very carefully in gingival locations to prevent inadvertent and undesirable removal of tooth structure.

Lingual areas

Lingual excess of composite is removed and a smooth surface is produced using a round 12-bladed carbide finishing bur at medium speed with air coolant and light intermittent pressure (Fig. 16-67, *B*). A bur of appropriate size and shape is used depending on the amount of excess and shape of the lingual surface. White stones in various shapes and sizes may also be used for final finishing of the lingual surface. If isolation is by the rubber dam, checking the occlusion and correcting (if indicated) follows removal of the dam (see Occlusion).

Proximal and embrasure areas

The gingival margin should always be examined for excess composite with an explorer. A sharp, gold finishing knife is well suited for removing excess material from the gingival proximal area. This instrument should be moved from the restoration to the tooth or along the margins, using light shaving strokes and keeping a portion of the cutting edge on the external enamel surface

*Moore Mandrel, EC Moore Co., Dearborn, Mich.
†Sof-Lex, 3M Company, St. Paul, Minn.
‡Pop-On, 3M Company, St. Paul, Minn.

*Super Snap, Shofu, Dental Corporation, Menlo Park, Calif.

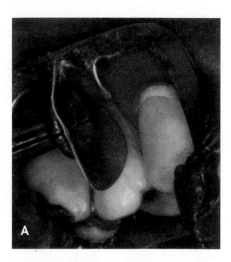

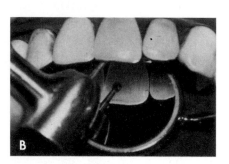

Fig. 16-67. Finishing composites. **A,** Abrasive disc mounted on mandrel can be used for finishing when access permits. **B,** Round carbide finishing bur is well suited for finishing lingual surfaces. **C,** No. 12 surgical blade in Bard-Parker handle can be used for removing interproximal excess. **D,** Abrasive strip should be curved over area to be finished.

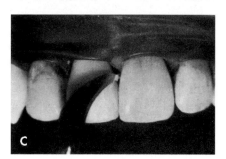

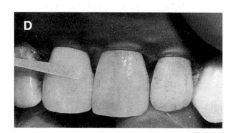

as a guide to prevent over-reduction. If a large amount of composite is removed with one stroke or in the wrong direction, it may fracture within the cavity margin and warrant a repair, because an irregular void that is left to collect plaque and debris invites discoloration or recurrent caries. Using the secondary cutting edges on the heel aspect of the blade in a scraping-pull mode is often preferred over using the primary cutting edge in the shaving mode. The knife blade design having these secondary edges in an arc is very helpful.

A carbon steel No. 12 surgical blade (not No. 12-B) in a Bard-Parker handle also can be used for removing interproximal excess (Fig. 16-67, *C*). The curved shape of the blade and the thin diameter make this instrument ideal for removing gingival overhangs. Gently shave away the excess to avoid removing a large chunk of material unintentionally.

Both the gold knife and No. 12 scalpel blade are made of carbon steel and may leave gray marks on the restoration. This discoloration is superficial and is easily removed during the final finishing by abrasive strips or discs (Fig. 16-67, *D*).

Special carbide finishing burs* and carbide hand instruments† can be used for removing excess and opening embrasure areas. Caution must be taken with all instruments not to remove too much contour or to produce a "ledged" contact (a ledge bordering the contact area).

Final contouring and finishing of proximal surfaces is completed with finishing strips. Some strips have two different types of abrasives (medium and fine) on opposing ends of the strip, with a small area between where no abrasive is present to allow easy and safe insertion of the strip through the contact area. The medium grit is zirconium silicate, and the fine grit is aluminum oxide. Different widths of the strips are available. A narrow width is usually more appropriate for contouring, since it allows more versatility for finishing specific areas. Wide strips tend to flatten the proximal contour, remove too much material at the contact areas, and extend too far gingivally. This results in a poor

*Esthetic Trimmers, Brasseler, U.S.A., Inc., Lombard, Ill.
†Carbide Carvers, Brasseler, U.S.A., Inc., Lombard, Ill.

contour and a weak contact or no contact, which must be corrected.

The strip should not be drawn back-and-forth across the restoration in a "sawing" manner. Rather, it should be curved over the restoration and tooth surface in a fashion similar to that which is used with a shoe-shine cloth, concentrating on areas that need attention (Fig. 16-67, *D*). To open the lingual embrasure or round the marginal ridge, the lingual part of the strip is held against the composite with the index finger of one hand while the other end of the strip is pulled facially with the other hand.

Occlusion

Remove the rubber dam if one was used. Evaluate the occlusion by having the patient close lightly on a piece of articulating paper and slide the mandibular teeth over the restored area. If excess composite is present, remove only a small amount at a time and re-check with articulating paper. It is sometimes helpful to recontour the adjacent and/or opposing natural teeth, although care must be taken not to remove a tooth's centric or functional contact.

Microfill composites

Although generally the same technique used for finishing conventional and hybrid composites applies to finishing microfill composites, certain differences do exist. Conventional and hybrid composites exhibit an opaque appearance during dry finishing, making the cavity margin easy to distinguish. Because microfill composites possess a surface luster similar to that of tooth enamel, it is more difficult to detect when the restoration has been finished back to the margin. Also, because less inorganic filler is present in microfill composites, finishing burs tend to clog and need periodic debridement.

Although conventional finishing techniques produce a smooth surface texture with microfill composites, a higher luster can be attained by using various discs, rubber points, or cups that are specifically made for polishing these materials.

GLASS IONOMER RESTORATIONS

As noted earlier, glass ionomers possess the favorable quality of releasing fluoride when exposed to the oral environment.[30,43] This property renders glass ionomer restorations more resistant to recurrent caries. Because of this anticariogenic quality, glass ionomer is often the ideal material choice for restoring root surface caries in patients with high caries activity and where esthetics is not so critical.

Both self-cured and light-cured versions of glass ionomers are available. Light-cured glass ionomers are pre-

ferred because of both the extended working time and their improved physical properties. Also, light-cured glass ionomers tend to be more resistant to dehydration and cracking during setting than are conventional self-cured versions.

Unfortunately, glass ionomers are not as esthetic as composite restorations. For this reason, glass ionomers are not recommended for use in areas of significant esthetic concern. However, newer light-cured "hybrid" (resin-modified) versions of glass ionomers contain some resin and possess much improved esthetic qualities, as well as other improved physical properties. In fact, this type of glass ionomer may be used even in the most esthetically demanding areas.

Because of their limited strength and wear resistance, glass ionomers are indicated generally for the restoration of low stress areas (not for typical Class I, II, or IV cavities) where caries activity potential is of significant concern. In addition to glass ionomers being indicated for root surface caries in Class V locations, slot-like preparations in either Class II or III cervical locations (not involving the proximal contact) may be restored with glass ionomers if access permits.

Class V preparation

The restoration of root carious lesions in elderly patients or those with high caries activity is the primary indication for the use of glass ionomer. Notched cervical defects of idiopathic, erosion, or abrasion origin (or any combination) also are well-suited for restoration with glass ionomers if esthetic demands are not critical. The cavity preparations for either of these clinical indications are the same as previously described for composite restorations. Review previous sections titled, Class V Cavity Preparations for Composite, and Class V Cavity Preparation for Abrasion/Erosion Lesions, especially noting Figs. 16-44, 16-50, and 16-52.

Classes II and III slot preparations

Elderly patients and those with high caries activity who have gingival recession may also experience carious lesions on the proximal root surfaces. Gingival recession frequently provides ready access to the carious lesion from the facial or lingual direction allowing a slot type of preparation to be used. The same slot preparation design used for amalgam is used for glass ionomers. The reader is referred to the section on slot preparations in Chapter 13 and Fig. 16-24 for specific details.

Insertion of the glass ionomer

With the exception of the matrix utilized (if needed), slot type preparations for Classes II and III cavities are restored in a similar manner to a Class V preparation.

Following preparation of the tooth, protect deeply

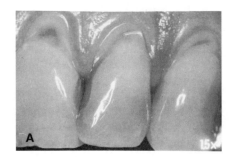
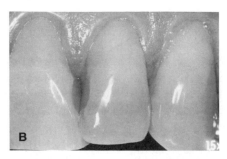

Fig. 16-68. Glass ionomer cement. Three typical light-cured glass ionomer restorations are shown before, **A,** and after, **B,** treatment.

excavated areas (within 0.5 mm of the pulp) with a calcium hydroxide liner/base. Glass ionomers should not be placed in close proximity to the pulp. Most glass ionomer systems require conditioning the dentinal surfaces to remove the smear layer, thereby effecting improved adhesion of the glass ionomer to the dentin. To condition the dentin, a mild acid such as 10% polyacrylic acid is placed in the cavity preparation for approximately 20 seconds, followed by rinsing and drying with clean, dry air. Dentin conditioning should be done only after placement of any needed calcium hydroxide liner or base. It should be noted that not all glass ionomer systems require dentin conditioning. Additionally, some new resin-modified glass ionomers use an intermediary bonding agent to facilitate bonding. *Each glass ionomer system should be used strictly according to the manufacturer's specific instructions.*

Most glass ionomer systems are quite technique sensitive. Original glass ionomers usually required carefully mixing a powder and liquid within 30 seconds to optimize powder incorporation (higher powder/liquid ratio). Currently, encapsulated versions for triturator mixing are available also. Such systems are recommended because they optimize and simplify the mixing procedure and facilitate insertion through direct injection into the cavity.

Place the glass ionomer material in slight excess and quickly shape it with a composite instrument. Clear plastic cervical matrices are also available for providing contour to the restoration. If a conventional type of glass ionomer is used, place a thin coat of light-cured resin bonding agent on the surface immediately after placement to prevent dehydration and cracking of the restoration during the initial setting phase. As noted earlier, new light-cured hybrid type glass ionomers are more resistant to dehydration and do not typically require this step. If a light-cured glass ionomer is used, cure for a minimum time of 40 seconds.

Contouring and finishing glass ionomers

Conventional versions of glass ionomers ideally require a polymerization period of 24 hours before final contouring and finishing. However, most light-cured glass ionomers presently available can be contoured and finished immediately after light curing. (The manufacturer's recommendations should be followed to optimize clinical performance of the material.) Once the material has set, the matrix, if used, is removed and the gross excess is shaved away with either a No. 12 surgical blade in a Bard-Parker handle or other appropriately shaped knives or scalers. As much as possible of the contouring and finishing should be accomplished with hand instruments, while striving to preserve the smooth surface that occurs upon setting. If rotary instrumentation is needed, care must be taken not to dehydrate the surface of the restoration. Micron finishing diamonds used with a petroleum lubricant to prevent desiccation are ideal for contouring and finishing. Also, flexible abrasive discs used with a lubricant can be very effective. A fine grit aluminum oxide polishing paste applied with a prophy cup is used to impart a smooth surface. Three typical light-cured glass ionomer restorations are shown before and after treatment in Fig. 16-68, *A* and *B*.

REFERENCES

1. Bowen RL: Adhesive bonding of various materials to hard tooth tissues. V. The effect of a surface active comonomer on adhesion to diverse substrates, *J Dent Res* 44:1369, 1965.
2. Bowen RL: Properties of a silica-reinforced polymer for dental restorations, *J Am Dent Assoc* 66:57, 1963.
3. Bowen RL: Dental filling material comprising vinyl-silane treated fused silica and a binder consisting of the reaction product of bis-phenol and glycidyl acrylate, U.S. Patent 3,06,112, Nov. 27, 1962.
4. Buonocore MG: A simple method of increasing the adhesion of acrylic filling materials to enamel surfaces, *J Dent Res* 34:849, 1955.
5. Buonocore M, Wileman W, Brudevold F: A report on a resin composition capable of bonding to human dentin surfaces, *J Dent Res* 35:846, 1956.
6. Byram JQ: *Principles and practice of filling teeth with porcelain,* New York, 1908, Consolidated Dental Manufacturing Co.
7. Calamia JR: High-strength porcelain bonded restorations: anterior and posterior, *Quint Inter* 20(10):717-726, 1989.
8. Charbeneau GT et al: *Principles and practice of operative dentistry,* ed 1, Philadelphia, 1975, Lea & Febiger.

9. Craig, RG: Chemistry, composition, and properties of composite resins, *Dent Clin North Am* 25(2):219, 1981.

10. Craig RG, editor: *Restorative dental materials,* ed 6, St Louis, 1980, Mosby.

11. Davis EL et al: Adhesion of dentin bonding agents after smear layer treatments, *Am J Dent* 5(1):29-32, 1992.

12. Davis WC: *Operative dentistry,* ed 5, St Louis, 1945, Mosby.

13. Dilts WE, Podshadley A, Neiman R: Effect of pins on some physical characteristics of composite resins, *J Am Dent Assoc* 87:595, 1973.

14. Farah JW, Dougherty EW: Unfilled, filled, and microfilled composite resins, *Oper Dent* 6(3):95, 1981.

15. Friedman MJ: The enamel ceramic alternative: porcelain veneers vs metal ceramic crowns, *CDA Journal* 20(8):27-32, 1992.

16. Garberoglio R, Cozzani G: In vivo effect of oral environment on etched enamel: a scanning microscopic study, *J Dent Res* 58:1859, 1979.

17. Heymann HO: The artistry of conservative esthetic dentistry, *J Am Dent Assoc* (special issue):14E-23E, 1987.

18. Heymann HO et al: Examining tooth flexure effects on cervical restorations: a two-year clinical study, *J Am Dent Assoc* 122:41-47, 1991.

19. Jaärvinen VK, Rytömaa II, Heinonen OP: Risk factors in dental erosion, *J Dent Res* 70(6):942-947, 1991.

20. Jorgensen KD, Matono R, Shimokobe H: Deformation of cavities and resin fillings in loaded teeth, *J Dent Res* 84:46-50, 1976.

21. Joynt RB et al: Dentin bonding agents and the smear layer, *Oper Dent* 16:186-191, 1991.

22. Lee WC, Eakle WS: Possible role of tensile stress in the etiology of cervical erosive lesions of teeth, *J Prosthet Dent* 52(3):374-380, 1984.

23. Leinfelder KF, Isenberg BP, Essig ME: A new method for generating ceramic restorations: a CAD-CAM system, *J Am Dent Assoc* 118:703-707, 1989.

24. Lorton L, Brady J: Criteria for successful composite resin restorations, *Gen Dent* 29(3):234, 1981.

25. Mair LH: Wear in dentistry—current terminology, *J Dent* 20:140-144, 1992.

26. Monteiro S Jr et al: Evaluation of materials and techniques for restoration of erosion areas, *J Prosthet Dent* 55:434-442, 1986.

27. Morin D, DeLong R, Douglas WH: Cusp reinforcement by the acid-etch technique, *J Dent Res* 63:1075-1078, 1984.

28. Mormann WH et al: CAD-CAM ceramic inlays and onlays: a case report after 3 years in place, *J Am Dent Assoc* 120:517-520, 1990.

29. Mormann WH et al: Chairside computer-aided direct ceramic inlays, *Quint Inter* 20:329-339, 1989.

30. Mount GJ: Adhesion of glass-ionomer cement in the clinical environment, *Oper Dent* 16:141-148, 1991.

31. Nelson RJ, Wolcott RB, Paffenbarger GC: Fluid exchange at the margins of dental restorations, *J Am Dent Assoc* 44:288, 1952.

32. Paffenbarger GC: Silicate cement: an investigation by a group of practicing dentists under the direction of the ADA research fellowship at the National Bureau of Standards, *J Am Dent Assoc* 27:1611, 1940.

33. Pashley DH: The effects of acid etching on the pulpodentin complex, *Oper Dent* 17:229-242, 1992.

34. Prevost AP, Fuller JL, Peterson LC: The use of an intermediate resin in the acid-etch procedure: retentive strength, microleakage, and failure mode analysis, *J Dent Res* 61(2):412-418, 1982.

35. Qualtrough AJE, Wilson NHF, Smith GA: The porcelain inlay: a historical view, *Oper Dent* 15:61-70, 1990.

36. Reinhardt JW, Chan DC, Boyer DB: Shear strengths of ten commercial dentin bonding agents, *Dent Mater* 3(1)43-45, 1987.

37. Retief DH et al: Tensile bond strengths of dentin bonding agents to dentin, *Dent Mater* 2(2):72-77, 1986.

38. Seltzer S: The penetration of microorganisms between the tooth and direct resin fillings, *J Am Dent Assoc* 51:560, 1955.

39. Silverstone LM, Dogan IL, editors: *Proceedings of the international symposium on the acid etch technique,* St Paul, Minn, 1975, North Central Publishing.

40. Skinner EW: Comparison of the properties and uses of silicate cement and acrylic resin in operative dentistry, *J Am Dent Assoc* 58:27, 1959.

41. Sockwell CL: Clinical evaluation of anterior restorative materials, *Dent Clin North Am* 20:403, 1976.

42. Sturdevant CM et al: *The art and science of operative dentistry,* ed 1, New York, 1968, McGraw-Hill Book Co.

43. Swift EJ: Effects of glass ionomers on recurrent caries, *Oper Dent* 14:40-43, 1989.

44. Tagami J, Hosoda H, Fusayama T: Optimal technique of etching enamel, *Oper Dent* 13:181-184, 1988.

45. Taleghani M, Leinfelder KF, Lane J: Posterior porcelain bonded inlays, *Compend Contin Educ Dent* 8(6):410-415, 1987.

46. Volker J, Bilkakis E, Melillo S: Some observations on the relationship between plastic filling materials and dental caries, *Tufts Dent Outlook* 18:4, 1944.

47. Welk DA, Laswell HR: Rationale for designing cavity preparations in light of current knowledge and technology, *Dent Clin North Am* 20(2):231, 1976.

48. Wilson AD, Kent BE: A new translucent cement for dentistry. The glass ionomer cement, *Brit Dent J* 132:133-135, 1972.

CHAPTER 17

Tooth-colored restorations for Classes I, II, and VI cavity preparations

Harald O. Heymann

John R. Sturdevant

Theodore M. Roberson

Clarence L. Sockwell*

*This author is inactive this edition; see Preface.

INTRODUCTION

For years, dentistry has strived to develop esthetic alternatives to dental amalgam and gold for the conservative restoration of posterior teeth. With the advent of the acid etch technique, including the conditioning of

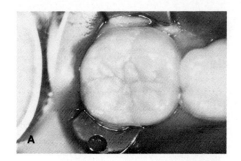
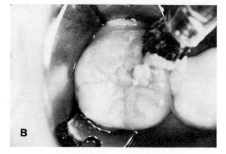
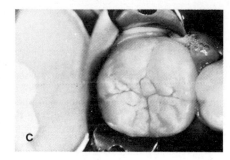
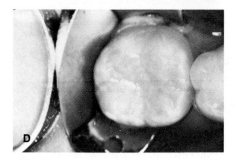

Fig. 17-1. Steps in application of sealant. **A,** Fissure in occlusal surface of mandibular molar with area isolated by rubber dam. **B,** Cleaning surface with pumice and bristle brush. **C,** Properly etched surface with lightly frosted appearance. **D,** Sealant inserted and finished. (Courtesy Dr. William Vann, Jr.)

both enamel and dentin, bonded restorations have become a reality.

This chapter presents the rationale and technique for the use of bonded tooth-colored materials on the occlusal and/or proximal surfaces of posterior teeth. Both sealants and tooth-colored restorations (including directly placed posterior composites, indirectly fabricated processed composite inlays/onlays, and indirect ceramic restorations) will be addressed. All of these materials offer one principal advantage over amalgam or gold—superior esthetics. They also conserve and strengthen tooth structure by virtue of being bonded. However, these restorative alternatives are not as technique friendly as dental amalgam nor offer the clinical longevity of a well-placed gold inlay or onlay (although recent improvements in dentin bonding and properties of tooth-colored materials offer a promising future). Nonetheless, esthetic alternatives presented in this chapter do offer specific advantages that make them a viable restorative option in many cases.

One of the first applications of the acid etch technique was with pit and fissure sealants. Recognizing the advantages of this technique, Buonocore[6] reported in 1955 that acid etching also could have other significant applications in restorative dentistry. Needless to say, the acid etch technique has found many uses in restorative dentistry; therefore, it seems most logical to begin discussing tooth-colored restorations involving the occlusal surfaces of posterior teeth with a review of pit and fissure sealants.

PIT AND FISSURE SEALANTS

As noted earlier in Chapters 2, 3, and 7, pits and fissures typically result from an incomplete coalescence of enamel and are particularly prone to caries. By using a low-viscosity fluid resin, these areas can be sealed following acid etching of the walls of the pits/fissures and a few millimeters of surface enamel bordering these faults.

Long-term clinical studies indicate that pit and fissure sealants provide a safe and effective method of preventing caries.[33,38] Sealants are most effective when they are applied in children to the pits and fissures of permanent posterior teeth immediately upon eruption of the clinical crowns. Adults also can benefit from the use of sealants if the individual experiences a change in caries susceptibility due to a change in their diet or medical condition (see Chapter 3).

Sealant materials (self-cured and light-cured) are based on urethane dimethacrylate or Bis-GMA resin. Tints are frequently added to sealants to produce color contrast for visual assessment.

Clinical studies show that sealants can be applied even over small, cavitated lesions with no subsequent progression of caries.[24,11] However, *it is recommended that sealants be used for the prevention of caries rather than for the treatment of existing carious lesions.* Therefore, a recent bitewing radiograph should be made and evaluated prior to sealant placement to ensure that no caries is evident that penetrates pulpally of the dentinoenamel junction (DEJ). Only caries-free pits and fissures or incipient lesions in enamel not extending to the DEJ are recommended for treatment with pit and fissure sealants.

Technique

Because there are variations in materials and techniques, it is important to follow the manufacturer's instructions for the sealant material being used. A standard method for applying sealants to posterior teeth is presented. Each quadrant is treated separately and may involve one or more teeth. The following discussion deals with a fissure present on a mandibular first permanent molar (Fig. 17-1, *A*). The tooth is isolated by a rubber dam (or cotton rolls) and cleaned with a slurry of pumice on a bristle brush (Fig. 17-1, *B*). Bristles reach into faulty areas better than a rubber prophy cup, which

Fig. 17-2. Typical failures of early composite restorations of occlusal and proximal surfaces. **A,** Color changes, no proximal contacts, and marginal leakage. **B,** Occlusal wear with loss of centric stops in central fossae.

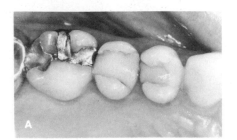
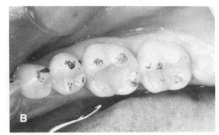

tends to burnish debris and pumice into the pits and fissures. The tooth is rinsed thoroughly while the explorer tip is used carefully to help remove residual pumice or additional debris. After the area is dried, a liquid acid etchant (35% to 50% phosphoric acid) is placed on the occlusal surface with a small sponge or brush for 30 seconds. Gel etchants, traditionally used for most restorative procedures, have less ability to effectively penetrate into the pits and fissures. Laser cleaning and etching is an alternative to traditional techniques, but lasing units are not yet widely available in general practice.

Next, the tooth is rinsed with water for 20 seconds while the area is evacuated with suction and then dried of all visible moisture. The properly acid-etched surface has a lightly frosted appearance (Fig. 17-1, *C*). Fluoride-rich, resistant enamel may need to be etched longer. Any brown stains that originally may have been in the pits/fissures may still be present and should be allowed to remain. The self-cured sealant is mixed and applied with a small applicator provided in the sealant kit. The sealant is gently teased to place to avoid entrapping air and it should slightly overfill all pits and fissures. Some operators prefer light-cured sealants, which also work well. After polymerization of the sealant, the rubber dam is removed, and the occlusion is evaluated using articulating paper. If necessary, a round 12-bladed carbide finishing bur or white stone is used to remove the excess. The surface usually does not require further polishing (Fig. 17-1, *D*).

HISTORY, DIAGNOSIS, AND TREATMENT PLANNING FOR DIRECT COMPOSITE RESTORATIONS INVOLVING OCCLUSAL SURFACES

There have been many attempts over the years to use various types of tooth-colored materials (synthetic resins and fused porcelain) as substitutes for amalgam or gold in restoring occlusal and proximal surfaces of posterior teeth. Many patients consider esthetics a major concern for these posterior restorations, even in areas that cannot normally be seen. Thus there is increasing patient demand for esthetic treatment of not only anterior teeth but also posterior teeth.

Many factors must be evaluated when selecting an esthetic restorative material, especially for use in high-stress areas. In a general practice it is not always possible to provide "ideal" dentistry because of limitations due to patient preferences, operator skill, laboratory support, economic considerations, and esthetics. As will be illustrated, *composite materials can be used successfully for restoring Classes I, II, and VI cavities when proper operative techniques are followed.*

History

The use of directly placed composite materials for Classes I and II cavity preparations was introduced in the mid-1960s.[22,23] Desirable features of these materials compared with metallic restorations were cited as better esthetics, fracture resistance, marginal integrity, wear resistance, low thermal conductivity, absence of tarnish or corrosion, low toxicity, and completion of the restoration in one appointment. Many of these initial claims were based on laboratory tests, and others were based on short-term clinical studies. Although the original clinical performance of early composite materials on occlusal and proximal surfaces seemed promising, failures began to occur in approximately 2 years.[17,29] Failures resulted from color changes, wear, microleakage, and recurrent caries (Fig. 17-2). It was apparent that laboratory tests were not totally effective in predicting the clinical behavior of composite materials, because the impact of the dynamic forces of mastication and other factors in the oral environment were not included.

Numerous improvements were made in the design of composite materials and their insertion techniques from 1970 to the 1990s.[2,14,37,40,41] Long-term clinical studies revealed encouraging improvements such as improved color stability, resistance to microleakage, reduced wear, and a lower incidence of recurrent caries. However, loss of contour in high-stress areas still presented a major problem (Fig. 17-3, *A* and *B*). Yet, some composite restorations of this same generation were observed to have shown very little surface loss when used in areas of the posterior teeth that had little or no occlusal contact (Fig. 17-3, *C* to *E*). Processes of composite wear are discussed in detail in Chapter 6.

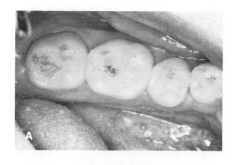
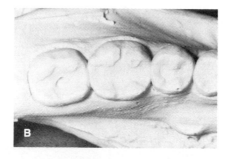
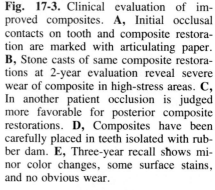
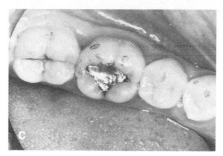
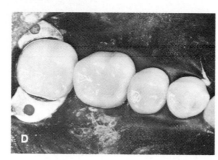
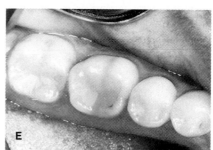

Fig. 17-3. Clinical evaluation of improved composites. **A,** Initial occlusal contacts on tooth and composite restoration are marked with articulating paper. **B,** Stone casts of same composite restorations at 2-year evaluation reveal severe wear of composite in high-stress areas. **C,** In another patient occlusion is judged more favorable for posterior composite restorations. **D,** Composites have been carefully placed in teeth isolated with rubber dam. **E,** Three-year recall shows minor color changes, some surface stains, and no obvious wear.

Present status

The search continues for an ideal tooth-colored material for high-stress areas. Newer formulations possess the following general composition features and improved properties: (1) radiopaque fillers, (2) smaller sizes of primary filler particles and the inclusion of dispersed microfillers, (3) increased amounts of filler and a corresponding decrease in the resin matrix, (4) greater strength and stiffness, (5) reduced porosity, (6) reduced water sorption, (7) compatibility with new enamel/dentin bonding agents, and (8) polymerization by visible light. More recent clinical studies of composite restorations in Classes I and II cavity preparations are in progress and long-term reports are encouraging.[3,4,20,21] In fact, the ADA Council on Dental Materials, Instruments, and Equipment has given Acceptance status to several composite materials for limited use in conservative Classes I and II preparations in the absence of significant occlusal stress. However, as of this writing, the ADA Council under its present Acceptance Program has not yet recognized any composite material as an amalgam substitute. Nonetheless, composite restorations involving the occlusal surface can provide a definite service when used appropriately. *Proper operative procedures and material manipulation are essential to ensure optimal results.*

Advantages

Advantages of bonded, direct, composite restorations (versus dental amalgam) for Classes I, II, and VI cavity preparations are as follows:
1. Esthetics
2. Conservation of tooth structure
3. Improved resistance to microleakage
4. Strengthening of the remaining tooth structure
5. Low thermal conductivity
6. Completion in one appointment
7. Economics—less expensive compared with gold or porcelain restorations
8. No corrosion

Disadvantages

The following features of present, direct posterior (Classes I, II, and VI) composites are considered disadvantages (compared with dental amalgam), some more so than others:
1. Very technique sensitive
2. Higher coefficient of thermal expansion than tooth structure
3. Low modulus of elasticity
4. Biocompatibility of some components unknown
5. Limited wear resistance in high-stress areas

Indications

A summary of primary indications for the use of direct composite materials in posterior teeth follows:
1. Classes I and II cavities that can be appropriately isolated and where some centric contact(s) on tooth structure is(are) present
2. Class V defects (see Chapter 16): (a) hypoplasia; (b) hypocalcification that is esthetically objectionable or is cavitated; (c) carious lesion that is cavitated; and (d) abrasion and erosion that is uncontrollably sensitive, excessively deep pulpally (threatening the integrity of the tooth), or esthetically objectionable

3. Class VI cavities (faulty pits on selected occlusal cusps)
4. Veneers for metal restorations (see Chapter 18)
5. Repair of fractured areas (teeth and/or restorations)
6. Interim restorations
7. Restoration of a weakened tooth that can be strengthened by a bonded restoration

Contraindications

Composite materials generally are *not* recommended for direct posterior (Classes I, II, and VI) restorations under the following conditions:

1. The operating site cannot be appropriately isolated
2. All occlusal contacts will be on the composite material
3. Heavy occlusal stresses
4. Deep subgingival areas that are difficult to prepare or restore

General considerations

During treatment planning the patient should be informed that (1) amalgam and/or gold posterior restorations provide an excellent service for many years, whereas posterior composite restorations may not serve as long, and (2) amalgam and/or gold posterior restorations have adequate strength and wear resistance to support occlusion in high-stress areas, whereas wear of a posterior composite restoration may be greater unless provisions are made to minimize this problem. These concerns about the use of composite should be addressed. Likewise, the benefits of a posterior composite restoration should be expressed. These would include the esthetics, the potential to bond the remaining tooth structure together, and the likelihood of "sealing" the tooth and thereby reducing microleakage. It should be mentioned that even the finest indirect gold restorations sometimes do not serve longer than 30 years, and that poor ones often do not serve as long as 10 years. High-quality posterior composite restorations made of the improved materials bonded to tooth structure in conservative cavity preparations should serve for 15 to 20 years in a relatively caries-free mouth.

It is important that the occlusion be evaluated preoperatively to determine the bite relationship and type of occlusal function. Patients whose teeth exhibit significant wear facets, craze lines, cracks, and/or fractures may not be good candidates for posterior composite restorations. Teeth that show little or no sign of occlusal abuse have a more favorable prognosis when using composites for restorations involving occlusal surfaces. To maintain proper vertical dimension, at least one centric holding contact should be located on sound tooth structure or on some type of restorative material that has

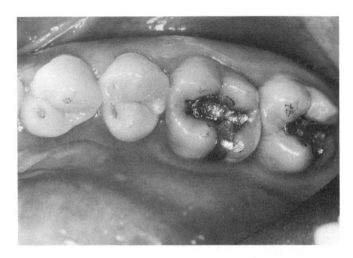

Fig. 17-4. During evaluation of occlusion, centric stops and functional patterns are marked with articulating paper. Classes I and II posterior composite restorations could be placed in selected areas of these premolar maxillary teeth.

a wear rate approximately that of tooth structure. Fig. 17-4 shows the preoperative location of centric contacts as marked with articulating paper. In this example, composite could be placed on the occlusal and proximal surfaces of the premolars without concern that wear would produce a change in the occlusion.

A very exacting technique is required to properly place a Class I or II posterior composite restoration. The operated tooth must be isolated to avoid contamination of the area from saliva or debris. If contamination occurs, the effectiveness of the composite's bonding to the tooth will be compromised, possibly resulting in loss of the restoration, recurrent caries, and/or sensitivity. Local anesthesia is usually indicated as described in Chapter 10. Extrinsic tooth stains and debris are removed with a slurry of pumice. The shade of the composite material must be selected preoperatively because color changes may occur in the teeth as a result of dehydration during operative procedures. An exact shade match is not as critical for the posterior teeth as for the anterior teeth. In fact, a slight mismatch makes postoperative evaluation easier. Isolation is best accomplished with a rubber dam; however, cotton rolls may be used in some instances.

CLASSES I, II, AND VI CAVITY PREPARATIONS FOR DIRECTLY PLACED COMPOSITES
Basic preparation designs

Cavity preparations involving the occlusal surfaces for directly placed composites are Classes I, II, and VI. Depending on the classification of cavity to be restored, *three basic designs of preparations* exist: (1)

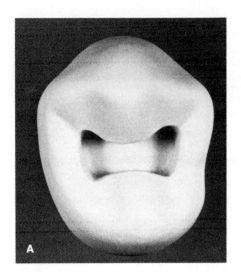
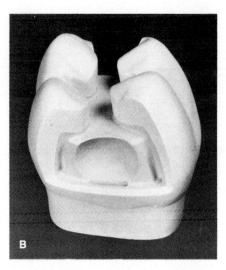

Fig. 17-5. Conventional cavity preparations for amalgam restorations: moderate-sized Class I cavity preparation (**A**); large Class II cavity preparation (**B**).

conventional, (2) *beveled conventional,* and (3) *modified.*

Conventional preparation design. Conventional cavity preparations are the types described in Chapters 12 and 13 for amalgam restorations. These box-like cavity designs have slightly converging (toward the occlusal) external walls, basically flat floors, and undercuts in dentin for retention form (Fig. 17-5, *A* and *B*). Recall that the cavosurface angle is as near to 90 degrees as possible when amalgam is used because of its limited edge strength and for Class II preparations, the margins of the proximal portion are extended to provide minimal clearance with the adjacent tooth. To meet these criteria, the tooth is weakened because sound tooth structure must be removed during cavity preparation. Unfortunately the amalgam restoration does not strengthen the remaining tooth structure if a bonding system is not used. Conversely, a bonded composite restoration has the capacity to strengthen the tooth. If an existing amalgam restoration is carefully removed, usually a conven-

tional preparation is noted. Although the conventional type of preparation can be used with posterior composites for Classes I, II, or VI cavities, it is usually not employed in its entirety because of the benefits of beveling most enamel walls. However, when a Class II cavity extends onto the root, the cavity preparation design of the root portion would be conventional.

Beveled conventional preparation design. As noted in Chapter 16, the incorporation of an enamel cavosurface bevel in preparations for composite is recommended, because it provides more surface area for bonding and it allows for the more preferred end-on etching of the enamel rods. These features increase retention, reduce leakage, and provide greater potential for strengthening the remaining tooth structure.[30] The bevel is prepared with a coarse, flame-shaped diamond instrument, approximately 0.5 mm wide, and at an angle of approximately 45 degrees to the external enamel surface (Fig. 17-6, *A*). Enamel rod direction largely determines where bevels are best placed. For instance,

Fig. 17-6. Marginal configuration for beveled conventional preparation (**A**). Occlusal bevels are less beneficial due to enamel rod orientation (**B**).

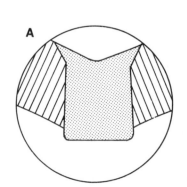
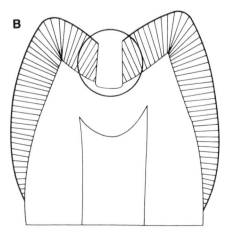

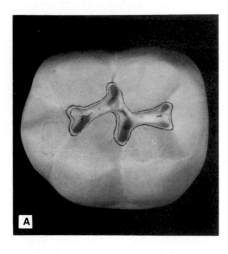

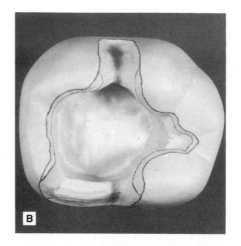

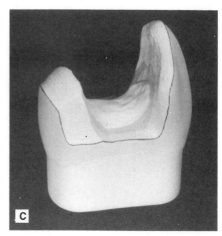

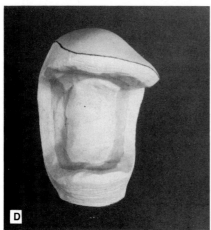

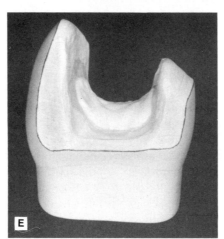

Fig. 17-7. Modified Class I cavity preparations for posterior composite restorations: conservative cavity preparation (**A**); extensive cavity preparation (**B**). Notice that some undermined enamel is maintained. Extensions strengthen remaining tooth structure. Modified Class II cavity preparation for posterior composite restoration: mesial view (**C**), occlusal view (**D**), and distal view (**E**). Note the reverse bevels, secondary flares, and brace-type "skirting" that enhance resistance and retention forms.

some beveling is particularly beneficial when placed along facial and lingual walls of a proximal box because the enamel rods run parallel to these cavity walls (see Fig. 17-15, *D*). Beveling these margins increases the surface area along the ends of the enamel rods, resulting in improved retention and resistance to leakage. However, due to the configuration of the enamel rods on an occlusal surface, occlusal bevels are less beneficial and are often not included in the preparation, especially if steep cuspal inclines exist (Fig. 17-6, *B*).

Although the beveled conventional cavity design may be used for Classes I and VI cavities, *it is most frequently used for the restoration of Class II cavities.* This design may be preferred over a modified Class II design when there is a need for increased resistance form to resist occlusal forces. Class II modified preparation designs, as described subsequently, often result in a proximal configuration that is dictated solely by the shape of the lesion and, thus, may not provide adequate resistance form features (flat floors and prepared walls parallel or perpendicular to occlusal forces). Studies suggest that modified cavity preparation designs for Class II restorations experience greater incidence of proximal failure due to fracture and dislodgement of the

restoration's proximal portion.[5,26,27] Whether the Class II preparation is for a posterior composite replacing an existing amalgam or for restoring a new carious lesion, a beveled conventional design is generally recommended. It should be noted, however, that conservation of tooth structure is of paramount importance. As will be noted later in this chapter, *Class II beveled conventional preparations should be prepared with as little faciolingual extension as possible and should not routinely be extended into all pits and fissures on the occlusal surface where sealants may be indicated.*

Modified preparation design. Recall from Chapter 16 that the design for most modified cavity preparations for composites is typically dictated by the extent of the lesion or defect. Emphasis is placed on conserving as much intact tooth structure as possible, and in some rare instances the preparation can be restricted entirely to enamel. "Extension for prevention" to so-called self-cleansing areas is not indicated.

Modified preparations are characterized by (1) the conservative removal of only the defective or carious tooth structure and (2) the establishment of a beveled configuration on all enamel cavosurface margins (Fig. 17-7, *A*). Along with the typical cavosurface bevel, ad-

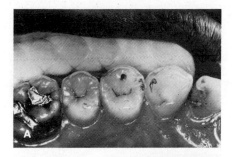
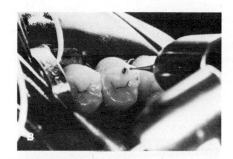
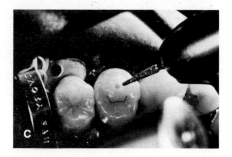

Fig. 17-8. Class VI cavity preparation for composite restoration. **A,** Class VI cavity on the facial cusp tip of maxillary premolar. **B,** Entry with small round bur. **C,** Preparation beveled with diamond instrument.

ditional beveling may extend the marginal outline conservatively to include pits, radiating fissures, or superficial defects (see Fig. 17-9). More extensive modified designs for Classes I and II cavities can incorporate unique preparation features such as reverse bevels, secondary flares, and brace-type "skirting" at the axial transitional tooth corners to enhance retention and resistance form (Fig. 17-7, *B* to *E*). However, these design features are used primarily when placing very large posterior composites for reasons of economics or when other factors preclude placement of a more permanent esthetic restoration. *Large preparations of this type should not be considered routine* and are contraindicated except in specific compromise situations.

Modified preparation designs primarily are recommended for Classes I and VI cavities where ultraconservative preparations can be made. However, beveled conventional preparations also may be used for Classes I and VI cavities when old, defective amalgams are being replaced or much caries is present.

Class VI cavity preparations

One of the most conservative indications for a directly placed posterior composite is a small faulty developmental pit located on a cusp tip. Fig. 17-8, *A,* is an example of a Class VI cavity on the facial cusp tip of a maxillary premolar and the occlusion in the area is minimal. Usually no anesthesia is required because the fault is entirely in enamel. The tooth is isolated with a cotton roll.

The usual modified Class VI cavity preparation should be as small in diameter and as shallow in depth as possible. Enter the faulty pit with a small, round bur (No. ¼ or ½) oriented perpendicular to the surface and extend pulpally to eliminate the lesion (Fig. 17-8, *B*). Visual examination and probing with an explorer often reveals that the fault is limited to enamel, since the enamel in this area is quite thick. Complete the preparation using either a coarse, flame-shaped or round diamond instrument to prepare a small bevel on the cavosurface margin (Fig. 17-8, *C*).

If a faulty restoration or extensive caries is present on the cusp tip, a round bur of appropriate size is used. Any stain that appears through the translucent enamel must be removed, otherwise it may be seen after the composite restoration is completed. Some undermined, but not friable, enamel may be left, and bonded to the composite.

Class I cavity preparations

When restoring small pits and fissures on an unrestored tooth, an ultraconservative, modified preparation design is recommended. This design allows for restoration of the lesion or defect with minimal removal of tooth structure and often may be combined with the use of composite or sealant to seal radiating non-carious fissures or pits that are at high risk for subsequent caries activity. This ultraconservative restoration is referred to as a ***conservative composite restoration.*** This general concept was developed and originally reported in 1978 by Simonsen and also is referred to as a ***preventive resin restoration.***[34,35] There is a distinction between these two types of restorations; namely, for the conservative composite restoration a diagnosis of carious cavitation has been made prior to cavity preparation, whereas for the preventive resin restoration, instrument intervention (exploration) may precede a possible diagnosis of cavitation.

An accurate diagnosis is essential prior to restoring the occlusal surface of a posterior tooth. The critical factor in this clinical assessment is whether or not the suspicious pit or fissure is cavitated, therefore requiring restorative intervention (see Chapter 3). After deciding that cavitation has occurred, it usually must be determined whether to use amalgam or composite. Important factors related to this decision include: (1) ability to isolate the tooth/teeth, (2) occlusal relationship, (3) esthetics, and (4) operator ability. (If environmental concerns regarding the use of amalgam result in its restriction in the future, then this also would be a factor.) *Usually, a conservative composite restoration is the treatment of choice for the small occlusal restoration.* The advan-

Fig. 17-9. Class I pit cavity preparations for composite restorations. **A,** Two small, faulty pits are often present on a mandibular first premolar. **B,** Each preparation and caries removal are accomplished with a No. ½ bur. **C,** Preparations are finished by placing a cavosurface bevel with a diamond instrument. Note bevel extension to include fissure.

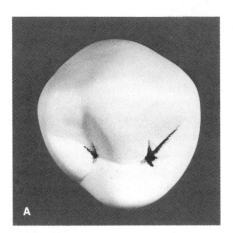

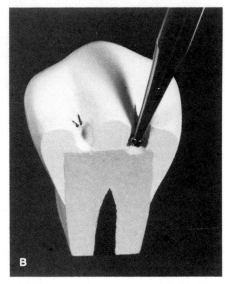

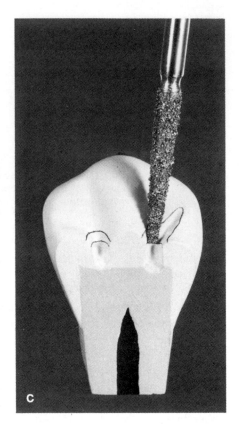

tages of composite over amalgam for such restorations are (1) conserving tooth structure, (2) enhancing esthetics, (3) bonding tooth structure together, (4) sealing the prepared tooth structure, and (5) including other suspicious areas on the occlusal surface with either the composite restorative material or a sealant material. Composite should not be used if the area cannot be properly isolated (resulting in an inadequate bond), the occlusion will be entirely on the composite restoration (resulting in increased wear), or the operator does not have the ability to place a composite restoration satisfactorily.

Mandibular premolars often have two separate faulty occlusal pits located in areas of minimal function as illustrated in Fig. 17-9, *A.* Assuming a diagnosis of active caries or that these pits are in a patient at high risk for caries (see Chapters 3 and 5), conservative resin restorations are indicated. The outline form and clinical procedures for the cavity preparation of each pit (Fig. 17-9, *B)* are similar to the Class VI modified preparation previously described with the possible exception of beveling. Any shallow fissure that extends laterally from the pit is incorporated in the preparation by an extended cavosurface bevel which is placed with a coarse, flame-shaped diamond instrument (Fig. 17-9, *C*). Normally the cavosurface bevel is 0.5 mm wide and placed at an angle of 45 degrees to the external enamel surface; however, when a fissure remains in the cavosurface area

the bevel is often extended to include the radiating fissure (Fig. 17-9, *C*). This extended bevel is similar to an enameloplasty procedure (Chapter 12) but is placed with a *coarse* diamond instrument. The entire bevel becomes part of the final cavity preparation (another difference from conventional enameloplasty), which is subsequently etched and restored with a posterior composite. Small radiating fissures also may be optionally filled with sealant.

A maxillary premolar may have a fissure in the occlusal surface as illustrated in the clinical example in Fig. 17-10, *A.* While every effort should be made to determine the presence of a cavitated lesion, if this diagnosis cannot be made, the *preventive resin restoration* may be considered. Fig. 17-10, *B* to *D* shows the initial, exploratory preventive resin cavity preparation of the fissure, using a No. ½ or No. 330 bur. The initial depth is kept in enamel at approximately 1 mm. The occlusal extension is complete when either the occlusal aspect of the fissure terminates or the opposite pit area is reached. Any pulpally directed remnants of pits and fissures are tested with a sharp explorer. If they are still defective as evidenced by a soft feel or "stick" of the explorer, the same bur is used to extend the preparation pulpally into these areas. *It is not necessary to extend the preparation in a pulpal direction if only a hard, dark line remains that cannot be penetrated by a sharp*

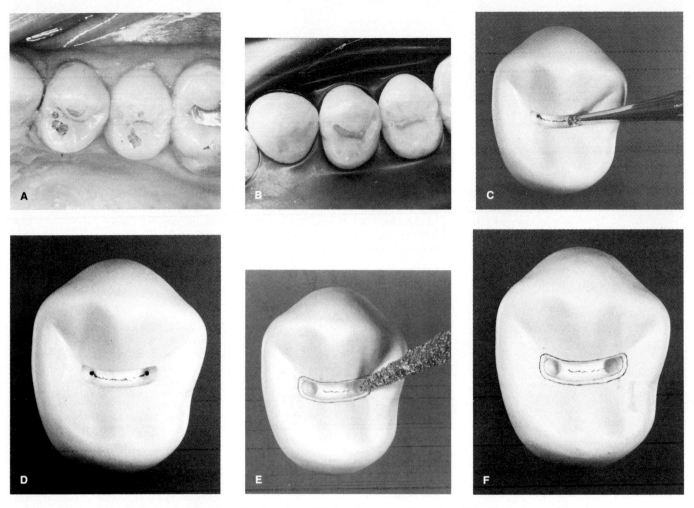

Fig. 17-10. Preventive resin Class I modified cavity preparation. **A** and **B,** Clinical examples of fissures and final exploratory cavity preparations. **C,** Preparation is made with a No. ½ bur. **D,** Initial extensions. Pit remnants "catch" a fine- tipped explorer. **E,** Caries suspicious pits excavated and bevel prepared. **F,** Completed preparation. The dark line on pulpal floor is hard and radiograph is negative for dentinal caries.

explorer, and the radiograph is negative for dentinal caries. The preparation is completed by using a coarse, flame-shaped diamond instrument to prepare a bevel on the cavosurface margin approximately 0.5 mm wide and 45 degrees to the external enamel surface (Fig. 17-10, *E*). This bevel may be widened to include any terminal ends of fissures. If no radiating fissures exist, the bevel may be considered optional due to the enamel rod direction in this area, especially if steep cuspal inclines are present. The completed preventive resin Class I modified cavity preparation on a maxillary premolar is illustrated in Fig. 17-10, *F*.

On molars the occlusion also must be carefully evaluated before a preparation is started, because centric holding areas are more likely to be involved. When possible, centric contacts on sound enamel should be maintained. The same procedures are followed in Class I

modified cavity preparations for molars as those described for premolars.

Clinical examples and models are used to illustrate conservative Class I modified cavity preparations for posterior composite restorations on maxillary and mandibular teeth. The maxillary molars are seen in Fig. 17-11, and the mandibular molars in Fig. 17-12. In Fig. 17-12, *A,* the occlusion is favorable as indicated by marks from articulating paper. The teeth are isolated by a rubber dam and preparations are made as previously described using a small, round bur. Only deep excavations into the dentin (within 0.5 mm of the dental pulp) are covered with calcium hydroxide. A light-cured glass ionomer base is recommended for restoring ideal pulpal wall contour (Fig. 17-12, *B*). The enamel cavosurface margins are beveled with a coarse, flame-shaped diamond instrument (see Fig. 17-7, *A*). Again, bevels on

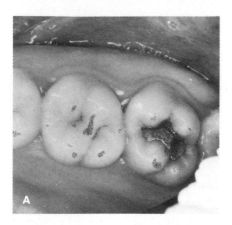
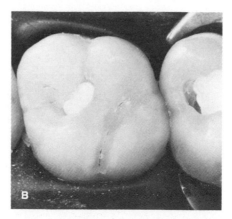
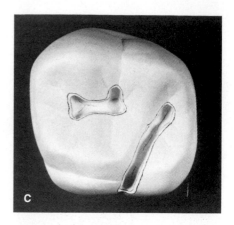

Fig. 17-11. Conservative Class I cavity preparations (maxillary first molar) for composite restorations. **A,** Occlusion marked with articulating paper. Note absence of centric contacts in area of proposed restoration. **B,** Completed preparations on maxillary first molar. Dark lines are hard and will not "catch" a fine-tipped explorer and radiograph is negative for dentinal caries. **C,** Final preparations on model with outlined cavosurface bevels.

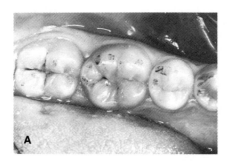
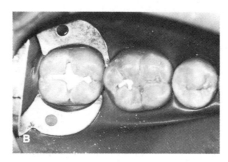

Fig. 17-12. Conservative Class I cavity preparations (mandibular molars) for composite restorations. **A,** Occlusion marked with articulating paper. **B,** Teeth isolated with rubber dam; conservative preparations with protective bases in place.

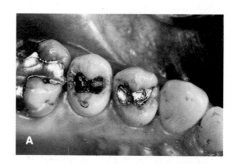

Fig. 17-13. Extensive Class I cavity preparation (maxillary second premolar) for composite restoration. **A,** Clinical examples of faulty existing occlusal amalgam restorations. **B,** A No. 245 bur is used for initial cavity preparation. **C,** Any remaining caries and/or faulty restorative material is removed with round bur. **D,** Completion of preparation by beveling with diamond instrument. Note liner in excavated area; however, use of new dentinal bonding systems favors having no liner/base except where within 0.5 mm of pulp. **E,** Final cavity preparation on model with outlined cavosurface bevel.

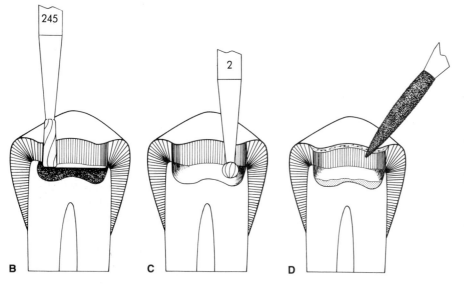
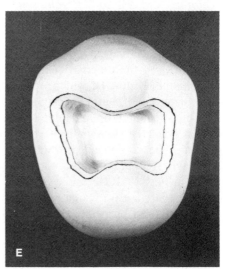

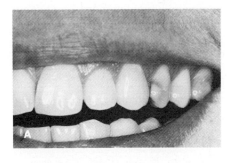
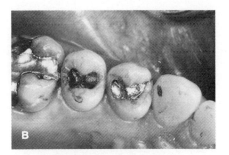
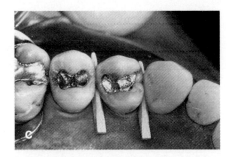
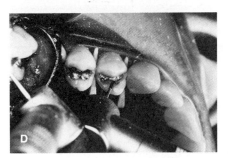
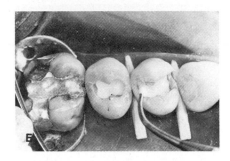
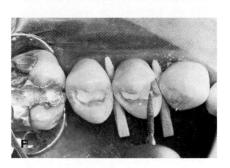

Fig. 17-14. Mesioocclusal Class II cavity preparation for posterior composite restoration in maxillary first premolar. **A,** Esthetic problem is caused by caries and existing amalgam restoration. **B,** In this patient mesial marginal ridge is not a centric holding area. **C,** Early wedging. **D,** No. 245 bur is used for initial cavity preparations on both premolars. **E,** Caries and stains are removed with round bur and protective base is inserted; use of new dentinal bonding systems favors having no liner/base except where within 0.5 mm of pulp. **F,** Preparations are completed by beveling cavosurface margin with diamond instrument.

the occlusal surface may be considered optional if no radiating fissures warrant inclusion in the preparation.

A No. 245 bur and a beveled conventional cavity preparation design may be used when a more extensive preparation is required because of caries or an existing faulty restoration (Fig. 17-13, *A* and *B*). After removal of the remaining faulty restorative material or caries with an appropriate round bur and/or spoon excavator (Fig. 17-13, *C*), a liner of calcium hydroxide and/or light-cured glass ionomer (depending on depth of excavation) is placed (Fig. 17-13, *D*). Where a marginal ridge is not completely supported by dentin, the remaining weakened enamel may be left if there is no heavy centric contact on the area. The unsupported marginal ridge will be strengthened by the composite restoration through the beveling, etching, and bonding procedures. The completed beveled conventional preparation is illustrated in Fig. 17-13, *D* and *E*.

Class II cavity preparations

Even though the ADA has not endorsed composite as a substitute for amalgam in posterior teeth, composite restorations in Classes I and VI (as already presented) are excellent when done properly. Similarly, composite may be used successfully when restoring Class II cavities. The same factors must be considered when selecting composite for Class II restorations. The potential to seal the tooth and strengthen the remaining tooth structure by bonding composite to the tooth, along with the obvious esthetic benefits, make composite a viable alternative in many Class II situations. Limiting factors for the use of composites in Class II applications are (1) the inability to isolate the area (the bond may be compromised), (2) deep subgingival extensions (preparation, insertion, and bonding may be compromised), and (3) occlusal contact entirely on the composite (increased wear may occur). This section will describe several uses of composite in Class II restorations.

Fig. 17-14 illustrates an esthetic problem seen on the mesiofacial corner of a maxillary first premolar as a result of caries and/or existing faulty restoration (Fig. 17-14, *A*). Preoperative occlusion is a consideration since the facial cusp of the opposing mandibular premolar usually occludes on the mesial marginal ridge of the maxillary premolar. In the patient shown in Fig. 17-14, *A,* articulating paper marks reveal no centric stop on the mesial marginal ridge (Fig. 17-14, *B*). The existing occlusal amalgam on the maxillary second premolar also is determined to be defective and will be replaced with a composite during the same appointment.

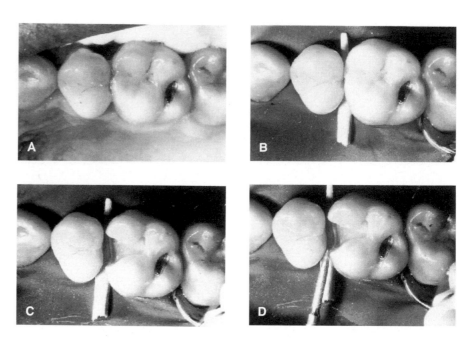

Fig. 17-15. Mesioocclusal Class II cavity preparation for posterior composite restoration in a maxillary molar. **A,** Carious lesion exists on mesial of maxillary molar in esthetically critical area. **B,** Rubber dam isolation and early wedging. **C,** Cavity walls are extended to nonfriable tooth structure and infected dentin excavated. **D,** Accessible proximal margins are beveled with coarse flame-shaped diamond instrument.

After the operator cleans the teeth, administers local anesthetic, selects the shade of composite, and isolates the area (preferably with a rubber dam), a wedge is placed in the gingival proximal region (Fig. 17-14, *C*). *Early wedging* helps in separating the teeth to compensate later for the thickness of the matrix band, thereby fulfilling one of several requirements for a good proximal contact of the finished composite restoration. The lack of pressure against the matrix during placement of composite, compared to pressure of amalgam during its condensation, explains the need not only for increased separation by early wedge insertion, but also for alertness of the operator to verify matrix apposition to the adjacent tooth before composite placement. The wedge also depresses and protects the rubber dam and gingival tissue when the proximal area is prepared. An additional, further tightening (insertion) of the wedge during cavity preparation may be helpful. The *presence of the wedge during cavity preparation* also is a guide to help prevent overextension of the gingival floor.

Recall that a conservative beveled conventional cavity preparation is recommended for most Class II composite restorations because of the need for adequate resistance form. A No. 245 bur is used to remove the existing amalgam restorations and to prepare the mesial surface of the first premolar in a conservative manner (Fig. 17-14, *D*).

A *notable difference* in Class II cavity design between the initial cavity preparation of an unrestored tooth for a composite restoration as opposed to that for an amalgam regards axial wall depth. When preparing the proximal box for a composite restoration, the axial wall initial depth usually is limited to a depth of 0.2 mm into dentin. This means that the tip of the No. 245 bur would be cutting less than one half in dentin and

more than one half in enamel to be most conservative. (The diameter of the bur's tip end is 0.8 mm.) This *decreased pulpal depth of the axial wall* allows greater conservation of tooth structure since retention locks will not be used. The occlusal walls are prepared to converge occlusally (due to the inverted shape of the No. 245 bur) and the proximal walls may be parallel or convergent occlusally. Convergent proximal walls may provide additional retention form, when needed.

With a round bur or spoon excavator, remove any remaining infected dentin and also any stains that show through the mesiofacial enamel. Apply a protective base/liner of calcium hydroxide and/or light-cured glass ionomer (depending on the depth of the excavation) (Fig. 17-14, *E*). Because of the removal of the amalgam and extensive caries, many areas of the enamel are unsupported by dentin, but not friable. This undermined enamel is *not removed*.

The beveled conventional preparations are completed by placing bevels on the occlusal and proximal cavosurface margins, access permitting, with a coarse, flame-shaped diamond instrument (Fig. 17-14, *F*). Recall that bevels on the occlusal surface may be considered optional (if not required for fissure treatment) due to enamel rod direction, especially in areas of steep cuspal inclines. Also, beveling of the proximal box enamel to cavosurface margins must be done judiciously. For a conservative (minimally extended) proximal box, the placement of bevels may necessitate undue extension, which may cause the operator to decide to either reduce or eliminate the proximal beveling.

For molars the same principles are followed for Class II beveled conventional cavity preparations as have been illustrated for premolars. Significant caries exists on the mesial of a maxillary first molar (Fig. 17-15, *A*).

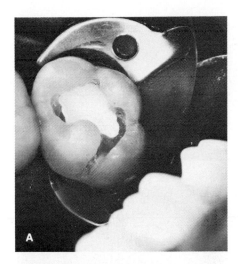
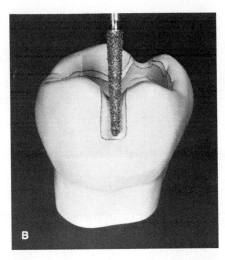
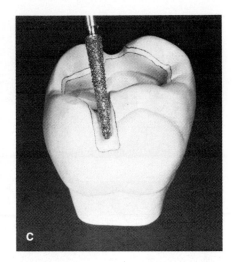
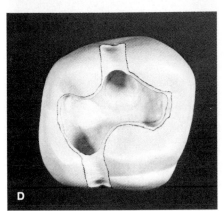

Fig. 17-16. Extensive modified Class I cavity preparation (maxillary molar) for composite restoration. **A,** Protective base is placed after removal of infected dentin and before completion of final cavity preparation. **B** and **C,** Model is used to illustrate splinting design obtained by preparing facial and lingual extensions in enamel with a diamond instrument. **D,** Occlusal view of completed preparation.

Isolation is achieved with a rubber dam. Early wedging with a short segment of a wooden toothpick initiates tooth separation which is critical to subsequently establishing a tight proximal contact (Fig. 17-15, *B*). Cavity walls are extended to sound tooth structure and infected dentin excavated (Fig. 17-15, *C*). Accessible proximal walls are beveled with a coarse flame-shaped diamond instrument (Fig. 17-15, *D*).

Although posterior teeth can be restored with composite materials, molars with severe occlusal and proximal involvement are best restored with amalgam, cast gold alloy, or with computer-generated ceramic restorations as noted later in this chapter.

Extensive Classes I and II preparations for posterior composites

Although large, extensive posterior composite restorations may have potential disadvantages when used routinely, "real world" dentistry sometimes necessitates esthetic treatment alternatives that, while representing a clinical compromise, may provide a needed service to the patient. Oftentimes patients simply cannot afford a more permanent esthetic restoration alternative or possess dental or medical conditions that preclude their

placement. In such instances, *large posterior composite restorations sometimes can be used as a reasonable alternative when more permanent options are not possible or realistic.* The patient must be informed of the possible limitations of these large posterior composite restorations; primarily excessive wear and increased recurrent caries potential. Most extensive Classes I and II composite restorations will utilize a beveled conventional cavity preparation design (see Fig. 17-13). Increased bevel widths may assist in both the retention of the material and strengthening of the weakened tooth structure.

Because some extensive restorations are very large, major cavity design variations may be indicated and, consequently, these preparations usually would be considered modified preparations. The following two sections present very modified approaches to cavity preparation for large composite restorations. Empirical clinical observations support their use, but there are no long-term clinical research results.

Class I extensive modified preparations. Because first molars erupt at an early age, they are sometimes neglected and extensive caries may develop. When infected dentin is removed, a severely weakened tooth with unsupported cusps may remain. Posterior composite restorations have the potential to strengthen these teeth and therefore offer a good service to the patient. Such a clinical situation is described.

Extensive involvement of a maxillary molar is shown in Fig. 17-16, *A*, after the existing restorative material and infected dentin have been removed and an appropriate liner placed. In an effort to splint the weakened facial and lingual cuspal elements together, facial and lin-

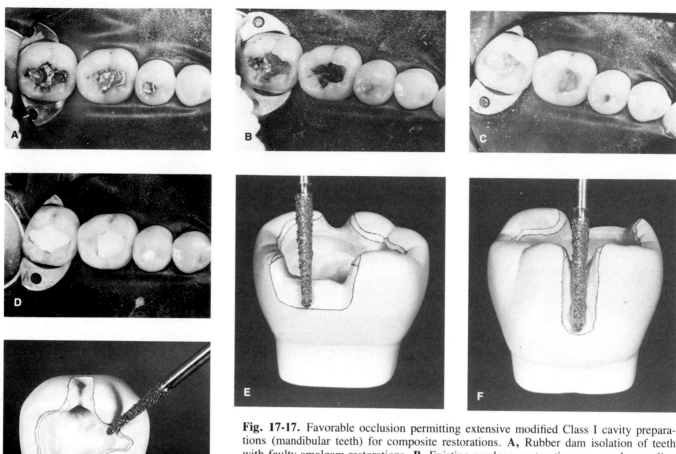

Fig. 17-17. Favorable occlusion permitting extensive modified Class I cavity preparations (mandibular teeth) for composite restorations. **A,** Rubber dam isolation of teeth with faulty amalgam restorations. **B,** Existing amalgam restorations removed, revealing secondary caries. **C,** Facial and lingual cusps undermined by removal of infected dentin. **D,** Bases inserted and preparations completed. **E to G,** Models illustrate extension and bevels prepared with diamond instrument.

gual extensions are made with a coarse, rounded-end diamond instrument as illustrated on a model in Fig. 17-16, *B* and *C*. The width and length of these extensions depend on the individual tooth and defect. The depth should be at least 1 mm into enamel as the extension crosses the cusp ridge and approximately 0.5 mm deep in the facial and/or lingual enamel (Fig. 17-16, *D*). Some unsupported, but not friable, enamel may be left because it will be reinforced by etching and bonding. When properly etched and restored, the composite material acts as a splint to lock the tooth together for resistance to fracture under masticatory forces.

Extensive modified cavity preparations for mandibular molars are illustrated in Fig. 17-17, *A* to *D*. Secondary caries is evident on removal of existing amalgams. Fortunately no exposure of the pulp is observed. Protective liners are inserted and the preparations completed. Models are used to illustrate extensions and bevels that will allow the weakened tooth to be strengthened by the

splinting action of the bonded composite restoration (Fig. 17-17, *E* to *G*).

Class II extensive modified cavity preparations. Fig. 17-18 illustrates an example of a very extensive Class II modified cavity preparation and restoration. A maxillary right first premolar is badly discolored from a large, faulty, corroded amalgam restoration and caries (Fig. 17-18, *A*). Esthetics and economics were factors in the decision to replace the amalgam with a composite restoration. The patient was reminded that the restoration may need to be replaced in a few years if excessive wear or inadequate bonding occurs. The preparation is shown with all of the old amalgam and infected dentin removed, leaving the facial and lingual enamel walls severely weakened (Fig. 17-18, *B*). Fortunately reparative dentin had obliterated the pulp horns. After placement of a protective liner (Fig. 17-18, *C*), a coarse, flame-shaped diamond instrument was used to reduce the severely undermined enamel of the lingual cusp approximately 1.5 mm

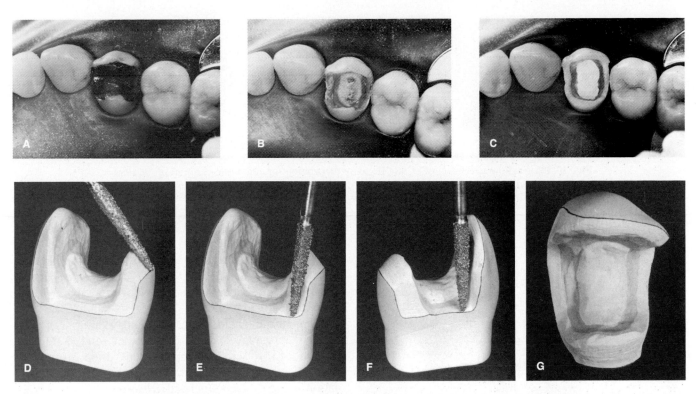

Fig. 17-18. Mesioocclusodistal Class II extensive modified cavity preparation for composite restoration. **A,** Esthetics, economics, and favorable occlusion are factors in decision to replace faulty restoration with posterior composite. **B,** Amalgam and infected dentin removed. **C,** Protective liner inserted. **D,** Diamond instrument used to reduce severely undermined lingual cusp and place reverse bevel. **E to G,** Skirting proximal axial corners with exception of mesiofacial, where a secondary flare is indicated.

and place a reverse bevel with a chamfered margin on the lingual surface (Fig. 17-18, *D*). The same instrument was used to reduce the facial cusp 0.75 mm and place a slight counterbevel. Next, skirts were placed on all of the axioproximal walls except the mesiofacial (Fig. 17-18, *E*), where a secondary flare was used (Fig. 17-18, *F*). This wraparound design in the enamel allows the bonded composite restoration to brace the tooth to resist fracture (Fig. 17-18, *G*). Again, this unique cavity preparation has been observed to be successful, but not from controlled clinical research studies. The completed restoration is shown in Fig. 17-29, *C*, and after 5 years of service (Fig. 17-29, *D* and *E*).

Pulp protection

If a composite restoration is satisfactorily bonded to the cavity preparation's walls, such as in preparations where all margins involve an adequate enamel wall for bonding, there should be little to no potential for microleakage and no need for a liner or base, unless a calcium hydroxide base (at least 1 mm thick) is indicated to treat a near exposure of the pulp (within 0.5 mm of the pulp), a possible microexposure, or an actual exposure. A liner or base generally is not indicated in mini-

mally extended Class II cavity preparations for composite (Fig. 17-19). Moreover, for such preparations it is desirable *not* to cover any portion of the dentinal walls with a liner, which would decrease dentinal bonding potential.

When satisfactory bonding is questionable, and there is the potential for some microleakage, such as when gingivally deep proximal boxes exist with little or no enamel along the gingival floor, a glass ionomer liner/base may be applied to provide its anti-cariogenic effect resulting from fluoride release. (Glass ionomer would be applied as a base over a calcium hydroxide liner in the situation of a near or actual pulpal exposure.) Even with the newer, improved enamel/dentin bonding systems, bonding can be suspect in cavity preparations having deeply extended gingival walls (and margins) because (1) isolation is more difficult and (2) the enamel walls (for etching and bonding) are minimal or nonexistent (in the crown but near the cementoenamel junction, or the root). In such cavity preparations a thin layer of a glass ionomer may be placed on the pulpal half of the gingival floor and the entire axial wall (Fig. 17-20). If subsequent leakage should occur along the gingival margin, the anti-cariogenic qualities of the

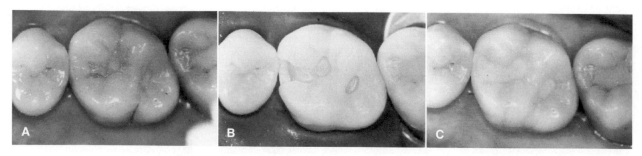

Fig. 17-19. Shallow mesioocclusal Class II cavity preparation for composite restoration, and not requiring protective liner or base. **A,** Mesial caries exists preoperatively. **B,** Conservative cavity preparation exhibiting full-thickness enamel walls. **C,** Completed restoration.

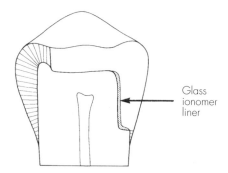

Glass ionomer liner

Fig. 17-20. Class II cavity preparation with deep gingival margin and thin enamel along gingival floor. Glass ionomer liner is placed on pulpal half of gingival floor and on the axial wall to help resist recurrent caries should leakage occur.

glass ionomer liner may offer protection against recurrent caries.

Preliminary steps for enamel and dentin bonding

As noted in Chapter 16, many enamel/dentin bonding systems presently condition both enamel and dentin simultaneously either with phosphoric acid or alternative organic etchants. Strict attention to the manufacturer's directions regarding use of the specific conditioner is imperative to ensure optimal results (see Chapter 16 for details of technique).

With any necessary bases/liners in place and the preparations completed, a phosphoric acid etching gel (or alternative conditioner) typically is applied with a brush (or other suitable applicator) or syringe to the enamel (and dentin) of the preparations and is allowed to remain undisturbed for 30 seconds (time is dependent on conditioner used). Typically, the etched (conditioned) area is rinsed with a copious stream of water for 10 to 15 seconds if a phosphoric acid-etching gel is used. Strictly follow manufacturer's instructions regarding etching (conditioning), rinsing, and drying the

enamel and dentin preparation walls. *Overdrying conditioned (etched) dentin surfaces may compromise dentin bonding* due to collapse of the collagen network of the conditioned dentin layer.[9,10,13]

The etched enamel areas should exhibit a lightly frosted appearance. Once the enamel (and dentin) is conditioned, rinsed, and appropriately dried, it must be kept clean and well isolated. Recall that rubber dam isolation is highly recommended. However, if cotton rolls are used for isolation, particular attention must be taken to prevent contamination. Any such contamination by saliva would necessitate repeating the conditioning procedure for a minimum of 10 seconds, followed by routine rinsing, minimal drying, and isolation. Also recall that sometimes it may be advantageous to condition the enamel and dentin *after* the matrix (with wedge) is applied, thereby enhancing the isolation of the area and allowing assessment of the gingival enamel for any fracture due to wedge placement.

DIRECT RESTORATION BY COMPOSITE OF CAVITY PREPARATIONS INVOLVING OCCLUSAL AND PROXIMAL SURFACES
Proximal matrix

Undoubtedly one of the most important steps in restoring posterior teeth with directly placed composite is the selection and proper placement of the matrix. Unlike amalgam, which can be laterally condensed to improve the proximal contact, posterior composites are almost totally dependent on the contour and position of the matrix for establishing appropriate proximal contacts. Care must be exercised in placing a matrix for a Class II restoration, because it is difficult to obtain good proximal contacts on posterior teeth when composite material is used. Early wedging and retightening of the wedge during cavity preparation aid in achieving sufficient separation of the teeth to compensate for the thickness of the matrix band. Also, as previously stated, prior to placing the composite material, the matrix band (strip) must be in absolute juxtaposition to (touching) the adjacent contact area.

An ultrathin metal matrix band is preferred for the restoration of a Class II cavity, because it is thinner and can be contoured better than a clear polyester matrix. Furthermore, a metal matrix offers greater resistance to condensation, which is especially important when a more viscous composite is used. No significant problems are experienced in placing and curing composite material when using a metal matrix so long as *small incremental additions are used* (each increment cured before adding the next).

A Tofflemire-type matrix can be used for restoring a two-surface cavity preparation but must be sufficiently wedged to compensate adequately for two thicknesses of matrix band (see Fig. 17-24, *A*). An ultrathin (.001 inch) universal metal matrix band* should be used in the Tofflemire retainer to aid in obtaining a good proximal contact. The metal matrix band for posterior composites first is burnished on a paper pad to impart proper proximal contour to the band (the same as a matrix for amalgam).

If the Tofflemire-type matrix band is open excessively along the lingual margins of the preparation due to the contour of the tooth, a "tinner's joint" can be used to close the matrix band. This joint is made by grabbing the lingual portion of the matrix band with No. 110 pliers and cinching the band tightly together above the height of contour of the tooth. The gathered matrix material can be easily folded to one side with a large amalgam condenser. By closing the open portion of the matrix band, significant time and effort are saved when contouring and finishing the restoration.

A customized, compound-supported metal matrix is an excellent matrix for a two-surface posterior composite restoration, because it is easier to obtain a good contact when the wedge has to compensate for only one thickness of metal matrix material. The materials needed for this matrix are shown in Fig. 17-21. A short length of thin, dead-soft or stainless steel metal matrix material† is cut, contoured, and burnished. Commercial, precontoured types‡ are also available. The small compound cones are made by softening green stick compound over a Bunsen burner as described in Chapter 13. The initial wedge placed during cavity preparation is removed, the matrix positioned, and a new wedge placed (Fig. 17-22, *A*). It is helpful to hold the strip against the adjacent tooth with a burnisher while the matrix is stabilized with the softened, compound cones (Fig. 17-22, *B* and *C*). If additional contouring is

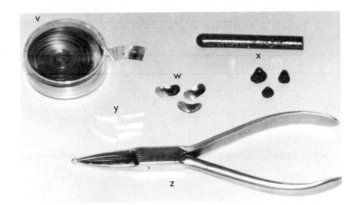

Fig. 17-21. Materials for application of matrix on two-surface preparations: thin, dead-soft strip metal *(v)* or preformed matrices *(w)*, green stick compound and cones *(x)*, wooden wedges *(y)*, and No. 110 pliers *(z)*.

needed, it can be accomplished with the back side of a warmed Black's spoon excavator.

When both proximal surfaces are involved, a Tofflemire retainer with an ultra-thin, burnishable matrix band as noted earlier is used. The band is contoured, positioned, wedged, and shaped as needed for proper proximal contacts and embrasures (Fig. 17-22, *D*). The use of compound to help support a matrix of this type is generally not necessary, since heavy condensing forces are not used when the posterior composite material is inserted.

Clear polyester matrices are available and may be used for the restoration of very small Class II preparations. Care must be taken to properly contour the polyester matrix strip, as described in Chapter 16, to impart sufficient convexity into the polyester band. Precontoured polyester matrices are also available for use in light-weight Tofflemire retainers* or as part of a unique circumferential matrixing system called the Translite Auto Matrix System.† Clear polyester matrices are typically thicker than metal matrices and must be firmly wedged to compensate for this additional thickness. Moreover, clear polyester matrices are not recommended for large posterior composite restorations, because they cannot be contoured as well as metal matrices nor do they provide adequate resistance to condensation if a viscous composite is used.

Insertion of composite

A two-step procedure (enamel/dentin bonding agent followed by posterior composite material) is followed

---

*Ho Dental Co., Goleta, Calif.
†Den-Mat Corporation, Santa Maria, Calif.
‡Palodent Matrix, Palodent Company, Portola Valley, Calif.

*Kulzer matrices and Tofflemire retainer, Kulzer, Inc. (USA), Irvine, Calif.
†Translite Auto Matrix System, L.D. Caulk/Dentsply, Milford, Del.

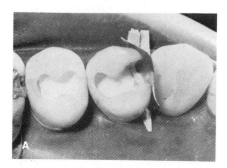

Fig. 17-22. Placement of proximal matrix for posterior composite restoration. **A,** Strip matrix positioned and wedged for two-surface preparation. **B** and **C,** Compound cones are softened and applied to matrix while a burnisher is used to stabilize the strip against adjacent tooth. **D,** Tofflemire matrix positioned and contoured for three-surface preparation.

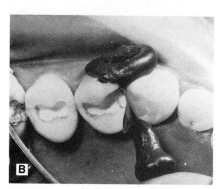

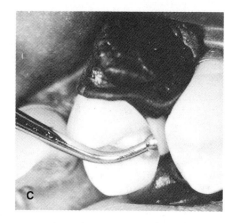

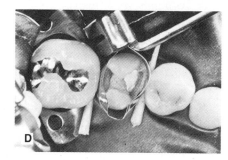

with either self-cured or light-cured composite materials. A light-cured system is used for restoring the Class II cavity preparation illustrated on the maxillary first molar shown in Fig. 17-24 and the maxillary left premolars in Fig. 17-25. These materials should not be dispensed until ready to use, because they will begin to polymerize from the available light in the room. Because of variations in materials, *each manufacturer's specific instructions should be followed.*

The enamel/dentin bonding agent(s) (including primers and adhesives) is placed over the entire preparation (conditioned enamel and dentin) with a brush, foam sponge, or other suitable applicator in accordance with the manufacturer's instructions (see Chapter 16 for details). Although bonding agents can be applied following matrix placement, remember these materials also may be applied prior to matrix placement, possibly preventing pooling of the adhesive, especially along the matrix/gingival margin junction. Often, it also is recommended that the adhesive layer be lightly blown with air to thin it and remove excess; however, manufacturer's instructions should be followed in this regard. The adhesive is polymerized with a visible light source, usually for 20 seconds.

Composite insertion hand instruments or a syringe may be used to insert the composite material (Fig. 17-23, *A* and *B*). The first type of syringe *(y)** shown can be used with a clear plastic tip for self-cured composites

or with a black or orange tip for light-cured composites. The second syringe *(z)** is designed by the manufacturer for use with preloaded compule tips. The tips on both types must be kept covered when not in use to prevent premature hardening of light-cured materials.

Following matrix and adhesive placement, small increments of composite material are added and successively cured (Fig. 17-24). It is important to place (and cure) the composite incrementally in order to reduce the effects of polymerization shrinkage, especially along the gingival floor. For this reason, the first *small* increment should be placed along the gingival floor and should extend slightly up the facial and lingual walls (Fig. 17-24, *B*). This increment should only be approximately 0.5 mm in thickness, since it is the farthest increment from the curing light and is most critical in establishing a proper gingival seal. This first increment should be cured with a light exposure of at least 40 seconds (Fig. 17-24, *C*). Subsequent additions are made and cured (never exceeding 2 mm in thickness at a time) until the preparation is filled to slight excess (Fig. 17-24, *D* and *E*). The restoration can be contoured and finished immediately after the last increment is cured. Another clinical example is illustrated in Fig. 17-25.

Light-cured composites work very well for the restoration of posterior teeth because of extended working time and the ease of incremental placement (and cure).

*Centrix, Inc., Milford, Conn.

*L.D. Caulk Dentsply, Milford, Del.

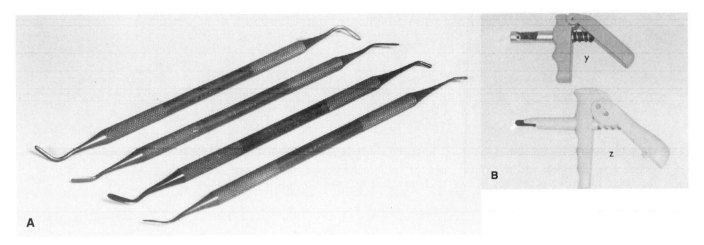

Fig. 17-23. Insertion instruments for composite. **A,** Anodized aluminum instruments. **B,** Two types of injection syringes: Centrix *(y)* and Caulk *(z)*.

Fig. 17-24. Insertion of light-cured composite material, maxillary molar. **A,** A thin Tofflemire-type matrix is positioned and wedged. Protective base and bonding agent have been placed. **B to E,** Composite is placed and cured in small increments until cavity is slightly overfilled.

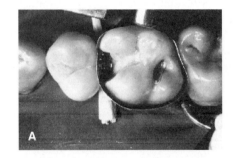
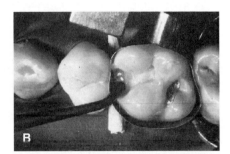
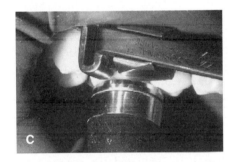
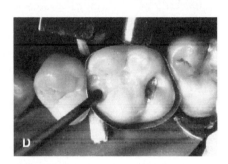
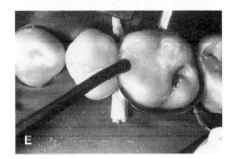

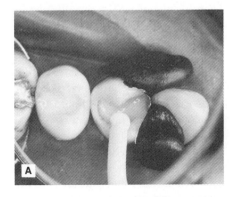
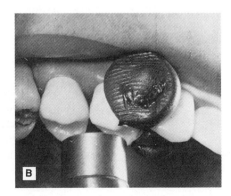
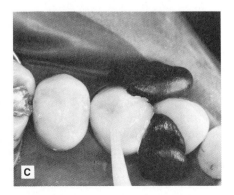

Fig. 17-25. Insertion of light-cured composite material, maxillary premolar. **A to C,** Compound-supported matrix has been positioned, wedged, and reinforced. Composite is inserted and cured in small increments until cavity is slightly overfilled.

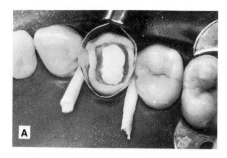
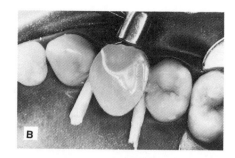

Fig. 17-26. A, Self-cured composite will be inserted into the three-surface preparation shown with matrix in place. B, Injected composite was covered by matrix strip and held under pressure during polymerization.

However, if a light-cured composite is not available, a self-cured composite can be used successfully.

A self-cured composite is used for restoring the extensive three-surface cavity preparation illustrated on a maxillary first premolar (Fig. 17-26, A). The enamel and dentin prepared surfaces already have been etched (conditioned), and the matrix is in place. Although the composite can be inserted with a hand instrument, an injection syringe is recommended for insertion of self-cured composites to prevent air entrapment (see Fig. 17-23, B). Before the self-cured material is mixed, the patency of the syringe tip should be verified, and the tip should be trial positioned in the preparation to verify access to the gingival floor. The resin bonding agent is mixed and applied according to the manufacturer's instructions, followed immediately by mixing and insertion of the self-curing composite material. As noted earlier, care must be taken when applying the adhesive after matrix application to avoid pooling. The preparation is filled to slight excess with one increment and left undisturbed until polymerization is complete. Some clinicians place a preformed occlusal index or polyester strip over the occlusal surface immediately after insertion to exert pressure for enhancing adaptation, minimizing excess, and reducing the need for finishing procedures (Fig. 17-26, B). The self-cured composite should not be disturbed for at least 3 minutes after a sample of the mixed material has hardened. Recall that an espoused advantage of self-cured composite, opposite to light-cured composite, is that the former cures first next to the warm cavity preparation walls and that polymerization shrinkage is directed toward these walls, thereby favoring maintenance of the bond between the composite and prepared tooth surfaces.

Following insertion and polymerization of the composite material, the matrix and wedges are removed, and the restoration is examined for voids or lack of proximal contact(s). If correction is needed, it should be accomplished at this time, because any additions will bond satisfactorily to the uncontaminated, oxygen-inhibited surface layer of the composite material.

Finishing procedures

Contouring can be initiated immediately after a light-cured composite material has been polymerized or 3 minutes after the initial hardening of a self-cured material. The occlusal surface is shaped with a round, 12-bladed carbide finishing bur (Figs. 17-27, A, and 17-28, A). Special carbide-tipped carvers* are useful for removing composite excess along occlusal margins (Fig. 17-27, B). Excess composite is removed at the proximal margins and embrasures with a flame-shaped, 12-bladed carbide finishing bur (Figs. 17-27, C, and 17-28, B) and abrasive discs (Fig. 17-28, C). Any overhangs at the gingival area are removed with a sharp amalgam knife or a No. 12 surgical blade mounted in a Bard-Parker handle. These instruments are used with light shaving strokes to remove the excess (Fig. 17-28, D). Narrow finishing strips are used to smooth the gingival proximal surface (Fig. 17-27, D). Care must be exercised to maintain the position of the finishing strips gingival to the proximal contact area to avoid inadvertent opening of the contact.

The rubber dam (or other means of isolation) is removed and the occlusion is evaluated for proper contact. Further adjustments are made if needed, and the restorations are finished with fine, rubber abrasive points and/or discs (Fig. 17-27, E). The restored teeth are illustrated in Figs. 17-27, F, and 17-28, E and F.

A series of preoperative and postoperative views is shown for a three-surface composite restoration on a maxillary right premolar (Fig. 17-29). In this example wear has been minimal during the 5-year service period. The following initial desirable conditions should be recalled: (1) favorable occlusal relationship, (2) no offending biting habits, (3) low caries activity, (4) good oral hygiene, and (5) careful operative procedures.

Another series is shown in Fig. 17-30. These two-surface composite restorations have been in service for 3 years. No centric contacts are located on the composite restoration.

*Carbide Carvers, Brasseler USA, Inc., Savannah, Ga.

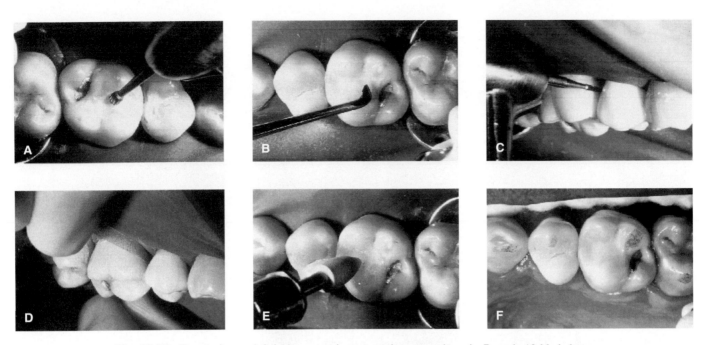

Fig. 17-27. Contouring and finishing posterior composite restoration. **A,** Round, 12-bladed carbide bur is used to contour occlusal surface. **B,** Carbide-tipped carver is useful for removing excess composite along occlusal margins. **C,** Flame-shaped carbide finishing bur is used to contour proximal areas. **D,** Narrow finishing strip smoothes proximal areas. **E,** Abrasive rubber point is used to smooth occlusal surfaces. **F,** Completed posterior composite restoration with articulation marks.

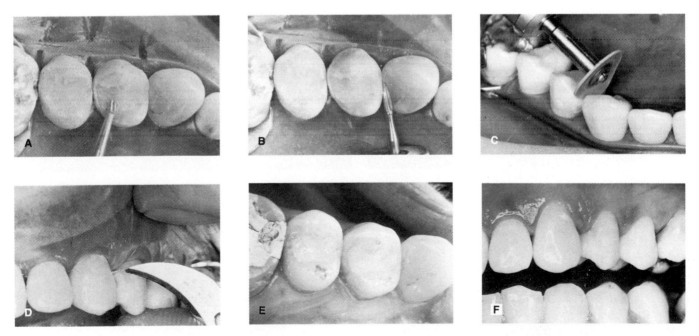

Fig. 17-28. Contouring and finishing posterior composite. **A,** Occlusal surface shaped with round, 12-bladed carbide bur. **B** and **C,** Proximal areas are shaped with flame-shaped bur and abrasive discs. **D,** Removing excess material at gingival area with a No. 12 blade (Bard-Parker handle). **E** and **F,** Occlusal and facial views after rubber dam removal, occlusal adjustments, and final finishing.

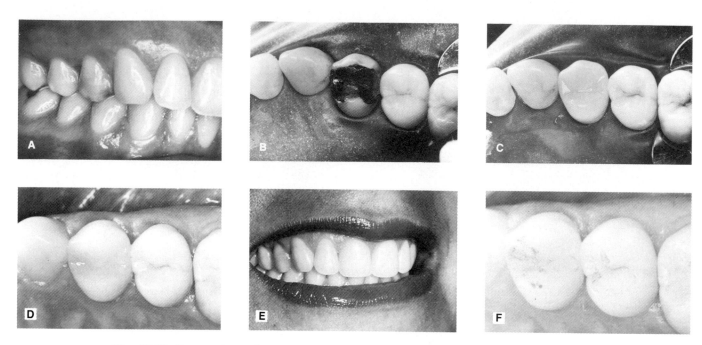

Fig. 17-29. Preoperative and postoperative views of posterior composite restoration. **A** and **B,** Preoperative facial and occlusal views. **C,** After inserting and finishing composite restoration. Occlusal (**D**) and facial (**E**) views after 5 years of service. **F,** Occlusion marked with articulating paper at 5-year recall appointment.

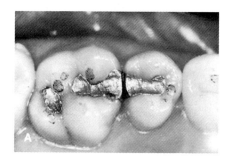
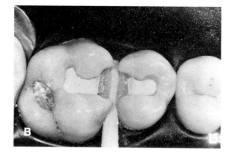
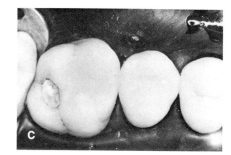

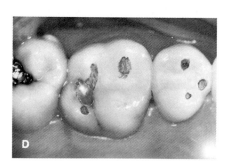

Fig. 17-30. Preoperative and postoperative views of posterior composite restorations. **A,** Failing amalgam restorations are not in centric holding areas. **B,** Isolation with rubber dam. Cavity preparations with protective bases in place. **C,** Initial appearance of composite restorations. **D,** After 3 years of service. Occlusion is marked with articulating paper.

INDIRECT TOOTH-COLORED INLAYS AND ONLAYS
Introduction and definitions

The previous sections describe the use of composites to fabricate tooth-colored restorations in the prepared tooth with *direct techniques.* Tooth-colored restorations also can be made using *indirect techniques,* in which restorations are fabricated outside of the prepared tooth. Most indirect restorations are made on a replica of the prepared tooth in a dental laboratory by a trained technician. Such systems include laboratory-processed composites or some type of ceramic, such as porcelain fired on refractory dies, or castable glasses. One new system, the *CEREC®* system,* allows indirect computer-generated ceramic restorations to be made chairside for more rapid delivery of the restoration, fewer patient visits, and reduced laboratory expenses (Fig. 17-31).

Advantages

Indirect tooth-colored restorations have the same *advantages* as those previously listed for direct composite restorations (except for cost and time), with the following additions:

Selection of materials; physical properties. A wide variety of high-strength tooth-colored restorative materials, such as laboratory-processed composites and ceramics, can be used with indirect techniques. Indirect restorations have better physical properties than direct restorations since they are fabricated in ideal laboratory conditions.

Increased resistance to abrasion and attrition. Ceramic restorations are *much* more wear resistant than direct composite restorations, an especially critical factor when restoring the occlusal surfaces of posterior teeth. Laboratory-processed composite restorations wear significantly more than ceramics, but less than directly inserted composites in laboratory studies.[7,39]

Reduced polymerization shrinkage stress. Since the bulk of the cavity is filled with the indirect tooth-colored restoration, very little composite is used during cementation. This small amount of composite has *relatively little shrinkage* upon polymerization, resulting in *less stress* on the restoration/cement/tooth interfaces, *fewer marginal voids, less microleakage,* and *reduced postoperative sensitivity.*[8,31,32]

Ability to strengthen remaining tooth structure. Tooth structure weakened by caries and/or cavity preparation(s) can be strengthened by adhesively bonding indirect inlays and onlays to conditioned tooth surfaces.[16,25] The reduced polymerization shrinkage stress obtained with the indirect technique is also desirable when restoring such weakened teeth.

*CEREC® system, Pelton & Crane, Siemens Product Division, Charlotte, NC.

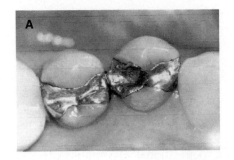

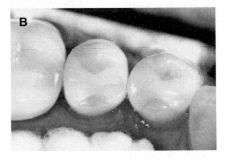

Fig. 17-31. A, Defective (MOD) amalgam restorations on mandibular premolars were replaced with ceramic inlays using the CEREC® system. **B,** Ceramic inlays (Dicor MGC®) after 3 years of service.

More precise control of contours and contacts. Indirect techniques usually result in better contours to restored tooth surfaces (especially proximal contours) and improved occlusal contacts, since there is greater access and visibility to all portions of the cavity preparation and restoration during fabrication in the dental laboratory.

Increased auxiliary support. Most indirect techniques allow the fabrication of the restoration to be totally or partially *delegated to dental laboratory technicians.* Such delegation allows for more efficient use of the dentist's time.

Disadvantages

The following are disadvantages of indirect tooth-colored restorations:

Increased cost and time. Most indirect techniques require two patient appointments, with the need for a temporary restoration. These factors, along with the bills from the dental laboratory, increase the cost. While indirect tooth-colored inlays and onlays are more expensive than direct composites, they are less costly than the next esthetic alternative, porcelain crowns.

Technique sensitive. Restorations made using indirect techniques usually require a high level of operator skill. A devotion to excellence is necessary during preparation, impression, seating, and finishing the restoration. Diligence is required during all stages of the process to obtain a high quality restoration.

Brittleness of ceramics. Ceramic restorations can fracture if the preparation does not allow adequate thickness to resist occlusal forces. Fractures may occur during try-in or post-cementation, especially in patients who generate unusually high forces.

Indications

The following are indications for Class I or II indirect tooth-colored restorations:

Esthetics. Indirect tooth-colored restorations are indicated for Class I or II cavities that are positioned so that esthetics is a major factor in the success of the restoration.

Large cavities or previous restorations. Indirect tooth-colored restorations should be considered for large Class I or II cavities or previous restorations, especially those that are wide faciolingually and require cusp coverage. Large cavities are best restored with adhesive restorations that strengthen the remaining tooth structure. The contours of large restorations are more easily developed when using indirect techniques. Indirect tooth-colored restorative materials are more durable than direct composites, especially in regard to maintaining occlusal surfaces and occlusal contacts. This ability to resist excessive occlusal wear is especially important in large posterior restorations which involve most or all of the occlusal contacts.[37] However, without sufficient bulk the extensive, bonded, indirect tooth-colored restoration may fracture under occlusal loads, particularly in the molar region.

Contraindications

Contraindications for indirect tooth-colored restorations are:

Heavy occlusal forces. Ceramic restorations may fracture when they do not have sufficient bulk or in patients who have bruxing or clenching habits. Heavy wear facets or a lack of occlusal enamel are good indicators of bruxing and clenching habits (Fig. 17-32).

Inability to maintain a dry operating field. Current adhesive techniques require near perfect moisture control.

Deep subgingival preparations. Bonding to enamel margins is greatly preferred, especially along gingival margins of proximal boxes.

Laboratory-processed composite inlays and onlays

The physical properties of composite restorations are improved when the composite is free of voids, and the resin matrix is maximally polymerized. Generating dense, well-cured restorations is best accomplished in the dental laboratory using devices that polymerize the composite under pressure, light, heat, vacuum, or a combination of these conditions. Several commercial systems utilize such techniques for optimizing the hard-

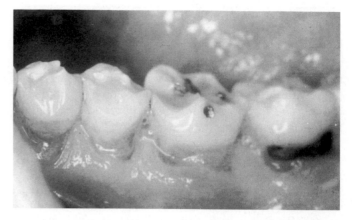

Fig. 17-32. Clenching and bruxing habits can create extensive wear of occlusal surfaces. This patient is not a good candidate for porcelain inlays.

ness and strength of their composite materials. Laboratory-processed composite inlays and onlays are more resistant to occlusal wear than direct composites, but much less than ceramic restorations.[7] They are indicated when: (1) maximum *wear resistance* is desired from a composite restoration, (2) more control is needed to achieve *proper contours and contacts,* and (3) the *cost* of the more expensive ceramic restoration is prohibitive. While there are unique aspects to each manufacturer's system, the *fabrication steps* for one system can be summarized as follows*:

1. The composite restoration is initially formed on a replica of the tooth (die) (Figs. 17-33 and 17-34).
2. The composite is initially light-cured for 1 minute on each surface with a hand-held curing light† (Fig. 17-35).
3. Final curing is accomplished by inserting the die/inlay into a curing oven that exposes the composite to additional light and heat for 7 minutes.‡ (Fig. 17-36) An alternative curing technique is to place the die/inlay into boiling water for 10 minutes.
4. The cured composite inlay is removed from the die and allowed to cool. It is then returned to the die for final trimming and finishing (Figs. 17-37 and 17-38).

Ceramic inlays and onlays

Ceramic inlays and onlays have become popular due to the public demand for esthetic, durable restorative materials, and due to improvements in materials, fabri-

---

*Herculite XRV™ Lab, Kerr Manufacturing Co., Romulus, Mich.
†Optilux™ 401 curing light, Demetron Research Corp., Danbury, Conn.
‡DI-500® Curing Oven, Coltene/Whaledent.

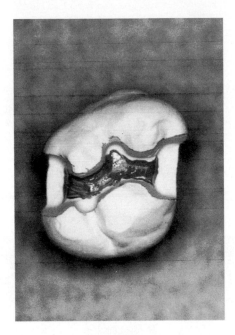

Fig. 17-33. Die prepared for making laboratory-processed composite inlay. Die spacer is usually applied to axial walls and pulpal floor. Sealing and release agents are applied to prevent composite from adhering to die surfaces.

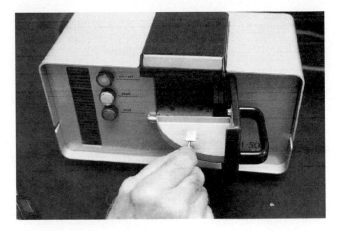

Fig. 17-36. Inserting die and inlay into curing oven for additional polymerization.

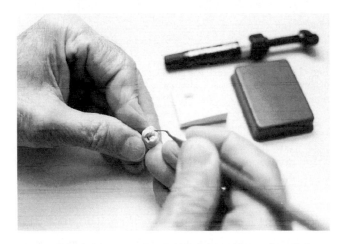

Fig. 17-34. Composite is added to the cavity to form inlay.

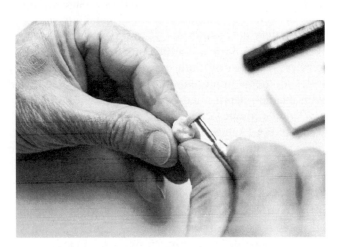

Fig. 17-37. Finishing composite inlay on die.

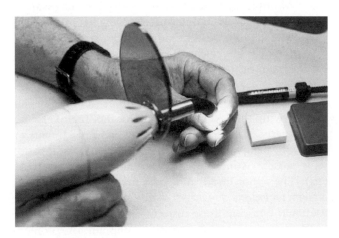

Fig. 17-35. Curing composite with hand-held curing light.

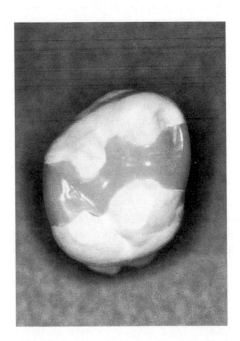

Fig. 17-38. Composite inlay polished, ready for delivery.

Table 17-1. Physical properties

	Enamel (1)	Dentin (1)	Composite (1)	Feldspathic porcelain (2)	Dicor® (2)	Dicor MGC®(2)
Hardness (KHN_{100})	343	68	30	460	362	340
Modulus of elasticity (PSI × 10^6)	12.2	2.6	2.4	12.0	10.2	9.9
Coefficient of expansion (10^{-6}/°C)	11.4	—	26-40	8.0	7.2	6.3
Occlusal wear resistance	High	Low	Low	High	High	High

(1)Restorative Dental Materials, Ed. By R.G. Craig, C.V. Mosby Co., 1980. From Craig RG, editor: *Restorative dental materials*, St Louis, 1980, Mosby.
(2)Physical Properties Department, Corning Glass Works, Corning, New York.

cating techniques, and bonding systems. Among the ceramic materials used today are feldspathic porcelain, castable ceramic *(Dicor®)*,* and a new machinable glass ceramic *(Dicor® MGC)*** for use with the CEREC® system. The physical and mechanical properties of ceramics come closer to matching those of enamel than do composites. They have excellent wear resistance and have a coefficient of thermal expansion very close to that of tooth structure. The physical properties of some representative ceramics are compared with enamel, dentin, and composite in Table 17-1.

Dental ceramics can be etched with acids to selectively remove some of the glassy matrix, exposing crystalline structures. Typically, hydrofluoric acid is used to etch feldspathic porcelain while ammonium bifluoride is used for etching Dicor® and Dicor MGC®. Such acid etching increases surface relief and therefore not only increases the surface area, but also results in micromechanical bonding of the composite cement to the ceramic restoration (see Fig. 6-68). As noted earlier, when cemented to acid-etched enamel surfaces, bonded ceramic restorations have considerable retention and are able to strengthen previously weakened tooth structures (see Fig. 6-69).

Porcelain inlays and onlays fired on refractory dies. Dental porcelains are partially crystalline minerals (feldspar, silica, alumina) dispersed in a glass matrix.[28] The porcelain restoration is made from finely ground ceramic powders which are mixed with distilled water or a special liquid, shaped into the desired form, then fired and fused together to form a translucent, toothlike material. Currently, *the majority of ceramic inlays and onlays are fabricated in the dental laboratory by firing dental porcelains on refractory dies.* The *fabrication steps* can be summarized as follows:

1. After cavity preparation, an impression is made and a "master" working cast is poured of die stone (Fig. 17-39).

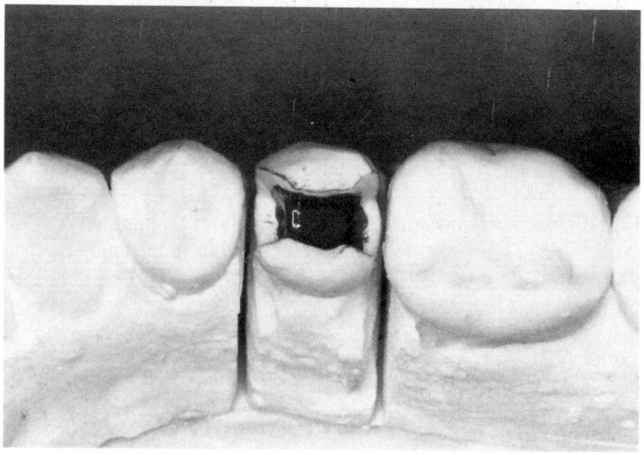

*Dicor®, Dentsply International Inc., York, Penn.
**Dicor MGC®, LD Caulk, A Division of Dentsply International, Milford, Del.

Fig. 17-39. Master cast for MOD ceramic inlay. Die spacer is usually applied to axial walls and pulpal floor prior to duplication.

2. The die is duplicated and poured of a refractory investment capable of withstanding porcelain firing temperatures. The duplication method must result in the master die and the refractory die being interchangeable regarding accuracy (Fig. 17-40).
3. Dental porcelains are added into the cavity preparation of the refractory die, and fired in an oven. Multiple increments and firings are necessary to compensate for sintering shrinkage (Fig. 17-41).
4. The ceramic restoration is recovered from the refractory die, cleaned of all investment, and then seated on the master die and working cast for final adjustments and finishing (Fig. 17-42).

Most dental laboratories fabricate ceramic inlays and onlays with this technique due to the relatively low start-up cost. The ceramic powders and investments are relatively inexpensive, and the technique is compatible with most existing ceramic laboratory equipment (ovens). The major disadvantage of this technique is that it is *very technique sensitive.* While some technicians can routinely fabricate these restorations with excellent marginal integrity, many dentists complain of problems with fit and strength. Inlays and onlays fabricated with

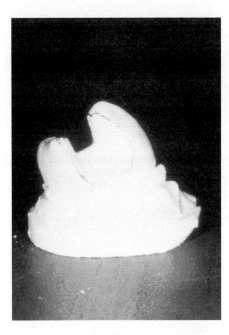

Fig. 17-40. "Master" die is impressed, then a duplicate die poured with refractory investment.

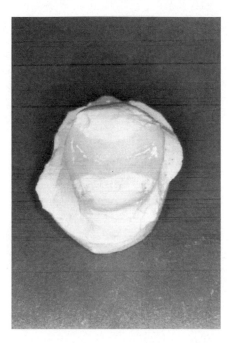

Fig. 17-41. Dental porcelains are added and fired in increments until inlay is the correct shape.

this technique must be *handled gently during try-in adjustments* to avoid fracture. Even after cementation, the incidence of fracture is higher for these restorations than with the other ceramic systems.

Castable glass (Dicor®). In 1968 it was discovered that certain glasses could be modified with nucleating

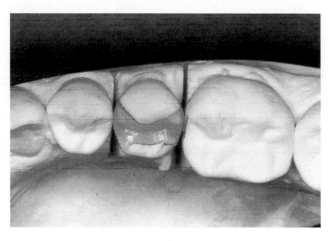

Fig. 17-42. Inlay is cleaned of all investment, then seated on master die for final adjustments and finishing. Ceramic inlay is now ready for delivery. (Photographs courtesy Dr. G. Sheen.)

agents and upon heat treatment changed into ceramics with organized crystalline forms. Such "glass-ceramics" were stronger, had a higher melting point, and had variable coefficients of thermal expansion.[18] In the beginning these glass-ceramics were primarily developed for cookware and other heat-resistant products. In 1984 the glass-ceramic material Dicor® was patented, and has become the most widely used *castable ceramic* in dentistry. The *fabrication steps* are summarized as follows:

1. After cavity preparation, an impression is made and a "master" working cast is poured of die stone.
2. A wax pattern of the restoration is made using conventional techniques (Fig. 17-43), invested in a special phosphate-bonded investment (Fig. 17-44), and then burned out using a conventional wax-eliminating furnace.
3. A special casting machine is used to melt the glass ingot and centrifugally cast the restoration (Fig. 17-45). After cooling, the inlay is recovered from the mold and cleaned of all investment (Fig. 17-46).
4. The fragile, transparent, glass casting is then heat treated (cerammed) at 1070°C for 6 hours, turning the casting into a whitish, opaque, semicrystalline material (Figs. 17-47 and 17-48). This heat-treating process increases the compressive and tensile strengths, and raises the modulus of elasticity.
5. The restoration is seated on the master die and working cast for final adjustments and finishing (Fig. 17-49).
6. After all fit and contour adjustments have been made, feldspathic "shading porcelains" are applied and fired onto the exterior surfaces for better color matching (Fig. 17-50).

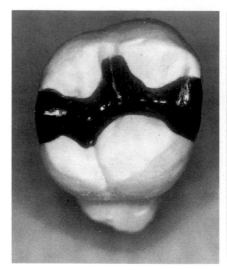

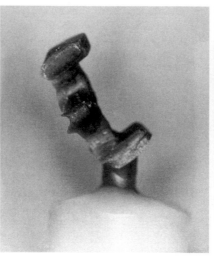

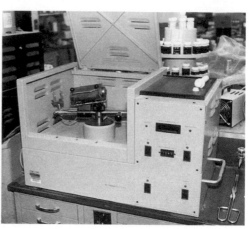

Fig. 17-45. Dicor® casting machine.

Fig. 17-43. Wax pattern for MOD Dicor® inlay.

Fig. 17-44. Wax pattern on sprue base, ready to be invested.

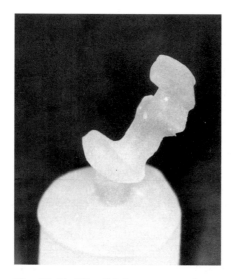

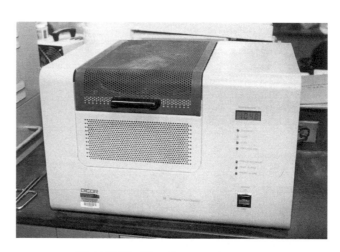

Fig. 17-47. Dicor® ceramming oven.

Fig. 17-46. Dicor® inlay as cast, prior to ceramming cycle.

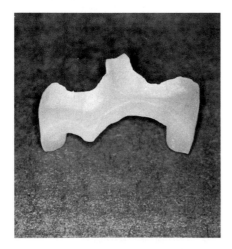

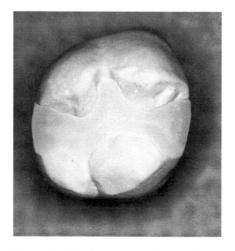

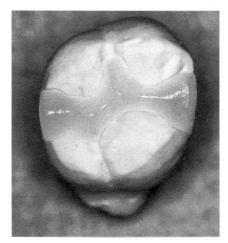

Fig. 17-48. Dicor® inlay becomes stronger, whiter, and more opaque after ceramming cycle.

Fig. 17-49. Cerammed Dicor® inlay seated on die.

Fig. 17-50. Shading porcelains are applied and fired onto exterior inlay surfaces for better color matching. The Dicor® inlay is now ready for delivery.

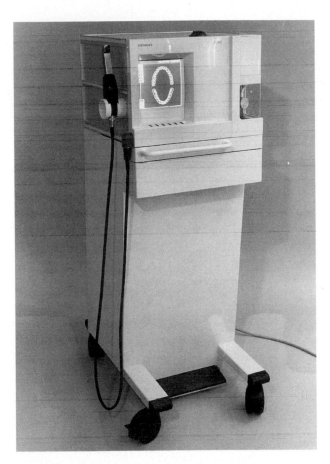

Fig. 17-51. CEREC® CAD/CAM device. Chairside unit is compact and mobile, allowing use in multiple operatories.

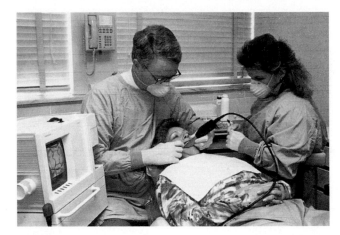

Fig. 17-52. "Optical impression" is made by placing a small video camera/scanner over the prepared tooth.

The *advantages of Dicor®* are (1) its compatibility with the lost-wax casting process, (2) its excellent marginal fit,[15] and (3) its relatively high strength. The surface hardness and occlusal wear of Dicor® are very similar to enamel. The primary *disadvantage of Dicor®* is that low-fusing feldspathic "shading porcelains" must be applied for good color matching. If the dentist has to adjust the inlay during try-in for occlusion or marginal fit, the external stains will be removed, marring the esthetics. While Dicor® inlays are stronger than porcelain inlays made on refractory dies, they are still quite fragile until cemented. The incidence of postcementation fracture for cast Dicor® inlays is lower than that for ceramic inlays made on refractory dies, but higher than for inlays made with the CEREC® system.

CEREC® System. *CAD/CAM* is an acronym for Computer Aided Design/Computer Aided Manufacturing. Rapid improvements in technology have spawned several computerized devices that can fabricate ceramic inlays and onlays out of very high-quality ceramics in a matter of minutes. Some CAD/CAM systems are very expensive *laboratory-based* units requiring the submis-

sion of an impression or working cast of the prepared tooth. The CEREC® system was the first commercially available CAD/CAM system developed for the rapid *chairside* design and fabrication of ceramic restorations (Fig. 17-51). The basic fabrication steps for restorations generated with the CEREC® system can be summarized as follows:

1. The dentist prepares the tooth, then uses a scanning device to collect information on the shape of the preparation (Fig. 17-52). This step is termed an "optical impression". A video image of the prepared tooth is displayed to ensure proper positioning of the scanning device. Most CAD/CAM systems, including the CEREC® system, use optical techniques such as Moiré fringe displacement and/or active triangulation to measure the height/depth of the preparation.

2. The system projects an image of the preparation and surrounding structures on a monitor, allowing the dentist or auxiliary personnel to use the CAD portion of the system to design the restoration. The operator must input and/or confirm the boundaries of the restoration, such as the position of the gingival margins and the proximal contacts (Fig. 17-53).

3. Once the restoration has been designed, the computer directs a micromilling device (CAM portion of the system), which mills the restoration out of a block of high-quality ceramic in a matter of minutes (Fig. 17-54).

4. The restoration is removed from the milling device, ready for try-in and cementation (Fig. 17-55).

As noted earlier, the CEREC® system is designed to be used chairside, which eliminates the need for a conventional impression, temporary restoration, and multi-

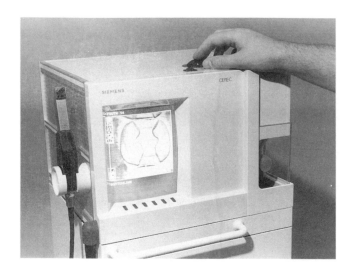

Fig. 17-53. Restoration is designed on computer screen by drawing position of gingival margins and proximal contacts. The device automatically finds the position of occlusal margins. Design time for experienced operator is 3 to 5 minutes.

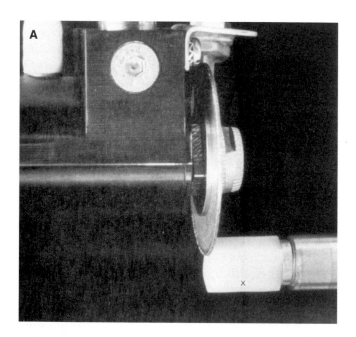

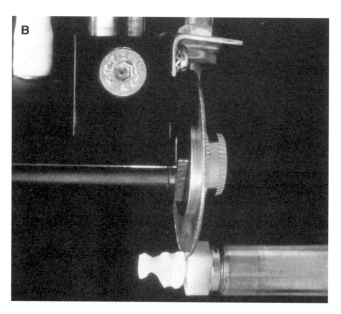

Fig. 17-54. A, Computer controls small milling device which cuts restoration out of block of high-quality ceramic, *(x)*. **B,** Ceramic block rotates as it moves forward into cutting wheel. Cutting wheel moves up and down as needed to form inlay.

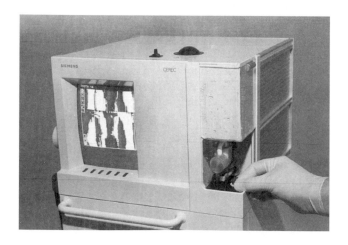

Fig. 17-55. Milling operation usually takes 5 to 7 minutes to complete. Inlay is then removed from milling chamber and is ready for try-in.

ple appointments. In addition to the speed of this system, *a major advantage is the quality of the ceramic restorative material*. Manufacturers make blocks of "machinable ceramics" specifically for computer-assisted milling devices. Since these materials are fabricated under ideal industrial conditions, they are among the strongest ceramics available for use in dentistry, and have many physical properties that closely match those of enamel. One such material is Dicor MGC® (see Table 17-1). Dicor MGC® is available in several shades, and is tooth-colored throughout the thickness of the ceramic block. This feature of Dicor MGC® eliminates the need to apply external shading porcelains for color matching. The major *disadvantages of CAD/CAM* systems are their high cost and the need for extended training. However, technology is changing rapidly, lowering costs and improving capabilities.

Clinical procedures for indirect tooth-colored inlays and onlays

The following sections describe the clinical procedures for laboratory-fabricated tooth-colored inlays and onlays. Many of the clinical steps described are common to both laboratory-fabricated inlays and onlays and CEREC®-generated restorations. However, for details of how the *chairside* CEREC® system differs from the following procedures, see the later section, Clinical Procedures for CEREC® CAD/CAM Inlays and Onlays.

Cavity preparation. *Cavity preparations* vary *for indirect tooth-colored inlays and onlays* due to differences in fabrication steps for each commercial system, and due to variations in the physical properties of the restorative materials. Prior to beginning any procedure, consult the manufacturer's literature and the dental laboratory to ensure the best results. In general, *cavity preparations for indirect tooth-colored inlays and onlays* are essentially the same as those described for cast metal inlays and onlays, minus beveling and secondary flaring (for a detailed description, see Cavity Preparation, in Chapter 19). Due to the physical properties of laboratory-processed composites and porcelains, the *occlusal reduction* for capping cusps should be approximately 1.5 to 2.0 mm. This amount of occlusal reduction will provide sufficient bulk of material for all ceramic and composite systems. The amount of *axial wall reduction* varies depending on the restorative material. Dicor® restorations need 1.2 to 1.5 mm of axial wall reduction, while other porcelain systems ask for 1 to 1.5 mm or more pulpal depth of the axial wall(s). A uniform axial reduction of 1.5 mm is adequate for all ceramic and composite systems. All margins should have a *90-degree cavosurface angle* for marginal strength of the restoration. *Line and point angles, internal and external, should be well-rounded* to avoid stress concentrations in the restoration and tooth, thereby reducing

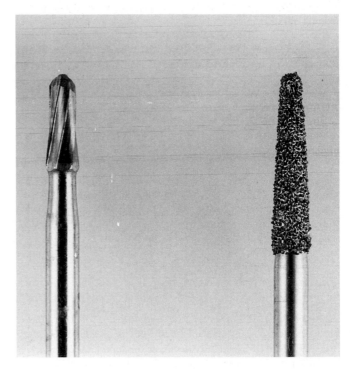

Fig. 17-56. Suggested instruments for cavity preparation: carbide bur No. 1172 and FG diamond No. 767.8C.

the potential for fractures (see Figs. 17-57, 17-58, and 17-59).[1]

The carbide bur used for initial cavity preparation should be a tapering instrument to make straight facial and lingual walls that diverge occlusally to allow for insertion and removal of the restoration, and a coarse diamond instrument similar in shape is used during final cavity preparation (Fig 17-56).* The junction of the side and tip of these instruments should be rounded to avoid sharp, stress-inducing internal angles in the preparation. The gingival to *occlusal divergence* of the cavity preparation may be increased from the 2° to 5° per wall for cast metal inlays and onlays to 6° 8°.[19] The divergence can be increased since the tooth-colored restoration will be adhesively bonded at cementation, and since very little pressure can be applied during try-in or cementation. Throughout cavity preparation the cutting instruments used to develop the longitudinal (vertical) walls are oriented to a single "draw" path, usually the long axis of the tooth crown (see Fig. 19-4). The occlusal step should be prepared 1.5 to 2 mm in depth. Most systems request that any isthmus and any groove extension be at least 1.5 mm wide to decrease the possibility

*Suggested instruments: Carbide bur No. 1172, Midwest Dental Products Co., DesPlaines, Ill. Two Striper® diamond No. 767.8C, Premier Dental Products Co., Norristown, Penn.

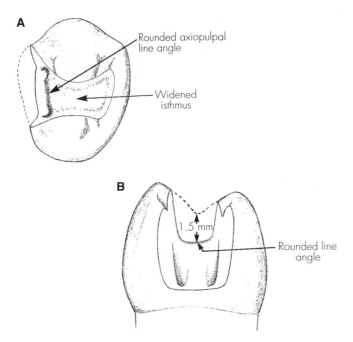

Fig. 17-57. A, MO inlay preparation for tooth-colored inlay in maxillary first premolar. Isthmus should be at least 1.5 mm in width to prevent inlay fracture. Axiopulpal line angle should be well-rounded to avoid seating errors and to lower stress concentrations. **B,** MOD inlay preparation for tooth-colored inlay in maxillary first premolar. Pulpal floor should be prepared 1.5 mm in depth, and axiopulpal line angles should be well-rounded. Interproximal margins should be extended to allow at least 0.5 mm clearance of contact with neighboring tooth. Gingival margins in enamel are greatly preferred. (Modified from Banks RG: J Prosthet Dent 63(6):619-626, 1990.)

of fracture of the restoration (Fig. 17-57). The facial and lingual walls should be extended to sound tooth structure, and should go around the cusps in graceful curves. Ideally, there should be no undercuts that would prevent the insertion or removal of the restoration. Small undercuts, if present, can be blocked out by the use of a glass ionomer cement. The pulpal floor should be smooth and relatively flat. Following removal of remaining infected caries or previous restorative material from any internal wall (pulpal or axial wall), the wall is restored to ideal position with a light-cured glass ionomer cement (see Fig. 19-9).

When extending up cuspal inclines to reach sound tooth structure, a cusp should be capped if the extension is two thirds or greater from any primary groove to the cusp tip (see Fig. 19-22, *A* and *B*). If cusps need to be capped, they should be reduced 1.5 to 2 mm, allowing for a 90-degree cavosurface angle (see Fig. 19-22, *C* to *F*). When capping cusps, especially centric holding cusps, it may be necessary to prepare a "collar" to move the facial or lingual cavosurface margin away from any possible contact with the opposing tooth, either in maximum intercuspal position or during mandibular move-

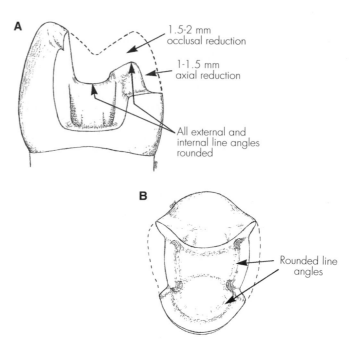

Fig. 17-58. A, Proximal view of a MODL inlay preparation on maxillary first premolar, capping lingual cusp. Lingual cusp has been reduced and lingual margin extended beyond any possible contact with opposing tooth by preparing a "collar." **B,** Occlusal view.

ments (Figs. 17-58 and 19-30, *A* to *C*). Such contacts directly on margins can lead to premature deterioration of marginal integrity. The axial wall of the collar should be prepared to allow for "draw" and be sufficiently deep to allow for 1 to 1.5 mm minimal thickness of the restorative material.

Proximal boxes are prepared identically as those for cast metal inlays (see Fig. 19-7). The facial, lingual, and gingival margins of the proximal boxes should be extended to clear the adjacent tooth by at least 0.5 mm. These clearances will provide adequate access to the margins during the impression and during finishing and polishing. For all walls, a 90-degree cavosurface margin is desired, since composite and ceramic inlays are fragile when in thin cross section. Take great care to have the minimum possible extension of the gingival margin, since margins in enamel are greatly preferred for bonding, and since deep gingival margins are difficult to isolate properly during cementation. When a portion of the facial (lingual) surface is affected by caries or other injury, it may be necessary to extend the preparation (with a gingival shoulder) around the transitional line angle to include the defect (Figs. 17-59 and 19-24, *I* to *J*). The axial wall of the shouldered extension should be prepared to allow for 1 to 1.5 mm minimum of restoration thickness.

A diamond instrument that has a similar shape as the carbide bur is used during final finishing of the cavity

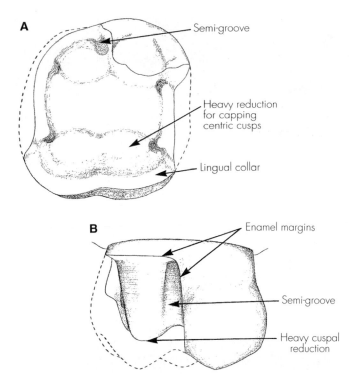

A

Semi-groove

Heavy reduction for capping centric cusps

Lingual collar

B

Enamel margins

Semi-groove

Heavy cuspal reduction

Fig. 17-59. MODFL inlay preparation on maxillary right first molar. Distofacial, mesiolingual, and distolingual cusps are reduced. **A,** Occlusal view. Shallow "semi-grooves," created by using ⅓ the diameter of diamond instrument, can be prepared when additional retention form is desired. **B,** Facial view. (From Banks RG: J Prosthet Dent 63(6):619-626, 1990.)

walls to *increase the surface roughness and the surface area for bonding.* During final finishing take care to remove all stains on the walls, such as those often left by corrosion products of old amalgam restorations. Such stains would later appear as black or gray lines at the margin after cementation. *It is especially critical to generously round all line and point angles, internal and external, to avoid areas of stress concentrations that could later fracture the tooth-colored restoration.*

Impression. Most tooth-colored indirect inlay/onlay systems require the dentist to make an impression of the prepared tooth and the adjacent teeth, which allows the restoration to be fabricated on a working cast in the laboratory (see Final Impression, in Chapter 19).

Temporary. A provisional restoration is necessary when using indirect systems that require two appointments. The temporary can be made using conventional techniques (see Resin Temporary in Chapter 19) but a *eugenol-free temporary cement* should be used to ensure proper setting of the final composite resin cement.*

Try-in and cementation. The try-in and cementation of tooth-colored inlays/onlays is more demanding than

*Temp-Bond NE℠, Kerr Manufacturing Co., Romulus, Mich.

that for cast metal restorations due to (1) the fragile nature of the ceramic or composite material, (2) the requirement of near perfect moisture control, and (3) the use of composite resin as a cement. The ceramic or composite inlay is relatively fragile until it is adhesively bonded in place with composite resin. *Very little pressure should be applied to the restoration during try-in. Due to this fragility, most clinicians delay checking and adjusting the occlusion until after cementation. Tooth-colored composite cements require excellent moisture control for adhesive bonding. Excess set composite cement is relatively difficult to visualize and remove compared with the conventional cements used for cast metal restorations.*

Preliminary steps for try-in and cementation. The use of the **rubber dam** should be considered mandatory to prevent moisture contamination of the conditioned tooth or inlay surfaces during cementation, as well as to improve access and visibility during all phases of delivery. Remove the temporary restoration, making sure that all the temporary cement has been dislodged from the cavity walls and cleared away.

Try-in of restoration and adjustment of the proximal contacts. Evaluate the fit of the inlay/onlay on the tooth. Use *very light* pressure. If the restoration does not seat completely, the most likely cause is an over-contoured proximal surface (Fig. 17-60). Using the mouth mirror where needed, view into the embrasures from the facial, lingual, and occlusal aspects. Judge where the proximal contour needs adjustment to allow final seating of the restoration, producing at the same time the *correct position and form of the contact.* Passing dental floss (or, better still, a separated thin strand of the floss) through the contact(s) will indicate the tightness and position, thus signifying to the trained operator the degree of excess contact and its location (see Seating the Casting and Adjusting Proximal Contacts, in Chapter 19). Use abrasive disks to adjust the proximal contour and to correct the contact relationship.* While adjusting the intensity and location of the proximal contacts, use successively finer grits of abrasive disks to polish the proximal surfaces since they will be inaccessible after cementation. After the restoration is completely seated, *verify the fit around the margins.* Slight excesses of contour can be removed if access allows using fine-grit diamond instruments or 30-fluted carbide finishing burs. The marginal fit of cast Dicor[R] restorations has been reported to be equal to that of gold castings.[15] Most of the other systems will typically produce restorations with slightly larger marginal gaps than for comparable gold restorations.[36]

Cementation. For proper adhesive bonding, *the cavity side of the inlay/onlay must be conditioned prior to*

*Soflex disks℠, 3-M, Dental Products Division, St. Paul, Minn.

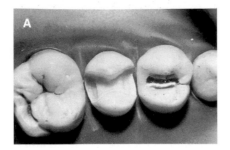
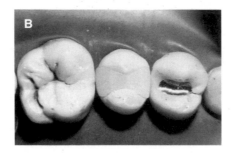
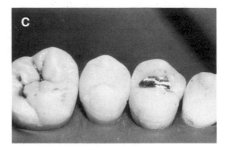

Fig. 17-60. A, MOD inlay preparation for ceramic inlay on maxillary right second premolar. **B,** Ceramic CEREC® inlay fails to seat due to tight interproximal contacts. **C,** Inlay seated after adjustments. Inlay proximal surfaces should be polished prior to cementation.

cementation. The techniques and materials vary depending on the specific restorative system used.

For most laboratory-processed composite inlays/onlays, the resin matrix has been polymerized to such an extent that few bonding sites are available for the cementing composite to chemically bond to the cavity side of the restoration. To improve the bond of the cement to the processed composite restoration, some systems require the use of a solvent (such as ethyl acetate) to soften the cavity side of the restoration prior to cementation. Other systems recommend sandblasting the cavity side of the composite restoration with aluminum-oxide abrasive particles to increase surface roughness and surface area for bonding. One particular system uses hydrofluoric acid to etch the cavity surface of the composite restoration.* This 10% solution of hydrofluoric acid purportedly etches the ceramic filler particles, providing further micromechanical retention.

For ceramic inlays and onlays, specific acids are used to *etch the cavity side of the ceramic restoration* (Figs. 17-61 and 6-68). After etching, the etched ceramic is treated with a **silanating agent**† to further improve the bond to the composite cement.

Clear *plastic matrix strips are applied* in each affected proximal, and *wedged* (Fig. 17-62).‡ The *preparation surfaces are conditioned with acid* etchants, and an enamel-dentin *bonding agent* applied.§ Unfilled bonding agent is applied to the cavity side of the restoration and blown to a thin film. A *dual-cured composite cement* is mixed and inserted into the cavity with a pad-

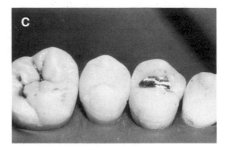

Fig. 17-61. Applying acid to cavity sides of ceramic inlay. After rinsing and drying, etched ceramic surfaces should have a "frosty" white appearance.

dle-shaped instrument or a syringe.* The cavity side of the restoration also is coated with composite cement (Fig. 17-63, *A),* and the inlay is immediately inserted into the cavity, using light pressure (Fig. 17-63, *B).* A ball burnisher applied with a slight vibrating motion is usually sufficient to *seat the restoration. Excess composite cement is removed* with thinly bladed composite

*Herculite XRV™ Lab, Kerr Manufacturing Co., Romulus, Mich.
†Scotchprime™, 3-M, Dental Products Division, St. Paul, Minn.
‡Polyester Matrix Tape, 3-M, Dental Products Division, St. Paul, Minn.
§Scotchbond™ Multipurpose Dental Adhesive, 3-M, Dental Products Division, St. Paul, Minn.

*Dual Cement™, Vivadent USA, Inc., Tonawanda, NY.

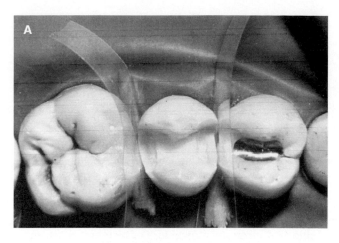

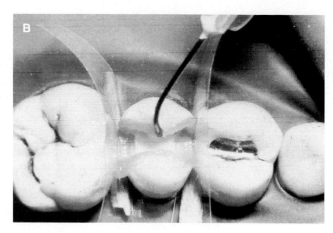

Fig. 17-62. A, Clear polyester matrix strips are applied and wedged prior to etching and cementation. **B,** Applying acid etchant to cavity surfaces.

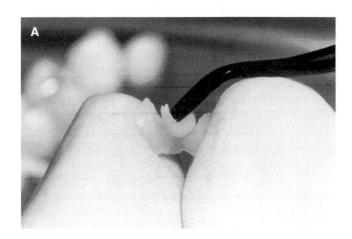

Fig. 17-63. A, Dual-cured composite cement is applied to cavity and to inlay. **B,** CEREC® ceramic inlay is seated into cavity preparation. **C,** Prior to curing, excess composite cement is removed with explorer, brushes, and IPC carver. **D,** Light-cure the composite cement from occlusal, facial, and lingual directions.

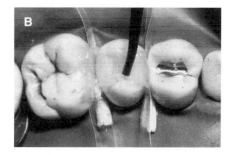

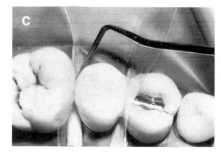

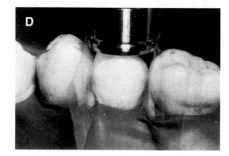

instruments, brushes, or with the tine of an explorer (Fig. 17-63. *C*). Take care not to remove composite from the marginal interface between the tooth and the inlay. The restoration is now *light-cured* from occlusal, facial, and lingual directions for a minimum exposure of 40 to 60 seconds each direction (Fig. 17-63, *D*).

Finishing and polishing procedures. Remove the plastic matrix strips and the wedges, and verify the setting of the composite cement. Inspect the margins in all areas with an explorer tine. In all regions, the composite should be hard. Since wedges and matrix were used interproximally, these difficult to finish areas should feel quite smooth, with little if any flash extending beyond the margins in a gingival direction.

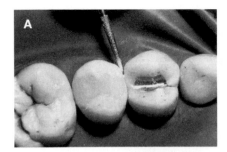

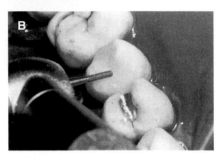

Fig. 17-64. A, Slender, fine-grit, flame-shaped, diamond instruments are used to remove flash along facial and lingual margins of CEREC® ceramic inlay. **B,** Cylindrical or oval shapes are used to remove flash on occlusal surface.

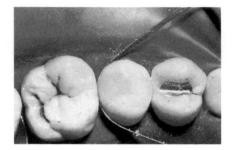

Fig. 17-65. Smoothing interproximal area with abrasive finishing strip.

Table 17-2. Instrumentation for finishing and polishing

Sequence	Instrument
1	Fine-grit diamond instruments
2	30-Fluted carbide burs
3	Rubber, abrasive, porcelain polishing points
4	Porcelain polishing paste

Fine-grit diamond instruments are used initially to remove any excess composite cement back to the margin. Care must be taken to preserve the glazed surface of ceramic restorations as much as possible. Slender flame shapes are used interproximally (Fig. 17-64, *A*), while larger oval or cylindrical shapes are used on the occlusal surface (Fig. 17-64, *B*). After using the fine-grit diamond instruments, 30-fluted carbide finishing burs are used to obtain a smoother finish.*

Interproximally, a No. 12 surgical blade can be used to remove excess composite cement when access permits (see Fig. 17-28, *D*).† Abrasive strips of successively finer grits also can be used to remove slight interproximal excesses (Fig. 17-65).‡ Much care must be used to avoid cutting the gingiva or scarring the root surfaces when using such instruments interproximally. After all excess composite cement has been removed and marginal integrity verified, the rubber dam is removed.

The occlusion is now checked and adjusted where

necessary. With good occlusal records and careful laboratory work, little if any correction should be necessary. Premature occlusal contacts can be adjusted using fine-grit diamond instruments followed by 30-fluted carbide finishing burs.

After occlusal adjustments are completed, the restoration must be repolished in all areas where corrections have been made, especially in areas on ceramic restorations where the glaze may have been disrupted. Indirect composite inlays/onlays can be polished using the same instrumentation and materials used for direct composites. (See in this chapter the previous section, Finishing Procedures.)

With care, ceramic restorations can be polished to a surface smoother than glazed porcelain using the abrasive sequence shown in Table 17-2.[12] Fine-grit diamonds are used for contour adjustments, followed by the use of 30-fluted carbide finishing burs (Fig. 17-66, *A*). Further smoothing is accomplished with a series of rubber abrasive points and cups used at slow speed with air-water spray (Fig. 17-66, *B* and *C*).* Final polishing of the ceramic restoration is achieved with a diamond polishing paste applied with a bristle brush or another suitable instrument (Fig. 17-66, *D*).† Ceramic restorations polished with this series of instruments can have a remarkably beautiful, smooth surface (Fig. 17-66, *E* and *F*).

*9803, 9406 carbide finishing burs, Kerr/Sybron, Romulus, Mich.
†Bard-Parker® No. 12 stainless steel surgical blade, Becton Dickinson AcuteCare, Franklin Lakes, NJ.
‡Enhance™ finishing and polishing strips, LD Caulk, A Division of Dentsply International, Milford, Del.

*Porcelain Laminate Polishing Kit, Shofu Dental Corp., Menlo Park, Calif.
†Truluster Porcelain Polishing System, Brassler USA Inc., Savannah, Ga.

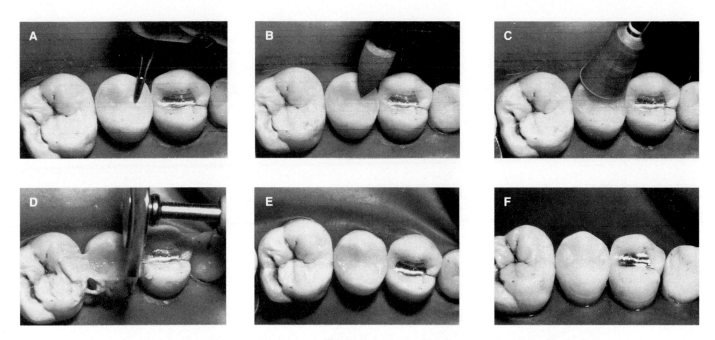

Fig. 17-66. Polishing sequence for ceramic inlays. **A,** 30-fluted carbide finishing burs can be used for fine contour adjustments or for minor corrections in the occlusal contacts. **B and C,** For further smoothing, rubber abrasive points and cups of successively finer grits are used at slow speed with air-water spray. **D,** Final polish imparted by porcelain polishing paste applied with bristle brush. Polished ceramic inlay; occlusal view, **E,** and view from lingual occlusal aspect, **F.**

Clinical procedures for CEREC® CAD/CAM inlays and onlays

The CEREC® CAD/CAM system has several differences in the clinical procedures previously described. Cavity preparations for CAD/CAM inlays must reflect the capabilities of the CAD (Computer Assisted Design) software and hardware, and the CAM machining devices (Computer Assisted Manufacturing) which fabricate the restorations. One example of how cavity preparations are modified when using the CEREC® system is in regard to "blocking out" undercuts. As previously described, most laboratory-fabricated indirect systems require the preparation to have "draw" so that the restoration can be inserted and removed without interferences from undercuts. The CEREC® system automatically "blocks out" any undercuts during the optical impression. This feature often results in a more conservative cavity preparation along the occlusal aspect, especially when replacing old amalgam restorations, which were prepared purposefully with undercuts for retention (Fig. 17-67). However, the facial and lingual walls of the proximal boxes should be prepared with draw to avoid excessively thick composite cement lines.

Using the CEREC® system, most dentists can prepare the tooth, fabricate, and deliver an inlay in about 1 hour. This system eliminates the need for a conven-

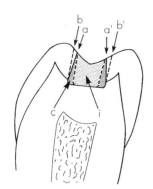

Fig. 17-67. Along occlusal aspect, margins at *a-a'* do not have to be extended to *b-b'* to make preparation draw when using CEREC® system. CEREC® inlay, *i,* will have internal clearance spaces with cavity walls. These spaces will be filled with composite cement, *c.*

tional impression, temporary restoration, and multiple patient appointments.

When delivering a CEREC® inlay, more adjustments are usually necessary when trying-in, finishing, and polishing. The CEREC® system initially mills the occlusal surface relatively flat without any significant surface detail, and does not take into account the opposing occlu-

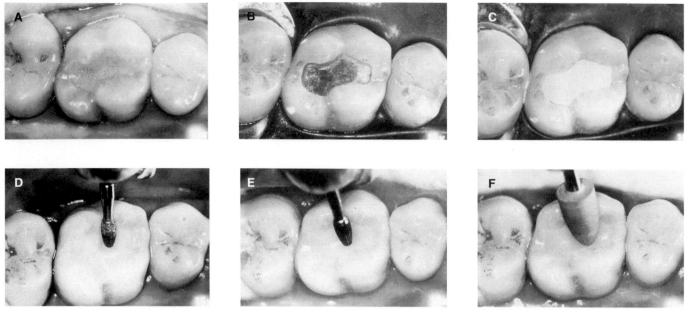

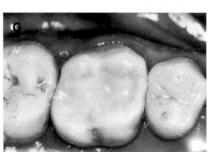

Fig. 17-68. Occlusal CEREC® inlay (Dicor MGC®) on maxillary first molar. **A,** Posterior composite restoration with excessive occlusal wear. **B,** Cavity preparation for CEREC® inlay. Note that occlusal preparation can have undercuts (does not have to draw). **C,** Initial try-in of inlay. Note that occlusal surface is relatively flat. **D,** Correcting occlusal contours of cemented inlay with medium-coarse diamond. **E,** 30-fluted carbide finishing bur is used for final contour corrections. **F,** Polishing inlay with abrasive rubber points. **G,** Completed inlay.

sion (Fig. 17-68). When adjusting the occlusion of a CEREC® inlay, it may be necessary to use coarse or medium-grit diamonds with air- water spray coolant for initial gross contouring of the occlusal surface, followed by the instrumentation previously discussed for finishing and polishing. Chairside CAD/CAM systems will soon have more capabilities relative to occlusal anatomy and occlusion, as well as the ability to manufacture more complex restorations that need fewer try-in adjustments. An arch containing several CEREC[R] CAD/CAM inlays is shown in Fig. 17-69.

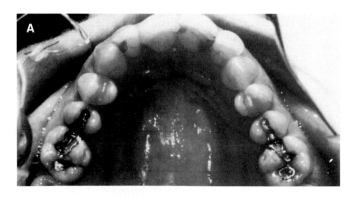

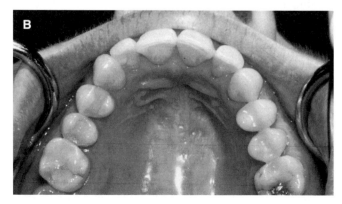

Fig. 17-69. A, Preoperative view. **B,** Postoperative view of dental arch containing several CEREC® inlays made of Dicor MGC®.

REFERENCES

1. Banks RG: Conservative posterior ceramic restorations: a literature review, *J Prosthet Dent* 63(6):619-26, 1990.

2. Barnes DM et al: A 5- and 8-year clinical evaluation of a posterior composite resin, *Quintessence Int* 22:143-151, 1991.

3. Bayne SC et al: Clinical longevity of ten posterior composite materials based on wear, *J Dent Res* 70:344, 1991 (abstract no. 630).

4. Bayne SC et al: Long term clinical failures in posterior composites, *J Dent Res* 68:185, 1989 (abstract no. 32).

5. Brunson WD et al: Analysis of modified retention for posterior composite restorations, *J Dent Res* 67(special issue):221, 1988 (abstract no. 865).

6. Buonocore MG: A simple method of increasing the adhesion of acrylic filling materials to enamel surfaces, *J Dent Res* 34:849, 1955.

7. Burgoyne AR, Nicholls JI, Brudvik JS: In vitro two-body wear of inlay-onlay composite resin restoratives, *J Prosthet Dent* 65(2):206-214, 1991.

8. Douglas WH, Fields RP, Fundingsland J: A comparison between the microleakage of direct and indirect composite restorative systems, *J Dent* 17(4):184-188, 1989.

9. Gwinnett AJ: Moist versus dry dentin: its effect on shear bond strength, *Am J Dent* 5:127-129, 1992.

10. Gwinnett AJ, Kanca JA: Micromorphology of the bonded dentin interface and its relationship to bond strength, *Am J Dent* 5:73-77, 1992.

11. Handelman SL et al: Clinical radiographic evaluation of sealed carious and sound tooth surfaces, *J Am Dent Assoc* 113:751-754, Nov 1986.

12. Haywood VB et al: Polishing porcelain veneers: an SEM and specular reflectance analysis, *Dent Mater* 4(3):116-21, 1988.

13. Heymann HO, Bayne SC: Current concepts in dentin bonding: focusing on dentinal adhesion factors, *J Am Dent Assoc* 124(5):27-36, May 1993.

14. Heymann HO et al: Two-year clinical study of composite resins in posterior teeth, *Dent Mater* 2:37-41, 1986.

15. Holmes JR et al: Marginal fit of castable ceramic crowns, *J Prosthet Dent* 67(5):594-9, 1992.

16. Jensen ME et al: Posterior etched-porcelain restorations: an in vitro study, *Compendium* 8(8):615-7, 1987.

17. Leinfelder KF et al: Clinical evaluation of composite resins as anterior and posterior restorative materials, *J Prosthet Dent* 33:407, 1975.

18. MacCulloch WT: Advances in dental ceramics, *Br Dent J* 124(8):361-365, 1968.

19. Malament KA, Grossman DG: The cast glass-ceramic restoration, *J Prosthet Dent* 57(6):674-683, 1987.

20. Mazer RB, Leinfelder KF: Evaluating a microfill posterior composite resin: a five-year study, *J Am Dent Assoc* 123(4):33-38, 1992.

21. Mazer RB, Leinfelder KF: Clinical evaluation of a posterior composite resin containing a new type of filler particle, *J Esthet Dent* 1:66-70, 1988.

22. McCune RJ, Cvar JF, Ryge G: Clinical comparison of anterior and posterior restorative materials, *Int Assoc Dent Res* p 161, March 1969 (abstract no 482).

23. McCune RJ et al: Clinical comparison of posterior restorative materials, *Int Assoc Dent Res* p 175, March 1967 (abstract no. 546).

24. Mertz-Fairhurst EJ et al: Cariostatic and ultraconservative sealed restorations: six year results, *Quintessence Int* 23(12):827-838, 1992.

25. Morin D, DeLong R, Douglas WH: Cusp reinforcement by the acid-etch technique, *J Dent Res* 63(8):1075-1078, 1984.

26. Oldenburg TO, Vann WF, Dilley DC: Composite restorations for primary molars:results after four years, *Pediatr Dent* 9(2):136-143, 1987.

27. Paquette DE et al: Modified cavity preparations for composite resins in primary molars, *Pediatr Dent* 5:246-251, 1983.

28. Phillips RW: *Skinner's Science of Dental Materials,* ed 8, Philadelphia, 1982, WB Saunders.

29. Phillips RW et al: Observations on a composite resin for Class II restorations: two-year report, *J Prosthet Dent* 28(2):164, 1972.

30. Schneider PM, Messer LB, Douglas WH: The effect of enamel surface reduction in vitro on the bonding of composite resin to permanent human enamel, *J Dent Res* 60:895, 1981.

31. Sheth PJ, Jensen ME, Sheth JJ: Comparative evaluation of three resin inlay techniques: microleakage studies, *Quintessence Int* 20(11):831-836, 1989.

32. Shortall AC et al: Marginal seal comparisons between resin-bonded Class II porcelain inlays, posterior composite restorations, and direct composite resin inlays, *Int J Prosthodont* 2(3):217-223, 1989.

33. Simonsen RJ: Retention and effectiveness of a single application of white sealant after 10 years, *J Am Dent Assoc* 115:31-36, July 1987.

34. Simonsen RJ: Preventive resin restorations: three year results, *J Am Dent Assoc* 100(4):535-539, 1980.

35. Simonsen RJ: Preventive resin restoration, *Quintessence Int* 9(1):69-76, 1978.

36. Sturdevant JR et al: Composite cement thickness of CEREC® CAD/CAM ceramic inlays, *J Dent Res* 70:296, 1991 (abstract no. 245).

37. Sturdevant JR et al: Five-year study of two light-cured posterior composite resins, *Dent Mater* 4:105-110, 1988.

38. Swift EJ Jr: The effect of sealants on dental caries: a review, *J Am Dent Assoc* 116:700-704, May 1988.

39. Wendt SL, Leinfelder KF: The clinical evaluation of heat-treated composite resin inlays, *J Am Dent Assoc* 120(2):177-181, 1990.

40. Wilder AD, May KN, Leinfelder KF: Three-year clinical study of UV-cured composite resins in posterior teeth, *J Prosthet Dent* 50(1):26, 1983.

41. Wilson NHF et al: Five-year findings of a multiclinical trial for a posterior composite, *J Dent* 19:153-159, 1991.

CHAPTER 18

Additional conservative esthetic procedures

Harald O. Heymann

Clarence L. Sockwell*

Van B. Haywood

*This author is inactive this edition; see Preface.

INTRODUCTION

Significant improvements in tooth-colored restorative materials and adhesive techniques have resulted in numerous conservative esthetic treatment possibilities. Although restorative dentistry always has enjoyed the distinction of being a blend of art and science, *conservative esthetic dentistry* truly emphasizes the *artistic component*. As Dr. Ronald E. Goldstein states, "Esthetic dentistry is the art of dentistry in its purest form."[23] As with many forms of art, conservative esthetic dentistry provides the individual a means of artistic expression that feeds on creativity and imagination. Because of this, dentists find performing conservative esthetic procedures to be most enjoyable. Furthermore, conservative esthetic dentistry is most rewarding, because patients typically appreciate the immediate esthetic improvements that are rendered, oftentimes without the need for local anesthesia.

One of the greatest assets a person can have is a smile that shows beautiful, natural teeth (Plate 18-1, *A* to *C*). When teeth are discolored, malformed, crooked, or missing, there is often a conscious effort to avoid smiling, and other defense mechanisms are used to "cover up" the teeth. Children are especially sensitive about unattractive teeth because of cruel remarks made by other children. Most teenagers are extremely concerned if their teeth are abnormal. Correction of these types of dental problems can produce dramatic changes in appearance, which often result in improved confidence, personality, and social life. The restoration of a smile is one of the most appreciated and gratifying services a dentist can render. In fact, the *positive psychological effects of improving a patient's smile* often contribute to an improved self-image and enhanced self-esteem. These improvements make conservative esthetic dentistry particularly gratifying for the dentist and represent a new dimension of dental treatment for patients.

In this chapter, many such conservative esthetic procedures, as well as other extended uses of the acid etch technique, are presented in the context of their clinical applications. The principles and clinical steps in acid etching and adhesive bonding for the treatment alternatives presented in this chapter are similar to those previously described in Chapter 16. Only specific conservative esthetic clinical procedures or variations from previously described techniques are presented in this chapter.

ARTISTIC ELEMENTS

Regardless of the final result desired, certain basic artistic elements must be considered to ensure an opti-

mally esthetic result. In conservative esthetic dentistry these include:

1. Shape or form
2. Symmetry and proportionality
3. Position and alignment
4. Surface texture
5. Color
6. Translucency

Some or all of these elements are common to virtually every conservative esthetic dental procedure. Therefore, a basic knowledge and understanding of these artistic elements is required to attain esthetic results consistently.

Shape or form

The shape or form of teeth largely determines their esthetic appearance. In order to achieve optimal dental esthetics, it is imperative that natural anatomic forms be achieved. Therefore, a basic knowledge of normal tooth anatomy is fundamental to the success of any conservative esthetic dental procedure.

When viewing the clinical crown of an incisor from a facial (or lingual) position, the crown outline is trapezoidal.[5] However, subtle variations in shape and contour produce very different appearances. For instance, a youthful, *feminine smile* typically is characterized by rounded incisal angles, open incisal and facial embrasures, and softened facial line angles. A more *masculine smile*, or a smile characteristic of an older individual having experienced attrition due to aging, typically exhibits incisal embrasures that are more closed as well as more prominent (less rounded) incisal angles. Frequently, minor modification of existing tooth contours, sometimes referred to as **cosmetic contouring**, can effect a significant esthetic change (see Alterations of Shape of Natural Teeth). As illustrated in Fig. 18-1, *A* and *B*, and Plate 18-1, *D* and *E*, reshaping enamel by rounding incisal angles, opening incisal embrasures, and reducing prominent facial line angles can produce a more feminine, youthful appearance.

Significant generalized esthetic changes are possible when treating all the anterior teeth (and also occasionally first premolars) visible in the patient's smile. This fact is particularly true when placing full coverage fa-

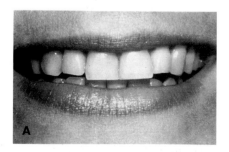
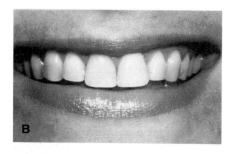

Fig. 18-1. Cosmetic contouring. **A,** Anterior teeth before treatment. **B,** By reshaping teeth, a more feminine, youthful appearance is produced.

cial restorations such as *laminate veneers* (see Veneers).[13,35,61] With this treatment method, the dentist can produce significant changes in tooth shapes and forms to yield a variety of different appearances.

Although less extensive, restoring an individual tooth rather than all anterior teeth simultaneously may, in fact, require greater artistic ability. Generalized restoration of all anterior teeth with full facial veneers affords the dentist significant control of the contours generated. When treating an isolated tooth, however, the success of the result is largely determined by how well the restored tooth esthetically matches the surrounding natural teeth. The contralateral tooth to that being restored should be closely examined for subtle characterizing features such as developmental depressions, embrasure form, prominences, or other distinguishing characteristics of shape or form. A high degree of realism must be reproduced artfully to achieve optimal esthetics when restoring isolated teeth or areas.

Illusions of shape or form also play a significant role in dental esthetics. The border outline of an anterior tooth (facial view) is primarily two-dimensional (length and width). However, the third dimension of depth is critical in creating illusions, especially those of apparent width and length.

Prominent areas of contour on a tooth typically are highlighted upon direct illumination, making them more noticeable, while areas of depression or diminishing contour are shadowed and less conspicuous. By controlling the areas of light reflection and shadowing, full facial coverage restorations in particular can be esthetically contoured to achieve various desired illusions of shape or form. Moreover, the *apparent size of a tooth* can be changed by altering the position of facial prominences or heights of contour without changing the actual dimension of the tooth. For example, when com-pared to normal tooth contours as seen in Fig. 18-2, *A*, a tooth can be made to appear narrower by positioning the mesiofacial and distofacial line angles closer together (Fig. 18-2, *B*). Developmental depressions also can be positioned closer together to enhance the illusion of narrowness. In like manner, greater apparent width can be achieved by positioning the line angles and developmental depressions further apart (Fig. 18-2, *C*).

Although more difficult, the apparent length of teeth also can be changed by illusion. When compared to normal tooth contours (Fig. 18-3, *A*), a tooth can be made to appear shorter by emphasizing the horizontal elements, such as gingival perikymata, and by positioning the gingival height of contour further incisally (Fig. 18-3, *B*). Slight modification of the incisal area, achieved by moving the incisal height of contour further gingivally, also enhances the illusion of a shorter tooth. The opposite tenets are true for increasing the apparent length of a tooth. The heights of contour are moved further apart inciso-gingivally, and vertical elements such as developmental depressions are emphasized (Fig. 18-3, *C*).

Used in combination, these illusionary techniques are particularly valuable for controlling the apparent dimension of teeth in procedures that result in an actual increased width of the teeth, such as *diastema closure* (see Correction of Diastemata). By contouring the composite additions in such a way that the original positions of the line angles are maintained, the increased widths of the restored teeth are less noticeable (Fig. 18-4, *A* and *B*). Furthermore, if full facial coverage restorations are placed in conjunction with a diastema closure, vertical elements can be enhanced and horizontal features de-emphasized to control further the apparent dimension of the teeth.

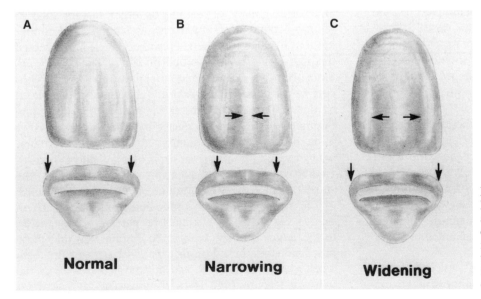

Normal   **Narrowing**   **Widening**

Fig. 18-2. Creating illusions of width. **A,** Normal width. **B,** A tooth can be made to appear narrower by positioning mesial and distal line angles closer together and by more closely approximating developmental depressions. **C,** Greater apparent width is achieved by positioning line angles and developmental depressions further apart.

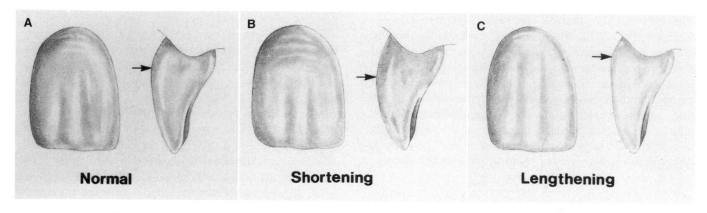

Fig. 18-3. Creating illusions of length. **A,** Normal length. **B,** A tooth can be made to appear shorter by emphasizing horizontal elements and by positioning the gingival height of contour further incisally. **C,** The illusion of length is achieved by moving the gingival height of contour gingivally and by emphasizing vertical elements such as developmental depressions.

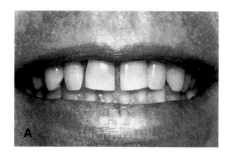
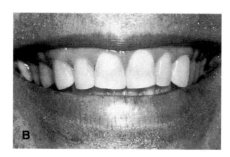

Fig. 18-4. Controlling apparent tooth size when adding proximal dimension. **A,** Teeth before treatment. **B,** By maintaining original positions of the facial line angles (see areas of light reflection), increased widths of teeth following composite augmentations are less noticeable.

Symmetry and proportionality

The overall esthetic appearance of a human smile is largely governed by the symmetry and proportionality of the teeth that constitute the smile. Asymmetrical teeth or teeth which are out of proportion to the surrounding teeth disrupt the sense of balance and harmony that are essential for optimal esthetics. Assuming the teeth are of normal alignment (i.e., rotations or faciolingual positional defects are not present), dental symmetry can be maintained if the sizes of the contralateral teeth are equivalent. A dental caliper should be used in conjunction with any conservative esthetic dental procedure that will alter the mesiodistal dimension of the teeth. This recommendation is particularly true for procedures such as diastema closure or other procedures involving augmentation of proximal surfaces with composite.[6,39] By first measuring and recording the widths of the interdental space and the involved teeth to be augmented, the appropriate amount of contour to be generated with composite resin addition can be determined (Fig. 18-5, *A* and *B*). In this manner, symmetrical and equal tooth contours can be generated (see Correction of Diastemata).

Particular attention also must be afforded to incisal and gingival embrasure form when dealing with restora-

tions of any type involving the midline. The mesial contours of both central incisors must be mirror images of one another to ensure an optimally symmetrical and esthetic result.

In addition to being symmetrical, anterior teeth must be in proper proportion to one another to achieve maximum esthetics. The quality of proportionality is relative and varies greatly depending on other factors such as tooth position, tooth alignment, arch form, and configuration of the smile itself. However, one long-accepted theorem of the relative proportionality of maxillary anterior teeth typically visible in a smile involves the concept of the *golden proportion*.[50] Originally formulated as one of Euclid's elements, it has been relied upon through the ages as a geometric basis for proportionality in the beauty of art and nature.[11] Based on this formula, when viewed directly from the front, a smile is considered to be esthetically pleasing if each tooth in that smile (starting from the midline) is approximately 60% of the size of the tooth immediately mesial to it. As seen in Fig. 18-6, *A,* the exact proportion of the smaller to the larger is .618. It must be emphasized that these proportions are based on the *apparent sizes* of the teeth when viewed straight-on and not the actual sizes of the individual teeth. Fig. 18-6, *B,* illustrates a typical es-

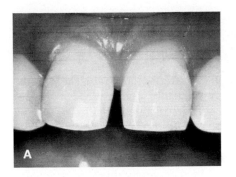

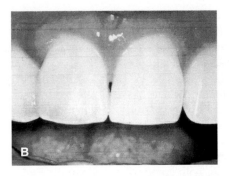

Fig. 18-5. Diastema closure. A, Teeth before composite additions. B, Symmetrical and equal contours are achieved in the final restorations.

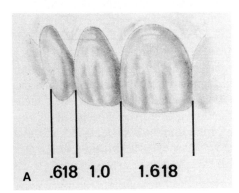

A   .618 1.0   1.618

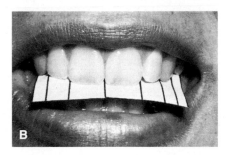

Fig. 18-6. The rule of the golden proportion. A, The exact ratios of proportionality. B, The anterior teeth of this patient are in "golden proportion" to one another.

thetically pleasing smile in which the maxillary anterior teeth are generally in golden proportion to one another. Although this theorem is not the absolute determinant of dental esthetics, it does provide a practical and proven guide for establishing proportionality when restoring anterior teeth.

Position and alignment

The overall harmony and balance of a smile are largely dependent on how well the teeth are in proper position and alignment in the arch. Malposed or rotated teeth not only disrupt the arch form, but also may interfere with the apparent relative proportions of the teeth. *Orthodontic treatment* of such defects should always be considered, especially if other positional or malocclusion problems exist in the mouth. However, if orthodontic treatment is either impractical or unaffordable, *minor positional defects* often can be treated with composite augmentation or full facial veneers indirectly made from composite or porcelain.[21] It must be emphasized that only those problems that can be conservatively treated without significant alteration of the occlusion or gingival contours of the teeth should be treated in this manner.

As illustrated in Fig. 18-7, *A* and *B, minor rotations* can be corrected by first reducing the enamel in the area of prominence followed by augmentation of the deficient area with composite material. Care must be taken to restrict all recontouring of prominent areas to enamel. If the rotation is to be treated with an indirectly

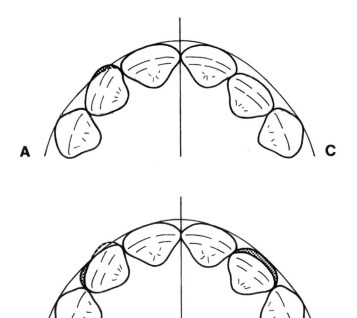

Fig. 18-7. Position and alignment. A, A minor rotation is first treated by reducing enamel in the area of prominence. B, The deficient area is restored to proper contour with composite. C, Maxillary lateral incisor is in slight linguoversion. D, Restorative augmentation of facial surface corrects malposition.

fabricated composite or porcelain veneer, an intraenamel preparation is recommended with greater reduction provided in the area of prominence to allow for subsequent restoration to appropriate physiological contours.

Malposed teeth are treated in a similar manner. As seen in Fig. 18-7, *C* and *D,* teeth in mild linguoversion can be treated by augmentation with full facial veneers either placed directly with composite or made indirectly from processed composite or porcelain. Care must be exercised to maintain physiological gingival contours that do not impinge on tissue or result in an emergence profile of the restoration that is detrimental to gingival health. Furthermore, a functional incisal edge should be maintained by appropriate contouring of the restoration. An excessively wide incisal edge should be avoided. If the occlusion allows, limited reduction of enamel on the lingual aspect can be accomplished to reduce the faciolingual dimension of the incisal portion of the tooth. However, lingual areas participating in protrusive functional contact should not be altered. It should be pointed out that individual teeth which are significantly displaced facially (facioversion) are best treated orthodontically.

Surface texture

The character and individuality of teeth are largely determined by the **surface texture** and characteristics that exist. Realistic restorations closely mimic the subtle areas of stippling, concavity, and convexity that typically are present on natural teeth. Young teeth characteristically exhibit significant **surface characterization** whereas teeth in older individuals tend to possess a smoother surface texture due to abrasional wear. However, even in older patients, restorations are rarely indicated that are totally devoid of surface characterizations.

The surfaces of natural teeth typically break up light and reflect it in many directions. Consequently, anatomical features such as developmental depressions, prominences, facets, and gingival perikymata should be closely examined and reproduced to the extent that they are present on surrounding surfaces. The restored areas of teeth should reflect light in a similar manner to adjacent surfaces which are unrestored. Also, as alluded to earlier, by controlling areas of *light reflection and shadowing,* various desired illusions also can be created.

Color

The artistic element of color and its role in conservative esthetic dentistry is undoubtedly the most complex and least understood. It is an area in which numerous interdependent factors exist, all of which contribute to the final esthetic outcome of the restoration. Although complex, a basic knowledge of color is imperative to producing consistently esthetic restorations.

Understanding the coloration of natural teeth is imperative to the accurate and consistent selection of appropriate shades of restorative materials. Teeth are typically composed of a multitude of colors. A *gradation of color* usually occurs from gingival to incisal with the gingival region being typically darker due to thinner enamel. The use of several different shades of restorative material may be required to esthetically restore a tooth. Exposed root surfaces are particularly darker (dentin colored) due to the absence of overlying enamel. Furthermore, in most individuals, *canines are slightly darker in coloration* than are the incisors.

Young patients with thick enamel characteristically exhibit lighter teeth. Moreover, patients who are more darkly complected usually will appear to have lighter teeth due to the contrast that exists between the teeth and the surrounding facial structures. In fact, female patients can enhance the apparent lightness of their teeth simply by using a darker shade of make-up and/or lipstick. By increasing the contrast between the teeth and the surrounding facial tissues, the illusion of lighter teeth can be created.

Color changes associated with *aging* also occur, primarily owing to wear. As the facial enamel is worn away, the underlying dentin becomes more apparent, resulting in a darker tooth. Incisal edges are often darker due to thinning of the enamel or frank exposure of the dentin as a result of normal attrition. Cervical areas also tend to darken due to abrasion.

An understanding of normal tooth coloration enhances the dentist's ability to create a restoration that appears natural. However, several clinical factors also must be considered to enhance the color-matching quality of the restoration. It should be recognized that most *shade guides* for composite materials are inaccurate. Not only are they usually composed of a material dissimilar to that of the composite, but also, they do not take into consideration color changes that occur from batch-to-batch or changes due to aging of the composite. *Accurate shade selection* is best attained by applying and curing a small amount of the composite restorative material in the area of the tooth anticipated for restoration. Shade selection also should be determined *prior to isolation of the teeth* to avoid color variations that can occur as a result of drying and dehydration of the teeth.

Problems in *color perception* also complicate selection of the appropriate shade of restorative material. Various light sources produce different perceptions of color. This phenomenon is referred to as **metamerism.**[67] Even the color of the room environment influences what is seen in the mouth. Color perception also is influenced by the physiological limitations of the eye. For example, upon extended viewing of a particular tooth site, the eyes experience *color fatigue* resulting in a loss of sensitivity to yellow-orange.[57] By looking away at a blue object or background (the complementary color), the eyes quickly recover and are once again able to distinguish subtle variations in yellow-orange. Because of the many indirect factors which influence color perception, it is recommended that the dentist, assistant, and especially the patient, all be involved in the decision-making process regarding shade selection.

Translucency

The property of translucency also affects the esthetic quality of the restoration. The *degree of translucency is related to how deeply light penetrates into the tooth or restoration before it is reflected outward*. Normally, light penetrates through the enamel into dentin before being reflected outward (Fig. 18-8, *A*). This affords the life-like **esthetic vitality** characteristic of normal, unrestored teeth. Shallow penetration of light often results in a loss of esthetic vitality. This phenomenon is a common problem encountered when treating severely intrinsically stained teeth, such as those affected by tetracycline, with direct or indirect veneers. Although opaque resin media can mask the underlying stain, a loss of esthetic vitality usually results due to reduced light penetration (Fig. 18-8, *B*). Indirect veneers of processed composite or porcelain fabricated to include inherent opacity also may experience this problem.

Illusions of translucency also can be created to enhance the realism of a restoration. Color modifiers (also referred to as tints) can be used to achieve apparent translucency, tone down bright stains, or characterize a restoration. Fig. 18-9, *A,* illustrates a maxillary right central incisor that warranted restoration due to intrinsic yellow staining resulting from trauma to the tooth. Bleaching treatments were unsuccessful. A direct composite veneer was utilized. Following an intraenamel preparation and acid etching, a blue color modifier (the complementary color of yellow) was applied to the prepared facial surface to reduce the brightness and intensity of the underlying yellow tooth. Additionally, a gray/violet mixture of color modifiers was used to simulate vertical areas of translucency. The final restoration is shown in Fig. 18-9, *B. Color modifiers* also can be incorporated in the restoration to simulate **maverick colors, check lines,** or **surface spots** *for further characterization.*

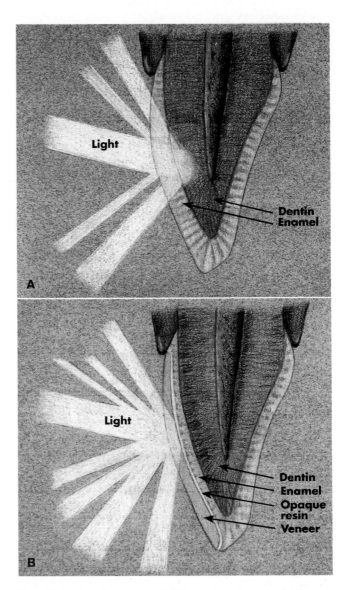

Fig. 18-8. Translucency and light penetration. **A,** Light normally penetrates deeply through the enamel and into dentin before being reflected outward. This affords life-like esthetic vitality. **B,** Light penetration is limited by opaquing resin media under veneers. Esthetic vitality is compromised.

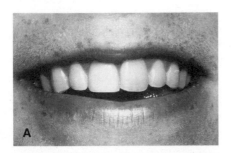
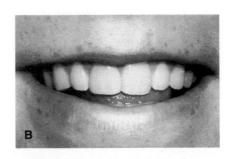

Fig. 18-9. Use of internally placed color modifiers. **A,** Maxillary right central incisor exhibits bright intrinsic yellow staining. **B,** Color modifiers under direct composite veneer tone-down brightness and intensity of stain and simulate vertical areas of translucency.

Clinical considerations

Although an understanding of basic artistic elements is imperative to esthetic restorations, certain clinical considerations must be addressed concomitantly to ensure the overall quality of the restoration. In addition to being esthetic, restorations also must be *functional*. As Dr. Peter Dawson states, "Esthetics and function go hand in hand. The better the esthetics, the better the function is likely to be and vice versa."[17]

The **occlusion** *must always be assessed prior to any conservative esthetic procedure*. Anterior guidance in particular must be maintained and occlusal harmony ensured when treating areas involved in occlusion.

As alluded to earlier, another requirement of all conservative esthetic restorations is that they possess **physiological contours** that promote good gingival health. Particular care must be taken in all treatments to finish gingival areas of the restoration adequately and to remove any gingival excess of material. *Emergence angles* of the restorations must be physiological and not impinge on gingival tissues.

CONSERVATIVE ALTERATIONS OF TOOTH CONTOURS AND CONTACTS

Many **unsightly tooth contours** and **diastemata** can be corrected or greatly improved by several conservative methods. Often these procedures can be incorporated into routine restorative treatment. The objective is to improve esthetics yet preserve as much healthy tooth structure as possible consistent with acceptable occlusion and health of the surrounding tissue. These procedures include reshaping natural teeth, correcting embrasures, and closing diastemata.

Alterations of shape of natural teeth

Some esthetic problems can be corrected very conservatively without the need for tooth preparation and restoration. Consideration should always be given to reshaping and polishing the natural teeth to improve their appearance and function (see Fig. 18-1, *A* and *B,* and Plate 18-1, *D* and *E*). In addition, the rounding of sharp angles also can be considered a prophylactic measure to reduce stress and to help prevent chipping and fractures of the incisal edges.

Etiology. Fig. 18-10, *A,* illustrates maxillary anterior teeth with worn incisal edges. Attrition of the incisal edges, such as in this case, often results in closed incisal embrasures and very angular incisal edges. Anterior teeth, especially maxillary central incisors, often also are fractured in accidents. Other esthetic problems which often can be corrected or improved by reshaping the natural teeth include *attrition and abnormal wear*

from habits such as biting fingernails or holding objects by the teeth.

Treatment. Consultation and examination are necessary before any changes are made in the shape of a tooth or teeth. Photographs, study models, line drawings, and/or esthetic imaging devices enable the patient to envision the potential improvement before any changes are made.

As noted earlier, cosmetic contouring to achieve *youthful, feminine characteristics* often includes rounding incisal angles, reducing facial line angles, and opening incisal embrasures. The opposite characteristics are typically considered more *masculine features*. However, cosmetic reshaping to smooth rough incisal edges and improve symmetry is equally beneficial to both women and men.

The patient must understand what is involved and want to have the alteration made. If reshaping is desired, it is helpful to mark the outline of the areas to be reshaped on the teeth in the mouth with a pencil or alcohol marking pen (Fig. 18-10, *B*). By marking the anticipated areas for enamel reshaping, the patient is provided some indication of what the postoperative result may look like (Fig. 18-10, *C*). Since all reshaping is restricted to enamel, anesthesia is not required. A cotton roll is recommended for isolation. Diamond instruments and abrasive discs and points are used for contouring, finishing, and polishing (Fig. 18-10, *D* and *E*). Through careful reshaping of appropriate enamel surfaces, a more esthetic smile characterized by youthful, feminine features is attained. Rounded incisal edges also will be less likely to chip or fracture (Fig. 18-10, *F*).

A second example involves irregular *fractured incisal surfaces* of the maxillary central incisors (Fig. 18-11, *A*). An esthetic result can be accomplished by slightly shortening the incisal edges and reshaping both teeth to a symmetrical form. Again, the use of photographs, line drawings, esthetic imaging, and/or marking the outline on the teeth in the mouth enables the patient to envision the potential improvement before any changes are made. Protrusive function always should be evaluated to prevent inadvertent elimination of this occlusal contact. Conservative treatment consists of using diamond instruments and abrasive discs and points for contouring and polishing the central incisors. The finished result is illustrated in Fig. 18-11, *B*.

As some *patients grow older* or have *bruxing habits,* the incisal surfaces often wear away, leaving sharp edges that chip easily. There is also an accompanying loss of the incisal embrasures (Fig. 18-12, *A*). To lessen the chance of more fractures and to create a more youthful smile, the incisal embrasures are opened and the incisal angles of the teeth are rounded (Fig. 18-12, *B*).

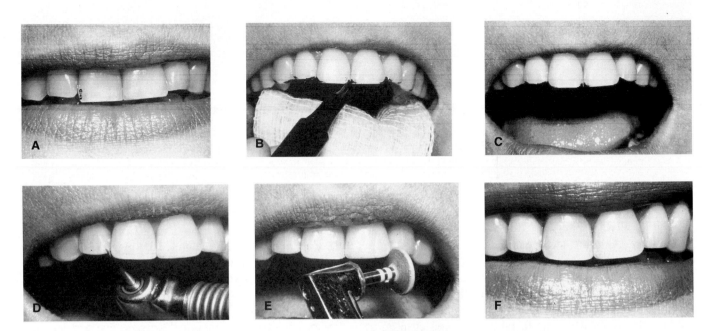

Fig. 18-10. Reshaping natural teeth. **A,** Maxillary anterior teeth with worn incisal edges. **B,** Areas to be reshaped are outlined. **C,** Outlined areas give the patient an idea of what the final result will look like. **D,** A diamond instrument is used to reshape incisal edges. **E,** A rubber abrasive disc is used to polish incisal edges. **F,** Reshaping results in more youthful, feminine smile.

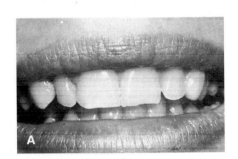

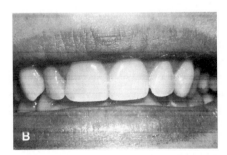

Fig. 18-11. Irregular incisal edges. **A,** Central incisors have rough, fractured incisal edges. **B,** Esthetic result is obtained by recontouring incisal edges.

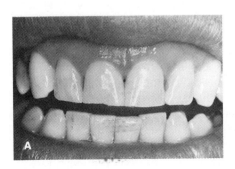

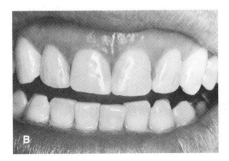

Fig. 18-12. Loss of incisal embrasures from attrition. Before **(A)** and after **(B)** recontouring teeth to produce a more youthful appearance and improve resistance to fracture.

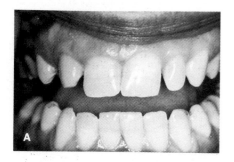 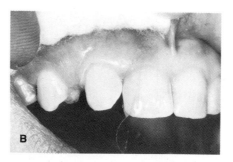 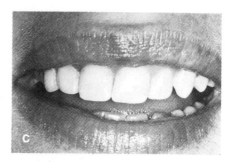

Fig. 18-13. Closing incisal embrasures. **A,** Maxillary canine moved to close space left by missing lateral incisor. Mesial incisal embrasure is too open. **B,** Etched final preparation (excess enamel contour was removed at midfacial area). A contoured strip is shown in the correct position. **C,** Canine reshaped to look like lateral incisor, and incisal embrasure of left lateral incisor was also corrected.

Alterations of embrasures

Etiology. Anterior teeth can have *embrasures that are too open* as a result of the shape or position of the teeth in the arch. For example, when the permanent lateral incisors are congenitally missing, the canines and posterior teeth may drift mesially or the space may be closed orthodontically. The facial surface and cusp angle of some canines can be reshaped to appear like lateral incisors. But in many instances, the mesioincisal embrasure remains too open (Fig. 18-13, *A*). Note that the left lateral incisor also has an open incisal embrasure.

Treatment. Composite can be added to *establish an esthetic contour and correct the open embrasures*. Evaluation of the occlusion before restoration determines if the addition will be compatible with functional movements. The patient should understand the procedures involved and must desire to have the change made. Line drawings, esthetic imaging, or photographs of similar examples are often helpful in explaining the procedure and allaying patient concerns. Another patient aid involves adding ivory-colored wax or composite to the teeth (unetched) to temporarily fill the embrasure in order to simulate the final result.

Preliminary procedures include cleaning the involved teeth, selecting the shade, and isolating the area. Local anesthesia is not usually required, because the preparation does not extend subgingivally and involves only enamel. A coarse, flame-shaped diamond instrument is used to remove overly convex enamel surfaces (if present) and to roughen the enamel surface area to be augmented with composite material. It may be necessary to place a wedge and use an abrasive strip to prepare the proximal surface. The final contour of the restoration should be envisioned before the preparation is made so that all areas to be bonded are adequately roughened.

A polyester strip is inserted to protect the adjacent tooth during acid etching. After etching, rinsing, and

drying, the contoured strip is positioned (Fig. 18-13, *B*). Either a self-cured or light-cured material is inserted, and the strip is closed during polymerization. The incisal embrasure of the left lateral incisor is corrected, and both restorations are finished by routine procedures (Fig. 18-13, *C*). The occlusion should be evaluated to assess centric contacts and functional movements, and any adjustments or corrections are made if indicated.

Correction of diastemata

Etiology. The presence of *diastemata* (spaces) between the anterior teeth is an esthetic problem for some patients (Fig. 18-14, *A*). Before treatment, a diagnosis of the etiology is made, including an evaluation of the occlusion. Probably the most frequent site of a diastema is between the maxillary central incisors. A prominent labial frenum with nonelastic fibers extending proximally often prevents the normal approximation of erupting central incisors.[25] Other etiological factors include congenitally missing teeth, undersized or malformed teeth, interarch tooth size discrepancies (Bolton discrepancy), supernumerary teeth, and heredity. Diastemata also may result from other problems such as tongue thrusting, periodontal disease, or posterior bite collapse. Again, *diastemata should not be closed without first recognizing and treating the underlying cause.* Treating the cause may correct a diastema.

Treatment. Traditionally diastemata have been treated by surgical, periodontal, orthodontic, and/or prosthetic procedures. These types of corrections can be impractical or unaffordable or do not result in permanent closure of the diastema. In carefully selected cases, a more practical alternative is use of the acid etch technique and composite augmentation of proximal surfaces (see Figs. 18-4 and 18-5). It is emphasized that all treatment considerations (including no treatment) should be studied before resorting immediately to composite augmentation. Line drawings, photographs, computer imaging, models with spaces filled, and/or direct tempo-

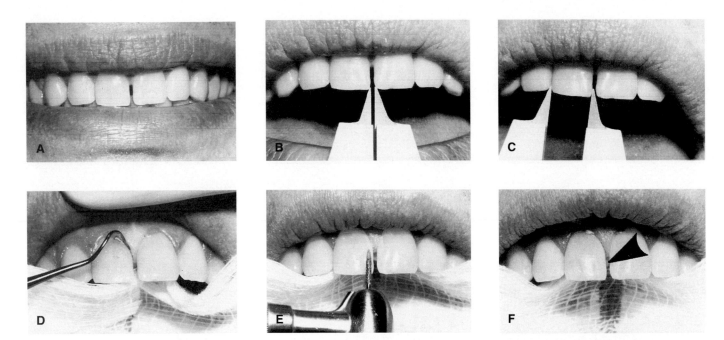

Fig. 18-14. Diastema closure. **A,** Esthetic problem created by space between central incisors. **B** and **C,** Interdental space and size of central incisors measured with caliper. **D,** Teeth isolated with cotton rolls and retraction cord tucked into gingival crevice. **E,** A diamond instrument is used to roughen enamel surfaces. **F,** Etched enamel surface indicated by arrow.   *Continued.*

rary additions of ivory-colored wax or composite material on the natural teeth (unetched) are important preliminary procedures.

The *correction of a diastema* between the maxillary central incisors is described and illustrated (Fig. 18-14). After the teeth are cleaned and the shade selected, a Boley gauge or another suitable caliper is used to measure the width of the diastema and the individual teeth (Fig. 18-14, *B* and *C*). Sometimes one central incisor will be wider than the other requiring greater addition to the narrower tooth. Assuming the incisors are of equal width, symmetrical additions can be ensured by using half of the *total* measurement of the diastema to gauge the width of the first tooth restored. Cotton rolls, instead of a rubber dam, are recommended for isolation because of the importance of relating the contour of the restoration directly to the proximal tissue. Usually, the restoration must begin below the gingival crest to appear natural and to be confluent with the tooth contours.

With cotton rolls in place, a gingival retraction cord of an appropriate size is tucked in the gingival crevice of each tooth from midfacial mesially to midlingual (Fig. 18-14, *D*). The cord retracts the soft tissue and prevents seepage from the crevice. In some instances, the retraction cord may need to be inserted for one tooth at a time to *prevent strangulation of the interproximal tissues* during preparation and restorative procedures. To enhance retention of the composite, a coarse, flame-

shaped diamond instrument is used to roughen the proximal surfaces, extending from the facial line angle to the lingual line angle (Fig. 18-14, *E*).[1] More extension may be needed to correct facial or lingual contours, depending on the anatomy and position of the individual tooth. The enamel is acid etched approximately 0.5 mm past the prepared roughened surface. The acid should not be allowed to flow into the gingival crevice. After rinsing and drying, the etched enamel should display a lightly frosted appearance (Fig. 18-14, *F*). A 2 × 2 inch (5 × 5 cm) gauze is draped across the mouth and tongue to prevent inadvertent contamination of the etched preparations by the patient. After both preparations are completed, the teeth are restored one at a time.

A polyester strip is contoured and placed proximally with the gingival aspect of the strip extending below the gingival crest. Additional contouring may be required to produce enough convexity in the strip. (For contouring a polyester strip, see Polyester Strip Matrix for Proximial Restorations, in Chapter 16.) In most cases a wedge cannot be used. The strip is then held on the lingual aspect of the tooth to be restored with the index finger while the facial end is reflected for access. Either self-cured or light-cured composite may be used for the restoration. After the resin bonding agent is applied, the composite material is inserted with a hand instrument (Fig. 18-14, *G*). Careful attention is given to pressing the material lingually to ensure confluence with the lin-

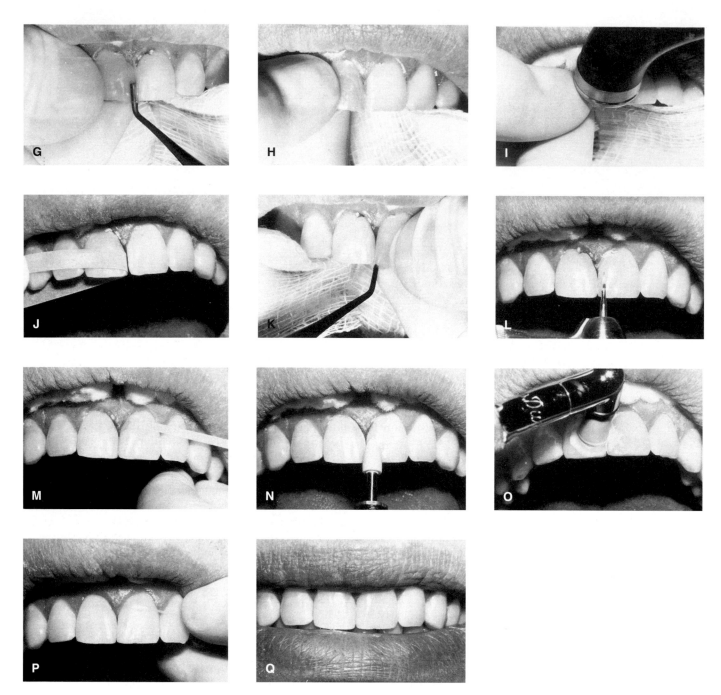

Fig. 18-14—cont'd. G, Composite inserted with composite instrument. **H,** Matrix strip closed with thumb and forefinger. **I,** Composite addition is cured. **J,** Finishing strip used to finalize contour of first addition. **K,** A tight contact is attained by displacing the second tooth being restored in a distal direction with thumb and forefinger while holding matrix in contact with adjacent restoration. **L,** Flame-shaped finishing bur used to contour restoration. **M,** Finishing strip used to smooth subgingival areas. **N,** Restoration is polished with rubber abrasive point. **O,** Final lustre attained with polishing paste applied with prophy cup. **P,** Unwaxed floss used to detect any excess composite. **Q,** Diastema closed with symmetrical and equal additions of composite.

gual surface. The matrix is then gently closed facially beginning with the gingival aspect (Fig. 18-14, *H*). Care must be taken not to pull the strip too tightly, because the resulting restoration may be undercontoured faciolingually and/or mesiodistally. If a light-cured material is used, it should be polymerized with the light from both facial and lingual directions for a *minimum* of 20 seconds from each direction for a total of 40 seconds (Fig. 18-14, *I*). It is better to initially overcontour the first restoration in order to facilitate finishing it to an ideal contour.

When polymerization is complete, the strip is removed. Contouring and finishing are achieved with appropriate carbide finishing burs or abrasive discs (Fig. 18-14, *L*). Finishing strips are invaluable for finalizing proximal contours (Fig. 18-14, *J* and *M*). Final polishing is deferred until completion of the contralateral restoration. It is imperative for good gingival health that the cervical aspect of the composite addition be immaculately smooth and continuous with the tooth structure. *Overhangs must not be present.* Removal of the gingival retraction cord will facilitate inspection and smoothing of this area. Flossing with a length of unwaxed floss will verify that the gingival margin is correct and smooth if no fraying of the floss occurs (Fig. 18-14, *P*). *It is important that the correct mesiodistal dimension of the first tooth be established before the second tooth is restored.*

After re-etching, rinsing, and drying, the second restoration is completed. A tight proximal contact can be attained by displacing the second tooth being restored in a distal direction with thumb and index finger while holding the matrix in contact with the adjacent restoration as seen in Fig. 18-14, *K*. As noted earlier, contouring is accomplished with a 12-fluted carbide bur and finishing strips (Fig. 18-14, *L* and *M*).

Articulating paper should be used to evaluate the patient's occlusion to ensure that the restorations are not offensive in centric or functional movements. Needed adjustments can be made with a carbide finishing bur or abrasive discs. Final polishing is achieved with rubber polishing points and polishing paste applied with a prophy cup in a low-speed handpiece (Fig. 18-14, *N* and *O*). Again, unwaxed floss is used to detect any excess material or overhang (Fig. 18-14, *P*). The esthetic result is seen in Fig. 18-14, *Q*.

More extensive diastemata between all the maxillary anterior teeth are shown in Fig. 18-15, *A*. Closing the spaces by orthodontic movement was considered; however, because the teeth were undercontoured mesiodistally, the spaces were filled by etching the teeth and bonding composite to the proximal surfaces. The teeth are shown 7 years after treatment (Fig. 18-15, *B*). A similar case is illustrated in Fig. 18-4.

When defective Class III restorations or proximal caries exists, it is recommended that they be restored with the same composite used for closing the diastema. Often these restorations can be restored at the same time the diastema is closed with composite additions (Plate 18-1, *F* and *G*).

Occasionally, diastemata are simply too large to esthetically close with composite augmentation alone. An example of an excessively large diastema is seen in Fig. 18-16, *A*. Closing a large space of this magnitude with composite would merely create an alternative esthetic problem, excessively large central incisors, which would further exacerbate the existing discrepancy in proportionality among the anterior teeth. In such cases, large spaces are best redistributed orthodontically among the anterior teeth so that symmetrical and equal composite additions can be made to both the central and lateral incisors (Fig. 18-16, *B* and *C*). The final result shown immediately after completion is shown in Fig. 18-16, *D*. This approach involving **space distribution** results in improved **proportionality** among the anterior teeth (see Artistic Elements).

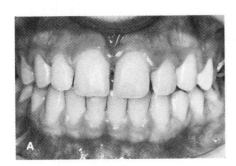
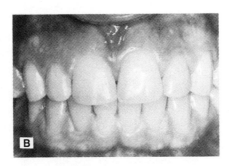

Fig. 18-15. Diastemata occurring between all maxillary anterior teeth. **A,** Before correction. **B,** Appearance after 7 years.

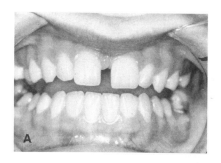
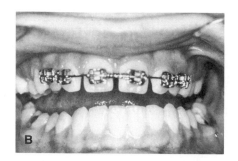
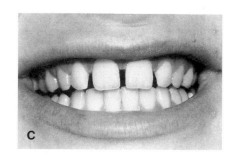

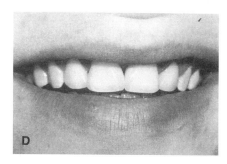

Fig. 18-16. Space distribution. A, Midline diastema too large for simple closure with composite additions. B and C, Space distributed among four incisors with orthodontic treatment. D, Final result following composite additions.

CONSERVATIVE TREATMENTS FOR DISCOLORED TEETH

One of the most frequent reasons for seeking dental care is discolored anterior teeth. Even persons having teeth with normal color often request to have them made whiter. Treatment options include removal of surface stains, bleaching, microabrasion or macroabrasion, veneering, and placement of porcelain crowns. Many dentists recommend porcelain crowns as the best solution for badly discolored teeth. If crowns are properly done, with the highly esthetic ceramic materials presently available, they have great potential for being esthetic and long lasting. On the other hand, there are increasing numbers of patients who do not want their teeth "cut down" for crowns and are electing an alternative, conservative approach, such as veneers, that preserves as much of the natural tooth as possible. This treatment is performed with the understanding that the corrective measures may be less "permanent."

Discolorations are classified as *extrinsic* or *intrinsic*. Extrinsic stains are located on the outer surfaces of the teeth, whereas intrinsic stains are internal. The etiology and treatment are discussed under each heading.

Extrinsic discolorations

Etiology. Stains on the external surfaces of teeth or restorations, referred to as *extrinsic discolorations,* are quite common. The etiology may be complicated by a number of factors. In young patients stains of almost any color can be found and are usually more prominent in the cervical areas of the teeth (Fig. 18-17, *A*). These stains may be related to remnants of Nasmyth's membrane, poor oral hygiene, existing restorations, bleeding gums, plaque accumulation, eating habits, or the presence of chromogenic bacteria or fungi.

In older patients stains on the surfaces of the teeth are more likely to be brown, black, or gray and occur on areas adjacent to the gingival tissue. Poor oral hygiene is a contributing factor, but coffee, tea, and certain types of food or medications can produce stains even on plaque-free surfaces. Tobacco stains also are observed frequently. Existing restorations may be discolored for the same reasons.

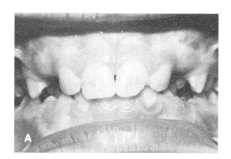
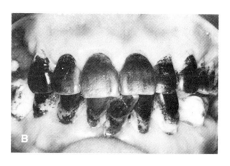

Fig. 18-17. Extrinsic stains. A, Surface stains on facial surfaces in young patient. B, Exotic decoration of anterior teeth by etching with citrus fruit juice and applying black pigment. (Courtesy Dr. Jeff Burkes.)

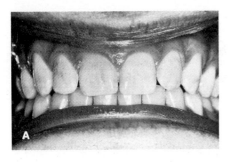
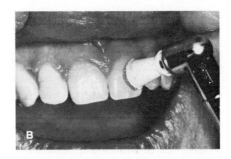
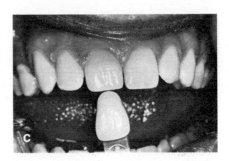

Fig. 18-18. Treatment of surface stains. **A,** Tobacco stains. **B,** Pumicing teeth with rubber cup. **C,** Shade guide used to confirm normal color of natural teeth.

An example of one of the most interesting and unusual types of external staining is illustrated in Fig. 18-17, *B.* In southeast Asia some women traditionally dye their teeth with beetlenut juice to match their hair and eyes as a sign of beauty.[19] Slices of lemon are held in contact with the teeth before applying the beetlenut juice to make the staining process more effective. This example was probably one of the first applications of the acid etch technique. A weak acid such as that found in citrus fruits is known to cause rapid decalcification of the enamel.

Treatment. Most surface stains can be removed by routine prophylactic procedures (Fig. 18-18, *A* to *C*). Some superficial discolorations on tooth-colored restorations and decalcified areas on the teeth cannot be corrected by such cleaning. Conservative correction may be accomplished by mild microabrasion or by surfacing the thin outer discolored layer with a flame-shaped carbide finishing bur or diamond instrument (macroabrasion), followed by polishing with abrasive discs or points to obtain an acceptable result. (See subsequent sections on microabrasion and macroabrasion for details of clinical technique.)

Intrinsic discolorations

Etiology. *Intrinsic discolorations* are caused by deeper internal stains or enamel defects and are more complicated to treat than external types. Teeth with vital or nonvital pulps can be affected, as well as root canal–treated teeth.

Vital teeth may be discolored at the time the crowns are forming, and the abnormal condition usually involves several teeth. Etiological factors include hereditary disorders, medications (particularly tetracycline preparations), excess fluorides, high fevers associated with early childhood illnesses, and other types of trauma. The staining may be located in enamel or in dentin. Discolorations restricted to dentin may still show through the enamel. Discoloration also may be *localized* or *generalized* involving the entire tooth.

Various preparations of the antibiotic drug **tetracycline** can cause the most distracting, generalized type of intrinsic discoloration (Fig. 18-19, *A*).[9] The severity of the staining depends on the dosage, duration of exposure to the drug, and the type of tetracycline analog used. Different types of tetracyclines induce specific characteristic discolorations varying from yellow-orange to dark blue-gray. Dark blue-gray tetracycline-stained teeth are considerably more difficult to treat than are those with mild yellow-orange discolorations.

The presence of excess fluoride in the drinking water at the time the teeth are forming can result in another type of intrinsic stain called **fluorosis,** and it usually is generalized. Because of the high fluoride content in the enamel, fluorosed teeth may be difficult to treat with acid etching and resin bonding.

Localized areas of discoloration may occur on individual teeth due to enamel and or dentin defects induced during tooth development. High fevers and other forms of trauma can damage the tooth during its development

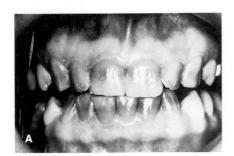
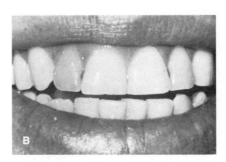

Fig. 18-19. Intrinsic stains. **A,** Staining by tetracycline drugs. **B,** Staining of maxillary right lateral incisor from tooth trauma and degeneration of pulp.

resulting in unesthetic hypoplastic defects. Additionally, localized areas of dysmineralization or failure of the enamel to properly calcify can result in hypocalcified *"white spots."* Following eruption, poor oral hygiene also can result in decalcified white spots. Poor oral hygiene during orthodontic treatment frequently results in these types of decalcified defects. However, white or discolored spots with intact enamel surface (surface not soft) are often evidence of intraoral remineralization, and such spots are not indications for invasive treatment unless for esthetic concerns. Additionally, caries, metallic restorations, corroded pins, and leakage or secondary caries around existing restorations can result in various types of intrinsic discoloration.

As noted earlier, aging effects also can result in yellower teeth. As patients grow older, the tooth enamel becomes thinner due to wear and thus allows the underlying dentin to become more apparent. This results in a yellowing effect depending on the intrinsic color of the dentin. Additionally, the permeability of teeth usually allows the infusion over time of significant organic pigments from foods, drinks, tobacco products, etc., which can result in a yellowing effect.

Non-vital teeth also can become discolored intrinsically. These stains usually occur in individual teeth after eruption has taken place. The pulp may become infected or degenerate as a result of trauma, deep caries, or irritation from restorative procedures. If these teeth are properly treated by root canal therapy, they usually will retain their normal color. If treatment is delayed, discoloration of the crown is more likely to occur. The degenerative products from the pulp tissue will stain the dentin and will be readily apparent because of the translucency of the enamel (Fig. 18-19, *B*). Trauma resulting in calcific metamorphosis—calcification of the pulp chamber and/or root canal—also can produce significant yellowing of the tooth that is extremely difficult to treat.

Treatment. Many persons have definite esthetic problems from intrinsic stains, whereas others worry needlessly about the overall color of their teeth. In the latter instance the dentist must decide if the color of the teeth can be improved enough to justify treatment even though the patient insists on having something done.

For example, persons with light complexions may believe that their teeth are too dark when actually they are normal in color (Fig. 18-20, *A*). Positioning a shade tab from a shade guide of tooth colors next to such teeth often will demonstrate to the patient that the color of their teeth is well within the normal range of shades. A suntan, darker makeup, or darker lipstick will usually make teeth appear much whiter by increasing the contrast between the teeth and the surrounding facial features (Fig. 18-20, *B*).

The patient should be told that many discolorations can be corrected or greatly improved through conservative methods such as bleaching, microabrasion/macroabrasion, or veneering techniques. Mild discolorations are best left untreated, bleached, or treated conservatively with microabrasion or macroabrasion, because no restorative material is as good as the healthy, natural tooth structure. Moreover, the *patient should be informed that the gingival tissue never will be as healthy when adjacent to restorative material as when next to normal tooth structure.*

Color photographs of previously treated teeth with intrinsic staining (before and after) are excellent adjuncts to help the patient make an informed decision. Esthetic imaging with modern computer simulation of the postoperative result also can be an effective educational tool. Patients appreciate knowing what the cause of the problem is, how it can be corrected, how much time is involved, and what the cost will be. They also should be informed of the life expectancy of the various treatment alternatives suggested. For example, vital bleaching usually will result in tooth lightening for only 1 to 3 years, whereas an etched porcelain veneer should last 6 to 8 years or longer. With continuous improvements in materials and techniques, a much longer lifespan may be possible with any of these techniques. The clinical longevity of esthetic restorations also is enhanced in patients who exhibit good oral hygiene, proper diet, a favorable bite relationship, and little or no contact with agents that cause discoloration or deterioration.

Correction of intrinsic discolorations caused by failing restorations entails replacement of the faulty portion or the entire restoration. Correction of discolorations

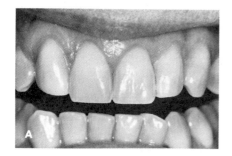
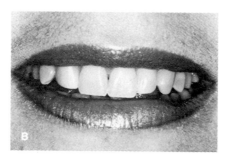

Fig. 18-20. Illusion of a lighter appearance of teeth by use of darker makeup. **A,** Before. **B,** After.

due to carious lesions requires appropriate restorative treatment. Conservative treatment methods are covered in the chapters on composite, amalgam, and cast restorations. Esthetic inserts for metal restorations are described later in this chapter. For the other types of intrinsic discolorations previously discussed, detailed treatment options are presented in the next three sections.

BLEACHING TREATMENTS

The lightening of the color of a tooth through the application of a chemical agent to oxidize the organic pigmentation in the tooth is referred to as **bleaching**. In keeping with the overall conservative philosophy of tooth restoration, consideration first should be given to bleaching anterior teeth when intrinsic discolorations are encountered. Bleaching techniques may be classified as to whether they involve vital or non-vital teeth, and whether the procedure is performed in the office, or with some outside-the-office component. Bleaching of non-vital teeth was first reported in 1848, while bleaching of vital teeth in-office was first reported in 1868.[30] By the early 1900s, in-office vital bleaching had evolved to include the use of heat and light for activation of the process. Although there are reports of a 3% ether-peroxide mouthwash used for bleaching in 1893, the "dentist prescribed-home applied" technique (also referred to as nightguard vital bleaching) for bleaching vital teeth outside the office began around 1968.[31]

Most bleaching techniques use some form or derivative of hydrogen peroxide in different concentrations and application techniques. The mechanism of action of bleaching teeth with hydrogen peroxide is considered to be oxidation of organic pigments, although the chemistry is not well understood. Bleaching generally has an approximate lifespan of 1 to 3 years, although the change may be permanent in some situations.

With all bleaching techniques, there is a transitory decrease in the potential bond strength of composite when it is applied to the bleached, etched enamel. This reduction in bond strength results from residual oxygen or peroxide residue in the tooth which inhibits the set of the bonding resin, precluding adequate resin tag formation in the etched enamel. However, *no loss of bond strength is noted if the composite restorative treatment is delayed at least 1 week after cessation of any bleaching.*[70]

Non-vital bleaching procedures

The primary indication for non-vital bleaching is to lighten teeth which have undergone root canal therapy. This discoloration may be a result of bleeding into the dentin from trauma prior to root canal therapy, degradation of pulp tissue left in the chamber after such therapy, and/or staining from restorative materials and cements placed in the tooth as a part of the root canal treatment. Most posterior teeth which have received root canal therapy require cast restorations which encompass the tooth to prevent subsequent fracture. However, anterior teeth needing restorative treatment and which are largely intact may be restored with composite rather than with partial or full coverage restorations without significantly compromising the strength of the tooth.[66] This knowledge has created a resurgence in the utilization of non-vital bleaching techniques.

Non-vital bleaching techniques include an in-office **thermocatalytic technique** and an out-of-the-office technique referred to as *"walking bleach."* (See next sections for details of these two techniques.)

Although non-vital bleaching is quite effective, there is a slight potential ($<1\%$) for a most deleterious side effect termed **cervical resorption**.[29] This sequela requires prompt and aggressive treatment. In animal models, cervical resorption has been observed most often when using the thermocatalytic technique.[53] Therefore, the "walking bleach" technique or an in-office technique which does not require the use of heat are preferred for non-vital bleaching. To reduce the possibility of resorption, immediately after bleaching a paste of calcium hydroxide powder and sterile water is placed in the operated pulp chamber as described in the following sections.[47] Also, sodium perborate alone, rather than in conjunction with hydrogen peroxide, may be used as the primary bleaching agent. Although sodium perborate may bleach more slowly, it is safer and less offensive to the tooth.[40] Periodic radiographs should be made post-bleaching to screen for cervical resorption, which generally has its onset in 1 to 7 years.[48]

In-office non-vital bleaching technique. The in-office bleaching for non-vital teeth is historically a *thermocatalytic technique* involving the placement of 35% hydrogen peroxide into the debrided pulp chamber and activation of the oxidation process by placement of a heating instrument into the pulp chamber.

A more recent technique utilizes a light-activated bleaching preparation of 35% hydrogen peroxide that requires no heat. This technique is frequently the preferred in-office technique for bleaching non-vital teeth. In both techniques, it is imperative that a sealing cement (polycarboxylate or light-cured glass ionomer cement is recommended) be placed over the exposed root canal filling prior to application of the bleaching agent.

Walking bleach technique. Prior to initiating the "walking bleach" technique, evaluate the potential for occlusal contact on the area of the root canal access opening. Place a rubber dam to isolate the discolored tooth. Now remove all materials in the coronal portion of the tooth (access opening). Remove gutta percha to approximately 2 mm apical of the clinical crown, and enlarge the endodontic access opening sufficiently to ensure complete debridement of the pulp chamber. Next, place a polycarboxylate cement or a light-cured glass ionomer to seal the gutta percha of the root canal filling from the coronal portion of the pulp chamber. After this seal has hardened, trim any excess material from the seal so the discolored dentin is exposed peripherally. Using a cement spatula with heavy pressure on a glass slab, blend one drop of 35% hydrogen peroxide with enough sodium perborate to form a creamy paste. Exercise caution in handling the material, since 35% hydrogen peroxide is a potent oxidizer and will chemically burn tissue upon contact. Should tissue be inadvertently contacted by the bleaching material, the affected area should be rinsed with copious amounts of water.

Use a spoon excavator or similar instrument to fill the pulp chamber to within 2 mm of the cavosurface margin with the bleaching mixture, avoiding contact with the enamel cavosurface margins of the access opening. Use a cotton pellet to blot the mixture to place. Now place a temporary sealing material such as IRM^R or Cavit^R to seal the access opening. The area should remain isolated for approximately 5 minutes after closure to evaluate the adequacy of the seal of the temporary restoration. If bubbles appear around the margins of the temporary material indicating leakage, the temporary restoration must be replaced. If no bubbles appear, remove the rubber dam and check the occlusion to assess the presence or absence of contact on the temporary restoration.

The bleaching mixture is very active for 24 hours, after which little potential for harm to tissue exists. The mixture may be changed every 3 to 5 days and usually 1 to 3 treatments are required. If sodium perborate is used alone, it should be changed bi-weekly. Upon successful bleaching of the tooth, rinse the chamber and fill it with a paste consisting of calcium hydroxide powder in sterile saline to within 2 mm of the cavosurface margin (keep the enamel walls and margins clean and free of the calcium hydroxide paste). The access opening is resealed with a temporary restorative material in a manner previously described. The calcium hydroxide material is allowed to remain in the pulp chamber for 2 weeks. Af-

terward, remove the temporary restorative material, rinse away the calcium hydroxide, and dry the pulp chamber. Next, condition the dentin and etch the enamel, and then restore the tooth with a light-cured composite. A typical non-vital bleaching case is shown before and after treatment following this technique in Fig. 18-21.

Occasionally a tooth which previously has been bleached by the walking bleach technique and sealed with a composite restoration will subsequently discolor. In this instance, the alternative treatment option should be an attempt to bleach the tooth externally with one of the external bleaching techniques (see Vital Bleaching Procedures, next).

Vital bleaching procedures

Generally the indications for the different vital bleaching techniques are similar, with patient preference, cost, compliance, and difficulty in removing certain discolorations dictating the choice of treatment or combination of treatments. Indications for vital bleaching include intrinsically discolored teeth from aging, trauma, or drug ingestion. As previously mentioned, alternative treatment options for a failed non-vital walking bleach are the external vital bleaching techniques. Vital bleaching also is often indicated before and after restorative treatments to harmonize shades of the restorative materials with the natural teeth.

Teeth exhibiting yellow or orange intrinsic discoloration appear to respond best to vital bleaching while teeth exhibiting bluish-gray discolorations often are difficult or impossible to treat in this manner. Other indications for external bleaching include single teeth which have darkened from trauma, but are still vital or have a poor endodontic prognosis due to the absence of a radiographically visible canal (calcific metamorphosis). Brown fluorosis stains also are often responsive to treatment, but white fluorosis stains are not effectively resolved.

Vital bleaching techniques include an in-office technique referred to as *"power bleaching,"*[18] and an outside-the-office alternative which is a dentist prescribed-home applied technique also referred to as *"nightguard vital bleaching."*[33] These techniques may be used sepa-

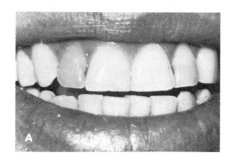

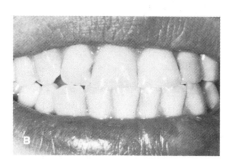

Fig. 18-21. Indication for bleaching root canal filled tooth. **A,** Before. **B,** After. Esthetics may be improved further by replacing defective mesial restoration.

rately or in combination with one another. (Details are described in the subsequent sections.)

Overall, vital bleaching has proven to be safe and effective when performed by, or under the supervision of, a dentist. There does not appear to be any appreciable effect on existing restorative materials, either in loss of material integrity or in color change. Because hydrogen peroxide has such a low molecular weight, it easily passes through the enamel and dentin. This characteristic accounts for the mild tooth sensitivity occasionally experienced during treatment. However, this effect is transient, and no long-term harm to the pulp has been noted.

Often the choice for the dentist is whether to use an in-office bleaching technique, or the dentist prescribed-home applied technique. The *advantages of the in-office vital bleaching technique* are that, while using very caustic chemicals, it is totally under the dentist's control, the soft tissue is generally protected from the process, and it has the potential for bleaching teeth more rapidly. *Disadvantages* primarily relate to the cost, the unpredictable outcome, and the unknown duration of the treatment. The features that warrant concern and caution include the potential for soft-tissue damage to patient and provider, the discomfort of a rubber dam and the potential for post-treatment sensitivity. The *advantages of the dentist prescribed-home applied technique (nightguard vital bleaching)* are the use of a lower concentration of peroxide (generally 10% to 15% carbamide peroxide), the ease of application, minimal side effects, and lower cost due to the reduced chair time required for treatment. The *disadvantages* are the reliance on patient compliance, the longer treatment time, and the (unknown) potential for soft-tissue changes with excessively extended use.

In-office vital bleaching technique. In-office vital bleaching requires excellent rubber dam technique and careful patient management. Place Vaseline™ or cocoa-cocoa butter on the lips and gingival tissues prior to the application of the rubber dam. Then isolate the anterior teeth, and sometimes the first premolars as well, with a heavy rubber dam to provide maximum retraction of tissue and an optimal seal around the teeth. Ensure a good seal of the dam by either ligation of the dam with waxed dental tape or the use of a sealing putty or varnish. Etching of the teeth with 37% phosphoric acid, previously considered a required part of this technique, now is considered unnecessary.[26] Place a 35% hydrogen peroxide–soaked gauze or a gel form of hydrogen peroxide on the teeth. The patient is instructed to note any sensations of burning of the lips or gingiva which would indicate a leaking dam and the need to terminate treatment. The oxidation reaction of the hydrogen peroxide can be accelerated by applying heat with either a heating instrument (2 minutes per tooth) set at the maximum tolerance of the patient, or with an intense light (30 minutes per arch).

As noted earlier, some bleaching gels do not require heat to potentiate the oxidation reaction, while others are accelerated with a composite curing light, usually in about 3 minutes. These latter light-activated bleaching materials change color upon completion of the oxidation reaction to allow visual monitoring of the bleaching process.

Upon completion of the treatment, rinse the teeth, remove the rubber dam, and caution the patient about postoperative sensitivity.

Bleaching treatments are generally rendered weekly for 2 to 6 treatments, with each treatment lasting 30 to 45 minutes. Patients may experience transient sensitivity of teeth between appointments, but again, no long-term adverse pulpal effects have been reported. Since the enamel is not acid etched, there is no need to polish the teeth post-treatment, nor is it essential to provide a fluoride treatment.

Dentist prescribed-home applied technique. The dentist prescribed-home applied technique (nightguard vital bleaching) is much less labor intensive and requires less in-office time. An alginate impression of the arch to be treated is made and poured in cast stone. The impression should be made free of bubbles on or around the teeth by wiping alginate onto the teeth and adjacent gingival areas prior to inserting the impression. After appropriate infection control procedures, rinse the impression vigorously, and then pour with cast stone. *Incomplete rinsing of the impression may cause a softened surface on the stone,* which may result in a guard which is slightly too small and irritates tissue. Trim the resultant cast around the periphery to eliminate the vestibule, and thin the base of the cast. The cast generally must be lifted from the table of the cast-trimming machine in order to successfully remove the vestibule without damaging the teeth. Allow the cast to dry, and block out any significant undercuts using a block-out material such as putty or clay.

The nightguard is formed on the cast using a heat/vacuum-forming machine. After the machine has warmed up for 10 minutes, a sheet of .020 to .035 inch nightguard material is inserted and allowed to soften by heat until it sags approximately 1 inch. Then close the top portion of the machine slowly and gently, and allow the vacuum to form the heat-softened material around the cast. After sufficient time for adaptation of the material, turn off the machine and allow the material to cool.

Next use a No. 11 surgical blade in a Bard-Parker handle to trim in a smooth straight cut about 3 to 5 mm from the most apical portion of the gingival crest of the teeth facially and lingually. This excess material is removed first. Then remove the horseshoe-shaped night-

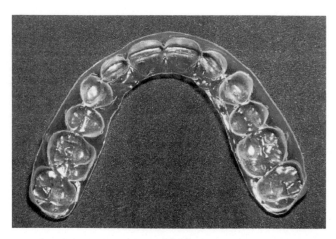

Fig. 18-22. Vacuum-formed clear plastic nightguard used for vital bleaching.

guard from the cast. Trim the edges of the nightguard to a smooth texture using sharp, curved scissors until only about 2 mm of tissue (apically of gingival crest) is covered, being sure the nightguard does not engage tissue undercuts. The nightguard is completed and ready for delivery to the patient (Fig. 18-22).

Insert the nightguard into the patient's mouth and evaluate it for adaptation, rough edges, or blanching of tissue. A properly fitting nightguard is shown in Fig. 18-23, *A* and *B*. Further shortening (trimming) may be indicated in problem areas. Evaluate the occlusion on the nightguard with the patient in maximum intercuspation. If the patient is unable to obtain a comfortable occlusion due to premature posterior tooth contacts, trim the nightguard to exclude coverage of the terminal posterior teeth as needed to allow optimal tooth contact in maximum intercuspation. Also, the edges of the guard on the palate should terminate in grooves or valleys where possible rather than on the heights of soft tissue contours such as in the area of the incisive papilla.

A 10% to 15% carbamide peroxide bleaching material generally is recommended for this bleaching technique. Ten percent carbamide peroxide degrades into 3% hydrogen peroxide (active ingredient) and 7% urea. Bleaching materials containing carbopol are recommended because it thickens the bleaching solution and

extends the oxidation process. Based on numerous research studies, carbamide peroxide bleaching materials appear to be *safe and effective when administered by or under the supervision of a dentist.*[32]

Instruct the patient in the application of the bleaching solution into the nightguard. Two to three drops of bleaching solution are placed into the area of each tooth to be bleached in the nightguard. Usually only the anterior 6 to 8 teeth are bleached. Review with the patient proper insertion of the nightguard. After inserting the nightguard, excess material is expectorated by the patient. Inform the patient not to drink liquids or rinse during treatment, but to remove the nightguard for meals and oral hygiene. The bleaching solution is usually replaced every 1½ to 2 hours during the day for a carbopol containing carbamide peroxide bleaching solution. If the nightguard is worn at night, a single application of bleaching material at bedtime is indicated. Total treatment time will usually be 2 to 6 weeks depending on how long the nightguard is worn each day. It is recommended that patients not exceed 12 hours total wearing time per day to allow teeth and soft tissues ample recovery time between bleaching applications. Also, tolerance to the nightguard and bleaching solution are improved if the patient gradually increases wearing time each day.

If either of the two primary side effects occur, sensitive teeth or irritated gingiva, the patient should reduce or discontinue treatment immediately, and contact the dentist so the cause of the problem can be determined.

It is recommended that *only one arch be bleached at a time,* beginning with the maxillary arch. Bleaching the maxillary arch first allows the untreated mandibular arch to serve as a constant standard for comparison. Moreover, restricting the bleaching to one arch at a time reduces the potential for occlusal problems which could potentially occur if the thicknesses of two mouthguards were interposed simultaneously. Fig. 18-24, *A* and *B*, and Plate 18-2, *A* and *B*, illustrate typical cases before and after treatment with nightguard vital bleaching.

Tetracycline-stained teeth typically are much more resistant to bleaching. Therefore, teeth stained with tetracycline require prolonged treatment times before any results are observed. Often, tetracycline-stained teeth are unresponsive to the procedure, especially if the

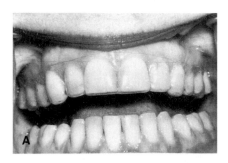
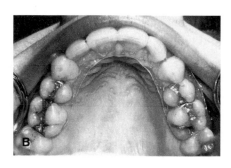

Fig. 18-23. Nightguard for vital bleaching. **A** and **B,** Clear plastic nightguard properly seated and positioned in the mouth.

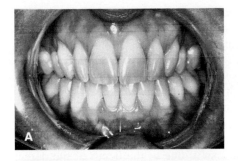
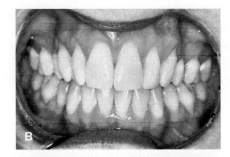

Fig. 18-24. Nightguard vital bleaching. A, Before bleaching treatment. B, After.

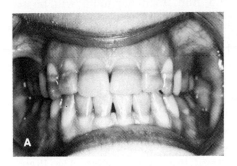
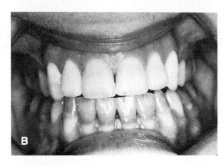

Fig. 18-25. Bleaching tetracycline-stained teeth. A, Before non-vital bleaching. B, After. (Courtesy Dr. Wayne Mohorn.)

stains are blue-gray in color. Tetracycline-stained teeth may approach but never seem to achieve the appearance of normal teeth. A single tetracycline-stained tooth with previous endodontic therapy or a different pulp size may respond differently from other teeth in the arch to the bleaching technique.

Due to the difficulty in bleaching tetracycline-stained teeth, some clinicians advocate intentional endodontic therapy, with the use of a non-vital bleaching technique in order to overcome this problem (Fig. 18-25, *A* and *B* and Plate 18-2, *C* and *D*). While the esthetic result appears much better than that obtained from external bleaching, this approach involves all the inherent risks otherwise associated with root canal treatment. External bleaching techniques offer a safer alternative, even though they may not be as rapid or effective. Veneers or full crowns are alternative treatment methods for the difficult tetracycline-stained teeth but involve irreversible restorative techniques. (See Indirect Veneer Techniques.)

No one bleaching technique is effective in every situation, and all successes are not equal. Often with vital bleaching, a combination of the in-office technique and the dentist prescribed-home applied technique will have better results than either technique used alone.

MICROABRASION/MACROABRASION

Microabrasion and macroabrasion represent conservative alternatives for the reduction or elimination of *superficial* discolorations. As the terms imply, the stained areas or defects are abraded away. These techniques do result in the physical removal of tooth struc-

ture and therefore are indicated only for stains or enamel defects that *do not extend beyond a few tenths of a millimeter in depth*. If the defect or discoloration still remains after treatment with microabrasion or macroabrasion, a restorative alternative is indicated.

Microabrasion

In 1984, McCloskey reported the use of 18% hydrochloric acid swabbed on teeth for the removal of superficial fluorosis stains.[55] Subsequently, in 1986, Croll modified the technique to include the use of pumice with the hydrochloric acid to form a paste applied with a tongue blade.[16] This technique was called *microabrasion* and involved the surface dissolution of the enamel by the acid along with the abrasiveness of the pumice to remove superficial stains or defects. Since that time, Croll further modified the technique, reducing the concentration of the acid to approximately 11% along with increasing the abrasiveness of the paste by using silicon carbide particles (in a water-soluble gel-paste) instead of pumice.[15] This product, marketed as Prema* compound, represents an improved and safer means for the removal of superficial stains or defects. It should be emphasized that this technique involves the physical removal of tooth structure and does not remove stains or defects through any bleaching phenomena.

Prior to treatment, evaluate the nature and extent of the enamel defect or stain.

First, differentiate between the non-hereditary developmental dysmineralization (abnormal mineralization) defects (e.g., white or light brown fluoretic enamel, and

*Premier Dental Products Co., Box 111, Norristown, PA 19404.

the idiopathic white or light brown spot) versus the incipient carious lesion. (Refer to Examination of Teeth and Restorations, in Chapter 5; Nomenclature, in Chapter 7; and Histopathology of Caries, in Chapter 3.)

Incipient carious lesions are usually located near the gingival margin. These lesions have a smooth surface (macroappearance), and appear opaque or chalky white when dried but are invisible when hydrated.

Incipient caries is reversible if treated immediately. Changing the oral environment by oral hygiene and dietary adjustments will allow remineralization to occur. If, however, the carious lesion has progressed to have a slightly roughened surface, microabrasion coupled with a remineralization program is an initial option, which if unsuccessful, can be followed by a restoration. Cavitation of the enamel surface is an indication for restorative intervention. As the location of smooth surface enamel caries nears the cementoenamel junction, the enamel is too thin to permit microabrasion or macroabrasion (see next section, Macroabrasion) as a treatment option.

The *developmental discolored spot* (opaque white or light brown) is the result of an unknown, local traumatic event during amelogenesis, and is therefore termed *idiopathic*. Its surface is intact, smooth, and hard. It is usually located in the incisal (occlusal) half of the enamel, which contributes to the unsightly appearance. The patient (or patient's parents) must be informed that an accurate prognosis for microabrasion cannot be given, but that microabrasion will first be applied; and if unsuccessful due to the depth of the defect exceeding 0.2 to 0.3 mm, then the tooth will be restored with a tooth-colored restoration.

Surface discolorations due to fluorosis also can be removed by microabrasion if the discoloration is within the 0.2 to 0.3 mm removal depth limit.

As seen in Fig. 18-26, *A,* a young patient presents with fluorosis stains on teeth 8 and 9. A rubber dam is placed to isolate the teeth to be treated and to protect the gingival tissues from the acid in the Prema paste or compound. Protective glasses should be given the patient to shield the eyes from any splatter. The Prema

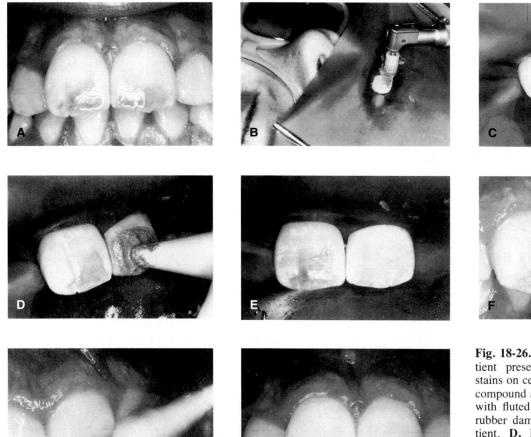
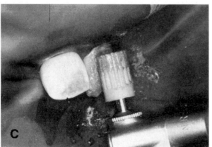
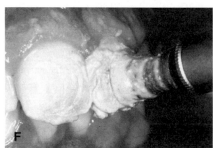

Fig. 18-26. Microabrasion. **A,** Young patient presents with unesthetic fluorosis stains on central incisors. **B** and **C,** Prema compound applied with special rubber cup with fluted edges. Protective glasses and rubber dam are needed for safety of patient. **D,** Hand applicator for applying Prema compound. **E,** Stain removed from left central incisor following microabrasion. **F,** Treated enamel surfaces polished with prophy paste. **G,** Topical fluoride applied to treated enamel surfaces. **H,** Final esthetic result. (Courtesy Dr. Ted Croll.)

paste is applied to the defective area of the tooth with a special rubber cup which has fluted edges (Fig. 18-26, *B* and *C*). The abrasive compound can be applied with either the side or the end of the rubber cup. A 10x gear reduction low-speed handpiece, similar to that used for placing pins, is recommended for application of the Prema compound to reduce the possibility of removing too much tooth structure and to prevent spatter. Moderately firm pressure is used in applying the compound.

For small localized idiopathic white or light brown areas, a hand application device is also available for use with the Prema compound (Fig. 18-26, *D*). Periodically, the paste is rinsed away to assess defect removal. The facial surface also is viewed with a mirror from the incisal aspect to determine how much tooth structure has been removed. Care must be taken not to remove excessive tooth structure. The procedure is continued until the defect is removed or until it is deemed imprudent to continue further (Fig. 18-26, *E*). The treated areas are polished with a fluoride-containing prophy paste to restore surface lustre (Fig. 18-26, *F*). Immediately following treatment, a topical fluoride is applied to the teeth to enhance remineralization (Fig. 18-26, *G*). Final results are seen in Fig. 18-26, *H*.

Macroabrasion

An alternative technique for the removal of localized superficial white spots (not subject to conservative, remineralization therapy) and other surface stains or defects is called *macroabrasion*. Macroabrasion simply utilizes a 12-fluted composite finishing bur or a micron finishing diamond in a high-speed handpiece to remove the defect (Fig. 18-27, *A* and *B*). Care must be taken to use light intermittent pressure and to carefully monitor removal of tooth structure in order to avoid irreversible damage to the tooth. Air-water spray is recommended, not only as a coolant, but also to maintain the tooth in a hydrated state to facilitate assessment of defect removal. Teeth that possess white spot defects are particularly susceptible to dehydration resulting in other apparent white spots that are not normally seen when the

tooth is hydrated. Dehydration exaggerates the appearance of white spots and makes defect removal difficult to assess.

Following removal of the defect or upon termination of any further removal of tooth structure, a 30-fluted composite finishing bur is used to remove any facets or striations created by the previous instruments. Final polishing is accomplished with an abrasive rubber point. The final results are seen in Fig. 18-27, *C*.

Comparable results can be achieved with either *microabrasion* or *macroabrasion*. However *advantages* and *disadvantages* exist with each. Microabrasion has the advantage of ensuring better control of the removal of tooth structure. High-speed instrumentation as used in macroabrasion is technique-sensitive to operator ability, and can have catastrophic results if extreme caution is not exercised. However, macroabrasion is considerably faster and does not require the use of a rubber dam or special instrumentation. Defect removal is also easier with macroabrasion compared to microabrasion if an air-water spray is used during treatment to maintain hydration of the teeth. Nonetheless, microabrasion is recommended over macroabrasion for the treatment of superficial defects in children because of better operator control and superior patient acceptance.

To accelerate the process, a combination of macroabrasion and microabrasion also may be considered. Gross removal of the defect is accomplished with macroabrasion followed by final treatment with microabrasion.

VENEERS

A veneer is a layer of tooth-colored material that is applied to a tooth for esthetically restoring localized or generalized defects or intrinsic discolorations (Plates 18-1, *B* and *C*; 18-2, *E* to *H*; and 18-3, *A* to *F*). Typically veneers are made of chairside composite, processed composite, porcelain, or cast ceramic materials.[10,12,35,49] Common indications for veneers include teeth with facial surfaces that are malformed, discol-

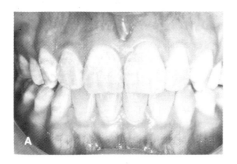
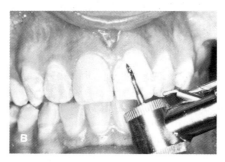
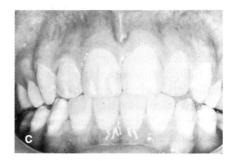

Fig. 18-27. Macroabrasion. **A,** Outer surface of teeth decalcified by high oral acidity during illness. **B,** Removal of discoloration by recontouring and polishing procedures. **C,** Completed treatment.

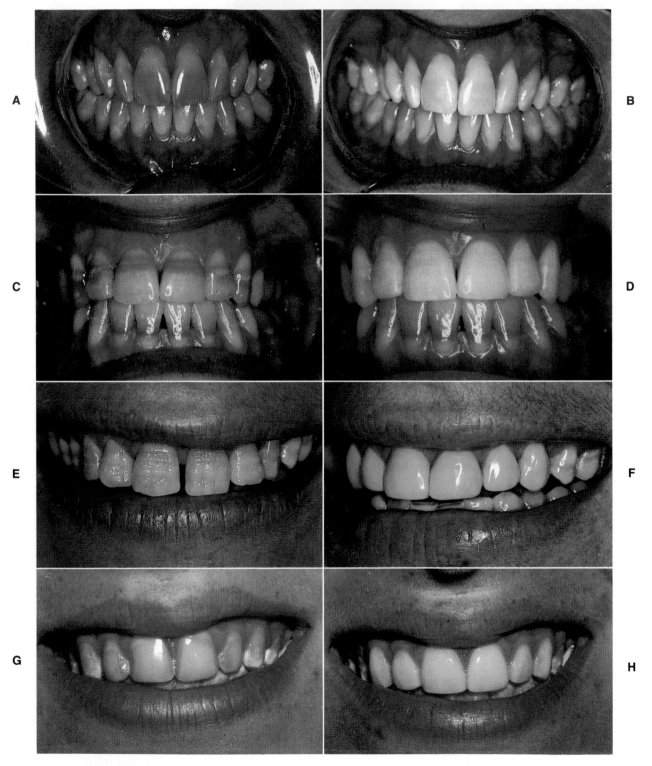

Plate 18-2. Examples of conservative esthetic procedures. **A** and **B,** Yellow discoloration is resolved through nightguard vital bleaching. **C** and **D,** Dark tetracycline stains can be treated through elective endodontic treatment and non-vital bleaching. **E** and **F,** Enamel hypoplasia and a midline diastema are corrected with direct composite veneers. **G** and **H,** Defective, discolored, direct composite veneers are replaced with indirect "etched resin" veneers. (**C** and **D,** courtesy Dr. H. Wayne Mohorn, Greensboro, NC.)

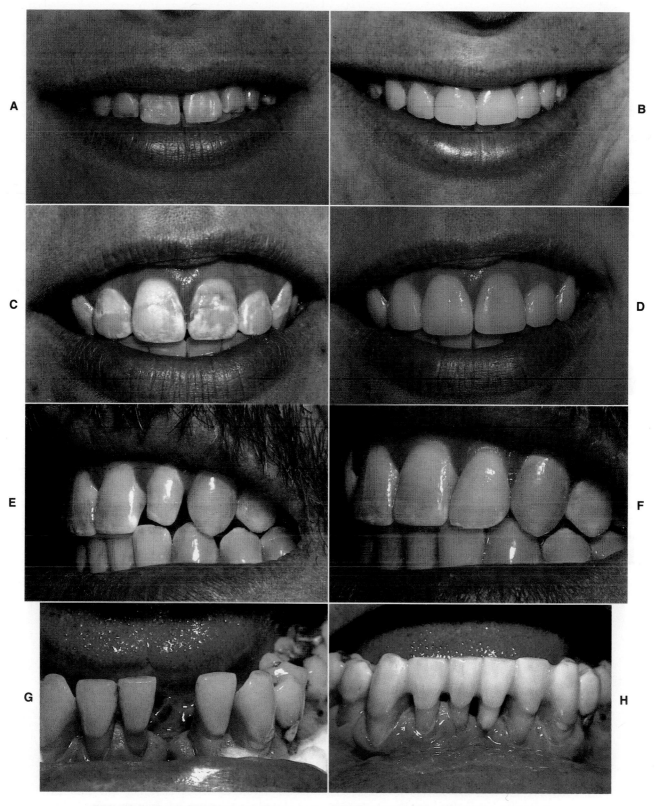

Plate 18-3. Examples of conservative esthetic procedures. **A** and **B,** Etched porcelain veneers. Enamel hypoplasia, discoloration, and a midline diastema are corrected with etched porcelain veneers. **C** and **D,** Etched porcelain veneers. Generalized hypocalcification defects unresolved with microabrasion are corrected with etched porcelain veneers. **E** and **F,** Etched porcelain veneer. A single etched porcelain veneer is used to conservatively restore a malformed lateral incisor. **G** and **H,** Splinting and natural tooth pontic. Periodontal disease resulted in the loss of the mandibular lateral incisor and mobility of the remaining anterior teeth. The crown was used as a bridge pontic, and the remaining teeth were splinted with composite.

chipped, discolored, or worn, it can usually be repaired or replaced.

Darkly stained teeth, especially those discolored by tetracycline, are much more difficult to veneer with full veneers than teeth with generalized defects, but normal coloration. The difficulty is further compounded when the cervical areas are badly discolored (see Fig. 18-33, *A*). Usually only the six maxillary anterior teeth require correction, since they are the most noticeable when a person smiles or talks. However, the maxillary first premolars also are included if they, too, are noticeably apparent upon smiling.

Discolored mandibular anterior teeth are rarely indicated for veneers, because the facioincisal portions are thin and usually subject to biting forces and attrition. Therefore, veneering lower teeth is discouraged if the teeth are in normal occlusal contact, because it is exceedingly difficult to achieve adequate reduction of the enamel to totally compensate for the thickness of the veneering material. Also, if porcelain veneers are placed, they may accelerate wear of the opposing maxillary teeth because of the abrasive nature of the porcelain. Fortunately these teeth are usually hidden by the lower lip, and esthetics is not as much of a problem. Most patients are satisfied with the conservative approach of veneering only the maxillary anterior teeth.

Direct veneer techniques

Direct partial veneers. Small localized intrinsic discolorations or defects that are surrounded by healthy enamel are ideally treated with direct partial veneers (Plate 18-1, *B* and *C*). All too often practitioners place full veneers when only partial veneers are indicated. Fig. 18-30, *A* illustrates four anterior teeth that had received direct composite veneers with no enamel preparation for the restoration of developmental white spot lesions. Ironically, the white spots still show through the veneers. The attendant problems of tissue incompatibility and contour inharmony associated with overcontoured veneers is readily apparent. Upon removal of the defective veneers, the localized white spots are evident (Fig. 18-30, *B*). Following preparation, etching, and restoration of the defective areas as described below, the finished partial veneers are seen (Fig. 18-30, *C* and *D*).

Six anterior teeth in Fig. 18-31, *A*, are used to illustrate the clinical technique for placing partial veneers. These can be restored in one appointment with either a self-cured or light-cured composite. Preliminary steps include cleaning, shade selection, and isolation with cotton rolls or rubber dam as described in Chapter 16. Anesthesia is usually not required unless the defect is very deep extending into dentin. The outline form is dictated solely by the extent of the defect and should include all of the discolored area as illustrated by models in Fig. 18-31, *B*. Use a coarse elliptical or round diamond instrument with air-water coolant to prepare the cavity generally to a depth of about 0.5 to .75 mm (Fig. 18-31, *C*).

Usually, it is not necessary to remove all of the discolored enamel in a pulpal direction. However, the preparation must be extended peripherally to sound, unaffected enamel. Use of an opaquing agent is described later for masking dark stains. In this example, no opaque is needed because the remaining stain is light and can be adequately hidden by the use of an appropriate composite restorative material. If the entire defect or stain is removed, then a microfill composite is recom-

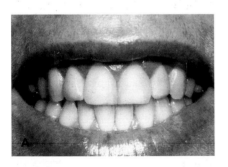
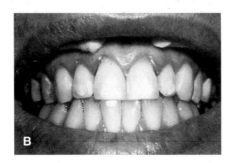
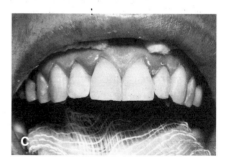
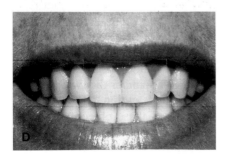

Fig. 18-30. Direct partial veneers. **A,** Patient with overcontoured direct full veneers. **B,** Following removal of old veneer, localized white spots are evident. **C,** Intraenamel preparations for partial veneer restorations. **D,** Conservative esthetic result of completed partial veneers.

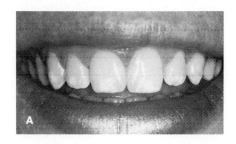
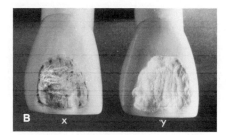
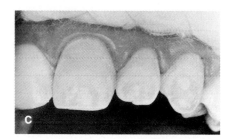

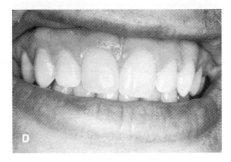

Fig. 18-31. Direct partial veneers. **A,** Small white hypocalcified spots. **B,** Models illustrate fault *(x)* and cavity preparation *(y)*. The chamfered margins are irregular in outline. **C,** Clinical appearance of etched preparations. **D,** Restoration of normal contour and color with partial veneers.

mended for restoring the cavity. If however a residual lightly stained area or white spot remains in enamel, an intrinsically less translucent composite can be used rather than extending the preparation into dentin to eliminate the defect. Most composites filled primarily with radiopaque fillers, such as barium glass, in addition to being radiopaque are also more optically opaque with intrinsic masking qualities. Use of these types of composites for the restoration of cavities with light residual stains is most effective and conserves tooth structure.

The procedures described in Chapter 16 are used to insert and finish the composite restorations (Fig. 18-31, *D*). In this example, all restorations are of light-cured composite.

Direct full veneers. Extensive enamel hypoplasia involving all of the maxillary anterior teeth was treated by direct full veneers and is illustrated in Fig. 18-32, *A*. Also see Plate 18-2, *E* and *F*. A diastema also exists between the central incisors. The patient desired to have both the hypoplasia and the diastema corrected. Examination indicated a good prognosis. A direct technique was used with a light-cured microfill composite. Although all six teeth can be restored at the same appointment, it is less traumatic for the patient and the dentist if the veneers are accomplished in two appointments. In this example, the central incisors were completed during the first appointment, and the lateral incisors and canines were completed during a second appointment.

After the teeth are cleaned and a shade selected, isolate the area with cotton rolls and retraction cords. Prepare the cavity preparations on both central incisors with a coarse, rounded-end diamond instrument. The "window" preparation is typically made to a depth

roughly equivalent to half the thickness of the facial enamel ranging from approximately 0.5 to .75 mm midfacially and tapering down to a depth of about 0.2 to 0.5 mm along the gingival margin, depending on the thickness of enamel (see Fig. 18-29). A heavy chamfer at the level of the gingival crest provides a definite cavity margin for subsequent finishing procedures. The margins are not extended subgingivally because these areas are not defective. The preparation for a direct veneer normally is terminated just facial to the proximal contact except in the area of a diastema (Fig. 18-32, *B*). To correct the diastema, the preparations are extended from the facial onto the mesial surfaces, terminating at the mesiolingual line angles (Fig. 18-32, *C* and *D*). (Refer to a previous section, Correction of Diastemata, for more complete instructions regarding restoration of this area.) The incisal edges were not included in the preparations in this example, because no discoloration was involved. Also, preservation of the incisal edges better protects the veneers from heavy functional forces as noted earlier for "window" preparations.

The teeth should be restored one at a time. After etching, rinsing, and drying procedures (Fig. 18-32, *E*), apply and polymerize the resin bonding agent. Place the composite on the tooth in increments, especially along the gingival margin, to *reduce the effects of polymerization shrinkage.* Place the composite in slight excess to allow some freedom in contouring. It is helpful to inspect the facial surface from an incisal view with a mirror to evaluate the contour before polymerization. After the first veneer is finished, restore the second tooth in a similar manner (Fig. 18-32, *F*). During a second appointment the remaining four anterior teeth are restored with direct composite veneers (Fig. 18-32, *G*).

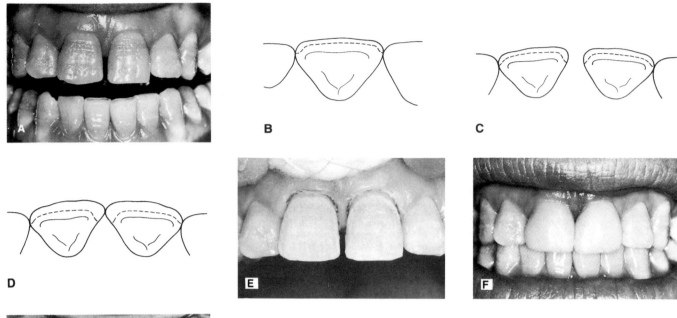

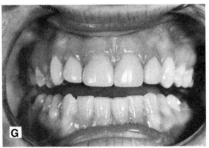

Fig. 18-32. Direct full veneers using light-cured composite. **A,** Enamel hypoplasia of maxillary anterior teeth. **B,** Drawing illustrates typical preparation of facial surface for direct full veneer. **C,** Preparation is extended onto mesial surface to provide for closure of diastema. **D,** Direct full veneers restore proximal contact. **E,** Etched cavity preparations of central incisors. **F,** Veneers completed on maxillary central incisors. **G,** Treatment completed with placement of full veneers on remaining maxillary anterior teeth.

As noted earlier, ***tetracycline-stained teeth*** are much more difficult to veneer, especially if dark banding occurs in the gingival third of the tooth (Fig. 18-33, *A*). In this example, time was a factor for the patient so all six maxillary anterior teeth were veneered in one appointment by using a *direct technique.* Veneer margins were placed subgingivally because of the dark discoloration in this area. This may indicate (along with other possible indications) local anesthesia. For reasons that have been stated previously, a light-cured composite is strongly recommended for veneers when the direct technique is used. Shade selection is more difficult because all of the anterior teeth are discolored. The posterior teeth usually have a more normal shade and can often be used as a guide. To obtain a natural appearance, it is helpful to make the cervical third of the teeth one shade darker than the middle or incisal areas. Additionally, the canines should be one shade darker than the premolars and incisors.

After cleaning and shade determination, mark the *gingival tissue level prior to isolation on the facial surfaces of the teeth to be veneered by preparing a shallow groove with a No. ¼ round carbide bur* (Fig. 18-33, *B*). Because the cervical areas are badly discolored and

the gingival tissue covers much of the clinical crown, isolation and tissue retraction is accomplished with a heavy rubber dam and No. 212 cervical retainer (Fig. 18-33, *C*). For details on application of the cervical retainer, see Chapter 11. Only one tooth is prepared and restored at a time. The outline form includes all of the facial surface, extending approximately 0.5 to 1 mm cervical to the mark indicating the gingival tissue level, and into the facial embrasures but not including the contact areas. The incisal margin includes the facioincisal angle in this instance because the discoloration involves this area. As much well-supported enamel as possible should always remain at the incisal ridge (surface) to preserve strength, wear resistance, and *functional occlusion on enamel.*

Prepare the tooth with a coarse, rounded-end diamond instrument (Fig. 18-33, *D)* by removing approximately half of the enamel thickness (0.3 mm in the gingival region to 0.75 mm in the mid-facial and incisal regions). Recall that the enamel is thinner in the cervical area. Some operators prefer to first make depth cuts to gauge the overall reduction. Although one preparation and restoration is completed at a time, if all veneers are to be completed in one appointment, the proximofacial

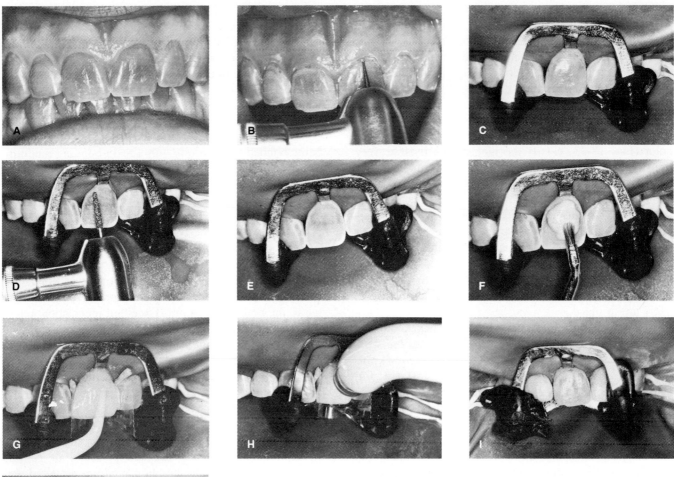

Fig. 18-33. Direct full veneers using light-cured composite for badly discolored teeth. **A,** Tetracycline-stained teeth. **B,** The level of gingival tissue on facial surface is scribed by cutting a shallow groove with a No. ¼ bur. **C,** Isolation with rubber dam and No. 212 cervical retainer. **D,** Diamond instrument used for making preparation. **E,** Etched surface of completed preparation. **F,** Application of resin opaquing material. **G,** Additions of composite completed. **H,** Curing the composite material. **I,** Retainer moved to next tooth and stabilized. **J,** All veneers completed.

line angles of the adjacent teeth can be reduced along with the tooth being prepared. This procedure makes the operation more efficient and helps to prevent damage later to the embrasure area of the restored tooth as the adjacent area is prepared.

After etching, rinsing, and drying, the completed cavity preparation is shown in Fig. 18-33, *E.* Now apply a thin layer of light-cured resin bonding agent to the etched enamel surface and lightly blow with air to leave a thin layer and to remove the excess; then light-cure (polymerize). Next, to mask the discolored area, apply a layer of opaquing agent (Fig. 18-33, *F*). Resin opaquing agents should be applied in thin layers (usually two), each layer being separately cured because of the

difficulty in light penetration through the opaque material. This will ensure complete polymerization of this intermediate layer. Care should be taken not to allow the opaque material to remain on the cavosurface margin, because it will appear as a definite opaque line along the margin of the final restoration. A stippled surface can be obtained by dabbing the partially cured opaque with the tip of a brush. This texturing will help reflect light rays in many directions outward through the veneer and result in a more natural appearance.

Now apply a gingival shade of composite with a hand instrument, starting with enough material to cover the gingival third of the tooth. An explorer tine, which first is touched to a sparing amount of bonding agent to prevent it from sticking to the composite, is used to adapt the composite to the margin. Excess composite should not be allowed to remain beyond the margin. The gingival shade of the composite is feathered out at the middle third, smoothed (lightly stroking with a small brush having fine bristles is helpful in smoothing the surface before curing), and cured.

Next, blend the incisal shade over the middle third and onto the incisal area to obtain proper contour and color (Fig. 18-33, G). If the incisal area itself is very translucent, special translucent shades of composite are available from most manufacturers and are recommended for restoration of this area. In this clinical example, the staining extended to the incisal edge, thus precluding significant translucency.

Evaluate the facial contour by inspecting from an incisal view with a mirror before the composite is polymerized (Fig. 18-33, H). General contouring is done at this time, but final finishing is delayed until all six veneers are in place.

The No. 212 retainer is moved to the next tooth and stabilized with compound (Fig. 18-33, I), and the steps for a direct veneer are repeated. This procedure is followed for each tooth until all veneers are inserted, finished, and polished (Fig. 18-33, J).

Indirect veneer techniques

Many dentists find that the preparation, insertion, and finishing of several direct veneers at one time is too difficult, fatiguing, and time-consuming. Some patients become uncomfortable and restless during long appointments. Also, veneer shades and contours can be better controlled when made outside of the mouth on a cast. For these reasons, indirect veneer techniques are usually preferable. Indirect veneers include those made of (1) processed composite,[8,35,58] (2) feldspathic porcelain,[2,12,20,41] and (3) cast ceramic.[49] Because of superior strength, durability, and esthetics, feldspathic porcelain is by far the most popular material for indirect veneering techniques used by dentists. Cast ceramic veneers offer comparable qualities, but require exacting laboratory technique and allow only limited chairside finishing and alteration of contours; however, excellent laboratory support and the superb marginal fit of these veneers can minimize or eliminate this disadvantage.

Although two appointments are required for indirect veneers, chair time is saved because much of the work is done in the laboratory. Excellent results can be obtained when proper clinical evaluation and careful operating procedures are followed. Indirect veneers are attached to the enamel by acid etching and bonding with either a self-cured, light-cured, or dual-cured resin bonding material.

Processed composite veneers. Composite veneers can be processed in a laboratory to achieve superior properties.[8,35,58] Using intense light, heat, vacuum, pressure, or a combination of these, cured composites can be produced which possess improved physical and mechanical properties compared to traditional chairside composites. Additionally, indirectly fabricated composite veneers offer superior shading and characterizing potential as well as better control of facial contours.

Because their composition is similar to chairside composite, indirect composite veneers are capable of being bonded to the tooth with a resin bonding medium. After acid etching, a bonding agent is applied to the etched enamel as with any composite restoration. A fluid resin bonding medium then is used to bond the veneer in place. A chemical bond is formed between the bonding agent and the bonding medium and to a lesser extent, between the bonding medium and the processed composite veneer. Because laboratory processing results in a greater degree of polymerization, fewer bond sites remain in the processed composite for subsequent bonding to the bonding medium. Excellent mechanical retention occurs at the interface of the bonding medium and tooth from the roughened tooth surface resulting from preparation with a coarse diamond instrument as well as from tag formation into the etched enamel.

Most processed composites presently are microfill composites. Although significant advantages exist over direct composite veneers, indirect veneers made of processed microfill composites possess limited bond strength because of the reduced potential to form a chemical bond with the bonding medium as noted earlier. Consequently, they should not be used in areas of high occlusal stress.

A newly developed processed composite of the hybrid type, filled with barium glass and colloidal silica, offers a significant improvement in bond strength.[69] Because this type of composite contains particles of barium glass, a relatively soft radiopaque filler, it can be sandblasted and etched in the laboratory with a mild concentration (9% to 10%) of hydrofluoric acid to produce numerous areas of microscopic undercuts, similar to the phenomenon that occurs when enamel is etched (Fig. 18-34). By producing a surface capable of micromechanical bonding, *"etched composite"* veneers (Herculite XRV Lab*) of this type can be strongly bonded to enamel without relying on significant chemical bonding. A typical case using "etched composite" veneers is illustrated in Plate 18-2, G and H.

Processed composite veneers are easily placed, finished, and polished. They also can be replaced or repaired easily with chairside composite (see Repairs of Veneers). For these reasons, indirect processed composite veneers are often recommended for placement in children and adolescents as interim restorations until the

---

*Herculite XRV Lab, Kerr/Sybron, Romulus, MI 48174.

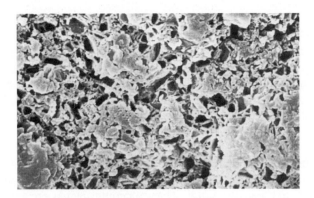

Fig. 18-34. Scanning electron micrograph (5000×) of sandblasted hybrid composite etched with mild concentration of hydrofluoric acid. (Courtesy Dr. James Hamilton.)

teeth have fully erupted and achieved their complete clinical crown length. At that time, usually at age 18 to 20 years, a more permanent alternative such as porcelain or castable ceramic veneers can be pursued.

Indirect processed composite veneers also are indicated for placement in patients who exhibit significant wear of their anterior teeth due to occlusal stress. However, only the "etched composite" type of veneers are recommended in cases of occlusal stress because of their superior bond strength. Because of their lower cost, indirect processed composite veneers also offer an esthetic, affordable alternative to more costly porcelain or castable ceramic types when economics is the primary consideration. However, it must be pointed out to the patient that processed composite veneers typically do not exhibit comparable clinical longevity.

The patient in Fig. 18-35, *A*, presents with six defective direct composite veneers that will be replaced with indirect processed composite veneers. Following shade selection, the teeth are isolated with bilaterally placed cotton rolls and gingival retraction cord. All existing defective Class III restorations or small carious lesions should be restored prior to preparation. *Multiple large existing restorations compromise the potential to bond the veneer to the tooth and may represent a contraindication.* Usually no anesthetic is required for tooth preparations for veneers. In fact, the patient's response is important in judging preparation depth, especially in the gingival third of the tooth. The preparations should be restricted entirely to enamel if at all possible.

A "window" preparation design as illustrated schematically in Fig. 18-29, *E*, is recommended for most indirect processed composite veneers due to the limited bond strength of the composite veneer. If the teeth require lengthening or if defects exist warranting involvement of the incisal edge, the "etched composite" veneer should be used with an "incisal lapping" design as shown in Fig. 18-29, *F*.

The window preparation is made with a rounded-end

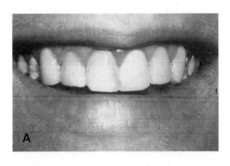
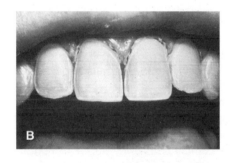
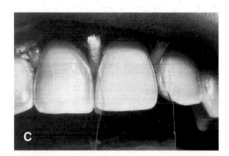
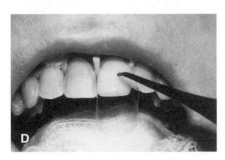
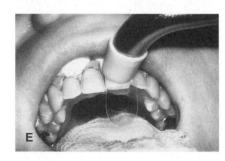
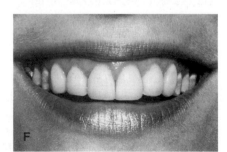

Fig. 18-35. Indirect processed composite veneers. **A,** Patient presents with six defective direct composite veneers. **B,** Finished "window" preparations for indirect processed composite veneers. **C,** Left central incisor isolated, etched, and ready for veneer bonding. **D,** Veneer is positioned and seated with blunt instrument or finger. **E,** Veneer bonding medium is light cured. **F,** Completed indirect composite veneers.

diamond instrument to a depth of approximately 0.5 to .75 mm midfacially diminishing to a depth of 0.2 to 0.5 mm along the gingival margin, depending on enamel thickness. As noted earlier for direct composite veneers, the gingival margin should be positioned just at or slightly above the level of the gingival crest unless defects, caries, or dark discoloration warrant subgingival extension. Also, the interproximal margins should extend into the facial and gingival embrasures, without engaging an undercut, yet should be located just facial to the proximal contacts. The finished preparations are seen in Fig. 18-35, *B*.

Generally, no temporary restorations are placed because the preparations are restricted to enamel. If a small amount of dentin is inadvertently exposed, a thin coat of a dentin bonding agent can be applied to the exposed dentin and cured to reduce the possibility for postoperative sensitivity. Patients always should be forewarned that the prepared teeth will be slightly rough during the interim until the final veneer restorations are bonded.

An elastomeric impression is made of the preparations. If the gingival margins are well isolated and spaced from the retraction cord, the cord may be left in place during impression making. If, however, the margins are subgingival or close to the gingival tissue, better access for recording the gingival margin is afforded by cord removal just prior to injection of the impression material. It also is recommended that the lingual aspect of the gingival embrasures be blocked out with soft wax (see Fig. 18-39, *B*). This step will prevent penetration and interlocking of the impression material through the gingival embrasure, which often results in torn impressions, especially along critical marginal areas.

A stone working cast is generated from the impression with individually removable dies to facilitate access to interproximal areas. Once the veneers are fabricated and returned, they should be closely inspected for fracture lines, chips along margins, or other significant defects that would preclude successful placement. Since the veneers are composed of composite, some intraoral recontouring is possible following bonding.

At the second appointment the teeth to be veneered are cleaned with a pumice slurry, the shade confirmed, and the operating site isolated. Frames are available that comfortably retract the lips for better access if needed. Routine isolation is accomplished by the placement of cotton rolls and insertion of retraction cords. A 2 × 2 inch cotton gauze is placed across the back of the patient's mouth to protect against aspiration or swallowing of a veneer if inadvertently dropped (see Fig. 18-35, *D*).

The fit of each veneer is evaluated on the individual tooth and adjusted if necessary. All of the veneers should fit closely to the tooth at the gingival area. The veneers should be tried in place both individually and collectively to ensure the fit of adjacent seated veneers. Veneers should be tried in place only on *clean, dry teeth* to eliminate any potential for contamination. If accidental contamination occurs, the veneer should be thoroughly cleaned with alcohol or acid etchant, rinsed, and dried prior to bonding. On removal, each veneer is placed tooth-side-up (concave side facing upward) on an adhesive pad or palette. Some processed composites (non-etched type) require that a priming agent be applied to the tooth side of the veneer following the manufacturer's instructions. These priming agents are typically adhesion-promoting materials that increase the bond strength of the veneer to the resin bonding medium. A thin layer of resin bonding agent is applied to the tooth side of the veneer with a brush or small sponge, *but not cured*. The veneers are stored under a jar lid or are placed in a container that is impervious to light to prevent premature curing of the bonding agent.

A light-cured resin bonding medium is recommended for bonding the veneer to the tooth. Shade selection of the bonding medium is determined once the fit of the individual veneers has been evaluated and confirmed. Shade selection is made by first placing a uniform layer of a selected shade of bonding medium, approximately 0.5 mm in thickness, on the tooth side of a single veneer. Typically, a central incisor veneer is used to facilitate shade determination of the bonding medium. The operatory light is turned away during shade assessment to prevent premature and inadvertent curing of the veneer to the tooth. The veneer is seated on a *clean, dry, unetched tooth,* the excess bonding medium removed with a brush, and the overall shade of the veneer evaluated. Following try-in, the veneer is quickly removed and stored under a jar lid or placed in a container that is impervious to light to prevent curing of the residual bonding medium. If the shade of the bonding medium is determined to be appropriate, more of the same shade of bonding medium is simply added to the veneer just prior to bonding. If a different shade is deemed necessary, the existing shade is wiped from the inner aspect of the veneer with a disposable brush and a new shade of bonding medium is placed in the veneer. In the meantime, the assistant can be removing residual bonding medium of the previous shade from the tooth with a cotton pellet or brush. The veneer loaded with the new shade of resin bonding medium is re-seated and evaluated as previously described.

It should be emphasized that the inherent shade of the veneer, characterization, and internal opaquing must be accomplished during fabrication of the veneer itself. Some additional opaque can be incorporated into the resin bonding medium at the time of bonding to achieve greater masking. Also, the overall shade of the veneer can be slightly modified by the shade of bonding medium selected. However, significant changes in shading cannot be accomplished chairside.

The retraction cords are evaluated to ensure that they are adequately tucked into the gingival crevice. A technique for the individual placement of each veneer is recommended. The tooth used for try-in to assess shade of the bonding medium should be cleaned again with a slurry of pumice to remove any residual resin which may preclude proper acid etching of the enamel.

Polyester strips are placed in the proximal areas of the first tooth to be restored. Wooden wedges can be used to secure the position of the strips, but care must be taken not to irritate the gingival papilla for risk of inducing hemorrhage. The acid etchant is artfully applied with a small brush, sponge, or etchant applicator. Acid should not be allowed to flow onto the retraction cord or soft tissue. The prepared tooth is seen in Fig. 18-35, *C,* ready for veneer bonding after acid etching, rinsing, and drying. A thin layer of resin bonding agent is applied to the etched enamel, lightly blown with air, *but not cured until placement of the veneer.* Premature curing of the bonding agent may preclude full seating of the veneer.

The selected shade of light-cured resin bonding medium is added to the tooth side of the veneer with enough material to cover the entire treated surface without entrapping air. The veneer is carefully placed on the appropriate tooth and lightly jiggled in place with a blunt instrument or light finger pressure (Fig. 18-35, *D*). A brush or explorer is used to remove excess bonding medium. Proper seating of the veneer should be evaluated with a No. 2 explorer. With the veneer properly positioned and excess bonding medium removed, a visible light-curing unit is used to polymerize the material with a minimum exposure time of 40 to 60 seconds each from the facial and lingual directions for a total exposure of 80 to 120 seconds (Fig. 18-35, *E*). Excess of cured bonding resin remaining around the margins is best removed with a No. 12 surgical blade held in a Bard-Parker handle (see Fig. 18-37, *F*). Each veneer again should be tried in place immediately prior to bonding to ensure full seating in the presence of the already bonded adjacent veneer. New polyester strips are positioned for each tooth as the other veneers (one at a time) are placed in a similar manner.

Once the veneers are all bonded, only a minor amount of finishing is required at the marginal areas. Removal of the retraction cord at this time allows access and visibility for finishing gingival margins. This step is accomplished as previously described for composite restorations. Unwaxed floss always should be used to assess the final smoothness of interproximal areas. If incisal areas have been involved, protrusive excursions should be evaluated to ensure occlusal harmony in the restored areas. Patients also should be cau-

tioned to avoid biting hard foods or objects to prevent fracturing the incisal edge, especially if an incisal lapping design was used. The completed veneers immediately after placement are shown in Fig. 18-35, *F.*

Etched porcelain veneers. The most frequently used indirect veneer type is the etched porcelain (feldspathic) veneer (see Plate 18-3, *A* to *F*).[2,12,20,41] Porcelain veneers etched with hydrofluoric acid are capable of achieving high bond strengths to the etched enamel via a resin bonding medium.[68] This porcelain etching pattern can be seen in Fig. 18-36. In addition to the high bond strengths, etched porcelain veneers are *highly esthetic, stain resistant, periodontally compatible, and appear to significantly outlast composite veneers.* The incidence of cohesive fracture for etched porcelain veneers is much less than for direct or indirect composite veneers.[45,64]

The patient in Fig. 18-37, *A,* presents with generalized discoloration of the anterior teeth along with facial and incisal hypoplastic defects. A midline diastema will be closed as well when porcelain veneers are placed.

The procedures for preparation, impression, try-in, and cementation are the same as for indirect processed composite veneers, with a few exceptions. The reader is referred to the previous section on indirect processed composite veneers for details of these basic techniques.

Following cleaning, shade selection, and isolation of the teeth, the intraenamel preparations are made with a rounded-end diamond instrument. A hemi-preparation as shown on the maxillary left central incisor in Fig. 18-37, *B,* is often used to assess tooth reduction. Unlike with processed composite veneers, an incisal lapping preparation design is generally used for porcelain veneers, especially if incisal defects warrant inclusion or

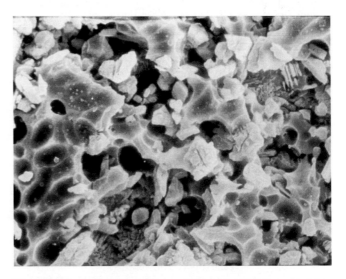

Fig. 18-36. Scanning electron micrograph (1000×) of feldspathic porcelain etched with hydrofluoric acid. (Courtesy Dr. Steven Bayne.)

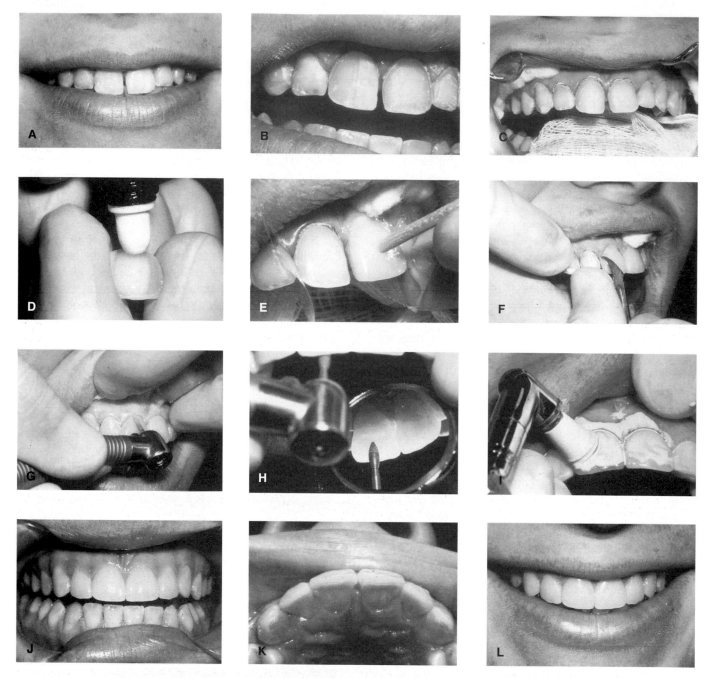

Fig. 18-37. Indirect etched porcelain veneers. **A,** Patient presents with generalized discoloration of the anterior teeth along with facial and incisal hypoplastic defects. **B,** A hemi-preparation is often used to assess tooth reduction. **C,** Completed incisal lapping veneer preparations. **D,** A thin layer of bonding medium is placed in the veneer. **E,** The etched porcelain veneer is carefully positioned and seated on the tooth. **F,** A No. 12 surgical blade in a Bard-Parker handle is ideal for removing excess cured bonding medium. **G,** A fine diamond instrument is used to finish rough gingival margins. **H,** Lingual areas are best finished with an oval-shaped diamond instrument. **I,** A final surface lustre is imparted through the use of porcelain polishing paste. **J to L,** Completed etched porcelain veneers.

the teeth need lengthening (see Fig. 18-29, *F*). As noted earlier, this preparation design facilitates seating of the veneer and enables the laboratory technician to produce a more esthetic incisal edge whose porcelain/resin margin is on the lingual surface. Because of the strength of the porcelain and excellent bond, incisal fractures are rarely encountered. Also, the preparations on the mesials of both central incisors are extended to the mesiolingual line angles to allow subsequent restoration of the proximal contacts (see Figs. 18-32, *C* and *D*).

After the preparations are completed (Fig. 18-37, *C*), an elastomeric impression is made. As noted earlier, no temporary restorations are required, because the preparations are shallow and involve only the enamel. The patient should be instructed to avoid biting hard objects, keep the area clean with a soft-bristled brush, and expect the possibility of some mild sensitivity to hot and cold.

Once completed by the laboratory, the porcelain veneers are returned to the dentist for cementation at the second appointment. The completed veneers must be inspected for cracks, overextended margins, and adequate internal etching as evidenced by a frosted appearance. Marginal areas in particular should be inspected for proper etching so that an adequate seal will occur in these areas. Overextended marginal areas interproximally may preclude full seating of adjacent veneers. These areas can be trimmed carefully with a micron finishing diamond instrument. *However, unless severe or inaccessible, most minor overextensions should be trimmed only after bonding the veneer to the tooth because of the risk of fracturing the porcelain.*

After the prepared teeth are cleaned with a pumice slurry, rinsed, and dried, isolation is accomplished with a lip retractor (optional), cotton rolls, and retraction cords. As noted earlier, the veneers are tried on the teeth to confirm proper contour and fit, and an appropriate shade of resin bonding medium is selected. The only difference in this procedure for porcelain veneers from the composite veneers is the need to condition the internal surface of each veneer with a **silane primer** just prior to applying the resin bonding agent. The silane acts as a **coupling agent** enabling a chemical bond to occur between the porcelain and the resin.[7] It also improves wettability of the porcelain. The primary source of retention with porcelain veneers still remains the etched porcelain surface itself. Only a modest increase in bond strength results from silanization of the porcelain, but is nonetheless recommended.

A technique is presented and recommended for applying the veneers *one at a time*. Polyester strips are placed interproximally to prevent inadvertent bonding to the adjacent tooth, followed by etching, rinsing, and drying procedures. It is recommended that the two central incisors be etched and their veneers bonded first,

because of their critical importance esthetically. A resin bonding agent is applied to the etched enamel and the tooth side of the silane-primed porcelain veneer. Next a thin layer (0.5 mm) of the selected shade of light-cured resin bonding medium is placed on the tooth side of the veneer, being careful not to entrap air (Fig. 18-37, *D*). The first veneer is placed on the tooth carefully and lightly jiggled to place with a blunt instrument or light finger pressure (Fig. 18-37, *E*). The margins of the veneer are examined with a No. 2 explorer to verify accurate seating. Next, the excess resin bonding medium is removed with a disposable brush or explorer, and the margins are once again evaluated before the veneer is exposed to the curing light. To ensure complete polymerization, the veneer should be cured for a minimum of 40 to 60 seconds each from facial and lingual directions for a total exposure time of 80 to 120 seconds. Following positioning and bonding of the first veneer, the second veneer is positioned carefully and bonded in like manner, followed individually by the remaining veneers.

As recommended earlier, a No. 12 surgical blade in a Bard-Parker handle is ideal for removing excess of cured resin bonding medium remaining around the margins (Fig. 18-37, *F*). Removal of the retraction cord at this point facilitates access and visibility to subgingival areas. If the marginal fit of the porcelain veneers is deemed acceptable and a favorable emergence angle exists, the marginal areas need only minimal finishing. This process is best accomplished with a rounded-end, 30-fluted carbide finishing bur (Midwest No. 9803) to remove any remaining excess resin bonding medium.

If the porcelain margins are overextended beyond the cavosurface angles, or if the marginal areas are too bulbous, recontouring of these areas is required, especially along gingival margins, to ensure proper physiological contours and gingival health. A fine diamond instrument is used to recontour these areas (Fig. 18-37, *G*). Marginal areas should be confluent with surrounding unprepared tooth surfaces when assessed with a No. 2 explorer. Lingual areas are best finished with an oval-shaped diamond instrument (Fig. 18-37, *H*). Because use of a diamond instrument breaks the glazed surface, a series of appropriate instruments are used to restore a smooth surface texture. Micron finishing diamonds are used to initiate the polishing sequence. Thereafter, a rounded-end, 30-fluted carbide finishing bur (Midwest No. 9803) is used to plane the porcelain surface and to remove the striations created by the diamond instruments. Studies show that the best results occur if the diamond instruments are used with air-water coolant while the 30-fluted bur should be used dry.[34] A final surface lustre is imparted through the use of a porcelain polishing paste applied either with a rubber prophy cup or a felt wheel (Fig. 18-37, *I*). Where access allows,

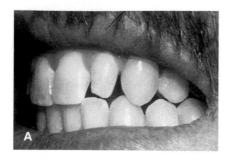 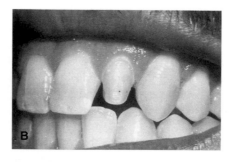 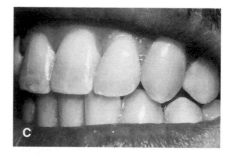

Fig. 18-38. Treatment of malformed tooth with porcelain veneer. **A,** Malformed left lateral incisor. **B,** An incisal lapping preparation much like a ¾ crown in enamel is used. **C,** Final esthetic result.

porcelain surfaces also may be smoothed using a commercially available porcelain polishing kit* consisting of a series of abrasive rubber points. The completed veneers are shown in Fig. 18-37, *J* to *L*. Also see Plate 18-3, *A* and *B*. A similar example of a completed case using etched porcelain veneers is seen in Plate 18-3, *C* and *D*.

Etched porcelain veneers also can be effectively used to conservatively restore malformed anterior teeth. A single malformed left lateral incisor is seen in Fig. 18-38, *A*. An incisal lapping preparation that is extended well onto the lingual surface is employed (Fig. 18-38, *B*). The resulting restoration is virtually comparable to a "three-quarter crown" in porcelain. The final esthetic result is shown in Fig. 18-38, *C*. See also Plate 18-3, *E* and *F*.

Darkly discolored teeth are more difficult to treat with porcelain veneers. However, several modifications in the veneering technique can be used to enhance the final esthetic result. First, the most important difference in technique is that opaque porcelain is incorporated in the fabrication of the veneers in order to induce more inherent masking. If the veneers are not inherently opaque, little chance exists for adequate masking of a darkly stained tooth. Typically 5% to 15% opaque porcelain is required to achieve optimal masking. Exceeding 15% opaque porcelain dramatically reduces light penetration and results in a significant loss of esthetic vitality. Recall that the esthetic vitality or life-like appearance of teeth depends on light penetration (see Translucency in the section on artistic elements).

Second, a slightly deeper cavity preparation can be used to allow greater veneer thickness. However, the preparation should always be restricted to enamel to ensure optimal bonding of the veneer to the tooth.

Third, the laboratory can be instructed to use several coats of a die spacing medium on the laboratory model in order to allow a slightly greater thickness of resin bonding medium. The die spacing medium must not be

extended closer than 1 mm to the margins to ensure adequate positioning of the veneer to the preparation during try-in and bonding and to provide for a slight internal space. A typical case is seen in Fig. 18-39, *A,* following preparation of the anterior teeth for etched porcelain veneers. A "window" preparation design was used for the canines to preserve the functional occlusal path on tooth structure. An incisal lapping preparation was used on the other teeth. An incisal view aptly illustrates the difference between the two designs (Fig. 18-39, *B*). As seen also in Fig. 18-39, *B*, soft wax is placed in the lingual embrasures to prevent interproximal tearing during impression making procedures. Incisal and facial views of the completed veneers are seen in Figs. 18-39, *C* and *D*. A similar case of darkly discolored teeth showing prepared teeth and post-operative result is seen in Figs. 18-40, *A* and *B*.

Patients who possess darkly stained teeth always should be informed that although porcelain (or composite) veneers can result in improved esthetics, they may not entirely eliminate or mask very dark stains. Moreover, due to the limited thickness of the veneers and the absolute necessity of incorporating intrinsic opacity, the life-like translucency or esthetic vitality of veneered teeth may never be comparable to that of natural, unaffected teeth (see Figs. 18-8, *A* and *B*). Full porcelain coverage with all-porcelain or castable ceramic crowns may be indicated in some patients with severe discoloration because of the crown's greater capacity to restore esthetic vitality. Nonetheless, porcelain veneers are a viable option in most cases for the patient who desires esthetic improvement without significant tooth reduction.

Castable ceramic veneers. Another esthetic alternative for veneering teeth is the use of castable ceramics such as Dicor®.*[49] Unlike etched porcelain veneers which are fabricated by stacking and firing feldspathic porcelain, castable ceramic veneers are literally cast using a lost wax technique. The castable Dicor® veneer

---

*Shofu Dental Corp., Menlo Park, CA 94025.

*Dentsply International, York, PA 17405-0872.

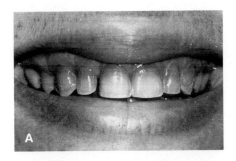
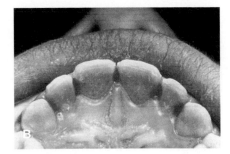
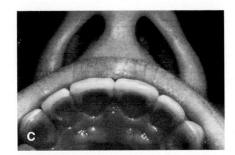

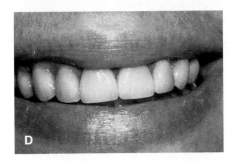

Fig. 18-39. Treatment of darkly discolored teeth with porcelain veneers. **A,** Tetracycline stained anterior teeth (including first premolars) shown following preparation for etched porcelain veneers. **B,** Incisal view shows "window" preparation design on canines and incisal lapping design on remaining prepared teeth. Soft wax is used to block out lingual embrasures to facilitate impression making. **C** and **D,** Incisal and facial views of completed etched porcelain veneers.

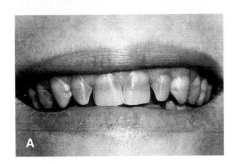
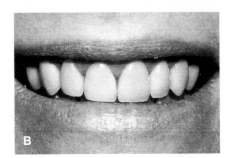

Fig. 18-40. Darkly stained teeth treated with porcelain veneers. **A,** Before treatment. **B,** After.

material itself is grayish in shade and very translucent. Low-fusing feldspathic shading porcelains fired onto the surface of the veneer provide the final coloration. Excellent esthetics are possible using castable ceramic materials for most cases involving mild-to-moderate discoloration. However, due to the limited amount of intrinsic opaquing possible with castable ceramic veneers, *dark discolorations are best treated with etched porcelain veneers.*

The procedures for tooth preparation, try-in, and bonding are the same as for etched porcelain veneers except that the margins of *castable ceramic veneers cannot be contoured and finished with rotary instrumentation.* Since shading of castable ceramic veneers is accomplished by surface coloration, the use of rotary instrumentation on the veneer surface would result in loss of this coloration revealing an unesthetic grayish appearance. Generally, however, little marginal finishing is necessary due to the excellent marginal fit possible with castable ceramic veneers. Only the excess bonding medium needs to be removed. A typical case showing

before prepared teeth and after treatment views is seen in Figs. 18-41, *A* to *C*.

Veneers for metal restorations

Esthetic inserts (partial or full veneers) of a tooth-colored material can be placed on the facial surface of a tooth previously restored with a metal restoration. For new castings, plans are made at the time of cavity preparation and during laboratory development of the wax pattern to incorporate a *veneer into the cast restoration.* After such a casting has been cemented, the veneer can be inserted as described in the next section, except that the portion of mechanical retention of the veneer into the casting has been provided in the wax pattern stage.

Veneers for existing metal restorations. Occasionally the facial portion of an existing metal restoration (amalgam or gold) is judged to be distracting (Fig. 18-42, *A*). A careful examination, including a radiograph, is required to determine that the existing restoration is sound before an esthetic correction is made. The size of the offensive area determines the extent of the prepara-

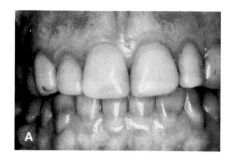

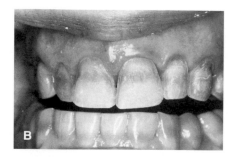

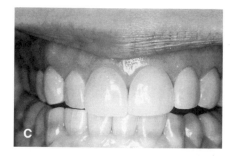

Fig. 18-41. Castable ceramic veneers. **A,** Before treatment. **B,** Prepared teeth. **C,** Esthetic result after completed veneers.

Fig. 18-42. Veneer for existing cast restoration. **A,** Mesiofacial portion of onlay is distracting to patient. **B,** Model of tooth and preparation. Note 90-degree cavosurface angle and retention prepared in gold and cavosurface bevel in enamel. **C,** Clinical preparation ready for composite resin. **D,** Completed restoration.

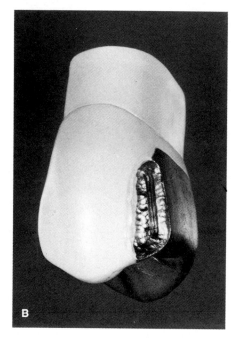

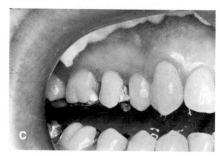

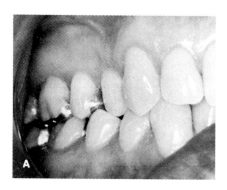

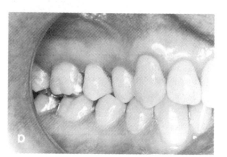

tion. Anesthesia is not usually required, since most of the preparation is in metal or enamel. Preliminary procedures consist of cleaning the area with pumice, selecting the shade, and isolating the site with a cotton roll. When the offensive metal extends subgingivally, the level of the gingival tissue is marked on the restoration with a sharp explorer, and a retraction cord is placed in the gingival crevice. Rubber dam isolation may be required in some instances.

A No. 2 carbide bur rotating at high speed with an air-water spray is used to remove the metal, starting at a point midway between the gingival and occlusal margins. The preparation is made perpendicular to the surface approximately 1 mm deep at a minimum, leaving a butt joint at the cavosurface margins. The 1 mm depth and a butt joint should be maintained as the preparation is extended occlusally. All of the metal along the facial enamel is removed, and the preparation is extended into the facial and occlusal embrasures just enough for the veneer to hide the metal. *The contact areas on the proximal or occlusal surfaces must not be included in the preparation.* To complete the outline form, the preparation is extended gingivally approximately 1 mm past the mark indicating the clinical level of the gingival tissue.

The final cavity preparation should have the same features as those described for veneers in new cast restorations. Mechanical retention is placed in the gingival area with a No. ¼ carbide bur (air coolant to enhance vision) 0.25 mm deep along the gingivoaxial and linguoaxial angles. Retention and esthetics are enhanced by beveling the enamel cavosurface margin (bevel approximately 0.5 mm wide) with the coarse, flame-shaped diamond instrument oriented at 45 degrees to the external tooth surface (Fig. 18-42, *B*). After it is etched, rinsed, and dried, the cavity preparation is complete (Fig. 18-42, *C*). New adhesive resin liners containing a chemical called 4-META, capable of bonding composite to metal, also may be used but are quite technique-sensitive.[14,54] Manufacturer's instructions should be followed explicitly to ensure optimal results with these materials. The composite material is inserted and finished in the usual manner (Fig. 18-42, *D*).

Repairs of veneers

Failures of esthetic veneers occur because of breakage, discoloration, or wear. Consideration should be given to conservative repairs of veneers if examination reveals that the remaining tooth and restoration are sound. It is not always necessary to remove all of the old restoration. The material most commonly used for making repairs is light-cured composite.

Veneers on tooth structure. Small chipped areas on veneers can often be corrected by recontouring and polishing. When a sizable area is broken, it can usually be repaired if the remaining portion is sound (Fig. 18-43, *A*).

For *direct composite veneers,* repairs ideally should be made with the same material that was used originally. After cleaning the area and selecting the shade, the operator should roughen the damaged surface of the veneer and/or tooth with a coarse, rounded-end diamond instrument to form a chamfered cavosurface margin (Fig. 18-43, *B*). For more positive retention, mechanical locks may be placed in the remaining composite material with a small round bur (Fig. 18-43, *C*). An etching solution is applied to clean the prepared area, which is then rinsed and dried (Fig. 18-43, *D*). Next, a resin bonding agent is applied to the preparation (existing composite and enamel) and polymerized. Chairside

composite material is then added, cured, and finished in the usual manner (Fig. 18-43, *E*).

Indirect processed composite veneers are repaired in a similar manner. However, in order to repair *porcelain veneers,* a mild hydrofluoric acid preparation, suitable for intraoral use, must be used to etch the fractured porcelain. Hydrofluoric acid gels are available in approximately 10% buffered concentrations which are intended for intraoral porcelain repairs. Although caution still must be taken when using hydrofluoric acid gels intraorally, the lower acid concentration allows for relatively safe intraoral use. Full-strength hydrofluoric acid should *never* be used intraorally for etching porcelain. Isolation of the porcelain veneer to be repaired should be accomplished with a rubber dam to protect the gingival tissues from the irritating effects of the hydrofluoric acid. The manufacturer's instructions must be followed regarding application time of the hydrofluoric acid gel to ensure optimal porcelain etching. A lightly frosted appearance, similar to that of etched enamel, should be seen if the porcelain has been properly etched. A *silane coupling agent* may be applied to the etched porcelain surface prior to the application of the resin bonding agent. Chairside composite material is then added, cured, and finished in the usual manner. Large fractures are best treated by replacing the entire porcelain veneer.

Faulty veneers in metal restorations. Fig. 18-44, *A,* illustrates two faulty acrylic resin veneers on gold crowns after 18 years of service that need replacing because of wear and discoloration. The teeth are cleaned with a slurry of pumice and the shade selected before isolation by cotton rolls and retraction cords. With superficial wear or staining, part of the old restoration (sil-

Fig. 18-43. Repairing veneer. **A,** Fractured veneer on maxillary canine. **B,** Preparation with round diamond instrument. **C,** Undercuts placed in existing veneer with No. ¼ bur. **D,** Completed preparation is shown isolated and etched. **E,** Veneer restored to original color and contour.

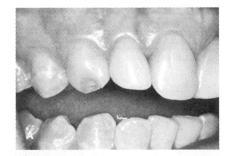
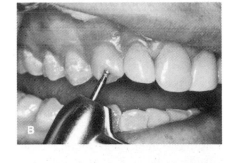
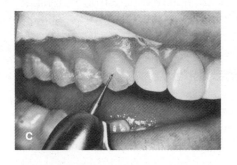
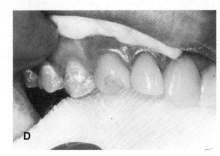
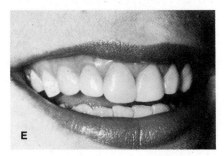

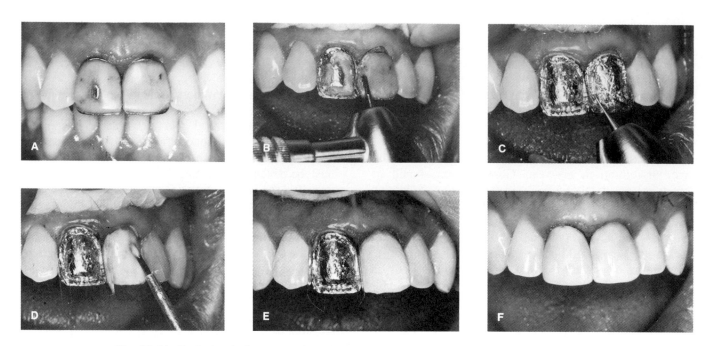

Fig. 18-44. Replacing faulty veneers in metal restorations with light-cured composite veneers. **A,** Acrylic resin veneers stained and worn after 18 years of service. **B,** Removal of existing veneers with a carbide bur. **C,** Mechanical retention is placed in metal with No. 33½ bur. **D,** Masking agent (opaquing resin) is needed to cover metal surface. **E,** Composite material is added and cured in the first preparation. The same steps are repeated for second veneer. **F,** Both veneers completed.

icate cement, acrylic, or composite) can be left to achieve some masking of the underlying metal. In this example, all of the old resin material is removed with an appropriate instrument such as a No. 1558 carbide metal cutting bur (Fig. 18-44, *B*). Both preparations are accomplished together. The outline of each preparation is extended gingivally by removing some of the gold. The operator should endeavor to create a chamfered finish line. Retention is placed with a No. 33½ carbide bur in selected areas in the metal along the line angles approximately 0.25 mm deep (Fig. 18-44, *C*).

Although the preparations are done simultaneously, it is usually better to place the veneers one at a time. A light-cured composite is recommended because of the extended working time. Polyester strips are placed between the proximal surfaces. The preparation is cleaned with acid etchant for 30 seconds, then rinsed and dried to remove debris and obtain a clean, dry surface. In this instance, the acid is used only to clean the surface, not to etch the metal. Wedges placed in the gingival embrasure may help to establish proper contour of the matrix. A masking material (opaquing resin) is artfully placed with a small brush over the metal areas of the preparation by applying and curing successive thin layers (Fig. 18-44, *D*). As noted earlier, adhesive resin liners containing 4-META, capable of bonding to metal, also may be used to achieve additional retention and to achieve some masking.[14,54] These materials should be placed

directly over the prepared metal surface. Manufacturer's instructions should be followed closely to ensure optimal results with these materials, as they are quite sensitive to proper technique.

Next, a small amount of composite material (gingival shade) is placed at the cervical area with a hand instrument, adapted with the tine of a No. 2 explorer, and cured with visible light. Now material of the preselected lighter shade is added to restore the middle and incisal portions. A small brush is helpful in smoothing the surface and obtaining the final contour before curing. Finishing is delayed except for removing any excess contour at the mesiofacial embrasure (Fig. 18-44, *E*).

Evaluation of the width of the teeth can be achieved with a Boley gauge or another appropriate caliper. The second preparation is cleaned and dried before the opaque or adhesive liner is added. Composite material is inserted and cured as described for the first veneer. The retraction cords are removed, and both restorations are finished together to obtain symmetrical contours (Fig. 18-44, *F*).

ACID-ETCHED, RESIN-BONDED SPLINTS

There are many causes for mobility of teeth: traumatic injury to the face, advanced periodontal disease, habits such as thumb-sucking and tongue-thrusting, and malocclusion.[22,23] In addition, teeth often need stabilization and retention after orthodontic treatment. In the past, clinical procedures for the stabilization of teeth either involved extensive loss of tooth structure or were poor in appearance. A conservative and esthetic alternative has been made possible by using acid-etched, resin-bonded splints.[24,43,59]

Certain criteria must be met when mobile teeth are splinted. Occlusal adjustment may be necessary initially. *The splint should have a hygienic design* so that the patient is able to maintain good oral hygiene. It also should allow further diagnostic procedures and treatment if necessary. The acid-etched, resin-bonded splinting technique satisfies these criteria. Light-cured composites are recommended for splinting, because they afford extended working time for placement and contouring.

Periodontally involved teeth

Loss of bone support allows movement of teeth, resulting in increased irritation to the supporting tissues and possible malpositioning of the teeth.[22] *Stabilizing mobile teeth is a valuable treatment aid before, during, and after periodontal therapy.* Splinting the teeth aids in occlusal adjustment and tissue healing, thus allowing better evaluation of the progression and prognosis of treatment.

A resin-bonded splint via the acid etch technique is a conservative and effective method of protecting the teeth from further injury by stabilizing them in a favorable occlusal relationship. If the periodontal problem is complicated by missing teeth, a bridge incorporating a splint design is indicated (see Conservative Bridges).

Techniques for splinting anterior teeth. In short-span segments subject to minimal occlusal forces, a relatively simple technique can be used for splinting periodontally involved teeth. Fig. 18-45, *A,* illustrates a maxillary lateral incisor that remains mobile because of insufficient bone support even after occlusal adjustment and elimination of a periodontal pocket. Esthetic recontouring with composite augmentation can be accomplished along with the splinting procedure.

Anesthesia is generally not required for a splinting procedure when enamel covers the clinical crown. However, when root surfaces are exposed and extreme sensitivity exists, local anesthesia is necessary. The teeth are cleaned with a pumice slurry, and the shade of light-cured composite is selected. A cotton roll and retraction cords are used for isolation in this instance.

With a coarse, flame-shaped diamond instrument the enamel on both teeth at the proximal contact area is reduced to produce an interdental space approximately 1 mm wide. This amount of space will enhance the strength of the splint by providing more bulk of composite material between the teeth. Other enamel areas of the tooth or teeth that need more contour are prepared by roughening the surface with a coarse diamond instrument. Where no enamel is present, such as on the root surface, a dentin bonding agent is used following the manufacturer's instructions. Otherwise, a mechanical lock is prepared with a No. ¼ round bur in the dentin at the gingivoaxial line angle of the box-like preparation. After the prepared enamel surfaces are acid etched, rinsed, and dried, a lightly frosted appearance should be observed (Fig. 18-45, *B*).

The enamel/dentin bonding agent is applied, lightly blown with air, and polymerized. A hand instrument is used to place a small amount of composite material in the gingival area. Additional shaping with a No. 2 explorer will reduce the amount of finishing necessary later. It is helpful to add and cure the composite in small increments, building from the gingival toward the incisal aspect. Finishing is accomplished with round and flame-shaped carbide burs and polishing discs and points. The retraction cord is removed, and the occlusion is evaluated to assess centric contacts and functional movements. Instructions on brushing and flossing are reviewed with the patient. Four-year results are illustrated in Fig. 18-45, *C.*

Another indication for splinting periodontally involved teeth is illustrated in Fig. 18-46, *A.* All of the maxillary incisors are mobile from lack of periodontal support. Typically, the incisors are weaker than the ca-

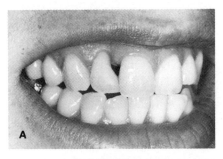
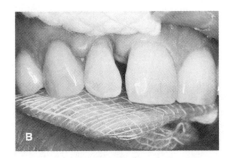
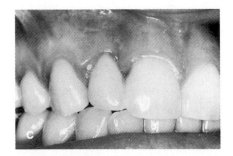

Fig. 18-45. Splinting and recontouring a mobile tooth using a light-cured composite. **A,** Maxillary right lateral incisor is loose from lack of bone support. **B,** Preparations completed and etched. **C,** Splinted and recontoured tooth after 4 years.

nines because of the difference in root length. To stabilize the incisors, a composite splint must include all of the maxillary anterior teeth. The same procedures are followed as before except that a rubber dam is used to isolate the teeth. After etching, rinsing, and drying procedures (Fig. 18-46, *B*), a light-cured composite is inserted, polymerized, and finished (Fig. 18-46, *C*). The completed splint is shown after 3 years of service (Fig. 18-46, *D*).

Splinting also can be used when the mandibular inci-

sors are mobile from severe bone loss. Fortunately the canines are firm (Fig. 18-47, *A*). Because the patient has several missing posterior teeth, the occlusion on the anterior teeth is abnormally heavy. *An orthodontic wire can be incorporated* into the splint to provide more strength. The same general steps are followed as with the maxillary teeth. In addition, horizontal grooves are prepared facially and lingually in the enamel with a coarse, rounded-end diamond instrument. The grooves are positioned at the junction of the cervical and middle

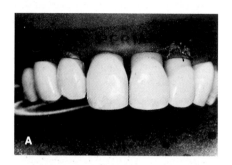
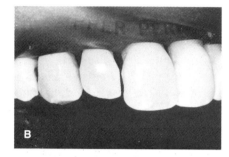
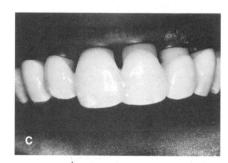

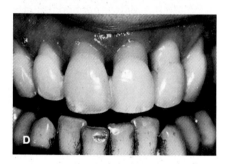

Fig. 18-46. Splinting maxillary anterior teeth. **A,** All maxillary incisors are loose and need splinting. **B,** Preparation consists of roughening proximal surfaces and creating slight diastemata to provide bulk to the connector areas of composite splint. **C,** Splint contoured and finished. **D,** Teeth and splint remain stable at 3-year recall.

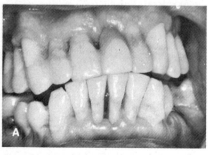
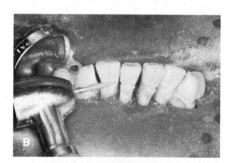
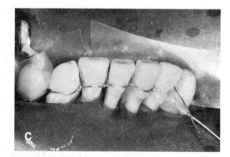

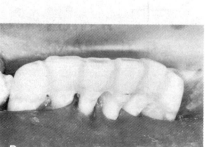
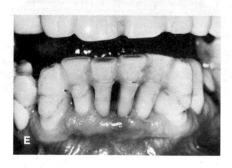

Fig. 18-47. Splinting of mobile mandibular incisors. **A,** Because of extreme mobility and heavy bite, an orthodontic wire will be incorporated into splint. **B,** Horizontal grooves are made 0.5 mm deep on the facial and lingual enamel surfaces of all mandibular anterior teeth. **C,** After enamel is etched, orthodontic wire is looped around teeth. **D,** Light-cured composite is contoured and finished to complete splint. **E,** Splint after 5 years of service.

thirds of the facial and lingual enamel and are cut approximately 1 mm wide incisogingivally and 0.5 mm deep (Fig. 18-47, *B*).

After etching, rinsing, and drying procedures, a continuous piece of orthodontic wire is threaded between the teeth and along the grooves in a figure-eight design (Fig. 18-47, *C*). A polyester strip is placed on the distal portion of each canine to prevent inadvertent bonding of the adjacent premolars. A thin layer of resin bonding agent is applied, lightly blown with air, and polymerized. The light-cured composite material is added and polymerized in increments to obtain the desired contour (Fig. 18-47, *D*). After finishing procedures, the rubber dam is removed, and the occlusion is evaluated.

Because the patient has high caries activity, the importance of proper diet and oral hygiene is carefully reviewed. In addition, daily fluoride rinses are recommended, and the need for recall evaluation is emphasized. With cooperative patients, excellent long-term results can be expected as shown in this example after 5 years of service (Fig. 18-47, *E*).

Alternatively, a stainless steel mesh (Splint-Grid, Ellman*) can be positioned and bonded to the lingual surfaces of the teeth to reinforce the composite splint (Fig. 18-48, *A* to *D*). Care must be taken to cover the wire mesh completely with composite to avoid rough irritating edges.

Stabilization of teeth after orthodontic treatment

Following orthodontic treatment, teeth may require stabilization using either fixed or removable appli-

*Splint-Grid, Ellman International Mfg., Hewlett, NY 11557.

ances.[25,72] The latter method allows continued minor movements for final positioning of the teeth. Once this position is reached, it is better to stabilize the teeth with a fixed retainer. Removable retainers tend to irritate the soft tissue. Also they may be damaged, lost, or not worn, which usually allows undesired movement of the teeth.

Fig. 18-49, *A*, shows a patient with a removable orthodontic retainer. Optimal positioning of the teeth has been achieved by orthodontic movement; however, stabilization of the teeth is required, and the unattractive spaces caused by undersized maxillary teeth need to be closed (Fig. 18-49, *B*). A carefully planned appointment is required to accomplish the following: (1) remove any fixed orthodontic appliance, (2) add composite to close the diastemata, and (3) stabilize the teeth with a *twisted stainless steel wire and composite*.

Technique. After the orthodontic appliance is removed and routine procedures followed for closing the diastemata (Fig. 18-49, *C*), the occlusion is carefully examined to determine the best position for locating the twisted wire, since it will be placed only on the lingual surfaces. A sufficient length of twisted stainless steel wire (0.0175 inch [0.45 mm] in diameter) is adapted to the lingual surface of the anterior teeth. A stone cast is helpful for adapting the wire. The wire must rest against the lingual surfaces passively without tension or interference with the occlusion. In the mouth, waxed dental tape is used to position the wire against the teeth and hold it in place while occlusal excursions are evaluated. The wire will be attached only to the lingual fossa of each tooth. After the position of the wire has been determined, it is removed, and the enamel in the fossae

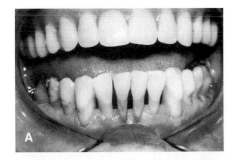
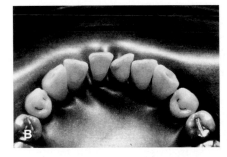
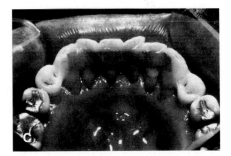
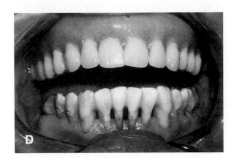

Fig. 18-48. Periodontal splint reinforced with wire mesh. **A,** Mobile periodontally involved teeth before treatment. **B,** Teeth isolated with rubber dam. **C,** Lingual view of completed splint. **D,** Facial view of splint after treatment.

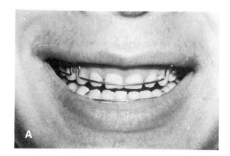

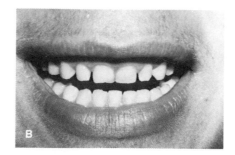

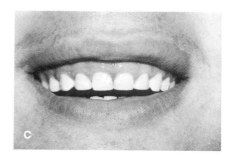

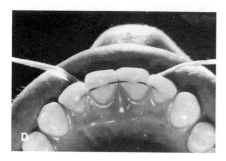

Fig. 18-49. Stabilizing teeth after orthodontic treatment. **A,** Patient with existing removable retainer. **B,** Residual spaces resulting from undersized teeth. **C,** Closure of spaces with composite additions is completed. **D,** Orthodontic wire is held in position with dental tape and bonded to place with composite.

only (not the marginal ridges or embrasures) is etched, rinsed, and dried.

A light-cured or self-cured composite can be used for attaching the fixed wire splint. The wire is repositioned and held in place with dental tape while a sparing amount of resin bonding agent is applied and lightly blown with air. After polymerization of the bonding agent, a small amount of composite material is placed to encompass the wire in each fossa and bond it to the enamel. The operator must be careful not to involve the proximal surfaces (Fig. 18-49, *D*). After polymerization of the composite, the occlusion is evaluated and adjusted as needed for proper centric contacts and functional movements.

This unique splint allows some physiological movement of the teeth, yet it holds them in the correct position. The splint should remain in place for at least 6 months to ensure stabilization. Longer retention may be necessary, depending on the individual situation and recommendations of the orthodontist.

Avulsed or partially avulsed teeth

Facial injuries often involve the hard and soft tissues of the mouth.[4,62] The damage may range from lacerations of the soft tissue to fractures of the teeth and alveolar bone. There can be partial or complete avulsion of teeth. Maxillary central incisors are involved more often than other teeth. A thorough clinical examination of soft tissue, lips, tongue, and cheeks should be made for lacerations and embedded tooth fragments and debris. Radiographic examination is necessary to diagnose deeply embedded fragments or root fractures.

Treatment of soft tissue lacerations should include la-

vage, conservative debridement, and suturing. Consultation with or referral to an oral surgeon may be necessary. A partially avulsed tooth is repositioned digitally and may or may not need splinting. *Traumatically avulsed teeth that are reimplanted immediately or within 30 minutes have a good prognosis for being retained.*[3,60] After 30 minutes the rate of success drops rapidly. Therefore the avulsed tooth should be repositioned as soon as possible. In the interim it should be placed in a moist environment such as saliva (held in the cheek or under the tongue), milk, saline, or a wet towel. The replacement of avulsed teeth has immediate psychological value and maintains the natural space in the event that a fixed prosthesis is required later.[71]

Technique. The maxillary right incisors that were completely avulsed in an accident (Fig. 18-50, *A)* are repositioned immediately. After the teeth are repositioned, radiographs reveal that no other complications exist. Isolation with cotton rolls or gauze is preferred to use of a rubber dam, which could cause malpositioning of the loose teeth. The occlusion should be evaluated to ensure that the teeth are properly positioned.

The facial surfaces of the crowns are quickly cleaned with hydrogen peroxide, rinsed, and dried by blotting with a gauze or cotton roll and/or by lightly blowing with air. The dentist should avoid blowing air into areas of avulsion or deep wounds to prevent the possibility of air emboli. If a crown is fractured, any deeply exposed dentin should be covered with calcium hydroxide to protect the pulp. A *twisted orthodontic wire* (0.0195 inch [0.49 mm]) must be long enough to cover the facial (or lingual) surfaces of enough teeth to stabilize the loose teeth. The wire is adapted and the ends rounded to

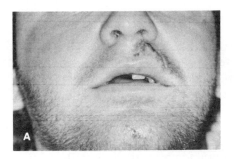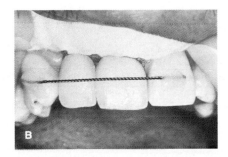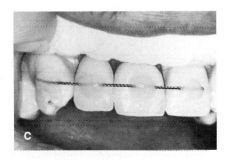

Fig. 18-50. Splinting avulsed teeth. **A,** Patient with traumatically avulsed maxillary right incisors. **B,** Orthodontic wire is positioned and bonded to adjacent uninvolved teeth with composite. **C,** Completed splint stabilizes repositioned incisors.

prevent irritation to the soft tissue. In an emergency, a paper clip can be used as a temporary splint.

No preparation of the enamel surface is necessary other than that provided by acid etching the enamel. The middle third of the facial surfaces are etched, rinsed, and dried of all visible moisture. Again, drying should be accomplished by blotting with a gauze or cotton roll and a light stream of air. A self-cured or light-cured composite may be used. The wire is positioned and held lightly in place while the ends are attached with the composite material (Fig. 18-50, *B*). Light pressure is applied to the repositioned teeth as the facial surfaces are bonded to the wire in succession (Fig. 18-50, *C*). Care is exercised not to allow the composite to flow into the proximal areas. Once the teeth are stabilized, any fractured areas can be conservatively repaired by the acid etch–resin bond technique. Finishing is accomplished by a flame-shaped carbide finishing bur and abrasive discs. The occlusion is evaluated carefully to ensure that no premature contacts exist.

The patient is advised of gentle care of the involved teeth. Antibiotic therapy may be required if the alveolar bone is fractured or significant soft tissue damage has occurred. Tetanus shots or boosters are advised if indicated by the nature of the accident. The patient's physician should be contacted regarding this need. Appointments are made for follow-up examinations on a weekly basis for the first month. The patient is alerted to the symptoms of pulpal necrosis and advised to call if a problem develops. If a root canal therapy is required, it is better accomplished with the splint in position.

Removal of the splint is accomplished in 4 to 8 weeks, provided recall visits have shown normal pulp test results and the teeth are asymptomatic. The wire is sectioned, and the resin material is removed with a flame-shaped carbide finishing bur at high speed with air-water spray and a light, intermittent application. Abrasive discs are used to polish the teeth to a high luster.

CONSERVATIVE BRIDGES

In selected cases conservative bridges can be made by acid etching and bonding a pontic to the adjacent natural teeth. These conservative bridges are classified according to the type of pontic: (1) natural tooth pontic; (2) denture tooth pontic; (3) pontic, either of porcelain-fused-to-metal or all metal, with metal retainers; and (4) all-porcelain pontic. Although the four types differ in the degree of permanency, they share a major advantage—conservation of natural tooth structure. In addition, they can be viable alternatives to conventional fixed bridges in circumstances where age, expense, or clinical impracticality are considerations.

It should be noted that because of the bonded nature of all of these bridge types, *retention is never as strong as for a conventional bridge.* As part of informed consent, patients should be told of the potential, although remote, for swallowing or aspirating bonded bridges that are dislodged. Furthermore, to reduce the risk of dislodgement, patients should be cautioned not to bite hard foods or objects with bonded bridge pontics.

The ideal site for a conservative bridge is where the edentulous space is no wider than one or two teeth. Other considerations include bite relation, oral hygiene, periodontal condition, and extent of caries, defects, and restorations in the abutment teeth. *Conservative bridges are especially indicated for young patients,* because the teeth usually have large pulp chambers and a short clinical crown. Many older patients with gingival recession and mobile teeth are prime candidates because *splinting can be incorporated with the bridge.* More specific indications and clinical procedures for each of the four types of bridges are presented in the following sections.

Natural tooth pontic

The crowns of natural teeth (primarily incisors) often can be used as acid-etched, resin-bonded pontics.[38,44] Considerations for this type of treatment occur when (1) periodontally involved teeth warrant extraction, (2) teeth have fractured roots, (3) teeth are unsuccessfully reimplanted following avulsion, and (4) root canal treatment has been unsuccessful. However lost, the immediate replacement of a natural anterior tooth has great psychological value for most patients, although the procedure may be temporary. Natural tooth pontics also can be placed as interim restorations until an extraction site heals if conditions require a conventional bridge.

Certain prerequisites must exist to ensure a successful result: (1) the extracted tooth, as well as abutments, must be in reasonably good condition, especially the pontic, since it may become brittle and more susceptible to fracture; (2) the abutment teeth should be fairly stable; and (3) the tooth to be replaced as a pontic must not participate in heavy centric or functional occlusion. Because of this third restriction, canines and posterior teeth are not usually good candidates for this procedure. If the adjacent teeth are mobile, it is frequently necessary to secure them as well by splinting with composite (see Acid-etched, Resin-bonded Splints).

Technique. A maxillary right central incisor must be extracted for periodontal reasons as seen in Fig. 18-51, *A* and *B*. Before the tooth is extracted, a small, round bur is used to place a shallow identifying mark on the facial surface to indicate the level of the gingival crest. Following extraction, a 2 × 2 inch (5 × 5 cm) sponge is held in the space with pressure for hemorrhage control.

By using a separating disc, the extracted tooth is transversely cut a few millimeters apical to the identification mark. When pontic length is determined, shrinkage of the healing tissue underlying the pontic tip must be anticipated. The root end is discarded.

If the pulp canal and chamber have completely calcified, the next procedure is shaping and polishing the apical end of the natural tooth pontic as described in the following paragraphs. If the chamber is calcified as disclosed on the radiograph and the canal is nearly calcified, the canal is opened from the apical end by using a No. 1 or No. 2 bur to the extent of the canal. The operator should be as conservative of tooth structure as possible, yet provide access for subsequent injection of composite material to fill the canal. A large chamber and canal are instrumented and debrided by using conventional endodontic procedures with *access from the apical end* (Fig. 18-51, *C*). Access is provided for subsequent injection of composite. Removal of the pulpal tissue in this manner prevents possible later discoloration of the tooth caused by degeneration products. Traditional lingual access for instrumentation is avoided to prevent weakening the pontic. Following these procedures the canal (and chamber, if present) is filled and closed with a self-cured composite. Light-cured materi-

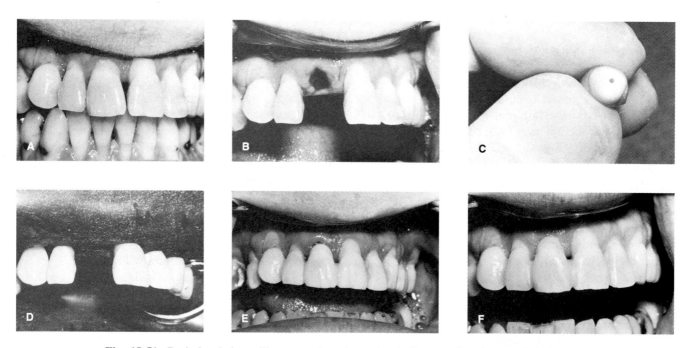

Fig. 18-51. Resin-bonded maxillary natural tooth pontic. **A,** Preoperative photograph before extraction of periodontally involved maxillary right central incisor. **B,** Extraction site immediately following removal of incisor. **C,** Enlarged apical opening ready to be filled with composite. Pontic tip has been contoured to ovate design. **D,** Abutment teeth isolated, roughened, and acid etched. **E,** Immediate postoperative photograph of natural tooth pontic bonded in place. **F,** Resin-bonded natural tooth pontic with healed residual ridge 6 weeks later.

als may be used, but must be placed incrementally to ensure complete polymerization.

After the composite has polymerized, the apical end is contoured to produce a bullet-shaped ovate design (Fig. 18-51, *C*). This design provides adaptation of the pontic tip to the residual ridge, yet it allows the tissue side of the pontic tip to be cleaned with dental floss. It is also by far the most esthetic pontic tip design that can be used. While being contoured, the tip is occasionally evaluated by trying the pontic in the space. In the maxillary arch, passive contact between the pontic tip and the healed residual ridge is considered ideal for maximal phonetic and esthetic potential. However, in the mandibular arch where esthetics is not generally a problem, the pontic tip is best shaped into the same bullet-shaped design, but positioned as a hygienic pontic type that does not contact tissue (Fig. 18-52, *B*).

The pontic tip is smoothed and polished, using a proper sequence of abrasive discs and/or polishing points. A polished pontic tip not only is easier to clean, but also retains less plaque.

A rubber dam is usually needed for isolation of the region to prevent seepage of blood and saliva. Isolation using cotton rolls and gingival retraction cords is acceptable if hemorrhage has been controlled. Any carious lesions or faulty proximal restorations on involved proximal surfaces of both the pontic and the abutments are now restored with light-cured composite (preferably the same material to be subsequently used for the bridge connectors) by using modified cavity designs. It is recommended that the resulting restored surfaces be undercontoured rather than overcontoured to facilitate positioning of the natural tooth pontic.

Next, the involved proximal enamel surfaces are roughened with a coarse, flame-shaped diamond instrument. Spaces of approximately 0.5 mm should exist between the pontic and the abutment teeth, because stronger connectors are provided by the additional bulk of

composite material. Now the operator should acid etch, rinse, and dry all prepared (roughened) enamel surfaces (Fig. 18-51, *D*).

A light-cured composite is preferred for bonding natural tooth pontics, because the extended working time allows the operator to contour the connectors before polymerization. First, the resin bonding agent is applied to the etched surfaces of the pontic and lightly blown with air to remove the excess. Then it is polymerized by application of light, and the pontic is set aside ready for bonding in the mouth. Next, the bonding agent is applied to the etched surfaces of the abutment teeth and cured. Then a small amount of composite material is placed on the proximal contact areas of the natural tooth pontic, and the pontic is carefully inserted in the proper position in the mouth. The composite is teased and shaped around the contact areas with an explorer tip. After final verification that the pontic position is correct, the composite is polymerized with light. Next, additional composite is applied in the proximal areas (more material is added on the lingual than on the facial surface), contoured, and cured. Adequate gingival embrasures must be provided to facilitate flossing and ensure gingival health. After sufficient material has been added and polymerized, the embrasure areas should be shaped and smoothed with carbide finishing burs and polishing discs or points. The rubber dam is removed, and the occlusion is evaluated for centric contacts and functional movements. Heavy contacts on the pontic or the connector areas must be adjusted. The finished bridge immediately after bonding is illustrated in Fig. 18-51, *E*. The patient should return in 4 to 6 weeks for evaluation of the relationship of the pontic tip to the tissue. Passive contact should exist between the pontic tip and the underlying tissue to prevent ulceration. If tissue ulceration is present, the pontic must be removed, recontoured, and rebonded. The finished bridge and healed residual ridge appear in Fig. 18-51, *F*.

As stated earlier, abutment teeth that are mobile can often be splinted with composite to afford stability to periodontally involved teeth. An example case in the mandibular arch is shown in Fig. 18-53. The abutments are isolated, roughened, and acid etched (Fig. 18-53, *A*). Because esthetics is not as critical, a hygienic-type pontic tip is recommended for mandibular incisors (Fig. 18-52, *B*). The finished bridge-splint is illustrated in Fig. 18-53, *B*. Also see Plate 18-3, *G* and *H*.

Denture tooth pontic

An acrylic resin denture tooth can be used as a pontic for the replacement of missing maxillary or mandibular incisors by using the acid etch–resin bonding technique (Fig. 18-54).[37,46,65] Although this type of bridge is sometimes used as an interim prosthesis and is called a *temporary bridge,* it can be a viable alternative to a

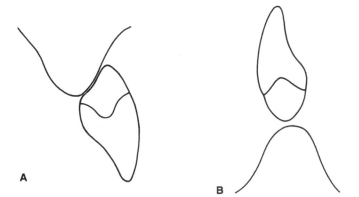

Fig. 18-52. Pontic tip design. **A,** Modified ridge lap-type pontic with slight concavity conforming to residual ridge. **B,** Hygienic-type pontic with ovate or bullet-shaped tip.

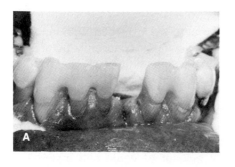

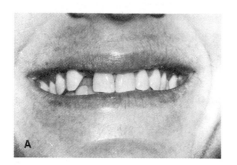

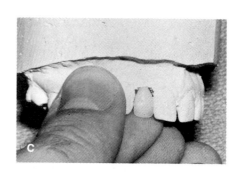

Fig. 18-53. Resin-bonded mandibular bridge-splint using natural tooth pontic. **A,** Anterior segment splinted with composite and abutment teeth isolated, roughened, and etched. **B,** Natural tooth pontic bonded in place.

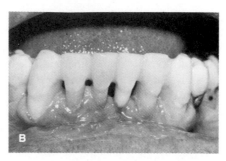

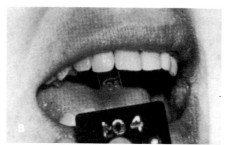

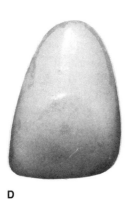

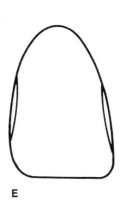

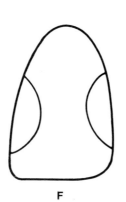

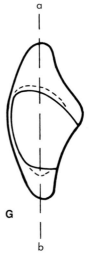

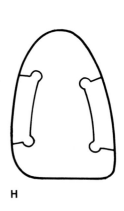

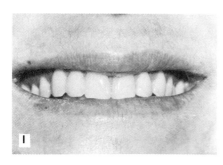

Fig. 18-54. Resin-bonded denture tooth pontic. **A,** Preoperative photograph showing missing maxillary lateral incisor. **B,** Shade and mould selection. **C,** Positioning pontic on working model while contouring. **D,** Contoured and polished pontic (lingual view). Outline form of Class III preparations: facial **(E),** lingual **(F),** and proximal **(G)** views. **H,** Cross section of denture tooth (longitudinal section) in plane *ab* as seen in **(G)** showing mechanical retention form incisally and gingivally as prepared with a No. ½ bur. **I,** Denture tooth pontic bonded in place with composite.

conventional bridge and may last for years in many circumstances. As with the natural tooth pontic, the major contraindications to this type of resin-bonded bridge are abutment teeth that have extensive caries, restorations, mobility, or a pontic area that is subjected to heavy occlusal forces.

In the illustrated example, the permanent maxillary right lateral incisor is missing, and the adjacent teeth are in favorable condition and position (Fig. 18-54, *A*). Further examination reveals an ideal situation for a conservative bridge that uses a ***denture tooth pontic.***

Technique. Although the entire procedure can be completed at chairside in one appointment, considerable time can be saved by an indirect technique. During the first appointment the shade (Fig. 18-54, *B)* and mold of the denture tooth are selected, and alginate impressions are made. In the laboratory, stone casts are poured and the ridge area is relieved slightly and marked with a soft lead pencil. As the pontic is trial positioned, the pencil markings will rub off onto its tip to facilitate contouring of this area (Fig. 18-54, *C*). Contouring is best accomplished with acrylic burs and a Burlew wheel in a straight handpiece. The tissue side of the pontic should be contoured to a modified ridge lap configuration that is convex mesiodistally and slightly concave faciolingually (Fig. 18-52, *A*). This type of design not only allows the pontic tip to adapt to the residual ridge, but also allows for effective cleaning with dental floss. After it is contoured, the pontic tip should be smoothed and highly polished with pumice and an acrylic polishing agent (Fig. 18-54, *D*).

Because composite does not normally bond to acrylic resin, provisions must be made to facilitate a strong connection between the pontic and the adjacent teeth. One provision may be completed in the laboratory by preparing large Class III conventional preparations in the pontic that will mechanically retain the composite material. The outline of the preparations must be large enough to provide adequate surface area of the composite restoration for bonding to the adjacent teeth (Fig. 18-54, *E* to *G*). An appropriate-sized round bur (No. 2 or No. 4) is used to cut each preparation to a depth of approximately 1.5 mm and extend the outline approximately 0.5 mm past the contact areas into the gingival, incisal, and facial embrasures. Even more extension should be made into the lingual embrasure to provide for bulk of composite material in the connector areas. The lingual extensions should not be connected, because this unnecessary step would unduly weaken the pontic. Mechanical undercuts are placed at the incisoaxial and gingivoaxial line angles with a No. ½ bur to mechanically lock the composite material (to be inserted later in the technique) in the acrylic resin pontic (Fig. 18-54, *G* and *H*).

During the next appointment the pontic is tried in place to confirm that the color and contours are correct. There should be approximately 0.5 mm of space between each proximal "contact" and the abutment tooth. The pontic is cleaned with acetone to remove dust and debris. Retention of the pontic by undercuts, as previously described, is augmented by a second provision, the conditioning of the proximal aspects of the pontic with two applications of ethyl acetate. A thin layer is applied in the Class III preparations and on the cavosurface areas and allowed to dry for 5 minutes. This process is repeated to ensure optimal bonding. The preparations are filled with the same light-cured composite material anticipated for bonding the pontic in place. The composite should be applied and cured in the retentive areas before the remainder of the cavity is filled. This step ensures complete polymerization. After the entire preparation is filled, it should be polymerized again with the light source. It is better to leave the contact areas slightly undercontoured in order for the pontic to fit easily between the abutment teeth. The pontic is set aside momentarily in a safe place.

Isolation of the abutment teeth should be accomplished with cotton rolls and retraction cords rather than with a rubber dam to better relate the pontic to the residual ridge area. Any caries or old restorations in the adjoining proximal areas of the abutment teeth should be removed at this time, and any indicated bases applied. The enamel on the proximal surfaces of the abutment teeth is roughened with a coarse flame-shaped diamond instrument. This step is followed by acid etching, rinsing, and drying. The resin bonding agent is applied, lightly blown with air, and cured. Cavity preparations, if present, are filled (again, with the same composite material). Care is taken not to overcontour the restoration(s).

The pontic is evaluated by positioning it temporarily in the edentulous space. If adjustments are made, the surfaces should be cleaned with acetone. Next, a small amount of composite is wiped onto the contact areas (mesial and distal) of the pontic, and the pontic is placed into the proper position between the abutment teeth. An explorer tip is helpful in teasing the material evenly around the contact area. Care must be taken to place the pontic so that it lightly touches the ridge but does not cause tissue blanching. The composite material used to position the pontic is polymerized. It is helpful to add and cure the additional composite in small increments to obtain the correct contour and minimize finishing procedures. The facial, incisal, and gingival embrasures should be defined with a flame-shaped finishing bur and polished with appropriate discs or points. The lingual aspect of the bridge is contoured with a round finishing bur without defining lingual embrasures because this could weaken the connectors. The retraction cords are removed from the gingival crevice. Articulating paper is used to mark the occlusion, and any offensive contacts are removed. The final restoration is shown in Fig. 18-54, *I*.

Pontic, either porcelain-fused-to-metal or all metal, with metal retainers

A stronger and more permanent type of acid-etched, resin-bonded bridge is possible by use of a cast metal framework.[36,42,51,63] In *anterior areas* where esthetics is a consideration, the design of the bridge includes a porcelain-fused-to-metal pontic with metal winged retainers extending mesially and distally for attachment to the proximal and lingual surfaces of the abutment teeth. In *posterior areas* where esthetics is not a critical factor, the bridge can have either a porcelain-fused-to-metal or an all metal pontic.

The technique is more complicated and time-consuming than the previously described methods, because it requires some initial tooth preparation, an impression, laboratory procedures, and a second appointment for etching and bonding. When compared with conventional bridges, resin-bonded bridges of this type offer several distinct advantages: (1) anesthesia is usually not required, (2) tooth structure is conserved (no dentin involvement), (3) gingival tissues are not irritated because margins usually are not placed subgingivally, (4) an esthetic result can be obtained more easily, and (5) the cost is less because not as much chair time is required and laboratory fees are lower.

Ideally this type of conservative bridge is used for short spans in the anterior or posterior areas with sound abutment teeth in good alignment. The most favorable occlusal relationship exists where little or no centric contact and only light functional contact are present. However, the teeth can be prepared and the bridge framework designed to withstand moderately heavy occlusal forces. Orthodontics may be required to improve tooth alignment. The bridge also can be extended to splint adjacent periodontally involved teeth. Crown lengthening procedures are sometimes indicated for teeth with short clinical crowns.

Although minimal, some preparation of enamel of the abutment teeth is mandatory in the retainer area of the bridge to (1) provide a definite path of insertion and/or seating, (2) enhance retention and resistance forms, (3) allow for the thickness of the metal retainers, and (4) provide physiological contour to the final restoration. The importance of tooth preparation design cannot be overemphasized. The success of these types of bridges depends on preparation design. The bridges must be independently retentive by design and cannot rely solely on the bonding resin for retention. Preparation design for these types of bridges is much like that for a cast three-quarter crown, only it is restricted to enamel.

The preparation for each abutment varies, depending on the individual tooth position and anatomy. Approximately the same amount of surface area should be covered on each abutment tooth. In some situations recontouring of the adjacent and opposing teeth may be indicated. The details of the preparations are described later.

Two primary types of retention designs have been used in the metal framework for the resin bonding: (1) *Rochette,*[63] *and (2) Maryland.*[51] A third "hybrid" design combining the features of both the Rochette and Maryland designs also has been suggested by Sockwell. Each type has advantages and disadvantages.

The Rochette type uses small perforations in the retainer sections for retention and is best suited for anterior bridges (Fig. 18-55, *A*).[63] Care must be exercised in placing the perforations to prevent weakening the framework. Perforations that are too large or too closely spaced will invite failure of the metal retainer by fracture. The perforations should be approximately 1.5 to 2 mm apart and have a maximum diameter of 1.5 mm on the tooth side. Each hole is countersunk so that the widest diameter is toward the outside of the retainer. When the bridge is bonded with a bonding medium, it is mechanically locked in place by microscopic undercuts in the etched enamel and the countersunk holes in the retainer (Fig. 18-56, *A*). Advantages of this design are as follows: (1) it is easy to see the retentive perforations in the metal; (2) if the bridge must be removed or replaced, the bonding medium can be cut away in the perforations to facilitate easy removal of the bridge; and (3) no metal etching is required. Disadvantages are as follows: (1) the perforations could weaken the retainers if improperly sized or spaced, (2) the exposed resin bonding medium is subject to wear, and (3) it is not possible to place perforations in proximal or rest areas.

A second type of cast metal framework, known as the Maryland bridge, is reported to have improved bonding strength (Fig. 18-55, *B*).[51,52] Instead of perforations, the tooth side of the metal framework is electrolytically or chemically etched, which produces microscopic undercuts (Fig. 18-55, *C*). The bridge is attached with a self-cured resin bonding medium that locks into the microscopic undercuts of both the etched retainer and the etched enamel (Fig. 18-56, *B*). It can be used for both anterior and posterior bridges. Although this design has been reported to be stronger, it is more technique-sensitive because the retainers may not be properly etched or may be contaminated before cementation. Because the retentive features cannot be seen with the unaided eye, the etched metal surfaces must be examined under a microscope to verify proper etching (minimum magnification).

Maryland bridges alternatively also can be fabricated with no electrolytical etching of the surface and chemi-

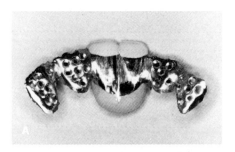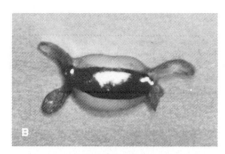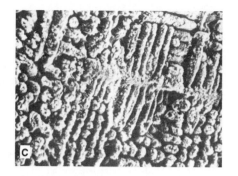

Fig. 18-55. Acid-etched, resin-bonded metal bridges. **A,** Rochette type. **B,** Maryland type. **C,** Scanning electron micrograph of etched-metal surface. (Courtesy Dr. John Sturdevant.)

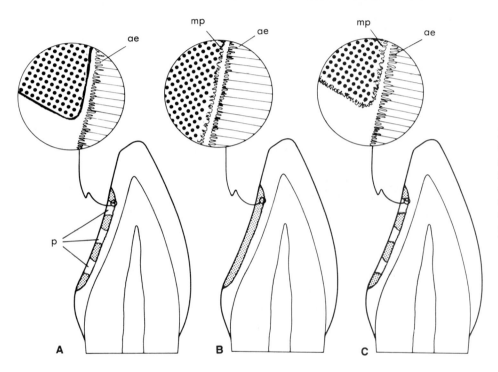

Fig. 18-56. Cross-sectional diagram of three types of resin-bonded bridges. **A,** In addition to acid etching prepared enamel surfaces *(ae),* the Rochette type uses small countersunk perforations *(p)* in retainer section. **B,** In Maryland type, tooth side of framework is etched to produce microscopic pores *(mp).* **C,** Hybrid type combines both types of retentive features.

cally bonded to the tooth either following a process called silicoating or with a 4-META–containing resin bonding medium.[27,28] Recall that resin materials containing 4-META are capable of strongly bonding to metal surfaces.[14,54] These types of Maryland bridges are referred to as ***adhesion bridges*** and differ only in the means of retention. The design of adhesion bridges is the same.

A hybrid design incorporating both perforations and etching of metal suggested by Sockwell is illustrated in Fig. 18-56, *C.* The perforated type (Rochette) can be etched on the tooth side of the metal retainer to provide microscopic undercuts for added retention. This is especially important in areas where perforations cannot be placed (such as the proximal surfaces). The etched-metal type (Maryland) often can be improved by adding perforations (design permitting) to provide both types of retention. If removal of the bridge is necessary, the resin bonding medium is easily removed from the countersunk holes before the bridge is tapped loose.

Perforations also can be added to Maryland type bridges that experience retention failures. This option is particularly valuable for salvaging bridges for which the metal type is unknown and the etching process therefore compromised.

Successes and failures have been observed with all three retentive designs of the metal framework. Because the procedures are technique-sensitive, it is emphasized that every step must be carefully followed.

Maxillary anterior bridge. In Fig. 18-57, *A,* a maxillary lateral incisor is congenitally missing, and the teeth on either side are sound. The occlusion is favorable, and there are no periodontal problems (Fig. 18-57, *B*). The patient has been wearing a removable partial denture that is undesirable. Radiographs and study casts are made to complete the diagnosis and to facilitate prepa-

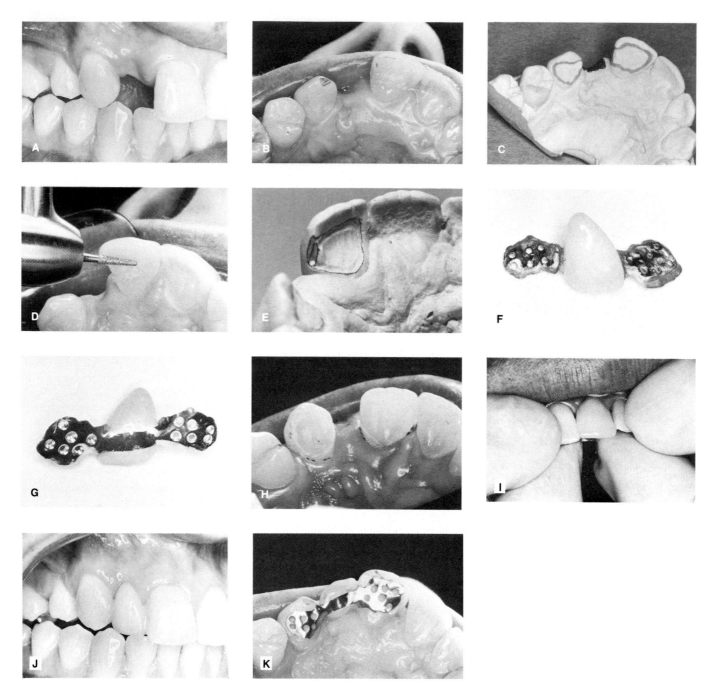

Fig. 18-57. Resin-bonded porcelain-fused-to-metal maxillary anterior bridge. **A,** Congenitally missing maxillary lateral incisor. **B,** Occlusion marked with articulating paper. **C,** Model with outline of preparations. **D,** Preparing lingual surface with diamond instrument. **E,** Working cast shows proximal groove prepared (a second groove is on mesial of canine) to establish path of insertion for prosthesis as well as provide positional stability and increase retention form. Completed Rochette-type bridge from facial view **(F)** and lingual view **(G). H,** Teeth isolated with gingival retraction cord and cotton rolls. Preparations are etched and ready for bonding. **I,** Holding bridge in place during polymerization. Bonded bridge: facial view **(J)** and lingual view **(K).**

ration design. The outline of the proposed preparation is penciled on the cast to cover as much enamel surface as possible for maximal bonding area, but with the following stipulations: (1) the lingual portions are extended neither subgingivally nor too far incisally, and (2) the proximal portions are not extended facially of the contact areas but enough to allow preparation of retention grooves (Fig. 18-57, *C* and *E*).

Before tooth preparation, clean the teeth, select the shade of the pontic, and mark the occlusion with articulating paper to evaluate centric contact(s) and functional movements. If adjustment or recontouring of the abutment teeth is indicated, it should be accomplished at this time. When a base metal alloy is used rather than high gold alloys for the bridge framework, less tooth structure is removed because the metal retainers can be made thinner. Base metal alloys have superior tensile strength.

Preparation. Make several depth cuts (0.3 to 0.5 mm) in the enamel with a small, round, coarse diamond instrument (1 to 1.5 mm in diameter). Join the depth cuts with the same instrument or a rounded-end diamond instrument (Fig. 18-57, *D*). A large surface area (outline form) is desirable to obtain maximum bonding and strength of the bridge. A *shallow* groove is cut *in the enamel* of each proximal portion of the preparations with a small, tapered cylindrical diamond instrument to establish a line of draw in the incisal direction.[36] This feature provides a definite path of insertion and positional stability for the prosthesis during trying-in and bonding. In addition, the retention of the bridge is improved because a shear force is required to unseat the bridge. Fig. 18-57, *E,* illustrates this groove on the working cast.

Take an elastomeric impression of the completed preparations and a bite registration. The patient continues to wear the partial denture as a temporary prosthesis. A small amount of self-curing acrylic resin is added to the mesial and distal portions of the removable partial denture tooth to maintain proximal relationships.

Laboratory phase. The impression, bite registration, patient information, and instructions are sent to the dental laboratory. A perforated retention design (Rochette) is specified in this instance, although the other types could be used. The bridge is fabricated in the laboratory (porcelain contoured but unglazed and perforations prepared in the retainers).

Try-in stage. During the initial try-in, the bridge is examined for proper color, contour, tissue compatibility, marginal fit, and occlusion. Adjustments are made, and the bridge is returned to the laboratory for corrections (if needed), glazing, and polishing of the metal framework. Fig. 18-57, *F* and *G,* shows the completed bridge from facial and lingual views.

Bonding steps. The steps in bonding require an ex-

acting coordination between the dentist and assistant. All of the equipment and materials needed for isolation, etching, and bonding must be available at the beginning of the appointment: prophylaxis angle handpiece, pumice slurry, a self-curing resin bonding medium kit with all accessories, plastic hand instrument, polyester strip, and cotton rolls.

The abutment teeth are cleaned with pumice slurry, rinsed, dried, and isolated with cotton rolls. If the cervical area of the retainer is subgingival, insert a retraction cord in the gingival crevice to displace the tissue and prevent seepage. The bridge should be carefully tried in place to review the path of insertion and verify the fit. On removal, place it in a convenient location near where the resin bonding medium will be mixed.

Artfully apply the etching gel or solution for 30 seconds to the prepared enamel and slightly past the margins. The acid must not be allowed to flow onto the unprepared proximal areas of the abutment or adjacent teeth. After rinsing the teeth, dry them of all visible moisture (Fig. 18-57, *H*). If a lightly frosted surface is not present, the etching procedure is repeated. It is emphasized that a *clean, dry* surface is absolutely essential. The slightest amount of saliva will contaminate the etched enamel and necessitate an additional 10 seconds of etching, followed by rinsing and drying. A rubber dam is preferred for isolation; however, cotton rolls and gingival retraction cord will provide adequate isolation in selected areas where salivary flow can be controlled.

The manufacturer's instructions for the bonding procedure should be read and followed. Usually equal parts of the resin bonding medium (base and catalyst) are placed on one mixing pad, and equal parts of the bonding agent (base and catalyst) are placed on another mixing pad. The operator mixes the bonding agent with a small foam sponge or brush and quickly paints a thin layer on the tooth side of the bridge and then onto the etched enamel. While the operator uses the air syringe to blow the excess bonding agent off the bridge and then the enamel, the assistant mixes the resin bonding medium and places a thin layer on the tooth side of the bridge retainers. The bridge is positioned on the abutment teeth and held in place with a polyester strip over the lingual surface. The retainers are seated and held firmly in place with the index fingers positioned on the strip over the lingual retainers, and the thumbs are held on the facial aspect of the abutment teeth to equalize the pressure (Fig. 18-57, *I*). The amount of resin bonding medium at the facial and gingival embrasures is quickly inspected. Sometimes the assistant may need to add more resin bonding medium or remove excess unpolymerized resin with an explorer or plastic instrument. Priority is given to the gingival embrasure, since later correction is more difficult in this area.

Finishing procedure. After the resin bonding medium has hardened, remove the polyester strip and inspect the lingual area. If voids are present, more resin is mixed and added. Additions will bond to the previously placed resin bonding medium without additional surface treatment. Remove excess resin along the lingual margins with a discoid-cleoid hand instrument, and evaluate the occlusion and adjust if necessary. Contouring and polishing are accomplished in the usual manner with carbide finishing burs, hand instruments, and discs. The completed Rochette-type bridge is shown as viewed from the facial and lingual aspects in Fig. 18-57, *J* and *K*. (Also see Plate 18-4, *A* and *B*.) The patient is instructed in how to use a floss threader and dental floss to clean under the pontic and around the abutment teeth. Another example of an anterior resin-bonded bridge replacing both central incisors is seen in Plate 18-4, *C* and *D*.

Mandibular anterior splint-and-bridge combination. An indication for a conservative bridge that incorporates a splint design of the porcelain-fused-to-metal framework is illustrated in Fig. 18-58. The mandibular central incisors were extracted because of advanced peri-

odontal disease. The weak lateral incisors are stabilized by including the canines in a splint-bridge design. These teeth are caries-free and have no restorations. An ill-fitting removable partial denture was uncomfortable and did not support the adjacent teeth (Fig. 18-58, *A* and *B*).

The preparations for the splint-and-bridge combination consist of removing approximately 0.3 mm of enamel on the lingual aspect of the lateral incisors and canines as outlined on the laboratory cast as well as preparing proximal retention grooves (Fig. 18-58, *C*). The perforated design of the winged retainers is of the Rochette type for ease of replacement or repair (Fig. 18-58, *D* and *E*). The splint-bridge is bonded by the method previously described (Fig. 18-58, *F* and *G*). Note that the gingival aspect of the pontic is free of tissue contact and has sufficient space for cleaning.

Mandibular posterior bridge with metal-porcelain pontic. In Fig. 18-59, *A,* a missing mandibular first molar needs to be replaced to maintain proper occlusal contacts and to preserve the integrity of the arch. A clinical examination with radiographs confirms that the

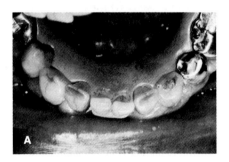
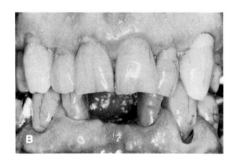
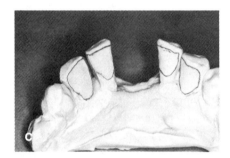

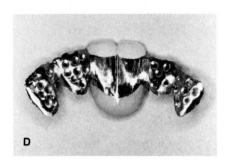
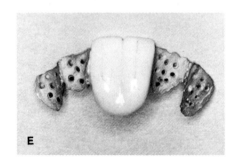
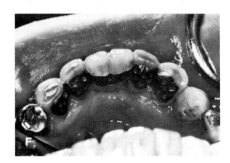

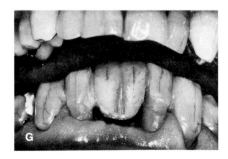

Fig. 18-58. Resin-bonded mandibular anterior porcelain-fused-to-metal bridge and splint. **A,** Patient wearing ill-fitting removable acrylic partial denture. **B,** Edentulous space resulting from missing mandibular central incisors. **C,** Laboratory model with preparations outlined. **D,** Lingual view of completed prosthesis (Rochette type with multiple countersunk perforations). **E,** Facial view of completed prosthesis. **F,** Lingual view of prosthesis bonded in place with composite resin. Anterior segment is stabilized by splinting effect of bridge retainers. **G,** Facial view of porcelain-fused-to-metal pontics bonded in place.

abutment teeth are in good alignment and are sound and that the occlusion is favorable. Conservative amalgam restorations have been inserted to correct occlusal fissures on the abutment teeth. Impressions and a bite registration are made for study casts. An acid-etched, resin-bonded cast metal bridge (Maryland type) including a porcelain pontic with metal occlusal centric stops will provide for optimal occlusal wear resistance while providing an acceptable esthetic result.

Use a surveyor to determine the most favorable path of draw, and mark the outline of the retainer area with a pencil (Fig. 18-59, *B*). The occlusal rest areas will provide rigidity and resistance form to vertical forces, while the extensions on the facial and lingual surfaces will provide a "wraparound" design for added retention and resistance against lateral forces. In this example the teeth have sufficient crown length to avoid subgingival margination.

Preparation. Prophylaxis, shade selection, and any needed occlusal adjustment are accomplished before the preparations are begun. As with the anterior teeth, some preparation is necessary to provide "draw," to increase retention and resistance forms, and to provide bulk to the retainers for strength without overcontouring. Preparation is minimal and involves only the enamel. Using the surveyed penciled cast as a reference, prepare the teeth with a coarse, rounded-end cylindrical diamond instrument (Fig. 18-59, *C*). Prepare the occlusal rests

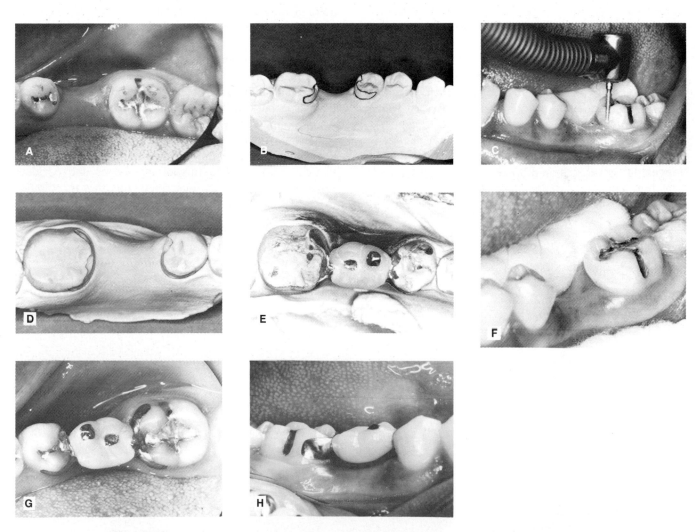

Fig. 18-59. Conservative mandibular posterior bridge with a combination metal and porcelain pontic. **A,** Missing mandibular first molar with occlusion identified by marks from articulating paper. **B,** Study model surveyed and outlines of the preparation marked with pencil. **C,** Preparation of axial surfaces with coarse, cylindrical diamond instrument. **D,** Laboratory model with margins outlined. **E,** Completed bridge on cast ready for try-in. Note centric contacts on metal to minimize wear of opposing teeth. **F,** Teeth cleaned, isolated, and etched. **G,** Occlusal view of bonded bridge. **H,** Facial view of bonded bridge.

with a round diamond instrument. Make an elastomeric impression and a bite registration for laboratory use.

Laboratory phase. Include a sketch of the bridge design with the laboratory instructions. The nonperforated, etched metal design (Maryland) is specified in this instance because the "wings" will be very thin and other areas of the bridge will be inaccessible for placing perforations. It is helpful to the technician if the margins of the preparation are marked with an indelible pencil (Fig. 18-59, *D*). Before any glazing of porcelain or polishing of framework or etching of metal, the bridge is returned to the dentist for the try-in stage (Fig. 18-59, *E*).

Try-in stage. Seat the bridge and evaluate for proper fit, occlusion, and color matching. After adjustments are made, the bridge is returned to the laboratory for corrections, final glazing, polishing of the metal framework, and etching procedures. The etched metal must be examined under a microscope to ensure that proper etching of the metal has occurred.

Bonding steps. Care must be exercised in handling the bridge, *since the etched area can be easily contaminated.* The bridge should not be tried in place (once again) until the teeth are isolated and the enamel has been etched (Fig. 18-59, *F*). Rubber dam isolation is preferred when bonding mandibular resin-bonded bridges. However, cotton roll isolation can be used with retraction cords if a rubber dam cannot be placed for whatever reason. Being careful not to touch or contam-

inate the etched metal, try-in the bridge to verify fit and path of draw. Everything must be "ready to go" as the manufacturer's instructions are followed for mixing and applying the bonding materials to the teeth and the bridge. Again, the preparations must be clean and dry to ensure proper bonding. Once the bridge is in place, a polyester strip is placed over the pontic, and finger pressure is used to secure the bridge until polymerization is complete. After removal of the excess resin, the occlusion is evaluated. The occlusal and facial views are esthetic with only the centric contacts in metal (Fig. 18-59, *G* and *H*). Another example of a posterior resin-bonded Maryland type bridge is seen in Plate 18-4, *E* and *F*.

Maxillary bridge with porcelain-fused-to-metal pontic. Fig. 18-60, *A*, illustrates a space resulting from the extraction of a maxillary second premolar. As with the mandibular bridge, resistance to lateral forces must be provided by the design of the preparations and resulting prosthesis. However, because esthetics is more critical in the maxillary arch, the wraparound design used in the mandibular arch cannot be employed to as great an extent, especially in the area adjacent to the facial aspect of the pontic. Therefore proximal grooves are prepared (in enamel) in the same occlusogingival orientation as the path of draw to provide additional resistance form to lateral forces. The lingual extensions and occlusal rests are prepared as described for the mandibular bridge (Fig. 18-60, *B* and *C*). For retention, perfora-

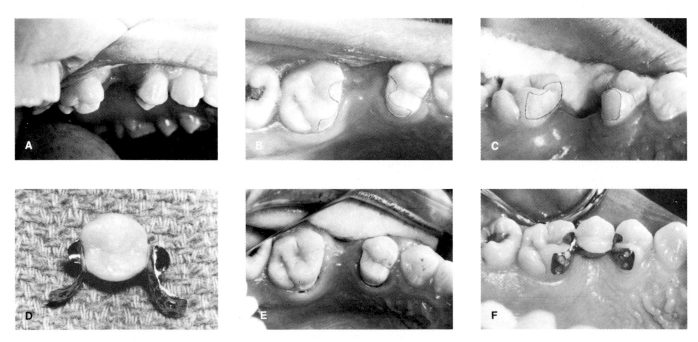

Fig. 18-60. Maxillary posterior resin-bonded bridge with porcelain-fused-to-metal pontic. **A,** Preoperative photograph of missing maxillary second premolar. Outlined final cavity preparations: occlusal **(B)** and lingual **(C)** views. **D,** Completed prosthesis. **E,** Etched preparations isolated and ready for bonding. **F,** Porcelain-fused-to-metal bridge bonded in place.

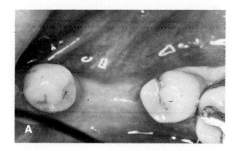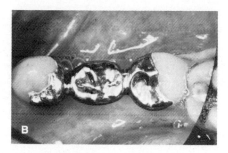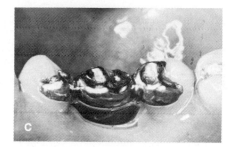

Fig. 18-61. Resin-bonded mandibular posterior all-metal bridge. **A,** Edentulous space resulting from loss of first molar and distal migration of second premolar. All-metal bridge with electrolytically etched retainers (Maryland type) bonded to place: occlusal view (**B**) and lingual view (**C**). Note nontissue-contacting hygienic-type pontic. (Courtesy Dr. William Sulik.)

tions in the retainer (Rochette design) are used in addition to acid etching the preparations. Perforations are placed in the accessible lingual extensions. This design aids in removing the bridge if replacement becomes necessary (Fig. 18-60, *D*). The etched preparations, which are ready for bonding, are illustrated in Fig. 18-60, *E*. The completed bonded bridge is illustrated in Fig. 18-60, *F*.

Mandibular posterior bridge with metal pontic. Fig. 18-61, *A*, illustrates a space between the mandibular premolars resulting from extraction of the permanent first molar at an early age and subsequent distal migration of the second premolar. Because esthetics was not a factor, an all-metal bridge (Maryland type) with a hygienically designed pontic was used. The steps are identical to those previously described for the mandibular posterior bridge with a porcelain-fused-to-metal pontic. The bridge is illustrated after several years of service (Fig. 18-61, *B* and *C*).

All-porcelain pontic

Improvements in dental porcelains along with the capacity to etch and bond strongly to porcelain surfaces have made all-porcelain pontics a viable alternative to pontics with metal "winged" retainers (Maryland and Rochette bridges).[56] Although all-porcelain pontics are not as strong as pontics with metal retainers, far superior esthetic results can be achieved because no metal substructure or framework is present. Moreover, all-porcelain pontics often can be used when tooth anatomy precludes or restricts the preparation and placement of a metal "winged" pontic. For example, long pointed canines with proximal surfaces exhibiting little occlusogingival height often lack adequate areas for the placement of retention grooves. Anterior teeth that are notably thin faciolingually also are not good candidates for metal resin-bonded bridge retainers, and often are esthetic failures due to metal showing through the tooth. In both instances, custom fabricated, etched porcelain

pontics frequently can provide an esthetic, functional alternative.

All-porcelain pontics are particularly indicated for placement in adolescents and young adults, in whom virgin, unrestored teeth are often encountered. However, because of their limited strength, all-porcelain pontics should be considered *provisional in nature,* similar to the natural tooth pontic and the acrylic denture tooth pontic.

Similar to the natural tooth and denture tooth pontics, certain prerequisites must exist to ensure a successful result. First, the abutment teeth must be in reasonably good condition with *proximal enamel surfaces* that are intact or contain very small composite restorations. Second, the abutment teeth should be stable with little mobility present. If the abutment teeth are mobile, it is frequently necessary to secure them as well by splinting with composite to adjacent teeth prior to placement of the bonded pontic (see Acid-etched, Resin-bonded Splints). Third, the pontic must not be placed in a position that will subject it to heavy centric or functional occlusal contacts. Because of these occlusion concerns, canines and posterior teeth are not usually good candidates for these types of resin-bonded bridges.

Technique. Fig. 18-62, *A* and *B*, illustrates a typical case of congenitally missing lateral incisors where tooth contours contraindicated the use of resin-retained bridges with metal retainers. The central incisors are very translucent and the mesial contours of the canines are deficient (Fig. 18-62, *C* and *E*). After assessing centric and functional occlusion, it was determined that all-porcelain pontics could be placed without subjecting them to heavy occlusal forces. At the first appointment, the involved abutments are cleaned with flour of pumice as previously described, and an accurate shade selection is made, noting any desired color gradients or characterizations.

No preparation of the teeth is recommended unless the proximal surfaces of the abutment teeth adjacent to

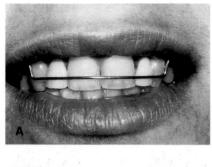

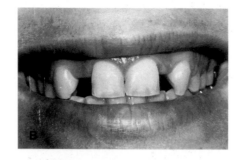

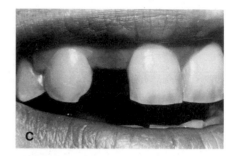

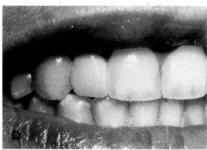

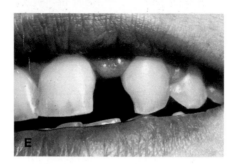

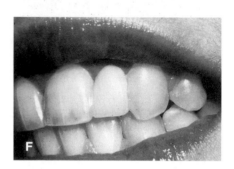

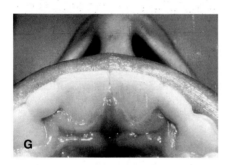

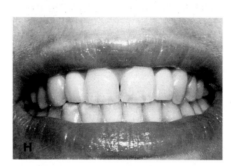

Fig. 18-62. All-porcelain pontics. **A** and **B,** Patient with congenitally missing lateral incisors. **C** and **D,** Right side before and after treatment. **E** and **F,** Left side before and after placement of all-porcelain pontic. **G,** Lingual view of completed bridges. **H,** Facial view of all-porcelain pontics.

the edentulous space are markedly convex. In such cases, slight flattening of the proximal surfaces with a diamond instrument will facilitate closer adaptation of the pontic to the abutment teeth, and thereby increase strength of the connectors. Otherwise, no retentive features are recommended for preparation in the abutment teeth, and thus the connector areas will be entirely made of composite.

Bridge connectors composed of porcelain are subject to eventual fatigue fracture, after which repair is made more difficult. Studies show in particular that "veneer bridges" (all-porcelain pontics retained by adjacent etched porcelain veneers) are the weakest design of all and should be avoided.[56] These types of bridges not only provide little bond strength to the pontic, but also needlessly cover adjacent healthy facial tooth surfaces. All-porcelain pontics whose connector areas consist only of the composite used for bonding to the abutment teeth are much like extracted natural tooth pontics in this regard. This design feature allows for easy repair and replacement of the composite connector should a fracture in this area be encountered.

It should be noted that if high-strength ceramics are

developed which are highly resistant to crack propagation and cohesive fracture, retentive features prepared in the adjacent abutment teeth may be desired. These features, *prepared in enamel,* would consist of proximal grooves or boxes, depending on the faciolingual dimension of the proximal surfaces. In the absence of totally fracture-resistant ceramics, all-porcelain pontics are best placed with composite connectors for ease of repair and replacement.

An elastomeric impression is made from which a working cast is generated. A modified ridge lap pontic tip design as previously described (see Fig. 18-52, *A*) is recommended. An occlusal bite registration should be made and forwarded to the laboratory so that the occlusal relationship can be considered during fabrication of the all-porcelain pontic. Proximal surfaces of the pontics are etched with hydrofluoric acid. Note that *the area etched must include all areas anticipated for bonding to the composite bonding medium.* The etched proximal surfaces should extend just beyond the lingual line angles so that additional composite can be placed in the lingual embrasure areas for additional connector strength.

At the next appointment, the teeth are isolated with cotton rolls. A 2 × 2 inch cotton gauze is placed across the back of the patient's mouth to act as a protective shield should the pontic be inadvertently dropped. A rubber dam is not recommended for this procedure, since it precludes accurate assessment of the adaptation of the pontic tip to the residual ridge.

Before the teeth dehydrate, each pontic is trial-positioned in the edentulous space to assess the shade and relationship of the pontic tip to the residual ridge. The pontic tip should contact the residual ridge passively with no blanching of the underlying tissue evident. Spaces of approximately 0.3 to 0.5 mm should exist between the pontic and the abutment teeth, because stronger connectors are provided by the additional bulk of composite material. Care must be taken not to allow contamination of the etched pontic from saliva to occur during the try-in phase. If saliva contamination occurs, the etched proximal surfaces of the pontic must be cleaned thoroughly with alcohol and dried. Following try-in, all etched proximal surfaces of the porcelain pontics are primed with a suitable *silane coupling agent* (see manufacturer's instructions for specific technique). The pontics are now ready for bonding.

Next, the involved proximal enamel surfaces of the abutment teeth are roughened with a coarse, flame-shaped diamond instrument. Thereafter, the operator should acid etch, rinse, and dry all prepared (roughened) enamel surfaces. Care must be taken to maintain clean, dry, uncontaminated etched surfaces until the pontic is positioned and bonded. The abutment teeth are now ready for bonding.

A light-cured composite is preferred for bonding all-porcelain pontics, because the extended working time allows the operator to initially contour the connectors before polymerization. First, apply the bonding agent to the etched surfaces of the porcelain pontic and the abutment teeth, and lightly blow with air to remove the excess. A 20-second application of light from the light curing unit is used to polymerize the bonding agent on each etched surface.

A small amount of composite material is placed on the proximal contact areas of the natural tooth pontic, and the pontic is carefully inserted into the proper position in the edentulous space. A stent, or index, made from bite registration material or fast-setting plaster can be used to position the pontic, if desired. However, positioning by hand is recommended so that optimal gingival pressure can be maintained for best tissue adaptation. Tease and shape the excess composite extruding from the connector areas around the contact areas with an explorer tip or small plugger end of a composite instrument. After final verification that the pontic position is correct, polymerize the composite with light for a minimum of 40 to 60 seconds each from facial and lingual directions for a total of 80 to 120 seconds.

Next, additional composite is applied in the proximal areas (more material is added on the lingual surface than on the facial surface), contoured, and polymerized. Adequate gingival embrasures must be maintained to facilitate flossing and ensure good gingival health. After sufficient material has been added and polymerized, shape and smooth the embrasure areas with carbide finishing burs and polishing discs. Facial embrasures are defined for esthetics, but lingual embrasures are closed with composite to strengthen the connectors (Fig. 18-62, *D, F,* and *G*). Evaluate the occlusion centric contacts and functional movements. Heavy contacts on the pontic or the connector areas must be adjusted. The finished bridges immediately after bonding are illustrated in Fig. 18-62, *D,* and *F* to *H.* (See also Plate 18-4, *G* and *H.*)

As with all resin-bonded bridges, patients must be advised to avoid biting hard foods or objects to reduce the potential for dislodgement. Also, as noted earlier, *the patient must be advised as part of informed consent that although the chances are remote, the potential for dislodgement exists with the possibility of swallowing or aspirating the pontic.* This possibility exists for all resin-bonded bridges and patients must be made aware of this hazard even though the risk is minimal.

ACKNOWLEDGMENT

Portions of the section on artistic elements were reprinted with permission from Heymann HO: The artistry of conservative esthetic dentistry, *J Am Dent Assoc* (special issue) 115(12E):14-23, 1987.

REFERENCES

1. Aker DA, Aker JR, Sorenson SE: Effect of methods of tooth enamel preparation on the retentive strength of acid-etch composite resins, *J Am Dent Assoc* 99(2):185, 1979.
2. Albers HF: *Tooth colored restorations,* Santa Rosa, Calif, 1985, Alto Books.
3. Andreasen JO: The effect of pulp extirpation or root canal treatment on periodontal healing after replantation of permanent incisors in monkeys, *J Endod* 7:245, 1981.
4. Antrim DO, Ostrowski JS: A functional splint for traumatized teeth, *J Endod* 8(7):328, 1982.
5. Ash MM: *Wheeler's dental anatomy, physiology, and occlusion,* Philadelphia, 1984, WB Saunders.
6. Banker CA, Berlocher WC, Mueller BH: Alternative methods for the management of persistent maxillary central diastemas, *Gen Dent* 20:136-142, 1982.
7. Bayne SC, Taylor DF, Zardiackas LD: *Biomaterials science,* Chapel Hill, NC, 1991, Brightstar.
8. Berge M: Properties of prosthetic resin-veneer materials processed in commercial laboratories, *Dent Mater* 5:77, 1989.
9. Bevelander G, Cohlan SQ, Rolle GK: The effect of the administration of tetracycline on the development of teeth, *J Dent Res* 40:1020-1024, 1961.
10. Black JB: Esthetic restoration of tetracycline-stained teeth, *J Am Dent Assoc* 104:846-852, 1982.

11. Borissavlievitch M: *The golden number,* London, 1964, Alec Tiranti.

12. Calamia JR: Etched porcelain facial veneers: a new treatment modality based on scientific and clinical evidence, *NY J Dent* 53:255-259, 1983.

13. Christensen GJ: Veneering of teeth: state of the art, *Dent Clin North Am* 29:373-391, 1985.

14. Cooley RL, Burger KM, Chain MC: Evaluation of a 4-META adhesive cement, *J Esthet Dent* 3(1):7-10, 1991.

15. Croll TP: Enamel microabrasion for removal of superficial dysmineralization and decalcification defects, *J Am Dent Assoc* 120:411-415, 1990.

16. Croll TP, Cavanaugh RR: Enamel color modification by controlled hydrochloric acid-pumice abrasion: (1) technique and examples, *Quintessence Int* 17:81-87, 1986.

17. Dawson PE: *Evaluation, diagnosis, and treatment of occlusal problems,* St Louis, 1974, Mosby.

18. Feinman RA, Goldstein RE, Garber DA: *Bleaching teeth,* Chicago, 1987, Quintessence Books.

19. Flynn M: Black teeth: a primitive method of caries prevention in southeast Asia, *J Am Dent Assoc* 95(1):96, 1977.

20. Friedman MJ: The enamel ceramic alternative: porcelain veneers vs metal ceramic crowns, *CDA Journal* 20(8):27-32, 1992.

21. Garber DA, Goldstein RE, Feinman RA: Porcelain laminate veneers, Chicago, 1988, Quintessence Publishing.

22. Goldman HM, Cohen WD, editors: *Periodontal therapy,* ed 6, St Louis, 1980, Mosby.

23. Goldstein RE: *Esthetics in dentistry,* Philadelphia, 1976, JB Lippincott.

24. Gomes BC et al: Importance of combined periodontal and acid etch composite treatment in restoration of anterior teeth and periodontal health, *J Am Dent Assoc* 99(5):834, 1979.

25. Graber TM: *Orthodontics principles and practice,* ed 3, Philadelphia, 1972, WB Saunders.

26. Hall DA: Should etching be performed as a part of a vital bleaching technique? *Quintessence Int* 22:679-686, 1991.

27. Hamada T, Shigeto N, Yanagihara T: A decade of progress for the adhesive fixed partial denture, *J Prosthet Dent* 54(1):24-29, 1985.

28. Hansson O: The Silicoater technique for resin-bonded prostheses: clinical and laboratory procedures, *Quintessence Int* 20(2):85-99, 1989.

29. Harrington GW, Natkin E: External resorption associated with bleaching of pulpless teeth, *J Endod* 5(11):344-348, 1979.

30. Haywood VB: History, safety, and effectiveness of current bleaching techniques and applications of the nightguard vital bleaching technique, *Quintessence Int* 23:471-488, 1992.

31. Haywood VB: Nightguard vital bleaching: a history and products update: part 1, *Esthetic Dentistry Update* 2(4):63-66, 1991.

32. Haywood VB, Heymann HO: Nightguard vital bleaching: how safe is it? *Quintessence Int* 22:515-523, 1991.

33. Haywood VB, Heymann HO: Nightguard vital bleaching, *Quintessence Int* 20:173-176, 1989.

34. Haywood VB et al: Polishing porcelain veneers: an SEM and specular reflectance analysis, *Dent Mater* 4:116-121, 1988.

35. Heymann HO: Indirect composite resin veneers: clinical technique and two-year observations, *Quintessence Int* 18(2):111-118, 1987.

36. Heymann HO: Resin-retained bridges: the porcelain-fused-to-metal 'winged' pontic, *Gen Dent* 32(3):203-208, 1984.

37. Heymann HO: Resin-retained bridges: the acrylic denture-tooth pontic, *Gen Dent* 32(2):113-116, 1984.

38. Heymann HO: Resin-retained bridges: the natural-tooth pontic, *Gen Dent* 31(6):479-482, 1983.

39. Heymann HO, Hershey HG: Use of composite resin for restorative and orthodontic correction of anterior interdental spacing, *J Prosthet Dent* 53(6):766-771, 1985.

40. Holmstrup G, Palm AM, Lambjerg-Hansen H: Bleaching of discolored root-filled teeth, *Endod Dent Traumatol* 4:197-201, 1988.

41. Horn H: Porcelain laminate veneers bonded to etch enamel, *Dent Clin North Am* 27:671-684, 1983.

42. Howe DF, Denehy GE: Anterior fixed partial dentures utilizing the acid-etch technique and a cast metal framework, *J Prosthet Dent* 37(1):28, 1977.

43. Iacono JV, Ceen R: An acid etch splint for periodontally involved teeth, *N Y State Dent J* 48(5):142, 1978.

44. Ibsen RL: Fixed prosthesis with a natural crown pontic using an adhesive composite, *J South Calif State Dent Assoc* 41:100, 1973.

45. Jordan RE, Suzuki M, Senda A: Clinical evaluation of porcelain laminate veneers: a four-year recall report, *J Esthet Dent* 1(4):126-132, 1989.

46. Jordan RE et al: Temporary fixed partial dentures fabricated by means of the acid-etch resin technique: a report of 86 cases followed for up to 3 years, *J Am Dent Assoc* 96:994, 1978.

47. Lado EA: Bleaching of endodontically treated teeth: an update on cervical resorption, *Gen Dent* 36:500-501, 1988.

48. Lado EA, Stanley HR, Weisman MI: Cervical resorption in bleached teeth, *Oral Surg* 55:78-80, 1983.

49. Lang SA, Starr CB: Castable glass ceramics for veneer restorations, *J Prosthet Dent* 67(5):590-594, 1992.

50. Levin EI: Dental esthetics and the golden proportion, *J Prosthet Dent* 40(3):244-252, 1978.

51. Livaditis G: Cast metal resin-bonded retainers for posterior tooth, *J Am Dent Assoc* 101:926, 1980.

52. Livaditis G, Thompson VP: Etched castings: an improved retentive mechanism for resin-bonded retainers, *J Prosthet Dent* 47(1):52, 1982.

53. Madison S, Walton R: Cervical root resorption following bleaching of endodontically treated teeth, *J Endod* 16:570-574, 1990.

54. Matsumura H, Nakabayashi N: Adhesive 4-META/MMA-TBB opaque resin with poly(methyl methacrylate)-coated titanium dioxide, *J Dent Res* 67(1):29-32, 1988.

55. McCloskey RJ: A technique for removal of fluorosis stains, *J Am Dent Assoc* 109:63-64, 1984.

56. Moore DL et al: Retentive strength of anterior etched porcelain bridges attached with composite resin: an in vitro comparison of attachment techniques, *Quintessence Int* 20(9):629-636, 1989.

57. Muia PJ: *The four dimensional tooth color system,* Chicago, 1982, Quintessence Books.

58. Nash RW: *Composite resin—indirect technique restorations*. In Dale B, Aschheim K: *Esthetic dentistry*, Philadelphia, 1993, Lea & Febiger.
59. Neaverth EJ, Goerig AC: Technique and rationale for splinting, *J Am Dent Assoc* 100(1):56, 1980.
60. O'Riorden MW et al: Treatment of avulsed permanent teeth: an update, *J Am Dent Assoc* 105(6):1028, 1982.
61. Pollack BF, Blitzer MH: Esthetic veneering: materials and techniques, *Gen Dent* 31:483-488, 1983.
62. Pulver F: Treatment of trauma to the young permanent dentition, *Dent Clin North Am* 26(3):525, 1982.
63. Rochette AL: Attachment of a splint to enamel of lower anterior teeth, *J Prosthet Dent* 30(4):418, 1973.
64. Rucker LM et al: Porcelain and resin veneers clinically evaluated: 2-year results, *J Am Dent Assoc* 121:594-596, 1990.
65. Sockwell CL: Clinical evaluation of anterior restorative materials, *Dent Clin North Am* 20:403, 1976.
66. Sorensen JA, Martinoff JT: Intracoronal reinforcement and coronal coverage: a study of endodontically treated teeth, *J Prosthet Dent* 51(4):780-784, 1984.
67. Sproull RC: *Understanding color*. In Goldstein RE, *Esthetics in dentistry*, Philadelphia, 1976, JB Lippincott Co.
68. Stangel I, Nathanson D, Hsu CS: Shear strength of the composite bond to etched porcelain, *J Dent Res* 66:1460-1465, 1987.
69. Swift EJ et al: Treatment of composite surfaces for indirect bonding, *Dent Mater* 8:193-196, 1992.
70. Titley KC, Torneck CD, Ruse ND: The effect of *carbamide-peroxide* gel on the shear bond strength of a microfil resin to bovine enamel, *J Dent Res* 71(1):20-24, 1992.
71. Urbanska DK, Mumford MJ: Autogenous transplantation of non-root filled maxillary canines: a long-term follow-up, *Int Endodont J* 13(3):156, 1980.
72. Zachrisson BU: Clinical experience with direct-bonded orthodontic retainers, *Am J Orthod* 71:440, 1977.

CHAPTER 19

Cast metal restorations for Class II cavity preparations

John R. Sturdevant

Clifford M. Sturdevant

The *cast metal restoration* is extremely versatile and is especially applicable to Class II preparations. To be satisfactory, the restoration procedure requires meticulous care both in cavity preparation and in proper manipulation of dental materials. Also, there must be a devotion to perfection on the part of the dentist and the laboratory technician. The high degree of satisfaction and service derived from a properly made cast metal restoration is a reward for the painstaking application that is required.

DEFINITIONS OF INLAY AND ONLAY

The Class II *inlay* involves the occlusal and proximal surface(s) of a posterior tooth and may cap one or more but not all of the cusps. The Class II *onlay* involves the proximal surface(s) of a posterior tooth and caps all of the cusps.

The procedure requires two appointments: The first for preparing the tooth and making an impression, and the second for delivering the restoration to the patient. The fabrication process is often referred to as an *indirect procedure,* since the casting is made on a replica of the prepared tooth in a dental laboratory.

INDICATIONS AND CONTRAINDICATIONS

The cast metal inlay is selected over an amalgam restoration when the *higher strength* of a casting alloy is needed or when the *superior control of contours* and contacts that the indirect procedure provides is desired. The cast metal onlay is the treatment of choice for the restoration of a tooth that has been greatly weakened by caries or by large, failing restoration(s) but the facial and lingual tooth surfaces are relatively unaffected by disease or injury. For such weakened teeth the superior physical properties of a casting alloy are desirable to withstand occlusal loads placed on the restoration; also, the onlay can be *designed to distribute occlusal loads* over the tooth in a manner that decreases the chance of tooth fracture in the future. *Moreover, conserving intact facial and lingual enamel (or cementum) is conducive to maintaining the health of contiguous soft tissues.* Additional indications and contraindications follow:

1. *Biocompatibility of the alloy.* The American Dental Association Specification No. 5 for Inlay Casting Golds was adopted in 1931 and established a minimum total gold plus platinum metals content of 75 weight percent.[29] Such traditional high-gold alloys are quite unreactive in the oral environment, and are some of the most biocompatible materials available to the restorative dentist.

   The preponderance of all cast restorations were made of high-gold alloys until the government stopped regulating the price of gold in 1968. Since then increases in the cost of gold and improvements in other materials and techniques have encouraged the use of alternative materials. Today over 80% of commercial U.S. dental casting alloys contain less than 75% of noble metals.[15] Similar changes have occurred in other countries as well.[3,6]

   At the present time there are *five distinct groups of alloys* in use for cast restorations: the traditional high-gold alloys; low-gold alloys; palladium-silver alloys; base metal alloys; and most recently, modified brasses or bronzes. Each of the alternatives to high-gold alloys has required some modification of technique or acceptance of reduced performance, most commonly in regard

to decreased tarnish resistance and decreased burnishability. *In general, the low-gold alloys have required fewer modifications in technique and auxiliary materials than the other alternative groups, and have excellent records in regard to clinical performance.*[26]

2. *Extent of proximal caries on the tooth.* When proximal surface caries is extensive, favorable consideration should be given to the cast inlay or onlay. The indirect procedure used to develop the cast restoration allows more control of contours and contacts (both proximal and occlusal). When the gingival margin is extremely subgingival and near the gingival attachment, as is often the case with extensive caries, the indirect cast metal restoration offers the finest possibilities for proper restoration at this difficult margin.

3. *Extent of facial and lingual caries or previous restorations.* Facial and lingual (especially lingual) smooth surface caries is indicative of a high caries activity that should be brought under control before expensive cast metal restorations are fabricated. If caries or previous restorations are present on the facial and lingual surfaces in addition to the occlusal and proximal surfaces, full crown restorations are usually indicated to restore all the lesions with one casting.

4. *Root canal fillings.* A molar or premolar with a root canal filling can be restored with a cast metal onlay providing the onlay has been thoughtfully designed to strengthen the remaining tooth (see Root Canal Filled Teeth).

5. *Fracture lines.* Fracture lines in enamel and dentin, especially in teeth having extensive restorations, should be recognized as cleavage planes for possible future fracture of the tooth. Restoring these teeth with a restoration that braces the tooth against fracture injury is a highly valued preventive service. Such restorations are cast onlays (with skirting) and crowns.

6. *Dental rehabilitation with cast metal alloys.* When cast metal restorations have been used to rehabilitate adjacent or opposing teeth, the continued application of the same material is favored to eliminate electrical and corrosive activity that sometimes occurs between dissimilar metals in the mouth, particularly when they contact each other.

7. *Diastema closure, occlusal plane correction.* Often the cast inlay or onlay is indicated when additional extension of the mesiodistal dimension of the tooth is desirable to form a contact with an adjacent tooth. When improvement in the occlusal plane of a tooth is desired during the course of treatment, a cast onlay rather than

an amalgam restoration offers the finest possibility for the desired result.

8. *Removable prosthodontic abutment.* Teeth that are to serve as abutments for a removable partial denture can often be restored with a cast metal restoration. The major advantages of a cast restoration versus amalgam are: (1) the superior physical properties of the cast metal alloy allow it to better withstand the forces imparted by the partial denture, and (2) the contours of the rest seats, guiding planes, and other aspects of contour relating to the partial denture are better controlled when the indirect technique is used.

9. *Economics and patient appreciation.* In some instances cost to the patient becomes a major consideration in the decision to restore a tooth with a cast metal restoration. The cast inlay or onlay requires more chairside time than an amalgam restoration, and the laboratory cost of fabrication must be included. Usually, however, this will not deter the discerning patient who has been educated to appreciate the merits of a well-made cast metal restoration.

10. *Age of the patient.* With younger patients amalgam or composite is usually the restorative material of choice for Class I and Class II cavities unless the tooth is severely broken down or root canal filled. Often younger patients will neglect oral hygiene, which results in additional caries.

11. *Esthetics.* The dentist must consider the esthetic impact (display of metal) of the cast metal restoration. This factor often limits the use of cast metal restorations to tooth surfaces which are not visible at a conversational distance. Composite and porcelain restorations are alternatives in esthetically sensitive areas (see Chapter 17 for tooth-colored restorations in Class II cavities).

OCCLUSION

Before an anesthetic is administered and before preparation of any tooth, evaluate the occlusal contacts of the teeth. As part of this evaluation, decide if the existing occlusal relationships can be improved with the cast metal restoration. An evaluation should include (1) the occlusal contacts in intercuspal position (IP) where the teeth are brought into full interdigitation, and (2) the occlusal contacts that occur during mandibular movements (Fig. 19-1). The pattern of occlusal contacts will influence the cavity design and the selection of interocclusal records and articulator. For information on how to evaluate and how to improve occlusal contact relationships, the reader is referred to the later sections in this chapter titled, Interocclusal Records, Forming the Occlusal Surface, and Occluding the Casting; as well as the section in Chapter 2 titled, Occlusion.

ANESTHESIA

Local anesthesia of the tooth to be operated on, as well as the adjacent soft tissues, usually is advocated. Anesthetizing these tissues eliminates pain and reduces salivation, resulting in a more pleasant operation for both the patient and the operator. (For details see Chapter 10, Pain Control.)

CONSIDERATIONS FOR TEMPORARY RESTORATIONS

Before preparation of the tooth, consideration must be given to the method that will be used to fabricate the temporary restoration. Most temporary restoration techniques involve using a preoperative impression to form the occlusal, facial, and lingual surfaces of the temporary restoration to the preoperative contours.

The technique involves making a *preoperative im-*

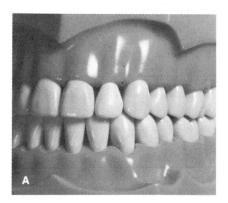 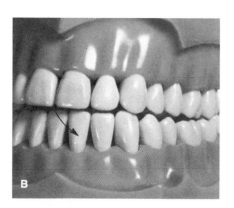 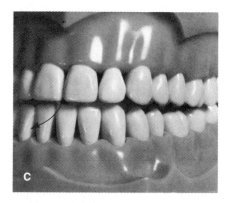

Fig. 19-1. Evaluate occlusal relationships in intercuspal position (**A**), and during mandibular movements (**B** and **C**). Be alert for problems with tooth alignment and contact position. Note the amount of posterior separation provided by the guidance of anterior teeth (working side) and articular eminence (non-working side).

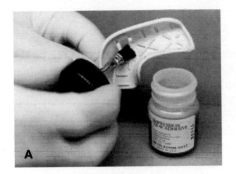
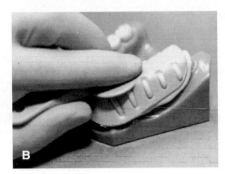
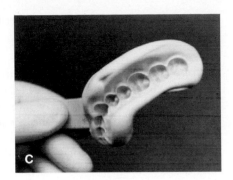

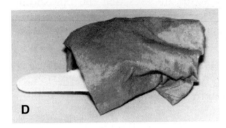

Fig. 19-2. **A,** Applying alginate tray adhesive to stock quadrant tray. **B,** Making preoperative alginate impression. **C,** Inspecting alginate impression for completeness. **D,** Wrap impression with wet paper towels to serve as a humidor.

pression with an elastic impression material. Alginate impression material is a common choice since it sets quickly and is relatively inexpensive. If the tooth to be restored has any large defects, such as a missing cusp, dry the tooth, and fill the large defects with utility wax. Smooth the wax, and make an alginate impression using a quadrant tray if no more than two teeth are to be prepared (Fig. 19-2, *A*). Use a full-arch tray for stability if more than two teeth are to be prepared. Apply by fingertip some alginate to the occlusal surfaces without trapping air; then seat the tray filled with alginate (Fig. 19-2, *B*). After the alginate has set, remove the impression and examine it for completeness (Fig. 19-2, *C*). Alginate impressions can distort quickly if they are allowed to gain or lose moisture, so wrap the impression in wet paper towels to serve as a humidor (Fig. 19-2, *D*). The preoperative impression may be made with a

polyvinyl siloxane impression material if additional accuracy, stability, and durability are required (such as when making multiple temporaries over an extended period of time). The preoperative impression is set aside for later use in forming the temporary. (Fabricating the resin temporary is described in the later section, Resin Temporary.)

CAVITY PREPARATION FOR CLASS II CAST METAL INLAYS

A small distal, cavitated, carious lesion in the maxillary right first premolar is used to illustrate the classic two-surface cavity preparation for an inlay (Fig. 19-3, *A*). Treatment principals for other defects are presented later in this section.

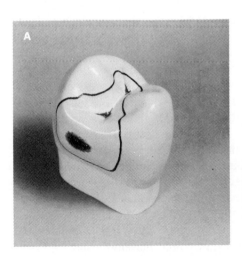
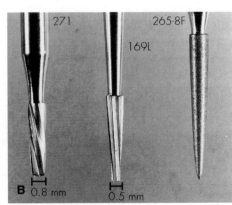
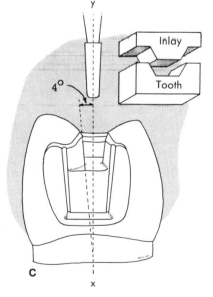

Fig. 19-3. **A,** Proposed outline form for distoocclusal cavity preparation. **B,** Dimensions and configuration of No. 271, No. 169L, and No. 265-8F instruments. **C,** Conventional 4-degree divergence from line of draw (line *xy*).

Initial cavity preparation

Convenience form. Carbide burs used to develop the longitudinal (vertical) internal walls of the preparation for cast metal inlays and onlays are plane-cut, tapered fissure burs. These burs are plane cut so the longitudinal walls will be smooth. The side and end surfaces of the bur should be straight to aid in the development of uniformly tapered walls and smooth pulpal and gingival walls. Recommended dimensions and configurations of the burs to be used are shown in Fig. 19-3, *B*. Suggested burs are the No. 271 and the No. 169L.* The operator is cautioned to verify the measurements of unfamiliar burs before they are used to judge depth into the tooth during cavity preparation. Note that the sides and end surface of the No. 271 bur meet in a slightly rounded manner so that sharp, stress-inducing internal angles will not be formed in the preparation.[23] The marginal bevels are placed with a slender, fine-grit, flame-shaped diamond instrument, such as the No. 265-8F† or No. 8862.‡

Throughout cavity preparation for a cast inlay the cutting instruments used to develop the longitudinal walls are oriented to a single "draw" path, usually the long axis of the tooth crown, so that the completed cavity will have draft (no undercuts) (Fig. 19-3, *C*). The gingival-to-occlusal divergence of these cavity walls may range from 2 to 5 degrees per wall from the line of draw. If the longitudinal walls are unusually short, a maximum of 2 degrees occlusal divergence is desirable to increase retentive potential. As the occlusogingival height increases, the occlusal divergence should increase because lengthy preparations with minimal divergence present difficulties during pattern withdrawal, trial seating and withdrawal of the casting, and cementing.

Outline, retention, and resistance forms, and enameloplasty

Occlusal step. With the No. 271 carbide bur held parallel to the long axis of the tooth crown, enter the fossa/pit closest to the involved marginal ridge, using a punch cut to a depth of 1.75 to 2 mm to establish the depth of the pulpal wall, the larger dimension when measured on the external walls, the smaller when related to the central groove/fissure location (Fig. 19-4, *A* and *B*). *In initial cavity preparation do not exceed this specified depth, regardless of whether the bur end is in dentin, caries, old restorative material, or air.* The bur should be rotating at high speed (with air-water spray) before application to the tooth and should not stop rotat-

ing until it is removed. This minimizes perceptible vibration and prevents breakage or chipping of the bur blades. Never should more than *very light pressure* be applied.[23] If heavy pressure is required, the bur is dull and should be discarded. *A general rule is to maintain the long axis of the bur parallel to the long axis of the tooth crown at all times* (Fig. 19-4, *B* and *C*). For mandibular molars and second premolars whose crowns tilt slightly lingually, this rule dictates that the bur should tilt slightly (5 to 10 degrees) lingually to conserve the strength of the lingual cusps (Fig. 19-4, *D*). It is emphasized that when the operator is cutting at high speeds, a properly directed air-water spray is used to provide the necessary cooling and cleansing effects.[23,24] A high-volume vacuum is constantly used to remove water and debris accumulation.

Maintaining the 1.75 to 2 mm limited depth and the same bur orientation, extend the cavity outline mesially along the central groove/fissure to include the mesial fossa/pit (Fig. 19-4, *E* and *F*). Ideally the faciolingual dimension of this cut should not exceed 1 mm when there is minimal or no caries. Exercise care to keep the mesial marginal ridge as strong as possible by not cutting away the dentin support of the ridge (Fig. 19-4, *F* and *H*). The use of light intermittent pressure will help minimize heat production on the tooth surface and reduce the incidence of enamel crazing ahead of the bur. Occasionally a fissure extends onto the mesial marginal ridge. This defect, if shallow, may be treated with enameloplasty, or it may be included in the outline form with the cavosurface bevel, which is applied in a later step in cavity preparation (Fig. 19-4, *G*).

Enameloplasty is the practice of removing the end of a developmental fault (fissure) with a suitable rotating instrument to create a smooth, saucer-shaped surface when the enamel fault is no deeper than one-third the thickness of the enamel. This procedure will occasionally reduce extension along the fissures, thereby conserving tooth structure vital for pulp protection and strength of the remaining tooth crown. The extent to which enameloplasty can be used usually cannot be determined until the operator is in the process of extending the cavity wall, when the depth of the fissure in the enamel wall can be observed (Fig. 19-5). When enameloplasty proves a fissure in a marginal ridge to be deeper than one-third the thickness of the enamel, then utilize the procedures described in the later section, Fissures in the Marginal Ridges.

Extend to include faulty facial and lingual fissures radiating from the mesial pit. During this extension cutting, the operator is cautioned again not to remove the dentin support of the proximal marginal ridge. To conserve tooth structure and the strength of the remaining tooth, the final extension up these fissures can be accomplished with the slender No. 169L carbide bur (Fig.

---

*No. 271 and No. 169L burs, SS White Inc., Lakewood, NJ.
†No. 265-8F diamond instrument, Den-Tal-EZ, Star Dental Division, Lancaster, Pa.
‡No. 8862 diamond instrument, Brassler USA, Inc., Savannah, Ga.

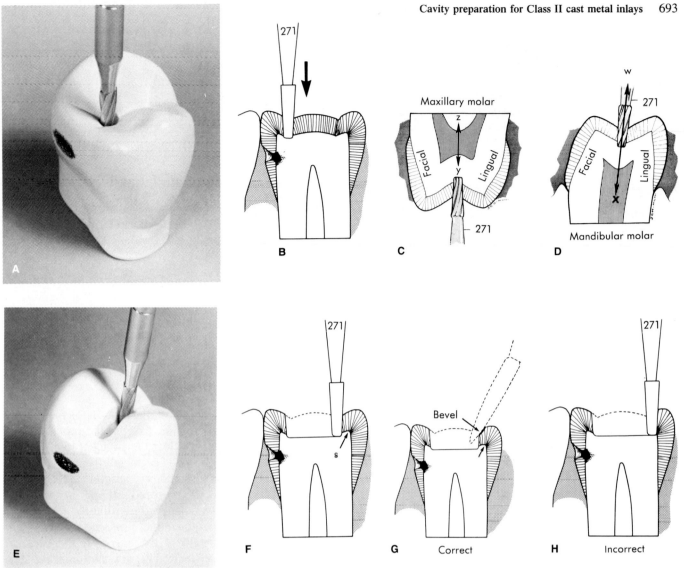

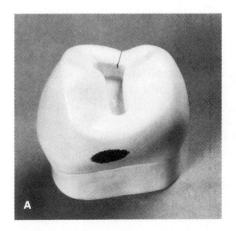

Fig. 19-4. A and B, Bur after punch cut to a depth of 1.75 to 2 mm. C, For maxillary posterior teeth, long axis of bur should parallel long axis of tooth crown (line *yz*). D, For molar and second premolar teeth of mandibular dentition, long axis of bur should tilt slightly lingually to parallel long axis of tooth crown (line *wx*). E and F, Extending mesial wall, taking care to conserve dentin that supports marginal ridge *(s)*. G, Marginal bevel can provide additional extension. H, Improper extension that has weakened the marginal ridge.

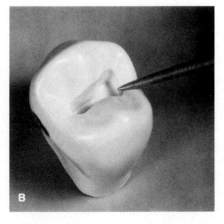

Fig. 19-5. A, Shallow enamel fault that is no deeper than one-third the thickness of enamel. B, Using fine-grit diamond instrument to remove enamel that contains shallow fault.

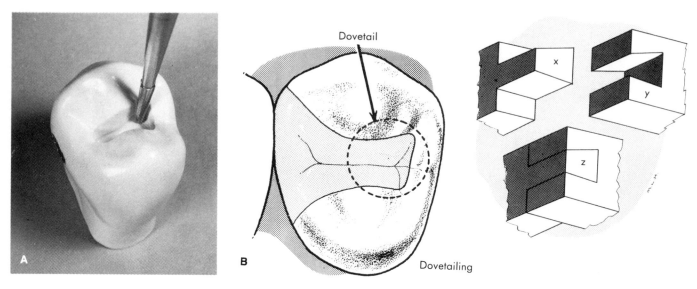

Fig. 19-6. A, Extending up the mesiofacial triangular groove using slender No. 169L bur. **B,** Dovetail retention form is created by extension shown in **A.** As *x* fits into *y* only in one direction resulting in *z*, similarly dovetail portion of inlay fits into dovetail portion of cavity preparation only in an occlusal-to-gingival direction.

19-6, *A*). Tooth structure and strength can be further conserved by remembering that (1) enameloplasty of the fissure ends should be employed when possible, and (2) the marginal bevel of the final cavity preparation often can be used to include (eliminate) the terminal ends of these fissures in the outline form. The facial and lingual extension in the mesial pit region should provide the desired *dovetail retention form,* which resists distal displacement of the inlay (Fig. 19-6, *B*). When these facial and lingual grooves are not faulty, sufficient facial extension in the mesial pit region should be made nevertheless to provide this dovetail retention form against distal displacement. Minor facial or lingual extension in the transverse ridge region to uncover caries may necessitate additional facial or lingual extension in the mesial pit to provide this dovetail feature. (Recall the principle that during such facial or lingual extensions to sound tooth structure the bur depth is maintained at 1.75 to 2 mm.) If major facial or lingual extension is required to remove undermined occlusal enamel, capping the weak remaining cuspal structure is indicated, as well as additional features in the cavity preparation to provide adequate retention and resistance forms. These considerations are discussed in the subsequent sections, Capping Cusps, and Enhancing Resistance and Retention Forms.

Continuing at the same depth, extend the occlusal step distally into the distal marginal ridge sufficiently to expose the junction of the proximal enamel and the dentin (Fig. 19-7, *A* and *B*). While extending distally, progressively widen the cavity to the desired faciolingual width in anticipation for the proximal boxing (described in the following section). The increased faciolingual width enables the facial and lingual walls of the boxing to project (visually) perpendicularly to the proximal surface at positions that will clear the adjacent tooth by 0.5 ± 0.2 mm (Fig. 19-7, *F*). The facial and lingual walls of the occlusal step should go around the cusps in graceful curves, and the prepared isthmus in the transverse ridge ideally should be only slightly wider than the bur, thus conserving dentinal protection for the pulp and maintaining strength of the cusps. If the occlusal step has been prepared correctly, any caries on the pulpal floor should be uncovered by facial and lingual extension to sound enamel (supported by dentin).

Proximal boxing. Continuing with the No. 271 carbide bur, isolate the distal enamel by cutting a *proximal ditch* (Fig. 19-7, *C* to *F*). Allow the harder enamel to guide the bur. Slight pressure toward the enamel is necessary to prevent the bur from cutting only dentin. If the bur is allowed to cut only dentin, the resulting axial wall will be too deep. The mesiodistal width of the ditch should be 0.8 mm (the tip diameter of the bur) and prepared approximately two-thirds (0.5 mm) at the expense of dentin and one-third (0.3 mm) at the expense of enamel. The gingival extension of this cut may be checked with the length of the bur by first measuring the depth from the height of the marginal ridge and then removing the bur and holding it alongside the tooth. A periodontal probe may also be used for this measurement. While penetrating gingivally, extend the proximal ditch facially and lingually beyond the caries to the desired position of the facioaxial and linguoaxial line angles. If the carious lesion is minimal, the ideal extension facially and lingually will be as previously de-

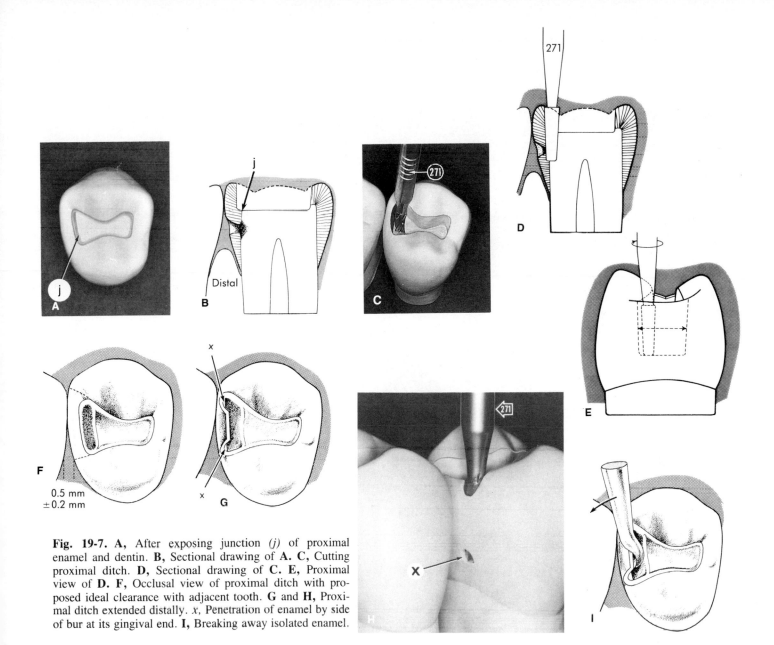

Fig. 19-7. A, After exposing junction *(j)* of proximal enamel and dentin. **B,** Sectional drawing of **A. C,** Cutting proximal ditch. **D,** Sectional drawing of **C. E,** Proximal view of **D. F,** Occlusal view of proximal ditch with proposed ideal clearance with adjacent tooth. **G** and **H,** Proximal ditch extended distally. *x,* Penetration of enamel by side of bur at its gingival end. **I,** Breaking away isolated enamel.

scribed (Fig. 19-7, *F*). *Ideal extension gingivally of a minimal, cavitated lesion will eliminate caries on the gingival floor, as well as provide 0.5 mm clearance of the unbeveled gingival margin with the adjacent tooth.* Moderate to extensive caries on the proximal surface dictates continued extension of the proximal ditch to the extent of the caries at the dentinoenamel junction, but *never pulpally* (Fig. 19-11, *D*). *When preparing the proximal portion of the cavity preparation, maintain the side of the bur at the specified axial wall depth regardless of whether it is in dentin, caries, old restorative material, or air.* Guard against overcutting the facial, lingual, and gingival walls, which would not conserve tooth structure and would result in overextension of the margins in the completed cavity preparation, a weakened tooth, and possible violation of the soft tissue. Because the proximal enamel diminishes in thickness from

the occlusal to gingival level, the end of the bur will be closer to the external tooth surface as the cutting progresses gingivally. The axial wall should follow the contour of the tooth faciolingually. *Any carious dentin on the axial wall should not be removed at this stage of cavity preparation.*

Proceeding with the No. 271 carbide bur, make two cuts, one at the facial limit of the proximal ditch and the other at the lingual limit, extending from the ditch perpendicularly toward the enamel surface (in the direction of the enamel rods) (Fig. 19-7, *G*). Extend these cuts until the bur is nearly through the marginal ridge enamel (the side of the bur may emerge slightly through the surface at the level of the gingival floor) as shown in Fig. 19-7, *H*. This weakens the enamel by which the isolated portion is held. Also, confirm the level of the gingival floor by observing where the end of the bur

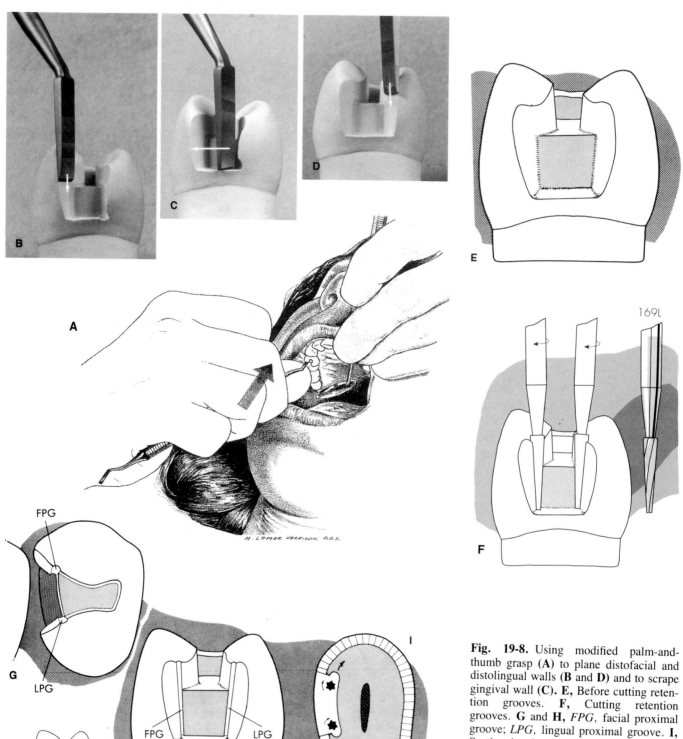

Fig. 19-8. Using modified palm-and-thumb grasp (**A**) to plane distofacial and distolingual walls (**B** and **D**) and to scrape gingival wall (**C**). **E,** Before cutting retention grooves. **F,** Cutting retention grooves. **G** and **H,** *FPG,* facial proximal groove; *LPG,* lingual proximal groove. **I,** Section in plane *x.* Larger arrows depict direction of translation of rotating bur. (Model of chisel courtesy American Dental Manufacturing Co.)

emerged through the proximal surface. If indicated, additional gingival extension can be accomplished while the remaining enamel still serves to guide the bur and prevent it from marring the proximal surface of the adjacent tooth. At this time, however, the remaining wall of enamel often breaks away during cutting, especially when high speeds are employed. If the isolated wall of enamel is still present, it is fractured out with a spoon excavator (Fig. 19-7, *I*). At this stage the ragged enamel edges left from breaking away the proximal surface may be touching the adjacent tooth.

Planing the distofacial, distolingual, and gingival walls by hand instruments to remove all undermined enamel may be indicated if minimal extension is needed to fulfill an esthetic objective. Depending on access, use a No. 15 (width) straight chisel, binangle chisel (Fig. 19-8), or enamel hatchet. For a right-handed operator the distal beveled binangle chisel is used on the distofacial wall of a distoocclusal preparation for the maxillary right premolar. Plane the wall by holding the instrument in the modified palm-and-thumb grasp, and use a chisel-like motion in an occlusal-to-gingival direction (Fig. 19-8, *A* and *B*). Plane the gingival wall by using the same instrument as a hoe, scraping in a lingual-to-facial direction (Fig. 19-8, *C*). In this latter action the axial wall may be planed with the side edge (secondary edge) of the blade. The distolingual wall is planed smooth by using the binangle chisel with the mesial bevel (Fig. 19-8, *D*). When proximal caries is minimal, ideal facial and lingual extension at this step in the preparation results in margins that clear the adjacent tooth by 0.5 ± 0.2 mm.

The experienced operator usually does not use chisel hand instruments during cavity preparation for inlays, inasmuch as the narrow, flame-shaped, fine-grit diamond instrument, when artfully used, will remove ragged, weak enamel during application of the cavosurface bevel and flares and will cause less apprehension on the part of the patient (Figs. 19-12 and 19-13). If the diamond instrument is to be used exclusively in finishing the enamel walls and margins, this procedure is postponed until after the removal of any remaining infected dentin and/or old restorative material, and the application of a base (see next section). This prevents any small hemorrhage (which occasionally follows the beveling of the gingival margin) from hindering (1) the suitable removal of remaining infected dentin and/or old restorative material and (2) the proper application of a base. Hand instruments are indispensable on the mesiofacial surfaces of the premolars and first molars of the maxillary dentition where minimal extension is desired to prevent an unsightly display of metal (see Modifications of Class II Cavity Preparation for Esthetics).

Shallow (0.3 mm deep) *retention grooves* may be cut in the facioaxial and linguoaxial line-angles with the No. 169L carbide bur (Fig. 19-8, *E* to *I*). These grooves are especially indicated when the prepared tooth is short and when retention form otherwise needs improvement. *When properly positioned, the grooves are in sound dentin near but not contacting the dentinoenamel junction.* The long axis of the bur continually must be held parallel to the line of draw. Preparing these grooves may be postponed until after any required bases are applied during final cavity preparation.

Final cavity preparation

Removal of infected carious dentin and application of bases. After the initial cavity preparation has been completed, evaluate the internal walls of the preparation visually and tactilely (with an explorer) for indications of remaining carious dentin (see Affected and Infected Dentin, in Chapter 7). If carious dentin remains and if it is judged to be *infected* and shallow or moderate (1 mm or more of remaining dentin between the caries and the pulp), satisfactory *isolation* for removal of such caries and the application of the base is attained by (1) the reduction in salivation resulting from *anesthesia,* and (2) the application of cotton rolls, saliva ejector, and *gingival retraction cord.* The retraction cord also serves to widen the gingival sulcus and slightly retract the gingiva in preparation for beveling and flaring the proximal margins (Figs. 19-9 and 19-12, *A* and *B*). For insertion of the cord refer to the later sections, Bevels and Flares, and Tissue Retraction. The removal of the remaining caries and placement of a base can be accomplished during the few minutes required for the full effect of the inserted cord. Use a slowly revolving round bur (No. 2 or No. 4) or spoon excavator to remove the carious *infected* dentin (Fig. 19-9, *F* and *G*). If the bur is used, improve visibility by cutting off the water in the coolant spray and use air alone. This excavation is done just above stall-out speed with light, intermittent cutting. Take care not to unnecessarily desiccate the exposed dentin during this procedure.

A light-cured *glass ionomer* cement may be mixed and applied with a suitable applicator to these shallow (or moderately deep) excavated regions to the level of the adjacent, unexcavated, prepared surface.* This takes very little time and results in working dies (subsequently in the laboratory phase) that have preparation walls with no undercuts, as well as "ideal" position and contour. *Also, applying a base at this time minimizes additional irritation of the pulp during subsequent procedures necessary for the completion of the restoration.* The light-cured glass ionomer adheres well to tooth structure and generally does not require retentive under-

*Vitrebond, 3-M Company, 3-M Center, St. Paul, Minn.

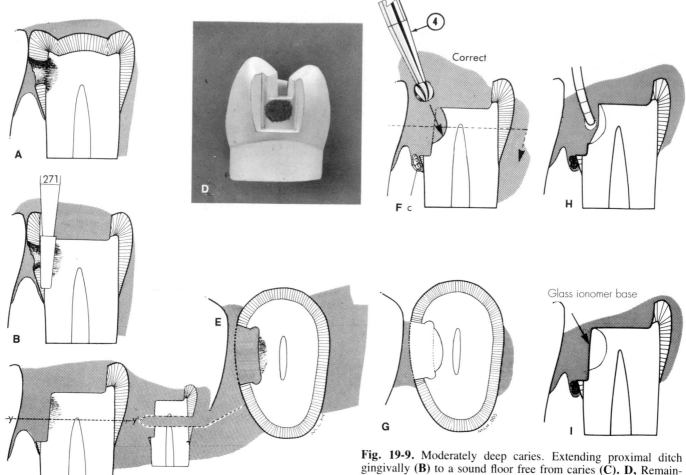

Fig. 19-9. Moderately deep caries. Extending proximal ditch gingivally (**B**) to a sound floor free from caries (**C**). **D,** Remaining caries on axial wall. **E,** Section of **C** in plane *yy'*. **F,** Removing remaining infected dentin. *c,* Inserted retraction cord. **G,** Section of **F. H,** Inserting glass ionomer base with periodontal probe. **I,** Completed base.

cuts when the base is small to moderate in size. The material is applied by conveying small portions on the end of a periodontal probe and is light-cured when the correct form has been achieved (Fig. 19-9, *H* and *I*). Any excess cement can be trimmed back to ideal position with the No. 271 carbide bur *after* the glass ionomer has hardened.

*If the carious lesion is judged to closely approach the pulp, a **rubber dam** should be applied before the removal of infected dentin.* This provides the optimal environment for the successful treatment of a pulp exposure should it occur. When excavating deep caries, attempt to remove only the *infected* dentin and not the *affected* dentin, since removal of the latter might expose a healthy pulp. (See Chapters 3 and 7 for descriptions of the principles governing the removal of carious dentin.) Ideally, caries removal should continue until the remaining dentin feels as hard as normal dentin; however, heavy pressure should not be applied with an explorer tip (or any other instrument) on what is judged

to be a thin layer of reasonably hard dentin next to the pulp, lest an unnecessary pulpal exposure be created. If removal of soft, infected dentin leads directly to a pulpal exposure *(carious pulpal exposure),* then a root canal filling should be accomplished before completing the cast metal restoration.

If the pulp is inadvertently exposed as a result of operator error or misjudgment *(mechanical pulpal exposure),* then a decision must be made whether to proceed with a root canal filling or to attempt a calcium hydroxide *direct pulp capping procedure.* A clinical evaluation should be made regarding health of the pulp. A favorable prognosis for the pulp after direct pulp capping may be expected if the following criteria are met:

1. The exposure is small (less than 0.5 mm in diameter).
2. The tooth has been asymptomatic, showing no signs of pulpitis.
3. Any hemorrhage from the exposure site is easily controlled.

4. The invasion of the pulp chamber was relatively atraumatic with little physical irritation to the pulp tissue.
5. A clean, uncontaminated operating field is maintained (i.e., a rubber dam).

If the excavation closely approaches the pulp or if a direct pulp cap is indicated, first apply a lining of *calcium hydroxide* using a flow technique (without pressure). This calcium hydroxide liner should cover and protect any possible near or actual exposure and also extend over a major portion of the excavated dentin surface (Fig. 19-10, *A*). Although undetected, there may be an exposed recessional tract of a pulp horn in any deep excavation. Calcium hydroxide treatment of an exposed, healthy pulp promotes the formation of a dentin bridge closing the exposure.[24] Leave the peripheral 0.5 to 1 mm of the dentin excavation exposed for bonding the light-cured glass ionomer cement base subsequently applied.

Although the light-cured glass ionomer cement is adhesive to dentin, *large cement bases can be subjected to considerable stresses during fabrication of the temporary, and try-in/cementation of the cast metal restoration.* Also, if a calcium hydroxide liner has been applied, less dentin is available for adhesive bonding. In these circumstances small undercuts can increase the retention of the glass ionomer base. If suitable undercuts are not present after removal of infected dentin, *retention coves* are cut with the No. 1/4 carbide bur (Fig. 19-10, *B* to *D*). These coves are cut in the peripheral dentin of the excavation and are as remote from the pulp as possible. The light-cured glass ionomer cement should be applied without pressure. It should completely cover the calcium hydroxide lining and some portion of the peripheral dentin excavation surface for good adhesion (Fig. 19-11). The cement base should be sufficiently thick in dimension to protect the thin underlying dentin

and calcium hydroxide liner from subsequent stresses. *Good resistance form dictates that the pulpal wall should never be formed entirely by a cement base;* rather, in at least two regions, one diametrically across the excavation from the other, the pulpal wall should be in normal position, flat, and formed by sound dentin (see region *s* in Fig. 19-11, *E*, depicting basing in a mandibular molar). One should consider the addition of other retention features such as proximal grooves if a major portion of a proximal axial wall is composed mostly of cement base, since this base should not be relied on for contributing to retention of the cast restoration (Fig. 19-8, *F*).

Remaining old restorative material on the internal walls should be removed if *any* of the following conditions are present: (1) the old material is judged to be thin and/or non-retentive, (2) there is radiographic evidence of caries under the old material, (3) the pulp was symptomatic preoperatively, or (4) the periphery of the remaining restorative material is not perfectly intact, (i.e., there is some breach in the junction of the material with the adjacent tooth structure that may indicate caries under the material). If none of these conditions is present, the operator may elect to leave the remaining restorative material to serve as a base, rather than risk unnecessary (1) removal of sound dentin or (2) irritation or exposure of the pulp. The same isolation conditions described previously for removal of infected dentin also apply for the removal of old restorative material.

After the cement has hardened, spread a thin coat of petroleum jelly over the base with a small cotton pellet. This serves to prevent the adherence of subsequently applied unpolymerized materials such as (1) the resin for the temporary restoration, or (2) the final impression material.

There is a possibility for the future need of root canal therapy for any tooth having been treated for deep car-

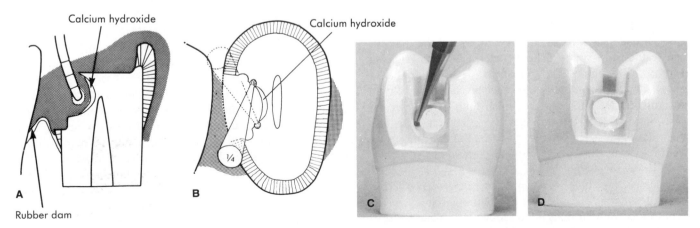

Fig. 19-10. A, Deep caries excavations are first lined with calcium hydroxide. Note rubber dam.
B to **D,** Cutting retention coves for retaining glass ionomer cement.

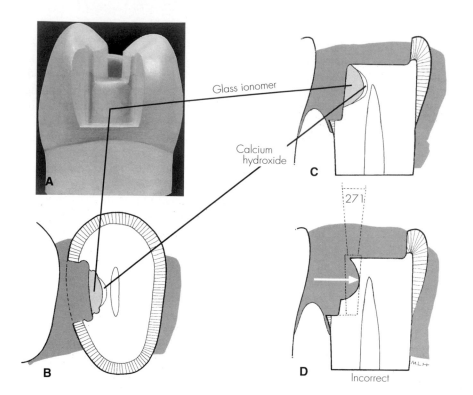

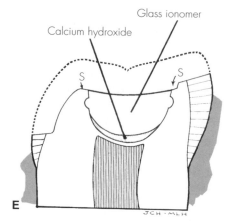

Fig. 19-11. A to **C,** Completed base for treatment of deep caries. **D,** *Never* deepen entire axial wall with side of fissure bur to remove caries because pulp will be greatly irritated from resulting closeness of gingivoaxial region of preparation. **E,** Cement base placed in deep excavation on mandibular molar. Note flat seats in sound dentin *(s)* that are required for adequate resistance form.

ies that approximates or exposes the pulp. When treating a tooth that has had such extensive caries, consider reducing all cusps to onlay the occlusal surface with metal for better distribution of occlusal loads, as well as adding skirts to augment resistance form, since teeth invariably are prone to fracture after root canal therapy. (See later sections, Cavity Preparation for Cast Metal Onlay, and Enhancing Resistance and Retention Forms.)

Preparation of bevels and flares. After the cement base (where indicated) is completed, the slender, flame-shaped, fine-grit diamond instrument is used to bevel the occlusal and gingival margins and to apply the secondary flare on the distolingual and distofacial walls. This should result in 30- to 40-degree marginal metal on the inlay (Figs. 19-12, *H,* 19-13, *J,* and 19-14, *B*). This cavosurface design helps to seal and protect the margins and results in a strong enamel margin with an angle of 140 to 150 degrees. A cavosurface enamel angle of more than 150 degrees is incorrect because it results in an indistinct enamel margin (finish line). The marginal cast metal alloy is too thin and weak if its angle is less than 30 degrees; conversely, the metal at the margins is too bulky and difficult to burnish if its angle is greater than 40 degrees (Fig. 19-14, *F*).

Usually it is helpful to insert a ***gingival retraction cord*** of suitable diameter into the gingival sulcus adjacent to the gingival margin and leave it in place for several minutes just before the use of the flame-shaped diamond instrument on the proximal margins (Fig. 19-12,

A to *C*). The cord should be small enough in diameter to permit relatively easy insertion and to preclude excessive pressure against the gingival tissue, yet it should be large enough to widen the sulcus to about 0.5 mm. Immediately before the flame-shaped diamond instrument is used, the cord is removed, resulting in an open sulcus that (1) improves visibility for beveling the gingival margin and (2) helps to prevent injury and subsequent hemorrhage of the gingival tissue.

Using the flame-shaped diamond instrument, rotating at high speed, prepare the lingual secondary flare (Figs. 19-12, *D* to *F,* and 19-13, *A*). Approach from the lingual embrasure, as shown in Fig. 19-12, *F,* moving the instrument mesiofacially. Compare the direction of the distolingual wall and the position of the distolingual margin before and after this extension (Figs. 19-8, *G,* and 19-13, *A*). Notice in Fig. 19-13, *A,* that the distolingual wall extends from the linguoaxial line angle into the lingual embrasure in two planes. The first is termed the lingual ***primary flare;*** the second is named the lingual ***secondary flare.*** During this (secondary) flaring operation the long axis of the instrument is held nearly parallel to the line of draw, with only a slight tilting mesially and lingually for assurance of draft (Fig. 19-12, *D* and *E*), and the direction of translation of the instrument is that which results in a *marginal metal angle of 40 degrees* (Figs. 19-12, *F,* and 19-13, *J*).

Now bevel the gingival margin by moving the instrument facially along the gingival margin (Figs. 19-12, *G,* and 19-13, *A*). While cutting the ***gingival bevel,*** re-

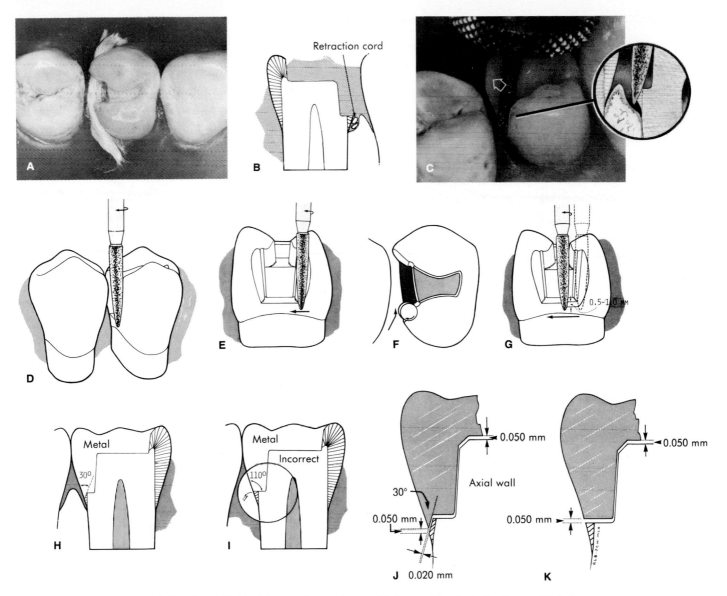

Fig. 19-12. A and **B,** Double-strand retraction cord is inserted in gingival sulcus and left for several minutes. **C,** "Open" gingival sulcus after cord shown in **A** is removed facilitates beveling gingival margin with diamond instrument. **D** to **F,** Diamond instrument preparing lingual secondary flare. Large arrow in **F** depicts direction of translation. **G,** Beveling gingival margin. Note in **C** the mesial tilting of diamond instrument to produce a bevel properly directed to result in 30-degree marginal metal as shown in **H. H,** Properly directed gingival bevel resulting in 30-degree marginal metal. **I,** Failing to bevel gingival margin results in weak margin formed by undermined rods (note easily displaced wedge of enamel) and 110-degree marginal metal, an angular design unsuitable for burnishing. **J,** Lap, sliding fit of prescribed bevel metal decreases 50 μm error of seating to 20 μm. **K,** A 50 μm error of seating will produce an equal cement line of 50 μm along unbeveled gingival margin.

duce the rotational speed to increase the sense of touch; otherwise overbeveling may result. The instrument should be tilted slightly mesially to produce a gingival bevel with the correct steepness to result in *30-degree marginal metal* (Fig. 19-12, *C, H,* and *J*). If the instrument is not tilted in this manner, the bevel will be too steep, resulting in gingival bevel metal that is too thin (less than 30-degree metal) and thus too weak. Although the instrument is tilted mesially, its long axis must not tilt facially or lingually (Fig. 19-12, *G*). The

gingival bevel should be 0.5 to 1 mm wide and should blend with the lingual secondary flare.

Complete the gingival bevel, and then prepare the facial secondary flare (Fig. 19-13, *A* to *F*). The long axis of the instrument during this secondary flare is again returned nearly to the line of draw with only a small tilting mesially and facially, and the direction of translation of the instrument is that which results in 40-degree marginal metal (Fig. 19-13, *E* and *J*). When the adjacent proximal surface (mesial of the second premolar) is

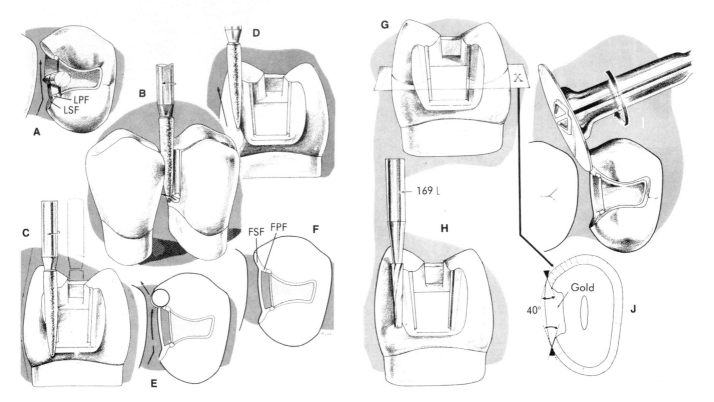

Fig. 19-13. A, Occlusal view of Fig. 19-12, *G. LSF* and *LPF* designate lingual secondary and lingual primary flares. **B** to **D,** Preparing facial secondary flare. Large arrows in **B, D,** and **E** depict direction of translation. **F,** Completed facial secondary flare. *FSF* and *FPF* designate facial secondary and facial primary flares. **G,** Distal view of **F.** *x,* Plane of cross section shown in **J.** Preparing secondary flare with the No. 169L carbide bur **(H)** or with paper disc **(I). J,** Secondary flares are directed to result in 40-degree marginal metal and 140-degree marginal enamel.

not being prepared, care must be exercised neither to abrade the adjacent tooth nor to overextend the distofacial margin. To help in preventing such abrasion or overextension, the instrument may be raised occlusally (thus using the narrower portion at its tip end) to complete the most facial portion of the wall and margin (Fig. 19-13, *D*). Also, the more slender No. 169L carbide bur may be used rather than the flame-shaped diamond instrument (Fig. 19-13, *H*). Moreover, the No. 169L bur produces an extremely smooth surface to the secondary flare and a smooth, straight distofacial margin. When access permits, the careful use of a fine-garnet disc followed by a medium-cuttle disc on the facial and lingual walls and margins of the proximal preparation is recommended, especially when minimal extension of the facial margin is desired (Fig. 19-13, *I*).* This produces smooth walls and helps to create respective margins that are straight (not ragged) and sound.

In the flaring and beveling of the proximal margins, as described in the previous paragraphs, the procedure

---

*Moores sandpaper discs, E.C. Moore Co., Inc., Dearborn, Mich.

began at the lingual surface and proceeded to the facial surface; however, the direction may be reversed, starting at the facial surface and moving toward the lingual surface. On the mesiofacial surface of maxillary premolars and first molars where extension of the facial margin should be minimal, it is usually desirable to use the lingual-to-facial direction.

The gingival bevel serves the following purposes:

1. *Weak enamel is removed.* If the gingival margin is in the enamel, it would be weak if not beveled because of the gingival declination of the enamel rods (Fig. 19-12, *I*).
2. *The bevel results in 30-degree metal that is burnishable* (on the die) because of its angular design (Fig. 19-12, *H*). Bulky 110-degree metal along an unbeveled margin is not burnishable (Fig. 19-12, *I*).
3. *A lap, sliding fit is produced at the gingival margin* (Fig. 19-12, *J*). This helps to improve the fit of the casting in this region. With the prescribed gingival bevel, if the inlay fails to seat by 50 μm, the void between the bevel metal and the gingival bevel on the tooth may be as small as 20 μm;

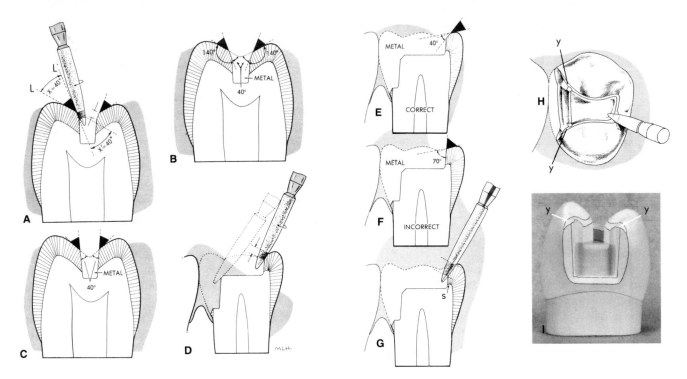

Fig. 19-14. A, Diamond instrument beveling occlusal margin when it is indicated to result in 40-degree marginal metal as shown in **B.** Angles *x* and *x'* are equal because opposite angles are equal when two lines (*l* and *l'*) intersect. Therefore diamond instrument is always directed so that an angle of 40 degrees is made by side of instrument and external enamel surface. **B,** Occlusal marginal metal is approximately 40 degrees in cross section, thus making enamel angle 140 degrees. **C,** When cuspal inclines are steep, no beveling is indicated inasmuch as 40-degree metal will result without beveling. **D,** Beveling mesial margin and axiopulpal line angle. **E,** Mesial bevel is directed correctly to result in 40-degree marginal metal. **F,** Unbeveled mesial margin is incorrect because it results both in weak enamel margin and unburnishable marginal metal. **G,** To conserve dentin support *(s)*, occlusal defects on marginal ridge are included in outline form by applying cavosurface bevel, which may be wider than conventional when necessary. **H,** Occlusal view of **G.** Preparing 140-degree cavosurface enamel angle at regions labeled *y* usually dictates that occlusal bevel be extended over marginal ridges into secondary flares. **I,** Distal view of **H.**

however, failure to apply such a bevel would result in a void (and a cement line) as great as the failure to seat (Fig. 19-12, *K*).

Uninterrupted blending of the gingival bevel into the secondary flares of the distolingual and distofacial walls results in the distolingual and distofacial margins joining the gingival margin in a desirable arc of a small circle; also, the gingivofacial and gingivolingual line angles no longer extend to the marginal outline. *If such line angles are allowed to extend to the cavity outline, early failure at these points usually follows because of an "open" margin, solution of exposed cement, and eventual leakage.*

There are several reasons for the secondary flare. First, the secondary flaring of the proximal walls extends the margins into the embrasures, making these margins more self-cleansing and more accessible to finishing procedures during the inlay insertion appointment, and does so with conservation of the dentin. Second, the direction of the flare results in 40-degree marginal metal (Fig. 19-13, *J*). Metal with this angular design is burnishable; however, metal shaped at a larger angle is unsatisfactory for burnishing; metal with an angle less than 30 degrees is too thin and weak, with a corresponding enamel margin that is too indefinite and ragged. Third, a more blunted and stronger enamel margin is produced because of the secondary flare.

In a later section, Modifications of Class II Cavity Preparation for Esthetics, the secondary flare is omitted for esthetic reasons on the mesiofacial proximal wall of cavity preparations on premolars and first molars of the maxillary dentition. In this location the wall is completed with minimal extension by using only hand instruments (straight or binangle chisel) followed by a medium-cuttle paper disc.

The flame-shaped, fine-grit diamond instrument is also used for *occlusal bevels*. The depth (width) of the cavosurface bevel on the occlusal margin should be approximately *one-fourth* the depth of the respective wall (Fig. 19-14, *A* and *B*). The exception to the rule is when a wider bevel is desired to include an enamel defect (Fig. 19-14, *G* and *H*). The resulting occlusal marginal metal of the inlay should be *40-degree metal; thus the occlusal marginal enamel is 140-degree enamel* (Fig. 19-14, *B* and *E*). Beveling the occlusal margins in this manner increases the strength of the marginal enamel and helps to seal and protect the margins. The marginal metal alloy is too thin and weak if the angle is less than 30 degrees; with an angle greater than 40 degrees the marginal metal is too difficult to burnish. While beveling the occlusal margins, a rule of procedure is to *always maintain a 40-degree angle between the side of the instrument and the external enamel surface.* This procedure will predetermine when an occlusal bevel is indicated, as well as create a bevel of the correct angle (Fig. 19-14, *A*). For example, if the cuspal inclines are so steep that the diamond instrument at a 40-degree angle to the external enamel surface is parallel with the enamel cavity wall, then no bevel is indicated (note in Fig. 19-14, *C*, how the rule for 40-degree marginal metal is satisfied without beveling). Observing the aforementioned procedure, the operator will realize that margins on the proximal marginal ridges always require a cavosurface bevel (Fig. 19-14, *D* and *I*). Failure to apply a bevel in these regions leaves the enamel margin weak and liable to injury by fracture, both before the inlay insertion appointment and during the try-in of the inlay when burnishing the marginal metal. Also, observe how the failure to bevel margins on the marginal ridges results in metal alloy that is difficult to burnish because it is too bulky (Fig. 19-14, *F*). Similarly, the importance of extending the occlusal bevel to include those portions of the occlusal margin that cross over the marginal ridge cannot be overemphasized (Fig. 19-14, *H* and *I*). These margins are beveled, as the rule of procedure indicates, to result in 40-degree marginal metal. Otherwise fracture of the enamel margin in such stress-vulnerable regions often occurs in the interim between the cavity preparation and the cementation appointment.

The diamond instrument also is used to lightly bevel the axiopulpal line angle (Fig. 19-14, *D*). Such a bevel provides a stronger wax pattern at this critical region.

Note: the desirable metal angle at the margins of inlays is 40 degrees, except at the gingival margins, where the metal angle should be 30 degrees. The completed cavity preparation is illustrated in Fig. 19-15, *A*.

Mesioocclusodistal cavity preparation

Before a two-surface Class II inlay is planned, a careful examination of the remaining untreated proximal surface must eliminate any possibility of that surface having caries or being liable to caries in the near future. To treat the remaining proximal surface of a premolar for caries at a subsequent time usually would indicate the removal of the previously inserted inlay. Thus it is more efficient and a greater service to the patient to restore both proximal surfaces in one operation when the probability exists that the other proximal surface will be affected by caries during the next few years (Fig. 19-15, *B* to *D*).

If a marginal ridge is severely weakened because of excessive extension into it, the cavity outline often should be altered to include the proximal surface. For

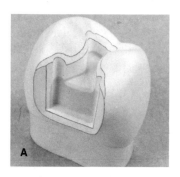
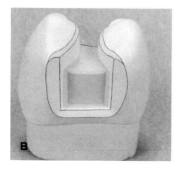
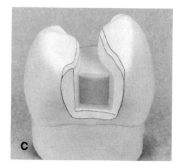
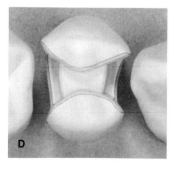

Fig. 19-15. A, Completed distoocclusal cavity preparation for inlay. **B,** Mesioocclusodistal cavity preparation for inlay on maxillary right first premolar, distoocclusal view. **C,** Same preparation as in **B,** mesioocclusal view. **D,** Same preparation as in **B,** occlusal view. Note absence, for esthetic reasons, of secondary flare on mesiofacial aspect and minimal extension of mesiofacial margin.

example, the distoocclusal cavity preparation illustrated in the previous section would be extended to a mesiooc-clusodistal preparation. The decision to extend the cavity in this manner calls for clinical judgment as to whether the remaining marginal ridge will withstand occlusal forces without fracture. A fortunate factor in favor of not extending the preparation is that such ridge enamel is usually composed of **gnarled enamel** and thus is stronger than it appears.

Class II cavity preparation for the mandibular first premolar

The Class II inlay cavity preparation on the mandibular first premolar is modified in several respects because of the dental anatomy peculiar to this tooth. To conserve the dentin protecting the large and tall facial horn of the pulp, as well as the dentin supporting the miniature lingual cusp, the pulpal wall should decline slightly lingually (Fig. 19-16). In Fig. 19-16, *D*, the No. 271 carbide bur is held so that its long axis *(ci)* is parallel with the bisector *(b)* of the angle formed by the long axis of the tooth *(la)* and a line *(p)* that is perpendicular to a plane *(de)* drawn through the facial and lingual cusp tips. This dotted line *(ci)* is then the line of draw of the cavity preparation.

Special attention is given to ensure that the depth of cutting in the occlusal step is no deeper than 2 mm (measured on prepared facial wall). This maximal depth is another factor that is emphasized to protect the facial horn of the pulp. Often, to minimize weakening the small lingual cusp, the occlusal step should be more at the expense of tooth structure facial to the central groove than lingual. However, capping the lingual cusp is frequently indicated.

Occasionally the transverse ridge is strong, smooth, without a faulty central groove. If this is true, and if the distal surface is carious and the mesial is not, and when the tooth is not too small, consideration should be given to preparing a distoocclusal cavity without crossing the transverse ridge (Fig. 19-16, *E* and *F*). This conserves tooth structure, and the restored tooth is stronger. To be satisfactory, however, such a small, two-surface cavity preparation requires diligent attention by a most careful operator. It is strongly suggested to first prepare the proximal boxing before cutting the occlusal dovetail. The tooth structure labeled *x* in Fig. 19-16, *F,* is necessary for the dovetail feature of retention form, and it can be easily and inadvertently lost in cavity preparation by the inexperienced operator if cutting the occlusal portion of the cavity is prematurely begun.

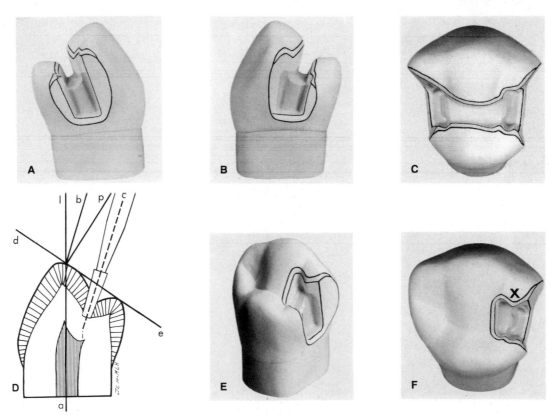

Fig. 19-16. Mandibular first premolar prepared for mesioocclusodistal inlay, distal view **(A)**, mesial view **(B)**, and occlusal view **(C). D,** Illustrating proper bur direction. **E,** If possible, preparation should not cross sound, transverse ridge. **F,** To prevent removal of tooth structure labeled *x,* prepare proximal boxing before cutting occlusal dovetail.

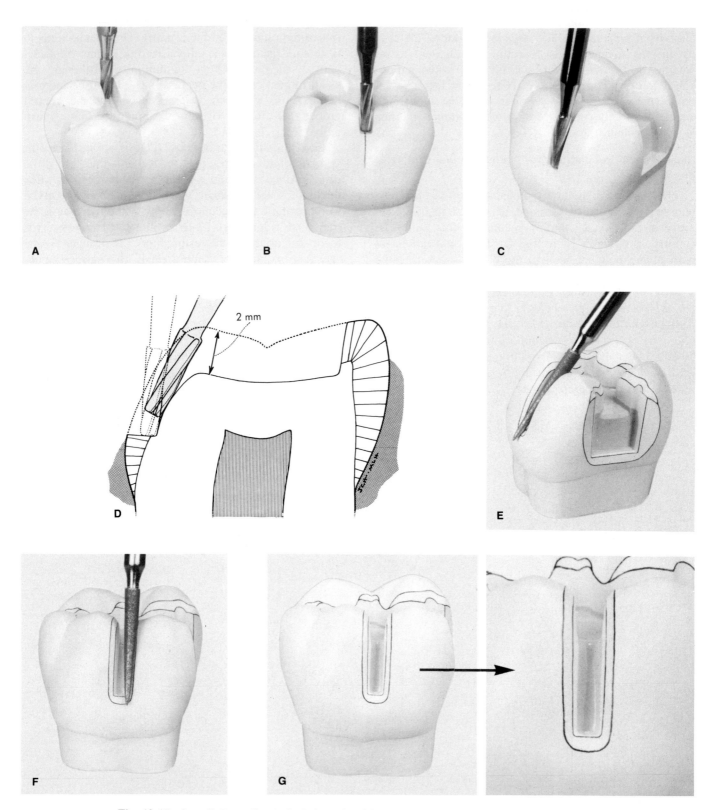

Fig. 19-17. A to **C,** Extending to include occlusal fissure that is continuous with facial fissure on facial surface. **D,** Section of **C.** Beveling gingival margin (**E**) and mesial and distal margins (**F**) of fissure extension. **G,** Beveling completed.

Modifications of Class II cavity preparation for esthetics

For esthetic reasons, minimal flare is indicated for the mesiofacial proximal wall in the maxillary premolars and first molars in Class II inlay cavity preparations (Fig. 19-15, *D*). The mesiofacial margin is minimally extended facially of contact to such a position that the margin is barely visible from a facial viewing position. To accomplish this, the secondary flare is omitted, and the wall and margin are developed with a chisel or enamel hatchet. Final smoothing with the medium-cuttle paper disc is recommended when access permits.

Facial or lingual surface groove extension

Frequently a faulty facial groove (fissure) on the occlusal surface is continuous with a faulty facial surface groove (mandibular molars), or a faulty distal oblique groove on the occlusal surface is continuous with a faulty lingual surface groove (maxillary molar). This indicates extension of the cavity outline to include the fissure to its termination (Figs. 19-17 and 19-19, *C*). Occasionally the operator may elect to extend even further gingivally than the fissure length to improve retention form because these groove extensions, when sufficiently long, are very effective for increasing retention. This extension may be indicated to provide sufficient retention form even though the facial or lingual surface grooves are not fissured.

For extension onto the facial surface, use the No. 271 carbide bur held parallel to the line of draw, and extend through the facial ridge (Fig. 19-17, *A* and *B*). The depth of the cut should be uniform and approximate 1.75 to 2 mm. The floor (pulpal wall) should be continuous with the pulpal wall of the occlusal portion of the cavity (Fig. 19-17, *D*).

With the bur still aligned with the path of draw, use the side of the bur to cut the facial surface portion of this extension (Fig. 19-17, *C*). The diameter of the bur serves as a depth gauge for the axial wall, which is in dentin. The blade portion of the No. 271 bur is 0.8 mm in diameter at its tip end and 1 mm in diameter nearest the neck; the axial wall depth should approximate 1 mm or slightly more. The bur should be tilted lingually as it is drawn occlusally, to develop the uniform depth of the axial wall (Fig. 19-17, *D*). The same principles apply for extension of the lingual surface groove.

With the flame-shaped, fine-grit diamond instrument, bevel the gingival margin (using no more than one third the depth of the gingival floor) to provide for 30-degree marginal metal (Fig. 19-17, *E*). Apply a light bevel on the mesial and distal margins that will be continuous with the occlusal and gingival bevels and will result in 40-degree metal at these margins (Fig. 19-17, *F* and *G*).

Class II cavity preparation for abutment teeth, and extension gingivally to include root surface lesions

Extending the gingival margin into the gingival sulcus is usually indicated on the proximal surfaces adjacent to connectors of removable partial dentures because of the difficulty in keeping these regions clean. For the same reason the facial and lingual proximal margins on such abutment teeth should be well extended. In addition, the occlusal outline form must be wide enough faciolingually to accommodate any contemplated rest preparation(s) without involving the margins of the restoration. The following modified cavity preparation is also recommended when further gingival extension is indicated to include a root lesion on the proximal surface.

The gingival extension should be accomplished primarily by lengthening the gingival bevel, especially when preparing a tooth that has a longer clinical crown than normal as a result of gingival recession. It is necessary to only slightly extend (gingivally) the gingival floor, and although the axial wall consequently must be moved pulpally, this should be only to a small extent. In addition, the gingival floor should not be as wide pulpally as when the floor level is at a normal position (Fig. 19-18, *A*). These considerations are necessary because of the draft requirement and because the tooth is smaller apically. *Extending the cavity preparation gingivally without these modifications would result in a dangerous encroachment of the axial wall on the pulp* (Fig. 19-18, *B*).

In relatively caries-immune mouths with moderate recession or in mouths with extreme recession (gingival attachment is more than 3 mm gingival to the cementoenamel junction) it is probably wise not to extend the gingival margin gingivally into the gingival sulcus. In such instances emphasis should be on the prophylactic attentions of both the dentist and the patient and period-

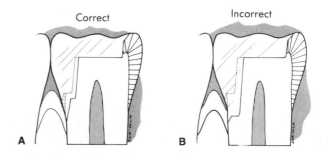

Fig. 19-18. Modifications of cavity preparation when extending to include proximal root surface lesions after moderate gingival recession. **A,** Correct. **B,** Incorrect. Note decreased dentinal protection of pulp, compared with management depicted in **A.**

ical topical application of fluoride to maintain the exposed proximal root surface free of caries.

Maxillary first molar with unaffected, strong oblique ridge

When a maxillary first molar is to be restored, consideration should be given to preserving the oblique ridge if it is strong and unaffected, especially if only one proximal surface is carious. A mesioocclusal cavity preparation for an inlay is illustrated in Fig. 19-19, *A* and *B*.

If a distal surface cavity appears subsequently to the insertion of a mesioocclusal restoration, the tooth should be prepared for a distoocclusolingual inlay (Fig. 19-19, *H* and *I*). The distoocclusolingual restoration that caps the distolingual cusp is preferable to the distoocclusal restoration because it protects the miniature distolingual cusp from subsequent fracture. The distoocclusolingual cavity preparation requires diligent application to develop satisfactory retention and resistance forms. Retention form is attained by (1) creating a maximum of 2-degree occlusal divergence of the longitudinal walls, (2) accentuating certain line angles, and (3) extending the lingual surface groove to create an axial wall in this extension of at least 2.5 mm occlusogingivally. Proper resistance form dictates (1) routine capping of the distolingual cusp and (2) guarding against the lingual surface groove extension being so close to the distolingual wall of the proximal boxing that it seriously weakens the intervening tooth structure.

To prepare the distoocclusolingual cavity, first reduce the distolingual cusp with the side of the No. 271 carbide bur. The cusp should be reduced a uniform 1.5 mm. Next prepare the remaining occlusal step of the preparation with the No. 271 carbide bur. Then prepare the proximal box portion of the cavity, giving special attention to achieve sufficient retention form. *Prepare the lingual groove extension only after the position of the distolingual wall of the proximal boxing is established.* This permits the operator to judge the best position of the lingual surface groove extension to maintain a minimum of 3 mm of sound tooth structure between this extension and the distolingual wall. If this is not possible because of extensive caries, then a more extensive type of cavity preparation is indicated (one that crosses the oblique ridge). Use the side of the No. 271 carbide bur to produce the lingual surface groove extension (Fig. 19-19, *C*). The diameter of the bur is the gauge for the depth (pulpally) of the axial wall in this extension, and the occlusogingival dimension of this axial wall is a minimum of 2.5 mm. With the end of this bur, also establish a 2 mm depth to that portion of the pulpal floor that connects the proximal boxing to the lingual surface groove extension. This should create a

definite 0.5 mm step-down from the reduced distolingual cusp to the pulpal floor.

Using the No. 169L carbide bur, increase retention form in the distoocclusolingual preparation by (1) creating mesioaxial and distoaxial grooves in the lingual surface groove extension (Fig. 19-19, *D*) and (2) preparing facial and lingual retention grooves in the distal boxing (Fig. 19-19, *E*).

Use the flame-shaped, fine-grit diamond instrument to bevel the proximal gingival margin and to prepare the secondary flares on the proximal enamel walls, as well as to bevel the lingual margins. A lingual *counterbevel* is prepared on the distolingual cusp that is generous in width and at an angle that will result in 30-degree metal at the margin (Fig. 19-19, *F*). The bevel on the gingival margin of the lingual extension should be 0.5 mm wide and should provide for a 30-degree metal angle. The bevels on the mesial and distal margins of the lingual extension are narrow and of such an angle as to result in 40-degree marginal metal.

Fissures in the facial and lingual cusp ridges

In the preparation of Class II cavities for inlays, facial and lingual occlusal fissures frequently extend nearly to or through the respective facial and lingual cusp ridges. Proper outline form dictates that the cavity preparation margin should not cross such fissures but should be extended to include them. For example, when preparing the occlusal step portion of the cavity, continue the extension along a lingual fissure with the No. 271 carbide bur until only 2 mm of tooth structure remains between the bur and the lingual surface of the tooth. Additional lingual extension in this manner is incorrect because it would remove the supporting dentin (Fig. 19-20, *A* and *B*). If the stipulated extension by the bur almost includes the length of the fissure, remember that additional extension is achieved later by virtue of the occlusal bevel; moreover, this bevel may be wider than conventional if the remaining fissure can be eliminated by such a wider bevel (Fig. 19-20, *C*). Also recall that enameloplasty sometimes may eliminate the end portion of the fissure and provide a smooth enamel surface where once there was a fault, thus reducing the extent of the required extension (Fig. 19-20, *D*). If possible, attempt to include the fissure in the cavity outline without extending the margin to the height of the ridge. If, however, the occlusal bevel places the margin on the height of the ridge, then the marginal enamel likely is weak because of both its sharpness and the inclination of the enamel rods in this region. Therefore the cavity outline should be extended onto the facial or lingual surface (Fig. 19-20, *I* and *J*). Also, such extension onto the facial or lingual surface would be indicated if the fissure still remains through the ridge after enameloplasty (Fig. 19-20, *E*).

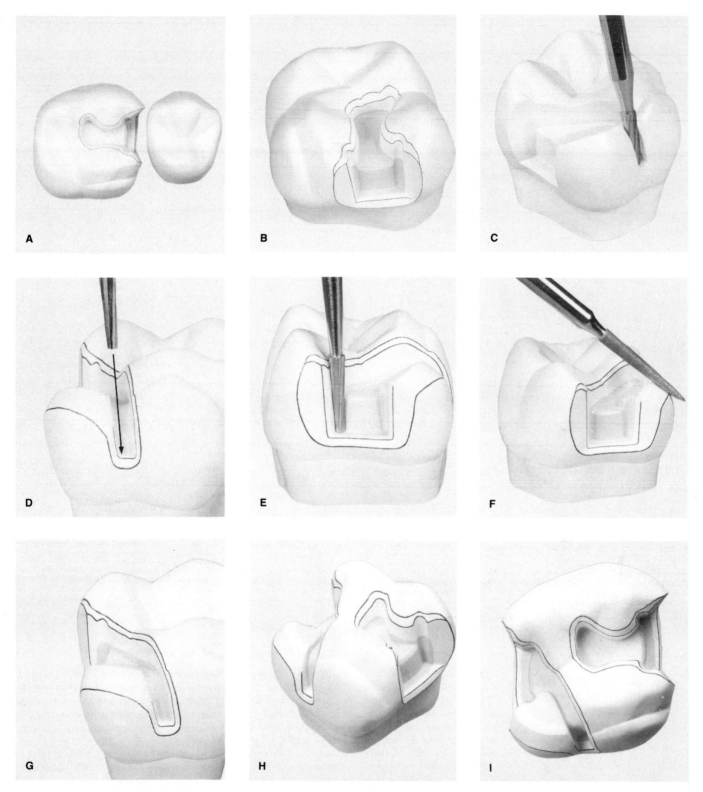

Fig. 19-19. A and **B,** Mesioocclusal cavity preparation on maxillary molar having unaffected oblique ridge. **C,** Preparing lingual groove extension of distoocclusolingual cavity preparation. Cutting retention grooves in lingual surface extension **(D)** and distal box **(E). F** and **G,** Completed distoocclusolingual cavity preparation on maxillary molar having unaffected oblique ridge. **H** and **I,** Cavity preparations for treating both proximal surfaces of maxillary molar having strong, unaffected oblique ridge.

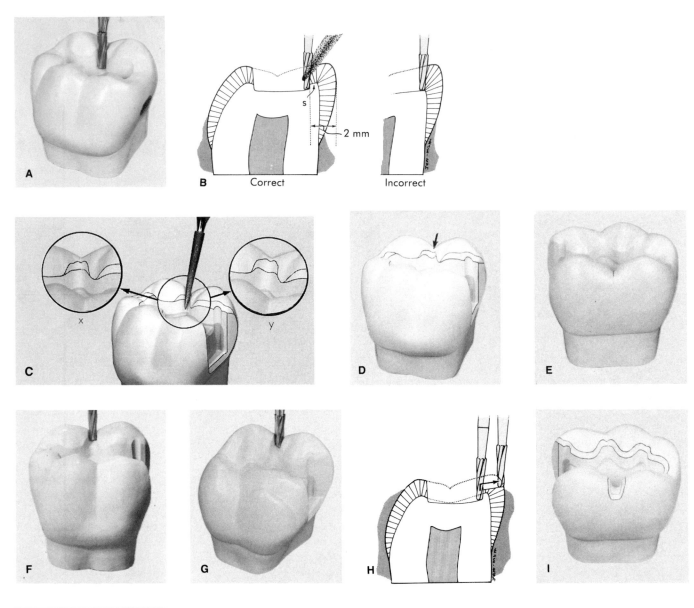

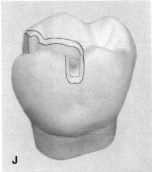

Fig. 19-20. A, Extending to include lingual (occlusal) fissure. **B,** Section of **A.** Dentin support *(s)* of lingual cusp ridge should not be removed. Bevel can provide additional extension to include fissure that does not extend to crest of ridge. **C,** Completed cavity preparations with standard width bevel *(x)* and with wider bevel to include groove defect that nearly extends to ridge height *(y)*. **D,** Completed cavity preparation illustrating enameloplasty for elimination of shallow fissure extending to or through lingual ridge height. (Compare smooth, saucer-shaped lingual ridge contour with **C,** where no enameloplasty has been performed.) **E,** Fissure remaining through lingual ridge following unsuccessful enameloplasty. *This indicates procedures subsequently illustrated.* Extending preparation if enameloplasty has not eliminated fissure in lingual ridge **(F)** or facial ridge **(G). H,** Section of **F.** Completed cavity preparations after beveling margins of extensions through lingual ridge **(I)** and facial ridge **(J).**

Extension through a ridge is accomplished by raising the No. 271 carbide bur half the depth of the occlusal preparation and cutting through the ridge (Fig. 19-20, *F* to *G*). This should make the extension approximately 1 mm deep. Bevel the margins of the extension with the flame-shaped, fine-grit diamond instrument to provide for the desired 40-degree marginal metal on the occlusal, mesial, and distal margins and for 30-degree marginal metal on the gingival margin (Fig. 19-20, *C, D, I,* and *J*).

Fissures in the marginal ridges

In the same manner as described in the preceding section, manage the fissures that sometimes extend into or through the proximal marginal ridge, assuming that the proximal surface otherwise was not to be included in the outline form and that such fissure management does not extend the cavity outline near the adjacent tooth contact. This treatment particularly applies to a mesial fissure of the maxillary first premolar (Fig. 19-21). If this procedure extends the margin near or into the contact, the outline form on the affected proximal surface must be extended to include the contact, as for a conventional proximal surface cavity preparation.

Capping cusps

The facial and lingual margins on the occlusal surface frequently must be extended toward the cusp tips to the extent of existing restorative materials and to uncover caries (Fig. 19-22, *B* and *C*). Undermined occlusal enamel should be removed because it is weak; moreover, removing such enamel provides access for proper excavation of caries and treatment of the cavity. When the occlusal outline is extended up the cusp slopes more than half the distance from any primary occlusal groove (central, facial, or lingual) to the cusp tip, capping the cusp should be considered. If the cavity outline is ex-

tended two-thirds this distance or more, capping the cusp is mandatory to (1) protect the weak, underlying cuspal structure from fracture caused by masticatory force; and (2) remove the occlusal margin from a region subjected to heavy stress and wear (Fig. 19-22, *A* and *B*). The following section describes the technique for capping less than all of the cusps of a posterior tooth. (For capping all of the cusps of a posterior tooth, see Cavity Preparation for Cast Metal Onlay.)

Reduce the cusp(s) for capping as soon as the indication for such capping is determined, since this improves access and visibility for subsequent steps in cavity preparation. If a cusp is in infraocclusion of the desired occlusal plane before reduction, then the amount of cusp reduction is less and needs only to be that which provides the required *clearance* with the desired occlusal plane. Before reducing the surface, cut **depth gauge grooves** with the side of the No. 271 carbide bur (Fig. 19-22, *D*). Such depth cutting should help to prevent thin spots in the restoration. With the depth grooves serving as guides, complete the cusp reduction with the side of the carbide bur (Fig. 19-22, *E*). The reduction should provide for a uniform 1.5 mm of metal thickness over the reduced cusp. On maxillary premolars and first molars the reduction should be only 1 mm (sometimes less) on the facial cusp ridge to satisfy the esthetic requirement. This thickness should increase progressively to 1.5 mm toward the center of the tooth to help provide rigidity to the capping metal (Fig. 19-23, *A* and *C*).

If only one of the two lingual cusps of a molar is reduced for capping, the reduction must extend to barely include the lingual groove that is between the reduced and unreduced cusps. This cusp reduction should terminate with a distinct longitudinal wall that is as deep as the prescribed cusp reduction. Applying the bur vertically, as shown in Fig. 19-22, *F*, should help to establish a longitudinal wall of proper depth and direction. Similar principles apply when only one of the facial cusps is to be reduced (Figs. 19-22, *L*, and 19-23, *B*).

A bevel of generous width is prepared on the facial (lingual) margin of a reduced cusp with the flame-shaped, fine-grit diamond instrument (with the exception of esthetically sensitive areas). This bevel is referred to as a **reverse bevel** or **counterbevel.** It should be at an angle that results in 30-degree marginal metal (Fig. 19-22, *G* and *H*). The exception is the facial margin on maxillary premolars and the first molar where esthetic requirements dictate only a blunting and smoothing of the enamel margin by the light application of a fine-garnet paper disc or the fine-grit diamond instrument (flame-shaped) held at a right angle to the facial surface (Fig. 19-23, *C*). The facial counterbevel on the mandibular posteriors should extend the margin gingivally beyond any occlusal contact (Fig. 19-26, *C*).

Cusp reduction appreciably decreases retention form

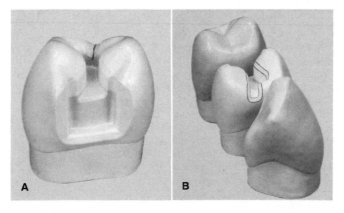

Fig. 19-21. Fissure that remains on mesial marginal ridge after unsuccessful enameloplasty (**A**) is treated (**B**) in same manner as lingual or facial ridge fissures (Fig. 19-20, *I* and *J*).

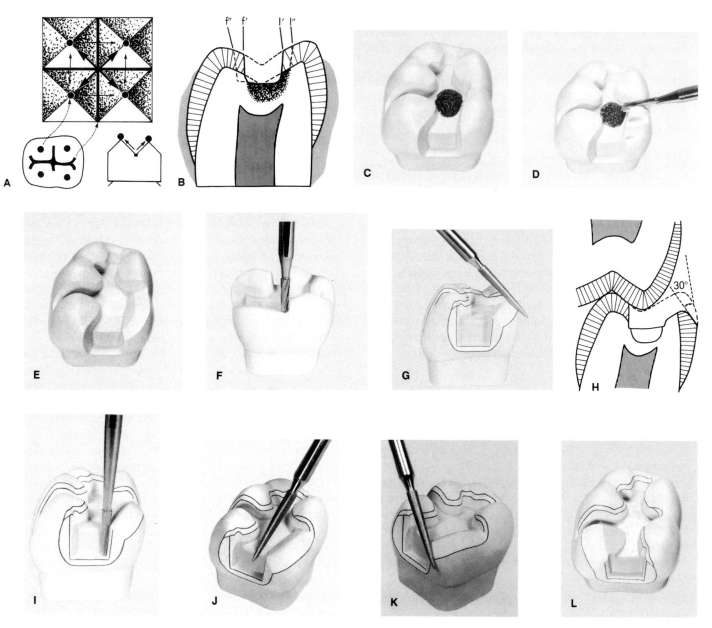

Fig. 19-22. A, When extension of occlusal margin is one-half the distance from any point on primary grooves *(cross)* toward cusp tip *(dot),* capping the cusp should be considered; when this distance is two-thirds or more, capping the cusp is definitely indicated. **B,** *l'* is midway between central groove and lingual cusp tip. *f'* is midway between central groove and facial cusp tip. When enamel at *l'* and *f'* is undermined by caries, respective walls must be extended to dotted lines *l''* and *f''* for caries to be uncovered. Then cusps should be reduced for capping. **C,** Extension to uncover caries indicates that mesiolingual cusp should be reduced for capping. **D,** Cutting depth gauge grooves. **E,** Reduced mesiolingual cusp. Note that caries has been removed and cement base has been placed. **F,** Applying bur longitudinally helps establish longitudinal wall that barely includes lingual groove. **G,** Counterbeveling reduced cusp. **H,** Section of counterbevel. **I,** Improving retention form by cutting proximal retention grooves. Cavity preparation is complete except for rounding axiopulpal line angle **(J)** and rounding junction of counterbevel and secondary flare **(K).** Facial surface groove extension improves both retention and resistance forms. **L,** Cavity preparation when reducing one of two facial cusps on mandibular molar.

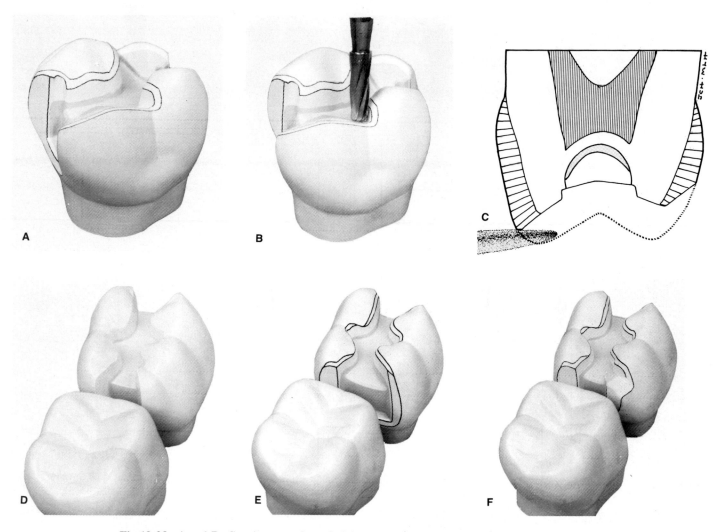

Fig 19-23. A and **B,** Capping one of two facial cusps on maxillary molar. **C,** Blunting margin of reduced cusp when esthetics is major consideration. **D** to **F,** Margin shown crossing distal cusp in **D** indicates treatment illustrated in either **E** or **F.**

because of decreasing the height of the longitudinal walls; consequently proximal retention grooves usually are recommended (Fig. 19-22, *I*). Often additional retention should be secured by the cutting of extensions in the facial and lingual groove regions of the respective surfaces, or by *collar* and *skirt* features presented in the later section, Enhancing Retention and Resistance Forms. *These additional retention features also provide the desired resistance form against forces tending to split the tooth* (Figs. 19-22, *K,* and 19-28).

Slightly round any sharp external corners to strengthen them and to reduce the difficulties these sharp corners foster in future steps (Fig. 19-22, *J* and *K*). Angles especially must never be in the marginal outline, since these are weak and subject to fracture before the inlay is completed.

The principles stated in the preceding paragraphs are frequently applied in the treatment of the distal cusp of

the mandibular first molar when preparing a mesioocclusodistal cavity (Fig. 19-23, *D*). Proper extension of the distofacial margin usually places the occlusal margin in a region subjected to heavy masticatory forces and wear. Satisfactory treatment dictates either (1) extending the distofacial margin (and wall) slightly mesial of the distofacial groove (Fig. 19-23, *E*) or (2) capping the remaining portion of the distal cusp (Fig. 19-23, *F*). The choice of treatment depends on the operator's judgment of local conditions.

Including portions of the facial and lingual smooth surfaces affected by caries or other injury

When a portion of a facial (lingual) smooth surface, as well as a proximal surface, is affected by caries or other injury (e.g., fracture) (Fig. 19-24, *A* and *I*), the treatment may be either an extended inlay, an onlay, a three-quarter crown, a full crown, or multiple amalgam

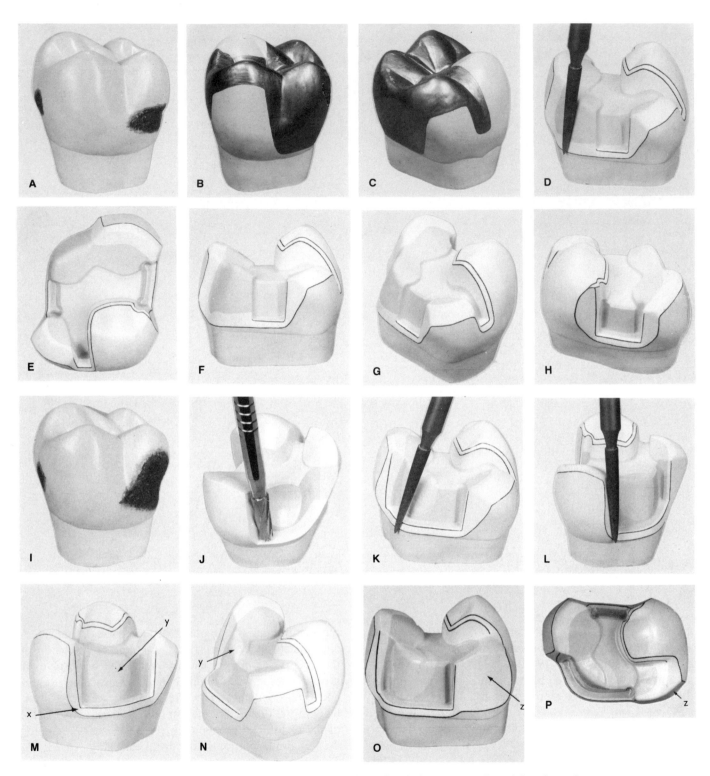

Fig. 19-24. A, Maxillary molar with caries on both distofacial corner and mesial surface. Completed MODFL inlay for treating caries shown in **A,** faciooocclusal view **(B)** and distolinguoocclusal view **(C).** Cavity preparation for treating caries illustrated in **A,** distoocclusal view with diamond instrument being applied **(D);** occlusal view **(E);** distal view **(F);** distolinguoocclusal view **(G);** mesioocclusal view **(H). I,** Maxillary molar with deeper caries on distofacial corner and with mesial caries. **J,** Cavity preparation (minus bevels and flares) for MODFL inlay to restore carious molar shown in **I.** No. 271 carbide bur is used to prepare gingival shoulder and longitudinal wall. **K** and **L,** Beveling margins. **M** and **N,** Completed cavity preparation for treating caries shown in **I.** Gingival and facial bevels blend at *x,* and *y* is cement base. **O** and **P,** When lingual surface groove has not been prepared and when facial wall of proximal boxing is mostly or totally missing, forces directed to displace inlay facially can be opposed by lingual skirt extension *(z).* (See Enhancing Retention and Resistance Forms.)

or composite restorations. Generally if carious portions are extensive, the choice between the previously listed cast metal restorations is determined by the degree of tooth circumference involved. A full crown is indicated if both the lingual and facial smooth surfaces are defective, especially if the tooth is a second or third molar and hygiene of the tooth is poor. When only a portion of the facial smooth surface is carious and the lingual surfaces of the teeth are conspicuously free of caries, an MODFL inlay or onlay with a lingual groove extension is chosen over the crown because the former is more favorable to the health of the gingival tissues. Often this is the treatment choice for the maxillary second molar, which so frequently exhibits caries on the distofacial surface as a result of poor oral hygiene in this region (Fig. 19-24).

In the preparation of the maxillary molar referred to in the preceding paragraph, usually the mesiofacial and distolingual cusps, as well as the distofacial cusp, are reduced for capping. If the caries on the distofacial cusp is not deep, the flame-shaped diamond instrument is used to reduce the involved facial surface and distofacial corner approximately the depth of the enamel and to establish the gingival margin of this reduction just apical to the affected area (Fig. 19-24, *D*). This instrument also is used to terminate the facial surface reduction in a definite facial margin running gingivoocclusally and in a manner to provide for 40-degree metal at this margin (Fig. 19-24, *E*).

If distofacial caries is more extensive and deeper into the tooth (Fig. 19-24, *I*), hence eliminating the opportunity for an effective distal boxing or groove (no facial wall possible), then the No. 271 carbide bur should be used to cut a shoulder extending from the distal gingival floor around to include the affected facial surface. This *shoulder* partially provides the desired resistance form. (A gingival floor, perpendicular to occlusal force, has been provided in lieu of the missing pulpal wall in the distofacial cusp region.) Use this instrument also to create a nearly longitudinal wall in the remaining facial enamel (Fig. 19-24, *J*). The width of the shoulder should be the diameter of the end of the cutting instrument. The longitudinal walls should have the degree of draft to contribute to retention form. Then the faciogingival and facial margins are beveled with the flame-shaped, fine-grit diamond instrument to provide 30-degree metal at the gingival margin (Fig. 19-24, *K*) and 40-degree metal along the facial margin (Fig. 19-24, *L*). These two bevels should blend together in an arc of a small circle (*x* in Fig. 19-24, *M*), and the faciogingival bevel is continuous with the gingival bevel on the distal surface. Additional retention and resistance form is indicated and can be developed by a lingual groove extension (Fig. 19-24, *N*), by a distolingual skirt extension (Fig. 19-24, *O* and *P*), or by pinholes placed in the lin-

gual structures. *These preparation features resist forces normally opposed by the missing distofacial wall and help to protect the restored tooth from fracture injury* (see Enhancing Resistance and Retention Forms).

CAVITY PREPARATION FOR CAST METAL ONLAY

The cast metal onlay restoration spans the gap between the inlay, which is primarily an intracoronal restoration, and the full crown, which is a totally extracoronal restoration. *The cast metal onlay, which by definition caps all of the cusps of a posterior tooth, can be thoughtfully designed to strengthen a tooth that has been weakened by caries or previous restorative experiences.* It can be designed to distribute occlusal loads over the tooth in a manner that virtually eliminates future tooth fracture.[7,25] It is more conservative of tooth structure than the full crown preparation and its supragingival margins are less irritating to the gingivae. Many times the prescription of an onlay for a tooth can be made preoperatively (such as a large failing amalgam that extends facially and lingually two-thirds of the distance from the central groove toward the cusp tips or gross occlusal attritional wear). The diagnosis for an onlay is at times deferred until extension of the occlusal step of an inlay preparation facially and lingually to the limits of the carious lesion demonstrates that cusp reduction is mandatory.

The mandibular first molar is used to illustrate a mesioocclusodistal cavity preparation for a cast metal onlay; other onlay preparations are presented subsequently.

Initial cavity preparation

Convenience form and occlusal reduction. *As soon as the decision is made to restore the tooth with a cast metal onlay, the cusps should be reduced, since this improves both the access and the visibility for subsequent steps in cavity preparation.* With the cusps reduced, the efficiency of the cutting instrument is greatly improved, as is the efficiency of the air-water cooling spray. *Also, once the cusps are reduced it is easier to assess the length of the remaining clinical crown of the tooth, which determines the degree of occlusal divergence for adequate retention form.* Using the No. 271 carbide bur held parallel to the long axis of the tooth crown, prepare a 2 mm deep depth cut along the central groove (Fig. 19-25, *A*). To verify the preoperative diagnosis for cusp reduction, this depth cut may be extended facially and lingually just beyond the caries to sound tooth structure (Fig. 19-25, *B*). The groove should not be extended farther than two-thirds the distance from the central groove to the cusp tips, since the need for cusp reduction is verified at this point. With the side of the No. 271 carbide bur, cut uniform 1.5 mm deep *depth gauge*

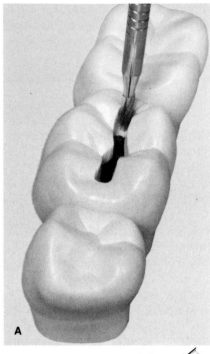

A

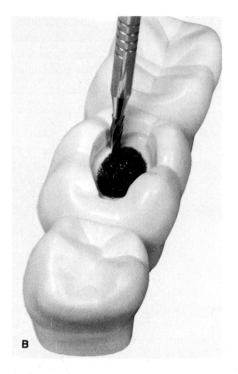

B

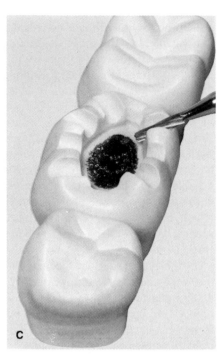

C

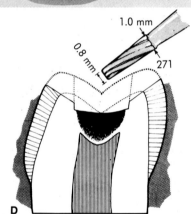

1.0 mm

0.8 mm

271

D

Fig. 19-25. A, Cutting 2 mm deep depth cut along central groove. **B,** Extending central groove depth cut facially and lingually to verify need for cusp capping. **C,** Cutting depth gauge grooves. **D,** Section of **C. E,** Completing cusp reduction. Note that small portions of mesial and distal marginal ridges are left unreduced to avoid scarring adjacent teeth. **F,** Occlusal step is extended facially and lingually past any carious areas and is extended to expose proximal dentinoenamel junctions (*j*) in anticipation of proximal boxing. **G,** Preparation with proximal boxes prepared. Note clearances with adjacent teeth.

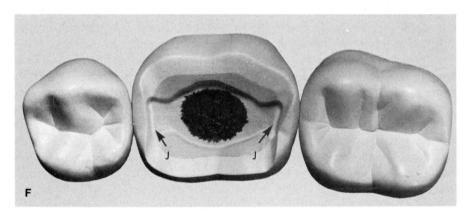

J   J

F

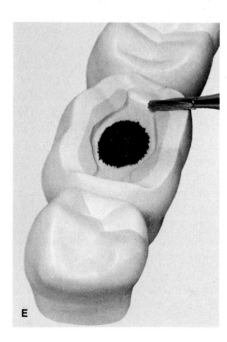

E

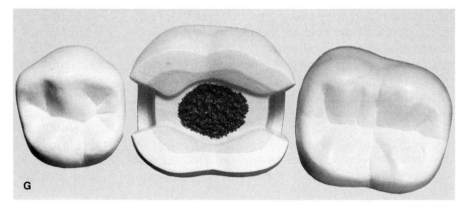

G

grooves on the remaining occlusal surface (Fig. 19-25, *C* and *D*). The grooves should be placed on the crest of the triangular ridges and in the facial and lingual groove regions. These depth grooves will help prevent thin spots in the final restoration. It should be remembered that if a cusp is in infraocclusion of the desired occlusal plane before reduction, then the amount of cusp reduction is less and needs only that which provides the required clearance with the desired occlusal plane. *Caries and/or old restorative material that is deeper in the tooth than the desired clearance is not removed at this step in cavity preparation.*

With the depth grooves serving as guides for the amount of reduction, complete the cusp reduction with the side of the No. 271 bur. This reduction, when completed, should reflect the general topography of the original occlusal surface (Fig. 19-25, *E*). Do not attempt to completely reduce the mesial and distal marginal ridges at this time if adjacent teeth are present, since the remainder of the ridges will be reduced in a later step when the proximal boxes are prepared.

Throughout the next steps in initial cavity preparation, the cutting instruments used to develop the longitudinal (vertical) walls are oriented continually to a single "draw" path, usually the long axis of the tooth crown, so that the completed cavity will have draft (i.e., no undercuts). For mandibular molars and second premolars whose crowns tilt slightly lingually, the bur should tilt slightly (5 to 10 degrees) lingually to help preserve the strength of the lingual cusps (Fig. 19-4, *D*). The gingival-to-occlusal divergence of these cavity walls may range from 2 to 5 degrees from the line of draw. If the longitudinal walls are unusually short, a minimum of 2 degrees occlusal divergence is desirable for retentive purposes. Cusp reduction appreciably decreases retention form because of decreasing the height of the longitudinal walls, so this minimal amount of divergence is often indicated in the preparation of a tooth for a cast metal onlay. As the gingivoocclusal height of the longitudinal walls increases, the occlusal divergence should increase, allowing as much as 5 degrees in the preparation of greatest gingivoocclusal length. The latter preparations present difficulties during pattern withdrawal, trial seating and withdrawal of the casting, and cementing unless this maximal divergence is provided.

Outline, retention, and resistance forms

Occlusal step. After cusp reduction there should be a 0.5 mm deep occlusal step in the central groove region. Maintaining the pulpal depth (0.5 mm) of the step, extend it facially and lingually just beyond any carious areas to sound tooth structure (or to sound base/restorative material if certain conditions have been met which will be discussed subsequently). Extend mesially and distally far enough to expose the proximal dentinoenamel junction (Fig. 19-25, *F*). Extend the step along any re-

maining facial (and lingual) occlusal fissures as far as they are faulty (fissured). The facial and lingual walls of the occlusal step should go around the cusps in graceful curves, and the isthmus should only be as wide as necessary to be in sound tooth structure or sound base/restorative material. Old restorative material or caries that is deeper pulpally than this 0.5 mm step is not removed at this stage of cavity preparation.

As the occlusal step approaches the mesial and distal surfaces, it should widen faciolingually in anticipation for the proximal boxing (Fig. 19-25, *F*). This occlusal step will contribute to the retention of the restoration[11] and will provide the wax pattern and cast metal onlay with the needed bulk for rigidity.

Proximal boxing. Continuing with the No. 271 carbide bur held parallel to the long axis of the tooth crown, prepare the proximal boxings as described in the inlay section, Proximal Boxing. Fig. 19-25, *G*, illustrates the preparation after the proximal boxes are prepared.

Final cavity preparation

Removal of infected carious dentin and/or defective restorative materials, and application of bases. If the occlusal step and the proximal boxes have been extended properly, any caries or previous restorative materials remaining on the pulpal and axial walls should be in view. For a detailed description of removing the remaining *infected* carious dentin and/or defective restorative material and the application of bases to restore ideal pulpal floor and axial wall positions, refer to the previous inlay section, Removal of Infected Carious Dentin and Application of Bases. Remaining old restorative material on the internal walls should be removed if *any* of the following conditions are present: (1) the old material is judged to be thin and/or non-retentive, (2) there is radiographic evidence of caries under the old material, (3) the pulp was symptomatic preoperatively, or (4) the periphery of the remaining restorative material is not perfectly intact (i.e., there is some breach in the junction of the material with the adjacent tooth structure that may indicate caries under the material).

Preparation of bevels and flares. After the cement base (when indicated) is completed (Fig. 19-26, *A),* use the slender, flame-shaped, fine-grit diamond instrument to place **counterbevels** on the reduced cusps, to apply the **gingival bevels,** and to create *secondary flares* on the facial and lingual walls of the proximal boxes. First insert a gingival **retraction cord** as described in the previous inlay section, Preparation of Bevels and Flares. During the few minutes required for the cord's effect on the gingival tissues, use the diamond instrument for preparing the counterbevels on the facial and lingual margins of the reduced cusps. The bevel should be of gen-

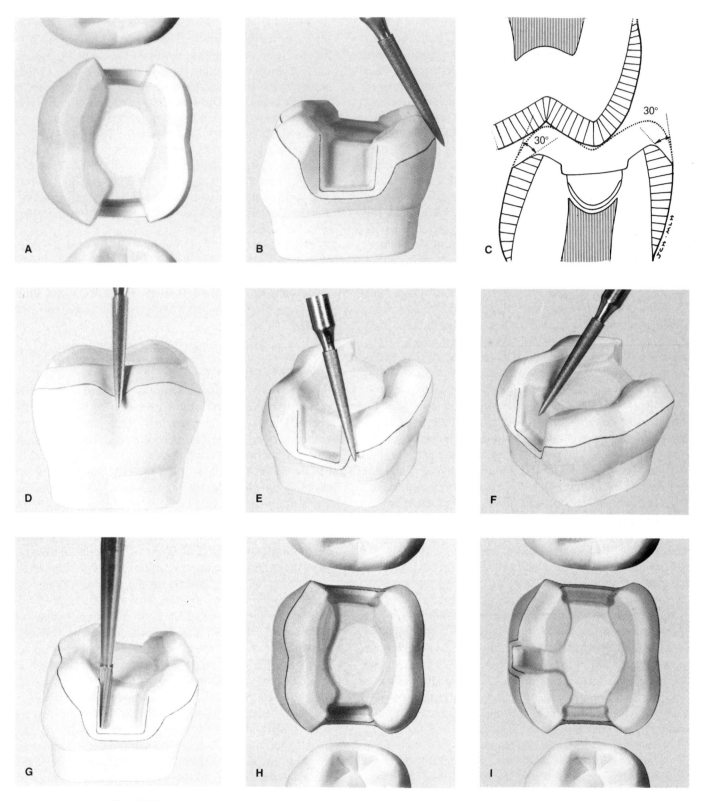

Fig. 19-26. A, Caries has been removed, and cement base has been inserted. **B,** Counterbeveling facial and lingual margins of reduced cusps. **C,** Section of **B. D,** Fissure that extends slightly gingival to normal position of counterbevel may be included by slightly deepening counterbevel in fissured area. **E,** Slightly round the junctions between counterbevels and secondary flares. **F,** Lightly bevel axiopulpal line angle. **G,** Improving retention form by cutting proximal grooves. **H,** Completed mesioocclusodistal onlay cavity preparation. **I,** Completed MODF onlay cavity preparation showing extension to include facial surface groove/fissure.

erous width and should be at such an angle that results in 30-degree marginal metal. The best way to judge this is to always maintain a 30-degree angle between the side of the instrument and the external enamel surface beyond the counterbevel (Fig. 19-26, *B* and *C*). *The counterbevel should be wide enough so that the cavosurface margin is beyond (gingival to) any contact with the opposing dentition.*

If a facial (lingual) surface fissure extends slightly beyond the normal position of the counterbevel, an option is to include (remove) the remaining fissure by deepening the counterbevel in the region of the fissure (Fig. 19-26, *D*). However, if the fissure extends gingivally more than 0.5 mm, then manage the fissure as described in the next section, Facial or Lingual Surface Groove Extension.

The counterbevel is not placed on the facial cusps of maxillary premolars and first molars where the esthetic requirement dictates only a blunting and smoothing of the enamel margin by the light application of a fine-garnet disc or the fine-grit diamond instrument (flame-shaped) held at a right angle to the facial surface (Fig. 19-23, *C*). The surface created by this blunting should be approximately 0.5 mm in width.

For beveling the gingival margins and flaring (secondary) the proximal enamel walls, refer to the inlay section, Bevels and Flares.

After beveling and flaring, slightly round any sharp junctions between the counterbevels and the secondary flares (Fig. 19-26, *E*). The fine-grit diamond instrument is also used to lightly bevel the axiopulpal line angles (Fig. 19-26, *F*). Such a bevel produces a stronger wax pattern at this critical region. Slightly round any sharp projecting corners in the preparation, since these projections are difficult to reproduce without voids when developing the working cast and often cause difficulties when seating the casting. *Note: the desirable metal angle at the margins of onlays is 40 degrees, except at the gingivally directed margins, where the metal angle should be 30 degrees.*

Shallow (0.3 mm deep) retention grooves may be cut in the facioaxial and the linguoaxial line angles with the No. 169L carbide bur (Fig. 19-26, *G*). These grooves are especially important for retention when the prepared tooth is short, which is often the case after reducing all the cusps. When properly positioned, the grooves are in dentin near the dentinoenamel junction, yet are not undermining the enamel at the expense of dentin that is immediately supporting the enamel. The direction of cutting (translation of the bur) is parallel to the dentinoenamel junction. The long axis of the bur continually must be held parallel to the line of draw.

The model showing the completed cavity preparation is illustrated in Fig. 19-26, *H*.

Facial or lingual surface groove extension

A facial surface fissure (mandibular molar) or a lingual surface fissure (maxillary molar) is included in the outline in the same manner as described in the inlay section, Facial or Lingual Surface Groove Extension. *This extension is sometimes indicated to provide additional retention form even though the groove is not faulty.* A completed MODF onlay preparation on a mandibular first molar is illustrated in Fig. 19-26, *I*.

Including portions of the facial and lingual smooth surfaces affected by caries, fractured cusps, or other injury

For inclusion of shallow to moderate lesions on the facial and lingual smooth surfaces, refer to the inlay section, Including Portions of the Facial and Lingual Smooth Surfaces Affected by Caries or Other Injury.

A mandibular molar with a fractured mesiolingual cusp is used to illustrate the treatment of a fractured cusp of a molar (Fig. 19-27, *A*). Use a No. 271 carbide bur to cut a shoulder perpendicular to occlusal force by extending the proximal gingival floor (adjacent to the fracture) to include the affected surface. This shoulder partially provides the desired resistance form by virtue of being perpendicular to gingivally directed occlusal force. Use this instrument also to create a longitudinal wall in the remaining lingual enamel (Fig. 19-27, *B*). The width of the gingival floor should be the diameter of the end of the cutting instrument. The longitudinal walls should have the degree of draft to contribute to retention form. If the clinical crown of the tooth is short, it is advisable to cut proximal grooves for additional retention with the No. 169L bur. The linguogingival and lingual margins are beveled with the flame-shaped, fine-grit diamond instrument to provide 30-degree metal at the gingival margin (Fig. 19-27, *C*) and 40-degree metal along the lingual margin (Fig. 19-27, *D*). These two bevels should blend together in the arc of a small circle (*x* in Fig. 19-27, *E*), and the linguogingival bevel is continuous with the gingival bevel on the mesial surface. Additional features to improve retention and resistance forms are indicated and can be developed by a mesiofacial skirt extension or by a facial groove extension. These preparation features, discussed in the following section, both (1) improve retention form and (2) resist forces normally opposed by the missing mesiolingual wall and help to protect the restored tooth from further fracture injury.

Enhancing resistance and retention forms

It has already been noted that when the tooth crown is short (which is often the case when all cusps are reduced), the operator must strive to maximize *retention form* in the preparation. Retention features that have al-

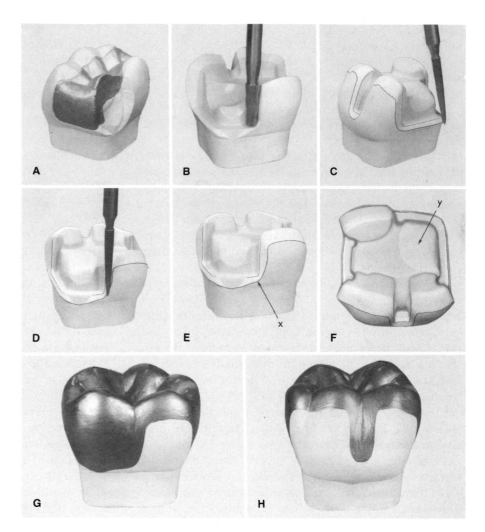

Fig. 19-27. A, Mandibular first molar with large mesioocclusodistal amalgam and fractured mesiolingual cusp. **B,** Cavity preparation (minus bevels and flares) for MODFL onlay to restore fractured molar shown in **A.** No. 271 carbide bur is used to prepare gingival shoulder and longitudinal lingual wall. Reducing cusps for capping and extending out facial groove improve retention and resistance forms. **C** and **D,** Beveling margins. **E** and **F,** Completed cavity preparation. Gingival and lingual bevels blend at *x,* and *y* is cement base. **G** and **H,** Completed onlay.

ready been mentioned follow:

1. The minimal amount of taper (2 degrees per wall) on the longitudinal walls of the preparation
2. The addition of proximal retention grooves
3. Preparation of facial (or lingual) surface groove extensions

If it is judged that the preparation needs *additional retention form,* then skirts, collars, or slots can be used.

In the preparation of a tooth that has been grossly weakened by caries or previous filling material and is judged to be prone to fracture under occlusal loads, the *resistance form* that cusp capping provides should be augmented by the use of skirts, collars, or facial (lingual) surface groove extensions. When properly placed, these features result in onlays that will distribute occlusal forces over most or all of the tooth and not a portion of it, thus reducing the likelihood of fractures of the teeth, as depicted in Fig. 19-28, *A* and *B. The lingual "skirt" extension(s)* (Fig. 19-28, *C* to *E*), *the lingual "collar" preparation* (Fig. 19-28, *F*), *or the lingual surface groove extension on a maxillary molar serve to*

protect the facial cusp(s) from fracture. The facial skirt extension(s), the facial collar preparation, or the facial surface groove extension on a mandibular molar serve to protect the lingual cusp(s) from fracture.

Skirt preparation. Skirts are thin extensions of the facial or lingual proximal margins of the cast metal onlay that extend from the secondary flare to a termination just past the transitional line angle of the tooth. The addition of skirt extensions is presented first, since it is effective as a conservative method of improving both the retention form and the resistance form of the preparation. It is relatively atraumatic to the health of the tooth, since it involves cutting very little (if any) dentin. Usually the skirt extensions are prepared entirely in enamel.

When the proximal portion of a Class II cavity preparation for an onlay is being prepared and the lingual wall is partially or totally missing, retention form normally provided by this wall can be developed with a skirt extension of the facial margin (Fig. 19-29, *A* to *C*). Similarly, if the facial wall is not retentive, a skirt extension of the lingual margin will supply the desired

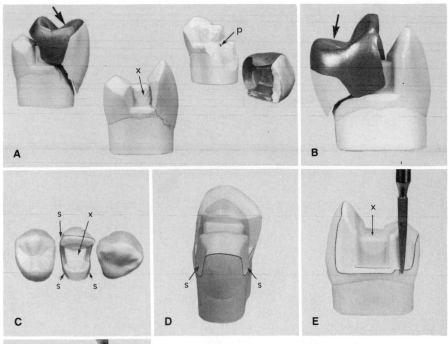

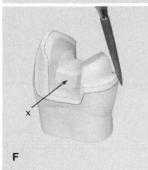

Fig. 19-28. Large cement base *x* indicates severely weakened tooth crown. Occlusal force *(heavy arrow)* may fracture facial cusp **(A)** or lingual cusp **(B),** which may expose pulp *(p)*. **C** and **D,** "Skirt" extensions *(s)* on mesiolingual, distolingual, and distofacial transitional line angles prevent fractures shown in **A** and **B**. Esthetic consideration contraindicates skirting mesiofacial line angle. **E,** Distal view of preparation shown in **D.** Skirt extensions are prepared with fine-grit diamond instrument. **F,** "Collar" preparation around lingual cusp prevents fracture shown in **A**.

retention form (Fig. 19-24, *O* and *P*). When both the lingual and facial walls of a proximal boxing are inadequate, skirt extensions on both the respective lingual and facial margins can satisfy retention and resistance form requirements. *The addition of properly prepared skirts to three of four line angles of the tooth virtually eliminates the chance of postrestorative fracture of the tooth, since the skirting onlay is primarily an extracoronal restoration that encompasses and braces the tooth against forces that might otherwise split the tooth.* The skirting onlay is often used successfully for many teeth that exhibit the **split-tooth syndrome** (see Examination of the Patient in Pain, in Chapter 5).

The addition of skirt extensions is also recommended when the proximal surface contour and contact are to be extended more than the normal dimension to create contact. Extending these proximal margins well on the respective facial and lingual surfaces *aids in recontouring the proximal surface to this increased dimension.* Also, when improving the occlusal plane of a mesially tilted molar by a cusp capping onlay, reshaping the mesial

surface to a satisfactory contour and contact is aided when the mesiofacial and mesiolingual margins are extended generously (see Restoring the Occlusal Plane of a Tilted Molar).

Skirting is also recommended when splinting posterior teeth together with onlays. The added retention and resistance form is very desirable, since the stress on each unit is increased. Because the facial and lingual proximal margins are extended generously, the soldering of the connector(s) and the finishing of the proximal margins are greatly aided.

A disadvantage of skirting is that it increases the display of metal on the facial and lingual surfaces of the tooth. For this reason skirts are not placed on the mesiofacial margin of maxillary premolars and first molars. Skirting the remaining three line angles of the tooth provides ample retention and resistance form.

The preparation of a skirt is done entirely with the slender, flame-shaped, fine-grit diamond instrument. Skirt preparations follow the completion of the proximal gingival bevel and secondary flares. The experienced

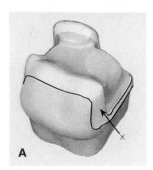

A

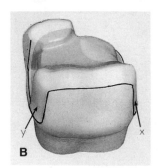

B

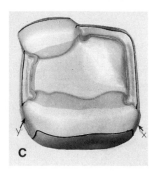

C

Fig. 19-29. For legend see facing page.

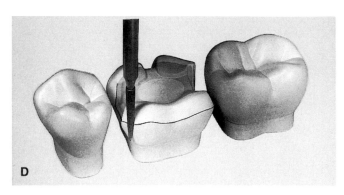

D

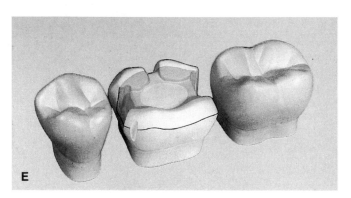

E

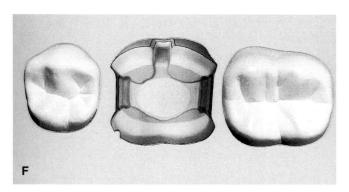

F

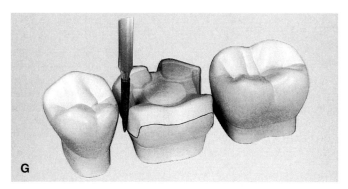

G

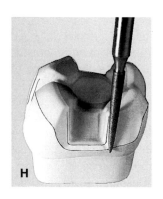

H

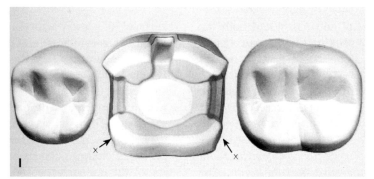

I

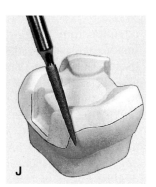

J

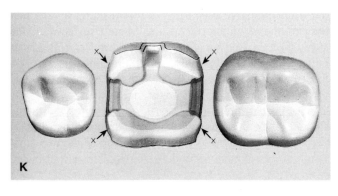

K

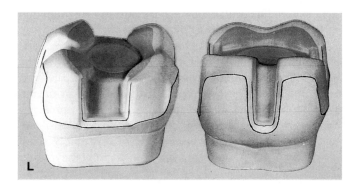

L

Fig. 19-29. A, When lingual wall of proximal boxing is inadequate or missing, retention form can be improved by facial skirt extension *(x)*. **B,** Faciooclusal view of **A.** Maximal resistance form is developed by skirting distofacial *(y)* and mesiofacial *(x)* transitional line angles. **C,** Occlusal view of **B. D** to **F,** Initial cut for skirt is placed just past transitional line angle of tooth. **G** and **H,** Blending skirt into secondary flare. **I,** Occlusal view showing mesiolingual and distolingual skirts. Caution is exercised to prevent over-reduction of transitional line angles *(x)*. Facial surface groove extension also improves both retention and resistance forms. **J,** Slightly round the junction of skirt and counterbevel. **K,** Skirting all four transitional line angles of tooth further enhances retention and resistance forms. Again, caution is exercised to prevent over-reduction of transitional line angles *(x)*. **L,** Mesial and facial views of preparation shown in **K.**

operator, realizing beforehand that the resistance and retention form of the preparation should be enhanced with skirts, will often prepare the skirt extensions at the same time that the secondary flares and gingival bevel are placed, working from the lingual toward the facial or vice versa. Maintaining the long axis of the instrument parallel to the line of draw, translate the rotating instrument into the tooth to create a definite longitudinal margin just beyond the line angle of the tooth, providing at the same time a 140-degree cavosurface enamel angle (40-degree metal angle) (Fig. 19-29, *D* to *F*). The occlusogingival length of this entrance cut will vary depending on the length of the clinical crown and the amount of extracoronal retention and resistance forms desired. *Extending into the gingival third of the anatomical crown is usually necessary for effective resistance*

form. Note that in most instances the gingival margin of the skirt extension is occlusal to the position of the gingival bevel of the proximal box (Fig. 19-29, *H* and *L*).

The operator must exercise caution to always use less than one half the tip diameter of the flame-shaped diamond instrument to avoid creating a ledge at the gingival margin of the skirt extension. Using high speed and maintaining the long axis of the diamond instrument parallel with the line of draw, translate the instrument from the entrance cut toward the proximal box to blend the skirt into the secondary flare and the proximal gingival margin (Fig. 19-29, *G* and *H*). *Be sure not to over-reduce the line angle of the tooth when preparing skirt extensions (x in Fig. 19-29, I and K).* If the line angle of the tooth is over-reduced, the bracing effect of the skirt will be greatly diminished.

Holding the diamond instrument at the same angle that was used for preparing the counterbevel, round the junction between the skirt and the counterbevel so that it has the radius of a small circle (Fig. 19-29, *J*). Be sure to slightly round any sharp angles that remain after preparation of the skirt, since these often lead to difficulties in subsequent steps of completing the restoration.

Collar preparation. To increase the retention and resistance forms when preparing a weakened tooth for a mesioocclusodistal onlay capping all cusps, a facial or lingual "collar," or both, may be provided (Fig. 19-30). To satisfy esthetics, however, the facial surfaces of maxillary premolars and first molars should not be prepared for a collar.

Use a No. 271 carbide bur at high speed parallel to

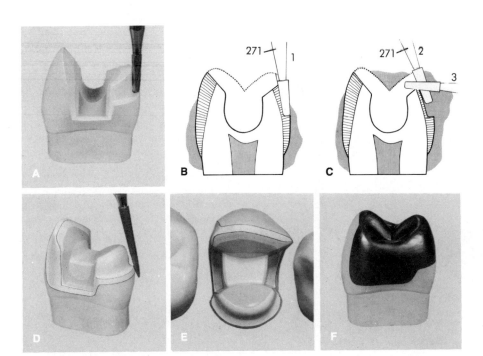

Fig. 19-30. A, First position of bur in preparing for lingual collar on weakened maxillary premolar. Section drawings of first position of bur (**B**) and second and third positions (**C**). **D,** Beveling lingual margin. Note distofacial skirt extension. **E,** Completed cavity preparation. **F,** Completed onlay.

the line of draw to prepare a 0.8 mm deep shoulder (equivalent to the diameter of the tip end of the bur) around the lingual (or facial) surface to provide for a collar about 2 to 3 mm high occlusogingivally (Fig. 19-30, *A* and *B*). To provide for a uniform thickness of metal, the occlusal 1 mm of this reduction should be "rolled in" to follow the original contour of the tooth (Fig. 19-30, *C*). Also, this rolling-in should round any undesirable sharp line angle formed by the union of the prepared lingual and occlusal surfaces. Complete this aspect of the preparation by lightly beveling the gingival margin of the shoulder with the flame-shaped, fine-grit diamond instrument to result in a 30-degree metal angle at the margin (Fig. 19-30, *D*).

Slot preparation. Occasionally the use of a slot in the dentin is helpful to provide the necessary retention form. An example is the mandibular second molar that has no molar posterior to it and that requires a mesioocclusal onlay restoration capping all of the cusps (Fig. 19-31, *A* to *C*). The distal, facial, and lingual surfaces are free of caries or other injury, and these surfaces are judged not to be prone to caries. After cusp reduction the longitudinal walls of the occlusal step portion of the cavity preparation have been so reduced as to offer very little retention form. The necessary retention can be achieved by cutting a distal slot. Such a slot is preferred over cutting a box in the distal surface because (1) the former is more conserving of tooth structure and of strength of the tooth crown, and (2) the linear extent of marginal outline is less.

To form this slot, use a No. 169L carbide bur whose long axis should parallel the line of draw (this must be reasonably close to a line parallel with the long axis of the tooth) (Fig. 19-31, *A*). The slot is cut in dentin so that if it were to be extended gingivally, it would pass midway between the pulp and the dentinoenamel junction (Fig. 19-31, *C*). Such a position and direction of the slot averts (1) exposure of the pulp, (2) removal of the dentin supporting the distal enamel, and (3) perforation of the distal surface of the tooth at the gingival termination of the slot. The slot should have the following approximate dimensions: (1) mesiodistally, the width (diameter) of the bur; (2) faciolingually, 2 mm; and (3) depth, 2 mm gingival of the normally positioned pulpal wall. To be effective, the mesial wall of the slot must be in sound dentin; otherwise different measures must be resorted to for sufficient retention form.

A comparable situation occasionally occurs in which the maxillary first premolar requires a distoocclusal onlay restoration capping the cusps and the mesial surface is noncarious and judged not prone to caries (Fig. 19-31, *D* to *F*). To satisfy esthetics and to conserve tooth structure, a slot similar to that described in the preceding paragraph, except that it is mesially positioned and 1.5 mm wide faciolingually, may be used for the production of adequate retention. The mesial occlusal marginal outline in this cavity preparation should be distal of the height of the mesial marginal ridge.

Modifications for esthetics on maxillary premolars and first molars

To minimize the display of metal on maxillary premolars and first molars, several modifications for esthetics are made to the basic onlay preparation. On the fa-

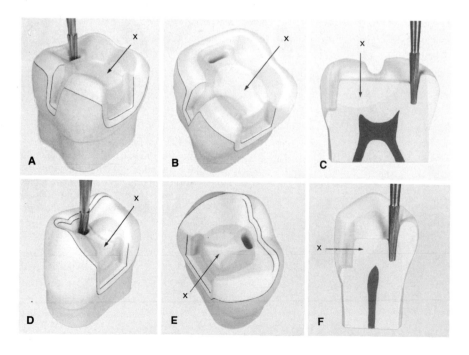

Fig. 19-31. **A** and **B,** Cutting distal slot for retention for mesioocclusal onlay to treat terminal molar having large cement base *(x)* resulting from extensive occlusal and mesial caries. **C,** Section of **A. D** and **E,** Preparing mesial slot for retention for distoocclusal onlay to treat maxillary first premolar that has large cement base *(x)*. **F,** Section of **D.**

cial cusps of maxillary premolars and on the mesiofacial cusp of the maxillary first molar the occlusal reduction should only be 1 mm on the facial cusp ridge to decrease the display of metal. This thickness should increase progressively to 1.5 mm toward the center of the tooth to help provide rigidity to the capping metal. Furthermore, these cusps do not receive a counterbevel but are "stubbed" or blunted by the application of a fine-garnet disc or the fine-grit diamond instrument held at a right angle to the facial surface (Fig. 19-23, *C*). The surface created by this blunting should be approximately 0.5 mm in width.

To further decrease the display of metal on maxillary premolars and first molars, the mesiofacial margin is minimally extended facially of contact to such a position that the margin is barely visible from a facial viewing position. To accomplish this, the secondary flare is omitted, and the wall and margin are developed with a chisel or enamel hatchet. Final smoothing with the medium-cuttle paper disc is recommended when access permits.

When more than ideal extension of the mesiofacial margin is necessary because of caries or previous restorations, and when the esthetic desires of the patient dictate, the operator may choose to place a composite resin insert at this margin. Many times this is a better and more conservative option than preparing the tooth to receive a porcelain-veneered metal crown. When preparing the mesiofacial margin, no attempt is made to develop a straight mesiofacial wall past the point of ideal extension. After caries excavation a glass ionomer cement base is inserted to temporarily form the missing portion of the wall. The cement is contoured to ideal form, and the cavity preparation can continue, terminating the mesiofacial onlay margin in ideal position in the cement. Following cementation, remove (with small round burs) the glass ionomer cement to a depth of 1 mm for a composite resin insert. Small undercuts should be prepared in the wall formed by the cast metal onlay (see Figs. 18-42, *B*, and 19-69, *A*). (It is always best to carve the undercut in the wall formed by the onlay during the wax pattern stage.) After beveling the enamel cavosurface margin and preparing a gingival retention groove where and if enamel is thin or missing, insert the composite veneer (see Figs. 18-42, *D*, and 19-77, *A*). (For more details on placing a composite insert, see Veneers for Existing Metal Restorations, in Chapter 18.)

Root canal filled teeth

Routinely teeth that have had root canal fillings are weak and subject to fracture from occlusal forces. These teeth require restorations that are thoughtfully designed to provide protection from this injury (Fig. 19-29, *K* and *L*). This particularly applies to the posterior teeth, which receive greater stress. The need for such protection is accentuated when much of the strength of the tooth has been lost because of extensive caries or previous restorations. When the facial and lingual surfaces of a root canal treated tooth are sound, it is advisable, for the health of the facial and lingual gingival tissues, not to prepare the tooth for a full crown but for a mesioocclusodistal onlay that has been designed with adequate resistance form to prevent future tooth fracture. Such features include skirt extensions and collar preparations. These features make the onlay more of an extracoronal restoration that encompasses the tooth, such that the tooth is better able to resist lateral forces that might otherwise fracture the tooth.

Before starting the preparation of a root canal treated molar, the pulp chamber should be excavated to the chamber floor and an amalgam foundation placed. This will give the onlay a firm base on which to rest. In the preparation of a root canal treated premolar for an onlay, the canal should first be prepared for a custom cast metal post, which is cemented in the canal before the onlay preparation is completed. This post will help the tooth resist forces that might otherwise cause a horizontal fracture of the entire tooth crown from the root. The cast post should extend roughly two-thirds the length of the root and should terminate leaving at least 3 mm of the root canal filling at the apical portion of the root.

Restoring the occlusal plane of a tilted molar

The onlay that caps all cusps is excellent for restoring the occlusal plane of a mesially tilted molar (Fig. 19-32). When the unprepared occlusal surface (mesial portion) is short of the desired occlusal plane, a corresponding decrease in occlusal surface reduction is indicated. To facilitate increasing the height of the tooth and yet maintain the desirable faciolingual dimension of the restored occlusal surface and good contour of the facial and lingual surfaces, the counterbevels on the latter surfaces often should be extended gingivally more than usual (Fig. 19-32, *B*).

Furthermore, often the mesiofacial and mesiolingual margins (on the "submerged" proximal surface) should be well extended on the respective facial and lingual surfaces to help in recontouring the mesial surface to desirable proximal surface contour and contact. This extension can be accomplished with a minimal loss of tooth structure by preparing facial and lingual skirt extensions on the respective proximal margins. Moreover, as previously cited, skirting improves retention and resistance forms. In comparison, achieving extension by cutting the mesiofacial and mesiolingual walls facially and lingually respectively does not improve retention or resistance forms and is less conservative of tooth structure.

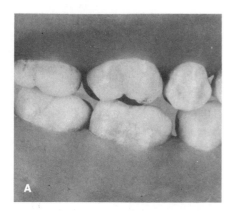
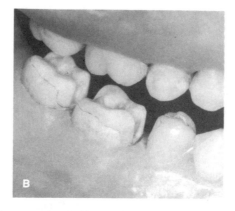
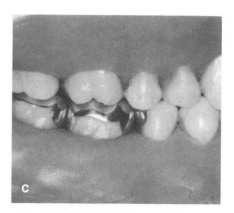

Fig. 19-32. A, Mandibular second and third molars tilted mesially, often the result of failure to replace lost first molar by bridgework. Note poor contact relationship between molars and between molar and second premolar. **B,** Second premolar is prepared for inlay, and molars are prepared for onlays. Margins of preparations are well-extended on facial and lingual surfaces to aid in recontouring teeth to improve occlusal relationship and to improve proximal contours and contacts. **C,** Completed restorations. Note improvement both in occlusal plane and in proximal contacts.

VERIFYING CUSP REDUCTION

After cusp reduction, visually verify that the occlusal clearances are sufficient. A *functionally generated paths (FGP)* interocclusal record is helpful when checking occlusal clearances, especially in areas difficult to visualize, such as in the central groove/lingual cusp regions. To make a FGP interocclusal record, first dry the preparation(s) free of visible moisture; do not, however, desiccate the dentin (Fig. 19-33, *A*). Next lightly press a portion of softened, low-fusing inlay wax over the *prepared* tooth (teeth); then immediately request the patient to close into the soft wax and slide the teeth in all directions (Fig. 19-33, *B* to *F*). During the mandibular movements, observe to verify that (1) the patient moves in right lateral, left lateral, and protrusive movements; (2) the adjacent unprepared teeth are in contact with the opposing teeth; (3) the wax in the cavity(ies) is stable (not loose and rocking); and (4) the wax is not in infraocclusion. Drying the cavity walls of visible moisture before applying the wax causes the wax to stick to the teeth just enough to prevent the patient from rocking the wax loose while registering the "functionally generated paths." Now cool and carefully remove the wax. Hold it up to a light, and note the degree of light transmitted. With experience, this is a good indicator of the thickness of the wax. An alternative method is to use wax calipers, or to section the wax to verify its thickness. Insufficient thickness calls for more reduction in the indicated area before proceeding.

INTEROCCLUSAL RECORDS

Before preparation of the tooth, the occlusal contacts in maximum intercuspal position and in all lateral and protrusive movements should have been carefully evaluated (see Figs. 2-47 through 2-60).

If the patient has sufficient canine guidance to provide disocclusion of the posterior teeth, then the necessary registration of the opposing teeth can be obtained by (1) making a *maximum intercuspal position (IP) interocclusal record* of wax or one of several commercially available bite registration pastes, or (2) making full-arch impressions and mounting the casts made from these impressions on a simple hinge articulator. The interocclusal record works well when preparing one tooth; the full-arch casts are preferred when more than two prepared teeth are involved. The IP interocclusal record can be made by drying the preparation with compressed air to remove visible moisture, and then pressing a portion of softened, low-fusing inlay wax over the prepared tooth. Immediately have the patient close completely into the soft wax. Observe to verify that the adjacent unprepared teeth are in maximum intercuspal position and that there is enough wax to fully record the opposing occlusal surfaces. The wax is chilled with a gentle stream of compressed air, carefully removed from the teeth, and set aside for later use in the laboratory.

The IP interocclusal record can also be made from one of several commercially available bite registration pastes used in conjunction with a disposable gauze-cov-

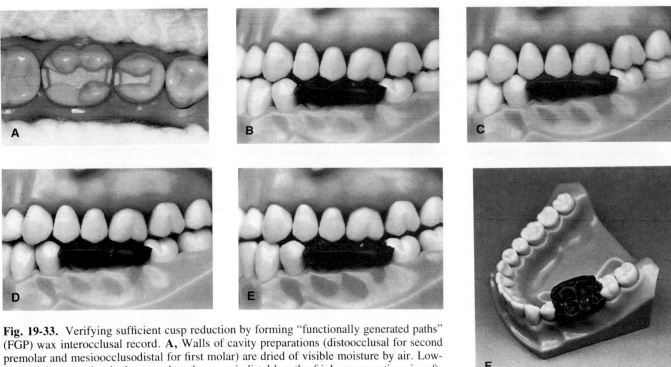

Fig. 19-33. Verifying sufficient cusp reduction by forming "functionally generated paths" (FGP) wax interocclusal record. **A,** Walls of cavity preparations (distoocclusal for second premolar and mesioocclusodistal for first molar) are dried of visible moisture by air. Low-fusing inlay wax that is the same length as mesiodistal length of inlay preparations is softened and pressed over prepared teeth; patient then registers "functionally generated paths" in soft wax. Patient moves mandible into all occlusal positions, left lateral **(B),** through maximum intercuspal position **(C),** to right lateral **(D),** and to protrusive **(E). F,** Completed FGP interocclusal record.

ered bite frame (Fig. 19-34, *A*). The most commonly used bite registration pastes are composed of heavily filled silicone or polyether impression materials. Several materials are available in cartridge systems that automatically mix the base and accelerator pastes together as they are expressed through a special disposable mixing tip. Other systems require the hand mixing of two pastes together on a paper pad. The mixed impression material is applied to both sides of a gauze-covered bite frame (Fig. 19-34, *B*). Usually a layer 2 mm thick on both sides of the frame is sufficient. The frame is positioned over the maxillary teeth so that no portion of the frame will interfere with closure, and then the patient closes completely (Fig. 19-34, *C*). Observe the teeth that are not hidden by the bite registration paste to verify that the teeth are in maximum intercuspal position. Once the material has set, remove the interocclusal record from the teeth and inspect it for completeness (Fig. 19-34, *D*). When held up to a light, there should be areas where the adjacent unprepared teeth have penetrated through the paste leaving only the thin gauze mesh intact. The interocclusal record is set aside for later use in the laboratory.

The IP interocclusal records described in the previous paragraph provide information on the shape and position of the opposing teeth in maximum intercuspal position. Such records give the laboratory technician some information on how to form the occlusal surface and position occlusal contacts on the restoration, but supply no data on how these structures and contacts might function during mandibular movements. *This is also true when **full-arch casts** are mounted on a **simple hinge articulator.*** Cast metal restorations made with these simple bite registration techniques often require major adjustments in the mouth to alleviate interferences during mandibular movements.

If information is desired in the laboratory about the pathways of cusps during mandibular movements (such as when the tooth is to be restored in group function), then a registration must be made of the opposing teeth and their functional paths by (1) making a **FGP** interocclusal record which will be used in the laboratory to make a cast of the functional pathways of the cusps (this cast is termed a **functional core),** or (2) making full-arch impressions and mounting the casts made from these impressions on a properly adjusted semi-adjustable articulator. The FGP interocclusal record works well when one or two teeth are prepared; the full-arch casts are preferred when more than two prepared teeth are involved. The FGP interocclusal record made when

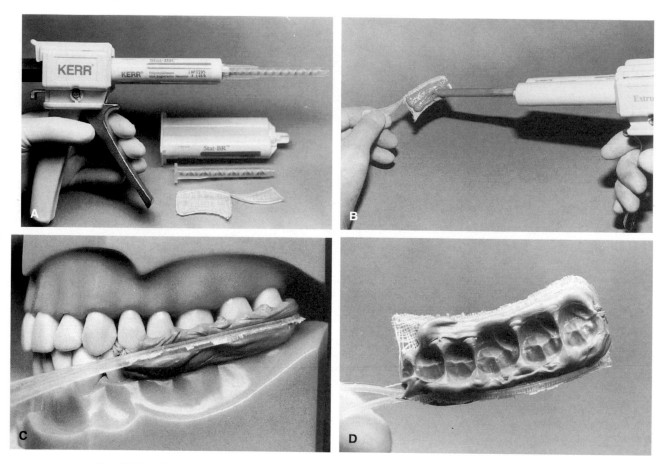

Fig. 19-34. *Maximum intercuspal position (IP) interocclusal record* made with polyvinyl siloxane bite registration paste. **A,** One of many commercially available bite registration pastes and gauze-covered bite frame used in this technique. **B,** Using cartridge dispenser and disposable auto-mixing tip, the base and accelerator pastes are automatically mixed and applied to both sides of bite frame (2 mm thick on each side). **C,** Seeing that no portion of bite frame interferes with closure, have patient close into maximum intercuspal position. Be sure that adjacent, unprepared teeth are touching in their normal relationships. **D,** Remove IP interocclusal record carefully after it has set, and inspect it for completeness. There should be areas where adjacent, unprepared teeth have penetrated through paste.

verifying clearance of the reduced cusps may be used for making the functional core in the laboratory if it was made carefully and was not sectioned or damaged when clearances were checked. The reader is referred to the previous section, Verifying Cusp Reduction, for details of how the FGP interocclusal record is made.

FGP interocclusal records can register the interactions of anterior guidance, horizontal condylar inclination, cusp inclines, and occlusal contact positions. Faciolingual, longitudinal cross sections through FGP records are depicted for four different occlusions in Fig. 19-35, *A* to *D*. Assuming a normal arrangement of teeth (no cross-bites), the inclined surfaces that can potentially contact during lateral mandibular movements on the non-working (nonfunction) side are the lingual inclines of the mandibular facial cusps and the facial inclines of the maxillary lingual cusps. In Fig. 19-35, *A*

to *C*, the pathways of the mandibular right molars during left lateral mandibular movements, *a*, have steeper inclinations than the cusp inclines that might contact during these movements, *b*. The inclinations of these non-working pathways are determined by the anterior guidance on the opposite (working) side and by the horizontal condylar guidance on the same (non-working) side. In the circumstances illustrated in Fig. 19-35, *A* to *C*, the centric holding (or supporting) cusps of the right maxillary molar wax pattern can be positioned on the opposing tooth with some assurance that they will not interfere (contact) during left lateral mandibular movements. Occasionally the non-working pathway is not as steep as the aforementioned cusp inclines (Fig. 19-35, *D*). When making the FGP record in this situation, the wax along the non-working pathway will be pushed aside and display a shiny, burnished surface. To prevent

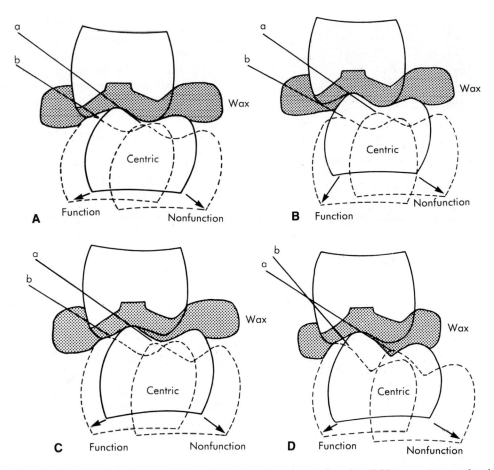

Fig. 19-35. A to **D,** Cross sections of *functionally generated paths (FGP) wax interocclusal records.* **A** illustrates FGP interocclusal record for "group function" occlusion where inclination of nonfunctional pathway *(a)* is steeper than nonfunctional cusp inclines *(b).* In this instance the centric holding cusps of the right maxillary molar wax pattern can be positioned on the opposing tooth with some assurance they will not interfere (contact) during left lateral mandibular movements (nonfunction). **B** is the same as **A** except that it shows steeper functional pathway seen in "canine guided" occlusions. **C** is an example of maxillary lingual cusp not originally in centric (IP) contact. However, because cuspal inclination *(b)* is less than angulation of nonfunctional pathway *(a),* potential nonfunctional interferences will not be recorded in FGP interocclusal record. **D** is an example of maxillary lingual cusp not originally in centric contact with mandibular fossa. Because of increased angulation and length of nonfunctional cusp inclines *(b),* nonfunctional contact potential will be recorded in FGP interocclusal record.

generating non-working contacts on the restoration in this circumstance, either: (1) the cusp must be repositioned to an alternate area where there is adequate disocclusion (where there were no burnished marks on the FGP interocclusal record), or (2) some adjustments to the opposing occlusal surface may be indicated to make the opposing cusp inclines less steep (raising opposing fossa by restoration and/or shortening opposing centric holding cusp). Obviously the cross-section diagrams in Fig. 19-35 cannot depict the intricacies of occlusal groove location and direction and how these factors affect the proper location of cusps and contacts. For maximal assurance that the centric holding cusps will not interfere on the non-working side, full-arch casts mounted

via a facebow transfer on a semi-adjustable articulator provide the necessary information in the laboratory on how to position the cusps so that such interferences do not occur (Fig. 19-36).

*The use of **full-arch casts** mounted on a **semi-adjustable articulator** is highly recommended when restoring a large portion of the patient's posterior occlusion with cast metal restorations.* It involves very little extra chair time and gives the laboratory technician much more information to work with (i.e., the general occlusal scheme, pathways of cusps, opposing cusp steepness and groove direction, and the anatomy of the other teeth in the mouth). The technique involves using a full-arch tray when making the final impression, and this in-

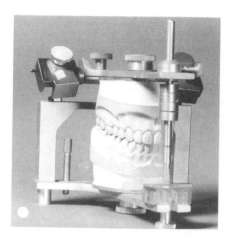

Fig. 19-36. Full-arch casts mounted via a facebow transfer on a semi-adjustable articulator provide maximal information in the laboratory on how to position cusps to prevent undesirable contacts.

volves mixing more material, especially when using stock trays. The opposing arch is impressed with alginate impression material, and the appropriate mandibular movement and face-bow transfer records are made. The reader is referred to Chapter 2 for principles regarding the use of the semi-adjustable articulator in developing proper occlusal relationships for cast metal restorations.

RESIN TEMPORARY

Between the time the tooth is prepared and the cast metal restoration is delivered, it is important that the patient be comfortable and the tooth be protected and stabilized with an adequate temporary restoration. The temporary restoration should satisfy the following *requirements:*

1. It should be non-irritating, and it should protect the prepared tooth from injury.
2. It should protect and maintain the health of the periodontium.
3. It should maintain the position of the prepared, adjacent, and opposing teeth.
4. It should provide for esthetic, phonetic, and masticatory function as indicated.
5. It should be easily cleaned by the patient.
6. It should have adequate strength and retention to withstand the forces to which it will be subjected.

When properly made, the custom resin temporary can satisfy the above requirements and is the preferred temporary restoration. Resin temporaries can be fabricated intraorally directly on the prepared teeth *(direct technique)* or outside of the mouth using a postoperative cast of the prepared teeth *(indirect technique).*

Technique for indirect temporary

The **indirect temporary technique** *has the following advantages:*

1. It has been shown that the marginal accuracy of indirect resin temporaries is significantly better than that of temporaries made by the direct technique.[8] Accurate marginal fit is desirable to prevent cement washout and pulpal irritation due to penetration of oral fluids and bacteria. Good marginal fit also promotes good oral hygiene and periodontal health.
2. The indirect technique avoids the possibility of "locking on" the set resin into undercuts on the prepared tooth or the adjacent teeth.
3. The indirect technique avoids placing polymerizing resin directly on freshly prepared dentin and investing soft tissue, thus reducing irritation to these tissues.[9,12,13]
4. The postoperative cast made in the indirect technique affords an opportunity to evaluate the preparation (before the final impression), and serves as an excellent guide when trimming and contouring the temporary.

To form the indirect resin temporary, first make an impression of the prepared tooth (teeth) with fast-setting alginate impression material. Use a stock, metal, perforated impression tray or a stock, plastic impression tray that has been painted with alginate tray adhesive (Fig. 19-37, *A*). Be sure that the teeth are slightly moist with saliva, and then apply some alginate over and into the preparation(s) with a fingertip to avoid or minimize trapping air (Fig. 19-37, *B*); then seat the alginate-filled tray over the region (Fig. 19-37, *C*). After the alginate has become elastic, remove the impression with a quick pull in the direction of draw of the cavity preparation(s) and inspect it for completeness (Fig. 19-37, *D*). Pour this impression with fast-setting plaster (Fig. 19-37, *E*).

As soon as the postoperative cast has been recovered from the impression, inspect the cast for any negative or positive defects (Fig. 19-37, *F*). Small voids on the cast may be filled in with utility wax. Large voids indicate repouring the impression. Positives (blebs) on the cast should be carefully removed with a suitable instrument.

Seat the postoperative cast into the preoperative impression (Fig. 19-38, *A* to *D*). Recall that the preoperative alginate impression has been wrapped in wet paper towels from the time it was made (see Fig. 19-2, *D*). Cut away the thin edges of alginate impression material that record the gingival sulcus (Fig. 19-38, *A*). If these thin edges are not removed, they may tear off and keep the postoperative cast from seating completely in the impression. Trial-seat the postoperative cast into the impression to verify that it seats completely. Usually much of the soft tissue areas registered on the impression and the cast should be removed by a knife or model trimmer

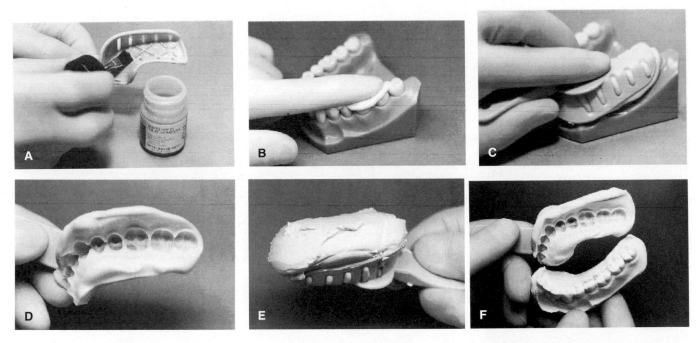

Fig. 19-37. Making a postoperative plaster cast for *indirectly* forming a resin temporary. **A,** Interior of tray is coated with alginate tray adhesive. **B,** Apply some alginate over and into preparations with fingertip to avoid trapping air. **C,** Alginate-filled tray in place. **D,** Alginate impression. **E,** Alginate impression is poured with fast-setting plaster. **F,** Plaster cast of preparations shown in Fig. 19-33, *A.*

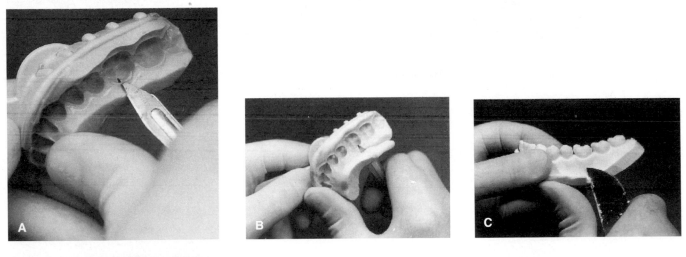

Fig. 19-38. Forming *indirect* resin temporaries for preparations initially shown in Fig. 19-33, *A.* **A,** Cut away thin edges of preoperative impression material that record gingival sulcus because these are apt to tear when seating postoperative cast in impression. **B** and **C,** Trimming away much of the soft tissue areas recorded by impression and cast also facilitates seating. **D,** Trial seating the postoperative cast into preoperative impression.

Continued.

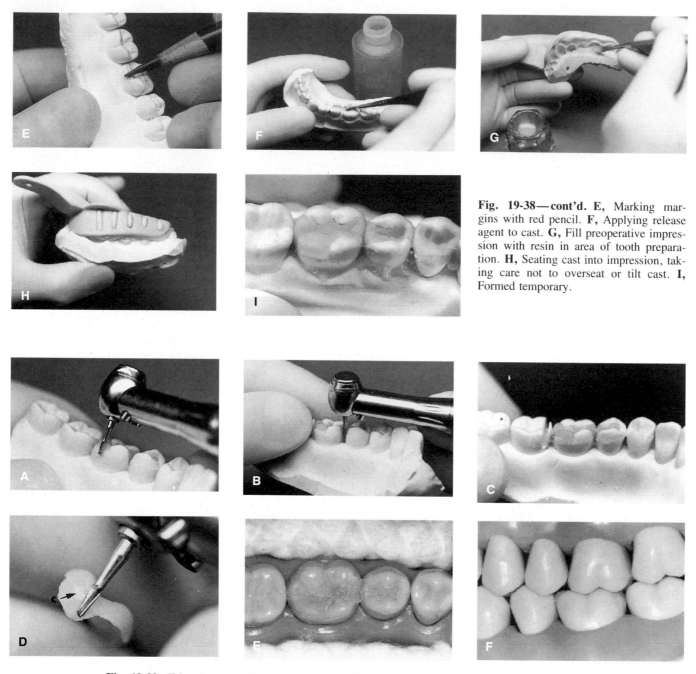

Fig. 19-38—cont'd. E, Marking margins with red pencil. **F,** Applying release agent to cast. **G,** Fill preoperative impression with resin in area of tooth preparation. **H,** Seating cast into impression, taking care not to overseat or tilt cast. **I,** Formed temporary.

Fig. 19-39. Trimming and adjusting *indirect* acrylic resin temporaries. **A,** Trim excess resin back to accessible facial and lingual margins (marked by red line on plaster cast). **B,** On multiple-unit temporaries, the slender 169L bur can be used to refine interproximal embrasure form. **C,** On cast, cut away any tooth adjacent to resin temporary. **D,** Trimming proximal surface of resin temporary to proper contour. Take care not to remove proximal contact, *c*. **E** and **F,** After final impression is made, resin temporary is cemented with zinc oxide–eugenol cement. Note anatomical contour and fit (**E**) and functional occlusion of temporary restoration (**F**).

to minimize seating problems (Fig. 19-38, *B* and *C*).

Once satisfied that the gypsum cast seats completely in the alginate impression (Fig. 19-38, *D*), remove the cast, and mark the margins of the preparations on the cast with a red pencil to facilitate trimming (Fig. 19-38, *E*). Brush a release agent on the preparations and adjacent teeth (Fig. 19-38, *F*). Mix tooth-colored temporary resin following the manufacturer's instructions. Allow some of the fluid resin to flow off the mixing spatula into the alginate impression in the area of the prepared teeth (Fig. 19-38, *G*). When adjacent teeth are prepared, the resin is continuous from one tooth to the next. Seat the cast into the preoperative impression, making sure it seats completely without tilting to one side or the other (Fig. 19-38, *H*). Do not apply too much pressure on the cast lest the temporary will be distorted and too thin in some areas. When the cast is seated, wrap the cast and the impression *passively* with a rubber band (too much pressure from the rubber band can distort the temporary), and submerge the assembly in hot water to accelerate the setting reaction. The formed temporary is shown in Fig. 19-38, *I*.

With suitable burs (No. 271 or a small acrylic bur), begin trimming away excess resin along the facial and lingual margins. The red line previously placed will help, especially if an auxiliary is trimming the temporary (Fig. 19-39, *A*). On multiple-unit temporaries, the slender 169L bur can be used to refine interproximal embrasures (Fig. 19-39, *B*). After the excess resin has been removed from the facial and lingual embrasures, cut through the adjacent unprepared tooth (teeth) 1 mm away from the proximal contact(s) (Fig. 19-39, *C*). Insert a knife into the cut, and pry off the temporary from the cast. Now improve the contour of the resin proximal surface that will contact the adjacent, unprepared tooth (Fig. 19-39, *D*). Do not disturb the contact area on the resin temporary that was accurately formed on the gypsum cast.

Try the resin temporary on the teeth (Fig. 19-39, *E*). It should fit well, make desirable contact with the adjacent teeth, and meet occlusal requirements with minimal adjustments (Fig. 19-39, *F*). If occlusal adjustments are indicated, alternately mark the prematurities with articulating paper and reduce these with a bur of suitable size. After correcting the occlusion, smooth any roughness or undesirable sharp edges with a rubber point or wheel. Remove the temporary from the mouth, and lay it aside for cementation with a temporary cement after the final impression has been made.

Technique for direct temporary

The **direct temporary technique** *involves forming the temporary restoration directly on the prepared tooth (teeth) and has the following* **advantages** (Fig. 19-40):

1. The direct technique requires no postoperative impression and gypsum cast.
2. The direct temporary can usually be completed in less time than the indirect temporary.

The main disadvantages of the direct temporary technique are: (1) there is a chance of "locking on" the hardened resin temporary into small undercuts on the prepared tooth and the adjacent teeth, (2) the marginal fit is somewhat worse than with the indirect technique,[4] (3) it is more difficult to contour the temporary without the guidelines offered by the postoperative cast, and (4) the technique involves placing unset resin directly on investing soft tissue and freshly prepared dentin. Acute pulpal and soft tissue irritation from the free monomer in the resin and thermal irritation from the resin's exothermic reaction are possible undesirable side effects.[10,16]

Forming the temporary directly on the prepared tooth requires the *preoperative* alginate impression (see Fig. 19-2, *C*). Trial seat the preoperative impression onto the teeth to verify that it seats completely. Usually some of the borders of the impression registering the soft tissues should be trimmed away to minimize seating problems (Fig. 19-40, *C*).

Since there is a potential for "locking on" the temporary when forming it directly, take great care to eliminate all undercuts in the preparation. Recall that undercuts in the preparation can and should be "blocked out" using a light-cured glass ionomer cement base (Fig. 19-40, *B*). Place a light film of petroleum jelly over any exposed cement bases to prevent them from adhering to the temporary resin. Some manufacturers recommend applying a light film of petroleum jelly over all exposed dentin surfaces to decrease pulpal irritation from unreacted resin monomers.

When using the direct technique with inlay and onlay preparations (preparations which gain their retention primarily through internal retention features), *it is helpful to select temporary resin systems which become elastic prior to final set, thus allowing removal from undercuts without permanent distortion.** Mix the temporary resin following the manufacturer's instructions. Flow some of the mixed resin into the alginate impression in the area of the prepared tooth, taking care not to entrap air (Fig. 19-40, *D*). Place the impression on the teeth, making sure it seats completely and does not tilt to one side or the other (Fig. 19-40, *E*). Follow the manufacturer's instructions for gauging the setting time of the resin. Most systems recommend monitoring the setting of the resin by rolling some excess resin into a small ball and holding it between two fingers. When the resin has set to a rubbery stage, remove the alginate im-

---

*Snap temporary resin, Parkell, Farmindale, NY.

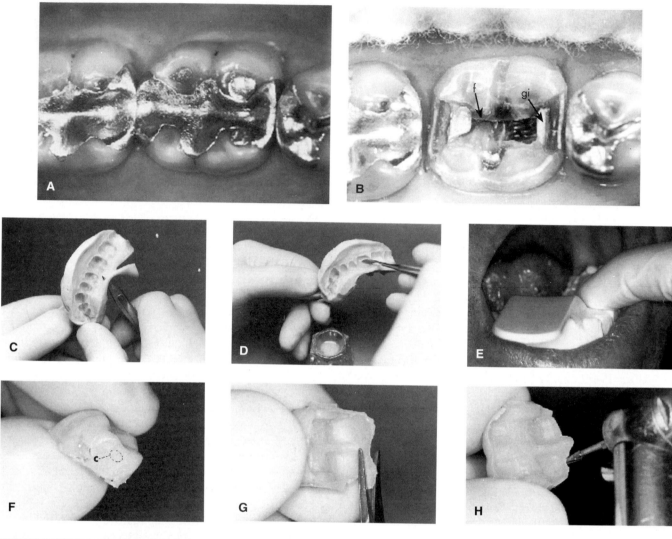

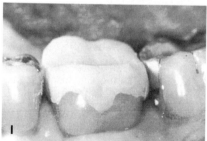

Fig. 19-40. Forming *direct* resin temporary with preoperative alginate impression. MODF onlay preparation for mandibular first molar is used for illustration. **A,** Preoperatively, patient had symptoms indicating incomplete fracture of vital tooth. **B,** After preparation for onlay, incomplete fracture *(f)* of dentin seen extending mesiodistally along pulpal floor. To maximize retention and resistance forms, all cusps are reduced for capping, a facial surface groove extension is prepared, and all four transitional line angles have skirt extensions. Glass ionomer cement bases were inserted into excavations on axial walls *(gi).* Cement bases and dentin walls should have light coat of petroleum jelly to prevent adhesion and reduce pulpal irritation from polymerizing resin. **C,** Trim away much of the border of preoperative alginate impression to facilitate seating. Trial seating of preoperative impression helps identify areas that interfere with seating. **D,** Flow mixed temporary resin into preoperative impression of prepared tooth. **E,** Seat preoperative impression with temporary resin onto prepared tooth. **F,** Formed temporary is removed from preparation (note contact area, *c,* which must not be removed during trimming). **G,** Thin excess can be removed with scissors. **H,** Internal surface of temporary has record of cavosurface margin which is used as guide for final trimming. **I,** After final impression is made, resin temporary is cemented with zinc oxide–eugenol cement. Resin over skirt extensions is left slightly overcontoured for additional strength.

pression. The formed temporary should remain on the prepared tooth. The reduced temperature of the alginate retards the setting time of most resin systems, so the temporary may not be fully elastic at this point. Test the temporary by pressing on the occlusal surface slightly, and when the resin becomes elastic and rebounds, remove it from the tooth using a Black spoon excavator. Place the temporary aside and allow it to cure completely (Figs. 19-40, *F*). When the temporary has hardened, trim away the excess resin (Fig. 19-40, *G*). The cavosurface margins of the preparation can be seen inside the resin temporary and must be used as a guide for trimming the critical external areas near the margins (Fig. 19-40, *H*). The techniques for try-in, adjustment, and finishing the direct temporary are identical as those described in the previous section (Fig. 19-40, *I*).

FINAL IMPRESSION

The indirect technique for making cast metal restorations is accurate and dependable. Fabrication of the cast metal restoration takes place in the laboratory, using a gypsum cast made from an impression of the prepared and adjacent unprepared teeth. The *impression material* used for the final impression *must* have the following *qualities:*

1. It must become *elastic* after placement in the mouth because it must be withdrawn from *undercut* regions that usually exist on the prepared and adjacent teeth. Note the shaded portions in Fig. 19-41, which are undercut areas with regard to the line of draw of the cavity preparation. A satisfactory impression must register some of this undercut surface to sharply delineate the margin and to signify the desirable contour of the restoration in regions near the margin.
2. It must have adequate strength to resist breaking

or tearing on removal from the mouth.

3. It must have adequate dimensional accuracy, stability, and reproduction of detail so that it is an exact negative imprint of the prepared and adjacent unprepared teeth.
4. It must have handling and setting characteristics that meet clinical requirements.
5. It must be free of toxic or irritating components.
6. It must be able to be disinfected without distortion.

In addition to the previously mentioned absolute requirements, the choice of impression material is usually made by comparisons of *cost, ease of use, working time, shelf life,* and *pleasantness of odor, taste, and color.* The most common impression materials used for the indirect casting technique at this time are the ***polyvinyl siloxanes*** (addition reaction silicones). The technique for the use of this material is discussed in detail in the following sections. Several other impression materials that are satisfactory for use with the indirect casting technique are discussed in Impression Materials, in Chapter 6.

Tissue retraction

Final impression materials will only make accurate impressions of tooth surfaces that are *visible, clean, and dry.* Therefore when margins are *subgingival,* it is necessary to use ***retraction cord*** to temporarily displace the free gingiva away from the tooth and to control the flow of any gingival hemorrhage and sulcular fluids. The objective of ***gingival retraction*** is to *widen* the gingival sulcus to provide access for the impression material to reach the subgingival margins in adequate bulk to resist tearing during impression withdrawal (Fig. 19-42). The objective of hemorrhage and moisture control is met by the use of retraction cord impregnated with appropriate *styptics* (such as aluminum chloride) and/or *vasoconstrictors* (such as epinephrine). *The use of vasoconstrictors in retraction cord is contraindicated in some patients,* especially those who have cardiac arrhythmias, severe cardiovascular disease, uncontrolled hyperthyroidism, diabetes, and those receiving drugs such as β-blockers, monoamine oxidase inhibitors, or tricyclic antidepressants.[14]

Anesthetize all sensory nerves to the region, apply cotton rolls, and insert the saliva ejector. *Profound local anesthesia substantially reduces salivation to facilitate a dry field and allows tissue retraction without patient discomfort.* Select and cut a retraction cord* of suitable diameter that is slightly longer than the length of the gingival margin. The cord may be cut long enough to extend from one gingival margin to another if

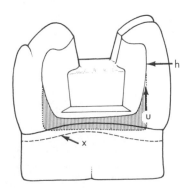

Fig. 19-41. Shaded area on prepared tooth is undercut in relation to line of withdrawal of impression. Impression material that is in position of greatest undercut (*u*) must be withdrawn in direction of vertical arrows and flexed over greatest heights of contour (*h*). Position of gingival attachment is indicated by *x*.

*Gingi-Pak retraction cord, Belport Company, Inc., Camarillo, Calif.

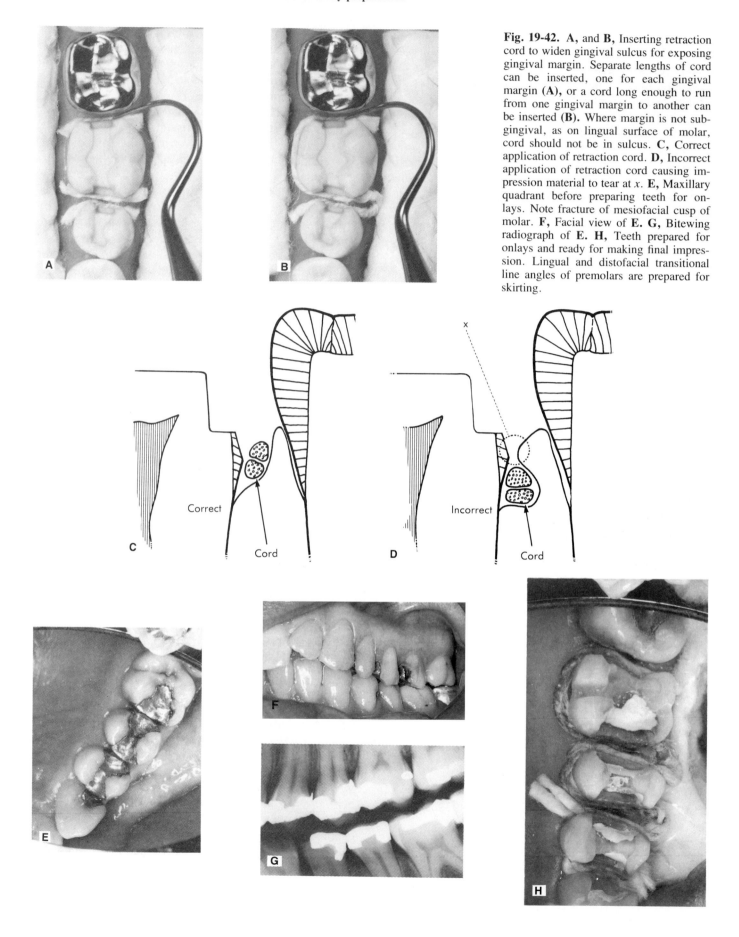

Fig. 19-42. **A,** and **B,** Inserting retraction cord to widen gingival sulcus for exposing gingival margin. Separate lengths of cord can be inserted, one for each gingival margin (**A**), or a cord long enough to run from one gingival margin to another can be inserted (**B**). Where margin is not subgingival, as on lingual surface of molar, cord should not be in sulcus. **C,** Correct application of retraction cord. **D,** Incorrect application of retraction cord causing impression material to tear at *x*. **E,** Maxillary quadrant before preparing teeth for onlays. Note fracture of mesiofacial cusp of molar. **F,** Facial view of **E. G,** Bitewing radiograph of **E. H,** Teeth prepared for onlays and ready for making final impression. Lingual and distofacial transitional line angles of premolars are prepared for skirting.

they are on the same tooth or on adjacent teeth. Note in Fig. 19-42, *A* and *B*, that the cord is inserted into the gingival sulcus only in areas where the cavosurface margin is prepared subgingivally. Moisten the retraction cord with the aqueous aluminum chloride solution,* and then squeeze the cord tightly between dry 2 × 2 inch (5 × 5 cm) cotton sponges to remove excess liquid. Using the edge of a paddle-tipped instrument or the side of an explorer, *gently* tuck one end of the cord into the sulcus about 2 mm facial to the point where the facial margin passes under the free gingiva. Then progressively work the cord into the sulcus, leaving the end of the cord exposed to grasp with tweezers later in the technique (Fig. 19-42, *A* to *C,* and *H*). *It is emphasized that the cord is placed to widen the sulcus and not to depress soft tissue gingivally* (although some temporary retraction does occur apically).

Occasionally, when the gingival margin is deep, it is helpful to insert a second cord of the same or larger diameter over the first. *When the free gingiva is thin and the sulcus is narrow (e.g., facial surface of the maxillary or mandibular canine), a cord of very small diameter must be selected to prevent undue trauma to the tissue.* When Gingi-Pak is used, a cord of small diameter can be obtained by separating the double-strand material into two single strands. The single-strand cord must be tightly twisted to minimize its diameter before use. Many times, when adjacent proximal surfaces are prepared, a similar small-diameter retraction cord must be used to avoid heavily pinching the interproximal tissue. *In instances when a small diameter cord is used, layering a second cord on top of the first may be necessary to keep the sulcus from narrowing at the gingival crest.*

In Fig. 19-42, *D,* the cord is incorrectly placed because it is tucked too deeply into a sulcus whose depth permitted such positioning. When the cord is withdrawn before the injection of the impression material, the sulcus will be open at the bottom but narrow at the top. If impression material is successfully injected into such a sulcus, the material is likely to tear in the region of *x* during the removal of the impression from the mouth. Correct application of the retraction cord is shown in Fig. 19-42, *C.*

Occasionally the retraction cord becomes displaced from the sulcus during its insertion if there is slight hemorrhage or seepage, but this can be controlled if an assistant repeatedly touches the cord with dry cotton pellets or dries the area with a gentle stream of air. When excessive hemorrhage from the interproximal tissue occurs, first wet a large cotton pellet with the aqueous aluminum chloride solution, and then wedge the pellet in between the teeth so that it presses on the

*Hemodent hemostatic solution, Premier Dental Products Co., Norristown, Pa.

bleeding tissue. Leave this pellet for a minimum of 5 minutes before removing it and inserting the cord. *Recall that the widening or opening of the gingival sulcus by the temporary insertion of retraction cord before the beveling of the gingival margin should minimize or eliminate hemorrhage of the gingiva.*

For retracting a large mass of tissue, first make a suitably shaped, large-diameter cotton pack by rolling cotton fibers between the fingertips; then wet the pack with a drop or two of aqueous aluminum chloride, and insert it into the sulcus.

The cords remain in place a minimum of 5 minutes. When hemorrhage or excessive tissue is present, a minimum of 10 minutes is recommended. The region must remain free of saliva during this interval, and the patient should be cautioned not to close or allow the tongue to "stray" on the teeth. Placing cotton rolls over the teeth and having the patient close lightly to relax while the teeth remain isolated is sometimes helpful.

It is suggested that the operator who is inexperienced in this work temporarily withdraw the retraction cord after 5 minutes and examine the region. The soft tissue should be standing away from the tooth, clearly exposing the gingival margin. This is an excellent time to reevaluate the gingival aspect of the cavity preparation and to make improvements where indicated. Reinserting the cord is easy and rapid. If hemorrhage occurs, the cord should again be moistened with the aqueous aluminum chloride solution before reinsertion.

Caution: Some brands of latex gloves and some hemostatic agents contain chemicals that can inhibit the setting of polyvinyl siloxane impression materials. Immediately prior to making the impression, thoroughly rinse the teeth and the retraction cord to remove any chemicals that could prevent the setting of the impression material. After rinsing, do not excessively dry the prepared teeth with compressed air. Have the patient close lightly on cotton rolls until the impression material is ready to be applied.

Polyvinyl siloxane impression

The polyvinyl siloxane impression is discussed in detail because it is widely used, and the technique for its use can be readily applied to most other "final" impression materials. Polyvinyl siloxane impression materials have many advantages over other impression materials used for final impressions. They have excellent reproduction of detail and excellent dimensional stability over time. They are enjoyable to work with since they are easy to mix and have no unpleasant odor or taste. Polyvinyl siloxane impressions can withstand disinfection routines without significant distortion. (See Chapter 4 for impression disinfection technique.) Most silicone impression materials come in the form of two pastes (base and catalyst) that are mixed prior to application to the teeth (Fig. 19-43, *A*). For even more convenience, most materials are available in disposable, auto-mix, cartridge dispensing systems. These auto-mix systems provide excellent mixing of the accelerator and base pastes as they are dispensed through a disposable injection tip (Fig. 19-43, *B*).

Tray selection and preparation. The impression tray must be sufficiently rigid to avoid deformation during the impression technique. If the tray bends or flexes at any time, the accuracy of the impression will be in doubt. Two types of trays, commercial stock and custom made, are suitable. The convenience and time saved with the use of stock, plastic trays is noteworthy. The custom resin tray made over a 2 to 3 mm wax spacer on the study cast is an excellent tray. A thickness of impression material greater than 3 mm increases shrinkage and the chance of voids; a thickness less than 2 mm may lead either to distortion or tear of the impression material or to breakage of narrow or isolated teeth on the cast during withdrawal from the impression. Adequate bonding of impression material to the tray is accomplished with the application of a special adhesive to the tray (Fig. 19-43, *C*).

Hand-mix technique. The technique for hand-mixing polyvinyl siloxane impression material is presented first. The items required are two mixing pads,* two spatulas,† a syringe,‡ a tray, heavy-bodied (high viscosity) materials, and light-bodied (low viscosity) materials (Fig. 19-44). Two viscosities of impression material are used because a double-mix technique, using a thicker viscosity in the tray and a thinner viscosity in

---

*Coe mixing pads, GC America, Inc., Chicago, Ill.
†No. 14R UNC spatula, Buffalo Dental Mfg. Co., Inc., Syosset, NY.
‡Coe syringe, GC America, Inc., Chicago, Ill.

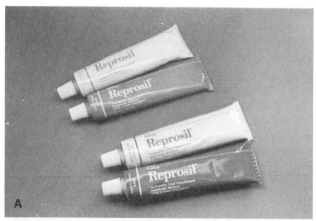

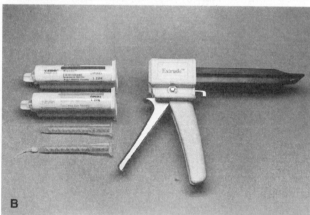

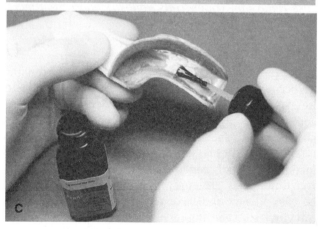

Fig. 19-43. A, Light-bodied (syringe-type) and heavy-bodied (tray-type) polyvinyl siloxane impression materials. **B,** Auto-mixing system for polyvinyl siloxane impression materials. **C,** Painting adhesive on stock tray.

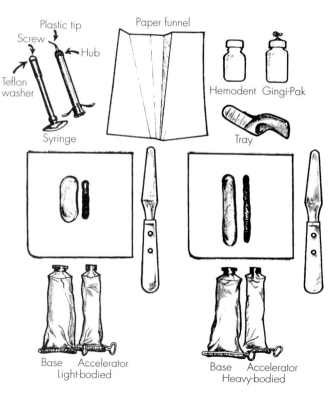

Fig. 19-44. Armamentarium for hand-mixed polyvinyl siloxane impression technique.

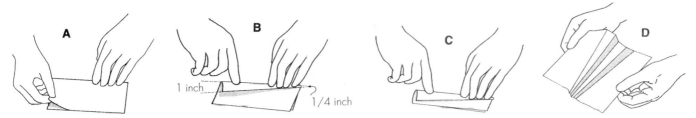

Fig. 19-45. A, To make a paper funnel, fold sheet of paper from mixing pad in half. **B,** Make second fold with one end ¼ inch (6 mm) wide and the other 1 inch (2.5 cm) wide. **C,** Make a third fold by folding over second fold. **D,** Unfolded paper.

the syringe, reduces the number and size of voids in the impression and improves accuracy.

Prepare a funnel using a sheet from the mixing pad. First, fold the sheet in half (Fig. 19-45, *A*). Then make a second fold by folding (from the folded edge created by the first fold) on an angle or bias (Fig. 19-45, *B*). One end of the second fold should be ¼ inch (6 mm) wide and the other end about 1 inch (2.5 cm) wide. Then fold again; this third fold should have the same measurements as the second (Fig. 19-45, *C*). Now unfold the sheet of paper (Fig. 19-45, *D*). It will be used to form a funnel that conveys the mixed, light-bodied, impression material into the syringe (Fig. 19-46, *G*).

Place on one pad the light-bodied impression material that will be used in the syringe. Following the manufacturer's instructions, place equal lengths of accelerator and base pastes on the pad (equal lengths, not equal volumes). On the other pad, place the heavy-bodied material that will be used to fill the tray. The amount varies depending on the fit of the tray, the extent of the region to be impressed, and the brand of material (Fig.

19-44). It is important to follow the manufacturer's instructions for dispensing and mixing the impression materials.

Now prepare the syringe for the light-bodied impression material. Assemble a plastic tip on the syringe by unscrewing the hub, placing the tip over the end of the barrel, and reapplying the hub. For injecting maxillary teeth, align the tip so that its curvature will be in a plane at right angles to the plane through the finger grips of the syringe. For mandibular impressions the curvature of the tip should be in line with the plane through the finger grips of the syringe. Try the piston in the barrel; the fit of the washer may be adjusted by turning the screw (clockwise to make a tighter fit). The piston should move in the barrel with about the same finger pressure customarily applied in using an anesthetic syringe. Now remove the piston.

Note the time and begin mixing the heavy-bodied material following the manufacturer's instructions (Fig. 19-46). Tilting the spatula so that the leading edge is always up away from the mix keeps the mix on just one

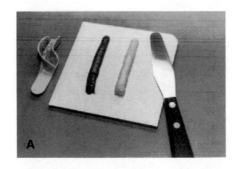

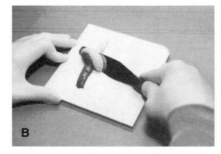

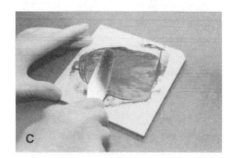

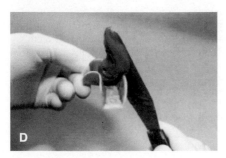

Fig. 19-46. Hand-mixing polyvinyl siloxane impression material and charging syringe. **A,** Separate mixing pad is used for each viscosity of impression material (injection-type and tray-type). **B,** Pick up both accelerator and base pastes from mixing pad and begin mixing. **C,** Keep one side of spatula free from material by tilting blade so that leading edge is always up out of mix. **D,** Convey mixed, heavy-bodied (tray-type) impression material into tray with spatula. *Continued.*

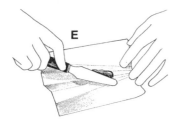

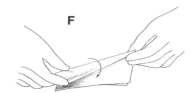

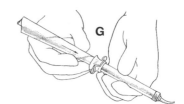

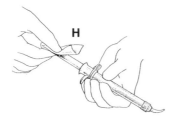

Fig. 19-46—cont'd. E, Place mix of light-bodied (syringe-type) impression material in center of unfolded sheet. **F,** Refold as originally folded, and roll into cone. **G,** Insert small end of funnel into back end of syringe barrel. **H,** Seal off back end of funnel by folding, and extrude material into syringe barrel by progressively squeezing from folded end of funnel toward syringe.

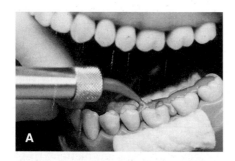

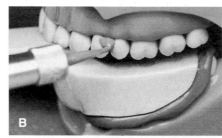

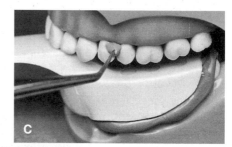

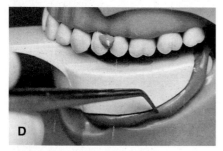

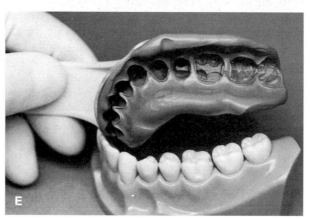

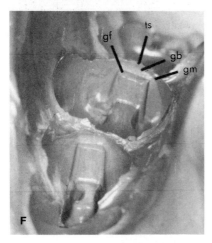

Fig. 19-47. Making and inspecting polyvinyl siloxane impression. **A,** Remove retraction cord and progressively fill opened sulci and preparations over and beyond cavosurface margins without trapping air. Note that occlusal surfaces of adjacent unprepared teeth are covered by light-bodied impression material. **B,** Injecting light-bodied material between and on posterior teeth not covered by impression. **C,** "Testing for set" the light-bodied impression material. **D,** "Testing for set" the heavy-bodied impression material. **E,** Completed polyvinyl siloxane impression. **F,** Close-up view of impression in **E** shows sharp detail of record of gingival floor *(gf),* gingival bevel *(gb)* and margin *(gm),* and a small amount of unprepared tooth surface *(ts)* beyond the margin.

side of the blade (Fig. 19-46, *C*). This is helpful and can be easily accomplished with practice. If the mix ever appears on the top side of the blade, both sides must be used during mixing by turning over the spatula at short intervals. Frequently interrupt the spatulation to gather the mix with the straight edge of the blade, lift it, and re-deposit it on the pad. *Thorough incorporation of the base and accelerator pastes is extremely important.* The mixing time suggested by the manufacturer should not be exceeded.

Immediately transfer this mix via the spatula blade into the tray, and temporarily set aside the filled tray (Fig. 19-46, *D*). Use care while transferring the material to minimize the incorporation of air.

With the second spatula, mix the light-bodied material on the second pad with the same mixing technique as described for the heavy-bodied material. Gather the mix onto the spatula blade and convey it to the center of the unfolded paper funnel (Fig. 19-46, *E*). Quickly re-fold the sheet in the same manner in which it was originally folded, and complete the funnel by rolling it into a cone (Fig. 19-46, *F*). Insert the small end of the cone into the back end of the syringe barrel (Fig. 19-46, *G*). Now fold over the wide part of the cone to confine the material, and extrude the light-bodied material into the syringe by progressively squeezing the funnel from the folded end toward the syringe (Fig. 19-46, *H*).

Quickly examine the teeth to be sure the field is still clean and dry. Remove any visible moisture on the teeth with compressed air. Gently remove the retraction cord with operative pliers. *All preparation surfaces should be clean, dry, and exposed to view.* Next, deliberately and progressively (moving from distal to mesial) fill the opened gingival sulci and cavity preparations over and beyond the margins with material from the syringe (Fig. 19-47, *A*). To avoid trapping air, keep the tip directly on the gingival and pulpal walls, thereby filling the cavities "from the bottom up," and regulate the movement of the piston so that material will not be extruded too fast ahead of the tip. Note in Fig. 19-47, *A*, that light-bodied material is also injected on the occlusal surfaces of the unprepared adjacent teeth; remembering to do this helps to eliminate the trapping of air on the occlusal grooves of these teeth.

After filling and covering the teeth with material from the syringe, immediately remove the cotton rolls, and seat the loaded tray over the region. While steadying the tray in the mouth for the first several minutes, inject some material from the syringe through the gingival embrasure between and on two dry teeth not covered by the tray (Fig. 19-47, *B*). Allow the cheek to cover this material and note when it can recover elastically from an indentation made by the tips of the operative pliers to determine the setting time of the light-bodied material (Fig. 19-47, *C*). Also, test the set of the

heavy-bodied material wherever it is accessible at the periphery of the tray (Fig. 19-47, *D*).

Auto-mix technique. Most dental manufacturers offer their polyvinyl siloxane impression materials in auto-mix dispensing systems. The *auto-mixing systems have many advantages,* including: (1) speed (the auto mixing technique is much faster than the hand-mixing technique); (2) the mixing of accelerator and base pastes is consistent and complete; (3) fewer air voids are incorporated during mixing and delivery to the teeth; and (4) fewer materials are required (no paper pads, funnel, spatulas, or syringe). The technique requires two viscosities of impression material, a light-bodied material to inject around the preparation, and a heavy-bodied material to fill the tray. Two dispensing guns are needed (Fig. 19-48, *A*). The dispensers are loaded with cartridges which contain the accelerator and base pastes (Fig. 19-48, *B*). A disposable auto-mixing tip fits onto the end of each cartridge (Fig. 19-48, *C*). The light-bodied mixing tip has an accessory curved tip that is small enough to gain access to the smallest, most remote areas of the cavity preparation (Fig. 19-48, *D*).

Use the first dispenser to mix and fill the impression tray with the heavy-bodied impression material (19-48, *E*). Keep the dispensing tip embedded in the impression material as it is expressed into the tray to decrease the chances of trapping air. Now use the second dispenser to mix and inject the light-bodied impression material on the prepared teeth (19-48, *F*). The methods of injecting the light-bodied material, seating the tray, and testing for final polymerization are identical to those described in the previous section, Hand-Mix Technique.

Removing and inspecting the impression. After the polyvinyl siloxane impression has properly polymerized, remove it from the mouth by a quick, firm pull that is directed as much as possible in line with the draw of the cavity preparation. Removal is aided by inserting a fingertip at the junction of the facial border of the impression and the vestibule fornix, disrupting the vacuum that occasionally occurs during withdrawal, especially with full-arch impressions. The impression should register every detail of the teeth (Fig. 19-47, *E* and *F*). Correcting a void by adding a small amount of newly mixed material to the impression and re-seating it is not recommended; the correct procedure is to make another impression. Rinse the impression clean under running water, and gently blow away the excess water. While individual impression materials vary, most can be permanently distorted if pressure is applied to the material for an extended period of time. Therefore, as a safety measure, do not allow the weight of the impression itself or any object to bear on the impression for an extended period of time (Fig. 19-49). Refer to Chapter 4 for information regarding the proper transport and disinfection of impressions.

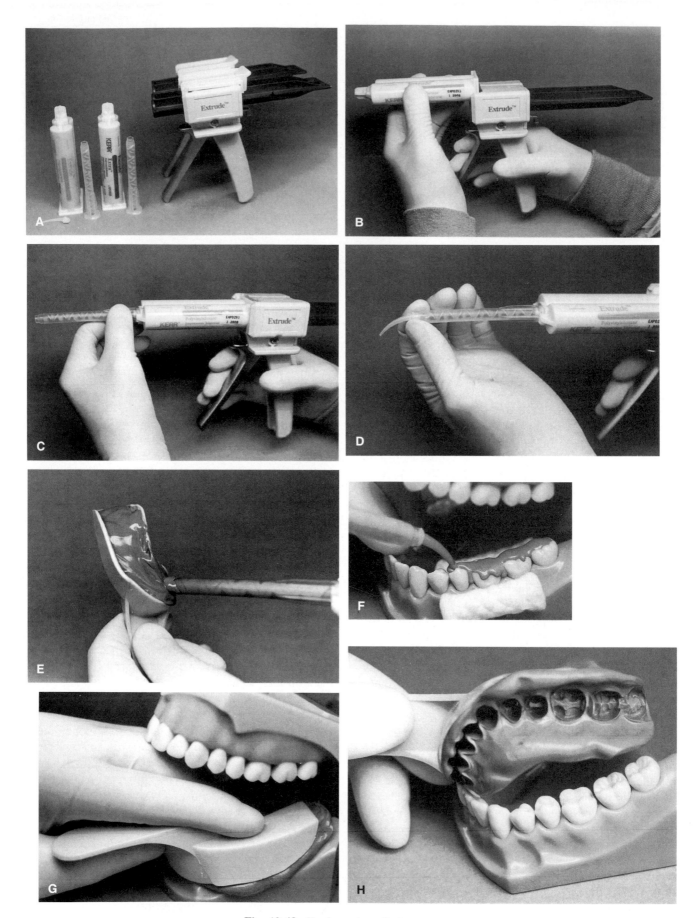

Fig. 19-48. For legend see facing page.

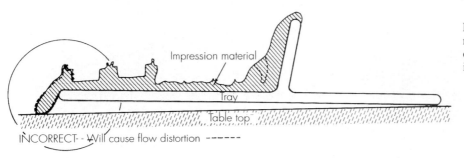

INCORRECT - - Will cause flow distortion - - - - - -

Fig. 19-48. A, Dispensers, cartridges, and mixing tips for auto-mixing polyvinyl siloxane impression materials. **B,** One dispenser is loaded with light-bodied impression material, while other dispenser is loaded with heavy-bodied impression material. **C,** Disposable auto-mixing tip fits onto end of cartridge. **D,** Accessory curved tip is added to end of auto-mixing tip for the light-bodied material. **E,** Impression tray is filled with heavy-bodied material. **F,** Remove retraction cord and progressively fill opened sulci and preparations over and beyond cavosurface margins without trapping air. Note that occlusal surfaces of adjacent unprepared teeth are covered by light-bodied impression material. **G,** Remove cotton rolls and seat impression tray. **H,** Completed auto-mixed polyvinyl siloxane impression.

WORKING CASTS AND DIES

The *working cast* is an accurate replica of the prepared and adjacent unprepared teeth that allows the cast metal restoration to be fabricated in the laboratory. During this fabrication procedure it is most helpful if the replicas of prepared and adjacent unprepared teeth, called *dies,* are individually removable. The most used methods for creating a working cast with removable dies from an elastic impression require two pours. The first pour is made to produce the removable dies, and the second pour is made to establish intraarch relationships. Working casts made in this manner are called *split casts.*

Several satisfactory methods are available for making a split cast with removable dies. The following *strip technique* is presented because it has proven to offer more control resulting in fewer difficulties, especially in the separation of those dies which are extremely close to one another.

Other advantages of the strip technique follow:
1. It provides landmarks so that dowel pins are positioned precisely in the center of the die base.
2. It provides a concave die base that helps index the die on the cast.
3. It allows speedy separation of dies without the use of rotary instruments or saws.

Stripping the final impression

Rest the impression on a loosely bunched cloth towel on the worktable (tray down) so the long axes of the greatest number of removable teeth (dies) are perpendicular to the tabletop. The impression shown in Fig. 19-47 is used to illustrate. Cut stainless steel strips from ribbon material that is ⁵⁄₁₆ inch (8 mm) wide and 0.002 inch (0.05 mm) thick, two strips for each tooth to be removable (Figs. 19-50, *A* to *C,* and 19-51).

Rule: The teeth to be removable are the prepared teeth with proximal gingival margins and any unprepared teeth adjacent to prepared proximal surfaces.

There are several advantages to making removable dies of unprepared teeth adjacent to prepared proximal surfaces: (1) the adjacent tooth will not interfere with removing the die that has the cavity preparation, as occasionally may happen otherwise; (2) there is less chance of distortion of the impression in the region of the gingival margins; and (3) adjusting the contacts is easier and more accurate, both when waxing and when finishing the castings.

Each strip, when tentatively held by tweezers exactly over the impression of the proximal gingival outline or margin, should be trimmed to follow but not quite touch the facial, lingual, and gingival contours of the impression. *It is emphasized that the strips do not touch the impression at any place.*

Note in Fig. 19-51 how the pairs of strips for each tooth to be removable slightly converge away from the impression, with the visualized bisector of this convergence perpendicular to the tabletop. Obviously if the dies of the teeth are to be removable from the completed cast, the pair of matrix strips forming each die must converge away from the impression. However, they must not converge so much that there is inadequate room for the head of the dowel pin subsequently placed. When a gingival margin is adjacent to an edentulous region, position the strip over the *edentulous* region about 1 to 2 mm away from the impression of the gingival margin (note the most distal strip in Fig. 19-52). *It is reemphasized that the bottom edges of the strips should directly overlie, but not quite touch, the gingival margins.*

Set aside the strips in their proper sequence. Next a 1

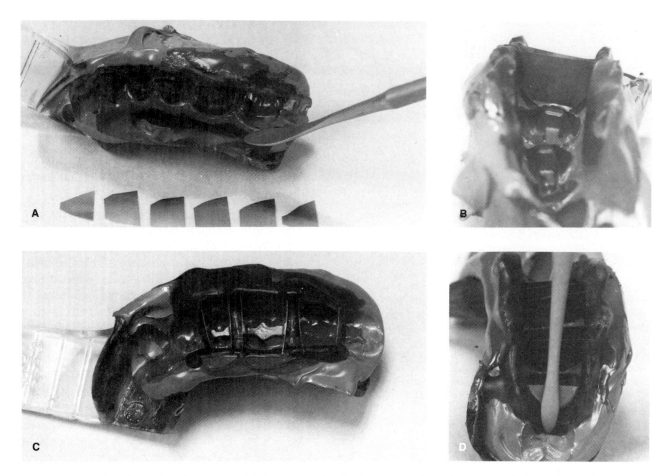

Fig. 19-50. A, After cutting stainless steel strips for impression shown in Fig. 19-47, flow utility wax on facial and lingual flange regions. **B,** Each strip is heated and inserted into wax. Two strips for unprepared second molar die and distal strip for prepared mesioocclusodistal first molar die are inserted. Note clearance of strip from impression material. **C,** Stripping is completed. **D,** Utility wax flowed from No. 7 spatula is applied to seal openings at end strips (*y* in Fig. 19-51).

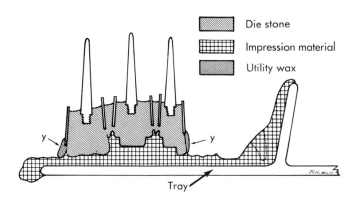

Die stone

Impression material

Utility wax

Fig. 19-51. Line drawing of stripping shown in Fig. 19-50, *C,* plus pouring of die stone and insertion of dowel pins. Note application of utility wax *(y)* to close small openings to confine die stone.

to 2 mm layer of utility wax is flowed on the facial and lingual flange regions of the impression (Fig. 19-50, *A*). This wax should not be extended closer than 2 mm to the important tooth record; it is placed only on the impression record of the facial and lingual mucosa.

Now take each strip in the tweezers, heat it in an open flame, and convey it to its proper position (Fig. 19-50, *B*). The strip should be hot enough that its edges will easily and readily enter and move in the wax. If after the strip is inserted its position is judged to be wrong, convey heat to the strip with warm tweezers and correct the position while the strip is warm enough to keep the wax soft; or the warm strip can be removed, wiped clean of wax while warm, reheated, and then reinserted in better position. *Never should pressure be exerted while inserting the strips.* Remember, also, that the strip comes close to the impression but never touches it. See that the convergence of each pair of strips is not so great as to bring the outer edges so close

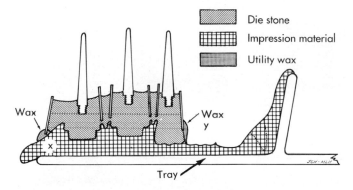

Fig. 19-52. Line drawing of stripping a final impression when two molars are prepared for mesioocclusodistal inlays and second molar is terminal tooth. Note that position of the most distal strip is 1 to 2 mm distal of distal gingival margin. Narrow bead of utility wax *(x)* is applied across this edentulous region (from previously applied facial wax to lingual wax) to receive edge of warm strip, hence sealing region and preventing escape of die stone.

to one another that there is inadequate space for the head of the dowel pin. Using the heated, small end of the No. 7 wax spatula, smooth and "seal" the wax at each strip-wax junction where it is not complete. *This assures the attachment of the strips to the impression during pouring and improves the smoothness and appearance of the cast.* With a warm spatula and utility wax, seal off any openings between the gingival edges of the *outside* strips and the impression (Fig. 19-50, *D,* and *x* and *y* in Figs. 19-51 and 19-52).

Pouring the final impression

Before mixing the die stone, have ready the required number of dowel pins. See that each pair of strips does not converge too much, thus reducing the width of the base of the die and interfering with the insertion of the pin. Special small-sized pins are available for narrow, small teeth.

Make a mix of high-strength die stone using a vacuum mechanical mixer and pour the dies with the aid of a vibrator and a No. 7 spatula. *Apply the first increments in small amounts, allowing the material to flow into the remote corners and angles without trapping air.* Surface tension-reducing agents* are available that allow the stone to more readily flow into the deep, internal corners of the impression. This die stone should be kept approximately 1 mm short of completely filling all the spaces between the metal strips. This leaves enough of each of the strips in view to aid in positioning the dowel pins and creating desirable, concave die bases. Moreover, overflowing the end strips may create "locks" that would prevent removing the dies from the cast.

Without delay, return the impression to the loosely bunched towel so the bisectors of the paired strips (long axes of the dowel pins to be placed next) are vertical. Gently insert the head portions of tapered brass dowel pins into the stone, one pin for each die to be removable on the completed cast (Fig. 19-53, *A*). Slightly "jiggling" the pin while inserting the knurled head aids in providing a complete and firm pin-to-stone attachment. Ensure that the head of the pin is completely inserted into the stone. Vertically align the dowel pins approximately parallel with the long axes of the teeth and parallel with one another while the die stone is still soft. They will stand without support if upright. Allow the die stone to set.

*Surfactant, Almore International, Inc., Portland, Ore.

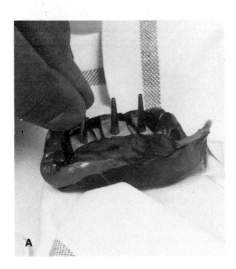
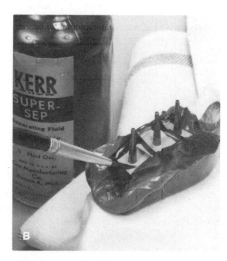
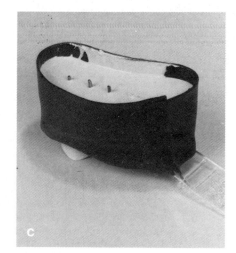

Fig. 19-53. A, Dies are poured, and impression is propped on loosely bunched towel at correct angle to result in dowel pins being upright. **B,** Separating medium is applied to die bases. **C,** Impression is boxed, and base portion of cast is poured in dental stone.

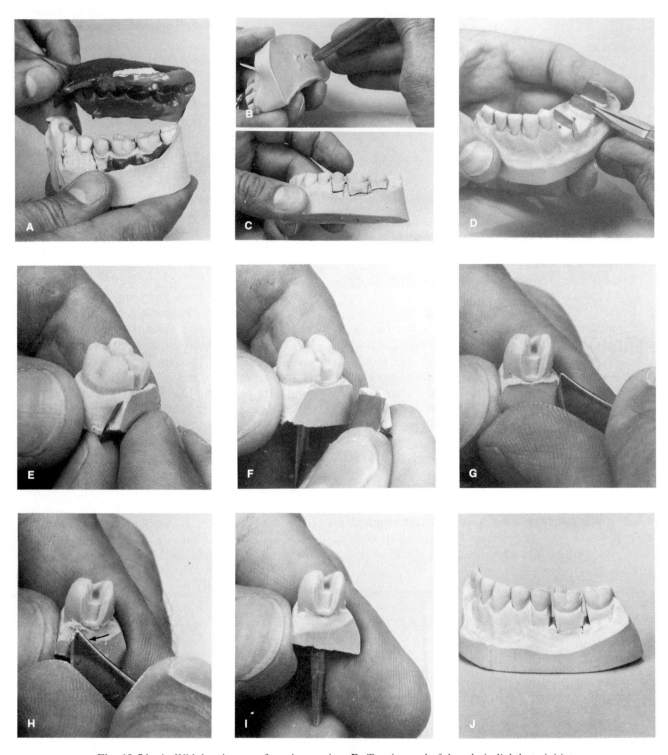

Fig. 19-54. A, Withdrawing cast from impression. **B,** Tapping end of dowel pin lightly to initiate removal of die. **C,** Initially dies should be moved conjointly, each die being moved from its seating the same distance as other dies. Removing and discarding metal strips **(D)** and stone wedges between dies **(E and F). G to I,** Trimming away any "extra-impression" die stone to fully expose gingival margin and recorded contour of tooth beyond gingival margin. Starting the trimming **(G).** Trimming across die slightly gingival of recorded gingival contour of tooth, thus both weakening "extra-impression" stone to cause it mostly to fall away and preventing knife from injuring recorded gingival contour of tooth **(H). I,** Trimming completed. **J,** Completed cast. Note accurate, close fit of dies to base portions of cast.

Completing the working cast

After the die stone has set, paint a separating medium on the stone, box the impression, and vibrate a mix of dental stone (30 ml/100 g) into the remainder of the impression (Figs. 19-53, *B* and *C*). Allow ⅛ inch (2 mm) of the ends of the dowel pins to protrude. To provide adequate strength, the base of the cast should not be less than 10 mm thick.

After the stone has hardened, remove the boxing wax and lift the cast out of the impression (Fig. 19-54, *A*). Tap the end of each dowel pin *lightly* with the end of an instrument handle until a different "ring" is heard; this indicates that the die has moved slightly from its seating (Fig. 19-54, *B*). Next, carefully tap or push the ends of the pins conjointly, causing the dies to move equally away from their seating (Fig. 19-54, *C*). After the dies are simultaneously removed in this manner, separating them with the fingers is an easy procedure. Discard the metal strips and the V-shaped wedges of stone that are between the dies (Fig. 19-54, *D* to *F*). To aid in carving the wax pattern and polishing the casting, carefully trim the gingival aspect of the dies to properly expose the gingival margins (Fig. 19-54, *G* to *I*). The dies should have a positive seating in the base portion of the cast (Fig. 19-54, *J*).

Caution: Do not allow even a trace of debris on the closely fitting surfaces of the cast or else the accuracy that is otherwise possible will be destroyed. This is especially true for the walls of the dowel pin holes. A small bit of wax or gypsum can be carelessly pressed onto the wall to ruin the seating of the pin, and such debris is difficult to detect and remove to regain accuracy.

Use of the Interocclusal records

A maximum IP interocclusal record or an FGP interocclusal record was made before making the final impression (see the previous sections, Verifying Cusp Reduction, and Interocclusal Records). From these interocclusal records, gypsum casts of the opposing teeth are made which can be accurately related to the working cast when forming the occlusal surface(s) of the wax pattern(s). This step can be omitted if full-arch casts are to be used in waxing. (See Chapter 2 for the principles of developing occlusion when using full-arch casts.)

Carefully fit the interocclusal record on the dies of the working cast (Fig. 19-55, *A*). The interocclusal record should and must seat completely without rocking. Interocclusal bite records must never touch registrations of soft tissue areas on the cast because these contacts usually interfere with complete seating. Such areas of contact on the interocclusal record can be easily trimmed away with a sharp knife. After ensuring that the interocclusal record is completely seated, lute the record to adjacent unprepared teeth with sticky wax to prevent dislodgment when dental stone is poured into the record.

Pouring the wax interocclusal record. Casts of opposing teeth made from *wax* interocclusal records are called *cores* since they are indexed to the adjacent unprepared teeth of the working cast. Cores made from wax IP interocclusal records are called *IP cores.* Cores made from wax FGP interocclusal records are called *FGP (or functional) cores.* Apply a separating medium for gypsum to the adjacent unprepared teeth of the working cast (Fig. 19-55, *B*). Make a regular mix of dental stone and apply the stone mix to the surface of the wax interocclusal record and to the occlusal surfaces of the adjacent teeth (or edentulous region), endeavoring not to trap air on these surfaces (Fig. 19-55, *C*). Load a suitable tray with stone and settle it on the stone previously placed (Fig. 19-55, *D*). Do not allow the stone to cover more than 1 or 2 mm of the facial and lingual surfaces of the adjacent unprepared teeth, since more coverage would cause difficulties when withdrawing and reseating the core. With experience, the stone can be applied without using a tray. After the stone has set, remove it from the working cast, remove the wax interocclusal record, and trim the facial and lingual aspects of the core nearly to the record of the occlusal surfaces of the unprepared teeth (Fig. 19-55, *E*).

After verification that the core accurately re-seats on the working cast, *the inherent stability of the core normally permits it to be hand-articulated while the operator establishes the occlusion of the wax patterns and subsequently of the cast metal restorations.* When relating a core to a working cast that has no unprepared tooth distal to the prepared teeth, it is helpful to index the stone core to the posterior land area of the working cast for a firm posterior vertical stop (Fig. 19-55, *G* to *J*). To make this posterior index, be sure that the posterior land area of the working cast is smoothly convex, or using a knife, it may be notched; then paint on a separating medium for gypsum (Fig. 19-55, *G*). Using sticky wax, attach the core to the working cast and add dental stone (Fig. 19-55, *H*) to form the posterior land index shown in Fig. 19-55, *I* and *J*.

An alternative technique of relating the working cast and stone core is to mount both on a small hinge articulator with fast-setting plaster (Fig. 19-55, *K* and *L*). First, properly position the core and cast together and temporarily secure this relationship by adding a small amount of sticky wax at appropriate places. Now, using plaster, mount the cast and the core on the opposing members of the hinge articulator. This articulator is only used in a pure hinge movement, which is the single requirement having formerly registered the "functionally generated paths" in the FGP core (made from the wax FGP interocclusal record). The IP core made from the wax IP interocclusal record is also related in

Fig. 19-57. To ensure optimal wax adaptation to cavity walls, first flow on a thin layer of wax **(A),** and then apply finger pressure for several seconds while wax cools **(B).**

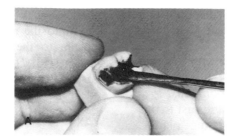 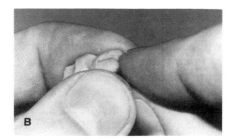

least several seconds on each increment of wax soon after surface solidification and before any subsequent wax additions (Fig. 19-57, *B*). In this incremental technique the wax that is flowed on the previously applied wax must be hot enough or else voids will be formed.

Forming the proximal contour and contact

The proximal contour and contact of the pattern are now formed upon the pattern base and deserve special attention (Figs. 19-58 and 19-59). The normal proximal contact relationship between teeth is that of two curved surfaces touching one another. Therefore the contact on each curved proximal surface is a point inside a small area of near approach. However, it must be realized that soon after eruption and the establishment of proximal contact, wear of the contact point through the individual movement of teeth will create a contact surface. Black[2] addressed the procedure for developing proper proximal contour and contact:

It is important that contact be of proper form and in the right position. The method of testing the extent of the near approach of the surfaces of the teeth about the contact is illustrated in [Fig. 19-58]. The ligature [dental floss] is first passed to the gingival of the contact; the two ends are then held parallel in the occlusal direction as shown for the contact between the premolars. This measures the faciolingual width of the contact or very near approach of the two surfaces. Without removing the ligature, the two ends should be held parallel in the facial direction as shown for the contact between the molar and premolar. This measures the occlusogingival width of the contact. In either position if the parallel strands are more than 1½ or 2 mm apart the contact is too broad.

Drawings of two maxillary premolars [Fig. 19-59] are used to illustrate forms of contact and mesiodistal widths of interproximal spaces. *A, B,* and *C* represent normal conditions. In *A,* the position of the contact is marked with an *x,* the area of near approach of the two surfaces is indicated with a broken line and the position of the crest of the gingiva with a continuous line. *B* is a mesiodistal section through the teeth at the point of contact and *C* is an occlusal view. If one will note first the slope of the surfaces from the marginal ridges to the contact in *B,* also the widening of the embrasures in *C,*

and will think of these in relation to the point of contact and the curvature of the gingiva in *A,* he should have a good understanding of the movements of food over these surfaces in chewing and their effectiveness in keeping them clean.

A broad contact faciolingually is illustrated in *D, E,* and *F.* In the proximal view *D,* the position of a normal contact is marked *x,* while the contact of this tooth is the outlined oblong area; the area of near approach is the broken line. As a rule, the crest of the gingiva is less arched, being almost horizontal along the area of near approach. Viewed from the facial in the mesiodistal section *E,* the contact appears to be the same as in *B,* but a comparison of the occlusal views *F* and *C* shows the extra breadth of this contact which prevents food from scouring the embrasures as far in as is the case when the contact is normal. [Also, the interproximal tissue will not receive the proper stimulative massage from the excursion of food. It is too protected.]

[Fig. 19-59, *H*] shows a contact that is too far to the gingival. Its position in comparison with normal is shown by the relation of the circle to the *x* in *G.* The

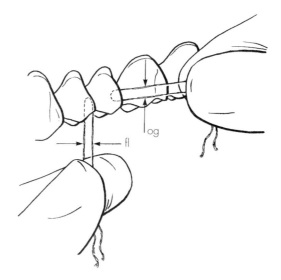

Fig. 19-58. Measuring diameters of proximal contact faciolingually *(fl)* and occlusogingivally *(og)* with dental floss. Two parallel strands should not be more than 1½ to 2 mm apart. (Modified from Black GV: *Operative dentistry,* ed 8, vol 2, Woodstock, Ill, 1947, Medico-Dental Publishing.)

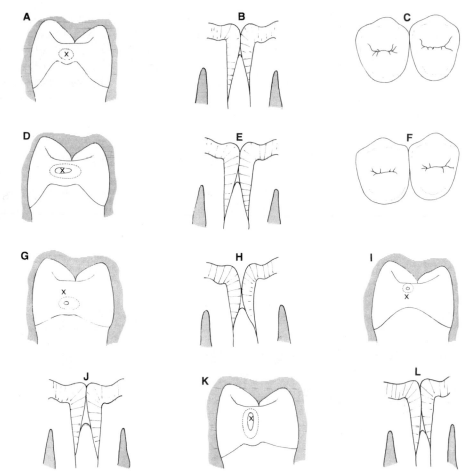

Fig. 19-59. A to **C,** Correct contact. Note position and form of contact and form of embrasures around contact. Also note that mesial and distal pits are below (gingival of) proximal marginal ridges. **D** to **F,** Contact too broad faciolingually. **G** and **H,** Contact positioned too far gingivally. **I** and **J,** Contact too close to the occlusal surface. **K** and **L,** Contact too broad occlusogingivally. (Modified from Black GV: Operative dentistry, ed 8, vol 2, Woodstock, Ill, 1947, Medico-Dental Publishing.)

danger in such a contact lies in the inclinations of the proximal surfaces from the occlusal marginal ridges to the contact. Stringy food is likely to become packed into this space and eventually force the teeth apart and injure the gingiva. [Also, such a contact often impinges on the interproximal tissue.]

[Fig. 19-59, *I* and *J*] illustrates a contact too close to the occlusal. This form is frequently observed in restorations (especially amalgams), seldom in the virgin teeth except in cases of [occlusal] abrasion. Such a contact prevents a proper amount of food from being forced into the embrasure, particularly close in where it is most effective; also the crest of the gingiva is far from the contact and invites caries of the proximal tooth.

[Fig. 19-59, *K* and *L*] illustrates a contact that is too broad in the occlusogingival direction. The principle objections to this form of contact are that stringy foods are likely to be caught and held; also that if proximal caries occurs it will be farther to the gingival requiring cavities to be cut very close to the cemental line.

In cases of excessive proximal wear of the teeth, the condition of the contact areas is similar to the combination of the areas illustrated in *D* and *K,* there being a facet of considerable dimensions. . . .

In a general way the conditions described for proximal surfaces of premolars and molars apply to the anterior teeth although their wedge form lessens the likelihood of injuries to the gum, and food which is forced through the contact is less likely to be held, or if held is more often noticed and removed.

R. E. Sturdevant[27] offered the following explanation of why the contact between posterior teeth generally is toward the facial with the lingual embrasure greater than the facial embrasure:

Nature has wisely provided the lingual embrasure greater than the facial in order that food in the process of closing the teeth will be forced by way of the lingual embrasures back over the tongue, which in turn conveys the food again between the teeth prior to the next closure of the jaws. If the facial embrasure were greater than the lingual, the greater portion of the bolus of food would be forced upon closing the teeth into the facial vestibule where it could not be so easily returned between the teeth.

Forming the occlusal surface

The fundamental principles in the following method of waxing were developed by Payne.[18] The technique is particularly applicable when capping cusps. With practice, it has proved to be faster than the old method of building up wax, cutting away, building up again, and so on. The amount of wax desired is added in steps until the occlusal surface of the pattern is completed (Fig. 19-60).

To obtain the faciolingual position of the cusp tips, divide the faciolingual width of the tooth in quarters. Facial cusps are located on the first facial quarter line. Lingual cusps will fall on the first lingual quarter line (Fig. 19-60, *B*). To obtain the mesiodistal position of the cusp tips, note the regions in the opposing tooth that should receive the cusp tips. Now wax to the pattern small cones of inlay wax to establish the cusp tips one at a time (Fig. 19-60, *C* and *D*).

Now wax the inner and outer aspects of each cusp, being careful not to generate premature occlusal contacts (Fig. 19-60, *D* to *F*). Again it is suggested to wax only one aspect of each cusp into occlusion at a time. For example, on the maxillary molar illustrated in Fig. 19-60, *D,* where all cusps are being restored, there are nine aspects, each one to be waxed separately before waxing another. Follow the proper angle on the inner and outer aspects as shown in Fig. 19-60, *E.*

Next, wax the distal slopes of the cusps (one at a time) into occlusal relation with the opposing teeth. Then wax the mesial slopes of the cusps (again, one at a

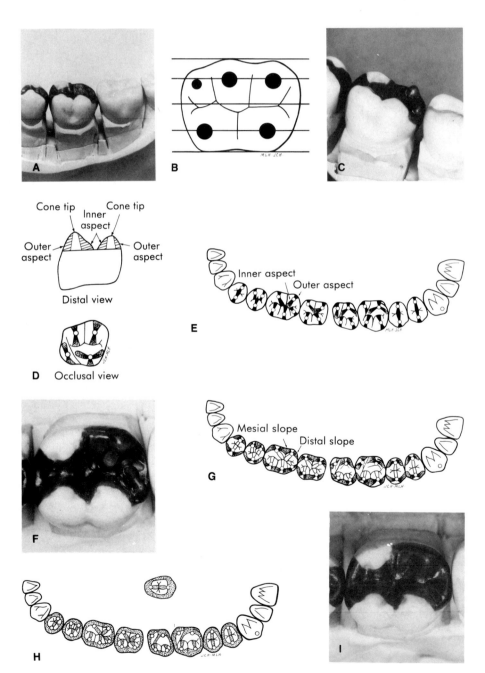

Fig. 19-60. A, Pattern base is completed and ready for waxing two reduced cusps (distolingual and distal) into occlusion by using Payne's waxing technique. **B,** Facial cusps are located on first facial quarter line, and lingual cusps will fall on first lingual quarter line. **C,** Distolingual and distal cusp tips are waxed into occlusion in the form of small cones. **D,** Cone tips and inner and outer aspects. **E,** Cone tips and inner and outer aspects of cusps of teeth. **F,** Inner and outer aspects of distolingual and distal cusps have been added to pattern base. **G,** Mesial and distal slopes of cusps of teeth. **H,** Marginal ridges of teeth. **I,** After marginal ridge is added to pattern base, fossae are waxed in, and grooves are carved to complete wax pattern. (Modified from Payne E: *Ney Tech Bull* 1(9): 1961.)

time) (Fig. 19-60, *G*). After the cusps are formed, wax in the proximal marginal ridge areas (Fig. 19-60, *H*). Develop the same level to adjacent proximal marginal ridges, even though occasionally this may sacrifice a contact on one of the two ridges. Restoring marginal ridges to the same level avoids a " food trap" that otherwise would be created. The mesial and distal pit regions should always be carved out enough to have them on a lower level than the respective marginal ridges.

To complete the occlusal wax-up, add wax (where appropriate) to the fossae until they contact the opposing centric holding cusps (Fig. 19-60, *I*). Establish spillways for the movement of food by carving appropriately placed grooves. Flat-plane occlusal relationships are not desired.

This technique is a systematical and practical method of waxing the occlusal aspect of the pattern into proper occlusion. Forming one small portion at a time allows waxing each portion into proper occlusion before confusing the situation by adding another. Moreover, building the occlusal aspect by such small increments should help to develop a pattern with minimal stress and distortion. Whenever a large portion of wax is added, there is an ever-present danger of pattern distortion caused by the large shrinkage of such an addition.

Using the FGP core to form the occlusal surface. When using a FGP core, several important changes must be made to the waxing technique described in the previous section. *The FGP core provides information regarding (1) the opposing teeth in maximum intercuspal position, and (2) the pathways of the opposing cusps during mandibular movements.*

Group function is attained by waxing the lingual inclines of the maxillary facial cusps into contact with the stone core (Fig. 19-61, +gf). If group function is not desired, relieve these inclines so that only the cusp tips and fossae are in contact (Fig. 19-61, −gf). The amount of clearance between these inclines will be the amount of disocclusion seen in the mouth during mandibular movement.

To ensure that undesirable non-working contacts are not generated in the restoration, some relief should be provided between the non-working slopes of the wax pattern and the stone core (Fig. 19-61, −nf).

Using the IP core/cast to form the occlusal surface. Either the IP core or the cast made from an IP interocclusal record (with bite registration paste) provides a dental stone replica of the opposing dentition against which occlusal contacts can be formed. For establishing stable occlusal relationships, take care to place cusp tips against flat plateaus or into fossae on the stone cast of the opposing teeth. In other areas the wax is shaped to simulate normal tooth contours, using adjacent teeth for references. Some relief between opposing cusp inclines should be provided inasmuch as these incline contacts

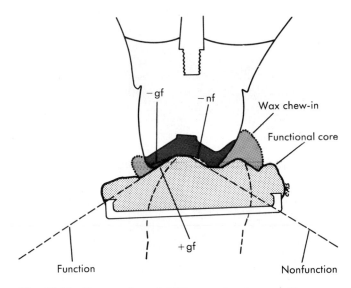

Fig. 19-61. Cross-section of FGP core related to maxillary wax pattern. Group function is attained by waxing lingual incline of facial cusps into contact with core *(+gf)*. If group function is not desired, these slopes are relieved *(−gf)*. To ensure that nonfunctional contacts do not occur, some relief is provided along nonfunctional inclines *(−nf)*.

often interfere during mandibular movements. *Remember, the IP record only provides information regarding the position of opposing teeth in maximum intercuspal position.* Therefore some adjustment to the casting may be necessary in the mouth to eliminate interferences during mandibular movements.

The previous sections described forming the occlusal surface of the wax pattern using a FGP core, an IP core, or a cast of the opposing teeth made from bite registration pastes. The reader is referred to Chapter 2 for the principles of cusp and fossa placement when using full-arch casts mounted on a semi-adjustable articulator.

Finishing the wax pattern

Extreme caution is mandatory for waxing the margins of the wax pattern. There must be a continuous adaptation of wax to the margins with no voids, folds, or faults. If adaptation is questionable, remelt the marginal wax to a distance into the pattern of approximately 2 mm. Apply finger pressure immediately after surface solidification and before subsequent cooling of the wax, maintaining this pressure for at least 4 seconds. This finger pressure helps to develop close adaptation to the die by offsetting the cooling shrinkage of the wax. Additional wax should be added during the remelting procedure to ensure a slight excess of contour and extension beyond the margin.

Wax that is along the margins is now carved back to the cavosurface outline with a warmed No. 7 wax spat-

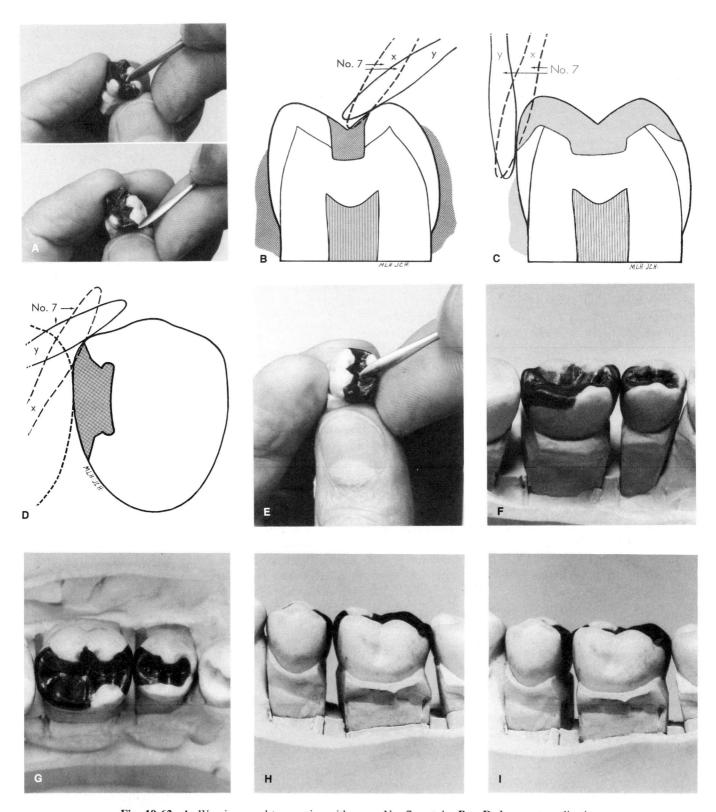

Fig. 19-62. A, Wax is carved to margins with *warm* No. 7 spatula. **B** to **D,** Incorrect application of No. 7 spatula to carve contour of marginal wax is shown by *x;* correct manner is labeled *y.* **E,** Carving occlusal groove and pit anatomy. **F,** Adjacent marginal ridges should be on same level as much as possible. **G,** Occlusal view of completed patterns. Note shape of facial and lingual embrasures and position of contact. **H** and **I,** Facial view of completed patterns. Note gingival and occlusal embrasures and position of contact.

ula (Fig. 19-62). This warming of the spatula permits carving the marginal wax with light pressure so that the stone margins will not be damaged. A little practice will help the user determine how much to heat the instrument to result in easy and effective carving. It must be emphasized that the No. 7 spatula should not have sharp edges; thus when it lightly touches the die, it will not abrade or injure the die surface. Use the die surface just outside the cavosurface margin to guide the position and direction of the carving instrument. *It is emphasized that the direction of the instrument is not dictated by the margin but by the contour of the unprepared tooth (die) surface just beyond the margin.* Hold the instrument blade parallel to this surface, thus using it as a guide for the contour of the pattern near the margin. This should result in a continuity of contour across the margin. This principle of carving is too often neglected, resulting in the contour errors depicted in *x* in Fig. 19-62, *B* to *D;* correct application of the carving instrument results in correct contours, exemplified by *y.*

Slightly overwax the proximal contact(s) so that the waxed die(s) will fail to seat on the cast by a slight amount. This provides a small excess of metal in the casting for polishing the contact (Fig. 19-63, *A*). However, an experienced technician can save much laboratory time by waxing the contacts without this slight excess contour and by being careful when finishing the casting.

On accessible surfaces of the carved pattern, satisfactory smoothness can be imparted by a few strokes with the end of a finger if surfaces have been carefully carved with the No. 7 spatula. Less accessible surfaces, such as grooves, may be smoothed by rubbing with cotton that has been twisted onto a round toothpick.

On the facial aspect of the pattern a small bleb or extension may be added to facilitate removal of the inlay after trying it in the tooth (Fig. 19-63, *B* and *C*) (see Removing the Casting).

Initially withdrawing and reseating the wax pattern

Care must be exercised when initially withdrawing the wax pattern from the die. Usually, if the pattern is of a mesioocclusodistal restoration, the wax can be dislodged by holding the die and pattern as shown in Fig. 19-64, *A*. When using this technique, extreme care must be used to avoid distorting the wax pattern, since one portion may be moving from its seating while the other portions are still lodged in position, resulting in a distorted pattern. Once this has occurred, the pattern usually cannot be reclaimed.

A good alternative technique for removing the wax patterns, especially for small inlay restorations, is to use a U-shaped wire (Fig. 19-64, *B* to *J*). To form the U-shaped wire, bend a 1¼ inch (3 cm) length of 24-gauge copper wire into a U shape having an attached loop; the length of the legs of the U-shaped wire should measure approximately ¼ inch (6 mm) each with their ends flattened (Fig. 19-64, *B* and *C*). Adjust the distance between the ends of the legs to that distance from mesial pit to distal pit. With operative pliers, hold the wire by the loop portion. Then warm the wire by passing it through a flame, and insert the ends of the legs into the wax pattern about ¾ mm deep in the mesial and distal pit areas. The heat of the wire should only be enough to melt the wax that immediately receives and surrounds the wire ends. Releasing the hold of the twee-

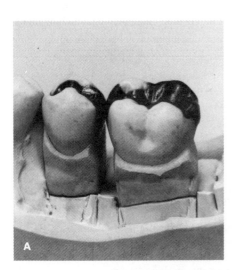
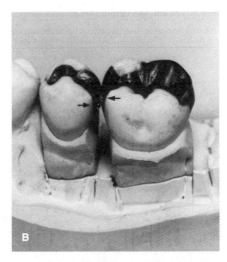
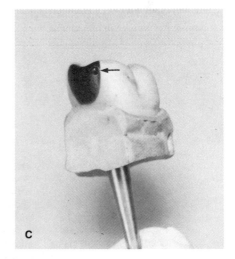

Fig. 19-63. A, After patterns are formed and just before their initial withdrawal, slightly overwax proximal contacts to provide metal in these areas for polishing. Waxed dies then should fail to seat on cast by approximately 0.3 mm. Wax a small bleb or extension for application of No. 48 chisel to aid in removing casting after trying it on tooth. **B,** Facial view. **C,** Proximal view.

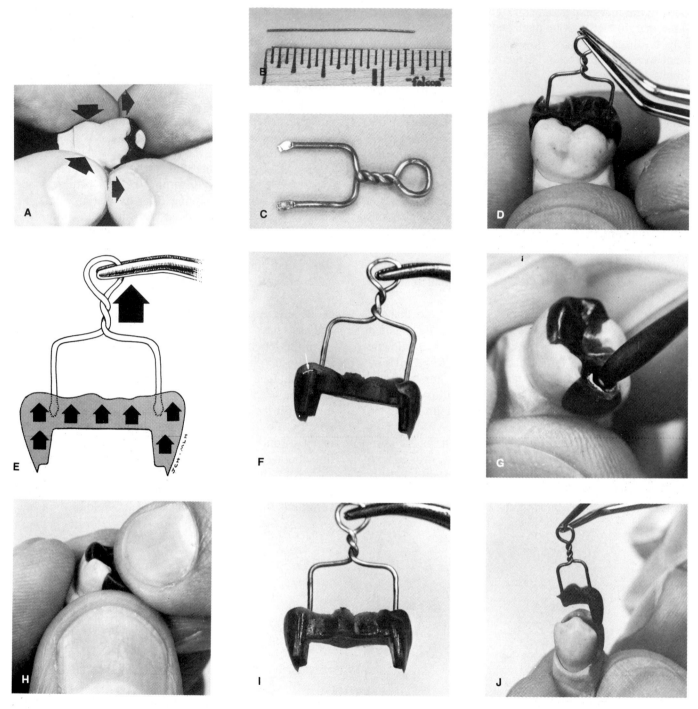

Fig. 19-64. A, Removing wax pattern by indirect finger pressure. Care must be used not to squeeze and distort wax pattern as it is initially withdrawn. U-shaped copper wire with a loop can be used to initially withdraw wax patterns with less chance of distortion. **B,** First cut 1¼-inch (3 cm) length of 24-gauge copper wire. **C,** After forming a loop in the middle, twist a few turns, and then form U shape with legs approximately ¼-inch (6 mm) long. Flatten ends of wire. Hold loop with tweezers, warm the wire, and insert it into pattern. **D** and **E,** With tweezers engaging loop, gently lift pattern without distortion. **F,** Incorrect waxing will result in air voids on cavity side of pattern as shown by arrow. **G,** Correcting air void shown in **F** by passing hot No. 7 spatula through pattern to unadapted region of die. **H,** Finger pressure is applied during cooling of reheated wax. **I,** After recarving wax pattern in corrected region, withdraw pattern to observe that void has been eliminated. **J,** U-shaped wire is especially helpful when withdrawing small two-surface inlay wax patterns.

zers but still steadying the wire subsequent to its insertion aids in the immediate cooling of the wire and hardening of the wax around the wire legs.

With operative pliers, lightly grasp the U-shaped wire by its loop and carefully (slowly) endeavor to attain uniform traction and movement of the entire pattern while lifting it from the preparation (Fig. 19-64, *D* and *E*). Frequently at the start of removal, one portion of the pattern may be seen to move slightly from its seating while the other portion remains lodged. In these instances, apply more or all of the lifting force to the portion of the pattern that has not moved by grasping the corner of the U-shaped wire directly over this lodged portion. When the stuck portion is freed slightly, the wire is again held by the loop to equalize the lifting force over the entire pattern, which is then lifted gently from the preparation. Inspect the cavity side of the pattern to see if there are any wrinkles or holes (Fig. 19-64, *F*). Such voids indicate poor wax adaptation and should be corrected, particularly if such voids are in critical regions of the preparation designed to provide retention form, if they are numerous, or if they are closer than 1 mm to the margin. To eliminate these voids, first relubricate the die and reseat the pattern on the die. Then pass a hot instrument through the wax to the unadapted region (Fig. 19-64, *G*). This usually results in the air (void) rising through the liquid wax to the pattern's surface as the wax takes the place of the air. As always, apply finger pressure on this remelted wax as it cools (Fig. 19-64, *H*). A consequence of this correcting procedure on the occlusal surface is the obliteration of the occlusal carving in the affected region, thus necessitating the addition of wax, recarving, and rechecking the occlusion. There is always the danger of pattern distortion because of the reheating of the wax.

Once satisfied with the pattern after its withdrawal and reseating, remove the U-shaped wire by holding it briefly with the heated beaks of the operative pliers while the pattern is in place on the die. In a second or two the wax holding the wire will melt sufficiently to permit lifting it from the pattern. The small holes left by the wire are easily corrected by touching them with a heated, small, pointed instrument such as a discarded explorer.

SPRUING, INVESTING, AND CASTING

If there is a delay of several hours or more between the forming of the wax pattern and the investing procedure, the pattern should remain on the die, and the margins should be inspected carefully once again before spruing and investing. When such a delay is contemplated, it is suggested to add the sprue to the pattern before the delay period. If the addition of the sprue caused the induction of enough stress to produce pattern distor-

tion, such a condition is more evident after the rest period, and corrective waxing can be instituted before investing. The reader is referred to textbooks on dental materials for the principles and techniques of spruing, investing, casting, and cleaning the casting. Be certain that all investment is removed from the casting and that it is properly pickled.

SEATING, ADJUSTING, AND POLISHING THE CASTING

It is critical to closely examine the casting, preferably under magnification, before testing the fit on the die. Closely examine the internal and external surfaces with good lighting, being alert for any traces of investment, any positive defects (blebs), or any negative defects (voids). Voids, if in critical areas, indicate rejection of the casting unless they can be corrected by soldering. Carefully remove any small positive defects on the internal surface with an appropriately sized round bur in the high-speed handpiece.

Try the casting on the die before removing the sprue and sprue button, which serve as a handle to remove the casting if removal is necessary. The casting should seat with little or no pressure (Fig. 19-65, *A*). *Ideally it should have the same feel when being placed on the die as the feel of the wax pattern when it was seated on the die.* If the casting fails to seat completely, remove it and inspect the die surface for small scratches to see where it is binding. Usually failure to seat is caused by small positive defects not spotted on the first inspection. Attempts at forcing the casting to place will cause irreparable damage to the die and foretell of later difficulties when trial-seating the casting in the mouth.

Once satisfied with the accuracy of the casting, separate the casting from the sprue as close to the inlay as possible using a carborundum separating disc. Make the cut twice as wide as the thickness of the disc to prevent binding, and do not cut completely through the sprue (leave a small uncut portion) (Fig. 19-65, *B*). If the cut is made completely through, control of the disc is sometimes lost, often resulting in damage to the casting or to the operator's fingers. The uncut portion should be so small that bending with the fingers will break it with very little effort (Fig. 19-65, *C*).

Having seated the casting on the die, hand *burnish* the marginal metal on a path about 1 mm wide adjacent to the total length of the margin using a ball or beavertail burnisher (Fig. 19-65, *D*). This improves marginal adaptation and begins the smoothing process, almost imparting a polish to this rubbed surface. While burnishing, continually assess the adaptation of the casting to the prepared "cavity wall" along the margin, using magnification as needed to see any marginal opening as small as 0.05 mm. Moderate pressure during burnishing is indicated only during closure of small marginal gaps.

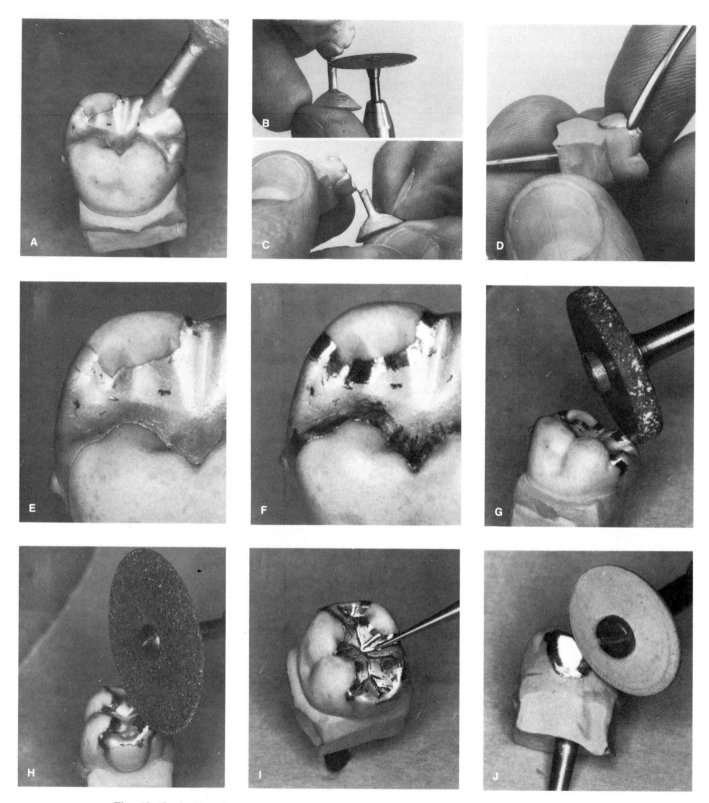

Fig. 19-65. A, Try cleaned casting on die to determine if it has a satisfactory fit. To remove sprue, first make a cut that is not quite complete and twice the width of the disc **(B),** and then bend-break the slim, uncut portion **(C). D,** Inlay is burnished with No. 2 burnisher along 1 mm path that is parallel with and adjacent to margin. **E,** Magnified view of casting before burnishing. **F,** Magnified view of same marginal region shown in **E** after burnishing. Removing remaining sprue metal with heatless stone **(G)** or with carborundum disc **(H). I,** Accentuating grooves with dull No. 1 round bur. **J,** Smoothing surfaces accessible to rubber polishing wheel.

Once the casting is well adapted, pressure is reduced to a gentle rubbing for continued smoothing of the metal surface. At this stage marginal openings and discontinuities should not be detectable even under ($\times 1.5$ or $\times 2$) magnification (Fig. 19-65, *E* and *F*). Care must be taken not to over-burnish the metal, since this can crush the underlying die surface. Such over-burnished metal will interfere with complete seating of the casting on the prepared tooth. Proper burnishing usually improves the retention of the casting on the die so that the casting does not come loose during subsequent polishing steps. *A casting must not be loose on the die if the inlay is to be properly polished.*

Carefully remove the remaining sprue metal with a heatless stone or a carborundum disc (Fig. 19-65, *G* and *H*). Accentuate the grooves by lightly applying a somewhat dull No. 1 round bur (Fig. 19-65, *I*). Next use the knife-edge rubber polishing wheel* on accessible surfaces (Fig. 19-65, *J*). Guard against the polishing wheel touching the margins or die because they can be unknowingly and quickly polished away, resulting in "short" margins on the tooth. Also, at this time, adjust the proximal contacts one at a time. For example, if the distal surface of a mesioocclusodistal casting on the first molar is being adjusted, only the first and second molar dies are on the cast. *Remember that proximal contacts are correct when they are the correct size, correct position, and are passive.* If a resin temporary restoration was properly made, these contact relationships will be the same in the mouth as on the cast. Thus chair time can be conserved by carefully finishing the contacts on the cast.

Now check the occlusion of the castings by marking the occlusal contacts with articulating paper. Correct any premature contacts and refine their locations by selective grinding. Often prematurities occur where the sprue was attached and insufficient sprue metal was removed. Now apply a smaller, rubber, knife-edge wheel,† which should reach some of the remaining areas not accessible to the larger disc (Fig. 19-66, *A* and *B*). The grooves, pits, and other most inaccessible regions are smoothed by a rubber, abrasive point‡ (Fig. 19-66 *C*). Exercise care when using the rubber discs and points not to touch the die surface and not to destroy anatomical contours by overpolishing. Keep these points and discs sharpened and true-running by "lathing" them on an abrasive stone whenever necessary (Fig. 19-66, *D*). When finished with the rubber abrasives, the surface of the casting should have a smooth, satin finish. Be sure that the contact relationships with the adjacent and opposing teeth have the correct size,

position, and intensity (Fig. 19-66, *E*).

Now brush the occlusal surface of the casting with a No. 11 (soft) Robinson bristle disc and tripoli (or BBC)* polishing compound, running the disc parallel with the grooves (Fig. 19-66, *F*). Use a small felt wheel with polishing compound on the proximal and other accessible surfaces (Fig. 19-66, *G*). *The metal should be so smooth before this application of polishing compound that a beautiful luster should develop in a few seconds.* A high sheen may be imparted, if desired, with a felt or chamois wheel and rouge (Fig. 19-66, *H* and *I*). Again as in the application of tripoli/BBC, only a few seconds of rouge application should be required. If more time were expended in the application of these polishing compounds, overpolishing (polishing away) of the margins and die would result. Also, such *overuse of polishing compounds is often an unsuccessful attempt to mask the fact that the preliminary stages of polishing were not thoroughly completed.*

Clean the polished casting of polishing compounds by immersing the die with its inlay in a suitable solvent for a minute or two or by scrubbing with a soft brush and soap and water. Rinse, and then remove the casting from the die. *No polishing compounds should be found on the cavity side of the casting or on the cavity walls of the die.* The presence of such materials on these surfaces indicates that marginal adaptation on the die is not as good as it should be.

When the casting is adapted well to the die, often it is not possible to remove it from the die by the fingers or by tapping the die. In this event the following procedure is advocated. Firmly grasp the dowel pin with a common slip joint pliers, with the corner of a cloth towel interposed between the pliers beaks and the dowel pin. The pin should be perpendicular to the jaws of the pliers; also, the die, as well as the head of the slip-bolt, faces up (Fig. 19-67, *D*). Now wrap the die in the remaining portion of the towel, leaving the head of the slip-bolt exposed. Using a hammer, sharply rap the slip-bolt head once, and once only (Fig. 19-67, *E*). This force should displace the die down and away from the casting, which now rests in the folds of the towel (Fig. 19-67, *F*). The towel over the die prevents the casting from flying onto the floor or tabletop with a force that would likely distort it. Rap the pliers with the hammer only once, for if the casting and die were separated by the first blow, a second might cause the loose casting to hit the die. If the first blow does not displace the die from the casting, then repeat the procedure using a heavier blow from the hammer.

---

*Burlew disc, J.F. Jelenko & Co., Armonk, NY.
†Sulci disc, J.F. Jelenko & Co., Armonk, NY.
‡Browne rubber point, Shofu Dental Corp., Menlo Park, Calif.

*BBC Buffing Bar Compound, J.F. Jelenko & Co., Armonk, NY.

tact and its location (Fig. 19-58). Apply the floss at an angle and with secure finger-bracing to pass it gently through the contact and not with a snap that is likely to injure the interproximal soft tissues. If the floss will not enter or tears on entering, the contact is excessive. *Caution: When adjusting a mesioocclusodistal restoration, adjust only one excess contact at a time (the stronger one) before trying again on the tooth and evaluating, unless both contacts feel equally strong.* This is done because one excessively strong contact can cause the other to feel strong, when in actuality the latter contact may be correct or even found to be weak (short of contact) after the excessively strong contact is properly adjusted.

Use the Burlew rubber wheel to adjust the proximal contour and to correct the contact relationship. This often requires several trials on the tooth, but it is best not to remove too much at a time. After each trial and removal the position of contact is visible in the form of a bright spot on the satiny surface left on the casting from previous surfacing by the rubber wheel. By noting the position of this bright spot in conjunction with observation in the mouth of the contact relationship, judgment can be rendered regarding the contact position and form and whether additional adjustment should be made to alter this position and form. (For removing the casting after each trial on the tooth, see Removing the Casting.)

Often the patient is able to testify whether the contact is strong, particularly when an anesthetic has not been given. The patient should not be aware of pressure between the teeth after the final adjustment of contact(s).

Remember: Proper proximal contact occurs when a visual inspection verifies that the adjacent proximal surfaces are touching, and the position and form of the contact relationship are correct; the correct "tightness" of the contacts is best judged with dental floss. This contact should be passive, since any pressure between the teeth would soon resolve and disappear in undesirable tooth movement.

If the contact is short of touching the adjacent tooth, a new contact area must be soldered to the casting. (The procedure for soldering contact is given in a later section, Soldering Contacts.) A short contact is best detected by visual inspection with the aid of the mouth mirror. The region must be isolated with cotton rolls and dried with the air syringe. Selection of the proper horizontal viewing angle will usually disclose the space between the teeth, small though it may be. Such an open contact will permit the passage of food that will impact on and irritate the interproximal gingiva.

When satisfied that the proximal contact(s) are correct and when hand pressure first positions the casting to within 0.2 mm of seating (Fig. 19-68, *A*), remove the

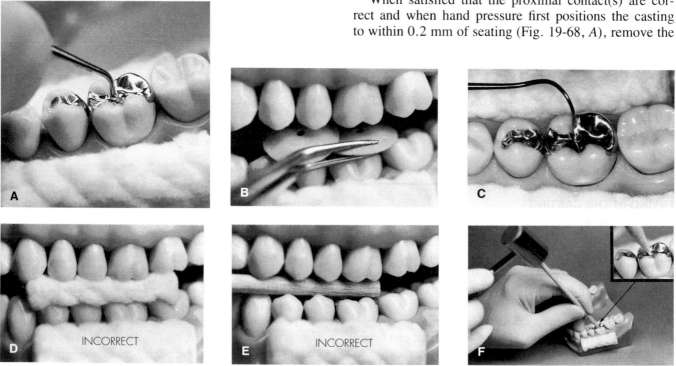

Fig. 19-68. A, Use hand pressure to initially seat casting on tooth by applying ball burnisher in pit anatomy. **B,** If casting fits to within 0.2 mm of seating, ensure complete seating using masticatory pressure by having patient close on Burlew wheel interposed between casting and opponent tooth (teeth). **C,** Inspect marginal fit of tried-in inlay. Do not use cotton roll (**D**) or piece of wood (**E**) in lieu of Burlew wheel method (**B**). **F,** *Only* when masticatory pressure cannot be applied by using Burlew wheel method (**B**), apply *light* tapping pressure with orangewood stick and leather-headed mallet.

3 × 3 inch (7.5 × 7.5 cm) gauze sponge and make sure the casting completely seats on the tooth by the application of masticatory pressure. This use of masticatory pressure should be a routine procedure. It is accomplished by positioning a Burlew disc (unmounted) on the occlusal of the restoration and requesting the patient to bite firmly; also request the patient to move the jaw slightly from side to side while maintaining this firm pressure (Fig. 19-68, *B*). At this time the operator must judge whether the restoration is satisfactory or should be rejected and another casting made. When evaluating the fit (seating) of the casting, view particularly the margins that are transversely (horizontally) directed (i.e., those that are perpendicular to the line of draw). Along at least half of the marginal outline the tip of the explorer tine should move from tooth onto the metal, and vice versa, with barely a catch or a bump (Figs. 19-68, *C*, and 19-69). If effective masticatory pressure is not possible, use the less satisfactory method of applying a few *very light* taps using a small leather-headed mallet and orangewood stick (Fig. 19-68, *F*). This tapping serves as a vibrating force to seat the casting. Exercise care to apply pressure only to the casting and to direct the force as close as possible to the long axis of the tooth.

Some operators advocate the use of a cotton roll or a piece of wood for the patient to bite on for seating pressure (Fig. 19-68, *D* and *E*). The cotton roll is too soft to be effective for seating *inlays,* and the piece of wood may not properly distribute the pressure, thus resulting in less effective seating or tooth fracture. Fig. 19-69 shows the castings tried on the teeth that were first shown in Fig. 19-42, *H*.

Occluding the casting

When the proximal contacts have been adjusted and the casting is satisfactorily seated on the tooth, have the patient *close into maximum intercuspal position (IP),* and inspect the unprepared adjacent teeth to see if there is any space between opposing wear facets. Usually the patient can indicate correctly if the casting needs occlusal adjustment; however, the dentist should verify the occlusal relationship objectively. After drying the teeth of saliva, insert a strip of articulating paper and request the patient to close and tap the teeth together (in IP) several times. Remove the paper, and examine it by holding it up toward the light for evidence of any areas of penetration caused by the restoration. Any holes can be matched with heavy markings on the casting, and there will be shiny, metal-colored spots in the center of the marks (Fig. 19-70, *A*). Such heavy contacts should be reduced with suitable abrasive stones while carefully observing the following fundamental **concepts for equilibration of occlusion.** The space observed between opposing wear facets of adjacent unprepared teeth (when the teeth are "closed") is an indication of the maximal amount of vertical reduction of the casting required. Often the "high" occlusal contacts are too broad and extend onto cusp or ridge slopes. When this occurs, *grind away the most incorrect portion of the incline contact (a deflective contact), leaving the most correct portion intact* (Fig. 19-70, *B*). *Occlusal contacts in maximum IP should be composed of supporting cusp tips placed against flat or smoothly concave surfaces (or into fossae) for stability. The force vector of occlusal contacts should be one that parallels the long axis of the tooth* (Fig. 19-70, *C*). *Contacts on inclines tend to deflect the tooth and are less stable* (Fig. 19-70, *D*). The use of articulating paper and stone is continued until (1) the heavy markings are no longer produced, (2) the contacts on the restoration have optimal position and form, and (3) there is an even distribution of contacts on the casting and the adjacent teeth. Visual inspection should verify that the adjacent unprepared teeth are absolutely touching.

Care must be used not to overreduce occlusal con-

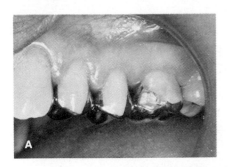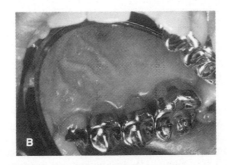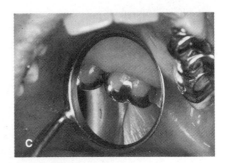

Fig. 19-69. **A** to **C,** Castings tried on teeth that were first shown in Fig. 19-43, *I*. Photographs were taken immediately after restorations were first seated on teeth before any dressing down or burnishing of margins. Neither occlusal adjustment nor contact adjustment was required. Extension of mesiofacial margin of second premolar was necessary because of extension of a previous amalgam restoration; extension of distofacial margins of premolars is caused by skirting (or bracing), which provides maximal resistance form to these weak teeth. Note area on mesiofacial margin of first molar that is to have composite insert placed after cementation.

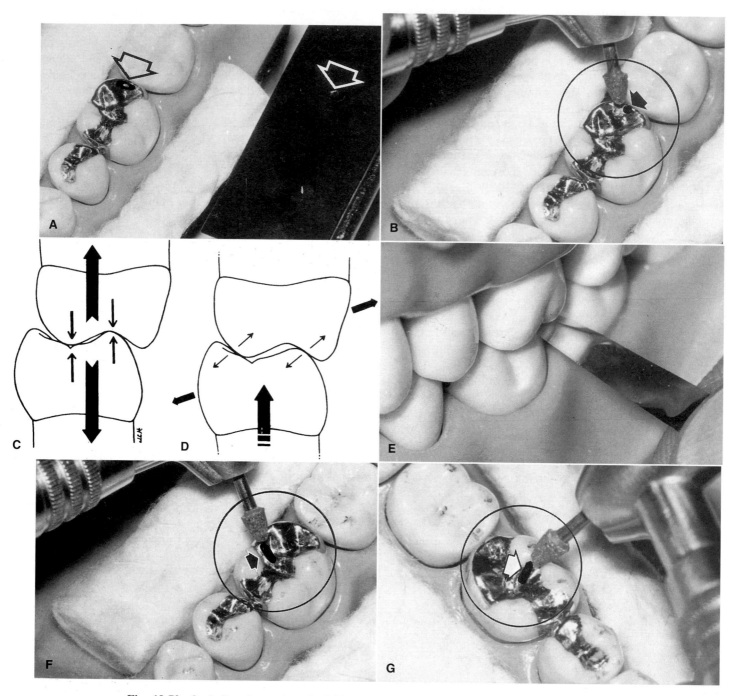

Fig. 19-70. Occluding the casting. **A,** Initial occlusal contact is high and produces heavy mark with metal-colored center. Note corresponding perforation in articulating paper. **B,** When adjusting occlusal contacts, remove most incorrect portion of contact, leaving most correct portion intact. **C,** Proper occlusal contacts in IP are composed of cusp tips placed against flat or smoothly concave surfaces (or fossae) for stability. **D,** Incline contacts are less stable and tend to deflect tooth. **E,** Testing intensity of occlusal contacts with thin (0.0005 inch [0.013 mm] thick) shim stock used as a "feeler gauge." **F,** Removing undesirable contact (lingual range) that may occur on working side during lateral mandibular movement. **G,** Removing undesirable contact that may occur on non-working side during lateral mandibular movement.

tacts. In the final phase of equilibration, the strength of occlusal contacts can be tested by using thin plastic shim stock* (0.0005 inch thick [0.013 mm]) as a "feeler gauge." Test the intensity of the occlusal contacts of the casting and the adjacent unprepared teeth to see if they hold the shim stock equally (Fig. 19-70, *E*). It may be helpful to test the occlusal contacts of the adjacent unprepared teeth with the casting out of the mouth for comparison.

Once the occlusal contacts have been adjusted in IP, check the casting for contacts that occur during lateral mandibular movements. Lateral *working (functional) contacts* on the casting are marked by (1) inserting a strip of articulator paper over the quadrant with the casting, (2) having the patient close into IP, and (3) then "sliding" the teeth toward the side of the mouth where the casting is located. Contacts between the lingual inclines of the maxillary lingual cusps and facial inclines of the mandibular lingual cusps are considered unusually stressful and should be eliminated (Fig. 19-70, *F*). Contacts between the lingual inclines of the maxillary facial cusps and the facial inclines of the mandibular facial cusps should remain only if they are passive and a group function pattern of occlusion is desired.

Insert a strip of articulating paper over the teeth with the castings, have the patient close into IP, and then slide the teeth laterally toward the opposite side. This will mark any lateral *non-working (nonfunctional) contacts* on the restoration. In a normal arrangement of teeth, contacts that might occur during the non-working pathway are positioned on the facial inclines of the maxillary lingual cusps and the lingual inclines of the mandibular facial cusps. These non-working contacts must be removed with a suitable stone (Fig. 19-70, *G*). Complete elimination of non-working contacts can be verified by using the plastic shim stock. Insert a strip of shim stock over the casting, and have the patient bite together firmly. As soon as the patient begins sliding the mandible toward the opposite side, the shim stock should slip out from between the teeth.

Now examine the casting for interferences in *protrusive mandibular movements* using the shim stock and articulating paper. The areas that may have to be adjusted to prevent contact are the distal inclines of the maxillary teeth and the mesial inclines of the mandibular teeth.

Finally, interferences that occur on the casting between centric relation (retruded contact position) and IP are identified and removed. Most patients have a small discrepancy between centric relation and maximum intercuspal position. Such a "skid" is considered normal for most patients, but the operator should be sure that the casting does not have *premature contact* at any

*Shim stock, Artus Corp., Englewood Cliffs, NJ.

point between centric relation and IP. The preferred technique for manipulating the mandible into centric relation is credited to Dawson.[5] Once the teeth have been marked in centric relation, observe the teeth to be sure the casting does not have premature contacts in centric relation, and that it does not exacerbate any centric relation-IP skid. If it does, the mesial inclines of maxillary restorations and the distal inclines of mandibular restorations will be the areas that may need adjustment.

Improving marginal adaptation

The next step is to "dress down" the margins, that is, to adapt the metal as closely as possible to the margins of the tooth. Regardless of how accurately a casting may seat in the preparation, the fit usually can be improved by using the following procedures.

With a ball or beaver-tail burnisher, improve marginal adaptation by burnishing the marginal metal with strokes that parallel the margin, the gingival margin excepted (Fig. 19-71, *A*). If the margin is inaccessible to the ball or beaver-tail burnisher (as sometimes at the termination of the casting in groove regions where possibly more enameloplasty or extension could have been employed), the edge of the discoid-type hand instrument serves well as a burnisher. The discoid is held perpendicular to the margin and is moved parallel with the margin (Fig. 19-71, *B*). The sharp edges of the discoid will also trim away any slight excess of metal at the margin. Continue with the discoid on other portions of accessible margins where a slight excess of metal is present.

If necessary, the marginal adaptation and continuity can be further improved by the application of a pointed, fine-grit carborundum stone, especially where the marginal enamel is slightly "high" and should be reduced or where more than just a slight amount of excess metal should be removed (Fig. 19-71, *C*). This stone should be used at low speed with light pressure and should rotate either parallel with the margin or from *metal to tooth across the margin* (never from tooth to metal). After this stoning, again burnish the margins to enhance marginal adaptation and to smooth the marginal metal.

Another instrument that can be used to improve marginal fit in accessible areas (such as the occlusal two thirds of the proximal margins) is a paper disc of medium-cuttle grit. Wherever possible, the disc should be revolved in a direction from the metal toward the tooth (Fig. 19-71, *D*). Sometimes these margins are inaccessible to the disc, and a gingival margin trimmer, a gold file, or a cleoid instrument may be helpful to remove a slight excess of metal (Fig. 19-71, *E*). It is moved in a scraping motion parallel to the margin and will burnish and trim the metal.

It is true that the experienced operator, if properly using the elastic impression material, *with care* can pro-

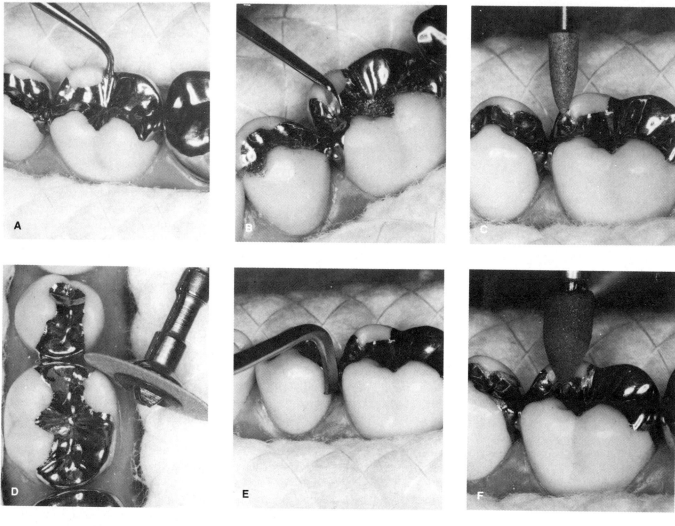

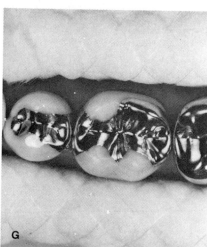

Fig. 19-71. A, Burnishing margins with No. 27s ball burnisher. Burnisher is moved parallel with margin. **B,** Using discoid on margins inaccessible to ball burnisher. It is moved parallel with margins. (Note small metal scrapings made by this instrument.) **C,** Dressing down margins with small carborundum stone, which is rotating from metal to tooth. **D,** Applying medium-cuttle disc to accessible supragingival proximal margins. Disc rotates, wherever possible, from metal to tooth. **E,** On facial or lingual margins on proximal surface that are inaccessible to paper disc, use gingival margin trimmer to remove any slight excess of metal. **F,** Using rubber point to smooth metal and tooth of scratches left by carborundum stone. **G,** Completed inlays ready for cementation.

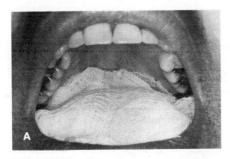
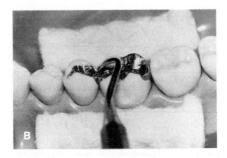
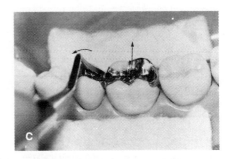

Fig. 19-72. Initiating removal of inlay before cementation. **A,** Place 3 × 3 inch (7.5 × 7.5 cm) gauze throat screen to prevent swallowing or aspiration of casting should it be accidentally mishandled. **B,** Tip of *sharp* Black spoon (15-8-14) is first inserted as deep as possible in occlusal embrasure with back of spoon against adjacent marginal ridge. **C,** Spoon is then pivoted in direction of arrow using adjacent tooth as a fulcrum. Note that casting has lifted from its seating. After only slight unseating, apply similar procedure to distal aspect.

duce restoration margins that require very little or no burnishing or dressing down. Certainly one of the significant advantages of the indirect procedure, when correctly applied, is the high degree of accuracy of the gingival margin adaptation.

At this time the margins should be such that the explorer tip can pass across the margins smoothly without jumping or catching. Use rubber polishing points of increasing fineness at low speed to smooth and polish the accessible areas of roughness left from adjusting procedures (Fig. 19-71, *F* and *G*). Attempt to preserve anatomical contour and detail. Take care to use light, intermittent pressure when using rubber points to prevent overheating the tooth. Now clean and dry the casting surface to verify that it is smooth and free of scratches.

Removing the casting

When preparing to remove a casting from a tooth, first place a 3 × 3 inch (7.5 × 7.5 cm) gauze sponge throat screen to prevent the patient from swallowing or aspirating the casting in the event that it is accidentally mishandled (Fig. 19-72, *A*). If the casting is very retentive, first initiate removal with the aid of a *sharp* Black spoon (15-8-14). The tip of the spoon is inserted as deep as possible in the occlusal embrasure with the back of the spoon resting against the marginal ridge of the adjacent tooth (Fig. 19-72, *B*). With the tip of the spoon firmly seated against the metal casting, pivot the spoon using the adjacent tooth as a fulcrum (Fig. 19-72, *C*). Repeat this procedure on the other occlusal embrasure if the casting is a mesioocclusodistal restoration. This should initiate the displacement of the casting, making complete removal thereafter easy.

Extremely retentive castings may be removed with the use of the No. 48 chisel and a small leather-headed mallet. One corner of the chisel's cutting edge is placed on the small bleb or extension formed during the completion of the wax pattern (Fig. 19-73). Without such an

extension the chisel's edge is placed on the proximal surface just under the facial "ear." The chisel's long axis is directed as nearly as possible parallel to the line of draw of the preparation, and a *very light tap* is delivered from the mallet to the chisel. (The cutting edge of the chisel must be sharp in order to "grab" the metal.) If the casting does not loosen slightly after this application of the chisel to one proximal surface of a mesioocclusodistal restoration, apply, if possible, the chisel to the other proximal surface for an additional light tap. *Obviously these taps by the mallet on a chisel could fracture a tooth if misdirected or too hard.* Moreover, extreme care must be given to placing the chisel lest the margin

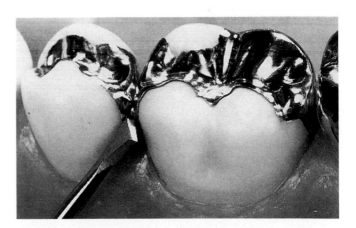

Fig. 19-73. When Black spoon technique fails or cannot be used, No. 48 chisel can be used to initiate removal. Long axis of No. 48 chisel is directed as much as possible with line of draw of cavity preparation with its blade edge engaging small bleb made for this purpose. A *very light* tap is delivered to the handle end of the No. 48 chisel with a *small* leather-headed mallet. Note that inlay is now displaced from its seating by a few tenths of a millimeter. After slight unseating, apply procedure shown in Fig. 19-72 on distal aspect.

be injured. Even with these stated hazards, this removal method is safe to use when care is exercised. The slight extension is easily removed after the casting displacement and before cementation, or it could be dressed down by paper discs after cementation.

Soldering contacts

When a casting is short of contacting the adjacent tooth, solder of 650 (or higher) fine is added to the proximal surface of the restoration to establish a proper contact. The difference between the solidus temperature of the inlay and the liquidus temperature of the solder should be 100° F (37.5° C) or more.

First, resurface the entire proximal surface of the casting with the Burlew wheel, thus cleaning the surface of any possible traces of antifluxes (e.g., tripoli/BBC, rouge) (Fig. 19-74, *A*). Next, cut a piece of strip solder that will extend approximately 1 mm in all directions beyond the contact near-approach surface and that, when positioned over the proposed contact position on the casting, will not extend closer than 1 mm to the margins or the marginal ridge. Apply a borax-type flux both to the proximal surface and both sides of the piece of solder. Do not apply too much flux; also, exercise care to keep flux from the occlusal surface or cavity side of the casting. These precautions prevent the solder from flowing onto these surfaces.

Holding the inlay in suitable soldering pliers (it is best not to have the pliers pressing on marginal metal), properly position the solder, and carry the casting into a clean-burning, blue, brush flame of a Bunsen burner for a second or two, and then remove it from the flame. Repeat this until the temperature of the parts slowly rises

to a point where the flux effloresces as it loses water of crystallization (Fig. 19-74, *B* and *C*). If the heating of the parts is too rapid, either the volatilization of the flux vehicle or the "flowering" of efflorescence will be violent and usually displaces the solder. Continue raising the temperature slowly until efflorescence stops. Then hold the casting with its solder in the flame until the solder flows, at which time immediately withdraw it from the flame. The solder will flow evenly outward from the contact over the proximal surface if, at the moment the solder flows, the casting is being held so that the proximal surface is level, with the proposed contact position being the highest elevation (Fig. 19-74, *D*). The proximal surface is tilted slightly only if it is desired that the new contact area be moved toward the direction of tilting.

The soldered casting is pickled clean, and the new proximal surface contour and contact are developed with sandpaper discs or rubber wheels. After the contact is adjusted and verified in the mouth, the surface is repolished with tripoli/BBC and rouge as before.

CEMENTATION
Cement selection

The selection of cement for permanent cementation is very important to the success of the final restoration. Presently there are four cements commonly used for permanent cementation of cast metal restorations: zinc phosphate, zinc polyacrylate, glass ionomer, and resin cements. Of these four cements, zinc phosphate and glass ionomer are the most popular. The advantages and disadvantages of each cement are discussed in detail in

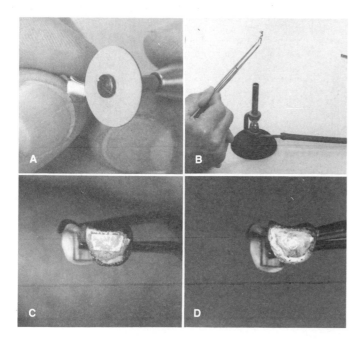

Fig. 19-74. Soldering the contact. **A,** Cleaning proximal surface of all traces of antifluxes by resurfacing with Burlew wheel. **B,** Bunsen burner is used for soldering procedure. **C,** Fluxed inlay and solder are heated slowly until flux gently effloresces. **D,** Soldered surface. Note how solder has spread evenly to cover most of proximal surface.

Chapter 6. Some of the properties of these cements are listed in Table 6-21.

Zinc phosphate cement has been used for the longest period and has "survived the test of time." When properly mixed, it has a *good working time* that allows the cementation of multiple castings from one mix. Once set, the excess material is fairly *easy to remove*. Zinc phosphate cements, as a group, display a *film thickness* as *low* as any of the cements, thus allowing complete seating of the restoration.[17] The major disadvantage of zinc phosphate cement is that it has initially a *low pH* (3.5 at cementation) which can irritate the pulpal tissues and cause transient pain during cementation. For this reason, some operators prefer to "seal" the dentin with copal varnish prior to cementation with zinc phosphate cement.

Polycarboxylate cements (zinc polyacrylates) were first introduced in 1968.[21] The primary advantage of these cements is that they are *less irritating to the pulpal tissues* than the previously mentioned cements because they are less acidic and the acid is only weakly dissociated. Unlike zinc phosphate cements, polycarboxylate cements have been shown to be *adhesive to enamel*, stainless steel, and certain properly prepared alloys.[1,20] For optimal adhesion the tooth surfaces and the casting must be absolutely clean and dry, and the metal casting should be sandblasted on the cavity side. Even so, laboratory tests have not demonstrated that polycarboxylate cements provide better retention of metal castings than zinc phosphate cement.[17]

The *working time of polycarboxylate cements is short*, so one should not attempt to cement more than two units with a single mix. Do not attempt to seat the restoration once the cement has lost its initial gloss. This cement must not be disturbed once it is in the rubbery stage for fear of pulling some of the cement out from under the casting. When set, this cement is more difficult to clean up than zinc phosphate cement.

Glass ionomer cements can also be used for the permanent cementation of metal castings. The material is basically a hybrid of silicate and polycarboxylate cements. These cements *adhere to enamel and dentin* because of the polyacrylic acid in the liquid.[19] The cement does *release fluoride* over time, which should inhibit recurrent caries.[28,30] *The setting reaction of glass ionomer cement is slow and is accompanied by a steady increase in strength.* The compressive and tensile strengths after 1 day become greater than those of zinc phosphate. The slow reaction time makes glass ionomer cements *technique sensitive, especially in regard to loss or gain of moisture during setting.* If glass ionomer cements are not mixed and handled properly (e.g., if they are contaminated by saliva during the first 10 minutes of setting) they are quite soluble and susceptible to marginal leakage, which may (in addition to the low pH

during setting) account for some reports of post-cementation sensitivity.[22]

For maximal adhesion the prepared tooth must be clean and dry, and the casting should be sandblasted on the cavity side. Mixing should be rapid and follow the manufacturer's instructions. The casting must be seated before the cement loses its initial gloss, and the excess should not be removed for 10 minutes. *Maintaining a dry field is essential, since this cement is susceptible to early water attack and subsequent loss of physical properties.* Some manufacturers provide a special waterproof varnish to coat the margins to reduce loss or gain of moisture from the setting cement.

The *resin-based (polymethacrylate) cements** have improved remarkably in the last decade. Their principle *advantages* are: (1) they have *good adhesion to tooth structure* and therefore provide good retention (even in cavity preparations which have less than ideal retention due to over-tapered and/or short longitudinal walls), (2) *microleakage is reduced* since they are used with dentin bonding agents, and (3) they are *virtually insoluble*. Their *disadvantages* are: (1) they are *technique sensitive*, (2) they are relatively *expensive*, and (3) *removal of excess set cement is more difficult*.

It becomes apparent that no cement is without shortcomings. Each product has specific requirements in regard to tooth surface conditioning, casting surface conditioning, and manipulation techniques. *To obtain optimal performance from the cement, carefully follow the manufacturer's instructions for dispensing, mixing, and application.*

Cementation technique with zinc phosphate cement

Zinc phosphate cement is a commonly used cement for inlay and onlay cementation because of low film thickness, good retention, good working time, and easy removal of set excess cement. Before cementing the casting, isolate the tooth from saliva with the aid of cotton rolls (and saliva ejector if necessary) (Fig. 19-76, *A*). With the air syringe, dry the cavity walls, but do not desiccate them. This air drying (approximately 3 to 5 seconds) should eliminate visible moisture from the walls, except possibly on the gingival bevel. With a very small cotton pellet, apply a thin coat of varnish to the dentin walls. This should reduce the irritation of the pulp by the acid in the zinc phosphate cement to be applied subsequently.

Before making the mix of zinc phosphate cement, be certain that the following items are ready for use: (1) a No. 2 beaver-tail burnisher; (2) a UNC Jiffy-tube, small, with curved tip; (3) two cotton pellets; (4) a small-sized cotton roll that has been prepared for cover-

*C&B Metabond, Parkell, Farmindale, NY.

ing the open end of the Jiffy tube (Fig. 19-75, *A*); (5) a large knife-edge Jelenko Burlew disc (two of these if two or more castings are to be cemented in one operation); (6) mouth mirror; (7) operating pliers; and (8) No. 26 ball burnisher. Now make a cementing consistency mix of zinc phosphate cement following the manufacturer's instructions. The dental assistant loads the Jiffy tube (Fig. 19-75, *B*), closes the back end of the tube with both the cotton pellets and the prepared cotton roll

(Fig. 19-75, *C* and *D*), and hands this to the dentist. While the dentist expels cement into the preparation by finger squeezing the tube (Figs. 19-75, *E,* and 19-76, *B*), the assistant covers the inside of the casting with cement using the beaver-tail burnisher (Fig. 19-76, *C*). During insertion of the cement into the tooth, the tip of the tube is kept directly on the gingival and pulpal walls, thereby facilitating the filling of the preparation from the bottom up without trapping air. Care is taken

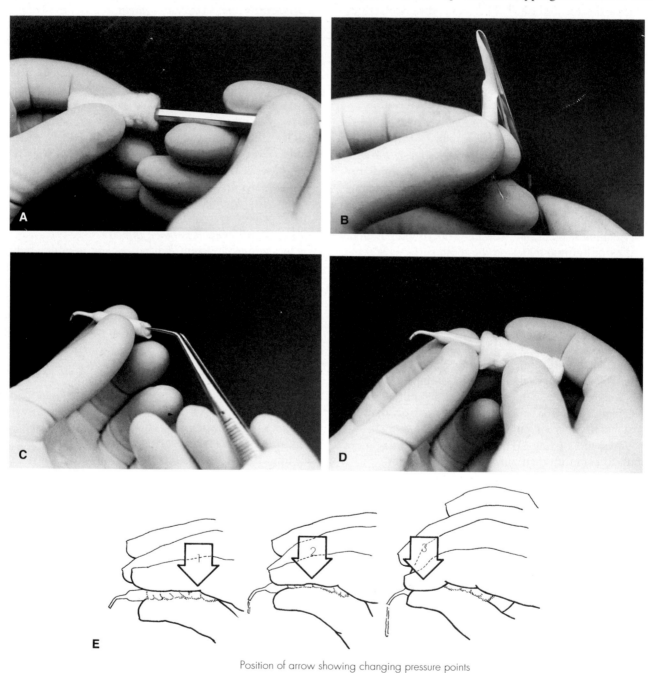

Position of arrow showing changing pressure points

Fig. 19-75. A, Punching a hole in end of cotton roll that will receive back end of UNC Jiffy tube. **B,** Conveying cement into tube. **C,** Cotton pellets are inserted into back end to tube. Prepared cotton rolls applied over tube **(D),** and cement is expelled into tooth by squeezing with thumb and forefinger progressively from back end of tube toward tip end, in three stages illustrated **(E).**

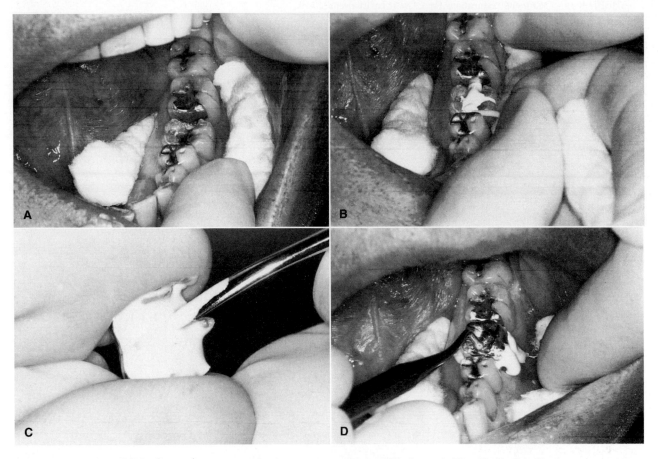

Fig. 19-76. Cementing cast metal onlay on preparation initially shown in Fig. 19-40, *B*, with zinc phosphate cement. **A,** Isolate tooth from saliva with cotton rolls. **B,** Using UNC Jiffy tube to expel zinc phosphate cement into cavity preparation without trapping air. **C,** Applying cement with No. 2 beaver-tail burnisher to cavity side of onlay. **D,** Seating onlay with ball burnisher and hand pressure. *Continued.*

by both the assistant and dentist not to trap air in the application of the cement. If the cement is not applied to both the cavity side of the casting and the preparation walls, the trapping of air is invited.

Without an assistant the dentist must work faster to (1) apply the cement to the casting, (2) fill the Jiffy tube, and (3) expel the cement that is in the tube into the preparation. This sequence must be adhered to. If the tube is filled first and set aside while the cavity side of the casting is covered, the mix in the tube will become too warm and consequently set too fast before its application. Unfortunately the Jiffy tube is a heat insulator; the cement mix is in bulk form and is developing exothermic heat. The result may be that the cement will be too viscous to permit complete seating of the casting. It is also incorrect to expel the cement from the tube into the preparation before applying the mix to the casting, inasmuch as the cement in the preparation may develop too much viscosity because of the increased rate of setting caused by mouth temperature and humidity. *It is emphasized that the Jiffy tube is loaded quickly and used immediately.*

If the cavity preparation includes a slot, the slot must be filled with cement before the Jiffy tube is loaded. To incorporate cement into the slot without trapping air, use a Lentulo spiral instrument in the contra-angle handpiece. After the tip of the spiral is placed in the cement mix on the mixing slab, the tip end is carried to the bottom of the slot and rotated. When it is turning in the proper direction, the cement is carried into the slot.

With the cement mix applied to the casting and the preparation, start the casting to place with the fingers or with operative pliers. Ideally two convex outward surfaces of cement should meet when the casting is started to place, thus preventing the trapping of air. Next, place the ball burnisher in the pit areas (first one and then another), exerting maximal hand pressure to seat the casting (Fig. 19-76, *D*). Then, using operative pliers, place the Burlew disc over the casting, remove the saliva ejector, and request the patient to close and exert heavy biting force on the disc (Fig. 19-76, *E* and *F*). Ask the patient also to move the mandible slightly from side-to-side while continuing to exert pressure. Ten seconds of this pressure is sufficient. When the disc is removed, much of the occlusal margin should be clean of the cement mix and visible to allow inspection and verification of complete seating of the casting. When the cusps are capped, complete seating of the casting is verified

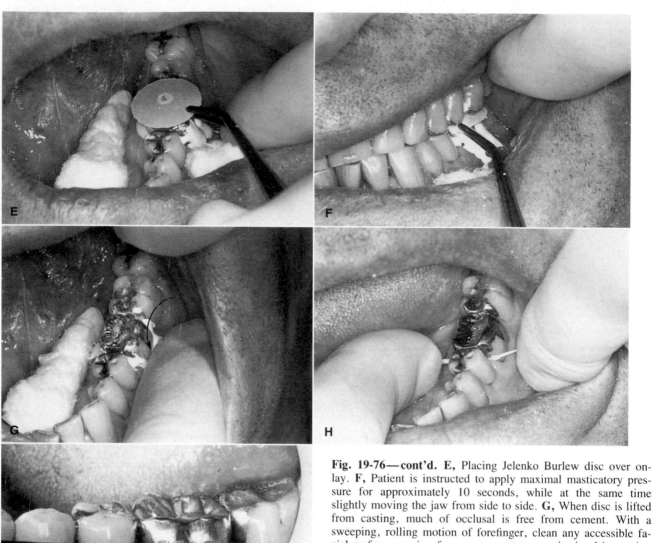

Fig. 19-76—cont'd. **E,** Placing Jelenko Burlew disc over on-lay. **F,** Patient is instructed to apply maximal masticatory pressure for approximately 10 seconds, while at the same time slightly moving the jaw from side to side. **G,** When disc is lifted from casting, much of occlusal is free from cement. With a sweeping, rolling motion of forefinger, clean any accessible facial surface margin of excess cement to permit visual inspection for verification of proper seating of onlay. Similarly clean any accessible lingual margin of excess cement. Full seating should also be verified tactilely with explorer tine. **H,** Remove excess set cement with explorer and air-water spray. Use dental tape with small knot to dislodge small pieces of interproximal cement. **I,** Onlay after cementation.

by inspection of the facial and lingual margins after wiping the excess cement away with a clean (of cement) finger or cotton roll (Fig. 19-76, *G*). Now while the cement is still soft, burnish all accessible margins. The saliva ejector is replaced in the mouth and the *region is kept dry during the setting of the cement.* Moisture that contacts setting zinc phosphate cement leaches out some of the phosphoric acid, which results in a weaker, more soluble cement. After the cement is hard, and not before, clear away the excess cement, *ensuring that all cement is removed along any subgingival margins.* When cementing has been properly accomplished, there should not be a visible cement line at the margins (Fig. 19-76, *I*).

Placement of a cotton roll over the occlusal surface of an *inlay* is not advocated in lieu of the rubber disc, inasmuch as the former does not concentrate enough seating pressure directly on the inlay (i.e., the cotton roll is likely to distribute much of the pressure over occlusal areas outside the inlay). Pieces of wood also should not be used for this purpose, since these are likely to exert high biting forces on occlusal areas outside of the inlay margins that do not serve to seat the inlay and may fracture the tooth.

After the cement has hardened it is easily cleaned off with an explorer and air-water spray. Dental tape should be passed through the contact, carried into the interproximal gingival embrasures and sulci, and pulled fa-

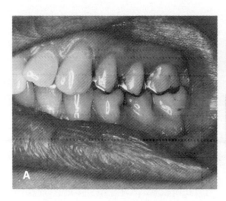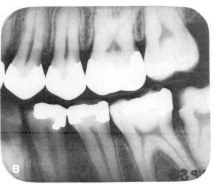

Fig. 19-77. A, Cemented castings on teeth first shown in Fig. 19-42, *E.* Photo was taken immediately after cementation and insertion of composite insert on molar. **B,** Bitewing radiograph of restored quadrant shown in **A.** Note fit of inlays at gingival margins and contour of proximal surfaces.

cially and lingually to help in the removal of cement in this hidden region (Fig. 19-76, *H*). Tying a small knot in the tape will help dislodge small bits of interproximal cement. Finally, directing a stream of air into the gingival sulcus will open it and reveal any remaining small pieces of cement, which then should be removed. If a facial surface composite insert is scheduled, the cement is easily removed from the preparation for the insert after the setting of the cement has progressed for a few minutes and before it is hard. A quadrant of inlays after cementation and insertion of a composite insert is illustrated in Fig. 19-77.

REFERENCES

1. Ady AB, Fairhurst CW: Bond strengths of two types of cement to gold casting alloy, *J Prosthet Dent* 29(2):217-220, 1973.
2. Black GV: *Operative dentistry,* ed 8, Woodstock, Ill, 1947, Medico-Dental Publishing.
3. Brockhurst PJ, Cannon RW: Alloys for crown and bridgework, *Aust Dent J* 26:287-294, 1981.
4. Crispin BL, Watson JF, Caputo AA: The marginal accuracy of treatment restorations: a comparative analysis, *J Prosthet Dent* 44:283-290, 1980.
5. Dawson PE: *Evaluation, diagnosis, and treatment of occlusal problems,* St Louis, 1974, Mosby.
6. Eichner K: Applications of metal alloys in dentistry—a review, *Int Dent J* 33(1):1-10, 1983.
7. Fisher DW et al: Photoelastic analysis of inlay and onlay preparations, *J Prosthet Dent* 33(1):47-53, 1975.
8. Fisher DW, Shillinburg HT, Dewhirst RB: Indirect temporary restorations, *J Am Dent Assoc* 82:160-163, 1971.
9. Grossman LI: Pulp reaction to the insertion of self-curing acrylic resin filling materials, *J Am Dent Assoc* 46:265-269, 1953.
10. Hume WR: A new technique for screening chemical toxicity to the pulp from dental restorative materials and procedures, *J Dent Res* 64(11):1322-1325, 1985.
11. Kishimoto M, Shillinburg HT, Duncanson MG: Influence of preparation features on retention and resistance. I. MOD onlays, *J Prosthet Dent* 49(1):35-39, 1983.
12. Kramer IRH, McLean JW: Response of the human pulp to self-polymerizing acrylic restorations, *Brit Dent J* 92(10):255-315, 1952.
13. Langeland K, Langeland L: Pulp reactions to crown preparation, impression, temporary crown fixation and permanent cementation, *J Prosthet Dent* 15(1):129-143, 1965.
14. Malamed SF: *Handbook of local anesthesia,* ed 3, St Louis, 1990, Mosby.
15. Moffa JP: Alternative dental casting alloys, *Dent Clin North Am* 27:733-746, 1983.
16. Moulding MB, Loney RW: The effect of cooling techniques on intrapulpal temperature during direct fabrication of provisional restorations, *Int J Prosthodont* 4(4):332-336, 1991.
17. Oilo G: Luting cements: a review and comparison, *Int Dent J* 41(2):81-88, 1991.
18. Payne E: Reproduction of tooth form, *Ney Tech Bull* 1(9):1961.
19. Phillips RW: *Skinner's science of dental materials,* ed 8, Philadelphia, 1982, WB Saunders.
20. Saito C et al: Adhesion of polycarboxylate cements to dental casting alloys, *J Prosthet Dent* 35:543-548, 1976.
21. Smith DC: A new dental cement, *Brit Dent J* 125:381-384, 1968.
22. Smith DC, Ruse ND: Acidity of glass ionomer cement during setting and its relation to pulp sensitivity, *J Am Dent Assoc* 112:654-657, 1986.
23. Sockwell CL: Dental handpieces and rotary cutting instruments, *Dent Clin North Am* 15(1):219-244, 1971.
24. Stanley HR: Pulpal response to dental techniques and materials, *Dent Clin North Am* 15(1):115-125, 1971.
25. Sturdevant CM: *Gold inlay restorations for Class II cavity preparations,* ed 1, New York, 1968, McGraw Hill.
26. Sturdevant JR et al: The 8-year clinical performance of 15 low-gold casting alloys, *Dent Mater* 3(6):347-352, 1987.
27. Sturdevant RE: *Personal communication,* 1955.
28. Swift EJ: An update of glass ionomer cements, *Quintessence Int* 19(2):125-130, 1988.
29. Taylor NO, Paffenbarger GC, Sweeny WT: Inlay casting golds: physical properties and specifications, *J Am Dent Assoc* 19:36-53, 1932.
30. van de Voorde A, Gerdts GJ, Murchison DF: Clinical use of glass ionomer cement: a literature review, *Quintessence Int* 19(1):53-61, 1988.

CHAPTER 20

Direct gold restorations*

Gregory E. Smith

Several types of dental restorative materials are currently available. They are generally grouped into categories such as silver amalgam materials, cast golds, tooth-colored materials, dental porcelains, porcelains fused to metal, and direct golds. *Direct golds* are those gold restorative materials that are manufactured for compaction directly into prepared cavities. Several types of direct golds are manufactured for dental use. Most are pure 24-karat gold, and they differ in their metallurgical structure.

Pure gold has been in use in dentistry in the United States for well over 100 years.[5,10,12,20,22] A variety of techniques have been advanced for its use in the restoration of teeth. It is generally agreed that this noble metal is a superior restorative material for treatment of

---

*Pure gold materials used for photography in this chapter were provided courtesy Williams Gold Refining Company, Inc.

many small lesions and defects in teeth, given sound pulpal and periodontal health. Success is achieved with direct gold restoration if meticulous care is given to an exacting technique in cavity preparation design and material manipulation. Direct gold restorations can last for a lifetime if attention is paid to details of restorative technique and to proper home care. The longevity of direct gold restorations is a result of both the superb biocompatibility of gold with the oral environment and its excellent marginal integrity.

It is the purpose of this chapter to discuss the various forms of direct gold presently available and explain the principles requisite to their manipulation. The principles of cavity preparation are reviewed as they are applied to direct gold restorations, and a detailed consideration is given to Class I, Class V, and Class III cavity preparations as well as to the manipulation of selected direct gold types.

DIRECT GOLDS AND PRINCIPLES OF MANIPULATION
Materials and manufacture

There are several physical types of direct-filling golds,[11] (Fig. 20-1). All are "compactible" in that they

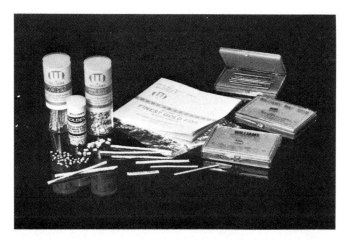

Fig. 20-1. Various forms of direct-filling gold available from the manufacturer. *Left,* samples of Goldent pellets and prerolled cylinders and ropes. *Center,* book of gold foil. *Right,* boxes of crystalline gold.

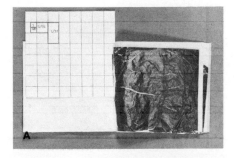

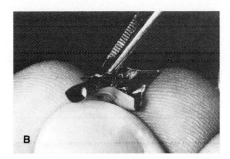

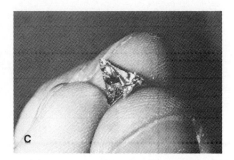

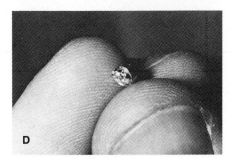

Fig. 20-2. **A,** 4 × 4 inch book of foil marked for cutting and rolling into pellets of various sizes. **B** and **C,** Corners of foil piece are tucked into center. **D,** Foil is rolled into a completed pellet. (**A,** courtesy Terkla and Cantwell.)

are inserted into cavity preparations under force and compacted or condensed into cavity line and point angles and against cavity walls. The six gold types currently manufactured* are gold foil, platinized gold foil, crystalline gold in three forms (as [1] mat gold, [2] mat gold wrapped in gold foil, and [3] mat gold alloyed with calcium and wrapped in gold foil [Electraloy R.V.]), and powdered gold.

Gold foil is manufactured by beating pure gold into thin sheets. The gold foil is cut into 4 × 4 inch (10 × 10 cm) sheets and sold in books of sheets separated by pages of thin paper. The books contain 1/10 or 1/20 ounce of gold. The sheets of foil which weigh 4 gr each are termed No. 4 foil; 4 × 4 sheets weighing 3 gr are termed No. 3 foil; and 4 × 4 sheets weighing 2 gr are termed No. 2 foil. Because the 4 × 4 inch sheets of foil are too large to use in restorative procedures, they are rolled into ropes, cylinders, or pellets before insertion into cavity preparations. Gold foil referred to in the restorative sections of this chapter is in pellet form.

Pellets of gold foil are generally rolled from 1/32, 1/43, 1/64, or 1/128 sections cut from a No. 4 sheet of foil. The book of foil is marked and cut into squares or rectangles (Fig. 20-2, *A*). Each piece is placed on clean finger tips, and the corners are tucked into the center (Fig. 20-2, *B* and *C*); then it is lightly rolled into pellet form (Fig. 20-2, *D*). Also, cylinders and ropes of gold foil may be rolled from segments of a sheet (see Figs. 20-1 and 20-4, *A*). Prerolled cylinders may be obtained into No. 4 or the thinner No. 2 gold foil, which is termed "Extraply," and may be purchased in 1/10- or 1/20-ounce vials.

*Williams Gold Refining Company, Inc., Buffalo, NY.

After pellets of gold are rolled, they may be conveniently stored in a *gold foil box* (Fig. 20-3), which is divided into labeled sections for various sizes of pellets. Cylinders of foil and/or selected sizes of other types of gold may also be stored in the box. Preferential contamination is suggested by placing a damp cotton pellet dipped into 18% ammonia into each section of the box. This will serve to prevent deleterious oxides from forming on the gold until it is used.

Platinized gold foil is recommended for use in areas of occlusal stress where increased restoration hardness is desired, such as in Class VI restorations in anterior teeth. This material is manufactured by sandwiching a sheet of platinum between two sheets of No. 4 gold

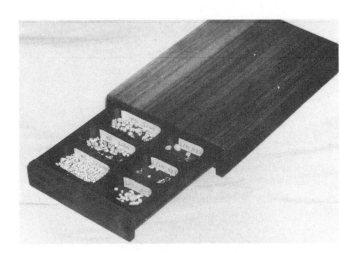

Fig. 20-3. Gold foil box. Compartments are labeled to show pellet size.

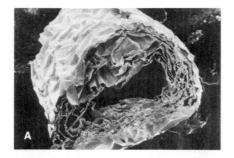
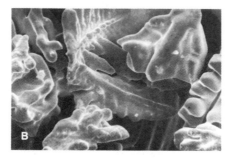
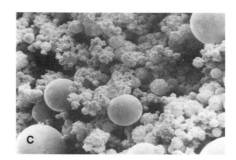

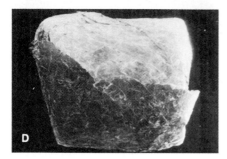

Fig. 20-4. Scanning electron photomicrographs of direct-filling golds. **A,** End view of machine-rolled pellet. **B,** Crystals of mat gold. **C,** Spheres of Goldent. **D,** Wrapped Goldent pellet that contains spheres. (Courtesy Williams Gold Refining Co, Inc.)

foil, and hammering the mass together until a final thickness of a No. 4 sheet of foil is obtained.[15]

Crystalline mat gold is made by electrolytic precipitation[4] (Fig. 20-4, *B*), and it is available (Fig. 20-1) in strips in either medium (2 mm) or wide (3 mm) widths. These strips are cut to preferred size just before insertion into a cavity preparation. Mat gold wrapped in No. 4 gold foil is called ***mat foil.***

Electraloy R.V. is mat gold alloyed with calcium 0.1% to 0.5% by weight and wrapped in No. 4 gold foil. The *purpose of the calcium is to give the product increased hardness and strength.*[16]

Powdered gold is made by a combination of chemical precipitation and atomization, with an average particle size of 15 microns[13] (Fig. 20-4, *C*). The atomized particles are mixed together in wax, cut into pieces, and wrapped in No. 2½ or No. 3 foil (Fig. 20-4, *D*). Several sizes of these pellets are available. Each pellet contains approximately 10 times more gold than a pellet of gold foil of comparable size. Two products (Easy Gold and Goldent) are commercially available.

Cohesion and degassing

Direct golds are inserted into cavity preparations under force. The purpose of the force is to weld the gold into restorations containing minimal porosity or internal void spaces.[7,8,18] Welding occurs because pure gold with an absolutely clean surface will cohere to itself as a result of metallic bonding. As the gold is forced and compressed into a cavity preparation, succeeding increments cohere to those previously placed. For successful welding to occur during restoration, *the gold must be in a cohesive state before compaction, and a suitable, bi-ologically compatible compacting force must be delivered.*

All of the forms of gold listed may be either ***cohesive*** or ***noncohesive.*** They are noncohesive if surface impurities are present that prevent one increment of gold from cohering to another. The manufacturer supplies books of gold foil in a cohesive or noncohesive state. Strips of mat gold, mat foil, and Electraloy R.V. are essentially cohesive when purchased but may have attracted some surface impurities during shipment. Goldent pellets are supplied with a wax coating that must be burned off before compaction.

Because gold attracts gases that render it noncohesive, such gases must be removed from the surface of the gold before dental compaction. This process is usually referred to as ***degassing*** or ***annealing*** and is accomplished by application of heat. Degassing is the preferred term, since the desired result is to remove residual surface contamination, although further annealing, resulting in additional internal stress relief or recrystallization, may also occur in this process. All direct-filling gold products are degassed immediately before use except when noncohesive foil is specifically desired. Underheating during degassing is to be avoided because it fails to render the gold surface pure. Overheating is also to be avoided, since it may cause the gold to become brittle or melt and render it unusable.

Degassing is accomplished by heating the gold on a mica tray over a flame or on an electric annealer, or each piece of gold may be heated over a pure ethanol flame (Fig. 20-5).

The advantage of the technique involving use of the *pure* ethanol flame is that each piece of gold is selected

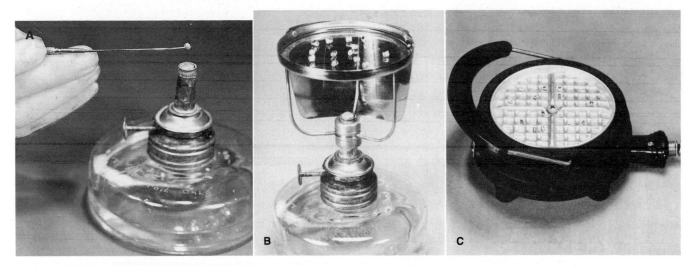

Fig. 20-5. A, Pellet of gold foil is degassed in *pure* ethanol flame. **B,** Mica tray mounted over alcohol lamp for degassing several increments of gold simultaneously. **C,** Gold foil degassed on an electric annealer. (Courtesy Terkla and Cantwell.)

and heated just before insertion, and waste of gold is avoided. A careful technique is needed to correctly degas an increment of gold in the flame. The gold is passed into the blue inner core of the flame on the tip of a foil passing instrument, held just until it becomes dull red, and then is withdrawn from the flame. After a few seconds are allowed for cooling, it is placed in the cavity preparation.

Any of the three degassing procedures is satisfactory for all golds except powdered gold. The powdered gold pellet is heated in the ethanol flame until a bright flame occurs (caused by ignition of the wax) and the pellet becomes dull red; then it is immediately withdrawn.

Principles of compaction

All direct-filling golds must be compacted during insertion into cavity preparations.[2] With the exception of powdered gold, the **compaction** takes the form of malleting forces, which are delivered either by a hand mallet used by the *assistant* or by an Electro-Mallet or pneumatic mallet used by the *dentist*. Powdered gold, because of its spheroidal powdered form, may be compacted by heavy hand pressure delivered in a rocking motion with specially designed hand condensers.[1,3] Successful malleting of the other golds may be achieved with any of the currently available equipment. Some operators prefer the Electro-Mallet or pneumatic mallet because a dental assistant is not required for the procedure.

A technique preferred by many uses a hand mallet to deliver light blows to a condenser held by the dentist (Fig. 20-6, *A*). This technique allows great control of malleting forces when variations are called for, and it allows for rapid change in condenser nibs, or tips, when

a multitude of condensers is required. In any case, a suitable condenser must be stepped over the gold systematically to achieve a dense, well-compacted restoration (see Fig. 20-9).

Condensers are designed to deliver forces of compaction to direct golds. Condensers used in the handpieces of the Electro-Mallet or pneumatic mallet consist of a *nib,* or working tip, and a short *shank* approximately 1 inch (2.5 cm) in length that fits into the malleting handpiece. Condensers used with the hand mallet are longer (approximately 6 inches [15 cm]) and have a blunt-ended *handle* that receives light blows from the hand mallet.

Condenser *nibs* are available in several shapes and sizes (Fig. 20-6, *B*). All have pyramidal serrations on the nib faces to prevent slipping on the gold. Those described in this chapter are (1) the round condensers, 0.4 to 0.55 mm in diameter, (2) the Varney foot condenser, which has a rectangular face that is approximately 1 × 1.3 mm, and (3) the parallelogram condensers, which are used only for hand pressure compaction and have nib faces that measure approximately 0.5 × 1 mm.

Condenser *shanks* may be straight, monangled, or offset, and their *nib faces* may be cut perpendicular to the long axis of the handle or perpendicular to the end portion of the shank (Fig. 20-7). *The smaller the nib face size (area) is, the greater the pounds per square inch delivered, given a constant malleting force.* For example, if the nib diameter is reduced by half, the effective compaction force in pounds per square inch is four times greater (since the area of a circle is proportional to the square of the diameter). For most compaction of gold foil and crystalline gold, the 0.4 to 0.55 mm diameter nibs are suitable. Smaller condensers tend

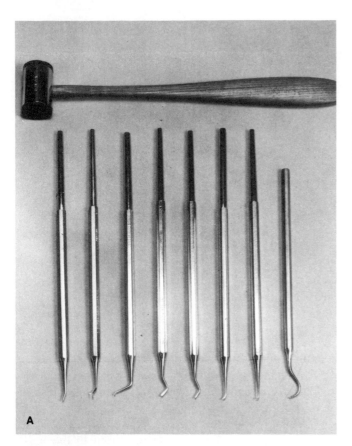

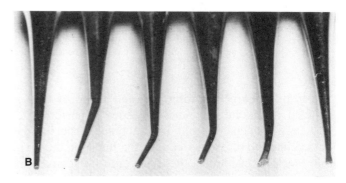

Fig. 20-6. A, Hand mallet and condensers used for hand mallet compaction of direct gold. **B,** A selection of variously shaped nibs. *Left to right:* Three round-faced nibs, oblique-faced nib, foot condenser, and rounded rectangular nib. (**A,** courtesy Terkla and Cantwell.)

to punch holes in the gold, whereas larger ones are less effective in forcing the gold into angles.

Two *fundamental principles involved in compaction* of cohesive gold are (1) to weld the gold into a cohesive mass and (2) to wedge as much gold as possible into the cavity preparation (minimal air inclusion).[14] Welding takes place primarily as a result of the coherence of a

noble metal to itself. Wedging results from careful compacting technique. Regardless of the technique used, some **bridging** will occur, resulting in void spaces not only in the compacted gold but also along the cavity walls. Success depends on minimizing these voids, particularly on the surface of the restoration and at the cavosurface interface where leakage to the internal aspects of the restoration might begin.

Gold foil compacts readily because of its thin form and produces a mass with isolated linear channels of *microporosity* (Fig. 20-8, *A*). Because the thin folds of the gold pellet weld to each other, the remaining channels of microporosity do not appear to be entirely confluent with one another. *It is for this reason that direct gold restorations are generally veneered with gold foil.*

Movement of either mat gold or Electraloy R.V. under compacting forces is different from that of gold foil because of the dendritic or fernlike structure of these crystalline golds. The crystals lock with each other under compacting forces, and movement of gold stops, resulting in a network of void spaces around the crystals (Fig. 20-8, *B*).

Compaction of powdered gold is frequently recommended to be done by hand pressure with a heavy rocking motion. As this is performed, the bag of atomized gold is opened and the spheres of gold powder move over one another and against the cavity walls. Very heavy pressure is required to compact this form of gold

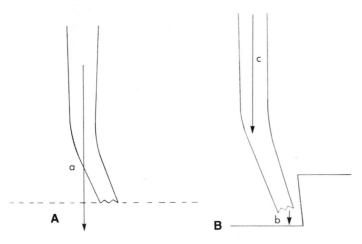

Fig. 20-7. A, Oblique-faced condenser with nib face established perpendicular to long axis of handle and perpendicular to line of force *(a)*. **B,** Conventional monangle condenser; nib face is not perpendicular to line of force *(b);* condenser nib face is established perpendicular to end portion of shank rather than perpendicular to handle *(c)*.

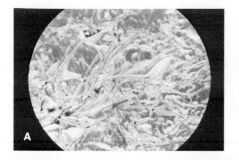
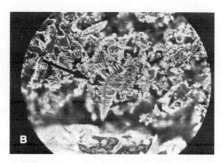

Fig. 20-8. A, Compacted gold foil. Linear channels are evident between creases in the foil pellet. Dark spots are void spaces in the compacted mass. **B,** Compacted mat foil. Intact crystal of gold is identified by arrow. Dark spots are void spaces between crystals. Remnant of foil wrapping is evident at bottom.

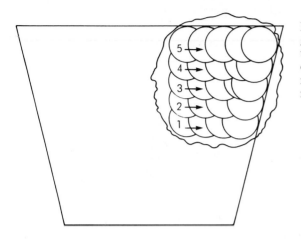

Fig. 20-9. Diagrammatic order of compaction for increment of direct-filling gold. Condensers are moved across surface of gold in an orderly stepping motion. Each succeeding step of the nib overlaps the previous one by at least half of the nib face diameter. Condensation begins at position *1* and moves to the right, resumes at *2* and repeats movement to the right, and then continues in rows *3, 4,* and *5.*

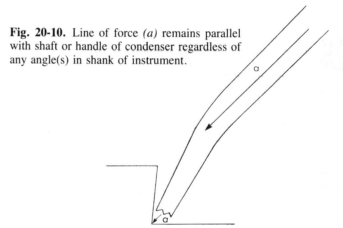

Fig. 20-10. Line of force *(a)* remains parallel with shaft or handle of condenser regardless of any angle(s) in shank of instrument.

effectively, and some prefer to augment the hand compaction with malleting.

Compaction technique

Compaction begins when a piece of gold is placed in a cavity preparation. The gold is first pressed to place by hand. Then while this first increment is often held steady in position by a holding instrument, a condenser of suitable size is used to begin malleting in the center of the mass. Each succeeding step of the condenser overlaps by half the previous one as the condenser is moved toward the periphery (Fig. 20-9). The gold moves under the nib face of the condenser, effecting compaction as malleting proceeds.

The most efficient compaction occurs directly under the nib face.[17] Some compaction also occurs by lateral movement of the gold against surrounding cavity walls. The result of compaction is to remove most of the void space from within each increment of gold, to compact the gold into cavity line and point angles and against walls, and to attach it to any previously placed gold via the process of cohesion.[9]

The line of force is important when gold is compacted. The line of force is that direction through which the force is delivered, that is, the direction in which the condenser is aimed (Fig. 20-10). Specific instructions regarding line of force are given in subsequent sections of this chapter as they relate to the restorations.

Research has shown that a biologically acceptable pulpal response occurs following proper direct gold procedures.[21] Care is required when condensing forces are applied to preclude pulpal irritation. The Electro-Mallet is an acceptable condenser if the manufacturer's instructions for mallet intensity are followed. Correct hand-malleting technique requires a light, bouncing application of the mallet to the condenser rather than the delivery of heavy blows.

PRINCIPLES OF CAVITY PREPARATION FOR DIRECT GOLD RESTORATIONS
Fundamentals of cavity preparation

The principles of cavity preparation for all direct gold restorations demand meticulous attention to detail for success. Failure to give attention to outline form may result in an unsightly restoration or, at the least, one in which cavosurface deficiencies are immediately obvious. Poor resistance form can result in tooth fracture. Inadequate retention form may result in a loose restoration that is frustrating to the dentist. Lack of detailed convenience form may render an otherwise excellent cavity preparation unrestorable. The cavity preparation must be smoothed and debrided to permit the first increments of gold to be stabilized.

The margins in *outline form* must not be ragged. They are established on sound areas of the tooth that can be finished and polished. Outline form includes an initial depth into dentin ranging from 0.5 mm from the dentinoenamel junction in Class I cavity preparations to 0.75 mm from the cementum in Class V cavity preparations (see Stages and Sites in Cavity Preparation, in Chapter 7). It must include all structural defects associated with the lesion except carious infected dentin that is deeper pulpally than the initial depth. The marginal outline must be designed to be esthetically pleasing because the final restoration may be visible.

Resistance form is established by orienting cavity walls to support the integrity of the tooth, such as a pulpal wall that is flat and perpendicular to occlusal forces. All enamel must be supported by sound dentin. Optimally placed axial or pulpal walls promote the integrity of the restored tooth, thus providing a suitable thickness of remaining dentin.

The *retention form* is established by parallelism of some walls and by strategically placed converging walls, as will be described in detail for each cavity preparation. In addition, walls must be smooth and flat where possible to provide resistance to loosening of the gold during compaction. Also, sharp internal line angles are required to resist movement.

Optimal *convenience form* requires suitable access and a dry field provided by the rubber dam. Access may additionally require the use of a gingival retractor for Class V restorations or a separator to provide a minimal amount of separation (0.5 mm maximum) between anterior teeth for Class III restorations. Sharp internal line and point angles are created to allow convenient "starting" of the gold as compaction begins.

Removal of remaining carious dentin, final planing of cavosurface margins, and debridement complete the cavity preparation for direct gold.

Indications and contraindications

Class I direct gold restorations are one option for the treatment of small carious lesions in pits and fissures of most posterior teeth and the lingual surfaces of anterior teeth (see Chapter 5 for Clinical Examination for Caries, in the section, Examination and Diagnosis, subsection, Examination of Teeth and Restorations). Direct gold is also indicated for treatment of small, cavitated Class V carious lesions or for the restoration, when in-

dicated, of abraded or eroded areas on the facial surfaces of teeth, although access to the molars is a limiting factor. Class III direct gold restorations are one option on the proximal surfaces of anterior teeth where the lesions are small enough to be treated with esthetically pleasing results. Class II direct gold restorations are one option for restoration of small cavitated proximal surface carious lesions in posterior teeth where marginal ridges are not subjected to heavy occlusal forces, such as the mesial or distal surfaces of mandibular first premolars and the mesial surface of some maxillary premolars. Incisal edges or cusp tips frequently prove to be suitable Class VI situations for use of direct golds. Margins of otherwise acceptable cast gold restorations may be restored with direct golds.

Direct gold restorations are contraindicated in some teeth with very large pulp chambers, in severely periodontally weakened teeth with questionable prognosis, when economics is a severely limiting factor, and in handicapped, elderly, or very young patients who are unable to sit for the longer dental appointment required. Root canal filled teeth are generally not restored with direct gold because these teeth are brittle, although in some cases gold may be the material of choice to close access preparations (for root canal therapy) in cast gold restorations.

CAVITY PREPARATIONS AND RESTORATIONS

Detailed consideration will now be given to cavity preparations and the restoration of Class I, Class V, and Class III lesions. The preparations for Class I and Class V lesions are designed to be restored with mat gold, mat foil, or Electraloy R.V. These are veneered with pellets of gold foil. The preparations described may be restored entirely with pellets of gold foil, or powdered gold may be used. If powdered gold is selected, heavy, rocking hand pressure compaction may be substituted for hand mallet or automatic mallet techniques.

The Class III cavity preparation in this chapter is that recommended by Ferrier, and only gold foil pellets are used for the restoration.

All cavity preparations and restorative procedures are accomplished after a suitable field of operation has been achieved by application of the ***rubber dam.***

Class I cavity preparation and restoration

Cavity preparation design. The marginal *outline form* for the Class I cavity preparation for compacted gold is extended to include the lesion on the tooth surface treated as well as fissured enamel; recall that outline form also implies a *limited depth* (only 0.5 mm pulpally of the dentinoenamel junction) *for this first step* in the initial stage of cavity preparation (see Chapter 7 for outline form and initial depth in section, Stages and Steps in Cavity Preparation). The marginal outline may

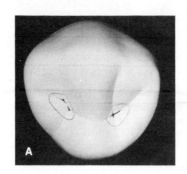

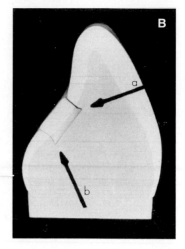

Fig. 20-11. A, Typical Class I occlusal marginal outlines for pit restorations with direct gold. B, Cross section of model of lingual Class I preparation on maxillary incisor. Undercuts (a and b) are placed in dentin incisally and gingivally for additional retention.

be a simple circular design for a pit defect, oblong, or triangular or may take on a more extensive form if needed to treat a defective fissure (Fig. 20-11, A). Cavity margins are placed out of the depth of pits and fissures. All noncoalesced enamel and structural defects are removed. The marginal outline is kept as small as possible consistent with provision of suitable access for instrumentation and for manipulation of gold.

For Class I cavity preparations the external walls of the preparation are parallel with each other, although in extensive occlusal preparations the mesial and/or distal wall(s) may diverge slightly occlusally to avoid undermining and weakening marginal ridges. The pulpal wall is of uniform depth, is parallel with the plane of the surface treated, and is established at 0.5 mm into the dentin. The pulpal wall meets the external walls at a slightly rounded angle created by the shape of the bur. Small undercuts may be placed in the dentin if additional retentive features are required to provide conve-

nience in beginning the compaction of gold (Fig. 20-11, B). Undercuts, when desired, are placed facially and lingually in posterior teeth or incisally and gingivally on the lingual surface of incisors at the level of the ideal pulpal floor position. These undercut line angles must not undermine marginal ridges. A very slight cavosurface bevel may be placed (1) to create 30- to 40-degrees metal at the margin for ease in finishing the gold and (2) to remove remaining rough enamel. The bevel is not greater than 0.2 mm in width and is placed with a white rotary stone or suitable finishing bur. The desired angle is sighted between the external tooth surface and the stone to determine where the bevel is needed, as described in Chapter 19.

Instrumentation. For description and illustration the preparation of a carious pit on the mandibular first premolar is presented (Fig. 20-12, A). By use of a high-speed handpiece with air-water spray, the No. 330 or No. 329 bur is aligned and the outline form (which in-

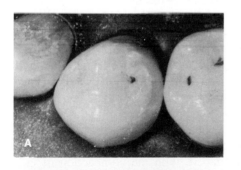

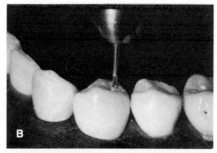

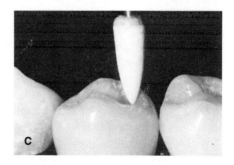

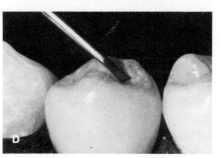

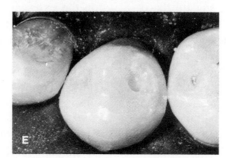

Fig. 20-12. Class I preparation for direct gold. A, Preoperative view of pit lesion. B, No. 330 bur is aligned properly for occlusal preparation. C, Occlusal cavosurface bevel is prepared with white stone. D, The bevel may be placed with an angle former. E, Completed cavity preparation.

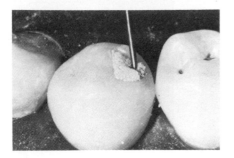

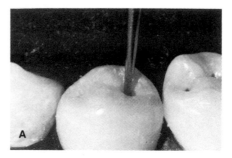

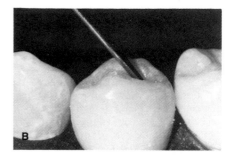

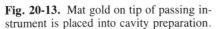

Fig. 20-13. Mat gold on tip of passing instrument is placed into cavity preparation.

Fig. 20-14. A, Compaction forces are delivered by condenser held at 90-degree angle to pulpal wall. **B,** Gold is condensed against external cavity walls by a condenser applied at 45-degree angle to pulpal wall.

cludes the limited initial depth) is established (Fig. 20-12, *B*). When the preparation is extensive due to including fissured enamel, a small hoe, 6½-2½-9, may be used to complete the desired degree of flatness of the pulpal wall; but do *not* remove by the hoe any carious infected dentin that may be remaining pulpally of the desired initial depth. Using the No. 33½ bur at low speed, small retentive undercuts are prepared into the dentin portion of the external walls at the initial pulpal wall depth; these also may be prepared using a 6½-(90)-2½-9 angle former excavator. Round burs of suitable size are used to remove any infected carious dentin that may remain on the pulpal wall. The preparation is completed by finishing the cavosurface with an angle former, a small finishing bur such as the No. 7802, or a flame-shaped white stone (Fig. 20-12, *C* to *E*).

Restoration. The *restorative phase* begins with application of cavity varnish, followed by insertion of a piece of *mat gold*. The gold is first degassed in the alcohol flame, cooled momentarily in air, and inserted into the preparation with the passing instrument (Fig. 20-13). The first increment of gold should be cut to be just slightly larger than the diameter of the preparation. The gold is pressed to place with the nib of a small round condenser, 0.5 mm in diameter. In larger preparations the pair of parallelogram condensers is used for this initial compaction of the gold. No malleting forces are yet delivered, because the purpose of this first step simply is to place the gold in the preparation and stabilize it. Next, malleting of the mat gold begins with a line of force directed against the pulpal wall (Fig. 20-14, *A*). As the condenser nib is stepped toward the periphery of the pulpal wall to compact the gold into the pulpal line angles and against the external walls, the line of force is changed to 45 degrees to the pulpal and respective external walls to best compact the gold against these walls (Fig. 20-14, *B*). The condenser nib is stepped over the entire increment twice. Additional increments of mat gold are added, and the procedure is repeated until the preparation is about half full of compacted gold.

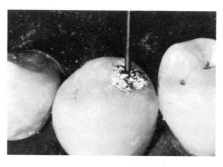

Fig. 20-15. Placement of pellet of gold foil and compaction into cavity preparation.

Next, *gold foil* is compacted into the preparation. Pellets of suitable size are selected; in larger preparations large pellets are convenient, whereas for small pit cavity preparations the operator should begin with ⅟₆₄-size pellets (Fig. 20-15). The pellet is degassed and carried to the prepared cavity. Hand pressure compaction first is used to secure the pellet against the compacted mat gold and to spread it over the surface; then mallet compaction is used. Likewise each succeeding pellet is hand compacted and then mallet compacted. The condenser point is systematically stepped over the gold twice as malleting proceeds. The line of force is generally perpendicular to the pulpal floor in the center of the mass and at a 45-degree angle to the pulpal floor as the external walls are reached. At this stage and during all building of the restoration, the compacted surface should be saucer shaped, with the compaction of gold on the external walls slightly ahead of the center. The surface should never be humped in the center because this sometimes results in voids and poor adaptation along the external walls when the condenser nib is "crowded out" along the wall by the center hump. Continue building the restoration until the cavosurface margin is covered with foil (Fig. 20-16). *Exercise extreme care that gold always lies between the condenser face and the cavosurface margin;* otherwise the condenser may injure (fracture) the enamel margin. Now fill in the

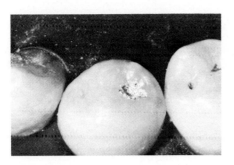

Fig. 20-16. Compaction of gold foil has proceeded sufficiently to cover all cavosurface margins.

central area of the restoration's surface to the desired level. Tooth surface contour of the gold is created to simulate the final anatomical form, and a slight excess of gold is compacted on the surface to allow for the finishing and polishing procedures.

The first step in the finishing procedure is to burnish the gold (Fig. 20-17, *A*). A flat beaver-tail burnisher is used with heavy hand pressure to harden the surface gold. A cleoid-discoid carver is used to continue the burnishing process and remove excess gold on the cavosurface margin. The cleoid, always directed so that a portion of the working edge is over or resting on enamel adjacent to or near the margins, is pulled from gold to tooth across the surface to smooth the surface and trim away excess gold (Fig. 20-17, *B*). If considerable excess gold has been compacted, a green stone may be used to remove the excess in Class I restorations. Care must be taken at this stage to avoid grinding on the surface enamel. Following use of the cleoid-discoid, a small round finishing bur No. 9004 is used to begin pol-

ishing (Fig. 20-17, *C*). It is followed in turn by the application of flour of pumice and tin oxide or white rouge (Fig. 20-17, *D*). These powdered abrasives are applied dry on a webless, soft rubber cup with a low-speed handpiece. Care is taken to use light pressure. Gentle blasts of air cool the surface during polishing. The completed restoration is illustrated in Fig. 20-18.

Class V cavity preparation and restoration

The operating field. As with all direct gold restorations, the *rubber dam* must be in place to provide a suitable, dry field for Class V restorative therapy. Furthermore, for lesions near the gingiva or that extend into the gingival sulcus, it is necessary to provide appropriate access to the cavity by placing a No. 212 retainer or gingival retractor. The punching of the rubber dam is modified to provide ample rubber between the teeth and to provide enough rubber for coverage and retraction of the soft tissue on the facial side of the tooth. The hole for the tooth to be treated is punched 1 mm

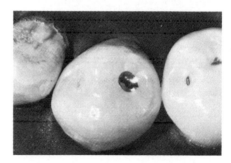

Fig. 20-18. Completed restoration.

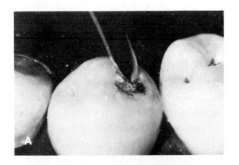
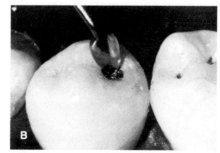
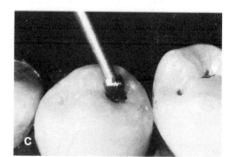
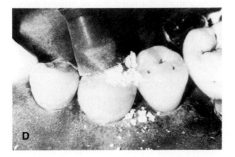

Fig. 20-17. Steps in finishing Class I direct gold restoration. **A,** Burnisher work-hardens the surface gold. **B,** Cleoid-discoid removes excess gold from cavosurface margins. **C,** No. 9004 bur is used to begin polishing phase. **D,** Polishing abrasives are applied with rubber cup.

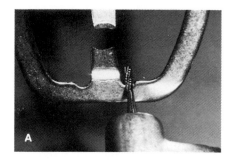
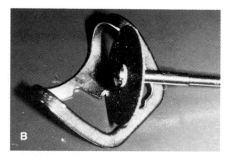

Fig. 20-19. A, Notches are deepened for secure holding of No. 212 retainer. **B,** Jaws may be modified with a disc to facilitate retainer placement on rotated teeth.

facial of its normal position, and an extra 1 mm of dam is left between the hole for the treated tooth and the holes for the immediately adjacent teeth.

Several modifications may be made to the No. 212 retainer to facilitate its use. If the notches that are engaged by the retainer forceps are shallow, they may be deepened slightly with a large, carbide fissure bur to provide a more secure lock for the forceps (Fig. 20-19, *A*). If the tips of the retainer jaws are very sharp, they may be dulled with a garnet disc to avoid scratching cementum during placement. For application to narrow teeth such as mandibular incisors, the facial and lingual jaws may be narrowed by grinding with a heatless stone or carborundum disc, followed by polishing with a rubber wheel. To expedite placement on rotated teeth, the jaws may be modified by grinding suitable contour to the tip edge (Fig. 20-19, *B*). The jaws may be bent for use on teeth where gingival access to lesions is difficult. This is done by heating the jaws to cherry red in a flame, then grasping the entire facial jaw and slightly bending it apically. The procedure is repeated for the lingual jaw, bending it slightly occlusally (Fig. 20-20).

The No. 212 retainer must be carefully applied to avoid damage to the soft or hard tissue. The retainer is secured in the retainer forceps and carried to the mouth after the rubber dam has been replaced. The lingual jaw

is positioned just apical to the lingual height of contour, and the index finger is placed against the jaw to prevent its movement. The retainer is rotated faciogingivally with the forceps while the thumb retracts the dam, and then the facial jaw is set against the tooth (Fig. 20-21, *A*). Next a ball burnisher is hooked onto one of the retainer notches and used to move the facial jaw gingivally (without scraping the jaw against the tooth) to the final position 0.5 to 1 mm apical of the expected gingival margin (Fig. 20-21, *B*). Gentle pressure is used to position the facial jaw so that only the free gingiva is retracted and the epithelial attachment is not harmed. The retainer is supported and locked into this desired position with red stick modeling compound, which is softened, molded by the fingers, and placed between the bows and the gingival embrasures (Fig. 20-21, *C*). The compound also serves to distribute compaction forces among all the teeth included in the retainer application. Also see application of the No. 212 retainer in Chapter 11.

Cavity preparation design. The typical *Class V cavity preparation* for restoration with direct gold is trapezoidal (Figs. 20-22, 20-23, and 20-24). This outline form is created to satisfy esthetic needs and requirements for retention and convenience forms in the treatment of lesions in the gingival third of the clinical crowns of teeth. The straight occlusal margin is esthetically pleasing, and by virtue of its straight design, excess gold is readily discerned and removed in the final stages of the restorative process. The gingival outline is shorter than the occlusal, since the tooth narrows in the gingival area; it is parallel with the occlusal margin for easy identification in finishing phases and, also, because there is no reason for orienting it in a different plane. The mesial and distal margins connect the gingival margin to the occlusal margin.

The occlusal margin is straight and parallel with the occlusal plane of the teeth in the arch. It is extended occlusally to include the lesion. (When several adjacent teeth are restored, some additional extension is permissible to create an esthetically pleasing uniform level.) Often the extension mesiodistally to the line angles of the tooth will place the junction of the occlusal and me-

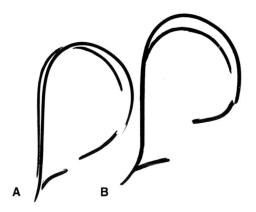

Fig. 20-20. A, No. 212 retainer as received from the manufacturer. **B,** Modified facial and lingual jaws.

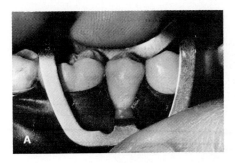
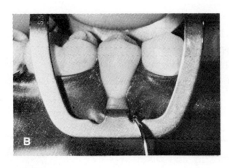
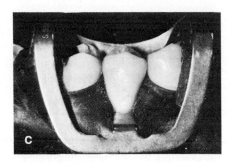

Fig. 20-21. Placement of No. 212 retainer. **A,** Initial placement of facial jaw after first placing lingual jaw. **B,** Use of ball burnisher to carry facial jaw to final position. **C,** Retainer stabilized with compound to distribute compaction forces, prevent tipping, and prevent either apical or occlusal movement of retainer.

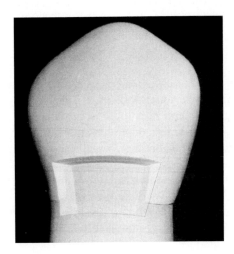

Fig. 20-22. Facial view of Class V cavity preparation for direct gold. Occlusal and gingival margins are straight, parallel with each other, and extend mesially and distally to respective mesiofacial and distofacial tooth crown line angles. Mesial and distal walls diverge facially and form obtuse angles with axial wall. Line angles and point angles are sharp. (See Fig. 20-24, *B.)*

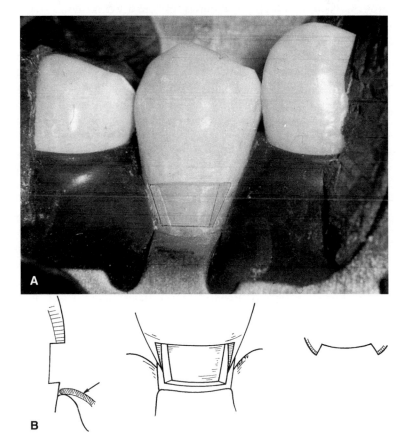

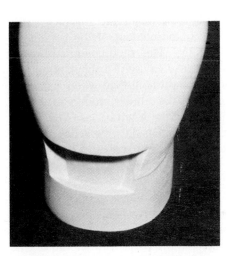

Fig. 20-23. Faciooclusal view of design of gingival wall in Class V preparation for direct gold. Axiogingival line angle is acute and was prepared at expense of gingival wall (note Fig. 20-28, *C).* This gingival margin is on cementum. If on enamel, the gingival cavosurface would be beveled slightly (note Fig. 20-28, *E).*

Fig. 20-24. A, Clinical Class V cavity preparation. Note proper isolation of operating field. This gingival margin is on cementum. **B,** Longitudinal section, facioocclusal view, and cross section. Line and point angles are sharp.

sial and distal margins under the crest of the free gingiva, rendering the most esthetic result. The gingival margin is also straight, is parallel with the occlusal margin, is placed only far enough apically to include the lesion, and extends mesiodistally to the line angles of the tooth.

The mesial and distal margins are parallel to the proximal line angles of the tooth and usually are positioned sufficiently mesially and distally, respectively, to be covered by the free gingiva. The mesial and distal margins are straight lines that meet the occlusal margin in sharp acute angles and meet the gingival margin in sharp obtuse angles to complete the trapezoidal form.

The depth of the axial wall varies with the position of the preparation on the tooth. The axial wall is approximately 1 mm deep in the occlusal half of the preparation. As the outline approaches the cervical line, the axial wall depth may decrease from 1 to 0.75 mm. The axial wall must be established in dentin, and occlusogingivally it should be straight and approximately parallel with the facial surface of the tooth (Fig. 20-24, *B*). Mesiodistally the axial wall is prepared approximately parallel with the surface contour of the tooth; this contour may create a slight curvature in the axial wall mesiodistally in both highly contoured teeth and where the preparation is proximally extensive. Mesiodistal curvature of the axial wall prevents encroachment of the cavity preparation on the pulp. Excessive axial curvature results in a preparation that is either too shallow in the center or too deep at the proximal extensions, and it further complicates restoration by failing to provide a reasonably flat wall against which to begin compaction. A subaxial wall may be created within the axial wall to remove infected caries that has progressed deeper than the ideal axial wall placement.

The axial wall meets the occlusal wall in a sharp right angle, and the occlusal wall forms a right angle with the external enamel surface, thus precluding undermining of the enamel. The axial wall meets the gingival wall in a sharp acute angle created at the expense of the gingival wall (Fig. 20-24, *B*). The axial wall meets the mesial and distal walls in sharp obtuse angles. These obtuse line angles are created to prevent undermining of the mesial and distal enamel while still providing some resistance to movement of the gold during compaction. They must never be acute angles.

The mesial and distal walls are flat and straight. They meet the occlusal wall in a sharp acute line angle and meet the gingival wall in a sharp obtuse line angle. The mesial and distal walls provide resistance for gold compaction; they provide no retention.

The orientation of the gingival wall is the key to the *retentive form* of the preparation. It is straight mesiodistally, meeting the mesial and distal walls in sharp line angles. Retention is provided by sloping the gingival

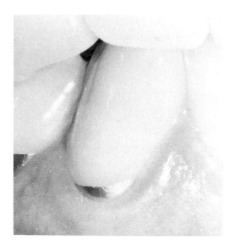

Fig. 20-25. Completed Class V gold restoration. Incisal margin curved to follow contour of gingival tissue for best esthetic result.

wall internally to meet the axial wall in a sharply defined acute line angle. Retention is thereby provided by the facial convergence of the occlusal and gingival walls. Gold wedged between these two walls is locked into the tooth.

If the gingival margin is established on enamel, the cavosurface is beveled slightly to remove the unsupported enamel (Fig. 20-28, *E*). When placed on cementum, the gingival cavosurface is not beveled (Fig. 20-24, *B*).

The outline of the cavity preparation may be modified. In those situations demanding restriction of display of gold, such as in anterior teeth, the incisal outline may be curved to follow the contour of the soft tissue mesiodistally (Fig. 20-25). This modification is made only when required because cavity instrumentation and finishing of gold are more difficult than when a straight marginal outline is created. A similar modification may be made in the occlusal outline when caries extends occlusally as the proximal extensions are reached. The mesiodistal extension (dimension) of the preparation may be limited in those instances where caries is only mesial or distal to the center of the facial surface in posterior teeth, thus conserving intact tooth structure. When access requires, the gingival wall may be modified to curve mesiodistally to include the gingival extent of advanced caries. The entire axial wall should not be extended pulpally to the depth of the lesion when deep cervical abrasion or erosion is treated; rather the axial wall is positioned normally, leaving a remaining V notch at its center to be restored with gold. When failing restorations are removed and restored with direct gold, the cavity outline is partially dictated by the previous restoration (Fig. 20-26).

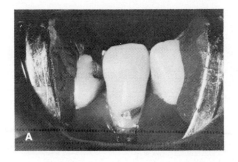
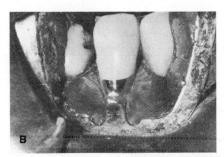

Fig. 20-26. A, Failing Class V amalgam restoration. B, Replacement direct gold restoration.

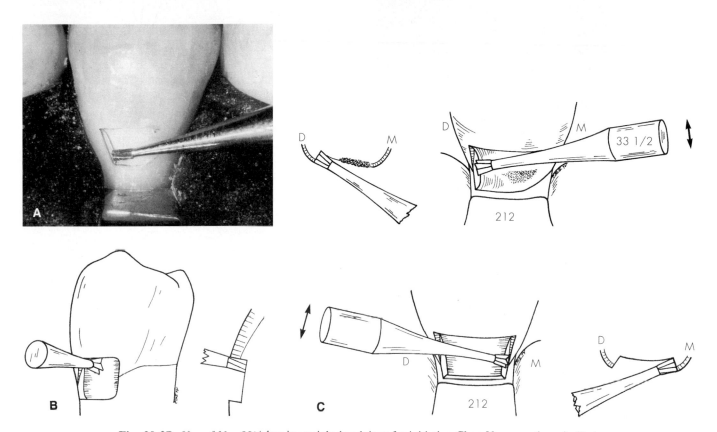

Fig. 20-27. Use of No. 33½ bur in straight handpiece for initiating Class V preparation. A, End of bur is used to establish distal wall. B, Side of bur is used to establish occlusal wall. C, End of bur prepares mesial wall if access permits.   *Continued.*

Instrumentation. The No. 33½ bur is used to establish the general *outline form* of the preparation. The *end* of the bur establishes the distal wall (Fig. 20-27, *A);* the *side* establishes the axial depth as well as the occlusal, gingival, and the mesial walls (Fig. 20-27, *B*). When access permits, the *end* of the bur may be used to establish the mesial and gingival walls (Fig. 20-27, *C* and *D*). The gingival and mesial walls may be prepared with the *side* of the bur if access so dictates (Fig. 20-27, *E* and *F*). The *end* of the bur is used to place the axial wall in dentin (Fig. 20-27, *G*).

The 6½-2½-9 hoe or the larger 10-4-8 hoe is useful for planing preparation walls, establishing sharp internal line angles (Fig. 20-28, *A),* and finishing margins. The Wedelstaedt chisel is used to finish the occlusal cavosurface margin (Fig. 20-28, *B*) and also may be used to plane the axial wall.

The acute axiogingival angle is established with the 6½-2½-9 hoe cutting from the cavosurface to the axial wall in a push-cut stroke (Fig. 20-28, *C*). The chips of dentin produced at the axiogingival angle may be removed with the tip of an explorer (Fig. 20-28, *D*) or the acute part of a 6½-(90)-2½-9 small angle former; care must be taken not to gouge the axial wall. When its use is indicated, the gingival bevel is prepared with the Wedelstaedt chisel or a hoe (Fig. 20-28, *E*).

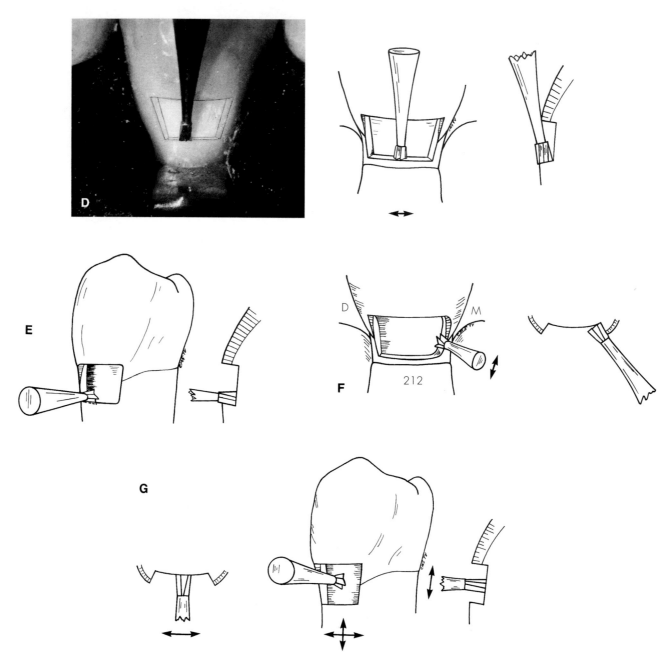

Fig. 20-27—cont'd. D, End of bur is used to establish gingival wall if access permits. **E,** Preparation of gingival wall with side of bur. **F,** Preparation of mesial wall with side of bur. **G,** The end of bur may be used to establish initial axial wall depth in dentin.

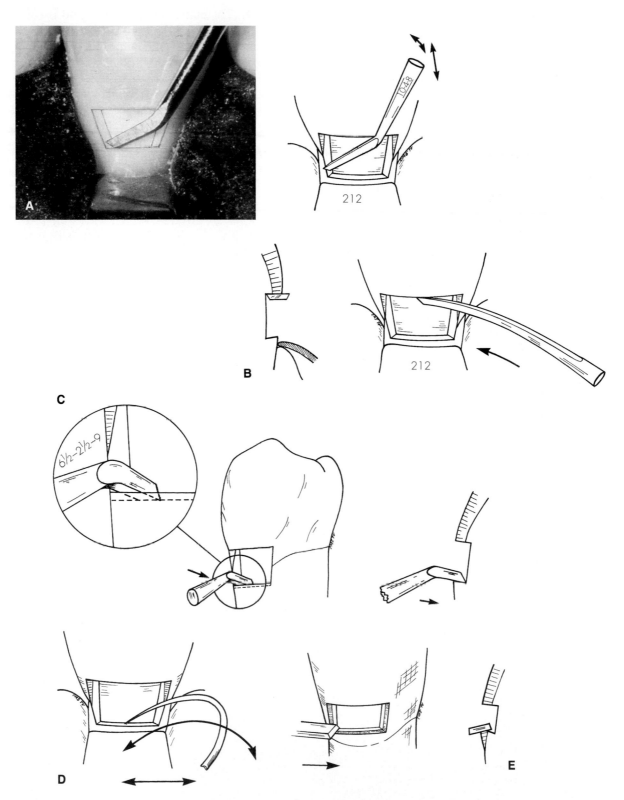

Fig. 20-28. Use of hand instruments in Class V cavity preparation. **A,** Small hoe planes preparation walls. **B,** Wedelstaedt chisel refines occlusal wall and margin. **C,** Small hoe creates acute axiogingival line angle in dentin. **D,** Explorer is used to remove debris from completed cavity preparation. **E,** Chisel blade bevels gingival cavosuface margin when indicated. (**E,** after Howard WC, Moller RC: *Atlas of operative dentistry,* St Louis, 1981, Mosby.)

Restoration. Restoration of the Class V cavity preparation begins with application of cavity varnish, followed by placing a piece of degassed *mat gold* into the preparation. The gold is first cut to a size and shape just slightly larger than the cavity preparation and carried to place in the preparation with the passing instrument (Fig. 20-29, *A*). A pair of parallelogram foil condensers is used to firmly force the mat gold against the axial wall and to wedge it into the line angles (Fig. 20-29, *B*). Then one instrument may be laid aside, and while the other is used as a holding instrument to prevent movement of the entire piece of gold, the compaction is begun by delivering malleting forces to the mat gold (Fig. 20-29, *C*).

Compaction begins in the center of the mass of gold with a 0.5 mm diameter, round, serrated condenser nib. Careful, methodical stepping of the gold proceeds outward toward the external cavity walls. The holding instrument is unnecessary as soon as the gold is stabilized. As the walls are reached, the line of force is changed from perpendicular to the axial wall to 45 degrees to the axial wall to drive the gold into the sharp line angles and against the external walls (Fig. 20-29,

D). The entire surface of the gold is condensed twice to complete compaction of the mat gold. Additional increments of mat gold are added until the preparation is filled to half its depth. *Gold foil pellets* are then used to complete the restoration.

Using medium-sized pellets, compaction of foil begins at the mesioocclusal or distoocclusal line angle and proceeds across the occlusal wall to cover the entire wall and occlusal cavosurface with compacted gold foil (Fig. 20-30, *A*). As previously mentioned, care should be exercised when approaching any enamel margin that gold covers and protects the margin from blows of the condenser face. Then the gingival, mesial, and distal walls are covered, which leaves the restoration concave at this stage (Fig. 20-30, *B*). It is essential that all cavosurface margins be covered at this time before the final convex surface of the restoration is formed.

Medium and large pellets ($\frac{1}{43}$ and $\frac{1}{32}$) are then compacted in the center of the restoration to complete the buildup of restoration contour. A slight excess contour is developed and is removed later as the gold is finished and polished. Any small remaining deficiencies in the surface contour are filled with small ($\frac{1}{128}$) pellets. A

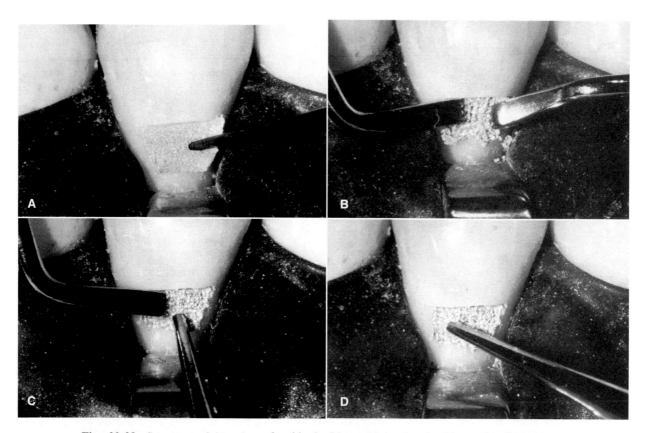

Fig. 20-29. Sequence of insertion of gold. **A,** Mat gold is placed with passing instrument. **B,** Parallelogram condensers are used with firm hand pressure to stabilize mat gold. **C,** Malleting compaction forces are delivered with small, round condenser nib. **D,** Line of force is changed as external walls are approached.

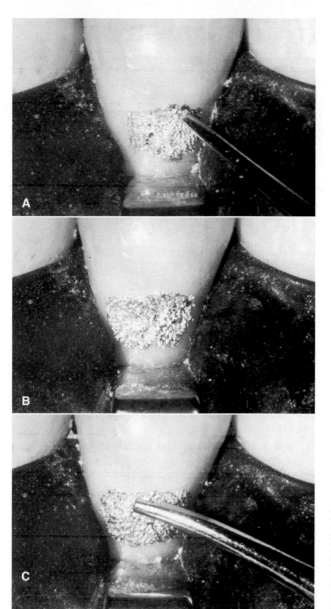

Varney foot condenser is applied to the entire surface to render it as smooth as possible at this stage and to assist in detection of any poorly compacted areas (Fig. 20-30, *C*).

Finishing begins with application of a beaver-tail burnisher to work-harden and smooth the surface (Fig. 20-31, *A*). Petroleum jelly may be applied to the dam to avoid abrasion from discs, and it also may be applied to the discs. Gross excess contour, if any, is removed with a fine garnet disc applied with a Sproule mandrel in a low-speed handpiece (Fig. 20-31, *B*). Excess gold is removed from the cavosurface margins with the cleoid-discoid instrument using pull-cut strokes or the gold knife by using only push-cut strokes from gold to tooth (Fig. 20-31, *C* and *D*). *When clearing away excess gold over the gingival margin, care is exercised not to remove cementum and not to "ditch" the root surface, especially when rotary instruments are used.*

Once final contour has been obtained, cuttle discs may be used in decreasing abrasiveness (coarse, medium, fine) to ready the surface for final polishing. These discs and the cleoid are helpful in removing very fine fins of gold from margins.

Polishing is performed with fine pumice followed by tin oxide or white rouge applied with a soft, webless

Fig. 20-30. Completion of compaction. **A,** Condensation of foil proceeds to cover cavosurface margins. A slight excess of gold has been condensed over mesial half of occlusal cavosurface margin. **B,** All cavosurface margins are covered with a slight excess of gold. Restoration at this stage of insertion is concave. **C,** After additional foil pellets are compacted in central area to form convex restoration surface with slight excess, a foot condenser is used to confirm condensation.

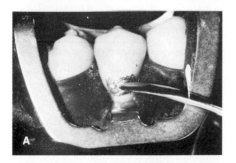
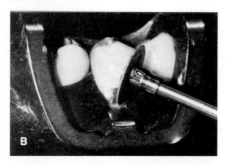
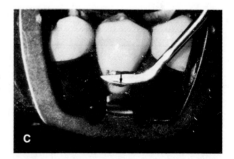
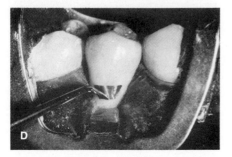

Fig. 20-31. Finishing the Class V restoration. **A,** Burnisher work-hardens surface. **B,** Small, fine garnet disc removes excess gold contour. **C,** Gold knife's secondary edge used with push-stroke *(arrow)* removes excess gold from gingival margin. **D,** After final surfacing with cuttle discs, any remaining marginal excess is removed with cleoid carver.

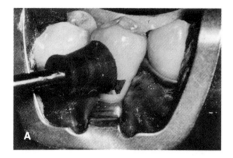

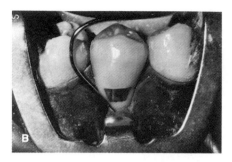

Fig. 20-32. A, Soft rubber cup is used to apply polishing abrasives. **B,** Explorer is used to remove any remaining polishing powder from site of completed restoration.

rubber cup. *Care is mandatory at this stage to avoid ditching the cementum with polishing abrasive.* The abrasives are therefore used dry so the field may be kept clean and the exact position of the rubber cup seen at all times (Fig. 20-32).

Following polishing, the No. 212 retainer and rubber dam are removed. Removal of the retainer is best accomplished with the forceps firmly locked into the notches on the retainer. The retainer jaws are sprung from the tooth with the forceps and carefully removed occlusally without scratching the restoration or the surface enamel of the tooth. The gingival sulcus is rinsed and examined to ascertain that it is free of debris. The soft tissue is massaged gently before the patient is dismissed.

Class III cavity preparation and restoration

There are many styles of Class III cavity preparation advocated for restoration with direct gold. Some preparations are based on the lingual approach and are restored with powdered gold. Others may be instrumented from either the facial or lingual surface and use gold foil as the restorative material. The outline form selected must provide adequate access for convenient res-

toration, as well as an acceptable esthetic result. The cavity design presented in subsequent sections was first described by Ferrier in the early years of the twentieth century[6] and has withstood the test of time. It has the advantage not only of conserving tooth structure but also of providing for compaction of gold foil directly against all cavity walls and cavosurface margins, thereby creating a dense, esthetically pleasing result, if careful attention is given to management of the outline. This cavity preparation is instrumented primarily from a facial approach, although some lingual instrumentation is performed in the maxillary treatment procedure. The preparation may be modified for lower anterior teeth or for the distal surface of maxillary canines as well as the distal surface of some lateral incisors.

Cavity preparation design for maxillary incisors. The *marginal outline* is most important. From a facial view the gingival four fifths of the facial margin is straight and generally parallel with the contour of the tooth (Fig. 20-33). The facial margin forms a gentle curve in its incisal one fifth to blend with the incisal margin. When viewed from a proximofacial aspect, the facial outline follows the general contour of the adjacent tooth (Fig. 20-34) and meets the gingival outline in a slightly ob-

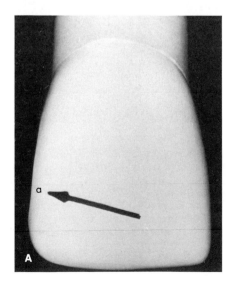

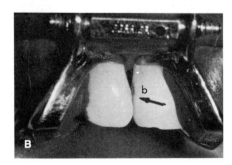

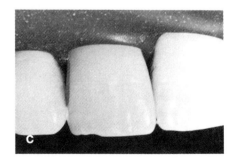

Fig. 20-33. Class III direct gold restoration. **A,** Model of preparation demonstrates esthetic marginal outline *(a)*. **B,** Central incisor *(b)* before distal cavity preparation. **C,** Completed Class III restoration.

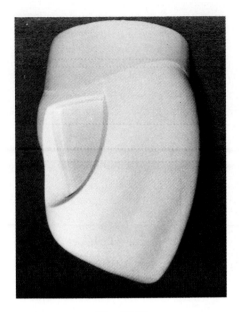

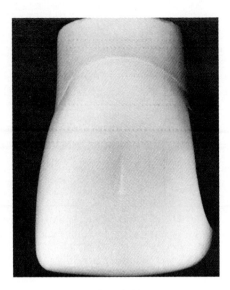

Fig. 20-34. Proximofacial view of Class III cavity preparation.

Fig. 20-35. Lingual view of Class III cavity preparation.

Fig. 20-34   **Fig. 20-35**

tuse angle. This juncture may be curved very slightly to enhance esthetics.

The gingival margin is critical to the entire preparation. Its faciolingual length controls the remainder of the preparation. Where possible, the gingival margin is established just apical to the crest of the free gingiva to enhance the esthetic result. It is straight faciolingually and is approximately at a right angle to the long axis of the tooth. It meets the facial margin in a sharply defined obtuse angle that may be rounded slightly as previously described, and it meets the lingual margin in a sharply defined acute angle.

Viewed from the lingual aspect, the lingual margin generally parallels the long axis of the tooth (Fig. 20-

35). However, it may diverge slightly proximally from the long axis to more nearly parallel the proximal contour. It meets the gingival margin in a sharply defined angle that is nearly 90 degrees when viewed from the lingual aspect (Fig. 20-36) but is acute when viewed from the proximal aspect. The lingual margin is straight in its gingival two thirds and then curves abruptly to meet the incisal margin.

The incisal margin is placed incisally from the contact area to provide access to the preparation, yet it is not so extended as to weaken the incisal angle of the tooth. It forms a smooth curve that connects the facial and the lingual margins of the preparation.

To provide suitable *resistance form,* the internal aspects of the preparation are carefully instrumented in every detail. The gingival wall is flat faciolingually. The axial wall is flat faciolingually and incisogingivally and is established 0.5 mm into the dentin. Resistance form is also created by establishment of sharp obtuse facioaxial and linguoaxial line angles in dentin. The facial and lingual walls diverge only enough to preclude undermined enamel, yet they provide firm, flat walls against which the gold can be compacted.

As in the Class V treatment, *retention form* is provided solely between the gingival and incisal walls. In the Class III preparation the *dentinal portion of the gingival wall* (as in the Class V gingival wall) slopes apically inward to create an acute axiogingival line angle (refer to Fig. 20-47, *B*). However, in the Class III preparation the incisal portion is undercut (Fig. 20-37). This undercut box is placed in *dentin facioincisally* to create a mechanical lock between the incisal and gingival walls. The increased retention form in the Class III

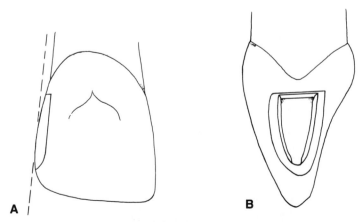

Fig. 20-36. Lingual marginal outline of Class III preparation. **A,** View of lingual outline. Note sharp linguogingival angle. **B,** Proximal view of preparation. Note linguogingival angle is sharp and acute in this view. (**A,** after Stibbs GD.)

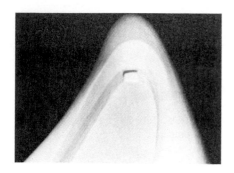

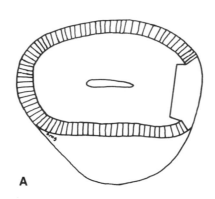

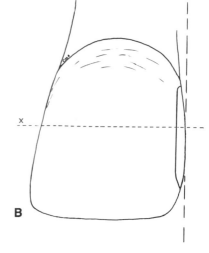

Fig. 20-37. View of incisal retention in Class III preparation. Undercut is placed in dentin but does not undermine enamel.

Fig. 20-38. Class III preparation internal form and facial marginal outline. **A,** Incisal view of cross section of preparation in plane *x* shown in **B.** Facial and lingual cavosurface bevels are shown placed in enamel. **B,** Facial view of facial marginal outline of cavity preparation. (After Stibbs GD.)

preparation is required because of the length of the preparation incisogingivally and because of the difficulty of access in compacting gold.

Provision for *convenience form* is made by the abrupt linguoincisal curve, which permits introduction of a condenser directed toward the gingival wall, by adequate clearance of all margins from the adjacent tooth, and by placement of sharp internal point angles suitable for beginning compaction of gold. The facioaxiogingival and linguoaxiogingival point angles may be enlarged slightly to assist in initial stages of foil compaction if desired.[19]

The *finish of enamel walls* creates a facial, incisal, and lingual cavosurface bevel to reach the final marginal outline. This bevel is made with hand instruments and is established totally in enamel. It is designed to create maximum convenience form, to remove all surface irregularities as well as any unsupported enamel, and to establish an esthetically pleasing result (Fig. 20-38).

Modifications of Class III preparations.. The *distal surface of maxillary canines* may require a modification in preparation design for convenience. Because of the highly convex surface generally present, it is often desirable to create a "straight line preparation" in which the facial outline appears as a slice. This modification provides clearance from the mesial marginal ridge of the first premolar and provides considerable convenience form to direct compaction gingivally from an incisal position; this type of preparation is also appropriate for the distal surface of highly contoured lateral incisors (Fig. 20-39).

The *mandibular incisors* are treated with a modified Class III preparation because of their small size and because access from a lingual position may be exceptionally difficult. The lingual wall is created in one plane,

and extension of both the lingual and incisal aspects is limited. The lingual wall meets the axial at a right or slightly obtuse angle. Care is taken to avoid overextending the lingual wall lingually, since this can result in removal of dentin support for the lingual enamel and thereby may render the preparation unrestorable by direct gold. Outline form is extended lingually only far enough to include the lesion and to allow access for finishing of gold. Incisal extension is restricted because the proximal contact area between mandibular incisors is often placed near the incisal angle and extension incisally beyond the contact may weaken this critical portion of the tooth. A mechanical separator is used to obtain clearance between the teeth for access and instrumentation. Facial extension is similar to the maxillary preparation (Fig. 20-40).

Internally the *incisal retentive angle* for the mandibular Class III preparation is placed directly incisally rather than facioincisally as in maxillary teeth. This modification is made to conserve thickness of tooth structure at the facioincisal angle where wear of mandibular anterior teeth frequently occurs.

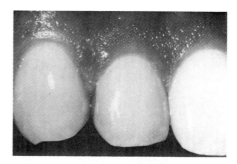

Fig. 20-39. Direct gold restoration of a clinical Class III preparation of "straight line" design on distal portion of maxillary lateral incisor.

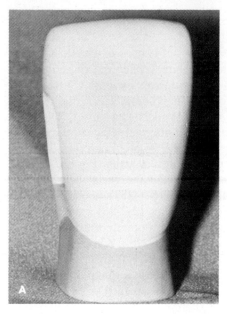

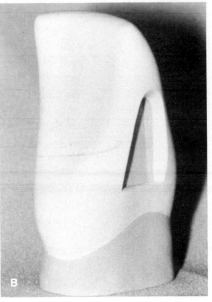

Fig. 20-40. Mandibular Class III preparation. **A,** Facial view. Facial margin is similar to that in maxillary preparation. **B,** Linguoproximal view.

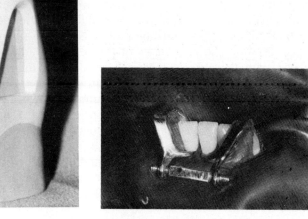

Fig. 20-41. Separator placed before clinical Class III cavity preparation for mandibular incisor.

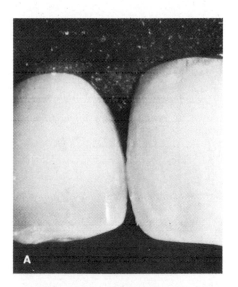

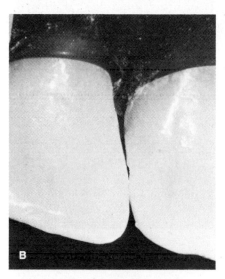

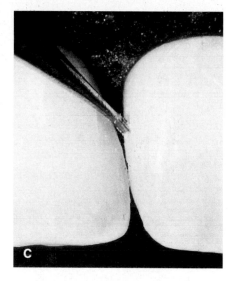

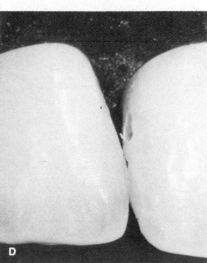

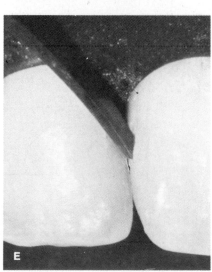

Fig. 20-42. A, Preoperative view of extracted maxillary central incisor that has been mounted in dentoform. Distal surface to be treated with Class III cavity preparation and restoration of compacted gold. **B,** Preoperative lingual view. **C,** Facial approach initial entry is made with No. 33½ bur. **D,** Initial bur entry. **E,** Wedelstaedt chisel begins to establish facial outline form.

Separation of teeth. Separation of teeth is frequently needed for instrumentation or finishing procedures performed on Class III direct gold restorations. The Ferrier separator is a convenient instrument for accomplishing this separation. It is applied and stabilized with compound, similar to stabilization of a No. 212 retainer (Fig. 20-41). The jackscrews of the separator are activated with the separator wrench to slightly draw the teeth apart, thus creating a maximum space of 0.25 to 0.5 mm. Care is used to create a minimum of separation and to remove the separator as soon as it is feasible, thereby preventing damage to periodontal structures.

Instrumentation. The No. 33½ bur (or a suitable Wedelstaedt chisel) is used to begin formation of the preparation (Fig. 20-42). The bur is used from the facial aspect to position the gingival outline and the facial wall. The Wedelstaedt chisel is used to establish the lingual extension, and the bur defines the linguogingival angle (Fig. 20-43) and completes the gingival floor. The marginal outline form is then completed as the cavosurfaces are beveled with a Wedelstaedt chisel. The internal dentinal aspects of the gingival, lingual, facial, and incisal walls are next planed. A small hoe (6½-2½-9) is used for the lingual and gingival walls (Fig. 20-44). An angle former is used to plane the facial dentinal wall (Fig. 20-45). An axial plane (8-1-23) smoothes the axial wall, and a bibeveled hatchet (3-2-28) establishes the incisal retentive angle with a chopping motion (Fig. 20-46). Small angle formers are used to complete the sharp facioaxiogingival and linguoaxiogingival point angles and complete the slightly acute axiogingival angle (Fig. 20-47). The point angles may be further enlarged with

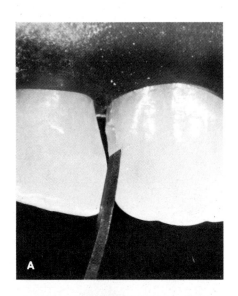

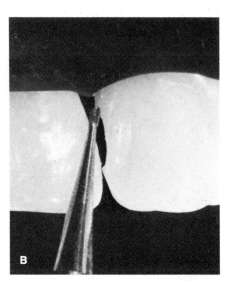

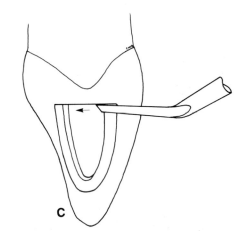

Fig. 20-43. Lingual view of cavity instrumentation. **A,** Wedelstaedt chisel planing lingual enamel wall. **B,** Inverted cone bur is used to establish sharp linguogingival shoulder.

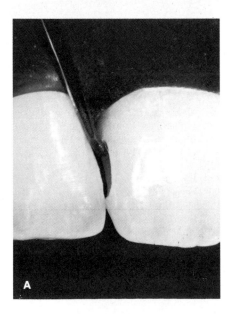

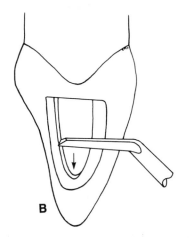

Fig. 20-44. Use of small hoe, facial approach, in cavity preparation. **A,** Hoe planes lingual dentinal wall from incisal to gingival aspect. **B,** Hoe also planes this wall from gingival to incisal aspect *(arrow)*. **C,** Hoe planes gingival cavosurface *(arrow)*. See Fig. 20-47, *D,* for direction of enamel portion of gingival wall for strong margin (full-length enamel rods).

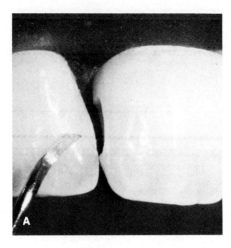
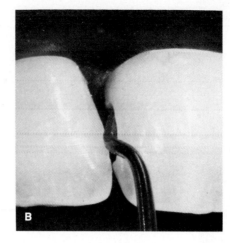
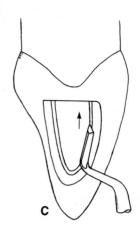

Fig. 20-45. Use of angle former to plane facial dentinal wall. **A,** Angle former before placement in preparation. **B,** Angle former in preparation. **C,** Angle former is directed apically *(arrow)* to plane facial dentinal wall.

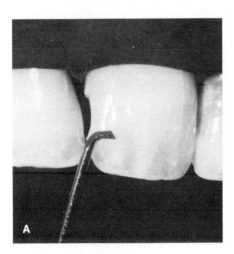
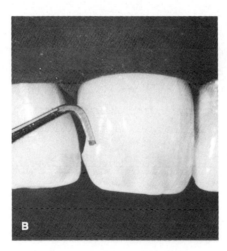
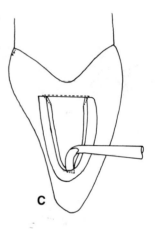

Fig. 20-46. A, Axial plane before placement in cavity preparation. **B,** Bibeveled hatchet before placement in preparation. **C,** Bibeveled hatchet is used to establish incisal retentive angle.

the No. 33S bur (end-cutting bur) for additional convenience form. The Wedelstaedt chisel may be used again to complete the final planing of the cavosurface margins (Fig. 20-48).

Restoration. Separation of 0.25 to 0.5 mm is attained by the separator. Compaction of gold begins at the linguoaxiogingival point angle (Fig. 20-49). A small (0.4 mm) monangle condenser is used to compact the gold, which is held by a small holding instrument. Pellets, size $1/64$ or $1/128$, are used in the beginning of the restorative phase. The line of force is directed from over the facial surface of the adjacent tooth and into the linguoaxiogingival point angle (Fig. 20-49, *B*). As soon as ample gold has been compacted into the linguogingival area to cover the linguogingival shoulder, compaction continues across the gingival wall (Fig. 20-50) and

into the faciogingival angle. The offset condenser, with a faciogingival line of force is used to fill the facioaxiogingival point angle (Fig. 20-51). Compaction of gold at the linguogingival aspect is next confirmed with the oblique-faced (0.5 mm) monangle condenser from the linguoincisal position (Fig. 20-52). Failure to provide dense gold in this linguogingival area at this stage may result in a void at the linguogingival angle and may lead to restoration failure.

The bulk of the restoration is now compacted with $1/43$- or $1/32$-size pellets mainly from the facial and occasionally from the lingual direction (Fig. 20-53).

The line of force is maintained in an axiogingival direction with the 0.5 mm monangle or oblique-faced monangle condenser (Fig. 20-53, *B*). This requires that the incisal surface of the growing restoration always slopes

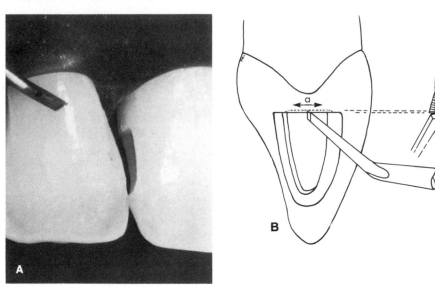

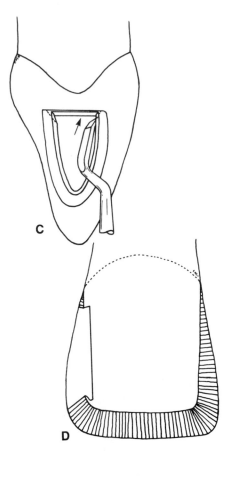

Fig. 20-47. A, Angle former before use in preparation. B, Angle former is moved faciolingually *(a)* to establish acute axiogingival line angle *(b)*. C, Offset angle former thrust faciogingivally establishes acute facioaxiogingival point angle. D, Completed incisal and gingivoaxial retention form. Also see Fig. 20-46, *C*. (D, after Stibbs GD.)

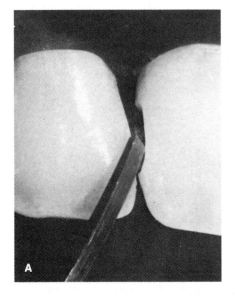

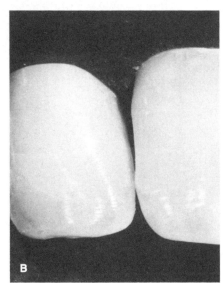

Fig. 20-48. A, Wedelstaedt chisel may be used again to plane margins. B, Completed facial margin of Class III cavity preparation viewed from facial position.

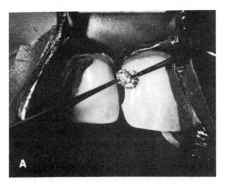

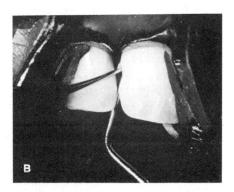

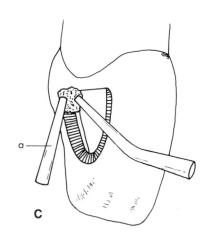

Fig. 20-49. A, First pellet of gold foil is placed from facial aspect into preparation. Note separation of teeth by 0.25 to 0.5 mm. B, Compaction of pellet into linguoaxiogingival point angle. Line of force is directed linguoaxiogingivally while holding instrument is placed from lingual position. C, Holding instrument *(a)* prevents dislodgment of foil during compaction.

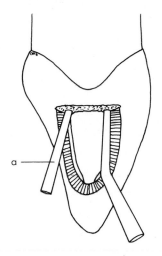

Fig. 20-50. Holding instrument *(a)* remains in position as gold foil is condensed across gingival wall toward facial portion of preparation.

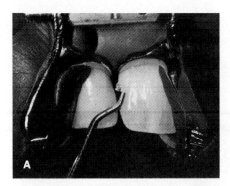

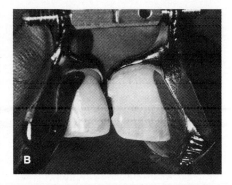

Fig. 20-51. A, Offset condenser before placement in cavity preparation. **B,** Compacted gold foil covering gingival wall and cavosurface.

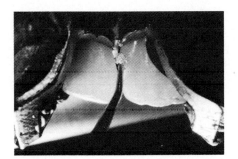

Fig. 20-52. Lingual view. Monangle condenser confirms compaction of gold at linguogingival aspect of restoration.

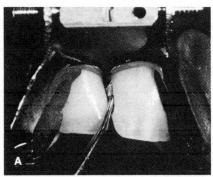

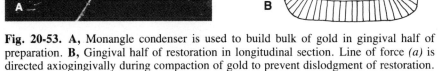

Fig. 20-53. A, Monangle condenser is used to build bulk of gold in gingival half of preparation. **B,** Gingival half of restoration in longitudinal section. Line of force *(a)* is directed axiogingivally during compaction of gold to prevent dislodgment of restoration.

apically, with the gold on the axial wall ahead of the proximal surface of the restoration. During the compaction procedure a vector of the line of force should always be toward the internal portion of the preparation to prevent dislodgment of the restoration. Gradually the incisal portion of the preparation is reached.

The next step is the restoration of the incisal portion of the preparation; this is termed "making the turn" and is accomplished in three steps. First, sufficient gold is built up on the lingual wall so that the gold is very near the incisal angle (Fig. 20-54). Second, the incisal area is filled by compacting $1/_{128}$-size pellets with the right-angle hand condenser (Fig. 20-55). Third, pellets of foil are compacted into the incisolingual area and directly into the incisal area with the offset condenser to fill the incisal portion, thus completely making the turn from lingual to facial (Fig. 20-56, *A*). The entire incisal cavosurface is covered with gold (Fig. 20-56, *B*).

All that remains is to compact gold to finish the facial one third of the restoration, and then the Varney foot condenser is used to "after-condense" the contour of the restoration.

A little more separation is now gained by slight activation of the separator before finishing and polishing the restoration. A sharp, gold foil knife is used to remove excess in the region of the contact, permitting a fine finishing strip or steel matrix strip to pass through the contact area. A pull-cut Shooshan file or gold knife may facilitate removal of excess gold facially (Fig. 20-57). Initial contouring of the contact area is performed with long, extra-narrow, extra-fine cuttle finishing strips to gain access to the proximal surface. Next, a wide, medium cuttle strip may be used for rapid removal of excess gold. Final contouring continues with the medium and fine, narrow strips. Finishing is performed with the extra-narrow, extra-fine cuttle strip (Fig. 20-58). Care is taken to finish *only* the facial or lingual contour with each insertion of the strip to avoid flattening the contact area. The gold knife or cleoid-discoid can be used to remove final excess gold from cavosurface margins. The separator is then removed.

Final polishing is accomplished with a worn-out extra-fine cuttle strip. Polishing powder may be used, but omitting this step results in a satin finish that is less

Fig. 20-54. A, Condenser is directed over facial surface of adjacent tooth as gold is built toward incisal aspect. **B,** Gold is compacted from facioincisal aspect to cover lingual cavosurface; however, compaction direction must continue to have a major vector *(arrow)* toward axial wall to prevent dislodgment. Therefore, at this stage the compacted foil on axial wall must be well ahead (incisally) of the "growing" proximal surface.

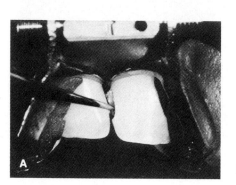

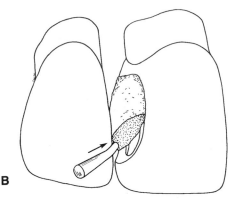

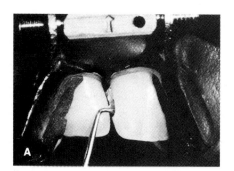

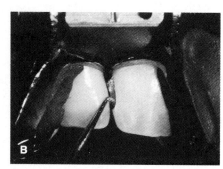

Fig. 20-55. A, Right-angle hand condenser begins to press gold into incisal retention. **B,** This condenser forces gold deeply into incisal retentive undercut.

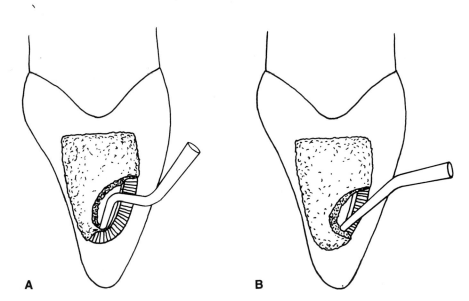

Fig. 20-56. Completing the compaction of gold into incisal region of preparation. **A,** Offset bayonet condenser condenses gold into incisal retention with mallet compaction. **B,** Incisal cavosurface is restored with gold foil condensed with small monangle condenser.

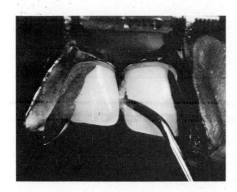

Fig. 20-57. A sharp, thin-bladed gold knife removes excess gold from facial surface.

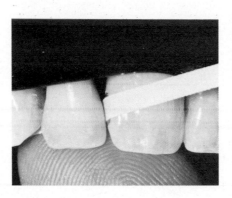

Fig. 20-58. Fine cuttle finishing strips polish proximal surface of gold foil restoration.

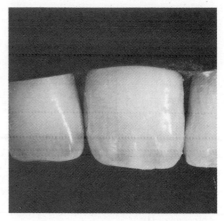

Fig. 20-59. Completed maxillary Class III gold foil restoration.

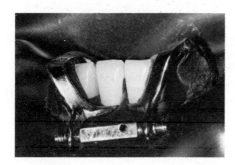

Fig. 20-60. Completed mandibular Class III gold foil restoration of lesion in Fig. 20-41.

reflective of light and may be of esthetic advantage (Fig. 20-59).

CONCLUSION

Direct-filling golds are useful in restorative dentistry. If carefully manipulated by a trained dentist, these restorative materials may provide lifetime service to patients and promote their oral health (Fig. 20-60). Direct-filling golds contribute to both the *art and science* of restorative dentistry and deserve a place in the armamentarium of the dentist.

REFERENCES

1. Baum L: Gold foil (filling golds) in dental practice, *Dent Clin North Am,* p 199, March 1965.
2. Black GV: The nature of blows and the relation of size of plugger points force as used in filling teeth, *Dent Rev* 21:499, 1907.
3. Cartwright CB: Powdered gold for single-surface restorations, *J Mich Dent Assoc* 47:122, April 1965.
4. Dwinelle WH: Crystalline gold, its varieties, properties, and use, *Am J Dent Sci* 5:249, 1855.
5. Ferrier WI: The use of gold foil in general practice, *J Am Dent Assoc* 28:691, 1941.
6. Ferrier WI: Treatment of proximal cavities in anterior teeth with gold foil, *J Am Dent Assoc* 21:571, 1934.
7. Hodson JT: Compaction properties of various pure gold restorative materials, *J Am Acad Gold Foil Oper* 12:52, Sept 1969.
8. Hodson JT: Structure and properties of gold foil and mat gold, *J Dent Res* 42:575, 1963.
9. Hodson JT, Stibbs GD: Structural density of compacted gold foil and mat gold, *J Dent Res* 41:339, 1962.
10. Hollenback GM: There is no substitute for gold foil in restorative dentistry, *J South Calif Dent Assoc* 33:275, 1965.
11. Ingersol CE, Williams Gold Refining Co., Inc.: Personal communication, 1982.
12. Lambert RL: A survey of the teaching of compacted gold, *Oper Dent* 5(1):20, 1980.
13. Lund MR, Baum L: Powdered gold as a restorative material, *J Prosthet Dent* 13:1151, 1963.
14. Medina JE: University of Florida College of Dentistry: Personal communication, 1982.
15. Medina JE et al: Compacted gold restorations. In Hardin JF: *Clark's clinical dentistry,* ch 25, vol 4, Philadelphia, 1991, Lippincott.
16. Phillips RD: *Skinner's science of dental materials,* ed 7, Philadelphia, 1973, WB Saunders.
17. Smith GE: Condenser selection for pure gold compaction, *J Am Acad Gold Foil Oper* 15:53, Sept 1972.
18. Smith GE: The effect of condenser design and lines of force on the dental compaction of cohesive gold, master's thesis, Seattle, 1970, University of Washington.
19. Smith GE, Hodson JT, Stibbs GD: A study of the degree of adaptation possible in retention holes, convenience points and point angles in Class III cavity preparations, *J Am Acad Gold Foil Oper* 15(1):13, 1972.
20. Stibbs GD: Direct golds in dental restorative therapy, *Oper Dent* 5(3):107, 1980.
21. Thomas JJ, Stanley HR, Gilman HW: Effects of gold foil condensation on human dental pulp, *J Am Dent Assoc* 78:788, 1969.
22. Trueman WH: An essay upon the relative advantage of crystallized gold and gold foil as a material for filling teeth, *Dent Cosmos* 10:128, 1868.

Index

Page numbers in italics indicate illustrations; *t* indicates table.